THE
THORACIC
SPINE

Edited by

Edward C. Benzel, M.D.

Professor and Chief, Division of Neurosurgery,
University of New Mexico School of Medicine,
Albuquerque, New Mexico

Charles B. Stillerman, M.D.

Clinical Associate Professor, Department of Neuroscience and Surgery,
University of North Dakota School of Medicine;
Director of Neurosurgery, Trinity Medical Center,
Minot, North Dakota

Quality Medical Publishing, Inc.

ST. LOUIS, MISSOURI
1999

PUBLISHER Karen Berger
EDITOR Beth Campbell
PROJECT MANAGEMENT Shepherd, Inc.
BOOK DESIGN Susan Trail
COVER DESIGN Diane M. Beasley
COVER ART Krista Osterberg

Quality Medical Publishing, Inc.
11970 Borman Drive, Suite 222
St. Louis, Missouri 63146
Telephone: 1-800-348-7808
Web Site: http://www.qmp.com

LIBRARY OF CONGRESS CATALOGING-IN-PUBLICATION DATA

The thoracic spine / edited by Edward C. Benzel, Charles B.
    Stillerman.
            p.   cm.
      Includes bibliographical references and index.
      ISBN 0-942219-75-9
      1. Thoracic vertebrae—Pathophysiology.   2. Thoracic vertebrae—
Surgery.   3. Spine—Diseases—Treatment.   I. Benzel, Edward C.
II. Stillerman, Charles B.
      [DNLM: 1. Thoracic Vertebrae—physiopathology.   2. Spinal
Diseases—diagnosis.   3. Spinal Diseases—therapy.   WE 725T4872
1999]
RD533.T49   1999
617.5'6—dc21
DNLM/DLC   98-30127
for Library of Congress   CIP

S/WW/WW
5   4   3   2   1

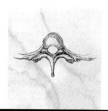

Contributors

Cary D. Alberstone, M.D.
Division of Neurosurgery, University of New Mexico
School of Medicine, Albuquerque, New Mexico

Felipe C. Albuquerque, M.D.
Clinical Instructor, Department of Neurological Surgery,
University of Southern California, Los Angeles,
California

John A. Anson, M.D.
Clinical Assistant Professor, Department of
Neurosurgery, University of Nevada School of Medicine,
Las Vegas, Nevada

Michael L.J. Apuzzo, M.D.
Department of Neurological Surgery, LAC/USC Medical
Center, Los Angeles, California

Nevan G. Baldwin, M.D.
Associate Professor of Surgery, University of New
Mexico School of Medicine, Albuquerque, New Mexico

Edward C. Benzel, M.D.
Professor and Chief, Division of Neurosurgery,
University of New Mexico School of Medicine,
Albuquerque, New Mexico

Mark H. Bilsky, M.D.
Assistant Attending, Department of Neurosurgery,
Memorial Sloan-Kettering Cancer Center,
New York, New York

Thomas A. Buchholz, M.D.
Assistant Professor, Department of Radiation Oncology,
University of Texas M.D. Anderson Cancer Center,
Houston, Texas

Natalie S. Callander, M.D.
Division of Hematology, University of Texas Health
Science Center at San Antonio, San Antonio, Texas

John R. Caruso, M.D.
Neurological Surgeon, Private Practice,
Haggerstown, Maryland

Thomas C. Chen, M.D., Ph.D.
Assistant Professor, Department of Neurological
Surgery, University of Southern California,
Los Angeles, California

Andrew G. Chenell, M.D.
Department of Neurological Surgery, University
of Virginia Health Sciences Center,
Charlottesville, Virginia

Bruce Chozik, M.D.
Private Practice, Albany, New York

Edward S. Connolly, M.D.
Professor of Neurosurgery, Louisiana State University
Medical School; Chairman (Emeritus), Department of
Neurosurgery, Ochsner Clinic and Alton Ochsner
Medical Foundation, New Orleans, Louisiana

William T. Couldwell, M.D., Ph.D.
Professor and Chairman, Department of Surgery,
New York Medical College, Valhalla, New York

Brian G. Cuddy, M.D.
Assistant Professor, Department of Neurosurgery,
Medical University of South Carolina, Charleston,
South Carolina

Steven Davis, B.S.
Research Assistant, Division of Neurosurgery,
Children's Hospital of Los Angeles, Los Angeles,
California

Kevin M. Deitel, M.D.
Resident, Division of Orthopaedic Surgery, University
of Toronto, Toronto, Ontario, Canada

Curtis A. Dickman, M.D.
Associate Chief, Spine Section; Director of Spinal
Research, Division of Neurological Surgery, Barrow
Neurological Institute, Phoenix, Arizona

Eldan Eichbaum, M.D.
Spine Fellow, Division of Neurosurgery, University
of New Mexico School of Medicine, Albuquerque,
New Mexico

Marc E. Eichler, M.D.
Assistant Professor, Department of Neurosurgery,
University of North Dakota, Grand Forks, North Dakota

Michael G. Fehlings, M.D., Ph.D.
Associate Professor, Department of Neurosurgery,
University of Toronto; Director, Spinal Program,
Department of Surgery, The Toronto Hospital, Toronto,
Ontario, Canada

Richard G. Fessler, M.D., Ph.D.
Dunspaugh-Dalton Professor of Brain and Spinal Surgery,
Department of Neurosurgery, University of Florida,
Gainesville, Florida

Kenneth A. Follett, M.D., Ph.D.
Associate Professor (Neurosurgery), Department of
Surgery, University of Iowa Hospitals and Clinics,
Iowa City, Iowa

Steven L. Giannotta, M.D.
Professor, Department of Neurological Surgery,
University of Southern California, Los Angeles,
California

John Go, M.D.
Assistant Professor, Department of Radiology,
University of Southern California,
Los Angeles, California

Ziya L. Gokaslan, M.D.
Assistant Professor, Department of Neurosurgery,
University of Texas M.D. Anderson Cancer Center,
Houston, Texas

David Greenwald, M.D.
University of Florida, Gainesville, Florida

Jeffrey D. Gross, M.D.
Fellow, Division of Neurosurgery, University
of New Mexico School of Medicine, Albuquerque,
New Mexico

Steven Haddy, M.D.
LAC/USC Medical Center, Los Angeles, California

Mark N. Hadley, M.D.
Associate Professor, Division of Neurological Surgery,
University of Alabama School of Medicine at
Birminghan, Birmingham, Alabama

Regis W. Haid, Jr., M.D.
Associate Professor, Department of Neurosurgery,
Emory University School of Medicine, Atlanta, Georgia

Robert W. Henderson, M.D.
Associate Professor of Clinical Radiology, Department
of Radiology, University of Southern California,
Los Angeles, California

James P. Hollowell, M.D.
Assistant Professor, Department of Neurosurgery,
Medical College of Wisconsin at Froedtert Memorial
Lutheran Hospital, Milwaukee, Wisconsin

James Huprich, M.D.
Associate Professor of Clinical Radiology, Department
of Radiology, University of Southern California,
Los Angeles, California

John A. Jane, M.D., Ph.D.
Professor and Chairman, Department of Neurosurgery,
University of Virginia School of Medicine,
Charlottesville, Virginia

Donald W. Larsen, M.D.
Associate Professor, Department of Neurological
Surgery, University of Southern California,
Los Angeles, California

Sanford J. Larson, M.D., Ph.D.
Associate Professor, Department of Neurological
Surgery, University of Southern California,
Los Angeles, California

Michael L. Levy, M.D.
Assistant Professor, Department of Neurosurgery,
Children's Hospital of Los Angeles; Assistant Professor,
Department of Neurological Surgery, University of
Southern California, Los Angeles, California

Geoffrey Shiu-Feng Ling, M.D., Ph.D.
Assistant Professor, Department of Surgery
(Neurosurgery), Uniformed Services University
of the Health Sciences, Bethesda, Maryland

Shari Miura Ling, M.D.
Assistant Professor, Department of Gerontology,
Johns Hopkins University School of Medicine,
Baltimore, Maryland

George H. Lum, M.D.
Assistant Professor, Division of Neurosurgery,
Uniformed Services University of the Health Sciences,
Bethesda, Maryland

Dennis J. Maiman, M.D., Ph.D.
Professor of Neurosurgery, Medical College of
Wisconsin; Medical Director, Model Spinal Cord Injury
Center; Medical Director, MCW SpineCare, Froedtert
Memorial Lutheran Hospital, Milwaukee, Wisconsin

David G. Malone, M.D.
Neurosurgery, Inc., Tulsa, Oklahoma

George J. Martin, Jr., M.D.
Emory Clinic, Crawford Long Hospital, Atlanta, Georgia

Paul Matz, M.D.
Chief Resident, Department of Neurological Surgery,
University of California–San Francisco, San Francisco,
California

J. Gordon McComb, M.D.
Head, Division of Neurosurgery, Children's Hospital
of Los Angeles; Professor, Department of Neurological
Surgery, University of Southern California School
of Medicine, Los Angeles, California

Bruce M. McCormack, M.D.
Assistant Professor, Department of Neurological
Surgery, University of California–San Francisco,
San Francisco, California

Paul C. McCormick, M.D.
Associate Professor of Clinical Neurosurgery,
Department of Neurosurgery, Columbia University
College of Physicians and Surgeons, New York,
New York

David M. McKalip, M.D.
Chief Resident, Division of Neurosurgery, University
of North Carolina at Chapel Hill, Chapel Hill,
North Carolina

Arnold H. Menezes, M.D.
Professor and Vice Chairman, Division of Neurosurgery,
University of Iowa Hospitals and Clinics, Iowa City,
Iowa

Michael A. Morone, M.D., Ph.D.
Neurosurgeon, Indianapolis Neurosurgical Group,
Indianapolis, Indiana

Wade M. Mueller, M.D.
Associate Professor, Department of Neurosurgery,
Medical College of Wisconsin, Milwaukee, Wisconsin

Sait Naderi, M.D.
Department of Neurosurgery, Marmara University,
Istanbul, Turkey

Richard K. Osenbach, M.D.
University of Iowa Hospitals and Clinics,
Iowa City, Iowa

Russell H. Patterson, M.D.
Professor, Department of Neurological Surgery,
New York Hospital–Cornell University Medical Center,
New York, New York

Bryan Payne, M.D.
Senior Resident, Department of Neurosurgery, Louisiana
State University, New Orleans, Louisiana

David Peace, M.S.
Chief of Medical Illustration, Department of
Neurosurgery, University of Florida, Gainesville, Florida

Noel I. Perin, M.D.
Associate Professor, Department of Neurosurgery,
Mount Sinai Medical Center, New York, New York

Phanor L. Perot, Jr., M.D., Ph.D.
Professor, Department of Neurosurgery, Medical
University of South Carolina, Charleston,
South Carolina

G. Jefferey Poffenbarger, M.D.
Senior Resident, Division of Neurosurgery, Walter Reed
Army Medical Center, Washington, D.C.

David Polly, M.D.
Chief Orthopedic Spine Section, Department of Surgery,
Walter Reed Army Medical Center, Washington, D.C.

Gregory J. Przybylski, M.D.
Instructor, Department of Neurosurgery, Medical
College of Wisconsin, Milwaukee, Wisconsin

Gerald E. Rodts, Jr., M.D.
Chief, Division of Neurosurgery, Grady Memorial
Hospital; Assistant Professor, Department of
Neurosurgery, Emory University School of Medicine,
Atlanta, Georgia

Michael K. Rosner, M.D.
Division of Neurological Surgery, University of Alabama
School of Medicine at Birmingham, Birmingham,
Alabama

Ranjan S. Roy, M.D., Ph.D.
Private Practice, Rowan Regional Medical Center,
Salisbury, North Carolina

Srinath Samudrala, M.D.
Assistant Professor, Neurological Surgery and
Orthopedic Surgery, LAC/USC Medical Center,
Los Angeles, California

John H. Schneider, M.D.
Division of Neurosurgery, Wilford Hall Medical Center,
Lackland Air Force Base, Texas

Leslie A. Sebring, M.D., Ph.D.
Associate Director, Neurosurgery Spine and Trauma
Program, Department of Neurologic Surgery, Henry Ford
Hospital, Detroit, Michigan

Christopher I. Shaffrey, M.D.
Departments of Orthopaedic Surgery and Neurological
Surgery, Henry Ford Hospital, Detroit, Michigan

Stephen N. Steen, Sc.D., M.D.
LAC/USC Medical Center, Los Angeles, California

Charles B. Stillerman, M.D.
Clinical Associate Professor, Department of
Neuroscience and Surgery, University of North Dakota
School of Medicine; Director of Neurosurgery, Trinity
Medical Center, Minot, North Dakota

George P. Teitelbaum, M.D.
Associate Professor, Department of Neurological
Surgery, University of Southern California,
Los Angeles, California

Richard M. Toselli, M.D.
Clinical Associate Professor, Division of Neurosurgery,
University of North Carolina at Chapel Hill,
Chapel Hill, North Carolina

Vincent C. Traynelis, M.D.
Associate Professor, Department of Surgery
(Neurosurgery), University of Iowa Hospitals and
Clinics, Iowa City, Iowa

Martin H. Weiss, M.D.
Professor and Chairman, Department of Neurological
Surgery, University of Southern California,
Los Angeles, California

Benjamin T. White, M.D.
Resident, Department of Neurosurgery, Wake Forest
University Shool of Medicine, Winston-Salem,
North Carolina

David M. Wildrick, Ph.D.
Department of Neurosurgery, University of Texas M.D.
Anderson Cancer Center, Houston, Texas

John A. Wilson, M.D.
Assistant Professor, Department of Neurosurgery,
Wake Forest University Baptist Medical Center,
Winston-Salem, North Carolina

Eric J. Woodard, M.D.
Instructor in Surgery, Division of Neurosurgery, Harvard
Medical School, Boston, Massachusetts

Julie E. York, M.D.
Neurosurgery Resident, Department of Neurosurgery,
University of Utah, Salt Lake City, Utah

Chi-Shing Zee, M.D.
Professor, Department of Radiology, University
of Southern California, Los Angeles, California

Seth M. Zeidman, M.D.
Assistant Professor, Department of Surgery
(Neurosurgery), Uniformed Services University of the
Health Sciences, Bethesda, Maryland

Vladimir Zelman, M.D., Ph.D.
LAC/USC Medical Center, Los Angeles, California

Mehmet Zileli, M.D.
MD Professor, Department of Neurosurgery, Ege
University Faculty Medicine, Bornova, Izmir, Turkey

To

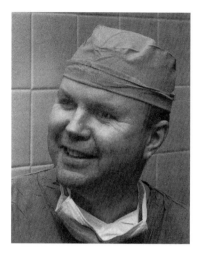

Sanford J. Larson

Without his foresight, ingenuity, and dedication to teaching,
this book would not have been possible, and the
advancement of spinal science deterred.

I cannot teach you anything.
The most I can hope to do is cause you to think.

— Socrates —

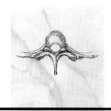

Preface

This book arose from the desire to address the specific nuances of the thoracic spine from a clinically relevant perspective. Historically, much attention has been paid to its neighbors, the cervical and lumbar regions. This attention has taken the form of chapters and books, as well as basic and clinical science research.

Although the thoracic spine may be affected less frequently by surgical pathology than the cervical and lumbar regions, its involvement with nonoperative pathology may rival that of its neighbors. It is time for greater attention to be paid to this pathology (both operative and nonoperative). Therefore it is hoped that this book will help readers understand the fundamentals of diagnosis and operative and nonoperative management, and that they will apply these fundamentals to their clinical practice.

Special thanks to Beth Campbell, Barbara Lopez-Lucio, and Jessica Leary for their endless energy and dedication to this project.

Edward C. Benzel, M.D.
Charles B. Stillerman, M.D.

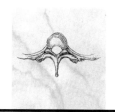

Contents

VII
Complications

Fundamentals

History

Cary D. Alberstone, M.D.

This chapter describes the history of the modern management of thoracic spinal disorders, beginning in the early nineteenth century with the evolution of the laminectomy and ending in the 1980s with the advent of spinal endoscopy. The chapter is organized into four sections. The first section comprises the history of the major surgical approaches to the thoracic spine, including the dorsal, dorsolateral, and ventral approaches. The three crucial developments that made the ventral approach possible—control of infection, control of pain, and thoracic anesthesia—are discussed at length to emphasize that the development of thoracic spinal surgery historically has depended on certain advances in perioperative surgical management.

The second section of the chapter, surgical stabilization and deformity correction, covers the technical innovations of spinal fusion and spinal instrumentation. Emphasized are the contributions of Holdsworth in spinal biomechanics and Harrington and Dwyer in spinal instrumentation. Nonoperative strategies, such as spinal bracing and spinal exercises, are addressed in the third section, and the fourth section discusses the emergence of spinal endoscopy.

SURGICAL APPROACHES AND SURGICAL DECOMPRESSION

Most of the major surgical approaches to the thoracic spine have attempted to provide for or improve upon a decompressive procedure. Thus in the nineteenth century, laminectomy was used for the decompression of traumatic fractures and later for spinal tumors and infection. Around the turn of the century, the dorsolateral, and later the ventrolateral, approaches to the thoracic spine were developed to decompress spinal tuberculosis. Decompression of thoracic disc disease, which began around the middle of the twentieth century, also played an important part in the evolution of these three approaches.

The Dorsal Approach
H. J. Cline and the Argument Against Spinal Surgery

In 1814 H. J. Cline, a British surgeon, performed a laminectomy that ended in disaster.[37] Although some form of laminectomy had been used since ancient times when Paul of Aegina[79] first attempted it, the repercussions of Cline's mortality served to dampen enthusiasm for the development of the procedure in the nineteenth century. Cline's case involved a thoracic fracture-dislocation that was treated with resection of the fractured spinous processes and laminae. On presentation, the patient revealed evidence of a complete transverse lesion of the spinal cord. Although Cline operated urgently, he was unable to reduce the dislocation. Shortly after surgery, the patient died.

Following this case, Cline's patient was used as evidence against the safety of performing spinal surgery. To be fair, Cline's operative mortality was not an isolated instance. For example, in 1827 Tyrell[98] reported a 100% mortality in his series of traumatic spinal injury operations. And Rogers,[87] in 1835, reported similarly discouraging results. But Cline's case remained a benchmark of sorts, over which surgeons would argue for or against spinal surgery. Looking back on this controversy, at least one observer was impressed by the vitriol it engendered, explaining,

> This [Cline's operation] precipitated and gave rise to widespread and vehement discussion as to its justification. This discussion, often degenerating into bitter and virulent personalities, went on many years. Astely Cooper, Benjamin Bell, Tyrell, South, and others favored it, while Charles Bell, John Bell, Benjamin Brodie, and others opposed it. The effect of so eminent a neurologist as Sir Charles Bell against the procedure retarded spinal surgery many years—the operation was described with such extravagant terms as "formidable," "well-nigh impossible," "appalling," "desparate and blind," "unjustifiable," and "bloody and dangerous."[5]

Of course, the surgical morbidities and mortalities in the nineteenth century were not attributable to surgical technique alone. Much more important were the septic and anesthetic complications that caused most attempts at surgery to end in failure. The lack of adequate pain control during surgery made speed essential and caused many disasters due to intraoperative shock. Furthermore, wound infection and septicemia occurred frequently after surgery and were often fatal. The solution to these problems came later in the century when general anesthetic agents such as nitrous oxide, ether, and chloroform were introduced in the mid 1840s, and when Listerian antiseptic techniques were adopted in the 1870s.

A. G. Smith and the First Successful Laminectomy

The risks and dangers of surgery aside, pioneer surgeons, throughout the nineteenth century, persisted in attempting to achieve surgical success. One such success came to a little-known Danville, Kentucky, surgeon named Alban G. Smith,[93] who performed a laminectomy in 1828 on a patient who had sustained a traumatic paraplegia after falling from a horse. Although the case attracted little attention at the time, it is remarkable because the patient not only survived the operation, but achieved a partial neurological recovery. In his 1829 report of the operation in the *North American Journal of Medi-*

cine and Surgery, Smith[93] wrote that the procedure involved a midline incision, removal of the depressed laminae and spinous processes, exploration of the dura mater, and closure of the soft tissue incision. Although the case does not appear to have been particularly influential, it may represent the earliest documented successful laminectomy.

Laminectomy for Extramedullary Spinal Tumor

During the half century that followed Smith's landmark operation, the primary indication for laminectomy was trauma. In the latter part of the century, however, the indication broadened. For example, in 1887 Victor Horsley performed perhaps the first successful removal of an intradural, extramedullary spinal cord tumor, through an exposure gained by a multilevel laminectomy[30] (Fig. 1-1). The patient was an English army officer named Captain Gilbey, who had lost his wife in a carriage accident in which he also was involved. Although Gilbey himself suffered no serious injury, he began to note a dull, nagging backache shortly after the accident. As the pain progressed, Gilbey was evaluated by multiple doctors who attributed his symptoms to neurosis.

Eventually, Gilbey was referred to the great London neurologist William Gowers (Fig. 1-2). However, in the approximately 3 years that had elapsed since the onset of symptoms, the patient had developed com-

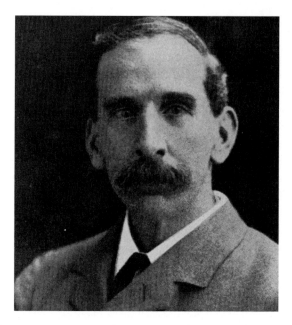

Fig. 1-1. Sir Victor Horsley. (From Stephen Paget's biography.)

plete paraplegia and loss of bladder control. For Gowers, Gilbey's case posed no diagnostic dilemma: Gilbey was suffering from a tumor of the spine causing compression of the thoracic spinal cord. Although no such case had ever been handled successfully with surgery, Gowers referred the patient to his eminent surgical colleague Victor Horsley. Gowers, after all, had asserted in his authoritative textbook, *Manual of Diseases of the Nervous System,* that removal of an intradural spinal cord tumor was "not only practicable, but actually a less formidable operation than the removal of intracranial tumors."

Horsley acted quickly. Within 2½ hours of meeting Captain Gilbey on June 9, 1887 at the National Hospital, Horsley had begun the operation. Despite the need for haste, Horsley was well prepared to undertake this dangerous operation. Although the Act of 1876 had made it a criminal offense to experiment on a vertebrate animal for the purpose of attaining manual skill, Horsley had prepared and practiced the proposed procedure during his experimental work [with the English neurologist Beevor]. Nevertheless, the initial exposure fashioned by Horsley failed to reveal the tumor, and only with the encouragement of his surgical assistant, Sir Charles Ballance, did Horsley decide to extend the

surgical exposure rostrally. Then, upon opening the dura, Horsley identified a round, dark, bluish mass compressing the spinal cord. Relieved to find the tumor, Horsley resected the almond-shaped mass in its entirety.

One year after the surgery, Captain Gilbey had recovered almost completely. He was ambulating and active and had resumed a 16-hour work day. Up until he died from an unrelated cause some 20 years later, the patient remained well with no evidence of tumor recurrence.

Laminectomy for Intramedullary Spinal Tumor

In 1890 Fenger made one of the earliest attempts to remove an intramedullary spinal neoplasm, but the patient died shortly after the operation.[16] In 1905, Cushing[18] likewise attempted to remove an intramedullary tumor, but after performing a myelotomy in the dorsal column, he decided the tumor was unresectable. To his surprise, the patient improved after surgery. Finally, in 1907, von Eiselsberg successfully removed an intramedullary tumor.[100]

Elsberg[26] described Cushing's technique, which he aptly named the "method of extrusion" (Fig. 1-3). The purpose of this technique was to achieve an adequate

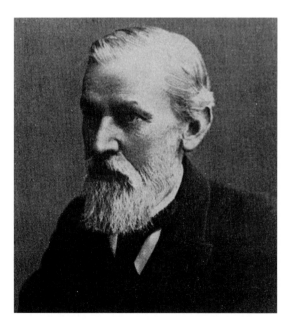

Fig. 1-2. William R. Gowers. (From Haymaker W, Schiller F. The Founders of Neurology, 2nd ed. Springfield, Ill.: Charles C Thomas, 1970, p 442. Courtesy Charles C Thomas, Publisher, Ltd., Springfield, Ill.)

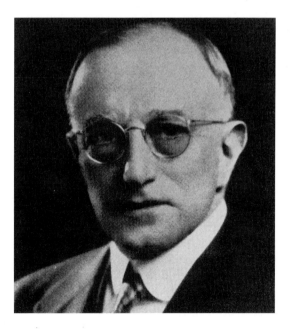

Fig. 1-3. Charles A. Elsberg. (From Haymaker W, Schiller F. The Founders of Neurology, 2nd ed. Springfield, Ill.: Charles C Thomas, 1970, p 553. Courtesy Charles C Thomas, Publisher, Ltd., Springfield, Ill.)

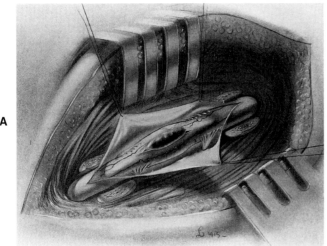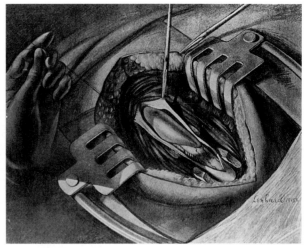

Fig. 1-4. A, The first stage in an intramedullary spinal cord tumor resection by the extrusion method. Note that the tumor is bulging through the myelotomy incision. The wound was subsequently closed. **B,** The second stage in an intramedullary spinal cord tumor resection by the extrusion method (1 week after the first stage). Note that the tumor has spontaneously extruded since the first operation and may now be easily removed. (From Elsberg CA. Diagnosis and Treatment of Surgical Diseases of the Spinal Cord and its Membranes. Philadelphia: WB Saunders, 1916, pp 274-275.)

resection of the tumor with a minimum amount of injury to the cord tissue. The premise was that an intramedullary neoplasm is associated with a local increase in intramedullary pressure. Thus a simple myelotomy brought down to the level of the tumor should provide an avenue through which the increased intramedullary pressure would spontaneously expel the substance of the tumor. Elsberg believed that the legitimacy of this method was confirmed in practice and that it was associated with minimum spinal cord tissue injury because it involved minimal surgical manipulation of the cord.

Because the process of spontaneous extrusion of the tumor was a slow one, Elsberg performed his operations for intramedullary tumor in two stages. In the first stage a myelotomy was performed in the dorsal column and was brought down deep to the level of the tumor (Fig. 1-4, *A*). After the tumor began to bulge through the myelotomy incision, the operation was concluded, with the dura left open; the muscles, fascia, and skin were then closed.

After about a week, the wound was reopened and the tumor identified. In most instances the tumor was outside the spinal cord and was removed by simply dividing the few adhesions remaining between the tumor and the cord (Fig. 1-4, *B*). When

the tumor had been removed, the wound, including the dura mater, was closed.

Dorsolateral Approaches

In 1779 Percival Pott[84] described the occurrence of spinal kyphosis associated with progressive paraparesis in the now-classic monograph, *Remarks on that kind of palsy of the lower limbs which is frequently found to accompany a curvature of the spine and is supposed to be caused by it; together with its method of cure; etc* (Fig. 1-5). Pott's recommended surgical treatment involved a paraspinal incision into the swelling of the trunk to drain pus. Other authors also recommended this early form of surgical therapy, which essentially involved draining pus from paraspinal abscesses. With the decrease in surgical mortality associated with Listerian methods beginning in the 1870s and the acceptance of the laminectomy in the late nineteenth century, surgeons naturally applied this decompressive procedure to the treatment of Pott's paraplegia.[15] However, disenchantment with the results of such attempts encouraged the development of new approaches. Thus in 1894 Ménard of France published a description of the so-called "costotransversectomy," which became a popular surgical approach for treating Pott's paraplegia.[68]

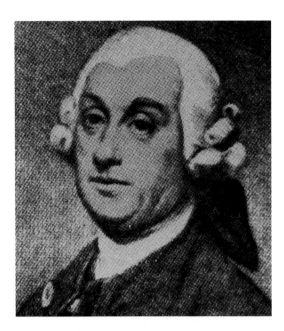

Fig. 1-5. Percival Pott. (From Garrison.)

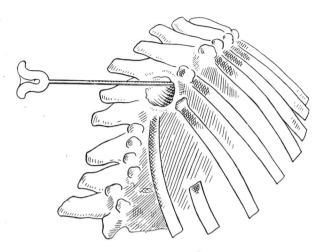

Fig. 1-6. Drainage of a tubercular abscess via the costotransversectomy of Ménard. (From Capener N. The evolution of lateral rhachotomy. J Bone Joint Surg 36B:178, 1954.)

Ménard's Costotransversectomy

The goal of Ménard's innovative surgical approach was not dissimilar to the goal of Pott's far simpler procedure, namely to drain the tubercular abscess. In a preface to the description of his new surgical exposure, Ménard explained that his invention had originated from his dissatisfaction with the surgical results obtained with the decompressive laminectomy. If the pathological lesion causing Pott's paraplegia was the tubercular abscess, then drainage of the abscess should be a primary surgical goal and one that the laminectomy was ill-designed to achieve. He thus proposed an alternative surgical approach that provided improved exposure of the lateral aspect of the vertebral column. This was the "costotransversectomy," also known as the *"drainage latéral,"* emphasizing that its goal was to drain the lateral, paravertebral tubercular abscess.

As described by Ménard, the costotransversectomy involves a transverse incision along the rib that corresponds to the apex of the kyphos. The rib is stripped subperiosteally and divided approximately 4 cm from its proximal tip. At its junction with the transverse process, the rib is then sectioned and removed. This provides access to the tuberculous focus, which may thus be decompressed directly (Fig. 1-6). For Ménard, it mattered little how much of the lesion had been removed, only that the abscess had been decompressed.

This operation gave much better results than the laminectomy. Among Ménard's first few cases were four successes, with significant improvements in motor function noted among his first 23 cases.[94] Unfortunately, along with these successes came increasing evidence that two major complications were adversely affecting the surgical results, namely the postoperative development of secondary infections and sinus tracts that occurred as a result of opening the abscess. Because the operation was performed in the days before antitubercular chemotherapy, these infectious complications were disastrous, frequently leading to the patient's death. As Calot[13] (1930) grimly put it, "The surgeon who, so far as tuberculosis is concerned, swears to remove the evil from the very root, will only find one result waiting him—the death of his patient." Ménard's operation thus fell into disrepute, and in time even he abandoned it.

Capener's Lateral Rhachotomy

Norman Capener of Exeter and Plymouth, England, took a different tack to the problem of Pott's paraplegia in a procedure that he developed and began using in 1933 and that was first reported by H.J. Seddon in 1935.[91] In a departure from the emphasis of both Pott and Ménard on the evacuation of the

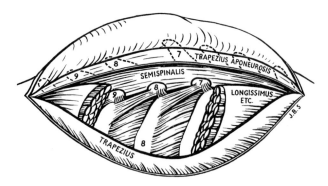

Fig. 1-7. Dorsolateral exposure via Capener's lateral rhachotomy. Note that the exposure requires a transverse division of the paraspinal muscles. (From Capener N. The evolution of lateral rhachotomy. J Bone Joint Surg 36B:174, 1954.)

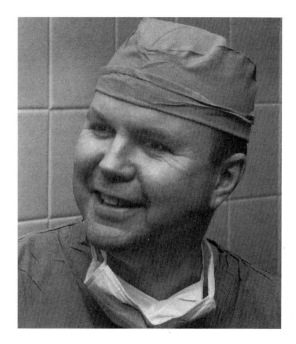

Fig. 1-8. Sanford J. Larson.

tuberculous abscess, Capener sought to directly remove the features causing spinal cord compression, which usually consisted of hardened material located ventrally. To accomplish this, the surgical exposure should provide a more lateral or ventral view of the vertebrae than was afforded by Ménard's costotransversectomy.

Capener's solution was to adopt the costotransversectomy with this difference: Capener[14] approached the vertebral column by transversely dividing the erector spinae muscles and retracting them rostrally and caudally, rather than developing a plane medial to them (Fig. 1-7). He named his new approach the "lateral rhachotomy" to distinguish it from Ménard's "costotransversectomy." The simple change in dissection planes that distinguishes the costotransversectomy from the lateral rhachotomy produces a significantly different trajectory and surgical exposure. Although the operation was designed to surgically treat Pott's paraplegia, Capener later drew attention to the versatility of the approach and its appropriateness for a variety of pathological processes, including "the exploration of spinal tumours, the relief of certain types of traumatic paraplegia, and the drainage of suppurative osteitis of the vertebral bodies."[14]

It was perhaps unfortunate that for 19 years the only description of Capener's lateral rhachotomy was in a single case report published by another surgeon.[91] Not until 1954 did Capener[14] himself describe his procedure, although he still chose not to publish the results of his 23 cases.

In the interval between these two reports on Capener's procedure, a major event in the history of the treatment of Pott's paraplegia occurred: the introduction of antitubercular chemotherapy. In 1947, streptomycin first became available for clinical use, followed by para-aminosalicylic acid and isoniazid in 1949 and 1952, respectively. The effect of these new chemotherapeutic agents on the treatment of tuberculosis was spectacular. The average relapse rate of tuberculosis with the addition of streptomycin alone was decreased by 30% to 35%. Although the effect of antitubercular chemotherapy was not as evident for the treatment of spinal tuberculosis as it was for the pulmonary form, its mere availability raised new questions about the indications for surgical intervention by creating several new limbs of rational therapy.

Larson's Lateral Extracavitary Approach

In 1976, Sanford J. Larson et al.[53] at the Medical College of Wisconsin published an influential article that helped popularize Capener's lateral rhachotomy, which they modified and renamed the "lateral extracavitary approach" (Fig. 1-8). This approach has been used more for trauma and tumor than for tuberculosis. The difference between the lateral rhachotomy and the lateral extracavitary approach is defined by the treatment of the paraspinous muscles. Whereas Capener's procedure

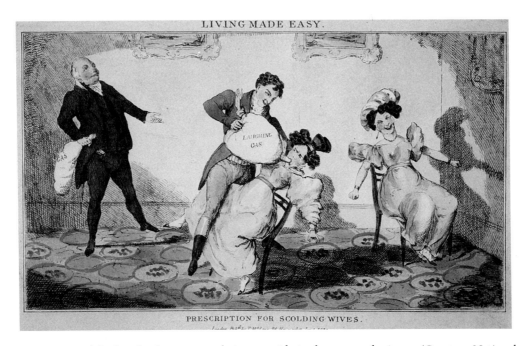

LIVING MADE EASY.

PRESCRIPTION FOR SCOLDING WIVES.

Fig. 1-9. One of the less laudatory uses of nitrous oxide in the preanesthetic era. (Courtesy National Library of Medicine, Bethesda, Md.)

involves dividing these muscles and reflecting them rostrally and caudally, Larson's procedure involves developing a plane that passes ventral to the paraspinous muscles, which are then reflected medially to expose the ventrolateral spine. Although neurosurgeons have always been involved in spinal decompressive surgery, a significant part of Larson's contribution lies in the fact that, as a neurosurgeon, he was a pioneer among the neurosurgical community in dedicating his career to the advancement of reconstructive spinal surgery.

Ventral Approaches

Like the dorsolateral approach, the ventral approach to the thoracic spine originated as a result of dissatisfaction with the approaches available for the management of tuberculous spondylitis. Although a ventral approach to the thoracic spine had obvious advantages, the technical obstacles to the procedure, including controlling pain and infection and administering anesthesia, were prohibitive. Finding solutions to these problems was a prerequisite to the successful development of thoracic surgery. Each of these developments—the control of pain, the control of infection, and thoracic anesthesia—has earned an important place in history, and each

will therefore be discussed before exploring the evolution of the ventral approach.

Three Crucial Developments

Control of Pain. The lack of an adequate means of pain control at the time of surgery severely limited the range of surgical possibilities. Speed, of course, was essential, and intraoperative shock greatly increased surgical mortality. Until the surgeon could adequately manage the problem of pain, no further advances in interventional procedures could be made.

In fact, the solution to surgical pain had long been available. Since the beginning of the nineteenth century, both ether and nitrous oxide had been known as agents of amusement at so-called frolics (Fig. 1-9). Although European scientists had suggested that these gases be used as anesthetic agents, the first documented clinical application was made by a Connecticut dentist named Horace Wells, who began anesthetizing his patients with nitrous oxide in 1844. Soon William Thomas Green Morton, also a dentist, became familiar with the work of Wells and began to administer ether as an anesthetic at the suggestion of his teacher, Charles T. Jackson (Fig. 1-10). Impressed by the results he

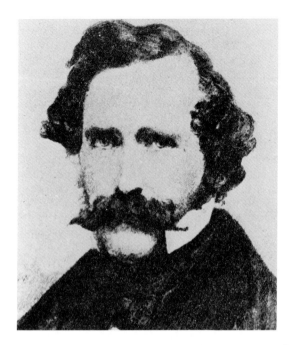

Fig. 1-10. William T.G. Morton. (From Selwyn-Brown A. The Physician Throughout the Ages, vol. 1. New York: Capehart-Brown, 1928.)

had obtained in his dental practice, Morton approached the eminent Boston surgeon John Collins Warren, suggesting that Warren test the efficacy of ether. On October 16, 1846, at the Massachusetts General Hospital, Warren successfully utilized ether anesthesia in a historic operation (Fig. 1-11). In 1847 an Edinburgh obstetrician named Sir James Simpson introduced chloroform as an alternative to ether, which it soon replaced (Fig. 1-12).

The effect of the discovery of general anesthesia was overwhelming. It allowed surgeons to work at a less breakneck pace, ameliorated the problem of intraoperative shock, and opened the gate to further developments in surgery. While these advantages benefitted spinal surgery in general, they proved especially important to the development of the ventral approach, which required greater operating time, greater soft tissue dissection, and (for the first time) the violation of the thoracic cavity compared with the dorsal and dorsolateral approaches.

Control of Infection. In the nineteenth century, the most feared complication of a surgical operation was infection. Few patients who entered the surgical wards of a hospital in those days did so with the

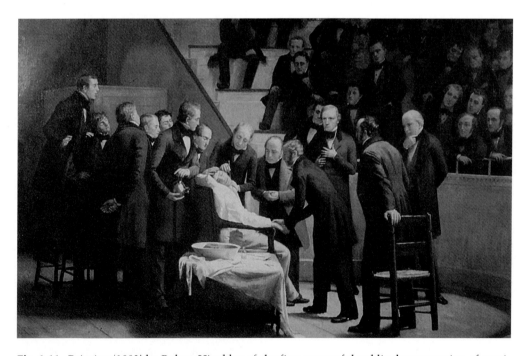

Fig. 1-11. Painting (1882) by Robert Hinckley of the first successful public demonstration of surgical anesthesia, October 16, 1846, at the Massachusetts General Hospital. (Courtesy Francis A. Countway Library of Medicine, Boston Medical Library, Cambridge, Mass; from Selwyn-Brown A. The Physician Throughout the Ages, vol. 1. New York: Capehart-Brown, 1928.)

hope of leaving alive. But by the turn of the century, all that had changed with the introduction of the Listerian principles of "antisepsis."

Joseph Lister, a Quaker physician, was appalled by the tremendous loss of life that naturally accompanied the practice of nineteenth-century surgery (Fig. 1-13). Lister observed that the mortality rates for cases of closed and open bony fractures differed markedly. He was familiar with the recent publications of Louis Pasteur, who had convincingly demonstrated the presence of bacteria in the air. Lister reasoned that the invasion of an open fracture by such bacteria could be responsible for the high incidence of infections in these patients. To deter this occurrence, Lister introduced the practice of decontaminating open fractures with carbolic acid, a disinfectant recommended by Jules Lemaire as early as 1860.

The results of the clinical trial by Lister,[55] which he began to publish in 1867, were astonishing. Lister capitalized on the success of his method and soon began applying it more widely in surgery. He named his principles antisepsis. This Listerian technique consisted of spraying the surgical wound and the operator's hands and instruments with carbolic acid (Fig. 1-14). Although at first the surgical world was skeptical of Lister's principles and reluctant to adopt his methods, by the 1870s surgeons in Germany had taken up his techniques, and surgeons in the United States, France, and eventually England then followed.

By the 1880s Lister's cumbersome methods of antisepsis were being replaced by simpler methods of "asepsis," in which the instruments were disinfected with steam and various agents were used to disinfect the surgical field and the surgeons' hands.

The effect of antisepsis and asepsis on the practice of surgery was remarkable, producing an overwhelming decrease in surgical morbidity and mortality that rejuvenated surgery. These techniques paved the way for the modern development of thoracic, abdominal, and cranial surgery, which up until the 1880s had comprised sanctuaries not to be entered, except by accident.

Thoracic Anesthesia. The most enduring obstacle for the would-be thoracic surgeon after the turn of the century was the problem of pressure relationships in the chest. Although pain and infection during surgery could be controlled, the peculiar problems associated with maintaining normal pressure relationships during surgery on an opened chest still needed to be overcome. Without a solution to this problem, no advances in thoracic surgery could be made.

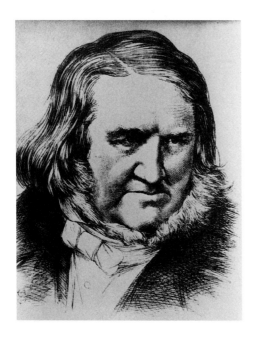

Fig. 1-12. James Y. Simpson. (Courtesy New York Academy of Medicine, New York, N.Y.; from Selwyn-Brown A. The Physician Throughout the Ages, vol. 1. New York: Capehart-Brown, 1928.)

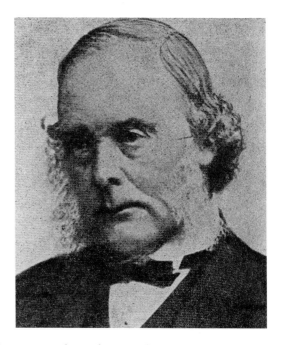

Fig. 1-13. Lord Joseph Lister. (From Selwyn-Brown A. The Physician Throughout the Ages, vol. 1. New York: Capehart-Brown, 1928.)

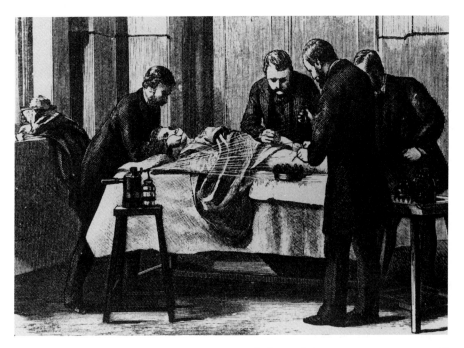

Fig. 1-14. The Listerian antiseptic technique using carbolic acid. (From Lyons AS, Petrucelli JR II. Medicine: An Illustrated History. New York: Harry N. Abrams, Inc., 1987.)

The technique of inserting a tube into the trachea to maintain respiration during surgical operations had been known for centuries. For example, in the sixteenth century Andreas Vesalius utilized this technique for open chest surgery on animals.[49] He maintained pressure gradients by blowing air through a tube of reed or cane placed in the trachea. In the eighteenth century, John Hunter invented a device that consisted of a double-chambered bellows connected to a tube in the nostrils, pharynx, or trachea.[73] Although the method was effective, it fell out of favor when it was discovered that forcing air into the lungs could result in a catastrophic pneumothorax.

In the nineteenth century, the development of endotracheal anesthesia was stimulated by the advent of general anesthesia. For example, in 1858 John Snow of London performed surgery on rabbits, using a tube inserted through a tracheotomy and attached to a bag of chloroform to simultaneously administer respiration and anesthesia.[10] A further advance was made by William Macewan[60] in 1880 when he described the insertion of endotracheal tubes through the mouth (Fig. 1-15). During the late nineteenth century, these techniques were used mainly to treat nonsurgical disease such as upper airway obstruction due to diphtheria.

A particularly effective apparatus was invented for this purpose in 1893 by George H. Fell of Buffalo,

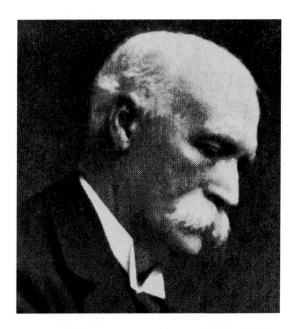

Fig. 1-15. Sir William Macewan. (From Walker AE. A History of Neurological Surgery. New York: Hafner Publishing Co., 1967, p 178.)

New York.[27] The Fell device consisted of a simple foot bellows connected to a face mask or endotracheal tube. A series of various-sized conical tubes was later designed by Joseph O'Dwyer, an American physician, and the Fell-O'Dwyer apparatus became a popular method of treating patients with diphtheria,

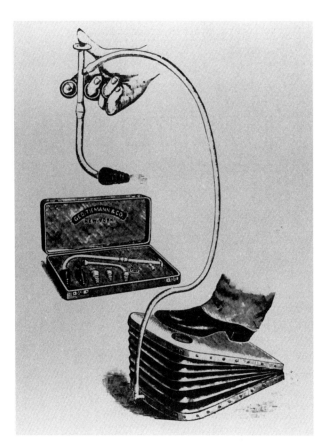

Fig. 1-16. The Fell-O'Dwyer apparatus. (Courtesy National Library of Medicine, Bethesda, Md.)

opium poisoning, and other nonsurgical diseases[49] (Fig. 1-16).

Still, the problem of thoracic anesthesia remained unsolved. In 1899, Rudolph Matas[62] defined the problem as follows:

> The sudden admission of air into the normal, healthy pleura, whether accidentally or as a result of deliberate purpose, in the course of an operation on the chest, is often a source of great peril to the patient and always of profound anxiety to the operator . . . it leads the surgeons of all time to dread the production of a traumatic or surgical pneumothorax as a great evil . . . in man acute traumatic pneumothorax, with pulmonary collapse and its attendant shock and asphyxia, is the rock that obstructs the otherwise open channel of the thorax.

Matas, an eminent New Orleans surgeon, was among the first American surgeons to demonstrate a special interest in thoracic surgery. Matas modified the Fell-O'Dwyer apparatus and used it in perhaps the first human intrathoracic operation performed in the United States. Matas's pleasure with his newly invented device was difficult to conceal:

> My colleague, Dr. F.W. Parham, has brilliantly confirmed the opinion . . . as to the value of the Fell-O'Dwyer apparatus, by successfully removing a large sarcoma of the upper chest wall . . . the collapse of the lung which would have inevitably followed, and the bad symptoms that were beginning to be noticed, were immediately corrected by the Fell-O'Dwyer apparatus.[78]

Despite these positive results, the apparatus failed to achieve widespread use.

However, in 1903 a series of experiments designed to solve the problem of thoracic anesthesia received world attention. In Breslau, Germany, Professor von Mikulicz wished to develop an operation for carcinoma of the esophagus. Hindered by the monumental problem of an open chest during surgery, von Mikulicz assigned his assistant, Ferdinand Sauerbruch, the challenging task of overcoming this problem,[74] and Sauerbruch succeeded brilliantly. His solution was to place the patient's thorax within an airtight chamber maintained at a negative pressure of −10 mm Hg. The patient's head was left outside the chamber with an airtight seal at the neck. A 500 cu ft chamber of glass and iron was built at the Trendelenburg Iron Works in Breslau, Germany and, after demonstrating its success, many similar chambers were built in Berlin, Cologne, Vienna, St. Petersburg, and throughout Europe (Fig. 1-17).

Further modifications of Sauerbruch's invention were soon developed, including a switch to positive pressure chambers that contained the patient's head. Later the chambers were eliminated completely and replaced by masks or intubation tubes. But the next major discovery was made in 1907 by Barthelemy and Dufour, who described the "insufflation principle" of endotracheal anesthesia. In 1909, Meltzer and Auer, two physiologists at the Rockefeller Institute, independently made the same discovery and devised an apparatus to administer endotracheal anesthesia (Fig. 1-18). Meltzer[67] described his discovery:

> The method of intratracheal insufflation consists of driving air, by means of external pressure, through a tube which has been introduced through the mouth and larynx deep into the trachea. The insufflated air, driven by the same external force, returns through the space between the tube and the wall of the trachea and escapes through the mouth and nose. The airstream has to be interrupted several times a minute for only about two seconds at a time. When the size of the tube, the rate of interruption, and the degree of pressure are properly

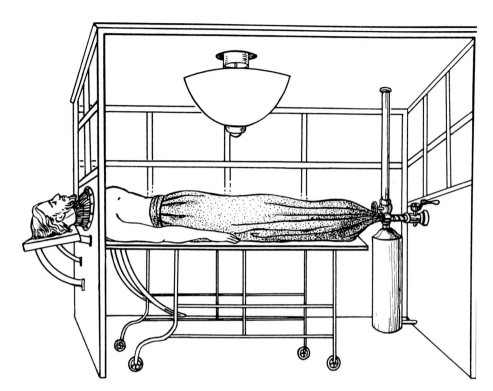

Fig. 1-17. An early version of Sauerbruch's negative-pressure chamber. (Courtesy National Library of Medicine, Bethesda, Md.; from Sauerbruch F. Zur Pathologie des offenen Pneu nothorax und die Grundlagen meines Verfahrens zu seiner Ausschaltung. Mitt Grenzgeb Med Chir 13:399, 1904.)

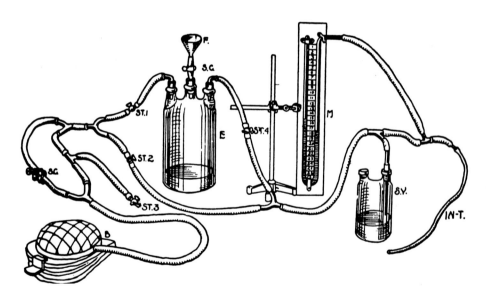

Fig. 1-18. Meltzer and Auer's insufflation apparatus. (From Johnson SL. The History of Cardiac Surgery, 1896-1955. Baltimore: Johns Hopkins Press, 1970, p 57.)

selected, the intratracheal insufflation is capable of maintaining properly the life of even completely curarized and anesthetized animals or individuals with a widely open double pneumothorax without any efficient respiration of their own.

The concept of insufflation anesthesia was new. It replaced the old inhalation principle that maintained respiration with an inflow and outflow of gases by providing a constant expansion through air flow under continuous external pressure.

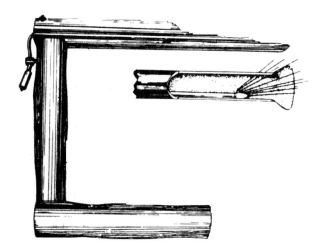

Fig. 1-19. Chevalier Jackson's direct laryngoscope. (From Johnson SL. The History of Cardiac Surgery, 1896-1955. Baltimore: Johns Hopkins Press, 1970, p 58.)

Charles A. Elsberg, a New York surgeon, was influential in popularizing insufflation anesthesia (see Fig. 1-3). In 1910, he reported the first application of insufflation endotracheal anesthesia to thoracic surgery. In the following years, Elsberg[24] performed hundreds of thoracic surgical operations in which he utilized insufflation endotracheal anesthesia. He introduced many important modifications of this technique, including a speculum that assisted in placing endotracheal tubes and a machine for administering anesthesia.

One of the major obstacles to the widespread use of endotracheal anesthesia was the technical difficulty involved in oral intubation. Thus direct laryngoscopy, developed by Alfred Kirstein[52] in 1895 and popularized by Chevalier Jackson[45] in 1913, represented an important milestone in the adoption of endotracheal anesthesia (Fig. 1-19). With the use of the endotracheal tube becoming standard, three major goals of anesthesia were achieved: An adequate airway was provided and maintained for respiration; a means for the removal of secretions was afforded; and the problem of coughing during surgery was resolved.

However, the aftermath of World War I revealed another problem. The sudden astronomical increase in surgical caseloads compounded the expense of anesthetic gases. To ameliorate this cost and improve ventilation, Rowbotham and Magill,[88] two anesthetists attached to the British Army Plastic Unit at Sidcup, England, abandoned the insuf-flation technique and resurrected the older inhalation principle.

The work of Rowbotham and Magill was highly influential, and by the early 1930s inhalation anesthesia had almost completely replaced the insufflation method. Although further advances such as the closed-system anesthesia machine and the introduction of cyclopropane in 1928[58] and sodium pentothal in the 1930s[59] continued to push back the frontiers of thoracic anesthesia, the problem of thoracic anesthesia had been overcome. By the 1930s, the time was ripe for the development of ventral approaches to the thoracic spine.

Hodgson and Stock

The first successful attempt to approach the spine ventrally is attributed to Müller,[72] who in 1906 performed a transperitoneal approach to the lumbosacral spine for a case of suspected sarcoma. At operation, Müller discovered tuberculosis. He fashioned a median suprapubic incision, curetted the bone, applied iodoform powder, and closed the wound. The surgical result was excellent, but despite this initial success, subsequent attempts to approach the spine ventrally ended in disaster, and Müller was forced to abandon the procedure.

In 1934, taking advantage of an aseptic method, more sophisticated anesthetic techniques, and the spinal fusion method of Albee and Hibbs, Ito et al.[44] performed a ventral approach for tuberculous spondylitis in 10 cases. In eight of the cases, the lumbar spine alone was involved, and in two cases the infection involved the thoracic spine and the thoracolumbar junction. In these latter cases, the costotransversectomy approach was used, and no attempt was made to approach the thoracic spine ventrally.

In 1956, Hodgson and Stock[39] of Hong Kong reported the first series of ventral approaches to the thoracic spine in 48 patients treated for Pott's disease. The authors acknowledged the contributions of Müller and Ito et al. (with whose work they had been unfamiliar at the time they commenced their study), and they duly signified the importance of the recent development of antitubercular chemotherapy. Their motivation for developing a ventral approach is stated clearly:

We were dissatisfied with the exposure afforded by costotransversectomy as we found the operation difficult and the field restricted. Through this approach it was impossible to determine the extent of the lesion or to evacuate it completely, neither could the graft be inserted with any accuracy.[39]

Hodgson and stock also expressed the aim of their new method:

> It appears to us that decompression of the abscess with removal of the pus, caseous material, granulation tissue, intervertebral disks, and sequestra is imperative to arrest further vertebral destruction where the disease is progressing. . . .[39]

It is noteworthy that the objects of decompression are carefully listed in this statement of purpose. Hodgson and Stock believed that undue importance had been attached to spinal stabilization in the treatment of Pott's paraplegia since 1911 when spinal fusion for this disease was introduced by Albee and Hibbs. To Hodgson and Stock, the emphasis on stabilization was maintained at the expense of an adequate infection operation, which required the complete extirpation of the tubercular abscess and its sequestra. Furthermore, the ventral approach provided an optimal exposure for insertion of a bone graft in compression, which offered the best chance for successful bony fusion. For all of these reasons, and given their excellent surgical results, Hodgson and Stock effectively advocated the ventral approach.

Their enthusiasm for this approach was corroborated years later when the Medical Research Council Committee for Research on Tuberculosis in the Tropics began to investigate the widely divergent forms of available treatment. Although recommending nonsurgical management in the majority of cases, the Council concluded that the "Hong Kong operation" allowed an earlier and more certain bony arthrodesis and a lower incidence of posttreatment kyphotic deformity.[65,66] Many other independent studies have supported these conclusions[4,31,48,51,92,103] and have also found a higher recovery rate in patients with neurological deficit.[6,28,54,61]

Interestingly, Hodgson and Stock made no mention of the lateral rhachotomy of Capener, which was first performed in 1933. As indicated previously, because Capener did not describe his procedure until 1954, few surgeons were familiar with his innovative approach.

Thoracic Discectomy

Before the publication of the landmark paper by Mixter and Barr in 1934, many reports of intervertebral disc rupture had been made. In 1932, Schmorl and Junghanns[90] published the results of their investigation of the condition of the ruptured intervertebral disc found at autopsy. The authors identified the pathological changes associated with dorsal prolapse of the intervertebral disc and attributed disc prolapse to weakness of the annulus fibrosus caused by degenerative changes.

However, many clinicians had reported cases involving ruptured intervertebral discs that were not recognized as such (usually mistaken for tumor) or were not held accountable for patients' symptomatology.[11,19,25,29,69] The landscape suddenly changed in 1934 when Mixter and Barr[70] published their classic description of the ruptured intervertebral disc, bringing together its anatomical, pathological, and clinical features (Fig. 1-20).

The early published series on the surgical treatment of thoracic disc disease were all based on a dorsal approach, and the results were astonishingly poor. Mixter and Barr[70] (1934) reported three cases, two of which developed a complete transverse lesion, while the third showed mild, delayed improvement. Hawk[36] (1936) reported on three patients, one of whom deteriorated after surgery, while the other two received no benefit. Müller[71] (1951) reported four cases, three of which developed a complete or almost complete transverse lesion postoperatively, while the fourth, after slight improvement, also developed a complete lesion. Logue[56] (1952) reported on a series of 11 patients, including three who developed total paraplegia postoperatively of whom two died, and two other patients who worsened after surgery but showed mild, incomplete recoveries. In 1969, Perot and Munro[80] summarized the literature as follows: Of 91 reported operative cases, 40 patients were not improved, and 16 of the 40 became paraplegic.

The uniformly poor results obtained by the dorsal approach were not lost on those spine surgeons who tried to tackle this difficult problem.[86] Of course, part of the problem was the difficulty of arriving at a correct diagnosis in a timely fashion. This was particularly true for laterally located disc herniations, which produced only radicular symptoms that were easily

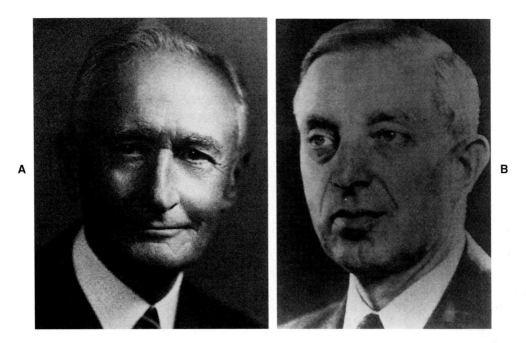

Fig. 1-20. A, William J. Mixter (1880-1958), Boston. **B,** Joseph S. Barr (1901-1964). (From Frymoyer JW. The Adult Spine: Principles and Practice. New York: Raven Press, 1991, p 27.)

misinterpreted as angina pectoris, intercostal neu-ralgia, or pain of an abdominal origin.[92] Love and Schorn[57] observed that a group of patients with a lateral disc herniation fared better than those whose herniation was located centrally. Left untreated, the natural course of central lesions was seen as an inexorable march to paraplegia.[103]

When the first lateral and ventrolateral approaches to thoracic disc herniation began to occur in the late 1950s, the surgical results were excellent.[17,43] Perhaps the first such report was by Crafoord et al.[17] in 1958, involving one patient with thoracic disc protrusion treated by "anterolateral disc fenestration" through the transthoracic approach. In the October 1969 issue of the *Journal of Neurosurgery*, two additional reports of a transthoracic approach to the thoracic disc appeared. Perot et al.[80] published the results in two patients, both of whom had undergone a transthoracic, transpleural approach with complete neurological recovery. Ransohoff et al.[85] reported equally good results in three cases.

Significantly, both Perot and Munro[80] and Ransohoff et al.[85] recognized the importance of leaving the artery of Adamkiewicz undisturbed. Animal studies had shown the catastrophic consequences of

disrupting this major artery.[104] Both reports recommended performing a preoperative spinal angiogram to localize this crucial structure.[20,21]

SURGICAL STABILIZATION AND DEFORMITY CORRECTION

The establishment of a transthoracic approach brought to a close an important chapter in the history of thoracic spine treatments. The application of these approaches to a wide variety of pathologies proved them to be versatile and clarified the advantages and disadvantages of the individual approaches. Aside from the development of the laminectomy, a nineteenth-century innovation, most of these approaches were developed during the first half of the twentieth century. At the same time, however, another series of developments was taking place that would change the face of spinal surgery entirely. This new idea in spinal surgery—"surgical stabilization"—has dominated spinal surgery in the second half of the twentieth century. The history of surgical stabilization and deformity correction has developed along two convergent lines: spinal fusion and spinal instrumentation. Early in their history, these two technical advances

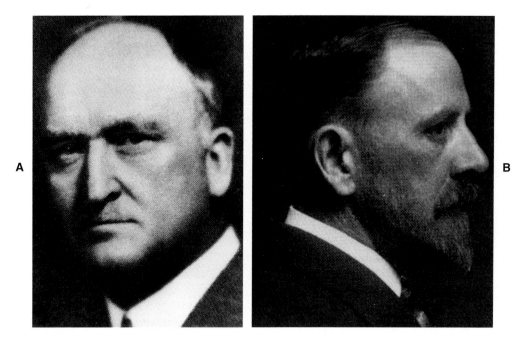

Fig. 1-21. A, Fred Albee (1876-1945). **B,** Russell Hibbs (1869-1932). (From Frymoyer JW. The Adult Spine: Principles and Practice. New York: Raven Press, 1991, p 29.)

were applied independently, often with an untoward outcome. Frequently, this was due to pseudoarthrosis.[97]

By the 1960s, a half century of experience with the problem of pseudoarthrosis had suggested the concept of the race between bony fusion and instrumentation failure. The improved surgical results obtained by combining spinal fusion with instrumentation supported this concept and ushered in the era of modern spinal stabilization.

Spinal Fusion

The first successful attempts at spinal fusion were independently reported by Albee[1] and Hibbs[38] in 1911 (Fig. 1-21). In both instances the fusion was performed to prevent the progressive deformity associated with Pott's disease. Soon thereafter, fusion techniques were applied to a wide variety of pathologies, including scoliosis and traumatic fracture. The method most frequently used was Hibbs's technique, which involved harvesting an autologous bone graft from the laminae and overlying the bone dorsally. Later modifications included harvesting the bone graft from the iliac crest. However, despite such improvements, the procedure was frequently complicated by pseudoarthrosis.[9]

Spinal Instrumentation and Clinical Biomechanics

Like spinal fusion, early efforts in spinal instrumentation began around the turn of the century. For example, in 1891 Berthold Hadra[32] of Galveston, Texas, employed an interspinous wiring technique in a case of pediatric cervical spine trauma (Fig. 1-22). Further efforts followed, but it soon became apparent that the metals employed in constructing the spinal instrumentation were subject to the corrosive effects of electrolysis.

In 1937, Venable, Stuck, and Beach[99] provided experimental evidence that using a combination of metals in the fixation of spinal fractures and other pathological processes resulted in electrolytic reactions that promoted metallic corrosion and inhibited the fusion of bone. In this same report they introduced the metal alloy vitallium, which they believed was associated with the least electrolytic reaction and with the least tissue reaction and bone change. Despite the importance of this technical advance and the innovative efforts of several pioneering spinal surgeons, progress in spinal instrumentation during the 1930s and 1940s was piecemeal.[50,102] In the 1950s, an increasingly sophisticated understanding of spinal biomechanics provided the necessary impetus for bringing spinal

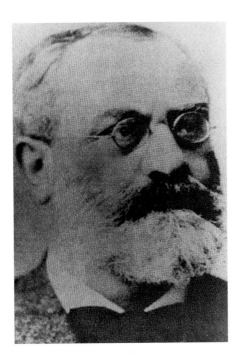

Fig. 1-22. Berthold E. Hadra (1842-1903). (From Hadra BE. Wiring of the spinoles process in injury and Pott's disease. Trans Am Orthop Assoc 4:206, 1981.)

instrumentation to a still higher level of performance. Among the most important individuals involved in this development was an orthopaedic surgeon from Sheffield, England, named F.W. Holdsworth.

F. W. Holdsworth

In 1953 Holdsworth and Hardy[42] published perhaps the first large systematic study of the treatment and surgical outcome of thoracolumbar fractures. In reviewing their experience, Holdsworth observed that most paraplegic patients die from the complications of bed sores and urinary tract infections. Of the 16 patients Holdsworth treated using external fixation by immobilization in plaster, all developed severe pressure sores that took at least 2 years to heal.

To identify the optimal treatment to prevent these complications, Holdsworth reviewed his experience with 68 patients. The methods of surgical stabilization utilized by Holdsworth, which consisted of bolting two plates to the spinous processes above and below the level of injury, were not in themselves exceptional. What was important, and *new*, about Holdsworth's management strategy was his method of patient selection.

Holdsworth[40,41] based his method of patient selection on a classification scheme of spinal fractures. His biomechanical definition of instability divided all fractures into two categories, stable and unstable. Further classification of fractures was based on mechanism of injury and mode of treatment. A two-column theory of spinal stability was the basis for Holdsworth's classification of fractures.

According to Holdsworth, the most critical group of structures for maintaining stability is the "posterior ligamentous complex," which comprises the facet capsule, the intraspinous and supraspinous ligaments, and the ligamenta flava. "It is upon this complex," Holdsworth states, "that the stability of the spine largely depends." Thus rupture of this ligamentous complex prohibits spontaneous healing, in contrast to an isolated vertebral body fracture, which tends to result in spontaneous fusion. Although both of these spinal injuries may be unstable initially, the former type requires operative intervention, whereas the latter, even in the presence of fracture of the articular processes, may be managed nonoperatively.

Using this approach, Holdsworth identified four mechanisms of spinal injury that correlate with fracture types and suggest an appropriate mode of treatment:[40]

1. *Pure flexion.* A pure flexion mechanism is usually associated with an intact posterior ligamentous complex and no evidence of spinal instability. The vertebral body absorbs the greater part of the impact, and the result is a wedge compression fracture. The recommended treatment is usually simple bedrest for 2 to 3 weeks, followed by active exercises for 6 to 8 weeks. In most cases reduction or immobilization is unnecessary.

2. *Flexion-rotation.* A rotation or flexion-rotation mechanism causes disruption of the posterior ligamentous complex and results in an unstable fracture-dislocation. Because it usually involves a horizontal fracture of the vertebral body in addition to fracture of the articular processes and rupture of all the major ligaments, this is the most unstable of all vertebral injuries. It is usually associated with paraplegia and requires either prolonged immobilization or surgical stabilization.

3. *Extension.* An extension mechanism, which is usually stable, most frequently occurs in the

cervical spine. It may be associated with a fracture of the dorsal elements, but is also associated with an intact posterior ligamentous complex.

    4. *Compression.* A compression or "burst" fracture is caused by forces transmitted directly along the line of the vertebral bodies. All of the ligaments are usually intact, and the fracture tends to be stable.

Holdsworth's classification was important, as he himself observed, not as a biomechanical theory (although it was this too), but because it had implications for treatment. Soon several alternative schemes were proposed by other authors, and a new era in spinal surgery had begun.[7,47]

Paul Harrington

Perhaps the best evidence that a new era in spinal surgery had begun was the pioneering work of a Houston, Texas, orthopaedic surgeon named Paul Harrington (Fig. 1-23). In 1945, after completing military service in World War II, Harrington entered into orthopaedic practice, where he soon faced the formidable task of providing care for an epidemic-sized population of poliomyelitis patients.[34] Many

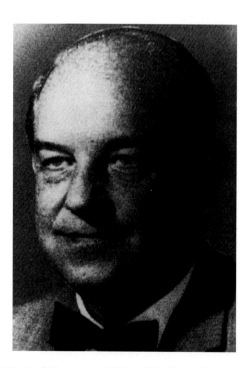

Fig. 1-23. Paul Harrington (1911-1980). (From Harrington PR. The history and development of Harrington instrumentation. Clin Orthop 93:110-112, 1973.)

of these patients developed scoliotic spinal deformity as a result of paraspinous muscle atrophy. Often these deformities resulted in cardiopulmonary compromise that prohibited the use of standard cast corrective measures (which were proving to be ineffective anyway).

In 1941, the American Orthopaedic Association reported the results of treatment in 425 cases of idiopathic scoliosis.[3] The report was quite discouraging. Among patients treated by exercises and braces but without spinal fusion, 60% experienced progression of their deformity, while 40% remained unchanged. In another group of patients who underwent surgical correction and fusion, 54 of 214 developed a pseudoarthrosis, and 29% lost all correction. Considering the entire group, the end result for 69% was deemed fair or poor, and only 31% were rated good to excellent. Such was the state of nonoperative treatment and dorsal spinal fusion against which the results of Harrington were to be compared.

At first Harrington attempted to achieve internal fixation with facet screw instrumentation. This was the first attempt to utilize internal fixation in the treatment of scoliosis. The initial results, though promising, were short-lived, and Harrington abandoned the method in favor of a combination of compression and distraction hooks and rods of stainless steel.[35] Never before had a single instrumentation system provided compression, distraction, and three-point bending capabilities, proving equally useful for deformity correction and maintenance of posttraumatic spinal stabilization. The advantages of the so-called Harrington rods, which possessed great versatility, soon became apparent, and over the next two decades Harrington dedicated himself to developing and investigating his instrumentation system.

Using a grant in aid for research awarded by the National Foundation for Infantile Paralysis in 1954, Harrington undertook a two-phase investigation that resulted in the manufacture of his instrumentation system in 1960.[34] In 1962, Harrington[33] published the results of the early phase of his investigations. In the first phase, Harrington proposed developing instrumentation on approximately 50 poliomyelitis patients over a 5-year period. During this time, a ratchet mechanism was added to the distraction rod, and the rod was lengthened to overcome the problem of frequent breaking. This problem was not observed with the compression system, which therefore remained essentially unchanged.

In the second phase of the investigation, Harrington produced experimental scoliosis in mice and observed the results before and after its correction. As he later observed, "The dramatic restoration to normal, seen when the scoliotic deformity was released, guided the next 3 years of instrument development into an unsuccessful channel."

Initially, the degree of deformity correction achieved with instrumentation appeared gratifying. However, a loss of the correction was almost invariably observed 6 months to 1 year after insertion of the implant. Frequently, such loss was attributed to instrumentation failure as a result of either rod breakage or disengagement of the hooks. More significantly, however, Harrington came to realize that his concept of a dynamic correction system was fundamentally flawed. Experience taught that spinal fusion, over the extent of the spinal instrumentation, would maintain the correction temporarily achieved with the spinal instruments alone. Thus the race between instrumentation failure and the achievement of spinal fusion was born. An understanding of this principle and its successful application comprises one of Harrington's most lasting and significant surgical achievements.

Meanwhile, between 1954 and 1959, repeated clinical observations indicated that metallurgic evaluation and redesign of the instruments were necessary to prevent instrument fatigue and failure. The instruments were made twice as strong by changing the hardness of the distraction rod and altering the design of the ratchet mechanism. In the 5-year study period, 47 changes in instrument materials and design were implemented. By the end of this time, despite persistent problems with disengagement of the lower hooks, the incidence of instrument failure had been dramatically reduced, and the modern era of spinal instrumentation had begun.

A.F. Dwyer

In essence, the Harrington method of scoliosis reduction was based on the principle of lengthening the short (concave) side of the curve. The Harrington system succeeded significantly once the concept of the race between instrumentation failure and the achievement of spinal fusion was recognized and respected by superimposing a bony fusion over the length of the instrumentation construct. Nevertheless, it soon became evident that despite its great promise, dorsal instrumentation was not without drawbacks. For example, the Harrington instrumentation system required that the construct extend at least two levels above and below the spinal curvature, thus forcing the hand of the surgeon to sacrifice mobility in otherwise normal spinal motion segments.

Furthermore, an uneven force application is borne by the two vertebrae attached to the upper and lower hooks, making disengagement of the lower hooks a not uncommon complication. Finally, the dorsal surgical approach provided inadequate exposure of the ventral spinal elements, which meant that to combine ventral decompression with dorsal stabilization required a two-stage operation involving two separate incisions and surgical exposures.

In 1969 an alternative to the Harrington dorsal instrumentation system was introduced by A.F. Dwyer. Dwyer was an orthopaedic surgeon from Australia, who developed his system of ventral instrumentation as an alternative to the Harrington system. In essence, the Harrington method of scoliosis reduction was based on the principle of lengthening the short (concave) side of the curve. In contrast, Dwyer, Newton, and Sherwood[22] described a method of ventral instrumentation in which compressive forces are applied to the *convex* side of the curve. The technique involves excising the discs at each of the levels involved and inserting screws into the convex side of the curve. A titanium cable is then threaded through the heads of the screws, and a tension force is applied, providing a corrective bending moment at the intervertebral spaces. The tension is maintained by swagging the cable on the screw heads (Fig. 1-24).

In 1974, Dwyer and Schafer[23] reported that their instrumentation procedure, performed in 51 cases of scoliosis, had demonstrated favorable results in deformity correction and only a 4% rate of pseudoarthrosis. What is more, the Dwyer device overcame several of the disadvantages of Harrington's dorsal instrumentation system, which had achieved a degree of popularity among spinal surgeons by this time. For example, the establishment of bony fusion could be restricted to the motion segments associated with the curve only. Furthermore, the load borne by the instrumentation device was evenly distributed over the length of the curve (multisegmental fixation). Finally, the exposure

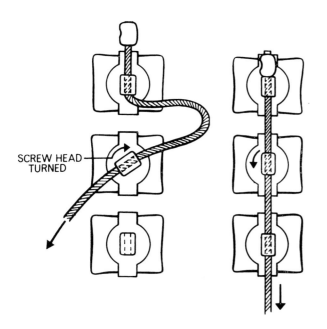

SCREW HEAD
TURNED

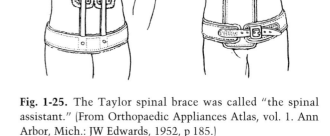

Fig. 1-24. Dwyer instrumentation system. The method of introduction of the cable. (From Dwyer AF, Schafer MF. Anterior Approach to Scoliosis. J Bone Joint Surg 56B:219, 1974.)

Fig. 1-25. The Taylor spinal brace was called "the spinal assistant." (From Orthopaedic Appliances Atlas, vol. 1. Ann Arbor, Mich.: JW Edwards, 1952, p 185.)

necessary for decompression, fusion, and instrumentation could all be achieved through a single incision and surgical approach.

Nevertheless, the disadvantages of the Dwyer instrumentation soon became apparent as many cases were complicated by progressive postoperative kyphosis, and no provision had been made for the construct to help accept an axial load. Although these disadvantages diminished the enthusiasm for the Dwyer device, its generally successful application in ventral instrumentation provided an impetus for the development of other ventral spinal implants, including those of Zielke[105] and Kaneda.[46]

NONOPERATIVE MANAGEMENT

Nonoperative strategies have always played an important role in treating thoracic spine disease. Among those strategies, spinal bracing and spinal exercises have been particularly important in the modern management of thoracic spinal disorders.

Spinal Bracing

Most spinal braces of American origin in the nineteenth century were developed to treat Pott's disease or scoliosis.[2] Numerous braces were designed for these purposes well into the twentieth century. For example, in his 1923 *Handbuch der Orthopä-*

dischen Technic, Schanz[89] described no less than 74 braces for the treatment of scoliosis. Among the most important innovations in nineteenth-century thoracic brace design was an understanding of the biomechanical principle of the "three-point bending force." This had an important influence on the design of many thoracic braces, including the Taylor and Milwaukee braces.

C.F. Taylor[96] was perhaps the first to recognize the importance of this biomechanical principle, which he applied in the design of a brace introduced in 1863. Taylor objected on mechanical grounds to the application of longitudinal forces, which was characteristic of most nineteenth-century designs. The Taylor brace, known as the "spinal assistant," instead utilized a horizontally applied, three-point bending force to produce hyperextension of the spine as a treatment for Pott's disease-related kyphotic deformity. Still used today in a modified form, this brace consists of a pelvic band with two dorsally attached longitudinal members that are fixed to a transverse bar behind the shoulders. Two axillary straps are attached to the transverse bar, and an abdominal pad is attached to the longitudinal members. This produces a three-point bending fixation in which horizontally directed forces are applied dorsally at the shoulders and hips and ventrally at the middle of the back (Fig. 1-25).

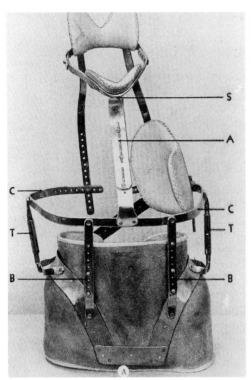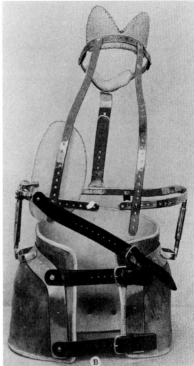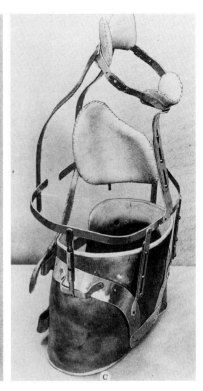

Fig. 1-26. The Milwaukee ventral **(A)** dorsal **(B)** and lateral **(C)** brace. The pictures show the uprights *(B)* extending between the horizontal band *(C)* and pelvic girdle only in front. These two uprights give sufficient stability in younger patients, but in older patients it is necessary to place two uprights dorsally also. (From Orthopaedic Appliances Atlas, vol. 1. Ann Arbor, Mich.: JW Edwards, 1952, pp 232, 233.)

Although the original Taylor brace served to remind the patient to resist excessive motion in flexion and extension, it provided little resistance to lateral bending or axial rotation. To correct these deficiencies, several modified models of the Taylor brace have been made over the years, including one with "lateral uprights." These uprights, which are anchored to the pelvic and thoracic bands, are intended to resist lateral bending. A model with the addition of "clavicular pads," attached to the lateral uprights, has been designed to resist axial rotation. Taylor also described a cervical support that could be readily attached to the spinal uprights dorsally. Further modifications of the original design have increased its efficiency by applying counterpressure ventrally against the upper chest and improving fixation at the pelvis.

At the 1946 meeting of the American Academy of Orthopaedic Surgeons, Walter Blount and Albert Schmidt from Milwaukee, Wisconsin, described a new spinal brace as a surgical adjunct for treating postpoliomyelitis scoliosis.[8] The "Milwaukee brace," as the brace came to be known, was devel-

oped as a refinement of the distraction plaster jacket (Fig. 1-26). At first the Milwaukee brace was used only to treat thoracic curves, which were fused after correction had been obtained. Later the brace was used to obtain correction only after an operative intervention. The rationale was that after contracted muscles and ligaments have been removed at surgery and congenital bars of bone have been osteotomized, the resistance to deformity correction can be improved. In 1958, 12 years after its original description, Blount et al.[8] reported the results of their experience with the Milwaukee brace.

When it was first introduced, the biomechanics of the Milwaukee brace were far more complex than any other available orthosis. That it was a highly effective treatment modality, particularly for the growing child, is corroborated by its survival 50 years after its original description. Essentially the brace was designed to treat thoracic deformity by applying a lateral force at the apex of the spinal curvature, coupled with a longitudinal force. The lack of a constrictive force on the thorax was an improvement over earlier orthoses, many of which tended to defeat the primary purpose of correcting a thoracic curve, which is the preservation of normal pulmonary function. What is more, the dynamic design of this sophisticated and elegant brace has appeared equally effective in applying corrective and immobilizing forces in both the kyphotic and scoliotic spine.

Spinal Exercises

Next to spinal bracing, the other major nonoperative treatment modality that has played an important part in the management of thoracic spinal disorders is "spinal exercises." In 1937, P.C. Williams,[101] an orthopaedic surgeon from Dallas, Texas, developed a set of spinal exercises based on his theory that low back pain and leg pain were the direct result of neural compression caused by spinal extension. Williams's solution was to create a set of spinal exercises that would encourage the reduction of the lumbosacral angle, causing the spine to assume a straight or slightly kyphotic posture. To achieve this, the Williams exercises involve a series of maneuvers intended to strengthen the flexor muscles of the spine and at the same time passively stretch the muscles and ligaments that tend to hold the spine in extension.

In contrast to Williams's negative view of spinal extension, Robin McKenzie, a New Zealand physical therapist, attributed the origin of low back pain to spinal flexion. In his 1981 mononograph, *The Lumbar Spine*, McKenzie[64] laid the groundwork of his nonoperative strategy for treating low back pain. McKenzie believed that with an intact annular wall, a bulge appearing in the dorsal annulus on extension is normal. According to McKenzie, this is because

> In extension the posterior annulus is not under tangential stress and, with the hydrostatic mechanism intact, the nucleus must move anteriorly. It is unlikely that annuluar tearing will occur under these circumstances. [On the other hand,] a bulge appearing in the posterior wall on flexion when the annular wall is damaged may be a threat, as it indicates a weakening posterior annulus. This time the bulge is under increased tangential stress and the nucleus has moved posteriorly.

Based on this theory, McKenzie devised a set of spinal exercises that were the converse of the Williams exercises in that they represented a series of extension maneuvers. To demonstrate the fervor

with which the battle over the optimal spinal posture was fought, McKenzie's defense of spinal extension is worth repeating:

> Insufficient understanding of the mechanics involved in the production of low back pain has led some people to condemn extension of the spine and those who advocate it. If a Higher Authority had decided that extension is undesirable or harmful, the facet joints in the spine would have been placed accordingly! In the absence of such an indication it appears impertinent for man to place such restrictions on the use of the human frame, which after all has evolved over millions of years.

Despite these polemics in defense of spinal extension, the McKenzie program was not limited to spinal extension exercises only. Rather, McKenzie advocated a pretreatment evaluation that included provocative testing of the patient with a variety of flexion, extension, lateral bending, and axial rotation movements to identify the movements that would reproduce the patient's pain. An individualized exercise program was then developed for each patient, based on the results of their pretreatment evaluation.

RECENT ADVANCES

Among the many recent advances in thoracic spinal surgery, one of the most important is the development of endoscopic surgery.

Spinal Endoscopy

In 1931, Burman[12] published the results of a series of cadaveric spine studies he had conducted with an arthroscope. Burman was interested in diseases of the cauda equina, and through innovative experimentation, which he termed "myeloscopy," he was able to visualize the dura mater and blood vessels coursing over the lumbar spine. Regrettably, the poor quality of visualization in those early days of endoscopy prohibited any practical clinical application.

In 1938, Pool[81-83] introduced an important technological advance that improved visualization with the endoscope. His so-called "hot-lamp system" was designed to allow intrathecal observations, which he documented in a collection of original drawings derived from over 400 cases (Fig. 1-27). Despite this remarkable achievement, the "myeloscope," as it was known, did not achieve widespread use because of its primitive visualization.

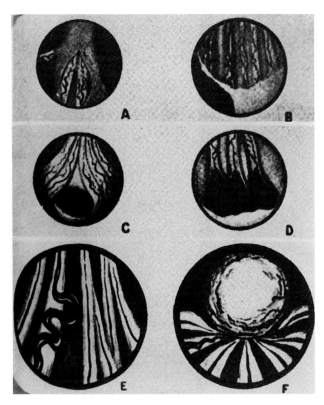

Fig. 1-27. Myeloscopy. Pool developed a hot-lamp system specifically designed for intrathecal observation. He hand-sketched in precise detail all the structures viewed through the endoscope. (From Pool JL. Myeloscopy: Diagnostic inspection of the cauda equina by means of the endoscope. Bull Neurol Inst NY 7:178-189, 1938.)

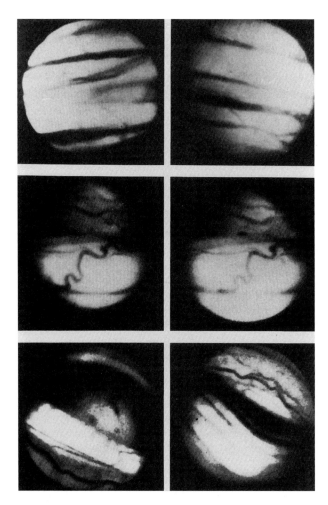

Fig. 1-28. Spinal endoscopy. Ooi, Mita, and Satoh described cases of chronic arachnoiditis, nerve root excursion during testing, and pathophysiological changes associated with claudication in lumbar spinal stenosis. (From Ooi Y, Satoh Y, Morisaki N. Myeloscopy. Int Orthop 1:107-111, 1977. Copyright © Springer-Verlag.)

The state of the art remained essentially unchanged until the 1970s, when Ooi, Satoh, and Morisaki[76,77] performed the first preoperative intrathecal myeloscopy. Several color photographs were obtained during this landmark procedure, providing anatomical detail that was later confirmed at surgery.

Also in the 1970s, important advances in medical engineering set the stage for progress in fiberglass and fiberoptics technology, which allowed the dissipation of heat and led to the development of a small-diameter cold-light system. This new system provided improved visualization, which facilitated the study of the lumbar spine. At least equally important was the change made in the outer diameter of the spinoscope from 5.6 to 0.35 mm. More recently, improved technology has demonstrated excellent visualization in cases of chronic arachnoiditis, nerve root excursion during testing, and pathophysiological changes associated with claudication in lumbar stenosis[75] (Fig. 1-28). With im-

provements in technology and an expanded scope of clinical applications, the spinoscope had finally come of age.

In 1989, epidural spinal endoscopy was performed in the United States using a flexible fiberoptic scope as an adjunct to open surgical procedures.[95] The scope was used both to demonstrate anatomy and to confirm the results of surgical manipulation. In 1991, Mathews[63] reported the use of percutaneous spinal endoscopy to create ventral and dorsolateral fusions. He presented his work at the First International Symposium on Lasers in Orthopedics. Further advances have created a system in which the fiberoptic image bundle is in the side wall of the cannula. This allows direct visualization of the area of pathology through the same cannula that houses the surgical instruments. An alternative, rigid wide-lens system, which provides a higher resolution image and a greater depth and field of view compared to the fiberoptic system, is also available.

CONCLUSION

This chapter reviews the evolution of modern spine surgery from its inception to the present. This evolution, as is the case with other disciplines as well, is based on a sequence of foundations, each of which depends on the acquisition of knowledge. Understandings of anatomy, both bony and soft tissue, and of the structure and function of the spine have played seminal roles in this process, culminating in the highly technical and superior-quality "state of the art" currently enjoyed by spine surgeons and their patients.

REFERENCES

1. Albee FH. Transplantation of a portion of the tibia into the spine for Pott's disease. JAMA 57:885-886, 1911.
2. American Academy of Orthopaedic Surgeons. Orthopaedic Appliances Atlas, vol 1. Ann Arbor, Mich.: JW Edwards, 1952, p 183.
3. American Orthopaedic Association Research Committee. End-result study of the treatment of idiopathic scoliosis. J Bone Joint Surg 23:963-977, 1941.
4. Arct W. Operative treatment of tuberculosis of the spine in old people. J Bone Joint Surg 50A:255-267, 1968.
5. Armour D. Surgery of the spinal cord and its membranes. Lancet 1:423, 1927.
6. Bailey HL, Gabriel SM, Hodgson AR, Shin JS. Tuberculosis of the spine in children, operative findings and results in one hundred consecutive patients treated by removal of the lesions and anterior grafting. J Bone Joint Surg 54A:1633-1657, 1972.
7. Bailey RW. Fractures and dislocations of the cervical spine: Orthopaedic and neurosurgical aspects. Postgrad Med 35:588-599, 1964.
8. Blount WP, Schmidt AC, Keever ED, Leonard ET. The Milwaukee brace in the operative treatment of scoliosis. J Bone Joint Surg 40A:511-525, 1958.
9. Boucher HH. A method of spinal fusion. J Bone Joint Surg 41B:248-259, 1959.
10. Bourne W. Avertin anaesthesia for crippled children. Can Med Assoc J 35:278, 1936.
11. Bucy PC. Chondroma of intervertebral disk. JAMA 94:1552, 1930.
12. Burman MS. Myeloscopy or the direct visualization of the spinal canal and its contents. J Bone Joint Surg 13:695-696, 1931.
13. Calot T. Sur Le meilleur traitement localdes tuberculoses doses articulations et ganglions lymphatiques. Acta Chir Scand 67:206-226, 1930.
14. Capener N. The evolution of lateral rhachotomy. J Bone Joint Surg 36B:173-179, 1954.
15. Chipault A. Une variete nouvelle de paraplegie pottique. Travaux de neurologie chirurgicale 1:190, 1896.
16. Church A, Eisendrath DW. A contribution to spinal cord surgery. Am J Med Sci 103:395-412, 1892.
17. Crafoord C, Hiertonn T, Lindblom K, Olsson SE. Spinal cord compression caused by a protruded thoracic disc. Report of a case treated with antero-lateral fenestration of the disc. Acta Orthop Scand 28:103-107, 1958.
18. Cushing H. The special field of neurological surgery. Bull Johns Hopkins Hosp 16:77-87, 1905.
19. Dandy WE. Loose cartilage from intervertebral disk simulating tumor of the spinal cord. Arch Surg 19:660-672, 1929.
20. DiChiro G, Doppman J, Ommaya AK. Selective arteriography of arteriovenous aneurysms of spinal cord. Radiology 88:1065-1077, 1967.
21. Doppman J, DiChiro G. The arteria radicularis magna: Radiographic anatomy in the adult. Br J Radiol 41:40-45, 1968.
22. Dwyer AF, Newton NC, Sherwood AA. An anterior approach to scoliosis: A preliminary report. Clin Orthop 62:192-202, 1969.
23. Dwyer AF, Schafer MF. Anterior approach to scoliosis: Results of treatment in fifty-one cases. J Bone Joint Surg 56B:218-224, 1974.
24. Elsberg CA. The value of continuous intratracheal insufflation of air (Meltzer) in thoracic surgery. Med Record 77:493, 1910.
25. Elsberg CA. Diagnosis and Treatment of Surgical Diseases of the Spinal Cord and its Membranes. Philadelphia: WB Saunders, 1916, p 238.
26. Elsberg CA. Diagnosis and Treatment of Surgical Diseases of the Spinal Cord and its Membranes. Philadelphia: WB Saunders, 1916, pp 271-278.
27. Fell G. Fell method—Forced respiration—Report of cases resulting in the saving of twenty-eight human lives—History and a plea for its general use in hospital and naval practice. Section of General Medicine, 1st Pan American Medical Congress, 1893, p 309.
28. Fellander M. Paraplegia in spondylitis: Results of operative treatment. Paraplegia 13:75-88, 1975.
29. Goldthwait JE. The lumbo-sacral articulation; An explanation of many cases of "lumbago," "sciatica," and paraplegia. Boston MS J 164:365, 1911.
30. Gowers WR, Horsley VA. A case of tumour of the spinal cord. Removal; recovery. Med Chir Tr 53:379-428, 1888.
31. Guirguis AR. Pott's paraplegia. J Bone Joint Surg 49B:658-667, 1967.
32. Hadra BE. Wiring the spinous processes in Pott's disease. Trans Am Orthop Assoc 4:206-210, 1891.
33. Harrington PR. Treatment of scoliosis. J Bone Joint Surg 44A:591, 1962.
34. Harrington PR. The history and development of Harrington instrumentation. Clin Orthop 93:110-112, 1973.
35. Harrington PR, Tullos HS. Spondylolisthesis in children. Clin Orthop 79:75-84, 1971.
36. Hawk WA. Spinal compression caused by enchondrosis of the intervertebral fibrocartilage: With a review of the recent literature. Brain 59:204-224, 1936.
37. Hayward G. An account of a case of fracture and dislocation of the spine. NENS/J Med Sci 4:1-3, 1815.
38. Hibbs RA. An operation for progressive spinal deformities. NY Med J 93:1013-1016, 1911.
39. Hodgson AR, Stock FE. Anterior spinal fusion: A preliminary communication on the radical treatment of Pott's disease and Pott's paraplegia. Br J Surg 44:266-275, 1956.

40. Holdsworth FW. Fractures, dislocations, and fracture-dislocations of the spine. J Bone Joint Surg 45B:6-20, 1963.

41. Holdsworth FW. Review article: Fractures, dislocations, and fracture-dislocations of the spine. J Bone Joint Surg 52A:1534-1551, 1970.

42. Holdsworth FW, Hardy A. Early treatment of paraplegia from fractures of the thoraco-lumbar spine. J Bone Joint Surg 35B:540-550, 1953.

43. Hulme A. The surgical approach to thoracic intervertebral disc protrusion. J Neurol Neurosurg Psychiatry 15:227-241, 1960.

44. Ito H, Tsuchiya J, Asami G. A new radical operation for Pott's disease. J Bone Joint Surg 16:499-515, 1934.

45. Jackson C. The technique of inserting of intratracheal insufflation tubes. Surg Gynecol Obstet 17:507, 1913.

46. Kaneda K, Abumi K, Fujiya K. Burst fractures with neurologic deficits of the thoraco-lumbar spine. Results of anterior decompression, and stabilization with anterior instrumentation. Spine 9:788-795, 1984.

47. Kelly RP, Whitesides TE. Treatment of lumbodorsal fracture-dislocations. Ann Surg 167:705-717, 1968.

48. Kemp HBS, Jackson JW, Jeremiah JD, Cook J. Anterior fusion of the spine for infective lesions in adults. J Bone Joint Surg 55B:715-734, 1973.

49. Keys TE. History of Surgical Anesthesia. New York: Dover, 1963.

50. King D. Internal fixation for lumbosacral fusion. J Bone Joint Surg 30A:560-565, 1948.

51. Kirkaldy-Willis WH, Thomas TG. Anterior approaches in the diagnosis and treatment of infections of the vertebral bodies. J Bone Joint Surg 47A:87-110, 1965.

52. Kirstein A. Autokopie des larynx und der trachea. Berliner Klin Wchnschr 32:476-478, 1895.

53. Larson SJ, Holst RA, Hemmy DC, Sances A Jr. Lateral extracavitary approach to traumatic lesions of the thoracic and lumbar spine. J Neurosurg 45:628-637, 1976.

54. Lifeso RM, Weaver P, Harder EH. Tuberculous spondylitis in adults. J Bone Joint Surg 67A:1405-1413, 1985.

55. Lister J. Six Papers. Selected by Sir Rickman J. Godley. London, 1912.

56. Logue V. Thoracic intervertebral disc prolapse with spinal cord compression. J Neurol Neurosurg Psychiatry 15:227-241, 1952.

57. Love JG, Schorn VG. Thoracic disc protrusions. JAMA 191:627-631, 1965.

58. Lucas GHW, Henderson BE. A new anaesthetic gas: Cyclopropane. Can Med Assoc J 21:173, 1929.

59. Lundy JS. Intravenous anesthesia: Preliminary report of the use of two new thiobarbituates. Proc Staff Meet Mayo Clin 10:536-543, 1935.

60. Macewan W. Introduction of tracheal tubes by the mouth instead of performing tracheotomy or laryngotomy. Br Med J 2:122, 1880.

61. Martin NS. Pott's paraplegia: A report of 120 cases. J Bone Joint Surg 53B:596-608, 1971.

62. Matas R. On the management of acute traumatic pneumothorax. Ann Surg 29:409, 1899.

63. Mathews H. First International Symposium on Lasers in Orthopedics. San Francisco: September 1991.

64. McKenzie RA. The Lumbar Spine: Mechanical Diagnosis and Therapy. Wellington, N.Z.: Spinal Publications, 1981.

65. Medical Research Council Working Party on Tuberculosis of the Spine. A controlled trial of anterior spinal fusion and debridement in the surgical management of tuberculosis of the spine in patients on standard chemotherapy: A study in Hong Kong. Br J Surg 61:853-866, 1974.

66. Medical Research Council Working Party on Tuberculosis of the Spine. A 10-year assessment of a controlled trial comparing debridement and anterior spinal fusion in the management of tuberculosis of the spine in patients on standard chemotherapy in Hong Kong. J Bone Joint Surg 64B:393-398, 1982.

67. Meltzer SJ. Anesthesia by intratracheal insufflation. In Keen WW, ed. Surgery, vol. 6. Philadelphia: WB Saunders, 1913, p 150.

68. Ménard V. Causes de la paraplégie dans le mal de Pott. Son traitement chirurgical par ouverture direct du foyer tuberculeux des vertèbres. Rev Orthop 5:47-64, 1894.

69. Middleton GS, Teacher JH. Injury of the spinal cord due to rupture of an intervertebral disk during muscular effort. Glasgow MJ 76:139, 1911.

70. Mixter WJ, Barr JS. Rupture of the intervertebral disc with involvement of the spinal canal. NENS/J Med 211:210-215, 1934.

71. Muller R. Protrusion of thoracic intervertebral disks with compression of the spinal cord. Acta Medica Scand 139:99-104, 1950.

72. Müller W. Transperitoneale freilegung der wirbelsaule bei tuberkuloser spondylitis. Deutsche Ztschr f Chir 85:128, 1906.

73. Mushin WW. Thoracic Anesthesia. Philadelphia: FA Davis, 1963, ch 20.

74. Nissen R, Wilson RHI. Pages in the History of Chest Surgery. Springfield, Ill.: Charles C Thomas, 1960.

75. Ooi Y, Mita F, Satoh Y. Myeloscopic study on lumbar spinal canal stenosis with special reference to intermittent claudication. Spine 15:544-549, 1990.

76. Ooi Y, Satoh Y, Morisaki N. Myeloscopy: The possibility of observing the lumbar intrathecal space by use of an endoscope. Endoscopy 5:901-906, 1973.

77. Ooi Y, Satoh Y, Morisaki N. Myeloscopy. Int Orthop 1:107-111, 1977.

78. Parham FW. Thoracic resections for tumors growing from the bony wall of the chest. Trans Southern Surg Gynecol Assoc 11:223, 1899.

79. Paul of Aegina. The Seven Books of Paulus Aegineta. Tr. Adams F. 3 vols. London: Sydenham Society, 1844.

80. Perot PL Jr, Munro DD. Transthoracic removal of midline thoracic disc protrusion causing spinal cord compression. J Neurosurg 31:452-458, 1969.

81. Pool JL. Direct visualization of dorsal nerve roots of the cauda equina by means of the myeloscope. Arch Neurol Psychol 39:1308-1312, 1938.

82. Pool JL. Myeloscopy: Diagnostic inspection of the cauda equina by means of the endoscope. Bull Neurol Inst NY 7:178-189, 1938.

83. Pool JL. Myeloscopy: Intrathecal endoscopy. Surgery 11:169-182, 1942.

84. Pott P. Remarks on that kind of palsy of the lower limbs which is frequently found to accompany a curvature of the spine and is supposed to be caused by it; together with its method of cure; etc. London: J Johnson, 1779.

85. Ransohoff J, Spencer F, Siew F, Gage L Jr. Cases reports and technical notes. Transthoracic removal of thoracic disc. Report of three cases. J Neurosurg 31:459-461, 1969.

86. Reeves DL, Brown HA. Thoracic intervertebral disc protrusion with spinal cord compression. J Neurosurg 28:24-28, 1968.

87. Rogers DL. A case of fractured spine with depression of the spinous processes, and the operation for its removal. Am J Med Sci 16:91-94, 1835.

88. Rowbotham ES, Magill L. Anesthetics in the plastic surgery of the face and jaws. Proc Roy Soc Med 14:17.

89. Schanz A. Handbuch der Orthopädischen Technik. Jena: Gustav Fischer, 1923.

90. Schmorl G, Junghanns H. Archiv und Atlas der normalen und pathlogischen Anatomie in typischen Rontgenbildern. Leipzig: Georg Thieme, 1932.

91. Seddon HJ. Pott's paraplegia—prognosis and treatment. Br J Surg 22:769, 1935.

92. Shaw NE, Thomas TG. Surgical treatment of chronic infective lesions of the spine. Br Med J 1:162-164, 1963.

93. Smith AG. Account of a case in which portions of three dorsal vertebrae were removed for the relief of paralysis from fracture, with partial success. In extracts from a letter to Dr BH Coates. North Am Med Surg J 8:94-97, 1829.

94. Sorrel-Dejerine Y. Contribution a l'Etude des Paraplegies Pottiques. Paris, 1925.

95. Stoll J, Watkins RG, Mathews H. FDA-IDE Study. Milwaukee: Midwest Spinal Center, 1989.

96. Taylor CF. On the mechanical treatment of Pott's disease of the spine—The "spinal assistant." Trans NY Med Soc 6:67, 1863.

97. Thompson WAL, Ralston EL. Pseudoarthrosis following spine fusion. J Bone Joint Surg 31A:400-405, 1949.

98. Tyrell F. Compression of the spinal marrow from displacement of the vertebrae, consequent upon injury. Operation of removing the arch and spinous processes of the twelfth dorsal vertebra. Lancet 11:685-688, 1827.

99. Venable CS, Stuck WG, Beach A. The effects on bone of the presence of metals: Based upon electrolysis. Ann Surg 105:917-938, 1937.

100. von Eiselsberg AF, Ranzi E. Ueber die chirurgische Behandlung der Hirn- und Rükenmarkstumoren. Arch Klin Chir 102:309-468, 1913.

101. Williams PC. Lesions of the lumbosacral spine. II. Chronic traumatic (postural) destruction of the lumbosacral intervertebral disc. J Bone Joint Surg 19:690-703, 1937.

102. Wilson PD, Straub LR. The use of a metal plate fastened to the spinous processes. American Academy of Orthopaedic Surgeons Instructional Course Lecture, Ann Arbor, Mich., 1952.

103. Wiltberger BR. Resection of vertebral bodies and bone grafting for chronic osteomyelitis of the spine. J Bone Joint Surg 34A:215-218, 1952.

104. Yoss RE. Vascular supply of the spinal cord: The production of vascular syndromes. U Mich Med Bull 16:333-345, 1950.

105. Zielke K, Pellin B. Neue Instrumente und Implantate zur Erganzung des Harrington Systems. Z Orthop Chir 114:218-224, 1976.

Anatomy

Jeffrey D. Gross, M.D., and Edward C. Benzel, M.D.

SKELETAL ANATOMY OF THE THORACIC SPINE
Segmental Features
Characteristic Features

Additional facet joints necessary for rib articulation make thoracic spinal vertebrae different from their cervical or lumbar siblings.[6,15,30] There are a total of 12 thoracic vertebrae, although the anomalic absence of the twelfth and possibly eleventh rib may be confusing when evaluating radiographs or performing surgical localization. Thoracic vertebrae have a typically small spinal canal (vertebral foramen) to transmit the thin thoracic spinal cord (Fig. 2-1).

Individual Vertebral Characteristics

The first thoracic vertebra is quite similar to its cervical neighbors except that there are no transverse foramina for the vertebral arteries and the costal facets are present.[6] In fact, the first thoracic vertebra contains an entire costal facet and the rostral portion

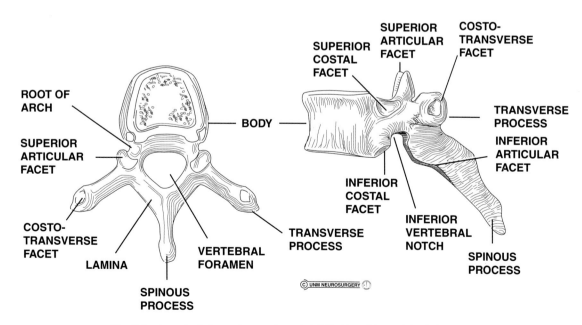

Fig. 2-1. A typical thoracic vertebra. Axial (*left*) and lateral (*right*) views.

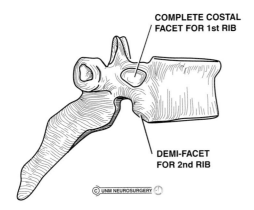

Fig. 2-2. The first thoracic vertebra (lateral view).

(demifacet) of the articulation for the second rib (Fig. 2-2).[6,15,30] This demifacet is the half-circular portion of the costovertebral articulation at one end of the vertebral body that, with the other semicircular demifacet from the neighboring vertebral body, makes a complete circular articular facet for the rib head. The vertebral body at this level also has two ventrolateral prominences on its lower border like the cervical vertebrae.[6] Additionally, the spinal canal is larger than more caudal thoracic segments to accommodate the caudal portion of the cervical enlargement of the spinal cord. The twelfth thoracic vertebra may be likened to the lumbar vertebrae in that the spinal canal is larger to allow the lumbar enlargement of the spinal cord, yet this body manifests costal facets unlike the lumbar bodies. The mean area of the spinal canal occupied by the thoracic spinal cord has been measured as 26.1% at T1 and 21.4% at T6.[11] Both the eleventh and twelfth thoracic vertebrae contain a single but complete costal facet on either side of the body, whereas all other thoracic vertebrae caudal to T1 contain a rostral and caudal demifacet on each side of the body (see Fig. 2-1). However, in some cases, the tenth thoracic vertebra contains a complete costal facet associated with the ninth vertebra having only a rostral articular costovertebral facet.[15]

Vertebral Body Anatomy

The thoracic vertebrae have rounded, triangular or heart-shaped bodies that harbor these costal facets on the lateral surfaces.[6,15,29,30] Typical thoracic vertebral bodies are somewhat shorter ventrally than dorsally (see Fig. 2-1). The degree of this "wedging"

varies with thoracic level.[10,12,14] The thoracic vertebral bodies increase in size, particularly in their transverse dimension, in a caudal direction after the third thoracic vertebra.[6,15,24] The body height also increases in this caudal trend.[4] In the lower thoracic spine, the lateral diameter of the body increases more rapidly than the ventrodorsal diameter.[5] The ventral aspect of the midthoracic vertebral bodies is concave, which forms a protective groove for the thoracic aorta.[6,15,29,30] This concavity is often off center to the left and is most marked at the T5 level. The thoracic vertebral body end plates are slightly convex toward the center of the bone.[30] Large vascular channels in the lateral portions of the bodies may be noted for the transmittal of draining medullary veins to the azygos system. Foramina may also be encountered in the dorsal aspect of each body, which allow the basivertebral vein to drain to the epidural spinal venous plexus.[6] Markings for the attachment of the anterior longitudinal ligament may also be seen on the rostral and caudal ventral surfaces of the body.[6]

Pedicle Anatomy

Thoracic pedicles are thick and leave the vertebral bodies near their rostral ends (see Fig. 2-1).[29] The T5 pedicle is the narrowest of the thoracic pedicles in the transverse plane.[19,31,36] In the sagittal plane, the T11 pedicle is the widest, and the first thoracic pedicle is the narrowest.[12] The longest rostrocaudal dimension is found in the T12 pedicle.[17,19] The outer diameter of the lower thoracic pedicles approaches 8 cm, and the internal diameter measures between 5 and 6 cm.[5] They can be extremely variable from level to level and within a single pedicle,[26] but the average transverse diameter ranges between 4.5 mm at T4 and 7.8 mm at T12.[5,33] In the upper thoracic segments, the pedicles are directed further rostral in their course. The medial pedicular cortical walls are between two and three times thicker than their lateral walls.[21] The infrapedicular spaces (inferior vertebral notches) are the largest of any of the spinal regions due to the relative rostral takeoff of the pedicle from the vertebral body.[6,15,29] The transverse pedicle angle decreases with increasing thoracic level number to become nearly directly sagittal in direction for the last two thoracic vertebrae.[4] Measurements of the transverse angle of the pedicles have been made: 30-40 degrees at T1-T2; 20-25 degrees at T3-T11; and 10 degrees at T12.[4,13] The sagittal pedicle angle remains relatively constant throughout the thoracic region about 15 degrees above the horizontal.[4]

Transverse Process Anatomy

Thoracic transverse processes arise from the dorsal aspect of the vertebrae, near the junction of the pedicle and lamina, dorsal to the facet joints (see Fig. 2-1).[4,6,15] At T1, the transverse process is found about 5.5 mm rostral to the pedicle, and this relationship changes as the spine descends.[23] Thus this landmark does not exactly predict the position of the pedicle.[17,23] This extremity of T11 and T12 may be very short.[4,15] They project somewhat dorsally as they extend laterally.[14] The transverse processes of the thoracic region are strong to provide support for the ribs, which also articulate with them from T1 to T10. These costotransverse articular facets are found on the ventral surface of the transverse processes from T1 to T7 (the sternal ribs), are located more rostrally on the transverse processes from T8 to T10 (the "false" ribs), and are not present on the transverse processes of T11 or T12 (the floating ribs), whose articulations are limited to the vertebral bodies. The costotransverse articulations slant more dorsally as the thoracic spine is descended, with the first thoracic level being directed most transversely. Additionally, this articulation is found more medially as the thoracic spine is descended. Tubercles, most notable on the twelfth and possibly eleventh thoracic transverse processes, function as muscular attachments.[6] Roughened and tuberculated areas on the processes are present for other muscular and ligamentous attachments.

Laminar and Spinous Process Anatomy

Midthoracic laminae and their spinous processes completely overlap the body and intervertebral disc of the next caudal segment[6,14,15] (Fig. 2-3). The laminae are taller than they are wide.[14] The seventh thoracic spinous process is commonly the longest and most caudally oblique. The spinous processes of the upper and lower thoracic spine are less obliquely directed. A linear ridge on the ventral surface of these laminae demarcates the rostral attachment of the interlaminar ligament (ligamentum flavum). There are prominent tubercles at the distal end of the tho-

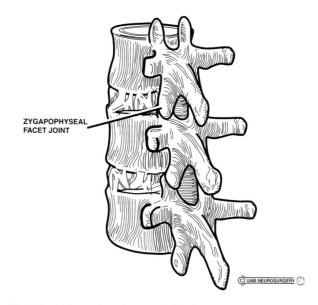

Fig. 2-3. Oblique dorsal view of the thoracic vertebral dorsal bony elements.

racic spinous processes for the origin of muscles and ligaments of the upper back.

Facet Joint Anatomy

Thoracic zygapophyseal facets are flat and nearly vertical, projecting from the pedicles (see Fig. 2-3). The superior articular facet projects slightly outward and rostral, and the inferior articular facet projects somewhat inward and caudal.[15] The slightly concave superior articular facets are angled 60 degrees from the horizontal plane and 20 degrees from the frontal plane[4,14,30] (Fig. 2-4). The facet joints are intermediate between the relatively coronally oriented cervical and sagittally oriented lumbar facet articulations.

Rib and Demifacet Anatomy

The typical configuration observed on thoracic vertebral bodies from T2 to T8 contains two demifacets per side, which together with the closest demifacets of the neighboring segments, makes the two complete articulations for two ribs on that side (see Fig. 2-1).[6,15,30] The costal facets are found closer to the rostral margin of the bodies and more caudal and dorsal on the bodies as the spine is descended.[24] These facets are near the root of the pedicle, dorsal on the vertebral body.[24] Bony markings around

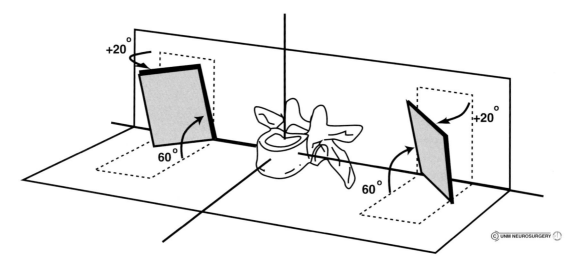

Fig. 2-4. Intermediate orientation of the thoracic facet joints.

these facets allow for the attachment of the radiate ligaments of the rib heads. The portion of the rib that articulates with the vertebrae is termed the head of the rib. Each rib head, except for the first, eleventh, twelfth, and often the tenth ribs, has two articular facets for articulation with the two demi-facets of two adjacent vertebrae.[6] These rib heads have a full single facet for individual articulation with the thoracic vertebral body for which it is named (Fig. 2-5). On ribs that articulate between two vertebral bodies, there is an intervening inter-articular crest between the two facets on the rib head for the attachment of ligaments to the inter-vertebral disc. These ribs may also be named by the caudal of the two vertebrae with which it articulates. The next portion of the rib, termed the "neck," contains a rough ridge, termed the "crest," where the costotransverse ligament attaches.[6] The pleural surface of the neck is smooth. The remaining distal portion of the rib is termed the "shaft" or "body." The point where the shaft joins the neck is called the "tubercle," because of a caudodorsal prominence for the articulation with the articular facet found on the transverse process of the vertebra for which it is named. Ribs are angled obliquely caudally; this oblique orientation increases with descending levels.

The first rib articulates only with T1. This rib is shorter and flatter than its siblings.[6,15] The second rib is the first to have two articular facets for vertebral articulation. It then articulates with the first and second thoracic vertebral bodies. The third through ninth ribs articulate with two adjacent ver-

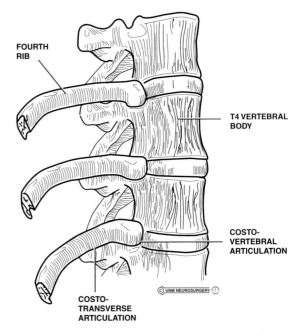

Fig. 2-5. Costovertebral and costotransverse articulations.

tebral bodies each, and with the transverse process of the caudal of the two vertebrae for which they are named.[6] The tenth through twelfth ribs typically articulate only with their corresponding vertebral bodies, and the eleventh and twelfth ribs do not articulate with transverse processes.[6,15,30]

The Thoracic Spinal Column

The primary curvature of the thoracic spinal column is normally slightly kyphotic, which corresponds to the lesser ventral vertical height of the

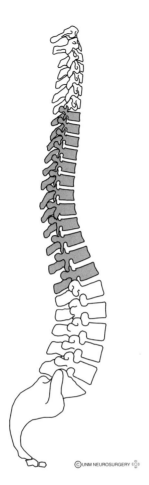

Fig. 2-6. The spinal column (sagittal view). The thoracic vertebrae are shaded.

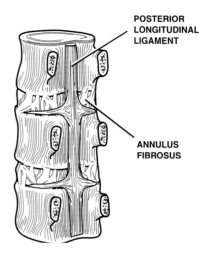

Fig. 2-7. Ligaments surrounding the thoracic vertebral body.

membranes).[16,30] The ligamentum flavum may be considered a syndesmosis (an immovable joint separated by connective tissue) between interposing laminae that is intimately attached to each articular facet capsule.[30] Other diarthroidial joints in the thoracic spine include the articular capsule of the rib head. This capsule is split into two independent capsules, divided by the interarticular ligament in cases where the rib articulates with two vertebrae.[14,16,30] Also, the costotransverse articulation is a diarthroidial joint.[16,30] Joints of the vertebral column are supplied by branches of the spinal nerve at each segment.[5,30]

SOFT TISSUES OF THE THORACIC SPINE
Ligamentous Anatomy of the Thoracic Spine
Ligaments of the Vertebral Body

The ligaments surrounding the thoracic vertebral bodies include the anterior longitudinal ligament, ventrally; the posterior longitudinal ligament, dorsally; and the annulus fibrosus of the intervertebral discs, rostral and caudal to each vertebral body[15] (Fig. 2-7). The anterior longitudinal ligament is a continuous band throughout the axial skeleton. It is found along the ventral portion of the vertebral bodies, attaching to each annulus fibrosus and to the vertebral end plates ventrally.[14,15] It is made of multiple layers of interlacing fibers oriented longitudinally. The most ventral fibers may span four or five segments, whereas the fibers most intimately associated with the vertebral bodies and discs are

bodies[6] (Fig. 2-6). The concavity peaks at the T7 level.[15] There may often be a slight lateral curve, often to the right, which is thought to be due to muscular asymmetry from favoring the dominant (right) arm.[6,15,30] The disc spaces in the thoracic region are somewhat short because the thoracic vertebral motions are limited by the thoracic cage made of the ribs, sternum, and spinal components. The spinal canal is thinnest in the thoracic region, except for the very upper and lower thoracic levels, owing to the cervical and lumbar enlargements of the spinal cord, respectively.[6]

Joints of the Thoracic Spine

The articular facet joints are diarthrodial (synovial-lined) joints between adjacent facets.[14,16,29,30] The bodies also articulate via the intervertebral discs, which are amphiarthrodial joints (without synovial

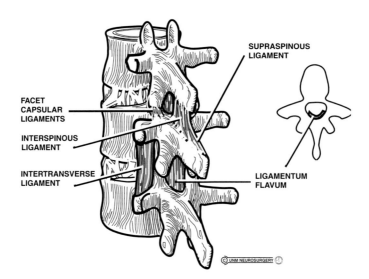

FACET
CAPSULAR
LIGAMENTS

INTERSPINOUS
LIGAMENT

INTERTRANSVERSE
LIGAMENT

SUPRASPINOUS
LIGAMENT

LIGAMENTUM
FLAVUM

© UNM NEUROSURGERY

Fig. 2-8. Dorsolateral view of the ligaments of the dorsal thoracic vertebral region.

shorter. The ligament is thickest in the thoracic region and intermittently thicker ventral to each vertebral body, where it fills in the concavity between the end plates.[15,24] In the upper thoracic region, the anterior longitudinal ligament blends with the tendon of insertion of the longus colli muscle. Laterally, the ligament transmits veins from the vertebral bodies destined for the azygos veins.[6]

The posterior longitudinal ligament also extends continuously throughout the spinal axis. Similarly, this ligament is also thickest in the thoracic region. It is broad and continuous where it attaches to the annulus fibroses and vertebral body end plates, and its fibers are organized like the anterior longitudinal ligament.[14,15,24] However, this ligament has significant narrowings over the center of the dorsum of each vertebral body. The basivertebral veins pass through this narrowing in the ligament at each level on their way to the epidural spinal venous plexus.[6,15] In general, the posterior longitudinal ligament is thicker than the anterior longitudinal ligament. The posterior longitudinal ligament is separated from the dura mater dorsally by loose connective tissue.[15]

The annulus fibrosus will be discussed later in this chapter. Lateral vertebral ligaments are made of short fibers that connect the anterior and posterior longitudinal ligaments around each intervertebral disc. They attach to the anterior and posterior longitudinal ligaments, the annulus fibrosus, and the end plates of the two vertebral bodies surrounding the disc space.[30]

Ligaments of the Laminae and Spinous Processes

The ligamentum flavum connects each overlapping lamina (Fig. 2-8). The ligament is bilateral and attaches laterally at the medial facet and dorsal aspect of the intervertebral foramen, rostrally along the midventral surface of the lamina above, medially along the base of the spinous process, and caudally to the dorsal surface of the lamina below.[15,24,30] Thus each lamina has a ventral interlaminar ligament extending to the next caudal segment and a dorsal interlaminar ligament extending to the next rostral segment (Fig. 2-9). This ligament is not very visible from the dorsal aspect due to the nearly overlapping laminae. There is a medial gap in this ligament complex for the passage of small vessels. These ligaments are thickest in the thoracic region.[14,15,30] The fibers of the ligamentum flavum are perpendicularly oriented to the laminae.[15] The thin interspinous ligaments similarly connect each adjacent spinous process and extend from the root to the dorsal margin of the spinous process, attaching to the interlaminar ligament laterally and to the supraspinous ligament dorsally. The fibers of these ligaments are also longitudinal.[28] The strong, fibrous supraspinous ligaments attach adjacent spinous process tips to the aponeurosis of the deep thoracic region (the thoracolumbar fascia) dorsally and to the interspinous ligaments ventrally.[15,24,28] The fibers of the supraspinous ligaments travel three to four segments dorsally and only a single segment ventrally.[15,28]

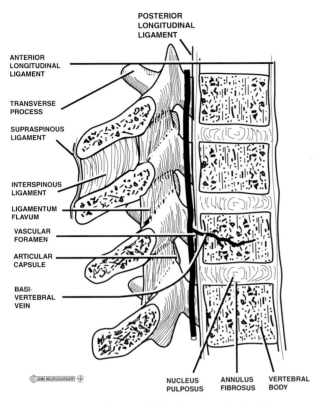

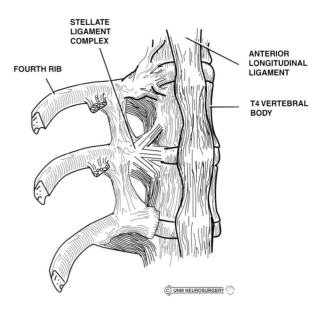

Fig. 2-9. Sagittal view of the thoracic spinal column.

Fig. 2-10. Ventral view of the thoracic vertebral column depicting the anterior costovertebral (stellate) ligament complex.

Ligaments of the Facet Joints

The capsular ligaments surround the facet joint capsule and attach to the interlaminar ligaments medially. They are thin, loose fibers that support the facet joints and attached ligaments. Intertransverse ligaments are interposed between adjacent transverse processes.[15,24] They are not true ligaments.[18]

Ligaments of Costovertebral Articulations

The anterior costovertebral (stellate or radiate) ligaments connect the ventral portion of the rib head to the lateral portion of the neighboring vertebral bodies with which they articulate.[15,30] They may be divided into three heads: (1) a rostral head that attaches to the rostral vertebral body; (2) a caudal head that articulates with the caudal vertebral body; and (3) a middle head that attaches to the annulus fibrosus of the intervening disc[15,24] (Fig. 2-10). These ligaments cannot be divided into three components when the rib of that segment articulates with only one vertebra, although fibers may extend to the next rostral level.

A loose costovertebral capsular ligament surrounds the costovertebral joint and attaches to the annulus fibrosus of the intervening disc. This ligament also attaches to the anterior costovertebral ligament. Some fibers attaching to the annulus extend through the intervertebral foramen to lie along the dorsal portion of the annulus.[15] A short interarticular ligament bridges the crest between the two articular portions of the rib head with the annulus fibrosus. Therefore this ligament does not exist where the rib head articulates with only one vertebra.

The anterior costotransverse ligament attaches the rostral portion of the rib neck to the caudal portion of the transverse process immediately above the rib (Fig. 2-11). Some dorsal fibers of this ligament attach to the base of the same transverse process and lateral margin of the inferior articular process of the vertebra, giving rise to this transverse process.[15] The intercostal neurovascular bundle passes through an opening in this ligament and then dorsal to it. Laterally, the anterior costotransverse ligament attaches to the external intercostal muscle and its aponeurosis.[15,30] This ligament is nonexistent at the first rib. A middle costotransverse ligament (interosseous ligament) attaches the dorsal portion of each rib neck to the ventral portion of the adjacent transverse process. Thus each rib has ligamentous attachments to the adjacent transverse process (middle costotransverse ligament) and the transverse process above (anterior costotransverse ligament).[24] A posterior costotransverse ligament passes obliquely lateral from the distal portion of

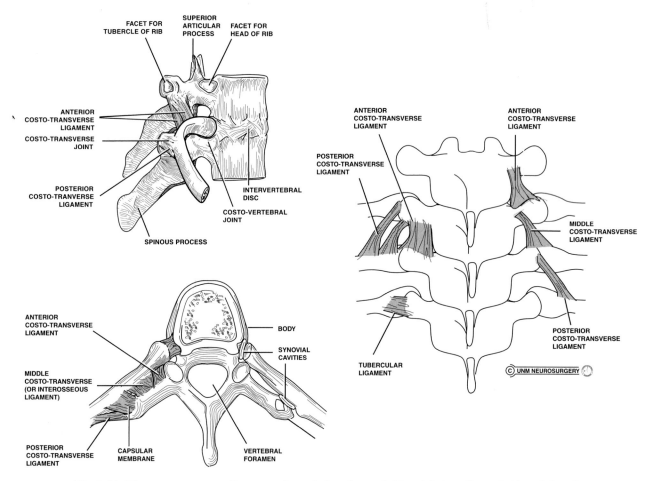

Fig. 2-11. The costotransverse ligaments: lateral view *(upper left)*; axial view *(lower left)*; and dorsal view *(right)*.

the transverse process to the tubercle of the rib of the same segment and the neighboring segment below. The middle and posterior costotransverse ligaments are often absent at the eleventh and twelfth ribs. The distal end of the transverse process also attaches to the nonarticular portion of the rib tubercle via the tubercular ligament, except on ribs eleven and twelve.[30] A capsular ligament surrounds the articular portion of the rib, where it attaches with the transverse process, except at the eleventh and twelfth thoracic levels.[15]

Intraspinal Ligaments

The meningo vertebral ligaments of Hoffmann bridge the dorsum of the vertebral bodies to the dural sac. They may play a role in back pain.[2]

Anatomy of Thoracic Intervertebral Discs

The intervertebral discs are shortest, yet possibly stronger, in the thoracic region.[14] The narrowest disc may be found at the T4-5 interspace.[27] The ratio of disc height to vertebral body height is 1:5.[14] The discs are slightly thicker dorsally than ventrally.[6,14,15,27] The surrounding annulus fibrosus is made of tough fibrous and cartilaginous tissue that attaches to the end plates of the two neighboring vertebral bodies.[14] Alternating fiber layers attach obliquely so that they are perpendicular.[14,15] Some superficial fibers extend beyond the end plate to the ventral and lateral surfaces of the vertebral body.[14] These fibers are termed Sharpey's fibers (Fig. 2-12).[14] The annulus is also intimately attached to numerous spinal and costovertebral ligaments. The confined nucleus pulposus is somewhat dorsally off

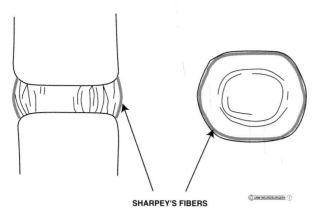

SHARPEY'S FIBERS

Fig. 2-12. The intervertebral disc. Note Sharpey's fibers at the periphery of the disc.

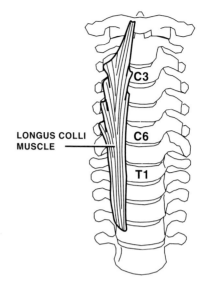

LONGUS COLLI MUSCLE

C3

C6

T1

Fig. 2-13. The ventral cervical and upper thoracic spine and longus colli muscle.

center.[3,8] It is separated from the vertebral end plates by articular cartilage.[14,15,24]

Thoracic Paravertebral Muscular Anatomy
Prevertebral Muscular Anatomy

The prevertebral muscles lie ventral to the thoracic spine. The longus colli inserts in the cervical spine and into the upper thoracic spine, often on to T3.[15] The inferior oblique portion of this muscle arises from the thoracic vertebrae, namely the ventral portion of the bodies, and ascends to the ventral tubercles of the transverse processes of the lower cervical vertebrae[15] (Fig. 2-13). The superior oblique portion pertains only to the cervical spine.[15] The vertical portion lies directly ventral to the spine and attaches to the vertebral bodies.[15] This muscle is immediately deep to the prevertebral fascia.

Paraspinal Muscular Anatomy

Dorsally, the erector spinae muscular group lies deep to the thoracolumbar fascia and fills in the vertebral grooves between the transverse and spinous processes bilaterally (Fig. 2-14). These paraspinal muscles are mostly longitudinal and are innervated by the dorsal divisions of the thoracic spinal nerves.[14] The origin of the iliocostalis thoracis muscle group, the most lateral of the crector spinae muscles, lies along the angles of the lower thoracic ribs, medial to the iliocostalis lumborum group. This muscle group ascends to the angles of the

upper ribs and to the transverse process of C7.[14] Rostral to the iliocostalis muscle lie the musculus accessorius and illiocostalem muscles, which extend from the rostral portion of the upper six rib angles to the dorsal portion of the seventh cervical transverse process.[15] Medial to the iliocostalis and musculus accesorius lies the longissimus thoracis group. This muscle begins at the dorsum of the transverse processes of the lumbar vertebrae and from the thoracolumbar fascia.[14] It extends to insert on the tips of the thoracic transverse processes. Some texts term the more medial fibers of the longissimus thoracis muscle as the spinalis thoracis muscle.[15] This spinalis thoracis muscle, which begins at the spinous processes of T11 to L2, inserts onto the spinous processes of the upper thoracic vertebrae.

The deeper erector spinae muscles include the semispinalis thoracis, the multifidus, the rotatores spinae, and the intertransversarii muscles (see Fig. 2-14). The semispinalis thoracis muscle arises from the transverse processes of the lower thoracic segments and attaches to the spinous processes of the upper thoracic and lower cervical segments.[14] It is just deep to the spinalis thoracis and the longissimus thoracis muscles. The multifidus muscle runs the entire course of the spine, filling in the groove at each side of the spinous processes and extending laterally in the thoracic region to the transverse processes. The

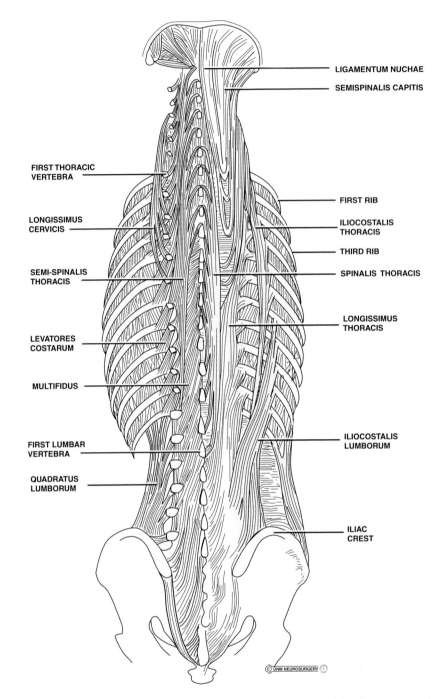

LIGAMENTUM NUCHAE

SEMISPINALIS CAPITIS

FIRST THORACIC VERTEBRA

FIRST RIB

LONGISSIMUS CERVICIS

ILIOCOSTALIS THORACIS

THIRD RIB

SEMI-SPINALIS THORACIS

SPINALIS THORACIS

LONGISSIMUS THORACIS

LEVATORES COSTARUM

MULTIFIDUS

FIRST LUMBAR VERTEBRA

ILIOCOSTALIS LUMBORUM

QUADRATUS LUMBORUM

ILIAC CREST

© UNM NEUROSURGERY

Fig. 2-14. The erector spinae muscle group of the dorsal thoracic spine *(left)* and deeper muscles of the erector spinae group of the thoracic spine *(right).*

fibers extend for a variable number of segments, with the more superficial fibers ascending more levels than the deeper fibers.[14] The rotatores thoracis longus and brevis muscles are the deepest muscles connecting the transverse processes and the dorsal portions of the spinal arches. Their origins are the root of each transverse process, and insertions are one to two laminae rostrally. The short intertransversarii muscles connect neighboring transverse processes.[14]

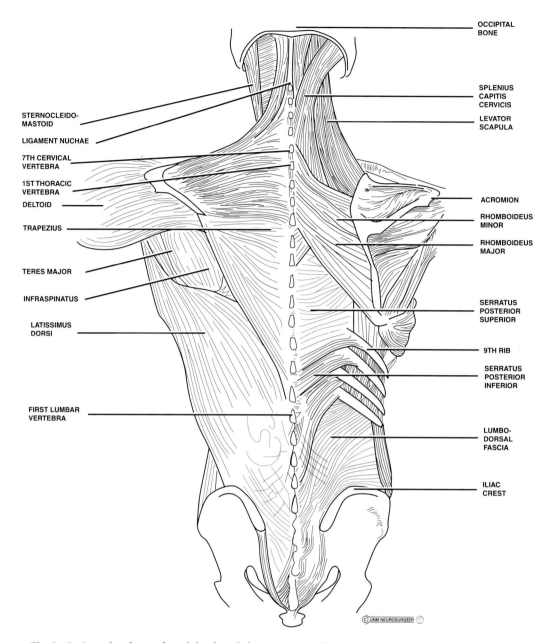

OCCIPITAL
BONE

SPLENIUS
CAPITIS
CERVICIS

LEVATOR
SCAPULA

STERNOCLEIDO-
MASTOID

LIGAMENT NUCHAE

7TH CERVICAL
VERTEBRA

1ST THORACIC
VERTEBRA

DELTOID

TRAPEZIUS

TERES MAJOR

INFRASPINATUS

LATISSIMUS
DORSI

ACROMION

RHOMBOIDEUS
MINOR

RHOMBOIDEUS
MAJOR

SERRATUS
POSTERIOR
SUPERIOR

9TH RIB

SERRATUS
POSTERIOR
INFERIOR

FIRST LUMBAR
VERTEBRA

LUMBO-
DORSAL
FASCIA

ILIAC
CREST

© UNM NEUROSURGERY

Fig. 2-15. Superficial muscles of the dorsal thoracic region *(left)* and the dorsal thoracic muscles deep to the trapezius and latissimus muscles *(right)*.

Nonparaspinal Muscular Anatomy

Muscles of the thoracic portion of the back also include nonparaspinal muscles. These muscles are not innervated by the dorsal divisions of the thoracic spinal nerves. The trapezius muscle is a flat, superficial muscle covering the neck and dorsal thorax (Fig. 2-15). It attaches from the spinous processes in the thoracic region and inserts onto the clavicle, the acromion of the shoulder, and the rostral portion of the spine of the scapula.[14] The lower border of the muscle attaches onto an aponeurosis that attaches to the caudal apex of the scapula. The innervation from this muscle comes mostly from the spinal accessory nerve (cranial nerve XI).

Superficial to the trapezius muscle is the latissimus dorsi muscle. It arises from the lower six

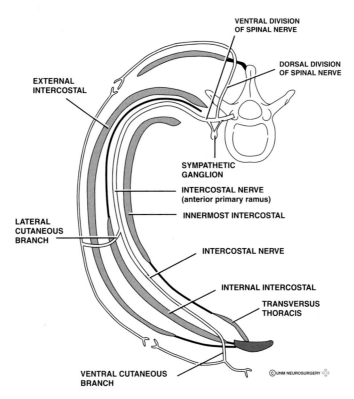

Fig. 2-16. Intercostal muscles and thoracic nerves.

thoracic spinous processes and from the lumbar fascia, which is attached to the supraspinous ligament. It has attachments to the scapula and humerus, but covers a significant amount of the caudodorsal thoracic region.[15] The laṭissimus dorsi muscle is innervated by the thoracodorsal nerve.

Deep to the trapezius lie the rhomboid muscles (see Fig. 2-15). The more rostral rhomboideus minor muscle arises from the cervical and first thoracic spinous processes. Its fibers travel obliquely to the spine of the scapula. It is parallel to the more caudal rhomboideus major muscle, which arises from the rostral four or five spinous processes and the supraspinous ligament. It inserts into the caudomedial border of the scapula.[15] The rhomboid muscles are innervated by the dorsal scapular nerve.

The serratus posterior inferior muscle is a quadrilateral-shaped thin muscle that has its aponeurotic origin from the lower thoracic and upper lumbar spinous processes (see Fig. 2-15). It lies deep to the caudal portion of the trapezius and deep to the latissimus dorsi muscle. Its aponeurosis blends with the thoracolumbar fascia. The serratus posterior inferior muscle inserts onto the lower four ribs near their angles. This muscle is the first of this list to be innervated by the ventral division of the thoracic spinal nerves from T9 to T12,[14] although some texts report the innervation of the serratus posterior or inferior as the dorsal divisions of these spinal nerves.[15]

Rostral to the serratus posterior inferior is the serratus posterior superior muscle (see Fig. 2-15). It arises from the lower cervical and upper thoracic spinous processes and from the supraspinous ligament. It fans out to the rostral borders of the second through fifth ribs beyond their angles, remaining superficial to the thoracolumbar fascia.[14] This muscle is supplied by branches from the dorsal divisions of the upper thoracic spinal nerves.

Also extending from the ends of the transverse processes (except T12) are the levatores costarum muscles. The levatores costarum brevis muscle inserts onto the rostrodorsal portions of the next caudal rib (Fig. 2-16). From T8 to T11 there is also a levatores costarum longus muscle that descends to insert two ribs caudal to its origin.[14] The internal and external intercostal muscles connect adjacent ribs, ventrally and dorsally, respectively (see Fig. 2-16).[14] Dorsally, the fibers of the internal intercostal muscle run medially from one rib to its caudal neighbor. The external intercostal muscle fibers are perpendicular

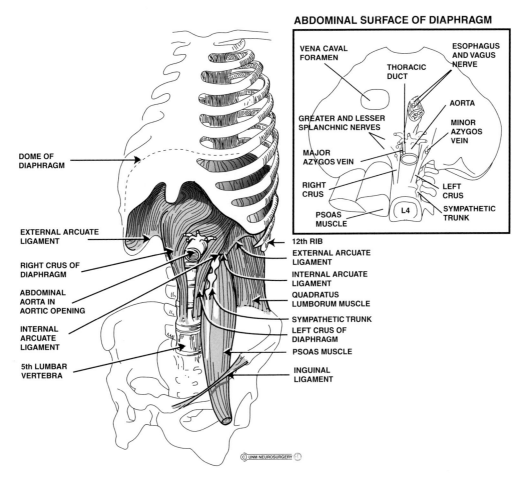

ABDOMINAL SURFACE OF DIAPHRAGM

Fig. 2-17. The diaphragm and associated structures.

to those of the internal intercostal muscle fibers. The external intercostal muscle is thicker than the internal intercostal muscle in the dorsal rib cage. The innervation of both intercostal muscles and the levatores is via the intercostal nerves.

The Diaphragm

Ventral to the thoracolumbar spine lies the diaphragm muscle. This muscle is thin and arises from the entire circumference of the thoracic cage, separating the thoracic and abdominal contents.[15] The diaphragm is innervated by the phrenic nerves. It attaches to the thoracolumbar spine its muscular attachments, the crura. The termination of these muscular extremities is the arcuate ligaments, which allow the great vessels and other anatomical structures to pass from the retropleural space to and from the retroperitoneal space, along the spinal column. The crura attach to the lumbar vertebral bodies, particularly the anterior longitudinal ligament, with the right being thicker and longer than the left. The right crus passes rostroventral to the left and ventral to the aortic opening. The right crus allows passage of the right-sided greater and lesser splanchnic nerves, and the left crus allows passage of the same nerves on the left, in addition to the minor azygos vein (Fig. 2-17).

The bilateral internal arcuate ligaments are tendinous arches extending from the first or second lumbar vertebral bodies and ventral portion of the transverse processes, to the more medial diaphragmatic crus, allowing passage of the psoas muscle and the sympathetic chain.[15] The external arcuate ligament extends from the ventral portion of the first lumbar vertebra to the twelfth rib. This bilateral opening is broader and longer than the internal arcuate ligament. It allows passage of the quadratus lumborum muscle and the last intercostal nerve. There is also an opening for the aorta ventral to the

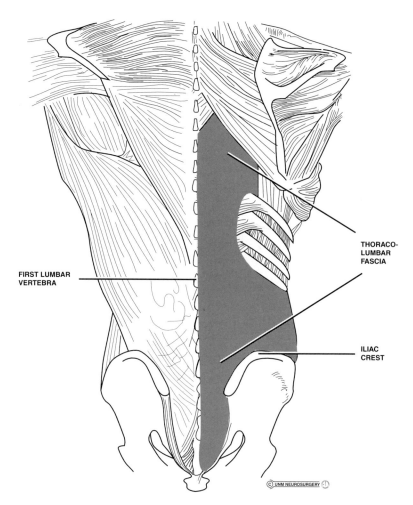

Fig. 2-18. The thoracolumbar fascia (shaded area).

vertebral bodies, although slightly to the left. This opening transmits the descending aorta, the major azygos vein, and the thoracic duct. Ventral to the aortic opening, the two crura cross. Therefore the contents in the aortic opening are technically dorsal to the diaphragm. Ventral to this muscular "cross" is the esophageal opening, which is in the axial plane of T10 (because the diaphragm ascends from dorsal to ventral). This opening transmits the esophagus, esophageal arteries, and vagus nerves. The ventral margin of this opening is the dorsal portion of the central tendinous portion of the diaphragm. Further ventral is the vena caval opening (T8 to T9), which allows passage of the inferior vena cava.

Fascial Planes of the Thoracic Spinal Region

A superficial thoracic fascial layer exists just deep to the dermis.[15] A deeper dorsal thoracic fascia cov-

ers the superficial muscles of the back. It contributes to sheaths for individual muscles. The paraspinal muscles of the thoracic region are covered by the thoracolumbar fascia (vertebral aponeurosis) (Fig. 2-18). It originates from the spinous processes of the thoracic vertebrae to attach to the angles of the ribs. A plane between the paraspinal muscles and the quadratus lumborum muscle leads directly to the transverse process and the intervertebral neuroforamen.[5] The prevertebral fascia is ventral to the longus colli muscle in the upper thoracic spine.[15]

NEUROANATOMY OF THE THORACIC SPINE
Membranes of the Spinal Nervous System

The thoracic spinal dura mater is a two-layer tubular membrane.[7] The space separating the vertebral periosteum from the dura is the spinal epidural

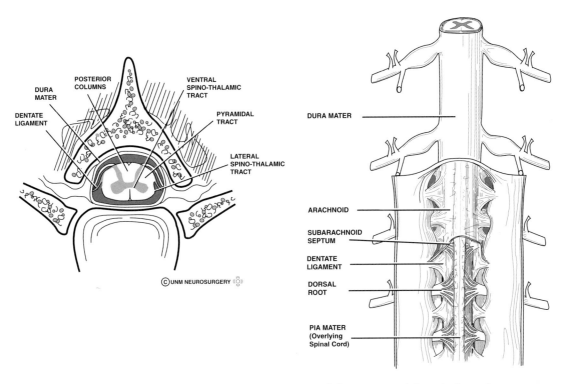

Fig. 2-19. An axial *(left)* and coronal *(right)* view of the contents of the spinal canal.

space. It contains epidural fat and the epidural spinal venous plexus[7] (Fig. 2-19). The dura mater has double openings for the bilateral segmental nerve roots at each level.[15] Deep to the dura is the spinal arachnoid mater. The arachnoid is trabecular connective tissue spanning from the dura to the pia mater. The thoracic subarachnoid space averages 12 to 13 mm in the sagittal diameter in the adult.[25] A thin dorsal longitudinal membranous partition in the arachnoid, the septum posticum, may be seen microscopically.[15,25] Some texts document the arachnoid as being a lymph space for this portion of the central nervous system.[15] The arachnoid combines with the dura mater at the level of the nerve root sleeves to become a significant absorptive area for cerebrospinal fluid (CSF).[1] The pia mater of the thoracic spine is also made of two layers: the intima pia and the more superficial epipial layer.[7] The intima pia is attached to the spinal cord, fills in the spinal cord fissures, and envelopes each spinal nerve root.[7,15,35] The blood vessels of the spinal cord lie in the epipial layer.[7] Flattened bands of this epipial layer form the denticulate ligaments. These triangular-shaped ligaments attach the pia to the spinal cord arachnoid tissue midway between the dorsal and ventral nerve roots bilaterally for the entire length of the thoracic spinal cord[7]

(see Fig. 2-19). There is also a ventral pial ligament termed the linea splendens.[15]

The Thoracic Spinal Cord

The thoracic section of the spinal cord is thinner than its cervical and lumbar counterparts, mostly because the ventral gray horns contain fewer motor neurons.[7] The thoracic spinal cord occupies 26.1% of the cross-sectional area of the spinal canal at T1 and 21.4% at T6.[11] The ventral surface of the cord is marked by the deep ventral median sulcus, which contains the central sulcal artery and vein[7,15] (Fig. 2-20). Dorsally, the spinal cord has a smaller dorsal median sulcus and the two dorsolateral sulci, which define the dorsal columns.[7] These columns, also termed the dorsal funiculi, represent the fasciculus gracilis, which conveys ascending dorsal column sensory fibers from the lower limbs, except in the highest thoracic levels. It may additionally harbor the fasciculus cuneatus (laterally), representing dorsal column sensory fibers from the upper limbs.[7] In this case the two dorsal fasciculi on each side are separated by a dorsal intermediate sulcus.[7] A lateral funiculus exists between the dorsal root entry zone (near the superficial extension of the dorsal gray horn) and the ventrolateral sulcus of the cord (the ventral root

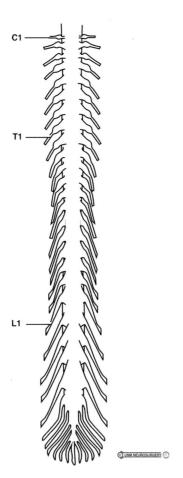

Fig. 2-20. The thoracic spinal cord and nerve roots. Note the increasing obliquity of thoracic spinal nerve roots as the thoracic spinal cord descends.

exit zone).[7] The anterior funiculus lies between the ventral median sulcus and the ventrolateral sulcus.[26] The thoracic lateral and anterior funiculi contain ascending and descending white matter fibers pertaining to the thoracic region and below.

The thoracic central gray matter is butterfly shaped and has the characteristic intermediolateral cell column that contains sympathetic fibers[7] (see Fig. 2-19). Also specific to the thoracic region is a medial bulge in the dorsal gray horn containing the dorsal nucleus of Clarke (nucleus thoracicus), particularly in lower thoracic segments.[7] There is less gray matter as a percentage of the spinal cord tissue in the thoracic region.[7]

Thoracic Spinal Nerve Roots
Proximal Nerve Root Anatomy

The 12 bilateral, segmental, ventral, and dorsal nerve roots of the thoracic spine exit more obliquely caudal as the spinal cord descends.[15] Because of the increasingly oblique descent of thoracic spinal nerve roots with more caudal spinal levels, they are longer with each descending spinal level. The lowest thoracic nerve root may pass the distance of two vertebral bodies before emerging from the spinal canal.[15] The spinal nerve roots take up 3.3% of the cross-sectional area of the spinal canal at T1 and 1.6% at T6.[11]

The thoracic dorsal nerve roots enter the spinal cord substance in the dorsolateral fissure, near the dorsal gray horns.[15] These roots contain mostly sensory fibers destined for the substantia gelatinosa, Lissauer's tract, and other dorsal gray laminae of the thoracic spinal cord. A few fibers cross to the contralateral dorsal gray, and some enter the ipsilateral ventral gray horn. Dorsal nerve roots have characteristic ganglionic enlargements termed the spinal ganglia and are located in the intervertebral foramina, lateral to the dura mater (Fig. 2-20). Ventral nerve roots exit the spinal cord near the ventral gray horn. They contain ipsilateral and contralateral fibers and are composed of four to eight filaments.[15] These roots are smaller than their dorsal siblings and are devoid of ganglionic enlargements.

Distal to the dorsal root ganglia, the ventral and dorsal spinal nerve roots combine into the spinal nerve. Thoracic spinal nerves are smaller than their cervical or lumbar counterparts. The spinal nerve immediately divides into a smaller dorsal and larger ventral division, each containing fibers from both roots. The spinal nerve gives off a small recurrent branch before dividing. This branch is joined by a sympathetic communicating branch, which then re-enters the intervertebral foramen to supply the spinal dura mater, vertebrae, and vertebral ligaments. The dorsal division supplies the paravertebral tissues, whereas the ventral division supplies the limbs and ventrolateral somatic structures. The ventral division is accompanied by a small sympathetic nerve.[15] Branches of spinal nerves and their sympathetic fibers are responsible for innervation of the disc space, local ligaments, and vertebral joints. The sinuvertebral nerve branch ascends to innervate the posterior longitudinal ligament and disc space, before the spinal nerve has exited the intervertebral foramen.[1,5] The ascending branch to the facet joint (recurrent nerve of Luschka) is responsible for sensation related to this joint[5] (Fig. 2-21). These nerves have a role in the pain associated with thoracic disc herniations and other spinal diseases.[1,5,30]

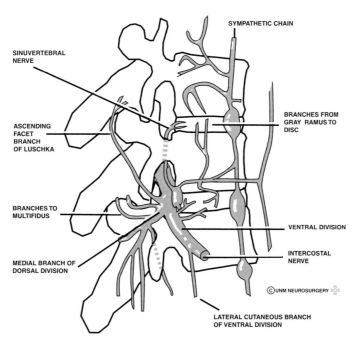

Fig. 2-21. Lateral view of the cutaneous and intercostal branches from the posterior divisions of thoracic spinal nerves.

Anatomy of Spinal Nerve Root Divisions

Dorsal divisions of thoracic spinal nerves branch into internal and external branches. For the upper six thoracic segments, the internal branch passes between and supplies the semispinalis dorsi and multifidus spinae muscles. They then pierce and supply the rhomboid and trapezius muscles and innervate the dorsal skin surface near the spinous processes. The remaining lower six internal branches have no cutaneous distributions, but supply the multifidus spinae muscles. The upper six external branches of the dorsal divisions penetrate and supply the longissimus dorsi muscle to reach the iliocostalis and levator costarum muscles. After piercing the serratus posterior inferior and the latissimus dorsi muscles, the lower six external branches of the thoracic dorsal divisions have cutaneous ramifications extending from the angles of the ribs.[15] They are larger than their rostral counterparts.

The ventral divisions of the thoracic spinal nerves join with sympathetic branches at each level to form the intercostal nerves. Before entering the subcostal spaces at each level, these nerves can be found between the pleura and the external intercostal muscles. They then enter the plane between the intercostal muscles. These nerves run under their segmental rib ventrolaterally and enter the chest and abdomen to innervate the somatic organs and the skin of the thorax[15] (see Figs. 2-16 and 2-21). The first thoracic spinal nerve enters the brachial plexus, destined for the chest and arm. A smaller branch from the first thoracic spinal nerve becomes the first intercostal nerve and ends as the first anterior cutaneous nerve of the thorax. The second thoracic spinal nerve also branches to give off an intercostal branch and an intercostohumeral branch. The latter has cutaneous distributions on the lateral thorax. The upper intercostal nerves supply the intercostal, infracostal, levatores costarum, serratus posterior superior, upper portion of the external oblique, and triangularis sterni muscles. Distal cutaneous branches of the intercostal nerves innervate the chest wall. The lower intercostal nerves supply the intercostals, serratus posterior inferior, abdominal muscles, and external oblique muscles, and innervate the skin of the lower thorax and upper abdomen. The last thoracic intercostal nerve is larger than its siblings and passes under the external arcuate ligament of the diaphragm to run ventral to the quadratus lumborum to join branches of the lumbar plexus. Its cutaneous distribution descends over the crest of the ilium toward the ventrolateral portion of the gluteal region.[15]

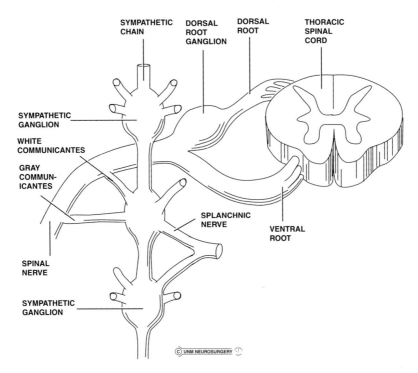

Fig. 2-22. Sympathetic chain, ganglia, and communicating fibers of the sympathetic nervous system of the thoracic region.

The Autonomic Nervous System

Nervous communication between the sympathetic chain and the spinal cord occurs via the white and gray communicantes. The white communicantes represents fibers traveling from the spinal nerve at each level to the sympathetic ganglion of the sympathetic chain at that level.[15] The gray communicantes represents fibers traveling back to the spinal nerve (Fig. 2-22). The sympathetic chain and its ganglia lie on each side of the vertebral bodies, ventral to the transverse processes, heads of the ribs, and intercostal bundle while remaining dorsal to the pleura.[5,15] The first thoracic ganglion is the largest in the thoracic sympathetic chain. The caudal two thoracic ganglia lie on the bodies of the eleventh and twelfth thoracic vertebrae. Sometimes segmental ganglia of the chain may coalesce. Branches from the ganglia are given back to the thoracic spinal nerves to reach the skin, joints, and muscles of the thorax. Internal branches supply the thoracic viscera, the vertebrae and its ligaments, and the aorta and its branches. These internal branches from the lower thoracic segments unite to form the greater, lesser, and smallest (renal) splanchnic nerves.[15]

Cerebrospinal Fluid

Cerebrospinal fluid (CSF) surrounds the spinal cord and intradural spinal nerve roots and is contained by the arachnoid. The CSF takes up 30.7% of the cross-sectional area of the spinal canal at T1 and 31.6% at T6.[11] Significant reuptake of CSF occurs in the arachnoid within the nerve root dural sleeves.[1]

VASCULAR ANATOMY OF THE THORACIC SPINE
Arterial Anatomy of the Thoracic Spine
Regional Arterial Supply to the Thoracic Spine

The arterial supply of the thoracic spinal cord is accomplished by radicular vessels that accompany each ventral root through the intervertebral foramina.[15] These radicular vessels are distributed by the subclavian artery and by the posterior intercostal arteries at each level. They arise directly from the aorta[3,15] (Fig. 2-23). Branches of these radicular vessels also supply the segmental nerve roots and the spinal meninges. These vessels bolster the descend-

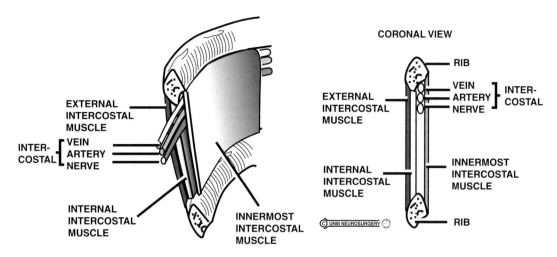

Fig. 2-23. Intercostal neurovascular and muscular anatomy.

ing vascular supply from the anterior spinal artery, with which they anastomose.[3] This connection of radicular vessels to the anterior spinal artery may be called the anterior spinal arterial network[1,32] (Fig. 2-24). Although this network is the major supply to the spinal cord, it is often discontinuous.[20] Not all radicular branches are large enough to contribute significantly to the spinal arterial plexuses.[3] There is also a posterior spinal arterial network, which is made up of smaller dorsal divisions of the radicular arteries that enter the spinal canal at each level and anastomose with the paired posterior spinal arteries that run in the dorsolateral sulci.[1,15,32] This network may also be discontinuous in the thoracic region.[7,20]

The upper thoracic spinal cord receives the majority of its blood flow from the anterior spinal artery, penetrating branches of the ascending vertebral arteries, and a branch from the costocervical trunk[3,15,20] (Fig. 2-25). The midthoracic region (T4 to T8) is mostly supplied by a single thoracic radicular branch (often from T7) and is poorly collateralized (and thus more susceptible to the effects of hypotension).[3,22] The lower thoracic region typically receives its major supply via a single larger radicular branch, most often on the left side. This vessel is termed the great radicular artery of Adamkiewicz. It most commonly enters via T10, although it may be found entering from T8 to L2.[1,3,8,20] The thoracic radicular vessels are more constant on the left side, possibly due to the proximity to the thoracic aorta.[7]

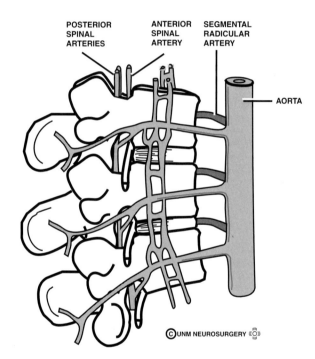

Fig. 2-24. Arterial source and distribution of the thoracic intercostal arteries.

Longitudinal watershed zones exist between the cervicothoracic and midthoracic vascular territories to the thoracic spinal cord, and between the midthoracic and thoracolumbar regions.[3] Radicular arteries run on the ventral surface of the nerve root for which they are partnered.[1] These vessels may divide to supply both the anterior and posterior arterial networks.[7]

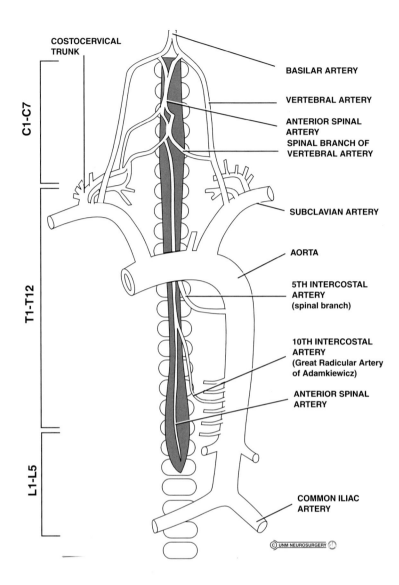

Fig. 2-25. Arterial supply to the thoracic spinal region.

Spinal Cord Arterial Blood Supply

Vessels (radicular) from these arterial networks travel the lateral surface of the spinal cord and give off many smaller branches that penetrate the spinal cord radially to supply the peripheral white matter tracts and dorsal gray horn[32] (Fig. 2-26). Note that these radicular vessels are not the same as the radicular arteries that enter the intervertebral foramen to supply the spinal arterial plexuses.[1] Those radicular branches, arising from the anterior spinal arterial plexus, are termed the ventral radicular arteries, and those arising from the posterior spinal arterial plexus are called the dorsal radicular arteries.[1] The remaining central gray matter and deep white matter are supplied by a large radial branch, the central

sulcal artery, which enters the ventral median sulcus of the spinal cord and then centrifugally distributes a branching network of smaller vessels.[1,3,32] This central sulcal arterial system is end-arterial in nature, whereas the penetrating radicular branches to the spinal cord have leptomeningeal anastomoses.[3,20,25,32] Thus peripheral white matter is often spared in cases of hypotension, whereas the central gray matter is more susceptible.[20] Based on pathological findings, the ventral two-thirds of the spinal cord is supplied ultimately by the anterior spinal arterial network and the remaining dorsal one-third by the posterior spinal arterial network.[20,32] An arterial watershed zone exists between the central sulcal and peripheral radicular system of the spinal cord[20] (see Fig. 2-26).

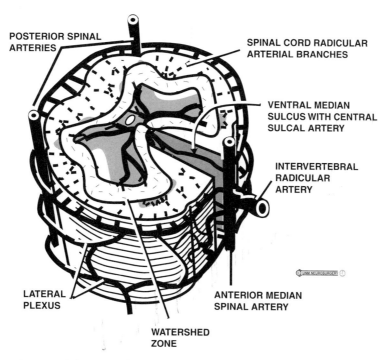

Fig. 2-26. Axial view of the arterial supply to the thoracic spinal cord (arterial watershed zone stippled).

Arterial Supply to Thoracic Spinal Elements

A collateral branch arising from each posterior intercostal artery runs along the rib of the same level to supply the dorsal portion of the rib, dorsal intercostal muscles, and later anastomoses with anterior intercostal arteries from the internal mammary arteries[15] (see Fig. 2-25).

Muscles and soft tissues of the thoracic paraspinous region are supplied by dorsal branches of the posterior intercostal arteries.[15] The posterior intercostal arteries emanate from the descending thoracic aorta at each level, and after giving off their radicular branch, they course along the ventral portion of the costotransverse ligament before dividing into superficial and muscular branches.[15] These arterial branches also supply the costovertebral and costotransverse articulations.[30] The intercostal vessels are enveloped by parietal pleura as they travel laterally in the subcostal space to reach the protection of the intercostal muscles. Branches from the posterior intercostal arteries also form a paravertebral arterial network on the lateral borders of the vertebral bodies, which supplies the vertebral bodies and intervertebral discs.[5] The intervertebral discs receive their vascular supply from the subchondral postcapillary venous network at each vertebral end plate.[9]

Venous Anatomy of the Thoracic Spine
Venous Drainage of the Spinal Cord

Venous drainage of the thoracic spinal cord is distinct from its vascular supply. A central sulcal tributary system drains the ventral spinal cord white matter and ventral gray horns to the anterior median spinal vein.[3,20,32] Unlike the arterial system, an anastomosis exists between the central sulcal and peripheral radial system of veins termed the centrodorsolateral anastomosis.[1,32] The spinal dorsal gray horns and ventrolateral, lateral, and dorsal white matter are drained radially to the pial veins known as the coronal plexus.[3,7,20,32] This pial venous plexus is richer dorsally, where longitudinal confluent veins may be found.[1] The surface venous pattern of the spinal cord is highly irregular and variable, except for the anterior median spinal vein. However, the veins are usually deep to the arterial plexuses. On the dorsal surface of the thoracic spinal cord lies the longitudinal posterior median spinal vein and the posterolateral spinal veins. These contribute to the venous network[9,32] (Fig. 2-27). The posterolateral spinal veins lie near the dorsal root entry zones.[9] Larger ventral and dorsal radicular veins at each level drain the coronal plexus, the posterior spinal vein, and the anterior median spinal vein.[1,3,7,22] A

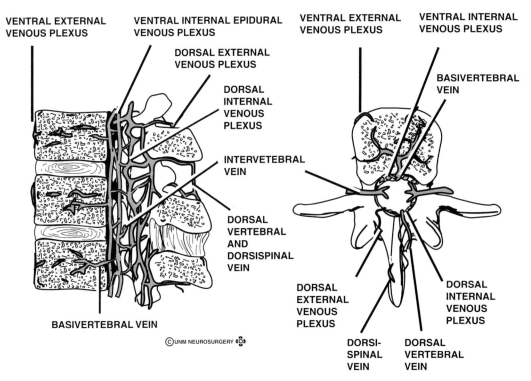

Fig. 2-27. Venous drainage of the spinal cord: sagittal view *(left)* and axial view *(right)*.

large "great anterior radicular vein" is usually found draining from the left side of the lower thoracic spinal cord.[7,20] These radicular veins often combine segmentally to become the lateral segmental veins that accompany each segmental nerve root and exit the dura mater.[1,3] The lateral segmental veins receive tributaries from the spinal dura mater.[1]

The Epidural Spinal Venous Plexus

The radicular veins and lateral segmental veins contribute to the (internal) epidural venous plexus (see Fig. 2-27). Two prominent venous channels that are integral to the epidural spinal venous plexus are the anterior longitudinal vertebral sinuses, which sit in the ventrolateral gutters of the spinal canal.[1,15,25,35] There are also dorsal longitudinal venous sinuses that are involved in the epidural plexus.[1] Transverse channels connect the longitudinal vessels within this plexus.[34] Veins drain the ventral portions of the laminae, and vertebral ligaments drain to the epidural venous plexus.[1] The vertebral bodies are drained by the basivertebral veins dorsally, into the ventral portion of the spinal epidural venous plexuses[1,15,25,35] (see Fig. 2-9). The basivertebral vein is a tributary from an elaborate venous grid within each vertebral body.[9] The veins

of the spinal venous network are without valves, and flow may be bidirectional.[1,7,20,34] The perivascular, particularly the perivenous spaces draining the spinal cord, have been described as surrounded by an arachnoid network that serves as the lymph space for the spinal cord.[1]

The epidural venous plexus drains via the intervertebral foramina to the (external) perivertebral venous plexus via the intervertebral veins[34] (see Fig. 2-27). This plexus is more significant dorsally, in the vertebral groove, aside the transverse and spinous processes.[34] The ventral portion is ventral to the vertebral bodies. Two portions of the perivertebral venous plexus anastomose through transverse channels.[34] The laminae, transverse processes, and spinous processes drain directly into the perivertebral venous plexus via dorsal vertebral veins.[32,35] The dorsospinal veins surround the spinous processes and drain to the perivertebral spinous plexus.[15] Prevertebral paraspinal tissues are drained via muscular veins into this plexus.

The Perivertebral Spinal Venous Plexus

The perivertebral venous plexus drains via the intercostal veins into the azygos-hemiazygous-superior vena caval system[15,20,35] (Fig. 2-28). The

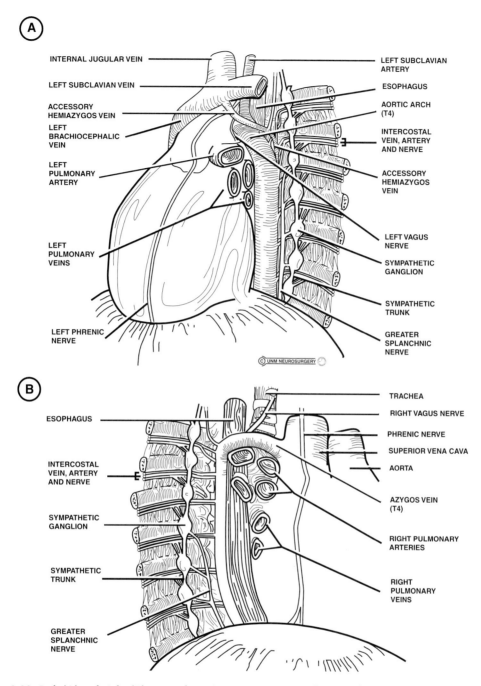

Fig. 2-28. Left (**A**) and right (**B**) upper thoracic cavity anatomy, showing the azygos and hemiazygos drainage systems.

right intercostal veins drain into the azygos vein, and the left intercostal veins drain into the hemiazygous or accessory hemiazygous veins.[34] The intercostal vessels are ventral to the anterior costotransverse ligament and lie with the intercostal nerve.[15] This neurovascular bundle lies in the subcostal groove, enveloped in parietal pleura dorsally, and is protected by intercostal muscular layers ventrolaterally.

REGIONAL THORACIC TISSUES

Ventral to the thoracic spine lies the thoracic cavity and its contents. Just dorsal to the pleura, the sympathetic chain (adjacent to the costovertebral articulations), the trachea, esophagus, and descending thoracic aorta caudal to T4 are found[5] (see Fig. 2-28). The aorta is just to the left of midline, and the ascending inferior vena cava is to the right.[5] The esophagus lies roughly in the midline, ventral to the upper thoracic spine.[11] Branches of the aortic arch, tributaries to the superior vena cava, and the vagus nerves lie ventral to the esophagus and trachea in the mediastinum.[5] Ventral to the midthoracic spine, the azygos vein may be found on the right side of midline.[5] The minor (hemi-) azygos vein is on the left side of the ventral thoracic spinal column in the retropleural space.[5,15] Also in this space run the intercostal vessels. Ventral to the lower thoracic region are the diaphragm and the peritoneal cavity and its contents.

Figures 2-1 to 2-28 used with permission of the University of New Mexico, Division of Neurosurgery, Albuquerque, New Mexico.

REFERENCES

1. Austin GM. The Spinal Cord, 3rd ed. New York: Igaku-Shoin, 1983.
2. Bashline SD, Bilott JR, Ellis JP. Meningovertebral ligaments and their putative significance in low back pain. J Manipulative Physiol Ther 19:592-596, 1996.
3. Benavente OR, Barnett HJM. Spinal chord infraction. In Carter LP, Spetzler RF, Hamilton MG, eds. Neurovascular Surgery. New York: McGraw-Hill, 1995.
4. Benzel EC. Biomechanics of spine stabilization: Principles and clinical practice. New York: McGraw-Hill, 1995.
5. Branch CL. Ventral thoracic and lumbar spine anatomy in surgical exposure of the spine: An extensile approach. In Benzel EC, ed. Park Ridge, Ill.: The American Association of Neurological Surgeons, 1995.
6. Breathnach AS. Frazer's Anatomy of the Human Skeleton, 5th ed. London: J&A Churchill, LTD, 1958.
7. Carpenter MB. Core Text of Neuroanatomy, 4th ed. Baltimore: Williams & Wilkins, 1991.
8. Champlin AM, Rael J, Benzel EC, Kesterson L, King JN, Orrison WW, Mirfakhraee M. Preoperative spinal angiography for lateral extracavitary approach to thoracic and lumbar spine. AJNR 15:73-74, 1994.
9. Crock HV, Yoshizawa H, Kame SK. Observations on the venous drainage of the human vertebral body. J Bone Joint Surg 55B:528-533, 1973.
10. Davies KM, Recker RR, Heaney RP. Normal vertebral dimensions and normal variation in serial measurements of vertebrae. J Bone Miner Res 4:341-349, 1989.
11. dePeretti F, Hovorka I, Ganansia P, Puch JM, Bourgeon A, Argenson C. The vertebral foramen: A report concerning its contents. Surg Radiol Anat 15: 287-294, 1993.
12. Ebraheim NA, Xu R, Ahmad M, Yeasting RA. Anatomic considerations of anterior instrumentation of the thoracic spine. Am J Orthop 16:419-424, 1997.
13. Ebraheim NA, Xu R, Ahmad M, Yeasting RA. Projection of the thoracic pedicle and its morphometric analysis. Spine 22:233-238, 1997.
14. Flynn RW, Greenman PE. The Thoracic Spine and Rib Cage: Musculoskeletal Evaluation and Treatment. Boston: Butterworth-Heinemann, 1996.
15. Gray H. Anatomy, Descriptive and Surgical. Pick TP, Howden R, eds. Revised American Edition from the Fifteenth English Edition. New York: Bounty Books, 1977.
16. Hamilton WJ, ed. Textbook of Human Anatomy, 2nd ed. St Louis: Mosby, 1976.
17. Hou S, Hu R, Shi Y. Pedicle morphology of the lower thoracic and lumbar spine in a Chinese population. Spine 18:1850-1855, 1993.
18. Jiang H, Raso JV, Moreau MJ, Russel G, Hill DL, Bagnall KM. Quantitative morphology of the lateral ligaments of the spine. Assessment of their importance in maintaining lateral stability. Spine 19:2676-2682, 1994.
19. Kim NH, Lee HM, Chung IH, Kim HJ, Kim SJ. Morphometric study of the pedicles of thoracic and lumbar vertebrae in Koreans. Spine 19:1390-1394, 1994.
20. Kim RC. Spinal cord pathology. In Nelson JS, Parisi JE, Schochet SS, eds. Principles and Practice of Neuropathology, St. Louis: Mosby, 1993.
21. Kothe R, O'Holleran JC, Liu W, Panjabi MM. Internal architecture of the thoracic pedicle. An anatomic study. Spine 21:264-270, 1996.
22. Lu J, Ebraheim NA, Biyani A, Brown JA, Yeasting RA. Vulnerability of great medullary artery. Spine 21: 1852-1855, 1996.
23. McCormack BM, Benzel EC, Adams MS, Baldwin NG, Rupp FW, Maher DJ. Anatomy of the thoracic pedicle. Neurosurgery 37:303-308, 1995.
24. Netter FH, Kaplan A. Anatomy of the Spine. CIBA Pharmaceutical Products,1950.
25. Osborn AG. Diagnostic Neuroradiology. St. Louis: Mosby, 1994.
26. Panjabi MM, O'Holleran JD, Crisco JJ, Kothe R. Complexity of the thoracic spine pedicle anatomy. Eur Spine J 6:19-24, 1997.
27. Prestar FJ, Frick H, Putz R. Ligamentous connections of the spinous processes. Anat Anz 159:259-268, 1985.
28. Pooni JS, Jukins DW, Harris PF, Hilton RC, Davies KE. Comparison of the structure of human intervertebral discs in the cervical, thoracic, and lumbar regions of the spine. Surg Radiol Anat 8:175-182, 1986.
29. Rothman RH, Simeone FA. The Spine, 3rd ed. Philadelphia: WB Saunders, 1992.
30. Schaeffer JP, ed. Morris' Human Anatomy. Philadelphia: The Blakiston Company, 1942.

31. Stanescu S, Ebraheim NA, Yeasting R, Bailey AS, Jackson WT. Morphometric evaluation of the cervicothoracic junction. Practical considerations for posterior fixation of the spine. Spine 19:2082-2088, 1994.

32. Thron AK. Vascular Anatomy of the Spinal Cord. Wien: Springer-Verlag, 1988.

33. Vaccaro AR, Rizzolo SJ, Allargyce TJ, Ramsey M, Salvo J, Balderston RA, Cotler JM. Placement of pedicle screws in the thoracic spine. I. Morphometric analysis of the thoracic vertebrae. J Bone Joint Surg 77A:1193-1199, 1995.

34. Vogelsang H. Intraosseous Spinal Venography. Baltimore: Williams Wilkins, 1970.

35. Willis WD, Grossman RG. Medical Neurobiology. St. Louis: Mosby, 1973.

36. Zindrick MR, Wiltse LL, Doornik A, Widell EH, Knight GW, Patwardhan AG, Thomas JC, Rothman SL, Fields BT. Analysis of the morphometric characteristics of the thoracic and lumbar pedicles. Spine 12:160-166, 1987.

Embryology

Andrew G. Chenell, M.D., Christopher I. Shaffrey, M.D.,
Mark N. Hadley, M.D., and John A. Jane, M.D., Ph.D.

Developmental disorders of the human thoracic spine represent a range of conditions that often result from disordered embryogenesis. Thus an understanding of normal development is imperative in order to understand the embryological miscues that result in the abnormal. Because much of what we have learned about spine embryology comes from the study of nonhuman vertebrates, there are gaps in our knowledge. Until recently, the embryogenetic mechanisms for many spinal disease processes have not been elucidated. However, with the advent of modern cell biology techniques, we are slowly filling the gaps in our understanding of human spinal embryology.

The first section of this chapter reviews human spinal embryology, with emphasis on the thoracic region. This is followed by a discussion of developmental abnormalities of the thoracic spine. For additional reference, several excellent reviews of spine embryology are available.[28,42,47,48,53,56,64]

EMBRYOLOGY OF THE SPINE

Spine development in the human embryo begins with the formation of the primitive streak at day 15 of embryonic life. The primitive streak is a thickened linear band of epiblast (the cellular layer that is the precursor to ectoderm), which appears caudally in the dorsal aspect of the embryonic disc. The primitive streak elongates by adding cells at the caudal end as the cranial end thickens to form the primitive knot. Concurrently, a depression forms in the primitive streak; this "primitive groove" is continuous with a depression in the primitive knot called the "primitive pit." The cranial-caudal axis of the embryo is defined with the development of the primitive streak.

Before the primitive streak is developed, the embryo is a bilaminar disc that consists of the epiblast (primitive ectoderm) and hypoblast (cellular layer that later forms part of the endoderm). At day 16 epiblastic cells invade the primitive groove, lose their attachments to the epiblastic tissue, and migrate between the epiblast and hypoblast. These cells form the embryonic mesoderm (Fig. 3-1, A). This migration of cells transforms the bilaminar embryo into a trilaminar embryo made up of the remnants of the epiblast forming ectoderm, the newly formed mesoderm, and the endoderm, which is composed of invading mesodermal cells and the laterally displaced remnants of the hypoblast. This process of transforming the bilaminar embryo into a trilaminar embryo is termed "gastrulation." Because many congenital disorders of the spine involve malformations of tissues derived from all three embryological layers, it is postulated that many congenital spinal disorders arise from defects in gastrulation, an embryological period when all three layers could be subjected to the same insult.[17]

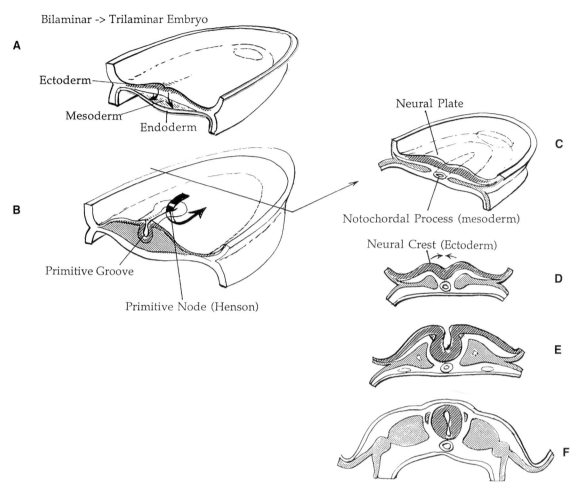

Fig. 3-1. A. The bilaminar embryo becomes a trilaminar embryo by the formation of mesodermal tissue between the ectoderm and endoderm in a process termed gastrulation. **B,** The notochordal plate forms in the region of the primitive knot and proceeds in a rostral direction. **C,** Three-quarter view of the developing embryo. **D, E,** and **F,** The infolding of the notochordal plate forms the neural tube (see text for details).

The primitive streak continues to make mesodermal cells until the fourth week of gestation when the primitive streak greatly diminishes in relative size and becomes an insignificant structure in the sacrococcygeal region of the embryo. The primitive streak normally undergoes degenerative changes and disappears. Teratomas can develop if remnants of the primitive streak remain and proliferate.

At day 16 the notochord begins to form. The notochord is formed in the midline at the rostral margin of the primitive knot. The notochord is formed by mesoblastic cells that migrate rostrally from the primitive knot between the ectoderm and endoderm (Fig. 3-1, *B*). The rostral ascent of these cells stops at the prochordal plate, a small collection of

endodermal cells destined to become the oropharyngeal membrane, which firmly adheres to the overlying ectoderm. The notochord runs rostrally to the prochordal plate and caudally to the cloacal membrane. As the notochord develops, the primitive pit extends into it to form a lumen known as the notochordal canal. Eventually, the floor of the notochordal canal disappears, and a notochordal plate is formed. The notochordal plate folds dorsoventrally, forming a solid rod of cells, the notochord. Defects in the folding of the notochord can result in diastomatomyelia.

As the notochord forms, it is probably involved in inducing the overlying ectoderm to form the neural plate (Fig. 3-1, *C*). The neural plate first appears rostral to the primitive knot. On day 18 the neural plate invaginates to form the neural groove with neural folds on either side (Fig. 3-1, *D* and *E*). The neural groove is closely associated with the underlying notochord, separated only by a basement membrane. By day 21 the neural folds have fused to form the neural tube. The neural tube then separates itself from the overlying ectoderm, and this ectoderm fuses to become continuous over the dorsal aspect of the embryo (Fig. 3-1, *F*). Obviously, if the ectoderm fails to fuse over the neural tube, spinal dysraphism results.

During the development of the notochord and the neural tube, the intraembryonic mesoderm on both sides begins to thicken and form paraxial mesoderm. At 20 days, the paraxial mesoderm divides into paired cuboidal structures (the somites) located laterally on both sides of the developing neural tube. The first pair of somites appears just caudal to the rostral end of the notochord. Additional somite pairs then propagate in a cranial to caudal sequence. By 30 days of gestation, 38 pairs of somites have formed. Eventually, 42 to 44 pairs of somites form (4 occipital, 8 cervical, 12 thoracic, 5 lumbar, 5 sacral, and 8-10 coccygeal). The first occipital and the last 5-7 coccygeal pairs eventually disappear. Somites must undergo normal formation and degradation, or excesses or shortages of one or more vertebrae may occur.

True development of the vertebral column begins when somites are formed. As the cells in the somite proliferate, they begin to demonstrate internal specializations when distinct cell masses are formed. The most lateral cell mass, called the dermatome, develops into the skin and subcutaneous tissue. The medial cell mass differentiates into two components: the dorsal aspect, the myotome (a cell aggregate that becomes striated muscle), and the ventral aspect, the sclerotome, which becomes the skeletal system.

It is clear that somites have regional specificity early in development. If thoracic region somites are transposed to the cervical region, they continue to form thoracic vertebral characteristics, including extrathoracic ribs.[32] It is believed that the regional specificity of the somites is conferred by expression of *Hox* genes.[30] Developmental abnormalities in the spine may arise due to mistakes in expression of these *Hox* genes or due to the influence of teratogens upon them.

Early fetal development results in a mesenchymal analogue of the vertebral column, which subsequently undergoes sequential overlapping steps of chondrification and ossification. By 35 days the cells of the sclerotome condense to surround the notochord and neural tube to form a mesenchymal vertebra. The ventral collection of mesenchymal cells condenses to form the mesenchymal centra, the primitive membranous vertebral body. The ventral aspect of the mesenchymal condensation occurs before the dorsal aspect is developed. Thus the vertebral body develops before the vertebral arch. Different mechanisms induce portions of the sclerotome to become the vertebral body or the neural arch. Differentiation of that portion of the sclerotome that becomes the vertebral body appears to be influenced by the neural tube, whereas the portion that becomes the neural arch appears to be influenced by the neural crest. Because the vertebral body and neural arch are under different inductive control and develop at different times, developmental abnormalities that occur during early gestation may affect the vertebral body or the developing neural arch independently. Timing differences in ventral/dorsal vertebrae development can result in malformations such as hemivertebrae or congenital bar-unilateral arch fusion.

The cells in each sclerotome form two distinct cell masses, a region of loosely packed cells in the rostral half and a region of densely packed cells in the caudal half (Fig. 3-2, *B*). The densely packed cells mature into the intervertebral discs, whereas the loosely packed cells develop chondrification centers and become the bony elements of the spine.

As the vertebral centra expand, the notochord gradually regresses within the expansions, and notochord cells tend to cluster in the eventual intervertebral spaces.[34,38,54] Notochord cells contribute significantly to the formation of the intervertebral disc, most notably the nucleus pulposus. Abnormal remnants of notochord can remain in the spinal axis, most commonly in the coccygeal or basosphenoid regions to form chordomas.

The actual mechanism by which the mesenchymal vertebrae are formed from somites is an area of some controversy. Resegmentation of the vertebrae had been a generally accepted theory since its presentation by Remak in 1855.[55] He theorized that vertebral bodies are formed by the joining of adjacent somites. The rostral half of one somite migrates

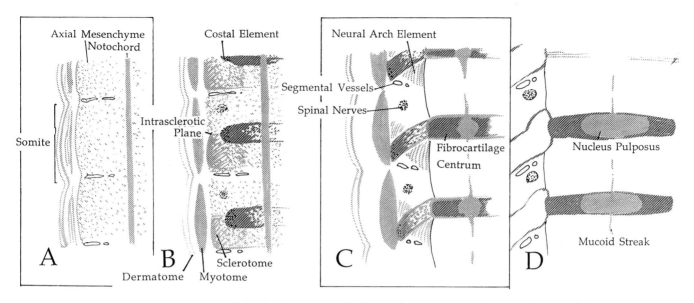

Fig. 3-2. A, Cross-section of the developing spinal column showing para-axial mesenchyme and the associated somites. **B,** Cross-section defining the loose rostral and dense caudal halves of each developing sclerotome (see text for discussion of resegmentation). **C** and **D,** Sagittal views of the developing spine defining the position of the spinal nerves and disc spaces.

superiorly and unites with the caudal half of the somite above. This theory is attractive because it explains how intersegmental arteries cross the vertebral body and nerve roots exit between the bodies.[31] (Fig. 3-2, *C* and *D*). It also helps explain developmental disorders of the spine such as hemivertebrae and congenitally fused vertebrae. Recent evidence supporting resegmentation includes Bagnall, Higgins, and Saunders,[1] using a chick-quail chimera model, and Ewan and Everett,[19] using retroviral-mediated transfer of the *lac Z* gene to trace migration of developing somites.

Recently, other theories regarding vertebral body formation have been reported.[16,29] In 1985 Verbout,[63] based on a histological study of serial sections, argued that the split between the dense (caudal) and loose (rostral) halves of the somite were artifacts. He proposed that the vertebral bodies are derived principally from an unsegmented perichordal tube and a loose column of axial mesenchyme, whereas the dorsal elements are derived from caudal condensed mesenchyme. Dalgleish,[16] made similar findings, by an autoradiographic study of the development of thoracic vertebrae in the mouse.

Currently, several investigators have advanced an integrated theory of vertebral formation in which the vertebral body is composed of the rostral and caudal halves of two adjacent somites while the

posterior elements derive from the caudal somite.[15] An advantage of the integrated theory is that it explains congenital malformations of the spine.

Relationships of the nerve roots and muscle connections of the vertebrae may be explained by considering the development of the dorsal elements. As described previously, dorsal element development is influenced by the neural crest and spinal ganglia. The neural arches develop between the spinal ganglia and are intersegmental with respect to the myotomes. Each neural arch is associated with two adjacent myotomal segments. This intersegmental orientation also explains the relationship of the nerve roots to the posterior elements.

The thoracic spine must develop ribs and rib articulations in addition to the usual vertebral elements. Experimental evidence reveals that the majority of each originates from its respective somite.[62] All vertebrae have the potential to form ribs, as evidenced by the rib process equivalents on each vertebrae, yet only the thoracic vertebrae have a full complement of ribs. Expression of *Hox* genes is believed to be responsible for the regional specificity of somite development. The costal elements are derived from the lateral aspect of the anatomical transverse processes.[11]

At day 42 of embryonic life, chondrification begins to occur[46] (Fig. 3-3). Chondrification centers

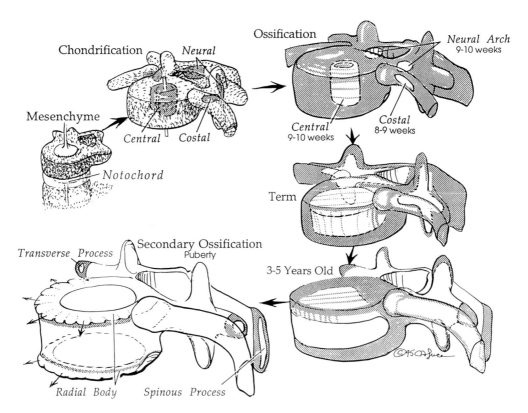

Fig. 3-3. Sequential diagrams of the chondrification and ossification of the typical vertebra. Chondrification begins in the central, costal, and neural centers. Ossification begins in the central, costal, and neural arch center at 72 days gestation and continues until puberty when the secondary ossification centers define the transverse and spinous processes.

appear on both sides of the small remnant of notochord in each mesenchymal vertebra and coalesce toward the center. A chondrification center also forms laterally in each vertebral arch and propagates dorsally to form a cartilaginous arch. This chondrification process expands dorsally to form the spinous process. Late chondrification centers are formed at the junction of the centrum and neural arch and extend laterally to form the transverse processes. At the same time, the dense mesenchymal part of the somite (which will form the intervertebral disc) condenses to form the annulus fibrosis.

Ossification of the spine begins about day 72. The process of converting the chondrous centrum to an osseous one is enhanced by embryonic movement[46] (see Fig. 3-3). Ossification of the vertebrae is not complete until age 25. Two primary ossification centers develop in the vertebral centrum after the invasion of pericostal vessels. These are dorsal and ventral to the notochord center, in contrast to the chondrification centers, which develop laterally.

The dorsal and ventral ossification centers fuse quickly to form a central vertebral body ossification center. Primary ossification centers also form in each half of the vertebral arch and develop into regions for the lamina, pedicle, and transverse process. By birth, each vertebra consists of three ossified bones connected by cartilage. The halves of the vertebral arch fuse between 3 and 5 years of age. The laminae first fuse in the lumbar region and then progress rostrally. At puberty, five secondary ossification centers appear: one at the tip of the spinous process, one at each tip of the transverse processes, and two rim epiphyses (superior and inferior) on the vertebral body. Ossification of the centrum resembles epiphyseal ossification in long bones, whereas ossification in the neural arch resembles diaphyseal long bone ossification.

Development of an adequate vascular supply to the vertebrae is essential to the development and proliferation of the ossification centers. The vertebral centrum has a vascular supply that runs in special

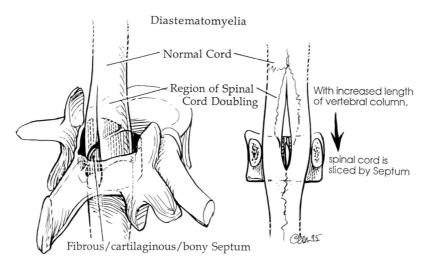

Diastematomyelia

Normal Cord

Region of Spinal
Cord Doubling

With increased length
of vertebral column,

spinal cord is
sliced by Septum

Fibrous/cartilaginous/bony Septum

Fig. 3-4. Three-quarter view of diastematomyelia showing the cartilaginous or bony spur separating the cord into two hemicords. Slicing of the spinal cord can result as the bony septum moves with growth in relation to the spinal cord.

structures called cartilage canals.[65] These canals grow into the centrum dorsally and ventrally. In contrast, the dorsal element vasculature enters from the peripheral periosteum.[12]

Each cartilage canal contains an artery, vein, and associated surrounding capillary network. These are end artery systems with little or no anastomosis across the epiphyses. Should a vascular network be compromised, rapid death of osteocytes occurs and can result in differential growth of the spine.

Disturbances of the normal embryological development of the human vertebral column are relatively uncommon. Several of the most frequent "errors" of embryological spinal maturation that manifest themselves as specific clinical disorders will be discussed next.

SPINAL DYSRAPHISM

"Spinal dysraphism" generally refers to the abnormal development of the spinal cord and the spinal column. Dysraphism refers to malformations that arise from a failure of normal embryological structures to fuse in the midline. Conventionally these malformations are somewhat artificially split into two groups. The first group, spina bifida aperta, involves midline lesions that are not covered by complete layers of dermis and epidermis and are termed spina bifida cystica (myelomeningocele, meningocele). The second group, spina bifida occulta, are malformations

that are hidden by complete layers of dermis and epidermis, such as lipomyelomeningocele, neurenteric cyst, and diastematomyelia[8,23] (Fig. 3-4).

The incidence of neural tube defects in the United States has declined from 1.3 per 1000 births in 1970 to 0.6 per 1000 births in 1989.[20,21,76] The worldwide incidence of neural tube defects varies greatly, approaching 8.7 per 1000 births in Belfast, Northern Ireland.[19] Many environmental causes have been implicated, including maternal age, maternal hyperthermia, maternal deficiencies in folate, calcium, vitamin C, and zinc, and either deficient or excessive amounts of vitamin A.[5,14,59,61] The level of the spinal dysplasia depends on the embryological age at which the malformation is initiated.

Malformations that begin before 28 days of gestation induce major defects in neurulation and cause higher-level defects than malformations that occur after 28 days of gestation when neurulation is complete. The higher the level of dysplasia, the less survivable the malformation. In a study of 510 infants with myelodysplasia who survived the first day of life, approximately 10% of lesions were cranial/cervical, 5% were thoracic, 25% were thoracolumbar, 33% were lumbar, and 32% were sacral.[3] Detailed anatomical studies suggest that the defect occurs 14 to 49 days postovulation.[43] Spina bifida aperta can range from myeloschisis or the exposure of the unfolded neural plate to a variety of meningoceles that involve either the spinal cord (myelomeningocele) or only the subarachnoid space (meningocele).

Several theories attempt to explain the embryological defects that cause spinal dysraphism. These theorists may be divided into two general groups: (1) those who postulate a defect in closure of the neural tube and subsequent malformation of overlying structures, and (2) those who postulate normal initial neural tube closure with late rupture of the closed neural tube and resultant malformation of associated structures. Experimental models have supported the possibility of both hypotheses.[58]

Von Recklinghausen proposed that myelodysplasia arises from an arrest of neural plate closure and a secondary failure of development of the posterior spinal elements.[39] In 1881 Ledeff suggested that the failure of the neural tube to close results from the overgrowth of neural tissue in the lateral folds.[39] The hydrodynamic theory proposed by Gardner hypothesizes that the neural tube initially closes normally, but is reopened by increased hydrostatic pressure within the central canal with subsequent malformation of posterior elements.[39] It is not likely that one hypothesis can explain the full range of spinal dysmorphism. However, the high incidence of dysraphism at the thoracolumbar junction is most likely due to failure of the dorsal neuropore to close normally.

The widening of the spinal column at the level of the defect is characteristic of spinal dysraphism. Abnormal neural tube development causes a failure of dorsal element formation and ventrolateral displacement of the pedicles and lateral elements of the spine. Rarely, other abnormalities of the vertebrae are associated with spinal dysraphism, such as wedge vertebrae and hemivertebrae. Some patients presenting with apparent idiopathic scoliosis may have some form of occult spinal dysraphism.[6] The inductive effects of spinal dysraphism can cause multiple rib anomalies.[35]

In the absence of normal neural tube development, the normal development of skin layers over the defect is also hindered. Dura mater arises ventrally to the deformed spinal cord but then stretches laterally over the expanded pedicles and facet joints to the lateral margins of the epidermis. The dorsal defect is covered by a thin layer of pia/arachnoid and an extremely thin layer of epithelium, the zona epitheliosa.

Spina bifida aperta most often occurs in the lumbar and sacral areas of the spinal column, but it can develop in the thoracic spine, particularly at the thoracolumbar junction. The morphogenesis of the dysraphism depends on the embryological period in which the malformation occurs. If the insult occurs before day 28, myeloschises (open exposure of the malformed spinal cord) occurs as a result of the neural tube failing to close. Myeloschises is common at the thoracolumbar junction. If the insult occurs after 28 days of gestation, various forms of meningocele and myelomeningocele can result. Occult spinal dysraphism includes a variety of spinal malformations not immediately visible on the skin surface. Of relevance to any discussion of the thoracic spine are spina bifida occulta, diastematomyelia/diplomyelia, neurenteric cyst, and lipomas.

Spina bifida occulta (malformations not readily visible at the surface due to overlying skin and soft tissue) occurs due to abnormal development of the posterior neural arch structures. This is believed to occur due to rupture of an already closed neural tube.[39] With increased pressure inside the central canal of the neural tube, a rupture can spill highly proteinaceous fluid from the canal into the surrounding tissue. The rupture relieves the pressure within the central canal, and the defect in the neural tube reanneals, but the extruded proteinaceous fluid inhibits normal development of the dorsal elements. Because the neural tube has closed, closure of the dermis and epidermis over the dorsal aspect of the spinal cord is not impeded.

Diastematomyelia and diplomyelia are embryological abnormalities that cause the spinal cord to develop into two hemicords, each surrounded by its own dural sheath and separated by a cartilaginous or bony septum.[40] (see Fig. 3-4). In a study of 60 patients, Hood et al.[27] found that diastematomyelia occurred from the third thoracic to the fourth lumbar vertebra; approximately 50% of the lesions were associated with thoracic vertebrae and 50% were associated with lumbar vertebrae. Pang[50] found that the lumbar spine was the most commonly affected region. He reviewed 39 cases and found six cervical lesions, two thoracic lesions, and 31 lumbar lesions. Diastematomyelia and diplomyelia can result in neurological compromise because the differential growth between the spinal cord and the spinal column causes progressive impingement of the caudal aspect of the septum against the spinal cord.

Theories abound about the embryology of diastematomyelia and diplomyelia. In 1940 Herren and Edwards[25] proposed the model of "twinning," in which the lateral neural folds may roll to the midline and fuse with the neural plate, rather than with each other. Two hemicords result. Each hemicord may induce mesodermal formation of a protective matrix, and the midline spicule results. Also in 1940 Lichtenstein[33] postulated that diastematomyelia was primarily a defect of mesoderm formation. He stated that the malformed midline septum splits the neural plate, and two hemicords develop.

In 1992 Pang et al.[51] proposed a unified theory of the embryogenesis of diastematomyelia and diplomyelia. They suggested that these lesions be characterized as "split cord malformation" (SCM). A type I SCM consists of two hemicords, each contained in its own dural tube and separated by a dural sheathed rigid, osseocartilaginous median septum. A type II SMC consists of two hemicords housed in a single dural sheath and separated by a nonrigid, fibrous midline septum.[51] In his study of 39 patients, Pang found 19 patients with type I SCMs, 18 with type II SCMs, and 2 with composite SCMs in tandem.[50]

The split cord malformation theory proposes that both types of SCMs originate from one embryological error around the time of neural tube closure. The basic error is in the formation of an accessory neurenteric canal through the midline of the embryonic disc that maintains communication between the yolk sac and the amnion and also between endoderm and ectoderm.[51] As this abnormal fistula develops, mesenchyme condenses around it, and the tract then splits the developing notochord and neural tube. The phenotype of the malformation depends on further development of the spinal column/cord. If the embryo is able to heal around the tract, a SCM results. If the tract picks up primitive cells from the mesenchyme, destined to become the meninges, the two hemicords will each be invested in dura. The dura mater can stimulate bone growth, and a midline spur results (SCM type I). If these precursor cells to dura mater are not contained in the tract, both hemicords are in the same dural sac, separated only by abnormal fibrous bands (SCM type II). If endoderm is retained in the tract, a neurenteric cyst can result.[51]

It was long believed that the presence or absence of medial nerve roots could help distinguish diastematomyelia from simple diplomyelia. However, Pang[51] found medial nerve roots in about three fourths of type I and type II SCMs. Notably, most medial nerve roots were dorsal; ventral medial nerve roots were exceedingly rare.

Neurenteric cysts are retained cystic structures derived from the embryological foregut and therefore ventrally located in the spinal canal.[7] These rare lesions occur most commonly in the thoracic and cervical spine.[26] Neurenteric cysts can cause spinal cord compression, and they usually present in childhood. In a meta-analysis of 23 reported cases, French found that 40% occurred in the cervical spine and 50% occurred in the thoracic spine.[22] The epithelium of these cysts varies from ciliated columnar lining (suggesting a respiratory origin) or gland-forming linings resembling the epithelium of gut mucosa. Neurenteric cysts tend to lie to the right of the vertebral column due to embryological gut rotation.[60] They most likely originate from communications between the yolk sac (eventual foregut) and the dorsal surface of the embryo. Normally a neurenteric canal is located in the region of the coccyx. However, accessory neurenteric canals can occur rostral to the coccyx, and if they persist with invaginated endoderm, neurenteric cysts result.[7] A persistent neurenteric tract may give rise to vertebral abnormalities such as a widened vertebral body due to increased bone formation around the tract.

Lipomas of the spine are relatively common in clinical practice and may be considered a developmental abnormality. Lipomas associated with occult spinal dysraphism are the most common form, and 90% occur in the lumbosacral area.[23] Lipomas associated with spinal dysraphism take three principal forms: terminal, dorsal, or transitional. In the dorsal form of the lesion, the lipoma extends from the subcutaneous space through incomplete neural arches and attaches to the dorsal cord. In this case it is rare for nerve roots to be contained within the substance of the lipoma. Terminal lipomas insert into the distal conus and may be entirely intraspinal. In this case nerve roots often run within the substance of the lipoma.[13] Transitional lipomas have characteristics of both dorsal and terminal lipomas.

In contrast, intraspinal lipomas not associated with spina bifida account for 1% of intraspinal tumors in adults and 4.7% of intraspinal tumors in children, showing a predilection for the thoracic spine.[57] In a meta-analysis of published cases, Caram et al.[10] found that 29 of 51 reported cases of intraspinal lipomas involved the thoracic spine.

These lesions most likely result when adipose cells from the overlying mesodermal tissue are included in the developing spinal canal or the folding neural tube.[10,18] Because these lesions often traverse both the bony and neural elements of the spine, tethering of the spinal cord results.[57]

TETHERED CORD

Usually the "tethered cord syndrome" defines a low-lying conus medullaris due to a short and thickened filum terminale. Recently the term has been used to denote either a spinal cord tethered by fibrous bands and adhesions or an intradural lipoma. The embryological origin of the short and thickened filum is not known. The pathophysiology of tethered cord syndrome has been postulated to involve hypoxic stress on the stretched spinal cord.[75] Tethering lesions produce traction on the spinal cord and nerve roots and may cause profound neurological deficits.

Pang and Wilberger[52] postulate that the degree of spinal cord traction, rather than the type or distribution of the tethering lesions, probably determines the age of symptom onset. Severe traction on the spinal cord results in presentation in childhood, whereas less severe traction is asymptomatic in childhood, but presents later in life due to repeated tugging of the conus during head and neck flexion or abnormal tension aggravated by trauma or spondylitic spinal canal stenosis.

CONGENITAL SCOLIOSIS

Congenital scoliosis is an abnormal curvature of the spine in the coronal plane that results from anomalous vertebrae present at birth. Although the vertebral abnormality in congenital scoliosis is present at birth, physical deformity is rarely found in newborns. The deformity often progresses with growth, and the scoliosis usually presents clinically during childhood, although it may be discovered incidentally and not until adulthood. Congenital scoliosis is distant from infantile idiopathic scoliosis (which also presents with deformity during childhood) because infantile idiopathic scoliosis has no structural vertebral abnormality. A variety of clinical presentations are possible because numerous types of congenital vertebral abnormalities exist. Some of these anomalies result in rapidly progressing scoliosis during early childhood that produces severe morbidity without treatment, whereas others cause little or no deformity at any time.[37]

Advances in radiographic imaging, including computed tomography (CT) and magnetic resonance imaging (MRI), have contributed greatly to the understanding of these disorders by allowing better classification of vertebral anomalies. Other recent advances in diagnosis and treatment have improved the understanding of the natural history of scoliotic deformities and helped clarify issues attendant to surgery, including indications and timing.

Normal growth occurs at the end plates of the rostral and caudal surfaces of the vertebral bodies.[4] Congenital vertebral anomalies can cause absence or functional deficiency of the growth plates on one or both sides of the spine. A spinal deformity will occur if there is asymmetrical growth, which occurs with a functional deficiency on one side compared with the other. The rate of angulation and the final severity of the congenital scoliosis are proportional to the degree of growth imbalance produced by the vertebral anomalies. The portion of the vertebra with deficient growth determines whether a pure scoliosis exists or some component of sagittal plane deformity (imbalance of growth ventrally or dorsally) is present, resulting in kyphoscoliosis or lordoscoliosis. Winter[74] evaluated the prognosis for scoliosis progression for different types of congenital vertebral abnormalities and devised a radiographic classification scheme.

The vertebral defects that result in congenital scoliosis can usually be classified by the abnormality in the developmental process during formation of the mesenchymal precursor of the vertebrae. This abnormality results in either a failure of segmentation between adjacent vertebrae or a failure of formation of all or a portion of the vertebrae (Fig. 3-5). Failure in formation can range from mild wedging to total absence of the vertebra. The complete absence of half of a vertebra results in a hemivertebra, which is one of the most common causes of congenital scoliosis. The hemivertebra consists of wedged vertebral body with a single pedicle and hemilamina.

Failure of segmentation results in abnormal bony fusion between adjacent vertebrae. The defect can involve ventral elements, dorsal elements, or both, and can be either unilateral or bilateral. The most common failure of segmentation is the unilateral

Defects of Segmentation

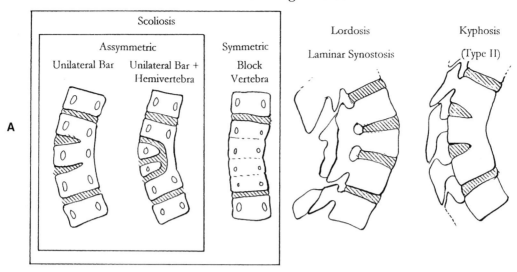

A

Defects of Formation

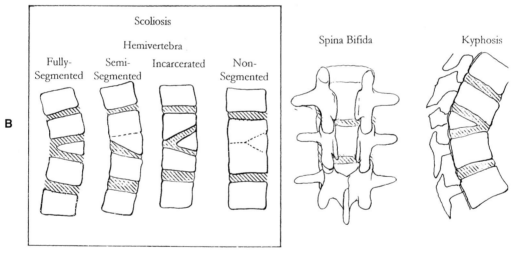

B

Fig. 3-5. Structural abnormalities in congenital spine deformity. **A,** Defects of segmentation result in congenital scoliosis, congenital lordosis, and congenital (type II) kyphosis. **B,** Defects of formation result in congenital scoliosis, spina bifida, and congenital (type I) kyphosis.

unsegmented bar that results in a solid fusion of the disc space and facet joint on one side of the vertebra (see Fig. 3-5, *A*). A combination of defects in formation and defects in segmentation in the same patient can negate or exacerbate the degree of scoliosis. For example, an unsegmented bar with a contralateral hemivertebra leads to severe progressive scoliosis because of a marked difference in potential growth between the two sides of the spine[37,44] (see Fig. 3-5, *A*).

There are three major types of hemivertebrae classified by their relationship to adjacent vertebrae and whether or not morphologically normal discs are associated (see Fig. 3-5, *B*). The potential for a hemivertebra to cause significant scoliosis depends on its type, its location, the number of hemivertebrae and their relationships (ipsilateral or contralateral), and the patient's age.[36] A hemivertebra in the thoracic region often has a rib associated with it that results in an unequal number of ribs.

A fully segmented hemivertebra has a normal disc space above and below the formed portion of the vertebral body that allows near-normal longitudinal growth on one side. A portion of the vertebral body is absent, and there are growth plates on the unformed side. Full growth potential exists on one side of the spine, and none on the other side; therefore a potential for significant deformity exists. (see Fig. 3-5, *B*). The hemivertebra acts like an enlarging wedge and is located at the apex of the convexity of the scoliosis in these cases. The rate of progression and need for treatment of the scoliosis caused by a fully separated hemivertebra depends on its location in the spine. A hemivertebra at the lumbosacral junction has the worst prognosis.[36] In general these scoliotic curves progress at one to two degrees a year, but some will progress more rapidly, requiring surgical intervention.[36,37] A variant of the fully segmented hemivertebra is the incarcerated hemivertebra. This more benign variant of fully segmented hemivertebrae is set into defects in the vertebrae above and below it. The incarcerated hemivertebra itself is small and oval shaped, with poorly formed disc spaces that have poor growth potential (see Fig. 3-5, *B*). The combination of defects in the adjacent vertebrae, which tend to compensate for the hemivertebra, and the poor potential growth of the malformed growth plates results in less scoliotic deformity than is associated with the standard, fully segmented hemivertebra.[36]

A semisegmented hemivertebra is fused to either the vertebra above or below it. This results in the absence of one disc space on the side of the hemivertebra, with obliteration of two growth plates (one from the hemivertebra and one from the adjacent vertebra) (see Fig. 3-5, *B*). Theoretically, this would result in similar growth on both sides of the spine because there are two active growth plates on each side. In fact, the wedge shape of the hemivertebra and differences in actual growth usually result in mild to modest scoliosis. Patients with a semisegmented hemivertebra usually do not require treatment.[36]

A nonsegmented hemivertebra is fused to the adjacent vertebrae above and below it with no disc spaces or growth potential. The wedge shape of the hemivertebra may cause some deformity, but it is not progressive. Some growth may occur on the opposite side of the spine, but this usually results in gradual correction of the deformity.

A unilateral unsegmented bar is another common cause of congenital scoliosis.[37,69] This condition results from a failure of segmentation of two or more vertebrae (see Fig. 3-5, *B*). The unsegmented bar contains no growth plates, but the unaffected, or less affected, side of the spine continues to grow. This imbalance in growth results in scoliosis with the unsegmented bar in the concavity. The number of vertebrae involved with the bar, the location, and the growth potential of the convex side of the spine determine the rate of angulation deformity and final severity of the scoliosis. On average, these curves deteriorate at a rate of 5 degrees or greater per year and will result in a significant deformity by puberty.[37] A bilateral failure of segmentation results in a block vertebra, which has little potential for asymmetrical growth because the disc spaces are either dysplastic or fused (see Fig. 3-5, *A*). In general, the reduction in growth between the two sides of the spine is equal, and significant scoliosis is unusual.[37] In the cervical spine, bilateral failure of segmentation is often present in the Klippel-Feil syndrome.

CONGENITAL KYPHOSIS

Congenital kyphosis is an uncommon sagittal plane spinal deformity that is often associated with neurological deficit if left untreated.[41,72] As with congenital scoliosis, the causes of congenital kyphosis are failure of formation and failure of segmentation of vertebrae. Winter, Moe, and Wang[72] classified congenital kyphosis into three types: type I, failure of formation of vertebral body; type II, failure of segmentation of vertebral body resulting in a ventral unsegmented bar; and type III, mixed failure of formation and segmentation (see Fig. 3-5). Type I deformity is the most common and the most likely to develop both a severe deformity and neurological compromise.[41,72] The severity of type I kyphosis is directly proportional to the amount of vertebral body or bodies that fail to form[72] (see Fig. 3-5, *B*). Type II deformity is less common, produces less severe deformity, and is associated more frequently with neurological compromise than type I. The amount of kyphosis produced is proportional to the discrepancy between the ventral vertebral growth and the growth of the dorsal elements (see Fig. 3-5, *A*). Type III deformity is very rare and most probably behaves like type I kyphosis. The natural history of congenital kyphosis is often one of progressive deformity that is unresponsive to nonoperative treatment.[70] Even type II deformities can progress significantly during the growth spurt at puberty. Once a significant deformity develops, the incidence of operative complications is high, and early surgery is often indicated.

CONGENITAL LORDOSIS

Congenital lordosis is less common than either congenital scoliosis or congenital kyphosis. This entity results from dorsal defects in segmentation with normal ventral growth.[73] (see Fig. 3-5, *A*). This condition often has some component of coronal plane deformity, leading to lordoscoliosis because of the dorsolateral location of the unsegmented bar. The most severe consequence of congenital lordosis is severe impairment of pulmonary function.[71,73] Early recognition and surgical treatment are necessary to prevent this complication.

SYRINGOMYELIA

Syringomyelia (fluid-filled cavitation of the spinal cord) occurs frequently in the thoracic spine. Although not directly a congenital malformation, it may be considered a developmental abnormality because of its frequent association with Chiari malformations.[39]

Chiari malformations manifest themselves as congenitally small dorsal fossas with herniation of hindbrain structures into the cervical canal. Chiari II malformations are associated with myelomeningoceles, whereas Chiari I malformations are usually not.

The embryological miscues that cause these conditions are not entirely clear. Overgrowth of the cerebellum and medulla has been postulated as one cause,[2] but differences in pressure between the cranial and spinal subarachnoid space causes Chiari I malformation. Patients who have undergone lumbarperitoneal shunting and have cranial and spinal pressure differences occasionally develop Chiari I-like malformations. It has been noted that among patients with Chiari I malformations there is a higher incidence of traumatic delivery and presumed subarachnoid hemorrhage.[45,66] This observation supports the hypothesis that the formation of subarachnoid adhesions impairs cerebrospinal fluid (CSF) flow, leading to a pressure gradient between the cranial

and spinal compartments. With regard to the pathophysiology of the hindbrain herniation in Chiari II malformations, the tethering of the spinal cord by the myelomeningocele is thought to result in the herniation of the hindbrain. Researchers have shown that the presence of the meningocele predates the formation of the hindbrain hernia.[49]

Chiari I malformations result in the herniation of the cerebellar tonsils into the foramen magnum and scarring of the dura to the tonsils. Cavitation (syrinx) within the spinal cord occurs in 50% to 75% of these patients.[39] The posterior fossa is foreshortened and small due to flattening of the squamous occipital bone. The foramen magnum is enlarged to accommodate the descended cerebellar tonsils.

The pathophysiology involved in syrinx formation in Chiari malformations is complex and still being debated.[66,68] The hydrodynamic theory, proposed by Gardner, states that the arterial pulse is transmitted to the central canal of the spinal cord, creating distention by a "water hammer" effect.[24] The cranial-spinal pressure dissocation theory of Williams[66] relies on herniated tonsils acting as a one-way valve that allows CSF to pass easily from the spinal subarachnoid space to the cranial subarachnoid space but preventing flow in the opposite direction. CSF in the fourth ventricle flows into the central canal via the obex due to the cranial-spinal pressure gradient. It is likely that a combination of these processes may produce the syringomyelia associated with Chiari malformations.

Syringomyelia may present with pain in the spine, limb, and trunk, dissociated sensory loss, and atrophy of musculature of the distal upper extremities. Radiographic features include widening of the spinal canal and erosion of the vertebrae.[67] Posterior fossa decompression without syrinx drainage is usually curative in patients with Chiari I malformations and spinal cord cavitation, lending support to the view that a cranial-spinal pressure gradient produces syringomyelia.[9]

CONCLUSION

The development of the human spinal column and its contents begins on day 15 from conception and continues through vertebral skeletal maturation to about the age of 25 years. It proceeds in an organized and systematic fashion. Discrepancies in embryological spinal cord and column development may result in important structural, physiological, and functional skeletal and neurological abnormalities. This chapter highlights the important embryological events in the development of the thoracic spine to give the reader better insight into congenital malformations of the thoracic spine.

REFERENCES

1. Bagnall KM, Higgins SJ, Sanders EJ. The contribution made by a single somite to the vertebral column: Experimental evidence in support of resegmentation using the chick-quail chimaera model. Development 103:69-85, 1988.
2. Barry A, Patten BM, Stewart BH. Possible factors in the development of the Arnold-Chiari malformation. J Neurol 14:285, 1957.
3. Barson AJ. Spina bifida: The significance of the level and extent of the defect to the morphogenesis. Dev Med Child Neurol 12:129-144, 1970.
4. Bick EM, Cogsel JW. Longitudinal growth of the human vertebrae: A contribution of human osteology. J Bone Joint Surg A:803-804, 1950.
5. Bound JP, Francis BJ, Harvey PW. Neural tube defects, maternal cohorts, and age: A pointer to aetiology. Arch Dis Child 66:1223-1226, 1991.
6. Bradford DS, Heithoff KB, Cohen M. Intraspinal abnormalities and congenital spine deformities: A radiographic and MRI study. J Pediatr Orthop 11:36-41, 1991.
7. Bremer JL. Dorsal intestinal fistula; accessory neurenteric canal; diastematomyelia. Arch Pathol 54:132-138, 1952.
8. Byrd SE, Darling CF, McLone DG. Developmental disorders of the pediatric spine. Radiol Clin North Am 29:711-752, 1991.
9. Cahan LD, Bentson JR. Considerations in the diagnosis and treatment of syringomyelia and the Chiari malformation. J Neurosurg 57:24-31, 1982.
10. Caram PR, Scarcella G, Carton CA. Intradural lipomas of the spinal cord. J Neurosurg 14:349-354, 1957.
11. Cave AJE. The morphology of the mammalian cervical pleurapophysis. J Zool 177:377-393, 1975.
12. Chandraraj S, Briggs CA. Role of cartilage canals in osteogenesis and growth of the vertebral centra. J Anat 158:121-136, 1988.
13. Chapman PH. Congenital intraspinal lipomas. Anatomic considerations and surgical treatment. Childs Nerv Syst 9:37, 1982.
14. Chatkupt S, Skurnick JH, Jaggi M, et al. Study of genetics, epidemiology, and vitamin usage in familial spina bifida in the United States in the 1990s. Neurology 44:65-70. 1994.
15. Christ B, Wilting J. From somites to vertebral column. Ann Anat 174:23-32, 1992.
16. Dalgleish AE. A study of the development of thoracic vertebrae in the mouse assisted by autoradiography. ACTA Anat 122:91-98, 1985.
17. Dias MS, Walker ML. The embryogenesis of complex dysraphic malformations: A disorder of gastrulation? Pediatr Neurosurg 18:229-253, 1992.
18. Ehni G, Love JG. Intraspinal lipomas. Arch Neurol Psychiatry 53:1-28, 1945.
19. Ewan KBR, Everett AW. Evidence for resegmentation in the formation of the vertebral column using the novel approach of retroviral-mediated gene transfer. Exp Cell Res 198:315-320, 1992.
20. Flood T. Spina bifida incidence at birth—United States 1983-1990. MMWR Morb Mortality Wkly Rep 41:497-500, 1992.
21. Flood T, et al. From the Centers for Disease Control. Spina bifida incidence at birth—United States. JAMA 268:708-709, 1992.
22. French BN. Midline fusion defects and defects of formation. In Youmans JR, ed: Neurological Surgery. Philadelphia: WB Saunders, 1990, pp 1081-1235.
23. French BN. The embryology of spinal dysraphism. Clin Neurosurg 30:295-340, 1983.
24. Gardner WJ. Hydrodynamic mechanism of syringomyelia: Its relationship to myelocele. J Neurol Neurosurg Psychiatry 28:247-259, 1965.
25. Herren RY, Edwards JE. Diplomyelia (duplication of the spinal cord). Arch Pathol 30:1203-1214, 1940.
26. Holcomb GW, Matson DD. Thoracic neurenteric Cyst. Surgery 35:115-121, 1954.
27. Hood RW, Riseborough EJ, Nehme A, et al. Diastematomyelia and structural spinal deformities. J Bone Joint Surg 62A:520-528, 1980.
28. Hori A. A review of the morphology of spinal cord malformations and their relation to neuroembryology. Neurosurg Rev 16:259-266, 1993.
29. Humphreys RP. Current trends in spinal dysraphism. Paraplegia 29:79-83, 1991.
30. Kessel M, Gruss P. Homeotic transformations of murine vertebrae and concomitant alteration of Hox codes induced by retinoic acid. Cell 67:89-104, 1991.
31. Keynes RJ, Stern CD. Mechanisms of vertebrate segmentation. Development 103:413-429, 1988.
32. Kieny M, Mauger A, Sengel P. Early regionalization of the somitic mesoderm as studied by the development of the axial skeleton of the chick embryo. Dev Biol 28:142-161, 1972.
33. Lichtenstein BW. Spinal dlysraphism, spina bifida and myelodysplasia. Arch Neurol Psychiatr 44:792-810, 1940.
34. Lohse CL, Hyde DM, Benson DR. Comparative development of thoracic intervertebral discs and intraarticular ligaments in the human, monkey, mouse and cat. Acta Anat 122:220-228, 1985.
35. McLennan JE. Rib Anomolies in myelodysplasia. Biol Neonate 29:129-141, 1976.
36. McMaster MJ, David CV. Hemivertebrae as a cause of scoliosis: A study of 104 patients. J Bone Joint Surg 68B:588-595, 1986.
37. McMaster MJ, Oktsuka K. The natural history of congenital scoliosis: A study of 251 patients. J Bone Joint Surg 64A:1128-1147, 1982.
38. Med M. Prenatal development of thoracic intervertebral articulation. Folia Morphol 25:175-177, 1975.
39. Menezes AH, Smoker WRK, Dyste GN. Syringomyelia, Chiari malformations, and hydromyelia. In Youmans JR, ed. Neurological Surgery. Philadelphia: WB Saunders, 1990, pp 1421-1459.
40. Miller A, Guille JT, Bowen JR. Evaluation and treatment of diastomatomyelia. J Bone Joint Surg 75A:1308-1317, 1993.
41. Montgomery SP, Hall JE. Congenital kyphosis. Spine 7:223-274, 1982.

42. Moore KL. The Developing Human Clinically Oriented Embryology. Philadelphia: W B Saunders, 1982.

43. Muller, F, O'Rahilly RO, Benson DR. The early origin of vertebral anomalies, as illustrated by a "butterfly vertebra." J Anat 149:157-169, 1986.

44. Nasca RJ, Stilling FH, Stul HH. Progression of congenital scoliosis due to hemivertebrae and hemivertebrae with bars. J Bone Joint Surg 57A:456-466, 1975.

45. Newman PK, Terenty TR, Foster JB. Some observations on the pathogenesis of syringomyelia. J Neurol Neurosurg Psychiatry 44:964-969, 1981.

46. Noback CR, Robertson GG. Sequences of appearance of ossification centers in the human skeleton during the first five prenatal months. Am J Anat 89:128, 1969.

47. O'Rahilly R, Muller F. Meyer DB. The human vertebral column at the end of the embryonic period proper 3. The thoracolumbar region. J Anat 168:81-93, 1990.

48. Ogden JA, Ganey TM, Sasse J, et al. Development and maturation of the axial skeleton. In Weinstein SL, ed. The Pediatric Spine: Principles and Practice. New York: Raven Press 1994, pp 3-69.

49. Osaka K, Tanimura T. Hiragoma A, et al. Myelomeningocele before birth. J Neurosurg 49:711-724, 1978.

50. Pang D. Split cord malformation: Part II: Clinical syndrome. Neurosurgery 31:481-500, 1992.

51. Pang D, Dias MS, Ahab-Barmada M. Split cord malformation: Part I: A unified theory of embryogenesis for double spinal cord malformations. Neurosurgery 31:451-480, 1992.

52. Pang D, Wilberger JE. Tethered cord syndrome in adults. Neurosurg 57:32-47, 1982.

53. Parke WW. Development of the spine. In Rothman RH, Simeone FA, eds. The Spine. Philadelphia: WB Saunders, 1992, pp 3-33.

54. Peacock A. Observations on the pre-natal development of the intervertebral disc in man. J Anat 85:260-274, 1960.

55. Remak R. Untersuchungen uber die Entwicklung der Wirbeltiere. Berlin: Reimer, 1855.

56. Roessmann U. The embryology and neuropathology of congenital malformations. Clin Neurosurg 30:157-164, 1983.

57. Rogers HM, Long DM, Chou SN, et al. Lipomas of the spinal cord and cauda equina. J Neurosurg 34:349-354, 1971.

58. Rokos J, Knowles J. An experimental contribution to the pathogenesis of spina bifida. J Pathol 118:21-24, 1976.

59. Sandford MK, Kissling GE, Joubert PE. Neural tube defect etiology: New evidence concerning maternal hyperthermia, health and diet. Dev Med Child Neurol 34:661-675, 1992.

60. Silvernail WI, Brown RB. Intramedullary enterogenous cyst. J Neurosurg 36:235-238, 1972.

61. Smith MT, Wissinger JP, Smith CG, et al. Experimental dysraphism in the rat. J Neurosurg 49:725-729, 1978.

62. Sweeney RM, Watterson RI. Rib development in chick embryos analyzed by means of tantalum foil blocks. Am J Anat 126:127-150, 1970.

63. Verbout AJ. The Development of the vertebral column. Adv Anat Embryol Cell Biol 90:1-22, 1985.

64. Vogter DM, Kaufman HH. Spinal dysraphism—A review. W V Med J 81:142-143, 1985.

65. Whalen JL, Parke WW, Mazur JM, et al. The intrinsic vasculature of developing vertebral end plates and its nutritive significance to the intervertebral discs. J Pediatr Orthop 5:403-410, 1985.

66. Williams B. Difficult labor as a cause of communicating syringomyelia. Lancet 2:51-53, 1977.

67. Williams B. Orthopaedic feature in the presentation of syringomyelia. J Bone Joint Surg 61B:314-323, 1979.

68. Williams B. On the pathogenesis of syringomyelia: A review. J R Soc Med 73:798-806, 1980.

69. Winter RB, Moe J H, Bradford DS. Congenital thoracic lordosis. J Bone Joint Surg 60A:806-810, 1978.

70. Winter RB. Scoliosis. In Bradford DMS, Lonstein JE, Moe JH, et al., eds. Moe's Textbook of Scoliosis and Other Spinal Deformities. Philadelphia: WB Saunders, 1987, p 282.

71. Winter RB, Leonard AS. Case report: Surgical correction of congenital thoracic lordosis. J Pediatr Orthop 10:805-808, 1990.

72. Winter RB, Moe JH, Wang JF. Congenital kyphosis: Its natural history and treatment as observed in a study of 130 patients. J Bone Joint Surg 55A:223-274, 1973.

73. Winter RB, Moe JH, Bradford DS. Congenital chronic lordosis. J Bone Joint Surg 60A:806-810, 1978.

74. Winter RB, Moe JH, Eiders VE. Congenital scoliosis: A study of 234 patients treated and untreated. J Bone Joint Surg 50A:1-47, 1968.

75. Yamada S, Zinke DE, Sanders D. Pathophysiology of "tethered cord syndrome." J Neurosurg 54:494-503, 1981.

76. Yen IH, Khoury MJ, Erickson JD, et al. The changing epidemiology of neural tube defects, United States, 1968-1989. Am J Dis Child 146:857-861, 1992.

Biomechanics

Nevan G. Baldwin, M.D.

The human thoracic spine is a highly specialized spinal region that is uniquely adapted to an erect posture and the load-bearing demands that result from the daily activities of biped (upright) creatures. The same anatomical features of the thoracic spine that give this region its unique biomechanical properties also provide for a particular set of responses to pathological processes, such as infection or trauma. The two transitional zones that adjoin the thoracic spine, the cervicothoracic junction and the thoracolumbar junction, each have a somewhat similar set of biomechanical properties. The biomechanical characteristics of the junctional zones are best described as a blending of the properties of the two adjacent spinal regions represented in the transition. Knowledge of the biomechanical characteristics of the cervicothoracic, thoracic, and thoracolumbar regions is crucial to understand how disease processes affect these areas and how to best establish appropriate diagnosis and provide appropriate treatment.

The predominant posture of the thoracic spine is a kyphotic curve.[33] Although the spine is nearly straight from T11 to L2, this straight segment is positioned in the sagittal plane at a slight diagonal from rostrodorsal to caudoventral (Fig. 4-1). This angled portion compensates for the thoracic kyphosis and keeps the axial load of the spine such that the body's center of gravity is positioned directly above the feet. The lumbar lordosis provides the remainder of the compensation for balance of posture. Spinal curvature may arise from postural or structural factors. Postural curves simply reflect positioning of the spine due to ligamentous tension and muscle tone, as well as the configuration of the disks, which is altered by spinal loading. The height of the vertebral bodies in the thoracic spine is less at the ventral aspect than at the dorsal aspect. The resulting kyphosis is therefore a structural curve rather than a postural one.

The kyphotic posture of the thoracic spine dictates that the axial load applied to this region (the weight of the head, neck, and shoulders) creates a bending moment that tends to produce further flexion. Therefore, disease processes that compromise the integrity of the thoracic spine tend to produce further flexion or forward angulation of the spine. In stabilizing this spinal region, it is important to ascertain that load-bearing capacity is adequate in the ventral bony structures (vertebral bodies) and that an adequate tension-band (the restrictive force exerted by the ligaments to prevent flexion) exists dorsally.[15] Dorsal tension-band stability and ventral weight-bearing integrity constitute the vital combination necessary for spinal stability and for the prevention of deformity in the thoracic spine (Fig. 4-2).

ANATOMY

The thoracic vertebrae are most immediately recognizable by their transverse processes and the articular surfaces that form the vertebral component of the costotransverse joints. The general configuration of the dorsal elements in the thoracic spine varies according to level. The pedicles vary both in

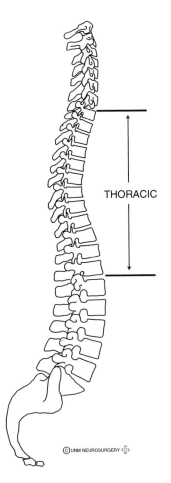

Fig. 4-1. A lateral view of the spine demonstrates the kyphotic posture of the thoracic region.

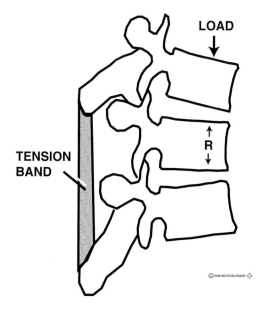

LOAD

TENSION
BAND

R

Fig. 4-2. Due to the kyphotic posture of the thoracic spine, there is a tendency for the normal curvature to progress into further kyphosis. To maintain stability and resist that progression, adequate weight-bearing capacity must exist ventrally to resist compression *(R)* and a tension-band force must be present dorsally. The spinous process of the middle vertebra shown is omitted for clarity.

size and in their angular relationships to the vertebral body. Thoracic pedicles have wide diameters in the sagittal plane but their coronal plane width is considerably narrower, significantly restricting the surgeon's ability to place bone screws in the pedicles at thoracic levels. Generally, pedicle size increases as the thoracic spine descends. In a detailed study of the thoracic pedicle, McCormack et al.[22] described the pedicle angles from cadaveric studies and also described an equation for the localization of the pedicles relative to the transverse processes. The equation is complex and not practical for clinical use, but its existence points out that this anatomy varies in a manner that is predictable according to spinal level.

The laminae of the thoracic vertebrae are broad in the rostrocaudal dimension and their lower margins are caudally located relative to the position of the vertebral bodies. This fact is particularly impor-

tant to consider in the design of spinal instrumentation constructs when the center of the construct is positioned at the level of injury. When laminar fixation is used, centering a construct at the injury level is usually best achieved by fixation of one segment fewer below the injury than is performed above the injury. This concept is also an important consideration for the proper identification of levels and maintaining orientation intraoperatively.

The facet joint angles vary throughout the thoracic spine. At the rostral end, and extending to the T5 or T6 level, the facet angles are oriented more in the coronal plane. Below these levels, the facet angles change, becoming almost completely oriented in the sagittal plane near the T12 or L1 level. The thoracic facets allow motion in all planes, but the ranges of motion are closely related to the facet joint angles. In flexion and extension, the upper thoracic region has very limited motion, whereas from T10 caudally, larger ranges of flexion/extension motion—similar to those of the lumbar spine—are commonly observed. The sagittal orientation of the facets in the lower thoracic region severely limits axial plane rotation and, to a lesser extent, lateral bending.

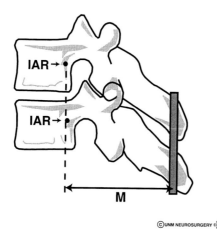

Fig. 4-3. The instantaneous axis of rotation *(IAR)* represents the imaginary line around which a vertebra rotates during movement. During flexion, the IAR is generally located near the dorsal portion of the vertebral body. It is represented here by a dot because the line of the axis would project directly out of the plane of the page. The dorsal ligamentous complex (shaded area) resists flexion effectively through the mechanical advantage afforded by a relatively long moment arm *(M)*.

The motion of the thoracic spine, in all planes, is limited by the spinal ligaments. The anterior longitudinal ligament (ALL) spans the entire length of the thoracic spine. It is a thick, strong ligament that attaches to the vertebral bodies of the spine. The posterior longitudinal ligament (PLL) is a thinner, less substantial structure that attaches to the intervertebral discs. The PLL contributes less to the stability of the spinal column. The ligamentum flavum, in conjunction with the interspinous ligament and supraspinous ligament, limits flexion movements. Flexion forces constitute the largest movement forces observed in the thoracic spine.

None of the structures of the dorsal ligamentous complex (ligamentum flavum, supraspinous ligament, interspinous ligament, and the capsular ligaments of the facet joints) are as robust as the ALL in terms of tensile strength. However, these structures are positioned far dorsal to the pivot point of each thoracic spinal motion segment. The pivot point of vertebral motion is known as the instantaneous axis of rotation (IAR). Dorsal to the IAR, the spinal elements move farther apart during flexion; ventral to the IAR, the vertebral elements move closer together during flexion. Because the dorsal ligamentous complex is located far dorsal to the IAR, a longer moment arm is created to resist flexion movements beyond the physiological range of motion (Fig. 4-3).

The transitional zones bordering the thoracic spine, the cervicothoracic and thoracolumbar junctions, possess anatomical and biomechanical properties that represent a blending of the characteristics observed above and below the thoracic spine. The facets of the upper thoracic spine are similar in orientation to those of the cervical region, and likewise the facets at the lower thoracic area are like those of the lumbar spine. The ranges of motion correspond to the facet joint anatomy in the transitional zones,[24] and therefore represent a blending of the ranges observed immediately adjacent to the thoracic area with those of the thoracic spine.

NORMAL MOVEMENT AND LOAD BEARING

The ranges of spinal movement in any given plane are divided into the neutral zone, the elastic zone, and the injury zone. The neutral zone is that portion of the range of motion wherein there is little resistance to movement in the osteoligamentous system. Movement in the neutral zone is most closely associated with ligamentous laxity. At the end of the neutral zone, the next portion of the range of motion is the elastic zone. The elastic zone is the range wherein the ligaments are drawn into resistance. In the elastic zone, the relationship between movement and the force required to produce that movement is relatively linear. Alternatively, the elastic zone can be viewed as the portion of the range of motion between the neutral zone and the point at which the system is stressed to its maximum tolerance. Together, the neutral zone and the elastic zone constitute the functional range of motion.

The injury zone is defined as movement beyond the maximum tolerance of the system. In this movement range, injury to the osteoligamentous structures occurs. The three zones of spinal movement are frequently altered by pathophysiological processes and they are used by some authors to describe the biomechanical changes that result from an injurious process[26] (Fig. 4-4).

Movement in the thoracic spine is limited by the facet anatomy and by the rib cage. The costotransverse articulations substantially limit the motion of the thoracic spine, providing a major degree of stability to the region. The costovertebral ligament and the costotransverse ligament provide a very strong, stable attachment of the thoracic vertebrae to the ribs. The interactions of the rib cage with the

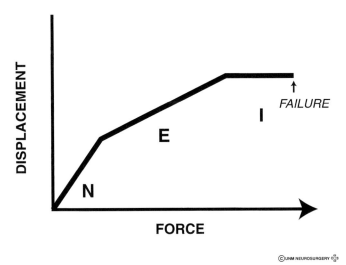

Fig. 4-4. In the neutral zone *(N)* a small increase in applied force leads to significant displacement of the spinal element. As the ligaments are drawn into tension, the elastic zone *(E)* begins. In the elastic zone there is a relatively linear association between the amount of applied force and the resulting displacement of vertebral elements. At the injury zone *(I)* a large increase in force results in relatively little displacement of the spinal elements, but structural damage occurs to the spinal elements in this zone and ultimately failure occurs.

dorsal elements also provide for a significant degree of load sharing.[25] Thoracic spinal motion increases dramatically when the costosternal junctions are divided, thereby removing the stabilizing point at the distal end of the ribs. The stabilized rib acts as a lever controlling (limiting) the movement of the thoracic vertebral body. When the distal stabilizer of the rib (the costosternal junction) is removed, the lever is then able to move freely with the vertebra and it no longer exerts its stabilizing influence.[29]

In an elegant biomechanical study of the interactions of the rib cage with the thoracic spine, Oda et al.[23] described the neutral zone and the range of motion (neutral zone plus elastic zone movement as determined by using nondestructive loads of 0.45 nm) of the thoracic spine with sequential sectioning of the dorsal elements, then the costovertebral joints, then destruction of the rib cage. With resection of the posterior elements of T6 to T7, they found a large increase in the range of motion in flexion-extension. After resection of the costovertebral joints bilaterally at T7, large increases in the neutral zones and ranges of motion in lateral bending and axial rotation were observed. After destruction of the rib cage, further increases in lateral bending and axial rotation were seen. The study concluded

that the state of the costovertebral joints and rib cage should be assessed to evaluate the stability of the thoracic spine.

A close correlation exists between deformities observed in the spines of scoliotic patients and deformities of the rib cages of these same patients. The Cobb angle measurement of a thoracic scoliotic curve correlates very closely with the lateral offset of the rib cage.[4] This phenomenon demonstrates the high degree of stiffness in the vertebral articulation with the ribs in the thoracic region. Because of this stiff articulation, the scoliotic spine exerts a displacing force on the ribs that corresponds closely to the degree of spinal deformity.

The stabilizing effect of the thoracic cage allows for nonsurgical treatment of a large proportion of thoracic spine fractures. The relatively abrupt change in stiffness from that observed in the thoracic spine to that of the lumbar region is thought by many to also explain the high incidence of fractures occurring at the thoracolumbar junction in comparison with the incidence of injuries in the midlumbar or midthoracic area. Another hypothesis is that the changes in facet joint orientation at the thoracolumbar junction may alter the stress distribution in the vertebrae, thereby producing stress patterns that are associated with spinal injury.[10]

As spinal movement occurs in axial rotation or lateral bending, the orientation of the facet joints dictates that motion must occur in another plane as well as that of the primary motion. This concept is described as the coupling of spinal movement.[19] The coupled movements caused by the facet joints allow altered patterns of load bearing to occur as the position of a given spinal segment changes.[30] In axial rotation, the facet joints cause lateral bending (coronal plane) and conversely, lateral bending causes axial rotation. Therefore patients with scoliosis demonstrate abnormalities of alignment in not only the coronal plane, but also in the axial plane. Because of the coupling of spinal motion, the only single-plane movement that occurs in the thoracic spine is that of sagittal motion (flexion or extension).

STABILITY AND INSTABILITY

Numerous concepts have evolved regarding what constitutes a stable spinal column and what degree of alteration is necessary to result in an unstable spine. The plethora of existing theories and systems for evaluating, measuring, and scoring clinical

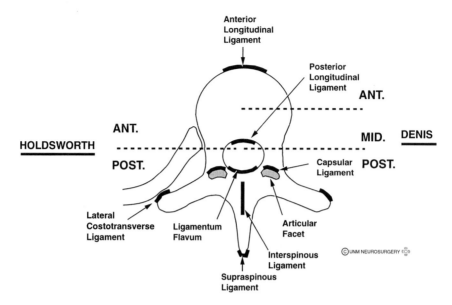

Fig. 4-5. The Holdsworth concept for spinal instability divides the spine into a ventral and a dorsal column. The Denis method for evaluating spinal stability subdivides the ventral column of Holdsworth into two columns relating to the ventral and dorsal halves of the vertebral body.

instability underscores the fact that no ideal theory or method exists. Conceiving of a sound definition for the term "spinal instability" is a goal that has eluded experts, researchers, and writers on the topic of spinal biomechanics. Perhaps the most widely quoted definition is that of White and Panjabi,[34] which states:

> Clinical instability is the loss of the ability of the spine under physiologic loads to maintain its pattern of displacement so that there is no initial or additional neurological deficit, no major deformity, and no incapacitating pain.

This definition provides a framework with which to develop the concepts necessary for the treatment of pathophysiology of the thoracic spine.

Historically, considerations of spinal stability and treatments for instability have advanced in parallel with refinements in neuroimaging technology and the development of spinal instrumentation. In 1963 Holdsworth[12] proposed a method of evaluating clinical instability in terms of a ventral and a dorsal column. The anterior column consists of the vertebral body and its associated ligamentous structures. The posterior column consists of the pedicles and the dorsal elements (Fig. 4-5). With Holdsworth's method, significant spinal instability is likely to be present if one column is severely compromised or if significant injury is observed in both columns. This two-column method was well-suited to plain radiograph technology and gained popularity in its time. The accurate diagnosis of injury to either of the two columns by plain radiographs was possible, and because treatment for thoracic spinal fractures was largely nonoperative in that era, the method was adequate.

Another method of assessing thoracic spine stability based upon radiographic measurements or displacement and angulation has been proposed. Panjabi, Hausfeld, and White[27] found that motion immediately prior to failure resulted in an average of 2.4 mm of horizontal displacement plus 4.1 degrees of angulation. They concluded that lateral radiographic motion of 2.5 mm or more, or angulation of 5 degrees or more, was indicative of a potentially unstable spine. The authors stressed that this information should be taken into consideration along with other clinical indicators of spinal instability. This method offered relatively limited clinical utility because the measurement of displacement with submillimeter resolution on plain radiograph studies is not possible. Furthermore, considerable judgement regarding the "other indicators of spinal instability" is required.

Denis[5] proposed a three-column model in the era of computed tomography (CT). This system considers the ALL and the ventral half of the vertebral body as the anterior column. The dorsal half of the vertebral body and the PLL are considered the middle column, and the dorsal elements (facet joints, ligamentum flavum, interspinous ligament, and the associated bony structures) constitute the posterior column (see Fig. 4-5). With this method a high likelihood of instability is considered to be present when disruption of two or more columns exists. The advent of CT scanning made the accurate assessment of middle column injury more achievable and perhaps played a role in the acceptance of the Denis system of classification. By CT imaging, small retropulsed bone fragments in the spinal canal and nondisplaced fractures through the vertebral body are more readily identified. The Denis method is simple to use and constitutes perhaps the most widely used clinical method at present.

Another three-column model is that proposed by Louis.[18] This method considers each facet joint complex to be a column and the vertebral body and its associated ligamentous structures are viewed as the third column (Fig. 4-6). This method has some clinical utility because it gives more in-depth consideration to the dorsal elements. It is deficient, however, because it gives less in-depth consideration to the extent of vertebral body injury.

Vertebral Body Stability

Benzel[2] has proposed a simple model for evaluation of clinical instability. In this model the vertebral body is viewed as a cubic arrangement of 27 smaller cubes (Fig. 4-7, *A*). There is considered to be a high likelihood of spinal instability when injury is such that nine or more cubes are deficient for spinal load bearing. The major limitation of this technique is that it is formulated only to evaluate injury to the vertebral body (ventral columns). It cannot be used to evaluate issues of stability relating to the dorsal bony elements or the ligaments. As with other spinal regions, the largest forces encountered by the thoracic spine are those involving flexion. The vertebral bodies bear the vast majority of a flexion load. After injury, if vertebral weight-bearing capabilities are compromised, progression of deformity is likely to result in kyphotic angulation. The naturally kyphotic posture of the thoracic area also tends to promote progression of a flexion deformity. Because the Benzel method focuses on the vertebral body, this technique is particularly well-suited to considerations for the thoracic region.

Some discussion of clinical examples of instability is warranted. A compression fracture involving

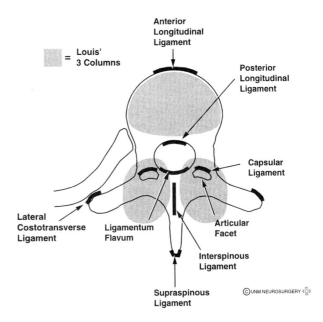

Fig. 4-6. The Louis system for determining stability involves three columns represented by the shaded regions in the figure.

the loss of one third of the vertebral body height (Fig. 4-7, *B*) is analogous to removal of nine cubes and the spine should be considered stable. If more than nine cubes are removed, such as in a fracture that results in a loss of 60% of vertebral height, the spine may be considered unstable and surgical stabilization should be entertained.

The concept applies to injury in other planes as well. In selected cases, a burst fracture may be relatively stable. A burst fracture is defined as a fracture that disrupts the ventral and dorsal margins of the vertebral body.[14] In a patient with a minimally displaced burst fracture and no significant loss of vertebral body height, weight-bearing capacity is likely to be maintained and simple external bracing may often be adequate for partial immobilization and satisfactory healing. If a partial corpectomy is needed to decompress the neural elements, such as in the case of a nerve sheath tumor or epidural abscess, this often entails resection of the dorsal third of the vertebral body (Fig. 4-7, *C*). If the remainder of the vertebral body is intact, the spine would be stable after such a resection. However, if the remainder of the vertebral body has also suffered injury, this should be considered equivalent to removal of more than nine cubes and spinal instability should be suspected. In such cases, surgical stabilization of the spine by fusion is indicated.

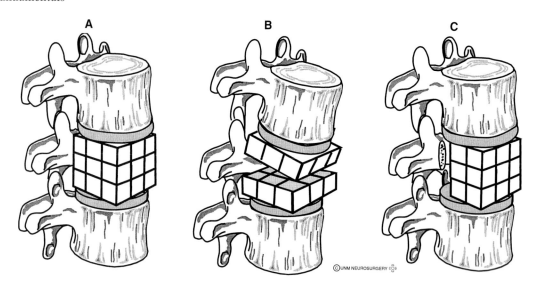

Fig. 4-7. A, Benzel's 27-cube model for evaluating spinal stability. The vertebral body is essentially evaluated as a theoretical cube consisting of 27 smaller cubes. **B,** Removal of the middle layer of cubes would result in only minor instability if one third or less of the vertebral body height is lost. **C,** In the case of a partial corpectomy to decompress the spinal elements, the dorsal layer of cubes might be removed from the coronal plane, creating a wide decompression while spinal stability is maintained. However, if the remaining bone tissue were compromised by the pathology that led to the decompression (such as a burst fracture), the spine should be considered unstable.

More recently, the concept of instability has been expanded to include slowly progressing spinal deformities. The terms "chronic instability" and "glacial instability" are used to describe the slow and constantly creeping nature of these disorders. Conditions such as progressive kyphosis and degenerative spondylolisthesis are commonly associated with this type of instability.[3] For surgeons, the identification of chronic or glacial instability can be crucial to the prevention of eventual neurological deficits.

Progressive kyphosis, chronic pain, and eventual neurological sequelae are indicative of chronic instability.[9,21] Because these are usually very slowly progressing problems, patients are often reluctant to undergo surgical treatment. However, if neurological deficits occur, surgery is usually advisable.

EFFECTS OF DISEASE PROCESSES ON SPINAL STABILITY

Spinal stability is altered by numerous disease processes. The essential feature of the instability is an increase in the neutral zone of spinal movement. If the osteoligamentous subsystem develops an expanded neutral zone, and if the musculotendinous subsystem is not able to compensate, then instability and abnormal spinal motion will occur. A common alteration of spinal stability results from degenerative changes in the spine. Other processes such as tumor, infection, trauma, and surgical decompression may also cause spinal instability. The proper surgical treatment of these problems relates largely to the degree of instability caused by them.

Minor instability may also exist in the absence of any initial insult. A significant degree of variation in the magnitude of the rotatory neutral zone at the thoracolumbar junction exists between individuals. Subjects with exaggerated motion demonstrate a greater likelihood of a mismatch between muscle coordination (in force application) and spinal segmental displacement, which may potentiate injury.[16]

The spinal musculature and the other muscles of the trunk are important in maintaining normal spinal function. These muscles generate all of the forces necessary for movement, lifting, and daily activities. It has been demonstrated that in painful conditions, these muscles cease to work in the normal, highly coordinated manner.[1] The loss of harmonious muscular activity may perpetuate the painful condition. The mismatch of desired motion and spinal muscle activity might also be a factor in progression of some disorders such as degenerative scoliosis.

BIOMECHANICS OF DEGENERATIVE DISEASE

The changes in spinal biomechanics resulting from degenerative disease are numerous and their relationship to spinal stability is highly complex. Degenerative changes in the intervertebral disc are extremely common. The primary process involved here is the loss of water content of the disc.[11] This is a normal physiological change of aging, but overuse or trauma can accelerate the process. Excess loading by these processes can rupture fibers in the inner portion of the nucleus with resultant fissure formation and progression of degenerative changes.[30] Tobacco smokers also have accelerated loss of disc hydration.

As the loss of disc hydration progresses, other processes take place within the disc. The content of various collagen subtypes is altered and the ability of the disc to absorb physical shock is decreased. Disc height also diminishes as shock-absorbing ability is lost. Although removal of the disc has little effect on the compressive properties of motion segments,[20] it has a greater effect on motion in other planes.[28] Bulging of the disc at the margins of the annulus fibrosis, which is associated with stretching of the annulus, also may occur. Stretching of the annulus at its insertion to the vertebral body also stretches the periosteum and results in osteophyte formation. In the early stages, there is probably an increase in mobility that results from these processes. The lowered stiffness of the degenerated disc has been demonstrated by numerous researchers.[11,17,32] With the loss of nucleus content, the facet joints become predisposed to bearing significantly larger loads.[13,30,31]

As degenerative changes become a more chronic condition, the spine tends to become more stable (restabilization). Osteophyte formation ultimately increases the amount of load-bearing surface of the vertebral body or facet joint. Chronically increased spinal mobility results in ligamentous thickening. The synovial capsules of the facet joints also thicken. All of these processes are responses to abnormal spinal mobility and their end result is enhancement of spinal stability.

Vertebral body changes due to aging and osteopenia cause an increase in the kyphotic curvature of the thoracic spine. Compression fractures due to osteoporosis are an extremely common cause of increased kyphosis. Eastell et al.[7] concluded that more than 20% of postmenopausal women had vertebral fractures of the lumbar or thoracic regions, with an average of two per individual. Neuromuscular disorders and conditions such as Parkinson's disease are also associated with degenerative changes that result in altered spinal curvature. Increased kyphotic thoracic curves can be compensated by an increase in the lordotic posture of the lumbar region. Such a compensatory posture serves to balance the distribution of spinal loading and maintain a normal center of gravity. It also predisposes to progressive worsening of the abnormal curves.

The facet joints respond to degenerative changes in much the same way as they do in the ventral portion of the spine. The normal purpose of the facet joints is to guide spinal motion. As degenerative changes progress in the spine, and specifically in the discs, the vertebral centrum changes in position (collapse). This process causes the facet joints to become axial load-bearing structures.[10,13] Abnormal spinal mobility causes an initial increase in movement at the facet joints. Osteophyte formation at the articular surfaces serves to increase the surface area of the joint. The angle of the articular surface can also change in association with joint hypertrophy, possibly resulting in an articular surface position that is more optimally suited to the loads borne by the joint. As mentioned previously, the ligamentous attachments of the facets and their synovial capsules also thicken in response to degenerative processes, with a tendency to increase spinal stability.

TRAUMA

Trauma to the thoracic spine results in a number of injury patterns that are indicative of the type and degree of instability that results. The lumbar spine, and more commonly the cervical spine, may suffer purely ligamentous injuries that lead to instability. In the thoracic spine, instability of a purely ligamentous nature is far less common. Unstable injuries in this region typically involve bony fractures of the vertebral body. Loss of height in the vertebral body indicates axial column loading in excess of the load-bearing capacity of the body. Asymmetry in spinal fractures identifies that the pattern was not produced by axial spinal loading alone. If the ventral loss of vertebral height is greater than the dorsal loss, a flexion component must also have been present. Fractures resulting in asymmetry in the coronal plane are caused by lateral bending during the injury with resulting asymmetrical load distribution. The extent of instability in any of these traumatic injuries can be determined by using the methods described previously. Shearing injuries that disrupt the annulus fibrosis and intervertebral disc are associated with disruption of the dorsal elements. These injuries are analogous to a three-column bony injury (Denis) method. They are grossly unstable and surgical stabilization should be advised.

INFECTION

Infections of the spine arise from direct extension of local infections or from hematogenous dissemination of systemic infections. The most common source of spinal infection is iatrogenic seeding of bacteria through surgery. The majority of these infections are caused by gram-positive bacteria representing skin flora, but they may be gram-negative, anaerobic, or fungal infections. Treatment of the infection itself is usually a straightforward matter. However, the biomechanical alterations resulting from surgery, and the potential disruptions arising from surgical debridement of infected tissues, may result in significant instability after spinal infection.

The common sites for spinal infection are the spinal canal (typically epidural abscess), the bony elements of the spine, and the discs. Although they may cause devastating neurological deficits, disease processes that are limited to the spinal canal, such as epidural abscess, usually do little damage with respect to the biomechanical properties of the spine. Some degree of ligamentous laxity may be noted after infection. This by itself, however, is not usually sufficiently disruptive to result in a significantly unstable spine.

Infections of bone or disc are quite different in terms of their biomechanical significance. The relatively avascular nature of the intervertebral disc creates an immunologically privileged site for infection to progress while protected from the normally vigorous response of the immune system. Therefore these infections are often detected after destruction of the disc has occurred and when the adjoining vertebral bodies are involved. The instability resulting from discitis is essentially a two-column disruption. Due to the limited vertical height of the disc space and the parallel surfaces of the adjoining end plates, an infection that destroys the disc often results in spontaneous fusion of the adjoining vertebral bodies. Due to the presence of the ribs and the relative stiffness of the thoracic spine, significant subluxation of the vertebrae in this region as a complication of isolated disc space infection is rare. The mainstay of therapy for this problem is the prompt treatment of the infection with appropriate antibiotics and percutaneous aspiration or surgical debridement if necessary. The mild degree of instability that may result from a thoracic spine infection involving only the disc space is usually adequately addressed by the use of an immobilizer device such as a thoracolumbosacral orthosis.

Infections that involve the vertebral body are more likely to result in instability. As described earlier, these infections may arise from an associated discitis or by direct inoculation by hematogenously spread infection. Vertebral body destruction results in two general patterns of abnormality. The vertebrae may simply collapse in a symmetrical fashion without angulation. This situation, although not reversed by treatment of the infection, will likely cease to progress with appropriate therapy. Obviously one must consider an exception to this approach when there is paraspinous involvement or if there are neurological deficits. Collapse of vertebral body height and angular deformities are common in cases of infection involving the vertebral bodies. Angular deformation may also have a tendency to progress over time. Therefore the need for surgical intervention may arise long after the initial infection has been successfully treated.

INFLAMMATORY DISEASES

The inflammatory diseases affecting the thoracic spine have the potential to dramatically alter the biomechanics of this region. They may also result in significant morbidity and mortality. The inflammatory diseases are numerous and each disease has associated characteristics. The pain of inflammatory spinal diseases is typically worse on rising in the morning and improves with activity. This feature helps differentiate inflammatory spinal pain from mechanical back pain.

Regardless of which specific spinal elements are affected by a particular inflammatory condition, these diseases share significant similarities in most instances. All tissues of the spine, including bone, ligament, disc, articular surfaces, and synovium, may be affected by inflammatory changes. Multiple tissues may be simultaneously involved by inflammatory diseases. Changes can also result from the treatments, such as steroid drugs, used for these diseases. Rheumatoid arthritis, for example, involves primarily the synovial joint capsules but it affects ligamentous tissue as well.

The inflammatory disorders of the spine are a highly heterogenous group of disorders, yet they affect the biomechanical functioning of the spine in two fundamental ways. The first is through destabilization of the spine. This is largely through the effects on soft tissues; repeated episodes of inflammation or chronic continuous inflammation will eventually alter articular surfaces at the facet joints. Joint hypertrophy, articular abnormalities, and ligamentous laxity are common sequelae of inflammatory processes. These changes may result in spinal deformity, instability, neurological deficits, and painful morbidity for the patient.

The second way in which inflammatory conditions alter spinal biomechanics is through spontaneous fusion. In patients with diseases such as ankylosing spondylitis or Reiter's syndrome, spontaneous fusion of multiple spinal levels results in long sections of solidly fused spine. When trauma is incurred—even episodes of minor trauma—these lever arms can then act to transmit focused and magnified forces that result in severe spinal fractures and spinal cord injuries.

The treatment of spine injuries in patients with inflammatory diseases generally follows conventional algorithms but there are some caveats to be considered. These patients, in many instances, have poorer healing capabilities than other trauma patients and are often poor operative risk patients. Therefore conservative nonsurgical methods are often preferable. When surgery is necessary it should be borne in mind that the existing autofused segments can be instrumented without any functional loss of mobility. Extending the instrumentation construct over additional levels is a simple alternative to gain additional points of segmental fixation and create a more solid construct. Also, the bone graft should only be applied to the mobile segments. This provides an opportunity to perform heavy onlay grafts at the fracture site without wasting valuable autograft on segments that are already fused. If interposition (interbody) grafts are used, an extremely rigid construct can be created by the use of long, multisegmentally fixed rods. With these "advantages," the impaired healing of patients with inflammatory diseases can be overcome and favorable results can be attained. The use of steroids or nonsteroidal anti-inflammatory medications should be minimized for several months after surgery in these patients.

TUMORS

The effects of tumors on spinal biomechanics and spinal stability are usually easily assessed. Tumors of the spine causing bony destruction, such as metastatic lesions, are most commonly discrete lesions involving the vertebral body. The need for spinal stabilization and/or reconstruction following resection or radiation treatment can be evaluated by the same methods used in cases of spinal trauma. Because the most common tumors of the thoracic spine are metastases, and because most metastatic tumors are disseminated by the hematogenous route, the ligamentous structures in these patients are usually not involved by the tumor. This makes the task of evaluating spinal stability in such patients easier.

Another biomechanical consideration in treating patients with spine tumors is the effect of radiation therapy on healing and reconstruction. In animals, it has been shown that preoperative radiation therapy did not substantially alter healing or the strength of the healed construct. This is in sharp contrast to the specimens receiving radiation therapy in the early postoperative period. Postoperatively irradiated specimens had reduced healing in terms of quality of healing, revascularization, and new bone formation.[8] These constructs were also significantly less stiff in biomechanical testing. The suggestion from this animal model is that if radiation therapy is needed it should be given preoperatively or postponed for several weeks (if possible) to allow graft incorporation.

SURGICAL DECOMPRESSION

After surgical decompression, iatrogenic spinal instability may be created. The degree of instability is dictated by the surgical approach and the amount of tissue resection performed. When a dorsal approach is chosen with the use of laminectomy and dorsal element resection the structures of the costotransverse articulation are usually left intact, allowing the stability afforded by the thoracic cage to remain unaltered. Surgical stabilization is therefore not required in most instances. After decompression by a transpedicular approach, instability may be an issue. This is most likely when the pathology, such as a tumor, for example, involves a substantial portion of the vertebral body. The choice of lateral or ventral approaches to the spine is usually dictated by the need for partial or complete vertebral body resection. With these approaches, significant instability is far more likely to occur after the decompressive procedure. The method of Benzel, described earlier, is highly applicable to these cases.

STABILIZING THE UNSTABLE SPINE

Choosing a construct to stabilize the thoracic spine is a complex consideration. With the plethora of spinal instrumentation devices and systems currently available, the surgeon is faced with the options of dorsal hook-rod constructs, ventral rod or plate devices, intervertebral devices such as titanium cages, or combinations of these. The use of bone screws in the pedicles, though they are not cleared for that application by the United States Food and Drug Administration (FDA), is also a useful technique. Placement of screws in the thoracic pedicles is technically difficult and should be undertaken only by spinal surgeons who are experienced and confident in this technique. Fluoroscopy is a useful adjunctive measure for thoracic pedicle screw placement.[15,22]

The author favors a sizable laminotomy with direct visualization of the pedicle during screw placement. With visualization of the spinal cord and the pedicle, screw placement can be achieved with both accuracy and safety. The key to successfully performing this procedure is choosing a screw that is as large as possible for load bearing but not so large as to risk fracture of the pedicle.

Dvorak et al.[6] have shown that bone screws may also be placed in a trajectory from lateral to the pedicles, coursing ventrally into the vertebral body. This technique has been shown to be biomechanically superior to the conventional pedicle screw in terms of pullout resistance. The Dvorak method is also, however, technically challenging. Experience and comfort on the part of the surgeon are key ingredients for successfully performing this procedure.

With the exception of the patient with a very short life expectancy, the objective in stabilizing the spine is to achieve bony fusion. The placement of a bone graft that restores load-bearing capabilities and leads to solid arthrodesis is therefore crucial. When the vertebral body is removed, the spine will tend toward a flexion deformity. The ideal graft position in such patients is therefore at the ventral aspect of the construct. Similarly, in the patient with a wedge-compression fracture, the ventral portion of the vertebral body has suffered the greatest degree of loss of weight-bearing strength. The reconstruction should therefore be aimed to restore the ventral column. If only the dorsal portion of a vertebral body is removed, the graft should be used to substitute for the missing bony element. Theoretically, if stability and load-bearing capacity are restored in two columns (Denis method), the spine will perform adequately under physiological loading conditions.

Figures 4-1 to 4-7 used with permission of the University of New Mexico, Division of Neurosurgery, Albuquerque, New Mexico.

REFERENCES

1. Anderson G. The function of the trunk muscles in health and with low back pain. Semin Spine Surg 5:3-9, 1993.
2. Benzel EC. Destabilizing effects of spinal surgery. In Benzel EC, ed. Biomechanics of Spine Stabilization: Principles and Clinical Practice. New York: McGraw-Hill, 1995, pp 97-102.
3. Benzel EC. Stability and instability of the spine. In Benzel EC, ed. Biomechanics of Spine Stabilization: Principles and Clinical Practice. New York: McGraw-Hill, 1995, pp 25-38.
4. Closkey R, Schultz A. Rib cage deformities in scoliosis: Spine morphology, rib cage stiffness, and tomography imaging. Orthop Res 11:730-737, 1993.
5. Denis F. The three column spine and its significance in the classification of acute thoracolumbar spinal injuries. Spine 8:817-831, 1983.
6. Dvorak M, MacDonald S, Gurr KR, et al. An anatomic, radiographic, and biomechanical assessment of extrapedicular screw fixation in the thoracic spine. Spine 18:1689-1694, 1993.
7. Eastell R, Cedel SL, Wahner HW, et al. Classification of vertebral fractures. J Bone Miner Res 6:207-215, 1991.
8. Emery SE, Brazinski MS, Koka A, et al. The biological and biomechanical effects of irradiation on anterior spinal bone grafts in a canine model. J Bone Joint Surg Am 76:540-548, 1994.
9. Farcy J, Weidedbaum M, Glassman S. Sagittal index in management of thoracolumbar burst fractures. Spine 15:958-965, 1990.
10. Goel V, Lim T, Gilbertson L, et al. Clinically relevant finite element models of a ligamentous lumbar motion segment. Semin Spine Surg 5:29-41, 1993.

11. Hansson T. The intervertebral disc: Dynamic changes during loading. Semin Spine Surg 5:17-22, 1993.

12. Holdsworth F. Fractures, Dislocations, and Fracture-Dislocations of the Spine. Bone Joint Surg 45B:6-20, 1963.

13. Kazarian LE. Creep characteristics of the human spinal column. Orthop Clin North Am 6:3-18, 1975.

14. King A, Nolte L. Spine trauma. Semin Spine Surg 5:51-58, 1993.

15. Krag MH. Biomechanics of thoracolumbar spinal fixation. A review. Spine 16:S84-99, 1991.

16. Kumar S, Panjabi MM. In vivo axial rotations and neutral zones of the thoracolumbar spine. J Spinal Disord 8:253-263, 1995.

17. Lin HS, Liu YK, Ray G, et al. Systems identification for material properties of the intervertebral joint. J Biomech 11:1-14, 1978.

18. Louis R. Spinal stability as defined by the three-column concept. Anat Clin 7:33-42, 1985.

19. Lovett R. The mechanism of the normal spine and its relation to scoliosis. Bos Med Surg J 153:349-358, 1905.

20. Markolf K, Morris J. The structural components of the intervertebral disc. A study of their contributions to the ability of the disc to withstand compressive forces. J Bone Joint Surg 56A:675-687, 1974.

21. McAfee P, Yuan HA, Lasda N. The unstable burst fracture. Spine 7:365-373, 1982.

22. McCormack BM, Benzel EC, Adams MS, et al. Anatomy of the thoracic pedicle. Neurosurgery 37:303-308, 1996.

23. Oda, I, Abumi K, Lu D, et al. Biomechanical role of the posterior elements, costovertebral joints, and rib cage in the stability of the thoracic spine. Spine 21:1423-1429, 1996.

24. Oxland T, Lin R, Panjabi M. Three-dimensional mechanical properties of the thoracolumbar junction. Orthop Res 10:573-580, 1992.

25. Pal GP, Routal RV. Transmission of weight through the lower thoracic and lumbar regions of the vertebral column in man. J Anat 152:93-105, 1987.

26. Panjabi M, Abumi K, Duranceau J, et al. Spinal stability and intersegmental muscle forces. A biomechanical model. Spine 14:194-200, 1989.

27. Panjabi M, Hausfeld JN, White AA III. A biomechanical study of the ligamentous stability of the thoracic spine in man. Acta Orthop Scand 52:315-326, 1981.

28. Panjabi M, Krag M, Chung T. Effects of disc injury on mechanical behavior of the human spine. Spine 9:1001-1007, 1984.

29. Panjabi M, White A. Physical properties and functional biomechanics of the spine. In Clinical Biomechanics of the Spine. Philadelphia: JB Lippincott, 1990, pp 1-83.

30. Shirazi-Adl A. Models of the functional spinal unit. Semin Spine Surg 5:23-28, 1993.

31. Shirazi-Adl A. Finite-element simulation of changes in the fluid content of human lumbar discs. Mechanical and clinical implications. Spine 17:206-212, 1992.

32. Shirazi-Adl SA, Shrivastava SC, Ahmed AM. Stress analysis of the lumbar disc-body unit in compression. A threedimensional nonlinear finite element study. Spine 9:120-134, 1984.

33. Stokes I. Biomechanics of the thoracic spine and rib cage. Semin Spine Surg 5:42-50, 1995.

34. White A, Panjabi M. The Problem of Clinical Instability in the Human Spine: A Systematic Approach. In Clinical Biomechanics of the Spine. Philadelphia: JB Lippincott, 1990, pp 278-378.

Imaging and Relevant Anatomy

Chi-Shing Zee, M.D., Robert W. Henderson, M.D.,
James Huprich, M.D., and John Go, M.D.

ANATOMY OF THE THORACIC SPINE AND ITS CONTENTS

The thoracic spine consists of twelve vertebrae that gradually increase in size from rostral to caudal. Each vertebral body is composed of an inner medullary portion of loose trabecular bone surrounded by an outer layer of dense cortical bone. The vertebral body end plates consist of dense trabecular bone. In the newborn, the vertebral body marrow is mostly red marrow (hematopoietically active). In young children, bone marrow is predominantly red (cellular) and appears to show isointensity to adjacent paraspinal muscle on T1-weighted images. With advancing age, the signal intensity of the vertebral bodies gradually increases on T1-weighted images as yellow marrow (fat) increases. The vertebral bodies show relatively high signal intensity compared to nucleus pulposus from late teens. By the approximate age of 70, the bone marrow consists of 60% yellow marrow and appears to show marked hyperintensity (due to fat content) on T1-weighted images.[172]

Focal fatty deposits in the vertebral bodies are frequently observed in adults. They are of high signal intensity on T1-weighted images and of intermediate signal intensity on T2-weighted images.[54]

The height of the thoracic intervertebral discs is less than cervical or lumbar discs. Each intervertebral disc consists of three distinct components:
(1) cartilaginous end plate, (2) annulus fibrosus, and (3) nucleus pulposus.[115]

The cartilaginous end plate is composed of peripheral fibrocartilage and central hyaline cartilage. The annulus fibrosus consists of fibrocartilaginous and collagenous fibers arranged in a circular and concentric fashion. The annulus serves as a limiting barrier for the nucleus pulposus. The fibrocartilaginous fibers (type II collagen) arise from the peripheral portion of the cartilaginous end plate and merge with the nucleus pulposus. The collagenous fibers (type I collagen) form the peripheral portion of the annulus and insert into the ring apophysis. In addition, they also insert into the vertebral cortex via Sharpey's fibers. The annulus has a strong and broad attachment to the anterior longitudinal ligament and less attachment to the posterior longitudinal ligament. On computed tomography (CT), the intervertebral discs are slightly hyperdense compared to adjacent muscle. On magnetic resonance imaging (MRI), the outer fibrous compact tissue is low signal on both T1- and T2-weighted images, whereas the nucleus pulposus is high signal on T2-weighted images.[169] Disc dessication and degeneration begins in the late teens and gradually increases with advancing age.

The pedicles arise from the dorsorostral, rostral aspect of each vertebral body. The broad, short laminae fuse in the midline, where the spinous process arises. The thoracic spinous process projects dorsally and caudally. Articular processes originate

80

from the rostral and caudal aspect of the laminae and form the facet joints. Transverse processes arise from the articular pillars between the rostral and inferior articular facets. The articulation of rib tubercles and tips of the transverse processes form the costotransverse joint.[42]

The anterior longitudinal ligament and posterior longitudinal ligament are thick, dense fibrous bands that extend along the midportion of the ventral and dorsal surface of all the vertebral bodies. Both ligaments are thicker in the thoracic region.[79] The ligamentum flavum also covers the facet joint capsule. Interspinous ligaments are seen between the adjacent spinous processes.

The spinal cord is the tubular portion of the central nervous system that occupies the rostral two thirds of the vertebral canal. It is continuous with the medulla at the level of the foramen magnum and caudally terminates as the conus medullaris, usually at the interspace between the first and second lumbar vertebrae. The caudal end may be as high as the caudal third of T12 or as low as the disc between L2 and L3; its position rises slightly in vertebral flexion. In the newborn, the spinal cord usually extends to the rostral border of L3, rising during the first few postnatal months. From the apex of conus medullaris descends the filum terminale. This is a connective tissue filament of about 20 cm long and is a derivative of the pia mater that extends to the dorsum of the first coccygeal segment. The approximate length of spinal cord in an adult person is about 45 cm. The transverse section of the spinal cord is elliptical in the cervical spine and round in the thoracic spine. There are two enlargements: the cervical enlargement from C3 to T2 and the lumbar enlargement from L1 to S3. The position of the enlargements corresponds to the innervation of the upper and lower limbs, respectively.[156]

Similar to any other part of the central nervous system (CNS), the spinal cord is covered by the meninges consisting of the dura mater, which anchors the spinal cord to the vertebrae, and the arachnoid and pia maters. Because it is important to describe a lesion in relation to the dura mater (i.e., extradural or intradural), one should visualize the dura in MRI sequences. Ordinarily meninges are obscured by the bright signal from fat in T1-weighted spin-echo images or cerebrospinal fluid (CSF) in T2-weighted spin-echo images. Dura can best be distinguished on T2-weighted gradient-echo MRI sequences. Dura and arachnoid maters are separated by the subdural space. On T1-weighted and proton density images, the spinal cord is surrounded by low-intensity CSF. The epidural space is the potential space outer to the dural mater. It contains vessels, connective tissue, and some fat. The pia mater attaches to the surface of the spinal cord. The lateral septa of the pia extending to the dura have a supportive function and are called ligamentum denticulatum. The ligamentum flavum lines the dorsal aspect of the vertebral canal.[78]

The spinal cord is shorter than the vertebral column. Therefore the segmental divisions of the spinal cord are determined arbitrarily by the spinal nerves. A series of paired dorsal and ventral roots of spinal nerves emerge from each spinal segment, cross the subarachnoid space, and transverse the dura mater separately, uniting in or close to their intervertebral foramina to form the spinal nerves. There are 31 pairs of spinal nerves, including eight cervical pairs, out of which the upper seven enter intervertebral foramina of corresponding vertebrae, rostral to that vertebral body. Because there is no C8 vertebra, the eighth pair and the remaining spinal nerves emerge through the intervertebral foramina caudal to their corresponding vertebrae. There are 12 thoracic pairs of spinal nerves, five lumbar and sacral pairs, and one coccygeal pair. It is of clinical importance to correlate a level of vertebral lesion that is evident on MRI to the segmental level of the spinal cord, which is lower than the corresponding vertebrae. The cauda equina (horse's tail) consists of the lumbar and sacral spinal nerve roots that encircle the filum terminale in the spinal theca.[30,159]

The external surface of the spinal cord exhibits a deep furrow in the midline of the ventral surface called the anterior median fissure. This fissure runs along the entire ventral surface and contains a reticulum of pia mater and perforating branches of the anterior spinal vessels that pass from the fissure to the anterior white commissure to supply and drain the central spinal region. The dorsolateral aspect of the spinal cord has many shallow grooves, or sulci. The posteromedian sulcus on the midline of the dorsal surface is shallower. From it a posterior median septum of neuroglia penetrates more than halfway into the spinal cord, almost to the central canal. A posterolateral sulcus exists 1.5 to 2.5 mm lateral to each side of the posterior median sulcus along which dorsal rootlets of spinal nerves enter the spinal cord. The white substance between the posterior median and each posterolateral sulcus is the paired posterior funiculus. In the cervical and upper thoracic segments, a longitudinal posterointermediate sulcus marks a septum dividing each posterior funiculus into two large tracts, the fasciculus gracilis (medial) and fasciculus cuneatus (lateral). Between the posterolateral sulcus and anterior medial fissure is the anterolateral sulcus, from which vertebral roots emerge.

On cross-section, gray matter of the spinal cord is butterfly shaped and centrally located. Anterior gray horns are the two short, broad, symmetrical ventrolateral projections from the gray commissure. The posterior gray horn is the dorsolateral projection of the gray matter. Both the anterior and posterior gray horns are located along the entire length of the spinal cord. The lateral gray horn, on the other hand, is an angular, small gray horn projection located between T1 and the conus medullaris. The butterfly-shaped gray matter can best be distinguished in cross-section on proton-density or T1-weighted images where gray matter has a brighter signal intensity than the surrounding white matter. The central canal, which transverses the entire spinal cord, begins rostrally at the caudal half of the medulla oblongata, caudal to the fourth ventricle, and extends caudally into the proximal 5 to 6 mm of filum terminale. It is lined by columnar, ciliated ependyma and contains CSF.[18]

The white matter is primarily composed of long descending and ascending fiber tracts. It is peripherally placed and surrounds the gray matter like a mantle. It may be divided into three parts: (1) the anterior white column, located between the anterior median fissure and the anterolateral sulcus; (2) the posterior white column, situated between the posterior median sulcus and posterolateral sulci; and (3) the lateral white column. The anterior white column contains the anterior corticospinal tract, tectospinal tract, and the vestibulospinal tracts that are ascending, the anterior spinothalamic tract that is ascending, and the anterior white commissure that is an intersegmental tract. The posterior white column contains the fasciculus gracilis and fasciculus cuneatus, which are ascending, and the posterior white commissure, which is an intersegmental tract. The lateral white column consists of the anterior spinocerebellar tract, the posterior spinocerebellar tract, the rostral spinocerebellar tract, the tectospinal tract, the posterolateral tract, and the rubrospinal tract. All are descending tracts.[143]

The blood supply of the spinal cord runs through a longitudinal anastomotic channel that is formed by a spinal branch of the vertebral, deep cervical, intercostal, and lumbar arteries, along with ventral and dorsal spinal arteries.

Only a few radicular arteries (usually four to nine) in the lower cervical, lower thoracic, and upper lumbar regions are large enough to reach the anterior median sulcus. They divide into slender ascending and large descending rami that anastomose with the ventral spinal arteries to form a single or partly double longitudinal vessel of uneven caliber along the anterior median sulcus. The largest anterior radicular spinal artery, anterior radicularis magna or Adamkiewicz's artery, varies in its location. It arises from an intersegmental aortic branch at the lower thoracic or upper lumbar level; about 65% arise on the left. Once reaching the spinal cord, it sends a branch to the anterior spinal artery below and another to anastomose with a ramus of the posterior spinal artery ventral to the dorsal roots. It is important to note that the anterior radicularis magna is occasionally the main supply to the lower two thirds of the spinal cord. The anterior spinal artery sends a central ramus that enters the anterior median fissure, turning right or left to supply the ventral gray column, the base of the dorsal gray column, and the adjacent white matter. Dorsal radicular branches of the spinal arteries supply the dorsal ganglia. Each posterior spinal artery contributes to a pair of longitudinal anastomotic channels ventral and dorsal to the dorsal spinal roots. These are reinforced by dorsal radicular arteries. They are variable in number and size but more numerous than the ventral radicular arteries. Central branches of the anterior spinal artery supply about two thirds of the cross-section of the spinal cord. The rest of the dorsal gray and white columns are supplied by numerous small radial vessels from dorsal spinal arteries and the pial plexus.[43]

Venous drainage of the spinal cord is through six tortuous, often plexiform, longitudinal channels located one each in the anterior and posterior medial fissures and four others, often incomplete. One pair is dorsal and the other ventral to the ventral and dorsal nerve roots. There are free anastomosies between these vessels and the cerebral veins and cranial sinuses.

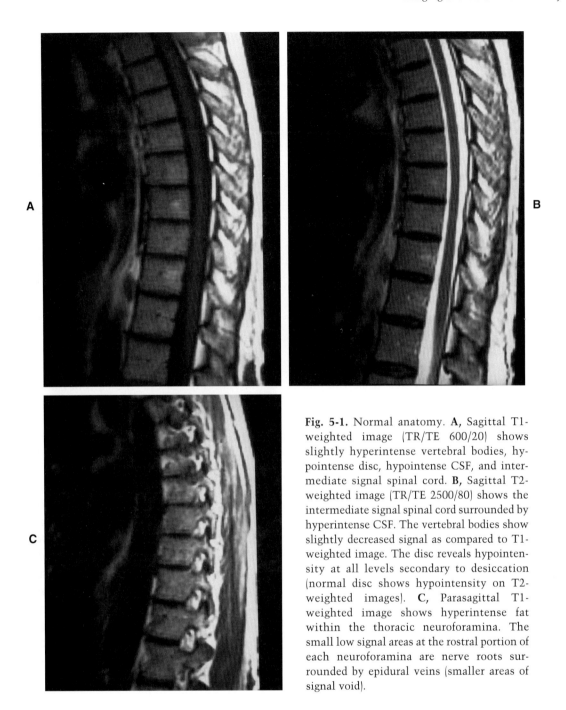

Fig. 5-1. Normal anatomy. **A,** Sagittal T1-weighted image (TR/TE 600/20) shows slightly hyperintense vertebral bodies, hypointense disc, hypointense CSF, and intermediate signal spinal cord. **B,** Sagittal T2-weighted image (TR/TE 2500/80) shows the intermediate signal spinal cord surrounded by hyperintense CSF. The vertebral bodies show slightly decreased signal as compared to T1-weighted image. The disc reveals hypointensity at all levels secondary to desiccation (normal disc shows hypointensity on T2-weighted images). **C,** Parasagittal T1-weighted image shows hyperintense fat within the thoracic neuroforamina. The small low signal areas at the rostral portion of each neuroforamina are nerve roots surrounded by epidural veins (smaller areas of signal void).

IMAGING TECHNIQUES
Magnetic Resonance Imaging

Since its introduction, MRI has improved dramatically in its image quality. MRI of the thoracic spine is associated with superb contrast resolution, the ability to include the entire thoracic spine in the imaging field, direct imaging in any desired plane at any angle of the primary othogonal planes, and direct visualization of the spinal cord. MRI is often the imaging modality of choice in the thoracic spine.[61,69,76,104,125,140,152,157]

For evaluation of thoracic spine diseases, MRI technique usually includes T1-weighted (short repetition time and short echo time) and T2-weighted (long repetition time and long echo time) images in the sagittal and axial planes (Fig. 5-1). Occasionally, coronal plane images may be useful (e.g., in patients with diastematomyelia). Slice thicknesses of 3 mm or less, with minimal interslice gap, are often used in the sagittal sequences. Slice thickness in the axial plane may vary from 5 to 10 mm, depending on the findings observed on sagittal plane imaging and the clinical history.

An adequate number of phase-encoding steps should be used to prevent the Gibb's artifact from appearing within the center of the spinal cord. A reasonable compromise should be achieved between image quality and reasonable imaging time. For sagittal imaging, the technologist should make all efforts to position the patient and coil in perfect alignment. For T2-weighted sequences, flow artifacts should be reduced, so that the spinal cord and surrounding high signal CSF can be adequately evaluated without interference from artifacts. Gradient moment nulling cardiac gating should be employed. In addition, a presaturation bond should be placed ventral to the thoracic spine on sagittal sequences to eliminate artifacts that could be created by the pulsation of the thoracic aorta and respiratory motion.

Gradient-echo sequences may be employed for the evaluation of spondylosis, intramedullary hemorrhagic or calcific lesions. The intravenous injection of paramagnetic contrast agents has been shown to be extremely useful for the imaging of certain spinal pathology. Their application for the evaluation of neoplastic diseases is essential, and their use for the evaluation of infectious and demyelinating disease may be quite helpful.[146]

Computed Tomography

CT of the thoracic spine is generally performed in the axial plane in 5 mm increments. These scans can be performed in a stacking method without angulation of the gantry. This method has the advantage of visualizing the entire thoracic spine. Reconstruction of the images in sagittal or coronal planes is feasible. Targeted images can increase the detail and resolution of the scans. Images should be acquired at two different window settings, one with a narrow window for evaluation of soft tissue and disc, and the other with a wide window for evaluation of the bony spine. When contrast material is observed in the thecal sac following a conventional myelogram, these two window settings should be wider.[57,85,120,127,128,153,163,171]

Conventional Myelography

Conventional myelography may be performed in a variety of situations, including overweight patients who cannot fit into MRI scanners, claustrophobic patients, and patients with MRI findings that do not correlate with clinical findings.[15,149,162,168] Thoracic myelography is generally performed in the prone position. A lumbar puncture is performed using a 22-gauge needle, usually at the L3-4 or L2-3 levels under aseptic conditions using local anesthesia. Nonionic contrast material is instilled into the subarachnoid space while the myelographic table is tilted to a 30- to 45-degree head up position. Following the instillation of the nonionic contrast material, the patient is turned into supine position and the myelographic table is tilted to approximately 20 degrees head down to move the contrast into the thoracic region. The table is then placed in the horizontal position. Anteroposterior (AP) and cross-table lateral views are obtained. If necessary, the patient may be placed in the lateral decubitus position. Cross-table AP and lateral views may be obtained on both sides to delineate a lateral lesion.

Spinal Angiography

In 1967 DiChiro, Doppman, and Ommaya[35] reported on the use of selective catheterization of individual arteries to demonstrate the circulation of the spinal cord. This method was soon adopted by others.[36] This procedure is considered to be safe and rarely results in complications. In the cervical region selective catheterization of the costocervical trunk and the vertebral arteries are performed. In the lumbar and thoracic region selective catheterization of intercostal arteries is performed from T9 to T12 bilaterally, then L1 to L2 bilaterally to visualize the artery of Adamkiewicz. If the artery is still not visualized, intercostal arteries above T9 may be catheterized bilaterally. Following catheterization of each intercostal artery or lumbar artery, only 1 to 2 ml of nonionic contrast material are injected with hand injection and high resolution (1024 matrix) digital subtraction angiograms are obtained. To visualize the entire angiographic phase, exposures are usually made for 15 seconds at two per second for 5 seconds, and one per second for the remaining 10 seconds. For evaluation of spinal arteriovenous malformations (AVMs) a faster rate of exposure (four to six per second) is recommended.

Spinal angiography is a useful procedure for the evaluation of spinal diseases, particularly spinal AVMs. It not only provides diagnostic information, but also provides access for the embolization of these lesions.

Usually, AVMs have dilated, tortuous feeding arteries that arise from an anterior or, less frequently, a posterior spinal artery. Venous drainage occurs through dilated medullary veins to radicular veins, and occasionally to the epidural plexus. If the feeding arteries to the AVM are of sufficient size, superselective catheterization and endovascular embolization may be performed. This could be an adjunct to surgery or the sole treatment. Because the blood supply to AVMs generally arises from spinal arteries, it is imperative that the embolic agent pass through the ventral and dorsal spinal cord blood supply and lodge within the nidus of malformation. It is also important that medullary perforations and draining veins be spared. Embolization may be performed with particulate emboli; polyvinyl alcohol of certain particle size.[25,84,144,155]

Recently, perimedullary arteriovenous fistulas and spinal dural arteriovenous fistulas have been recognized. Spinal angiography plays a significant role in their diagnosis and management. They can be effectively treated with surgical clipping or embolization with particulate or liquid adhesive agents.[55,100,130]

Scintigraphy

The conventional bone scan is performed 2 hours following intravenous administration of about 20 mCi of a (99m-Tc) labeled phosphate compound, such as methylene diphosphate (MDP). High-resolution collimation and high count images (e.g., 750,000 per view) are needed for optimal thoracic spine imaging. Single photon emission computed tomography (SPECT) is helpful to clarify equivocally increased uptake, to localize uptake to the vertebral body versus dorsal elements, and to differentiate primary vertebral disease from disc disease. Gallium scintigraphy is a useful adjunct when infection is a consideration. The examination is reviewed and compared with the conventional bone scan. Imaging is performed 24 hours after the intravenous adminis-

tration of about 5 mCi of 67 gallium citrate with medium-energy collimation.

The primary role of scintigraphy for the evaluation of thoracic spine disease is the differential diagnosis of thoracic pain and the clarification of radiographic findings. The diphosphanate bone scan is highly sensitive for processes that provoke new bone formation. The intensity parallels the rate of accretion of calcium and phosphate on the hydroxyapatite crystal lattice.

Acute fracture provokes an intense reparative response. Typical vertebral compression fractures produce a banded pattern of intense pathological activity spanning the width of the vertebral body within 24 to 72 hours of its occurrence. The usual axial loading/hyperflexion mechanism should produce a compression from side to side whether bone density is normal or diffusely osteoporotic (insufficiency fracture). Partial end plate compressions should raise suspicion of underlying focal bone disease (pathological fracture). Activity decreases with time more variably than in the appendicular skeleton, especially in older patients. This is probably related to further compression with daily activities. Pinpointing the date of injury without sequential radiographs or scans is difficult, other than to state it as recent when intense, subacute when moderate, and old (many months) when inactive.

Malignant tumor involvement of the thoracic spine is also variably expressed, depending on the degree of new reparative bone formation. The most prevalent tumors, such as breast, prostate, and lung carcinoma, are predictably active. An entire skeletal survey has a sensitivity that is 30% greater than radiography. This makes bone scintigraphy the mainstay of clinical oncology staging. However, there are certain uncommon histological types (e.g., oat cell lung cancer, inflammatory breast cancer) and tumor types (e.g., multiple myeloma, lymphoma) that are notoriously diffuse and limited in osteoblastic reaction. MRI is far more effective in evaluating symptoms or planning therapy in these marrow packing and predominately osteoclastic diseases.

Thoracic spine infection is rare and potentially devastating. The pattern of two adjacent vertebral end plates with increased activity is more difficult to appreciate in the thoracic spine than in the lumbar spine. The role of bone scintigraphy is to exclude the diagnosis or to localize the level, when positive, for further evaluation with CT or MRI. Gallium scintigraphy is better than labeled white cells, but is limited regarding diagnosis. When positive, it is the best parameter to assess the subsequent success or failure of therapy.

Degenerative disc disease is usually quiescent on scintigraphy. On rare occasions, severe disc disease can be seen as a band of modest intensity at the interspace level. Osteophytes are also modest by comparison to radiographic appearance. The chief value of bone scintigraphy in most cases is to indicate the nonaggressive nature of the process when radiographs are striking.

In summary, bone scintigraphy is a unique indicator of the metabolic activity of diseases that affect thoracic vertebral bone. It is a highly sensitive, but a nonspecific, indicator and localizer of pathology. Liberal use of correlative radiographs, CT, and MRI is necessary when focal disease is detected. Specific diagnoses are frequently possible when combined imaging studies are correlated.

CONGENITAL MALFORMATIONS
Meningocele

Congenital meningocele is a relatively rare developmental anomaly. Clinically, meningoceles present as subcutaneous masses that change size and tension with the Valsalva maneuver. More than 80% of meningoceles are located in the lumbosacral spine. Imaging (CT or MRI) shows spina bifida with the dorsal extension of a sharply demarcated CSF-filled sac.[13]

Thoracic meningoceles are quite rare. They may herniate outward from the spinal canal laterally and ventrally. In contrast with meningoceles elsewhere in the spine, two thirds or more of lateral meningoceles are associated with neurofibromatosis (Fig. 5-2). Occasionally, a neurofirbroma may be present within the wall of a meningocele. Ventral meningoceles, which project through or between the dorsal vertebral bodies, are not associated with neurofibromatosis. Associations with other congenital anomalies may be found.

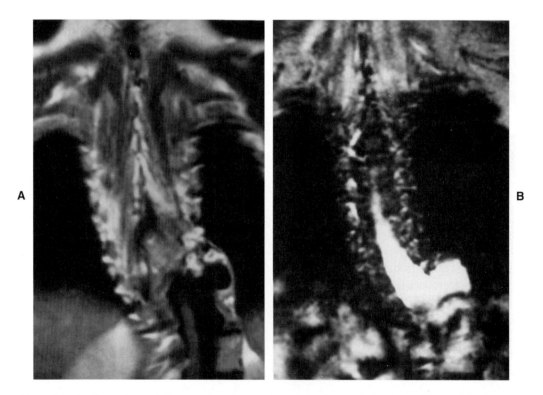

Fig. 5-2. Lateral meningocele in patient with neurofibromatosis type 1. **A,** Coronal T1-weighted image shows scoliosis of the thoracic spine with a lateral meningocele seen on the left side, which contains low signal intensity CSF. **B,** Coronal T2-weighted image confirms the presence of a lateral meningocele on the left side, which contains high signal intensity CSF.

Dorsal Dermal Sinus

Dorsal dermal sinuses are thought to result from faulty disjunction between the superficial and neural ectoderm. A focal segmental adhesion persists as an elongated epithelial-lined tube connecting the spinal cord with the skin. Infection is a common complication of the dermal sinus, and the thoracic spine is the third most common site of dermal sinuses, preceded by the lumbosacral spine and occipital area. Imaging (CT or MRI) shows a sinus tract that traverses the subcutaneous fat and passes through a dysraphic lamina into the spinal canal (Fig. 5-3). The tract may merge with the dura mater and terminate in the subarachnoid space, the conus medullaris, or filum terminale. The sinus tract shows a low intensity band traversing the high signal subcutaneous fat on T1-weighted images and a high signal band traversing the low signal subcutaneous fat on T2-weighted images.[12]

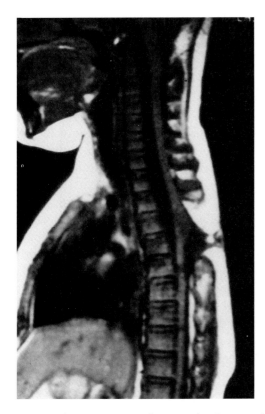

Fig. 5-3. Dermal sinus. A sagittal T1-weighted image shows a sinus tract extending from the subarachnoid space through a defect in the dorsal elements and subcutaneous fat to the skin surface.

Spinal Lipomas

There are three major types of spinal lipoma: (1) lipomyelomeningocele, (2) filum terminale fibrolipoma, and (3) intradural lipomas. Lipomyelomeningocele is a closed neural tube defect. Most patients present before the age of 6 months. Plain radiographs show focal spina bifida, a widened spinal canal, and segmentation anomalies. MRI shows a low-lying spinal cord that ends in the neural placode, similar to myelomeningocele. The lipoma is outside the dura mater and contiguous with the subcutaneous fat.[23] Syringohydromyelia is seen in 25% of the cases (Fig. 5-4). Filum terminale fibrolipomas are incidental findings in up to 6% of the MRIs of the spine. They are usually asymptomatic and of no clinical significance.

Intradural lipomas are intradural, subpial-juxtamedullary lesions. Most lipomas are located in the cervical and thoracic spine. The T1-weighted image demonstrates a characteristic high signal intensity mass over the dorsal aspect of the spinal cord. Intradural lipomas commonly extend extradurally as well, but the bony spinal canal is often normal or shows minor defects. Pure intramedullary lipomas are extremely rare.[173]

Diastematomyelia

Diastematomyelia is characterized by focal splitting of the spinal cord by a fibrous, bony, or osteocartilaginous septum. The spinal cord above and below the cleft is single. The two hemicords each contain a central canal, one set of dorsal and ventral horns and nerve roots. In about half of the cases, the two hemicords share a single dural sac; in the other half, the hemicords are enclosed in separate dural sacs. Females are affected more often than males. Cutaneous stigmata, such as hair patches and nevi lipomas, are seen in up to 75% of patients with diastematomyelia. The cleft is located between T9 and S1 in 85% of the cases. Plain radiographs demonstrate widening of the interpedicular distance, hemivertebra or butterfly vertebra, and a bony spur (when present). Hemicords and adjacent subarachnoid spaces, along with the fibrous or bony spur, can be demonstrated by myelography, CT-myelography, or MRI (Fig. 5-5). Many other conditions can exist with diastematomyelia. A thickened filum terminale and a low conus medullaris, hydromyelia, meningocele, dermal

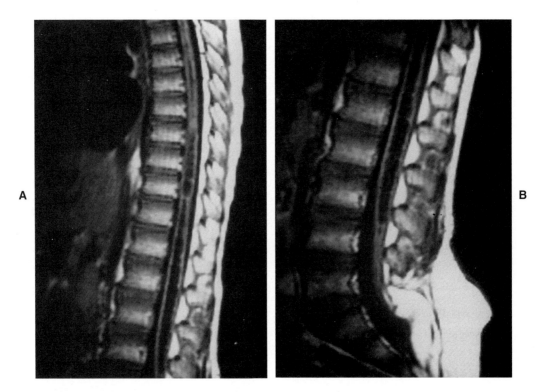

Fig. 5-4. Lipomyelomeningocele associated tethered cord and syrinx. **A,** Sagittal T1-weighted image shows a syringohydromyelia involving the entire thoracic spinal cord. **B,** Sagittal T1-weighted image demonstrates the presence of a lipomyelomeningocele associated with tethered cord and syrinx.

sinus, lipoma, Klippel-Feil syndrome, and Chiari malformations may be seen on imaging studies in association with diastematomyelia.[59,118]

Enterogenous Cyst

Enterogenous cysts are formed due to the failure of notochord and foregut separation during formation of the alimentary canal. They are thin-walled, fluid-containing masses with a fibrous wall lined by a single layer of columnar or cuboidal epithelial cells. The most common location is the thoracic spine, followed by the cervical spine, posterior fossa, and craniovertebral junction. Most are located ventral to the spinal cord or brain stem.

Imaging studies show a sharply marginated intradural extramedullary mass ventral to the spinal cord. The mass is low density on CT and slightly hyperintense to CSF on both T1-weighted and T2-weighted images of MRI.[22,115] Extension of the cyst through a ventral bony defect, with a cyst ventral to the spine, may be seen (Fig. 5-6).

Syringohydromyelia

Hydromyelia is an ependymal-lined dilatation of the central canal, whereas syringomyelia is a CSF dissection through the ependymal lining to form a paracentral cavity. On imaging studies, it is impossible to distinguish the two entities. They are grouped under the term syringohydromyelia. They can be congenital or acquired. A minority of syringohydromyelias communicate with the fourth ventricle via the obex, whereas the majority are noncommunicating. The cervical spinal cord and cervicothoracic cord are frequently involved. Classic clinical findings include sensory (pain and temperature) disturbances, muscular weakness, and spastic paraparesis. Associated scoliosis is common.

MRI demonstrates an enlarged spinal cord with a central cavity that contains fluid of CSF singal intensity. A beaded configuration of syringohydromyelia channels, containing multiple septations within them, are frequently shown on sagittal MRI (Fig. 5-4, *A*). These are due to circumferential gliotic bands.[63,138] Occasionally, syringohydromyelia

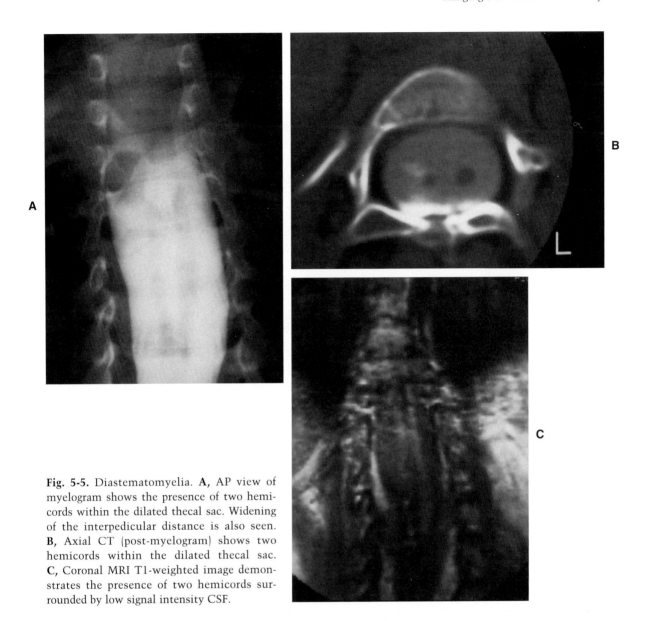

Fig. 5-5. Diastematomyelia. **A,** AP view of myelogram shows the presence of two hemicords within the dilated thecal sac. Widening of the interpedicular distance is also seen. **B,** Axial CT (post-myelogram) shows two hemicords within the dilated thecal sac. **C,** Coronal MRI T1-weighted image demonstrates the presence of two hemicords surrounded by low signal intensity CSF.

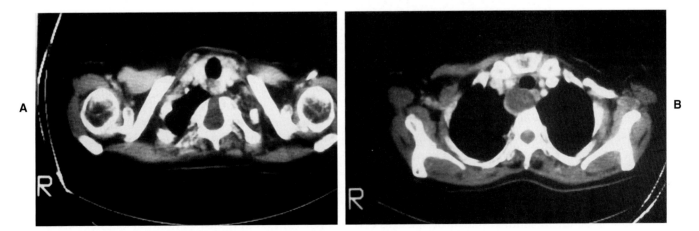

Fig. 5-6. Enterogenous cyst. **A,** Axial CT shows a bony defect through the midvertebral body with soft tissue density seen within it. **B,** Axial CT (lower level than *A*) shows a cystic mass ventral to the thoracic spine, dorsal to the trachea and to the right side of the esophagus.

may be associated with a spinal cord neoplasm. Gadolinium enhanced MRI may be useful to exclude the underlying neoplasm.

DEGENERATIVE DISEASES

Degenerative diseases of the spine are among the most common afflictions of mankind. Because these conditions can occur at any joint, clinical signs are likely to be distributed as defined by anatomical relationships, and symptomatology is governed by the level of involvement. The most common levels of degenerative changes occur at C5-6 in the cervical spine and L5-S1 in the lumbar spine.

Disc Degeneration

Disc degeneration is common in asymptomatic patients and presents as decreased signal on T2-weighted images with disc space narrowing. Another sign of disc degeneration is gas within the disc, the so-called vacuum phenomenon. There may be associated changes in signal intensity in the vertebral body marrow, which are associated with degenerative disc disease. These changes are classified as follows:

1. *Type 1 change.* The bone marrow adjacent to the vertebral body end plates shows decreased signal intensity on T1-weighted images and slightly increased signal intensity on T2-weighted images. Disruption and fissuring of end plates and vascularized fibrous tissues are seen histologically.

2. *Type 2 change.* Increased signal intensity on T1-weighted images and slightly increased or isointense on T2-weighted images. This actually represents fatty marrow replacement.[103]

Degenerative changes of the spine may be categorized as follows:

- Intervertebral osteochondrosis is an injury to the nucleus pulposus. The radiographic features include vacuum disc phenomena centrally, disc space narrowing, osteophyte formation, and marginal eburnation of the vertebral bodies.

- Spondylosis deformans is due to injury at the attachment of the disc to the end plate. Findings include asymmetrical vacuum disc near the end plate attachment, normal height of disc space, osteophyte formation and osteoarthrosis of the apophyseal and costovertebral joints.

Vertebral body osteophytes probably result from weakening of annular fibers with disc bulging and traction on Sharpey's fibers. Schmorl's nodes, herniation of the disc material through the end plate into the vertebral body, may be observed in spondylosis. Spondylosis occurs with increasing age and there is a male predominance. The thoracic spine is less frequently and less severely involved, compared to the cervical and lumbar spine.

Plain radiographs demonstrate osteophyte formation, end plate sclerosis, Schmorl's nodes, and facet hypertrophy. CT and MRI show the above findings. In addition, the bony spinal canal and neuroforamina narrowing are better assessed with CT and MRI.

Spinal Stenosis

Spinal stenosis occurs less frequently in the thoracic spine than in the cervical and lumbar spine. This is probably due to the large size of the thoracic spinal canal relative to the spinal cord. Bony or ligamentous hypertrophy must be in a quite advanced stage to significantly compromise the spinal canal, resulting in spinal cord compression. Spinal stenosis can be congenital, acquired, or a combination of both. Congenital spinal stenosis is due to congenitally short pedicles. These short pedicles are thick, causing a narrow spinal canal. When mild spondylotic changes are superimposed with congenital spinal stenosis, severe neurological manifestations may occur. Congenital spinal stenosis may occur in patients with achondroplasia, Morquio syndrome, and Hurler's syndrome.[58]

Acquired spinal stenosis is caused by spondylosis, ligamentous degeneration, and hypertrophy. Disc bulge and herniation can further exacerbate spinal stenosis. Decreased stability of the disc and facet joints, in conjunction with ligamentous laxity, can lead to progressive degenerative changes of the spine. Ossification of the posterior longitudinal ligament may be seen in the thoracic spine (Fig. 5-7), but is more common in the cervical spine.

MRI, CT, myelography, or CT-myelography all demonstrate decreased size of the spinal canal with a small thecal sac. Exaggerated narrowing may be seen at the level of disc space secondary to osteophyte formation or disc herniation. Serpiginous and edematous nerve roots may be observed in the thecal sac due to compression.

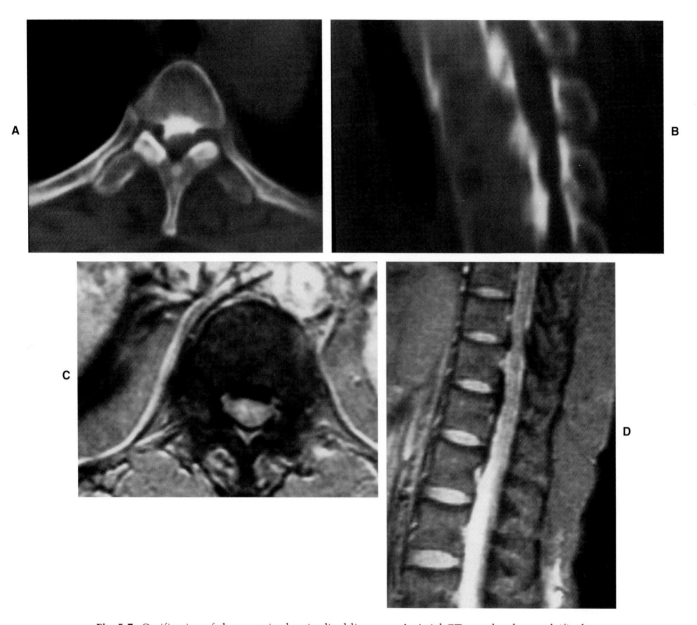

Fig. 5-7. Ossification of the posterior longitudinal ligament. **A,** Axial CT reveals a large calcific density extending from the dorsal margin of the vertebral body in the region of the posterior longitudinal ligament. **B,** Sagittal reformatted CT at midsagittal level demonstrates the extent of the ossified posterior longitudinal ligament. Compromise of the bony spinal canal is obvious. **C** and **D,** Axial and sagittal MRIs show the ossified posterior longitudinal ligament to be of low signal intensity.

LESIONS

Pathology involving the thoracic spine, spinal cord, and nerve roots can be divided into three major categories regarding location: intramedullary, intradural extramedullary, and extradural. Intramedullary lesions are enveloped completely within the spinal cord parenchyma or filum terminale. Exophytic growth of intramedullary lesions may involve both the intramedullary and extramedullary compartments. Intramedullary lesions of the filum terminale usually appear as intradural extramedullary lesions by myelography. Intradural extramedullary lesions are located within the dura with displacement of the spinal cord. Extradural lesions consist of lesions external to the dural compartment and lesions of the osseous spine.

Intramedullary Lesions
Intramedullary Neoplasms

Intramedullary tumors comprise 6% to 10% of CNS neoplasms in children and overall approximately 20% of intraspinal neoplasms.

Ependymoma. Ependymoma is the second most common spinal glioma of childhood and the most common spinal glioma for all age groups. In a large series of 273 spinal intramedullary gliomas, Slooff, Kernohan, and MacCarty[141] found 169 (61.9%) to represent ependymomas of the spinal cord and filum terminale.

Approximately 70% of spinal ependymomas occur between the ages of 30 and 60 years and only about 10% occur before the age of 19 years. There is a slight male predominance in myxopapillary ependymomas of the cauda equina.

The myxopapillary ependymoma is the most common histologic variant found in the regions of the conus medullaris and filum terminale (95%). However, the more classical epithelial, cellular, and papillary types are also observed at these sites.[98] The cellular or mixed ependymomas are most commonly observed in the cervical region. Microscopic evidence of previous hemorrhage is frequently seen in myxopapillary ependymomas. Ependymomas can occasionally be a source of subarachnoid hemorrhage (SAH). Malignant ependymomas and subependymomas are uncommon lesions in the spinal canal.

Using radiography, localized enlargement of the spinal cord may occasionally manifest as widening of the interpediculate distance and increased AP diameter of the spinal canal with dorsal scalloping of the vertebral bodies.

With myelography, ependymomas located within the spinal cord cause focal fusiform widening of the spinal cord and a decrease in the surrounding subarachnoid space. Occasionally, blockage of the flow of the contrast may be observed. It is not uncommon for ependymomas of the filum terminale and conus medullaris to demonstrate a sharply delineated rounded defect at the interfaces of the lesion and contrast medium, simulating an intradural extramedullary mass, and frequently a block of the subarachnoid space, since these lesions may go unrecognized until late in their course.

CT-myelography demonstrates focal widening of the spinal cord or filum with obliteration of the adjacent subarachnoid space. Reformatted sagittal and coronal images reveal findings similar to those demonstrated by conventional myelography.

MRI demonstrates focal enlargement of the spinal cord or filum terminale and typically is hypointense/isointense on T1-weighted, iso/hyperintense on proton density–weighted, and hyperintense on T2-weighted images. Subacute hemorrhage within the tumor is identified as focal high signal intensity on T1-weighted images, and hemosiderin deposition in chronic hemorrhage is identified as areas of marked hypointensity on T2-weighted images. Intense, homogeneous contrast enhancement typically occurs (Fig. 5-8). Associated cystic cavitation of the spinal cord or syringohydromyelia may be observed. Contrast-enhanced MRI clearly delineates the extent of the neoplasm and is useful in distinguishing tumor cyst from benign syrinx.[147]

Astrocytoma. Astrocytoma accounts for approximately 25% to 30% of intramedullary gliomas of the spinal cord for all age groups and is the most common intramedullary tumor in children. Overall, spinal astrocytomas are more common in adults. There is no gender predilection. Over 80% of spinal astrocytomas are located in the cervical and upper thoracic cord. Long segments of the spinal cord may be involved.[43]

Spinal cord astrocytomas are usually of low grade and of the fibrillary type, with a common conversion to the pilocytic variety. Malignant astrocytomas are less common and comprise approximately 25% of spinal intramedullary astrocytomas in adults and 10% to 15% of spinal intramedullary astrocytomas in children.

Except for location preferences, the myelographic and CT-myelographic appearances of ependymomas are indistinguishable from astrocytomas. On MRI, contrast enhancement is less intense and inhomogeneous.[26] Cyst formation is commonly observed (Fig. 5-9). Cyst fluid may contain various concentrations of protein, exhibiting higher signal intensity, compared to CSF, on both T1-weighted and T2-weighted images. Astrocytomas are unlikely to contain hemorrhage, whereas ependymomas often hemorrhage. Astrocytomas often show multisegmented spinal cord enlargement.

Hemangioblastoma. Hemangioblastomas constitute approximately 3% of spinal intramedullary tumors. Approximately 60% are intramedullary, 11% both intramedullary and intradural extramedullary, 21% intradural extramedullary, and 8% extradural in location. Spinal hemangioblastomas are observed with cerebellar hemangio-

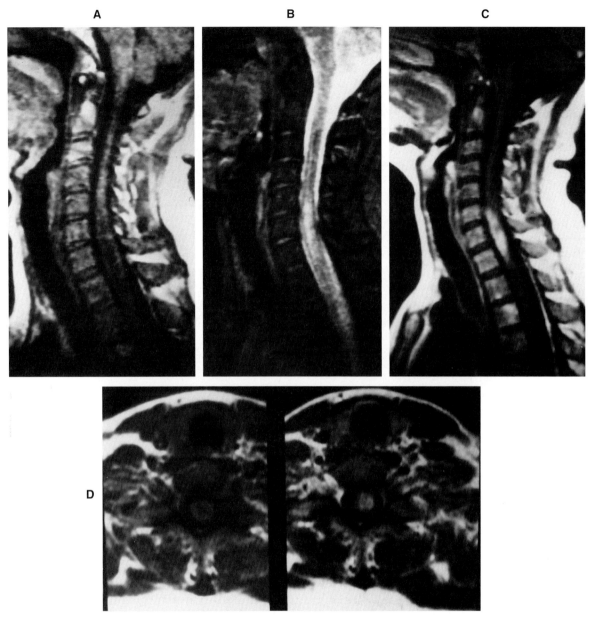

Fig. 5-8. Ependymoma. **A,** Sagittal T1-weighted image shows focal widening of the spinal cord at the cervicothoracic junction with a low signal intensity area seen within the spinal cord. **B,** Sagittal T2-weighted image exhibits a high signal intensity lesion within the spinal cord. **C,** Sagittal, post-contrast T1-weighted image reveals an enhancing mass with a small syrinx distal to the enhancing lesion. **D,** Axial T1-weighted images confirm the presence of the enhancing mass and the syrinx at different levels.

blastomas in patients with von Hippel-Lindau syndrome.[9]

The majority of hemangioblastomas occurs between the ages of 25 and 50 years, although they may be seen in any age group. The incidence in males and females is about equal. The majority of spinal intramedullary hemangioblastomas are located from the cervical spine to the middle third of the thoracic spine, and are more common in the dorsal aspect of the spinal cord.

The majority (80%) of spinal intramedullary hemangioblastomas are solitary. Intramedullary hemangioblastomas are usually cystic (70%). Microscopically, reticular (common) and cellular

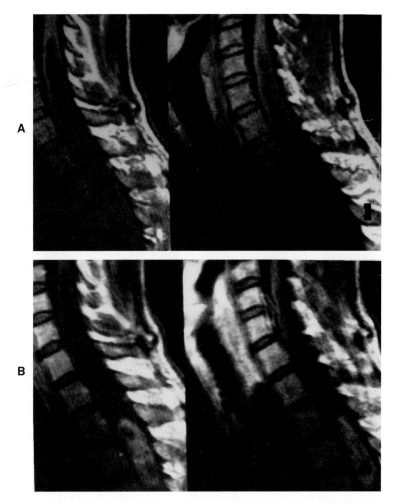

Fig. 5-9. Astrocytoma. **A,** Sagittal T1-weighted image shows focal widening of the spinal cord with inhomogeneous low signal intensity. **B,** Sagittal, post-contrast T1-weighted image shows enhancement of the mass with small cystic areas seen within the mass. In addition, an associated syrinx is seen above the tumor.

variants are noted and both variants may coexist in the same tumor. Like its intracranial counterparts, the tumor is usually attached to the adjacent pia mater. There is a high incidence (50% to 70%) of associated syringohydromyelia.[107]

Radiographic, myelographic, and CT findings are similar to other intramedullary tumors. Serpentine filling defects on the spinal cord surface, secondary to meningeal varicosities, exist in 50% of cases on myelography or CT-myelography.[67] Contrast-enhanced CT usually demonstrates dense contrast enhancement of the solid component of the lesion. Fluid in the associated cavity may be similar or slightly hyperdense compared to CSF.

With MRI, T1-weighted images demonstrate spinal cord enlargement and heterogeneous areas of mixed signal intensity. T2-weighted images show

hyperintensity secondary to tumor, cyst, and edema. Contrast-enhanced images show marked enhancement of the solid component of the tumor. Cyst fluid may be similar or slightly hyperintense to CSF on both T1-weighted and T2-weighted images.

Spinal angiography demonstrates an intense prolonged tumor stain with dilated feeding arteries and draining veins.

Lipoma. Intradural intramedullary lipomas include subpial-juxtamedullary lipomas and fibrolipomas of the filum terminale. Subpial-juxtamedullary lipomas comprise approximately 4% of spinal lipomas. Fibrolipomas of the filum terminale occur in about 6% of asymptomatic adults.[113] In the absence of neurological symptoms and spinal cord tethering, fibrolipomas of the filum terminale should be considered a normal variant.

Approximately 80% present by the age of 30 years, with about 25% presenting during the first 5 years of life. Subpial lipomas most commonly occur in the thoracic and cervical regions.[115]

Pure intramedullary lipomas are exceedingly rare. Technically, neither subpial-juxtamedullary lipomas nor fibrolipomas are intramedullary because neither are completely surrounded by the spinal cord. Subpial-juxtamedullary lipomas arise in the dorsal midline cleft of the spinal cord. Spinal cord rotation is present when these lipomas are in ventral and ventrolateral positions. The outer surface of these lipomas is covered by pia mater. These lipomas consist of mature fat cells containing variable amounts of collagen that penetrate neural tissue in variable degrees.[164] Malignant degeneration occurs in about 1%.

The myelographic findings are similar to those previously mentioned for intramedullary lesions. CT and CT-myelography can identify the lipomatous lesions by their characteristic negative Hounsfield units associated with fat density.

In MRI findings, the high signal intensity of fat on T1-weighted images identifies the lesions in their appropriate locations. Fat suppression techniques render the fat hypointense.[173] The fat displays decreased signal intensity on T2-weighted images (Fig. 5-10).

Oligodendroglioma. Oligodendrogliomas constitute approximately 3% of spinal gliomas. Most spinal oligodendrogliomas present between the ages of 10 and 50 years. There is no apparent gender predilection.

Intramedullary oligodendrogliomas have a predilection for the cervicothoracic spine. The typical microscopic picture of oligodendroglioma shows honeycomb-like compact masses of swollen cells containing clear cytoplasm and rather uniform round to oval nuclei interspersed within a scanty, delicate supporting structure of blood vessels and collagen.[154] The findings by radiography, myelography, CT, and MRI are indistinguishable from those of other intramedullary masses.

Ganglioglioma. Gangliogliomas of the spinal cord constitute approximately 1% of spinal tumors. There is no known age or gender predilection. The most common site is the cervical spinal cord, but involvement of the entire spinal cord has been reported. In the pediatric age group the tumor tends to involve long segments of the spinal cord.

Gangliogliomas of the spinal cord, like gangliogliomas of the brain, are mixed neurogliogenic tumors with an admixture of mature ganglion cells and relatively mature glial cells. The usual glial component consists of pilocytic or gemistocytic astrocytes, but oligodendrocytes may be involved. Microscopic calcifications have been noted in oligodendroglial components of spinal gangliogliomas.[29,154]

Using myelography and CT, the findings are similar to those of other intramedullary masses. MRI findings are expansion of the spinal cord, associated with hypointensity on T1-weighted images and hyperintensity on T2-weighted images.

Melanoma. Primary melanoma of the spinal cord constitutes less than 1% of spinal tumors.[154] Spinal melanoma is primarily a disease of adulthood and there is no apparent gender predilection. Common locations are the middle and lower portions of the thoracic spinal cord. Primary melanoma of the spinal cord consists of a black or dark blue poorly marginated tumor mass situated eccentrically in the thoracic spinal cord.[82]

Using myelography and CT-myelography, the findings are similar to other intramedullary masses. The only known reported case with MRI findings demonstrated a heterogeneous, hyper/isointense mass with adjacent decreased signal on T1-weighted images, decreased signal intensity on T2-weighted images, associated syrinx cavities above and below the lesion, and homogeneous, dense contrast enhancement.[166]

Teratoma. Intramedullary teratomas are very rare lesions that comprise about 0.7% of intramedullary tumors. They are more commonly observed in the lower thoracic spinal cord.

Teratomas are masses composed of a mixture of mature tissues derived from all three germ layers, which together do not resemble any recognizable structure although they are composed of mature tissue elements.

Calcifications and fat within the lesion may be detected on CT. MRI findings are an intramedullary thoracic mass demonstrating increased signal secondary to fat and decreased signal secondary to calcium on T1-weighted images.[154]

Dermoid and Epidermoid Tumors. Dermoids and epidermoids each represent about 1% of intramedullary tumors. Dermoids and epidermoids together comprise about 10% of spinal tumors in

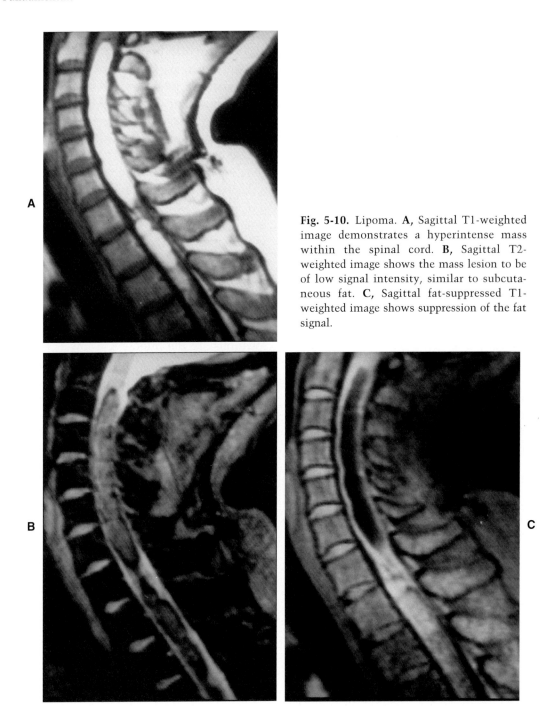

Fig. 5-10. Lipoma. **A,** Sagittal T1-weighted image demonstrates a hyperintense mass within the spinal cord. **B,** Sagittal T2-weighted image shows the mass lesion to be of low signal intensity, similar to subcutaneous fat. **C,** Sagittal fat-suppressed T1-weighted image shows suppression of the fat signal.

patients less than 15 years of age. Dermoid and epidermoid tumors are more common in intradural extramedullary locations. Dermoids usually cause symptoms before the age of 20, whereas epidermoids usually produce symptoms after the age of 20.

Only about 20% of dermoids occur above the level of the cauda equina. Intramedullary epidermoids most commonly occur between T5 and T8, followed by the upper and lower thoracic and lumbar regions.

Dermoids are usually cystic masses composed of dermal elements consisting of squamous epithelium, hair follicles, sweat glands, and sebaceous glands and their products. Epidermoids are cystic masses lined by a membrane of superficial (epidermal) layers of the skin. Some epidermoid cysts are thought to be secondary to previous spinal surgery, lumbar puncture, or other penetrating injuries to the spine.

Radiography reveals bony anomalies such as spina bifida or block vertebrae may be present. The myelographic and CT findings are usually the same as with other intramedullary masses. Low density fat within the mass may be demonstrated by CT.

The MRI signal of dermoid cysts is variable and dependent upon the fat content and chemical composition of the cyst fluid. The lesion may be isointense to hyperintense on T1-weighted images and hyperintense on T2-weighted images. The MRI signal of epidermoids is usually isointense to CSF in both T1-weighted and T2-weighted images. Contrast enhancement usually does not occur with epidermoids, but may occasionally occur in dermoid lesions.[10,51,133]

Metastases. The peak ages for metastasen are 40 to 70 years and gender predilection is related to the primary tumor. The thoracic spinal cord is most commonly involved (50%), followed by the cervical spinal cord (35%).

Lung carcinoma is the most common primary site for metastases, followed by breast cancer. Other less common primary tumors are melanoma, kidney, colorectal, and lymphoma. The primary site is unknown in approximately 5% of cases.

Radiographs may demonstrate associated bony metastases, which may be osteolytic or, less likely, osteoblastic. Myelography, CT, and MRI findings are nonspecific, that is, a low signal on T1-weighted images and a high signal on T2-weighted images. The degree of spinal cord enlargement is quite variable. MRI shows marked contrast enhancement of the lesions.[46]

Intramedullary Inflammatory Lesions

Transverse Myelitis. Diagnosis of transverse myelitisis is one of exclusion and the imaging findings are nonspecific. The set of diagnostic criteria established by Berman et al.[17] are as follows:

1. Acute development of paraparesis affecting motor and sensory systems, in addition to sphincter disturbances.
2. Complete spinal segmental level sensory disturbance (excluding patients with cord hemisection syndromes and patchy sensory deficits).

3. Stable, nonprogressive clinical course.
4. No clinical, laboratory, or imaging evidence of spinal cord compression.
5. Absence of any known neurological disease, including trauma, syphilis, metastatic malignancy, encephalitis, and prior spinal radiation therapy.
6. A preceding viral infection or vaccination has been commonly associated in children. In adults, AIDS, collagen vascular disease, sarcoidosis, multiple sclerosis, and paraneoplastic syndrome have been associated. The precise etiology in most cases remains unknown.[8,11,16]

Neuromyelitis optica, or Devic's syndrome, presents as paraplegia and blindness due to progressive fulminant demyelination of the spinal cord and optic nerve. Disorders associated with Devic's syndrome, in addition to those already known for transverse myelitis, include infectious mononucleosis, acute disseminated encephalomyelitis, and systemic lupus erythematosus.

The spinal cord levels below which all sensory functions are lost fall predominantly in the thoracic spinal cord (80%).

Histopathology demonstrates distortion of normal spinal cord architecture with hemorrhage, necrosis, perivascular inflammation, and demyelination. The length of spinal cord involvement is variable but is usually at least one to three segments in length.

Myelography and CT-myelography findings may vary from normal to the nonspecific findings of spinal cord enlargement. The MRI appearance of transverse myelitis is variable and ranges from normal to focal or diffuse cord hyperintensity on T2-weighted images and focal contrast enhancement[8] (Fig. 5-11).

AIDS Myelopathy. The clinical history of AIDS in combination with clinical findings of myelopathy and in conjunction with intrinsic spinal cord neoplasia/inflammation and extrinsic spinal cord compression enables the diagnosis of AIDS myelopathy. Approximately 20% to 30% of AIDS patients at autopsy reveal a vacuolar myelopathy, probably related to direct injury of neurons by the HIV virus. Findings also include demyelination in the white matter, predominantly in the lateral and dorsal columns of the thoracic cord, in association with lipid-laden macrophages.[135]

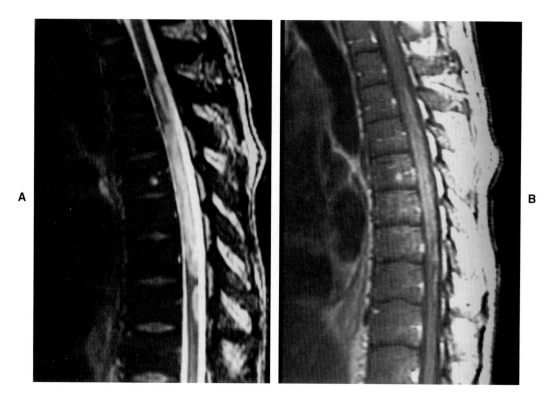

Fig. 5-11. Transverse myelitis. **A,** Sagittal T2-weighted image shows abnormal high signal intensity involving a long segment of thoracic spinal cord. **B,** Sagittal post-gadolinium T1-weighted image demonstrates abnormal enhancement within the thoracic spinal cord.

The vacuoles are surrounded by a thin myelin sheath and appear to arise from swelling within myelin sheaths. Axonal disruption may occur in areas of severe vacuolation. These histological findings are similar to the pathological findings of subacute combined degeneration due to vitamin B_{12} deficiency. The clinical manifestations of vitamin B_{12} deficiency are very similar to those of AIDS myelopathy. The imaging findings of AIDS myelopathy are similar to those for transverse myelitis.[11] Contrast enhancement may be seen on gadolinium-enhanced images.

Tuberculosis. Tuberculomas of the spinal cord usually occur in association with tuberculosis in the lungs or elsewhere in the body. Due to the increasing incidence of AIDS, the incidence of spinal cord tuberculomas will likely increase. Tuberculomas have been known to be evenly distributed throughout the entire spinal cord. The imaging characteristics are nonspecific and indistinguishable from those of other intramedullary lesions (Fig. 5-12).

Abscesses. Intramedullary abscesses are extremely rare. Preoperative diagnosis on imaging studies is unusual. MRI shows an intramedullary mass that is hypointense on T1-weighted images and hyperintense on T2-weighted images with hyperintense surrounding edema. Contrast enhancement could be nodular or ring-like, depending upon the stage of the abscess (similar to intracranial abscesses).[137]

Intramedullary Vascular Lesions

Arteriovenous Malformations. Vascular malformations of the spine are rare. Intramedullary AVMs of the spinal cord consist of type II (glomus AVMs) and type III (juvenile type AVMs) spinal vascular malformations. Intramedullary AVMs present with symptoms at a mean age of approximately 20 years. There is no known gender predilection. Glomus AVMs are comprised of a compact vascular nidus buried within a relatively short segment of spinal cord parenchyma, fed by one or more branches of the anterior or posterior spinal arteries, and drained by enlarged, tortuous arteriolized veins. Glomus AVMs are usually located

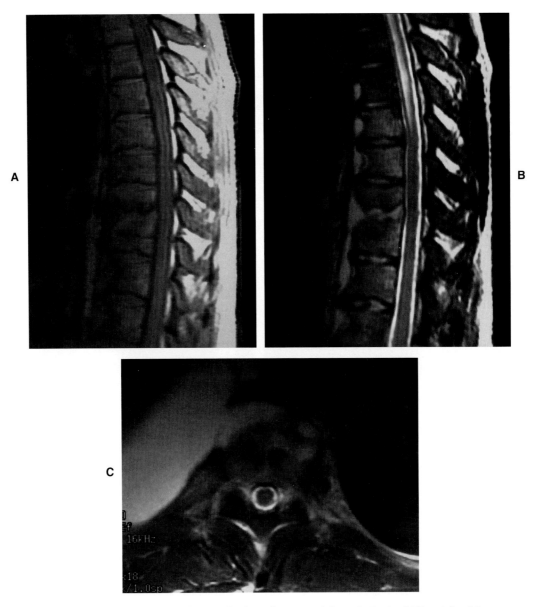

Fig. 5-12. Intramedullary tuberculosis and tuberculous spondylitis. **A,** Sagittal T1-weighted image reveals narrowing of the disc space at T7-8 with irregular vertebral body end plates. Note the presence of a ventral paraspinal mass extending from T4 to T10. **B,** Sagittal T2-weighted image demonstrates irregular vertebral body end plates with disc space narrowing. The ventral paraspinous abscess shows high signal intensity. Note the intramedullary high signal intensity seen above the level of T5 secondary to intramedullary disease. **C,** Axial T2-weighted image shows bony destruction of the vertebral body with a large high signal right paraspinal abscess extending ventral to the vertebral body.

dorsally in the cervicomedullary region.[3] Associated aneurysms of the feeding arteries are present in approximately 20% of cases. Juvenile AVMs are more common in children and adolescents and are generally larger than glomus AVMs. Juvenile AVMs occur in both the intramedullary and extramedullary compartments. Extraspinal extension may occur. Multiple arterial feeders are common.[111,115]

Myelography reveals the presence of serpentine filling defects secondary to dilated vessels. Hematomyelia may cause spinal cord enlargement. Spinal cord atrophy may also be observed.

On MRIs, curvilinear flow voids may be noted within the spinal cord parenchyma and on the surface of the spinal cord on all sequences, but are more clearly seen on proton-density weighted

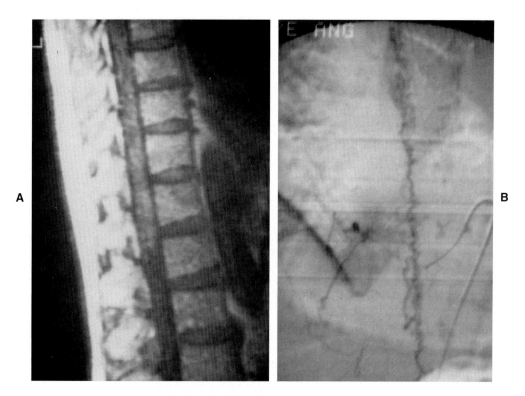

Fig. 5-13. Spinal AVM. **A,** Sagittal T1-weighted image shows multiple curvilinear filling defects surrounding the lower spinal cord and cauda equina. **B,** AP view of spinal angiogram demonstrates the AVM, with dilated feeding arteries and draining veins.

sequence. The spinal cord is sometimes atrophic and may exhibit a high signal intensity on T2-weighted images[94] (Fig. 5-13, *A*).

Spinal angiography demonstrates one or more dilated feeding arteries to an intraparenchymal nidus of tangled blood vessels associated with one or more dilated, tortuous early draining veins (Fig. 5-13, *B*). An associated aneurysm may be observed.[19]

Cavernous Angiomas. Cavernous angiomas of the spinal cord are extremely rare (less than 1% of intramedullary tumors). There is a slight female predominance.[4] They commonly occur in the thoracic and cervical spinal cord.[112] Spinal cavernous angiomas are histologically similar to their intracranial counterparts. Microscopically, they consist of blood-filled endothelial-lined spaces lined by thickened, hyalinized walls with little or no interspersed parenchyma.[112] They present sensorimotor symptoms between the third and sixth decades. These lesions have a propensity for intramedullary hemorrhage and have been reported to occasionally cause massive hematomyelia.

MRI typically shows mixed high and low signal intensity on both T1-weighted and T2-weighted images, corresponding to the residue of subacute and chronic hemorrhage. On T2-weighted or gradient-echo images, a very low signal intensity rim (hemosiderin) is characteristically observed.[45,160] Angiography is typically normal.

Infarction. Spinal cord infarction apparently constitutes approximately 1% of cases of central nervous system ischemic infarction. In the absence of associated pathology such as necrotizing myelopathy due to vascular malformations, systemic lupus erythematosus, spinal cord phlebothrombosis, radiation therapy, etc., spinal cord infarctions probably occur due to compromised blood flow in the anterior spinal artery.[102] The single anterior spinal artery has an extensive vascular territory with limited anastomotic channels. The paired posterior spinal arteries have somewhat limited vascular territories with a much more plentiful supply of anastomotic channels. A spinal cord infarction is much more likely to result from anterior spinal artery flow compromise than from posterior spinal artery involvement.[170] Prior to the advent of MRI, the sequelae of acute and subacute spinal cord infarction could not be directly imaged in vivo. The MRI findings in ischemic spinal cord infarction are similar to those of ischemic brain infarction.[48,60] Acute and subacute infarcts demonstrate the involved segment of the spinal cord to be hypointense/isointense on T1-weighted images and hyperintense on T2-weighted images. During the middle and late subacute phases contrast enhancement is commonly observed.[102,150] During the chronic phase, spinal cord atrophy and myelomalacia may be present.[60] Atherosclerosis, herniated disc, osteophytes, displaced vertebral body fragment, aortic dissection and aortic aneurysmal surgery, and disruption of intercostal arteries with radicular branches to the anterior spinal artery may be underlying causes of spinal cord infarction.

Intramedullary Trauma

Spinal Cord Injury. Only since the advent of MRI has the direct imaging of intramedullary spinal cord injuries been possible. Spinal cord injuries may present various MRI findings, ranging from normal, to edema, to hemorrhage, to cord transection.[53,72] Obviously, injuries with initial physiological spinal cord transection carry a poor prognosis. Incomplete spinal cord injuries are classified relative to clinical findings as follows:[154]

1. *Anterior cord syndrome.* Flexion injuries and central disc herniations
2. *Central cord syndrome.* Hyperextension injuries
3. *Brown-Sequard syndrome.* Cord injury to lateral half of the spinal cord
4. *Posterior cord syndrome.* Dorsal column injury (rare)
5. *Conus medullaris syndrome.* Compression fracture of T12 or L1.

Plain radiographs may demonstrate the results of an associated bony injury. There is often no correlation between the extent of bony and soft tissue injury with the extent of spinal cord injury.

Sagittal and coronal MR images demonstrate the presence or absence of spinal cord swelling or transection. The findings of edema and blood in the spinal cord are the same as those involving the brain. Spinal cord edema is hypointense/isointense on T1-weighted images and hyperintense in T2-weighted images. The appearance of blood is related to the age of the blood clot and the volume of the clot.[68,93,97,99,114,115]

During the acute (deoxyhemoglobin) phase, blood appears hypointense/isointense on T1-weighted images and markedly hypointense on T2-weighted images. During the early subacute (intracellular methemoglobin) phase blood appears hyperintense on T1-weighted images and very hypointense on T2-weighted images. During the later subacute (extracellular methemoglobin) phases blood is hyperintense on both T1-weighted and T2-weighted images. During the chronic (extracellular methemoglobin/hemosiderin) phase, blood varies from early hyperintensity with peripheral hypointensity on T1-weighted images and hyperintensity with peripheral marked hypointensity on T2-weighted images, to late hypointensity on T1-weighted images and hypointensity to marked hypointensity on T2-weighted images. Regions of myelomalacia and cystic cavitation remain hypointense on T1-weighted images and hyperintense on T2-weighted images.[21]

Spinal Cord Compression. Obviously, spinal cord compression results in varying degrees of injury to the spinal cord. The spectrum of injuries includes normal, edema, and hemorrhage in addition to necrosis, gliosis, and demyelination. The contour abnormalities of spinal cord compression are best demonstrated by sagittal and axial MR images obtained in planes in the direction of and perpendicular to the compressing force. When the spinal cord is compressed, it is wider in the plane perpendicular to the force and narrower in the plane in the direction of the force.

Miscellaneous Intramedullary Lesions

Multiple Sclerosis. Multiple sclerosis (MS) is the most common demyelinating disease of the spinal cord. Patients with known intracranial disease and spinal cord symptoms have been reported to have detectable spinal cord lesions on MRI in up to 75% of cases. Isolated spinal cord involvement is uncommon and occurs in less than 10% of patients.[41]

MS has a peak incidence in the third and fourth decades, but the disease may be seen in the pediatric group. There is a female predilection of 2:1. In the pediatric age group the female preponderance is approximately 10:1.[116]

Approximately two thirds of spinal MS plaques are located in the cervical spinal cord with most of these in the mid- and lower cervical spinal cord.

Thoracic spinal cord involvement is less common. In the late stages of the disease, any segment of the spinal cord may be involved.

Spinal MS plaques are the same as those of the brain. They involve areas of selective demyelination with axonal sparing and a tendency toward perivenous locations. Most MS plaques are detected in the lateral columns of the spinal cord and abut the lateral pial surface. The second most common site involves the posterior columns near the midline.

Imaging of MS of the spinal cord has become possible with the advent of MRI. The spectrum of findings may vary from focal spinal cord widening to spinal cord atrophy. The typical MRI findings of spinal MS are vertically elongated areas of hyperintensity involving the lateral or dorsal aspect of the spinal cord on T2-weighted images.[86,92] Occasionally, homogeneous contrast enhancement is seen.[82] Brain MRI has been reported to be abnormal in up to 50% of patients with spinal disease presenting only with spinal symptoms. The imaging findings of MS are nonspecific, and correlation with clinical and laboratory findings is essential to making the definitive diagnosis.

Syringohydromyelia. Syringohydromyelia refers to cystic cavitation of the spinal cord. Since neither imaging studies nor histopathological examinations can clearly differentiate between hydromyelia and syringomyelia, the term "syringohydromyelia" is frequently used in the radiologic literature. Syringohydromyelia may be either congenital or acquired. The congenital form is usually associated with the Chiari I and II malformations, as well as other congenital anomalies such as diastematomyelia. Acquired syringohydromyelia may be related to trauma, spinal cord neoplasms, spontaneous intramedullary hemorrhage, ischemia, arachnoiditis, and inflammatory disease (Fig. 5-14).

Syringohydromyelia presents from childhood through adulthood but is more common in adulthood. There is no known gender predilection.

In classical hydromyelia, which is the result of dilatation of the central canal of the spinal cord, the cyst is lined by ependyma. A cyst associated with syringomyelia is located eccentrically in the spinal cord and lined by reactive glial tissue. However, this distinction cannot be made by imaging studies and is commonly not made by histopathology. It is not uncommon for the wall of a hydromyelic cavity to split, allowing the fluid to

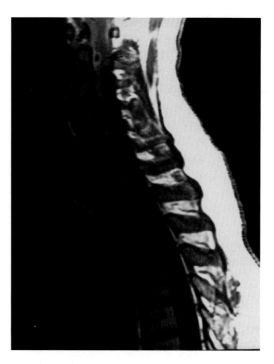

Fig. 5-14. Syringohydromyelia associated with cysticercosis. Sagittal post-gadolinium, T1-weighted image demonstrates the presence of a syrinx and a small ring-like enhancing lesion in the upper cervical region (arrow).

dissect into the spinal cord parenchyma. The reverse process could also occur with syringomyelia. Both of these processes may lead to cavities lined partially by ependyma and partially by reactive glial tissue.

With regard to imaging, MRI is the modality of choice. Sagittal and axial T1-weighted images show hypointense cystic cavitation within a dilated spinal cord. Sagittal and coronal T2-weighted images demonstrate rather uniform hyperintensity of the spinal cord cavity. Internal septa within the syrinx cavity are frequently observed.[115,154]

Acute Disseminated Encephalomyelitis. Acute disseminated encephalomyelitis is a monophasic demyelinating disease that affects children following a recent vaccination or viral infection. The histopathological findings of foci of perivenous white matter demyelination are indistinguishable from those of MS. Similarly, the imaging findings are indistinguishable from those of MS.

Radiation Myelitis. Radiation myelitis is usually a self-limiting disease that occurs a few weeks or months following radiation therapy during which the affected segment of spinal cord was included within the treatment ports. Occasionally, a progressive myelopathy leading to progressive or permanent paralysis may occur as well. MRI is the imaging modality of choice, and may reveal a normal or slightly swollen spinal cord, with hypointensity on T1-weighted images and hyperintensity on T2-weighted images, shortly following the initial onset of disease. Focal spinal cord enhancement may be observed following the administration of contrast material.[101,161,174] Spinal cord atrophy without associated signal abnormality may be seen in patients who have had the disease for more than 3 years. The vertebral bodies included in the radiation ports characteristically show marked hyperintensity on T1-weighted images due to fatty replacement of the irradiated marrow.

Subacute Necrotizing Myelopathy. Subacute necrotizing myelopathy (SNM) is a progressive disease with clinical deterioration, in contrast to the relatively benign clinical course of transverse myelitis. The exact etiology of SNM is uncertain. The current theory is spinal cord ischemia secondary to local venous hypertension, causing disturbed spinal cord perfusion and venous drainage in association with a spinal dural arteriovenous fistula (AVF). SNM with spinal cord ischemia secondary to venous thrombosis is termed the Foix-Alajouanine syndrome.[32] SNM is a rare disorder with an unknown incidence. Surgical resection and/or therapeutic embolization of the dural AVF may occasionally prevent the clinical progression of the disease. The Foix-Alajouanine syndrome has a peak incidence between the ages of 50 and 70 years. There is a slight male preference.

Most spinal dural AVFs are located at or below the midthoracic level. Therefore SNM related to this entity should produce spinal cord lesions in similar locations, although spinal cord lesions above the AVF can occur.

The histopathological findings of SNM are quite variable. Eventually, focal necrosis is observed. SNM related to AVF demonstrates hyalinization and mural thickening within the venocapillary network of the spinal cord. Idiopathic SNM is associated with striking focal necrosis with a relative paucity of inflammatory cells.

MRI findings are similar to those of transverse myelitis. Superselective spinal angiography may demonstrate the presence of an associated dural AVF.

Intradural Extramedullary Lesions
Intradural Extramedullary Neoplasms

More than half of all primary spinal tumors are located in the intradural extramedullary compartment. The majority of these lesions are nerve sheath tumors and meningiomas.

Nerve Sheath Tumors. Nerve sheath tumors consist of schwannomas and neurofibromas. Even though schwannomas and neurofibromas have different histopathological features, they have often been discussed together in the radiologic literature because their radiologic features are indistinguishable from one another.

Nerve sheath tumors constitute approximately 15% to 30% of primary spinal tumors. An association exists between neurofibromatosis type I and neurofibromas and between neurofibromatosis type II and schwannomas.[56] The peak incidence is between the ages of 20 and 50 years. There is no gender predilection.

Nerve sheath tumors usually involve the dorsal nerve roots. The most common site is the thoracic spine (43%) followed by the lumbar spine (34%). Approximately 70% are intradural extramedullary; about 15% each of combined extradural/intradural and extradural, and less than 1% intramedullary in location.[154]

Schwannomas are firm circumscribed and encapsulated lesions arising from Schwann cells, which are comprised mostly of compact cellular Antoni type A tissue intermingled with loosely textured myxoid stroma of Antoni type B tissue. Cyst formation is common. Malignant schwannomas are rare and cannot be differentiated from their benign counterparts (Fig. 5-15). Neurofibromas are soft, nonencapsulated lesions consisting of loosely textured mixtures of Schwann cells and fibroblasts with wide separation of nerve fibers by poorly cellular tissue lacking orderly architecture. Schwannomas are slightly more common than neurofibromas.

Large tumors may show evidence of localized enlargement of the spinal canal or neuroforamen using plain x-ray films.

In the cervical and thoracic regions well circumscribed, sharply marginated filling defects causing displacement of the spinal cord are noted in myelographic findings. They are typical of an intradural extramedullary lesion. Displacement of the spinal cord results in widening of the subarachnoid space on the same side and narrowing on the opposite

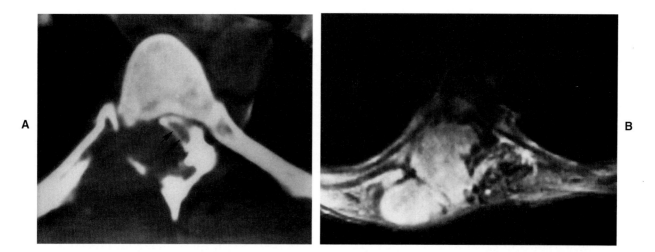

Fig. 5-15. Malignant schwannoma. **A,** Axial CT-myelogram shows a large mass lesion in the spinal canal, as well as outside the canal, with evidence of bony destruction. The spinal cord, surrounded by contrast, is compressed and displaced to the left (arrows). **B,** Axial T2-weighted MRI shows the extent of the tumor better than CT. The neoplasm shows higher signal intensity than the adjacent muscle.

side. Total blockage of the subarachnoid space may be present when the lesion is large. A small lesion arising from a nerve root may present as a solitary grape-like filling defect attached to the nerve root. Multiple lesions may be seen (Fig. 5-16).

CT-myelography demonstrates a soft tissue mass, producing findings similar to conventional myelography. Bony erosion with enlargement of the spinal canal or neuroforamen may be observed.

In MRI findings, typically both schwannomas and neurofibromas are isointense/hypointense to cord on T1-weighted sequences and hyperintense on T2-weighted sequences. When located in the cervical or thoracic region, nerve sheath tumors often displace the spinal cord (Fig. 5-17). When located in the lumbar region, these tumors may be difficult to detect without the usage of a contrast agent. Both lesions typically demonstrate homogenous, intense contrast enhancement. Ring-like enhancement may be seen in schwannomas due to cystic changes within the schwannoma itself.[49,62,89,157]

Meningioma. Meningiomas comprise 25% to 45% of intraspinal tumors and typically present in the fifth and sixth decades. There is a 4:1 female preference.[142] Meningiomas are rare in children and account for only 3% of pediatric spinal tumors. Multiple spinal meningiomas are also rare and are usually associated with neurofibromatosis type I.[28]

The marjority of spinal meningiomas (80%) occur in the thoracic region, followed by cervical region (15%), lumbar region (3%), and at the foramen

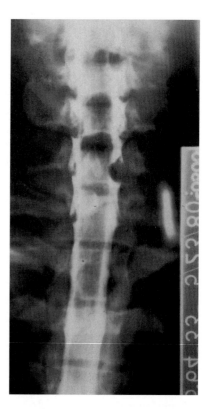

Fig. 5-16. Neurofibromatosis. AP view of myelogram shows multiple small filling defects bilaterally along the nerve roots at the cervicothoracic junction.

magnum (2%).[154] Thoracic meningiomas tend to be located dorsal or lateral to the spinal cord (Fig. 5-18). Cervical and foramen magnum meningiomas tend to be located ventral to the spinal cord. Spinal

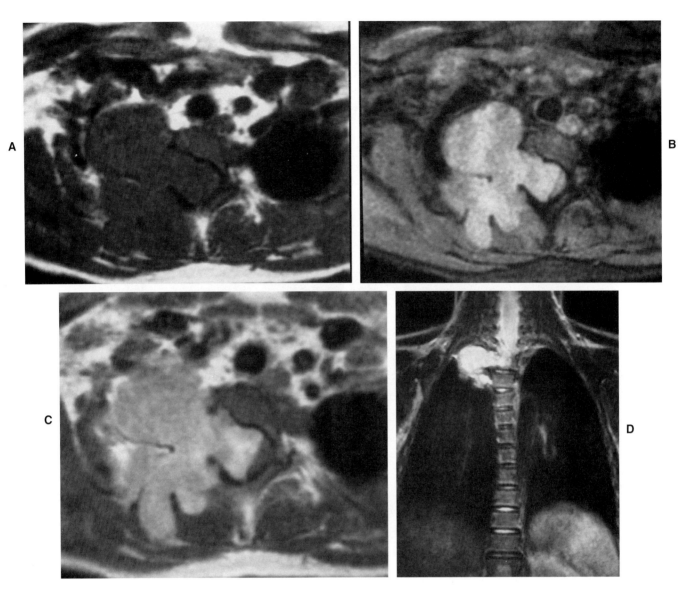

Fig. 5-17. Schwannoma. **A,** Axial T1-weighted image shows a large, lobulated mass lesion over the right side of the spinal canal, extending through the enlarged neuroforamen to the right paraspinal region. The tumor cannot be clearly separated from the spinal cord. **B,** Axial T2-weighted image reveals a large, lobulated hyperintense mass with compression and displacement of the spinal cord to the left. **C,** Axial contrast-enhanced, T1-weighted image demonstrates relatively homogeneous enhancement of the large, lobulated tumor. Note the compressed and displaced spinal cord on the left shows no enhancement. **D,** Cornoal T2-weighted image shows the lobulated mass at the right pulmonary apex.

meningiomas are histologically the same as their intracranial analogue.

Radiographic findings may include localized widening of the spinal canal and calcification. The myelographic findings are similar to those for nerve root tumors. With CT findings the mass may be hyperdense, possibly secondary to psammomatous calcifications or dense tumor tissue. Homogeneous contrast enhancement is usually observed. The typical MRI findings are similar to their intracranial analogue. The majority of meningiomas are broad dural based masses that are isointense to the spinal cord on both T1-weighted and T2-weighted sequences. Less frequently, meningiomas may be hypointense on T1-weighted images and hyperintense on T2-weighted images. Following contrast administration, homogeneous, intense contrast enhancement is observed.[7,96]

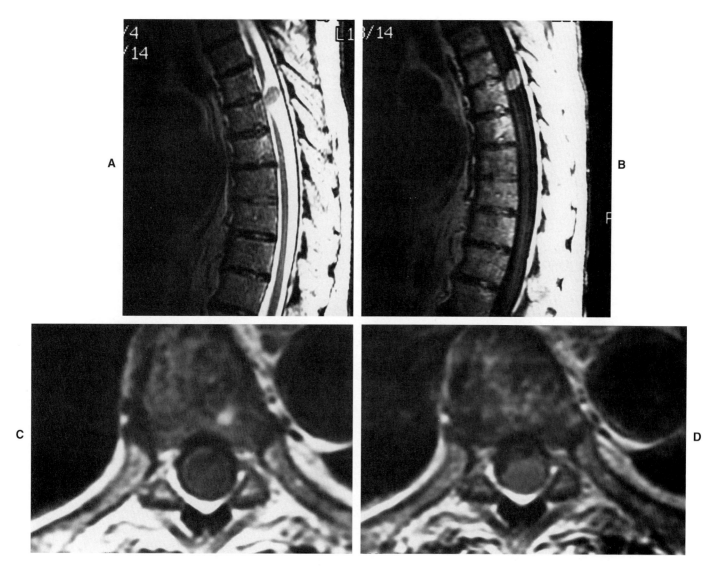

Fig. 5-18. Thoracic meningioma. **A,** Sagittal T2-weighted image shows a round, iso- to slightly hyperintense lesion in the upper thoracic spine displacing the spinal cord ventrally. **B,** Sagittal Gd-enhanced, T1-weighted image shows the round, enhancing mass in the upper thoracic spine. **C,** Axial T1-weighted image demonstrates an isointense mass hardly separable from the spinal cord. **D,** Axial Gd-enhanced, T1-weighted image shows the enhancing mass dorsally and the spinal cord displaced ventrally and to the right.

Epidermoid and Dermoid Cysts. About two thirds of both epidermoids and dermoids are intradural extramedullary in location. The myelographic, CT, and MRI findings are the same as previously discussed, except for their location in the intradural extramedullary compartment.

Teratoma. Teratomas were previously discussed under intramedullary lesions. The imaging findings are the same as previously discussed, but applied to the intradural extramedullary compartment.

Ependymoma and Astrocytoma. Sloof, Kernohan, and MacCarty[141] reported the incidence of intradural extramedullary ependymomas (3.4%) and astrocytomas (2.7%) among 301 intraspinal gliomas. These lesions probably originate from heterotopic glial tissue. The MRI findings of an encapsulated extramedullary thoracic ependymoma or astrocytoma are similar to their intramedullary counterparts, except for the intradural extramedullary compartment.

Paraganglioma. More than 50 intraspinal paragangliomas have been reported. There is a slight male predilection (55% to 60%). Most of the paragangliomas are found in the cauda equina and filum terminale. At least one intradural thoracic paraganglioma has been reported. Paragangliomas are usually firm, encapsulated masses attached to the filum terminale. They can be completely resected. Conventional and CT-myelography demonstrate the typical findings of a lumbar intradural extramedullary mass, often with blockage of the subarachnoid pathway and dilated intradural vessels. Spinal angiography demonstrates highly vascular lesions, exhibiting an intense angiographic tumor stain. MRI findings indicate isointensity to the spinal cord on T1-weighted images and hyperintensity on T2-weighted images.[6,87]

Leptomeningeal Metastases. Leptomeningeal metastases (LMM) occur from either "seeding" through the CSF from intracranial neoplasms or from hematogenous spread of non-CNS neoplasms. Obviously, LMM is more common in patients above the age of 50, though leptomeningeal spread is not uncommon in the pediatric age group. Gender predilection is dependent upon the primary tumor.

LMM is most commonly observed in the lumbosacral region (75%). In the cervical and thoracic regions, LMM is mainly observed dorsal to the spinal cord. This is probably due to the CSF flow dynamics, with flow away from the brain running primarily dorsal to the spinal cord and towards the brain running primarily ventral to the spinal cord. The lumbosacral preponderance could probably be explained by gravity.

LMM may present with a variable appearance, possibly as nodules or sheets of tumor cells coating the nerve roots and spinal cord. Involvement may be localized or diffuse. Diffuse thickening of the thecal sac also occurs. LMM arising from primary central nervous system tumors are referred to as "drop" metastases or "seeding." The usual sources of origin of "drop" metastases, in descending order of frequency, are medulloblastoma, glioblastoma multiforme, ependymoma, oligodendroglioma, astrocytoma, and retinoblastoma. Other less common sources of origin are germinoma, pineoblastoma, and choroid plexus papilloma. The two most common systemic sources are carcinomas of the breast and lung, followed by melanoma, non-Hodgkin's lymphoma, leukemia, and carcinomas of the genitourinary tract.[154]

Conventional radiography is very useful for the evaluation of associated osseous metastatic disease. Conventional CT and CT-myelography remain very useful for the evaluation of LMM, especially when a high-resolution MRI is not available. Typical findings include nerve root irregularity, nodular filling defects involving the spinal cord and nerve roots, clumping of thickened nerve roots, irregular narrowing of the subarachnoid space with thickening of the thecal sac, and varying degrees of blockage of the subarachnoid space.[73]

With MRI, noncontrast images demonstrate nodules or irregular lesions that are hyperintense with respect to CSF on T1-weighted images and hypointense to CSF on T2-weighted images. Contrast-enhanced MRI shows enhancement of nodular lesions, irregularly thickened nerve roots, and irregularly thickened meninges. Contrast enhancement usually presents as focal, nodular areas of enhancement and/or an enhancing coating on the surface of the spinal cord and nerve roots and along the thecal sac.[75]

Intradural Extramedullary Inflammatory Lesions

Arachnoiditis. "Arachnoiditis" is a descriptive term for arachnoidal inflammation associated with adhesive changes resulting in the adherence of nerve roots, variable degrees of obliteration of the subarachnoid space, intradural cyst formation, and intramedullary cavitation presumably secondary to ischemia. Various reported causes of arachnoiditis include (1) infection, (2) trauma, (3) subarachnoid hemorrhage, (4) surgery, (5) lumbar puncture, (6) intradural neoplasms (7) granulomatous disease such as tuberculosis or sarcoidosis, (8) idiopathic, and (9) intrathecal injections of contrast agents and various therapeutic agents.[27,33,47,50] Arachnoiditis most commonly occurs in the thoracic region; the lumbar region is the next most common site.

Due to the presence of a fibrinous exudate, the fibrin-covered nerve roots and thecal sac become adherent. The reparative production of collagen adhesions causes multiple loculations of CSF occur, resulting in intradural cyst formation. Obliteration of the subarachnoid space and changes in CSF flow patterns follow. Neurological symptoms may be produced secondary to direct spinal cord or nerve root pressure by the intradural cysts or from the generalized fibrosis producing vascular occlusion resulting in spinal cord ischemia.

Myelographic findings include clumping of nerve roots, absence of filling of the nerve root sheath, irregular loculations of contrast, irregular contour of the subarachnoid space, and an empty thecal sac

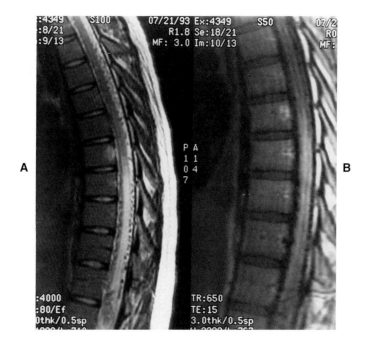

Fig. 5-19. Arachnoiditis. **A,** AP view of the myelogram shows marked irregularity of the thecal sac with clumping of the nerve roots. **B,** Axial post-myelogram CT shows clumping of the nerve roots, with an irregular thecal sac delineated by contrast material in the subarachnoid space.

apparently devoid of nerve roots. The "empty" thecal sac is due to the nerve roots adhering to the thecal sac. On CT-myelography, it may present as peripheral, small filling defects. The combination of conventional CT and CT-myelography probably is still the most definitive method for diagnosing arachnoiditis[65] (Fig. 5-19).

On MRI, T1-weighted images demonstrate the thickening of nerve roots clumped centrally within the thecal sac or adherence to the walls of the thecal sac. Contrast enhancement of the thickened nerve roots may or may not be present. Associated intramedullary cavitation is demonstrated by MRI.[64,77]

Subdural Empyema. Spinal subdural empyema is exceedingly rare. The empyema is usually slightly hyperintense to CSF on both T1-weighted and T2-weighted images.[14]

Intradural Extramedullary Vascular Lesions

Vascular Malformations. Symptomatic vascular malformations are responsible for about 10% of spinal pathology among the combined group of symptomatic patients with neoplasms and vascular malformations. Spinal AVMs have been subdivided into four general categories[115]:

Type I	Dural arteriovenous fistula (AVF)
Type II	Intramedullary AVM (glomus type)
Type III	Large AVM that involves the spinal cord with extramedullary extension (juvenile type)
Type IV	Intradural extramedullary arteriovenous fistula

Dural AVFs present in older patients with a mean age of approximately 50 years, whereas intramedullary vascular malformations present in a younger age group with a mean age of approximately 20 years. Men are affected more often than women at a 3-4:1 ratio. Nearly all intradural type I and type IV spinal vascular malformations occur at or below the midthoracic level.

Intradural extramedullary vascular malformations are of the type I (dural AVF), type III (juvenile type AVM) and type IV (intradural extramedullary AVF) varieties. Type III vascular malformations are large lesions that involve both the intramedullary and extramedullary compartments. Type IV vascular malformations are AVFs with the anterior spinal artery feeding directly into a draining vein on the ventral surface of the spinal cord. Occasionally, type IV vascular malformations involve posterior

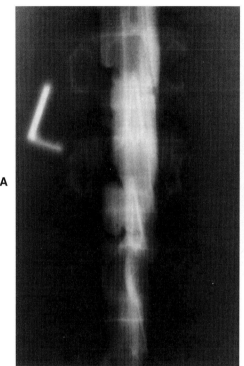

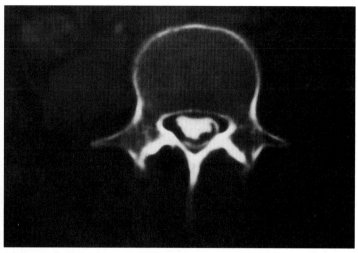

Fig. 5-20. Spinal arteriovenous malformation. **A,** Sagittal T2-weighted image shows multiple curvilinear filling defects surrounding the thoracic spinal cord, consistent with an AVM. The high signal intensity seen within the thoracic spinal cord is due to ischemia and edema. **B,** Sagittal Gd-enhanced, T1-weighted image shows curvilinear filling defects surrounding the spinal cord (not as obvious as T2-weighted image). The high signal intensity within the spinal cord is enhancement secondary to ischemia.

spinal arteries and veins. Type I vascular malformations are AVFs in which arteries located on the spinal cord surface or within nerve root sleeves shunt directly into perimedullary draining veins causing perimedullary venous hypertension. This may result in spinal cord edema.[130,145]

Conventional CT and CT-myelography remain quite useful in demonstrating the presence of abnormal serpentine filling defects, which indicate the presence of enlarged vessels.[37] Myelography may be performed as a guide to spinal angiography.

With MRI, dilated perimedullary veins are best visualized as curvilinear areas of flow void on proton-density or T2-weighted images (Fig. 5-20). Occasionally, contrast enhancing perimedullary veins may be seen, consistent with the presence of slow flow.[39,81]

Spinal angiography is the only definitive imaging modality to demonstrate the site of AVF. This demonstrates direct arteriovenous shunting without an intervening nidus of vessels.

Intradural Extramedullary Trauma

Nerve root/sheath avulsions, severe spinal dislocation injury, and penetrating injuries due to surgery, needle puncture, stab wound, gunshot wound, or bone splinter are various causes of trauma to the

dura mater. Pseudomeningocele formation may result from these injuries. Penetrating injuries could also result in the formation of posttraumatic arachnoid cysts. Most nerve root/sheath avulsion injuries involve the brachial plexus and, less likely, the lumbosacral region. Thoracic region involvement is very unusual.

Dural trauma may be demonstrated by conventional CT, CT-myelography, and MRI. Postsurgical pseudomeningoceles usually appear as dorsal bulging of the thecal sac at sites of previous laminectomy. The nerve root/sheath avulsions usually demonstrate bulbous or cylindrical, somewhat irregular collections of CSF. On myelography posttraumatic arachnoid cysts may initially present as intradural defects that may later be filled with contrast material.[158] Posttraumatic arachnoid cysts are more readily detected by MRI as intradural regions of hyperintensity (usually slightly hyperintense to CSF) on T2-weighted images, frequently with a thin line of hypointensity at the cyst margin. Usually there is no significant mass effect.[151]

Spinal subdural hematomas are rare lesions. They are usually associated with trauma, anticoagulation therapy, bleeding diasthesis, or vascular malformations. MRI is the imaging modality of choice. It has the ability to detect the subdural mass and identify the hemorrhagic nature of the mass. A mass situated between the hypointense dura mater and the adjacent subarachnoid space allows for MRI localization of the lesion within the subdural space. The imaging characteristics of hematoma on MRI are the same as previously described. Spinal subdural and epidural hematomas may occasionally coexist.

Miscellaneous Intradural Extramedullary Lesions

Arachnoid Cyst. Arachnoid cysts are defined as diverticula of the subarachnoid space. Communication between the arachnoid cyst and subarachnoid space through a relatively narrow neck may occur. Arachnoid cysts may be primarily intradural, extradural, or combined intradural/extradural in location. Intradural arachnoid cysts may be congenital or acquired. The acquired type is usually secondary to arachnoiditis.

Arachnoid cysts comprise approximately 1.3% of intraspinal mass lesions. Extradural arachnoid cysts are more common than intradural ones. Because most arachnoid cysts are believed to be of congenital origin they may produce symptoms from childhood through late adulthood. There is no gender predilection. The Nabors classification of arachnoid cysts is as follows:[108]

Type I   Extradural cysts that arise directly from the dura mater and contain no nerve tissue

Type II   Tarlov cysts (usually sacral in location, contain neural tissue in cyst wall, and arise at or distal to dorsal root ganglion) and meningeal diverticula (arise proximal to dorsal root ganglion, nerve tissue within cyst but not in cyst wall) (Fig. 5-21); both are extradural cysts

Type III Intradural cysts

Excluding Tarlov cysts, approximately 65% of extradural cysts are thoracic in location, 20% lumbosacral, 10% thoracolumbar, and 5% cervical.[154] The majority (85%) are dorsal or dorsolateral, and the minority (15%) are located lateral to the thecal sac. Approximately two thirds of both congenital and acquired intradural arachnoid cysts occur in the upper- to midthoracic region. Congenital intradural arachnoid cysts are usually dorsal to the spinal cord, whereas acquired cysts are commonly ventral in location.[109]

Plain radiographs frequently demonstrate bony erosion of the spinal canal and neural foramina. Widening of the spinal canal may occur in intradural cysts.

On conventional CT and CT-myelography congenital intradural and extradural arachnoid cysts demonstrate filling or delayed filling of smoothly marginated lesions (Fig. 5-22). Findings of arachnoiditis are usually observed in addition to the filling defect with acquired intradural arachnoid cysts.

On MRI, arachnoid cysts are loculations of fluid that are usually isointense to CSF. As with CT, the congenital varieties demonstrate smooth margination, whereas irregularity is usually present in the acquired forms.

Extradural Lesions
Extradural Neoplasms

Nonmetastatic epidural tumors are comprised mostly of lipomatous lesions, lymphomas, sarcomas, and neuroblastomas. Extramedullary hematopoiesis has been rarely associated with betathalassemia and myelofibrosis, which, although not neoplastic, can present with compression of the thoracic spinal cord and imaging findings similar to those of neoplasms in the same location.

Lipomatous lesions consist of lipomas, angiolipomas, and lipomatosis. Approximately 40% of spinal lipomas are extradural in location. These lesions usually cannot be differentiated by imaging. Epidural lipomatosis and lipomas are most common in the dorsal aspect of the thoracic spinal canal.[38,124] The majority of epidural lipomatoses are asymptomatic. Epidural lipomatosis is frequently associated with steroid therapy.[44] A significant reduction in epidural fat has been noted to accompany weight loss. Angiolipomas are usually located in the thoracic region (80%) and are differentiated from lipomas and lipomatosis by the presence of vascular elements.[123] Even though epidural lipomas, epidural lipomatosis, and angiolipomas are frequently asymptomatic, symptoms ranging from nonspecific back pain to paraplegia can occur. The imaging findings are the same as previously discussed for the intradural lipomatous lesion, but here the lesion is located in an extradural site.[95,117]

Lymphoma with involvement of the extradural compartment most likely results from extension from retroperitoneal lymph nodes or from osseous lymphoma (Fig. 5-23). Intradural lymphoma usually

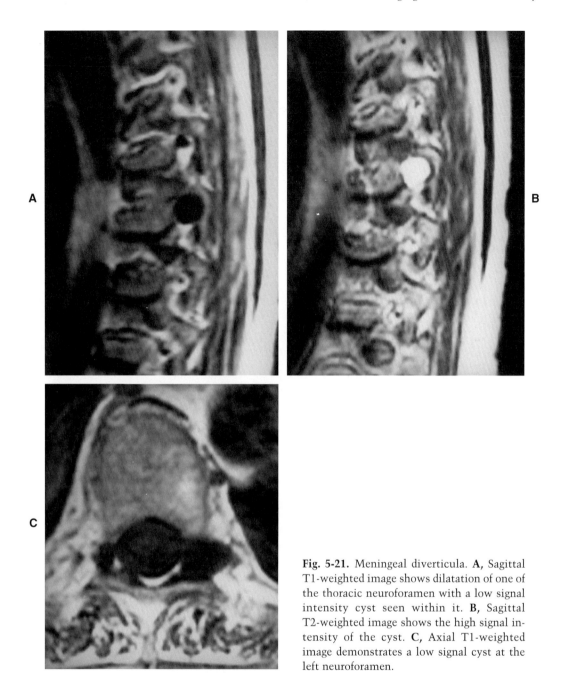

Fig. 5-21. Meningeal diverticula. **A,** Sagittal T1-weighted image shows dilatation of one of the thoracic neuroforamen with a low signal intensity cyst seen within it. **B,** Sagittal T2-weighted image shows the high signal intensity of the cyst. **C,** Axial T1-weighted image demonstrates a low signal cyst at the left neuroforamen.

occurs from hematogenous spread or spread via lymphatics. Extradural lymphomas present as mass lesions that are hypointense to isointense on T1-weighted images and predominantly hyperintense on T2-weighted images. A moderate degree of contrast enhancement is usually observed.[90]

Neuroblastoma constitutes approximately 10% of all neoplasms in children. Approximately 15% of neuroblastomas extend into the spinal canal through the neural foramina. Extension of neuro-

blastomas through abdominal and thoracic neural foramina to involve the spinal canal is well demonstrated by MRI. Calcifications are frequently (>25%) observed on plain radiographs. Neuroblastomas are associated with low to intermediate signal on T1-weighted images and high signal on T2-weighted images. Heterogeneous contrast enhancement is the rule. Sarcomatous lesions tend to exhibit signal intensities similar to neuroblastomas with fairly homogeneous contrast enhancement.

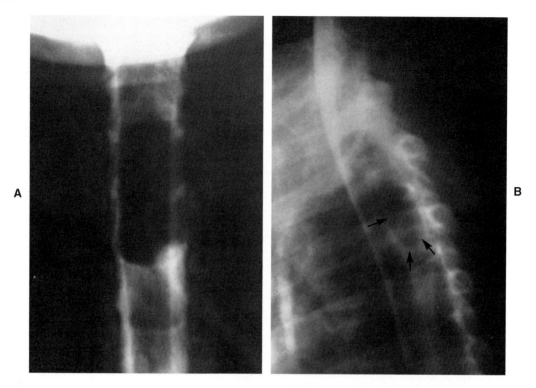

Fig. 5-22. Intradural arachnoid cyst. **A,** AP view of a myelogram shows the presence of a mass lesion with compression of the upper thoracic spinal cord. **B,** Lateral view of the myelogram reveals an intradural mass lesion (arrows) dorsal to the spinal cord.

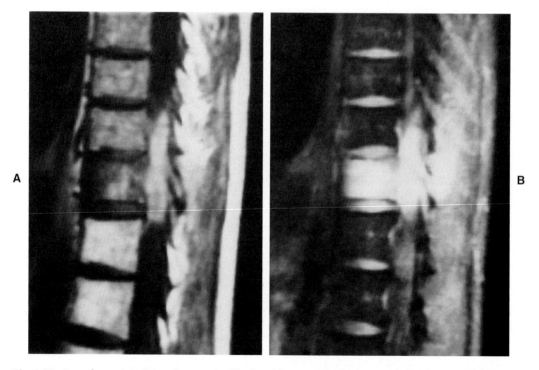

Fig. 5-23. Lymphoma involving the vertebral body with an epidural mass. **A,** Sagittal post-gadolinium T1-weighted image demonstrates an enhancing mass in the parasagittal region with an adjacent low signal vertebral body, which shows patchy enhancement. **B,** Sagittal fat-suppressed, post-gadolinium, T1-weighted image shows enhancement of the epidural mass and the involved vertebral body.

Disc Disease

Thoracic Disc Herniation. Thoracic disc herniations are the least common type of disc herniation. They constitute only about 0.3% of all symptomatic disc herniations. Most thoracic disc herniations are located at the T9-10, T10-11, and T11-12 levels where there is greater mobility of the thoracic spine. Thoracic herniated discs often show calcification.[131]

Disc herniations are associated with defects in the annulus fibrosus, which allows herniation of nuclear material through the defects. The annular defects are most commonly dorsal or dorsolateral, where the annulus fibrosus is thinner and the restraining posterior longitudinal ligament is weaker as compared to the anterior longitudinal ligament. In bulging discs the annulus fibrosus is intact. There are three types of herniated discs:

1. *Protrusion.* The displaced nuclear material remains attached to the nucleus pulposus and herniates through the annular defect, but is contained by the posterior longitudinal ligament. It presents as a small paracentral ventral epidural mass.
2. *Extrusion.* A more advanced protrusion produces a larger ventrolateral epidural mass that may extend above or below the level of disc space, yet is still contained to some degree by the posterior longitudinal ligament.
3. *Sequestration or free fragment.* The nuclear material becomes detached from the original nucleus pulposus and herniates through the annular defect to a position ventral or dorsal to the posterior longitudinal ligament. Migration of herniated nuclear material to a location dorsal to the posterior longitudinal ligament indicates ligamentous disruption. Free fragments may migrate above or below the affected disc space.

Myelography usually exhibits compression of the spinal cord, a nerve root, or both. CT may demonstrate obliteration of epidural fat, as in the lumbar area when sufficient fat is present. Herniated thoracic discs are more likely to be calcified than cervical and lumbar discs. CT without intrathecal contrast may be useful in detecting thoracic herniations, particularly when the disc is calcified. CT-myelography, however, is frequently needed to confirm the diagnosis of thoracic herniations.

MRI is the imaging modality of choice for the evaluation of thoracic disc herniations because anatomical detail can be obtained directly in multiple planes by a noninvasive technique. The entire spine can be imaged with MRI. Herniated disc material is usually of relatively low to intermediate signal on T1-weighted images and low, intermediate, or high signal on T2-weighted images, depending on the degree of hydration of the disc[20,122] (Fig. 5-24).

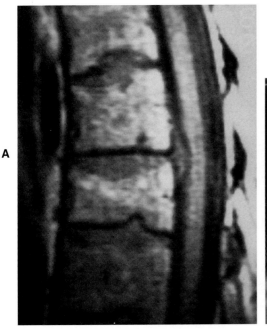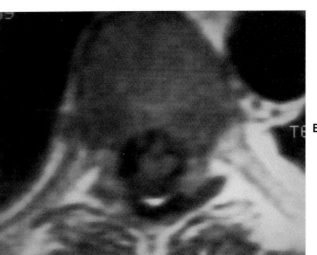

Fig. 5-24. Thoracic disc herniation. **A,** Sagittal T1-weighted image shows disc herniation at the T7-8 level with compression of the thoracic spinal cord. Slight compression of the T8 vertebral body is observed. **B,** Axial T1-weighted image demonstrates herniated disc fragments ventrally, with compression and dorsal displacement of the thoracic spinal cord.

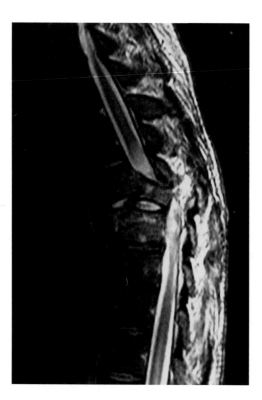
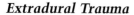

Fig. 5-25. Combined fracture and dislocation. Sagittal T2-weighted image shows combined fracture and dislocation of the spine and transection of the spinal cord.

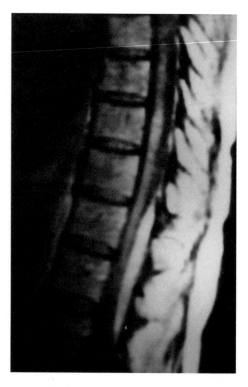

Fig. 5-26. Epidural hematoma. Sagittal T1-weighted image shows a dorsal extradural high signal intensity collection with mild compression of the thoracic spinal cord, consistent with a subacute epidural hematoma.

Extradural Trauma

Epidural hematomas, disc herniations, encroachment by parts of the osseous spine, and residual foreign bodies (usually metallic fragments from gun shot wounds) are common manifestations of trauma involving the extradural compartment.[122]

Thoracic vertebral body "burst" fractures can occur secondary to severe axial loading. Thoracic spine fractures are usually stable, unless multiple rib or sternal fractures are present.

Thoracolumbar junction fractures frequently occur between T12 and L2. The majority are compression fractures with ventral wedging of the vertebral bodies. The dorsal arches are usually intact. Only a minority of thoracolumbar injuries consist of combined fracture and dislocation[91] (Fig. 5-25).

Spinal epidural hematomas occur in conjunction with approximately 1% to 8% of spinal fractures. Because of the large number of veins in the epidural space, their disruption is a plausible cause. Some consider bleeding to be most likely to arise from higher pressure small and delicate arterial systems, due to the rapid progression of symptoms of spinal cord compression. Myelography and CT demonstrate nonspecific varying degrees of extradural compression of the thecal sac. MRI is the imaging modality of choice, as long segments of the spinal canal can be imaged in the sagittal plane (Fig. 5-26). MRI can localize the lesion and characterize it as a hematoma in different stages. The signal intensity of the hematoma varies depending on the presence of various blood by-products. The presence of bony encroachment upon the epidural space may result in pressure upon the spinal cord and/or nerve roots, producing myelopathy and/or radiculopathy.[52,132]

Extradural Infections

Epidural abscesses have increased in recent years, secondary to increased intravenous drug abuse and the increased sensitivity of detection by modern imaging modalities. Epidural abscesses may result from hematogenous spread or direct spread from paraspinal, osseous spinal, and disc space infections (Fig. 5-27). The average age reported has been in the mid sixties, with a range from childhood to the elderly. In light of the increased incidence of intra-

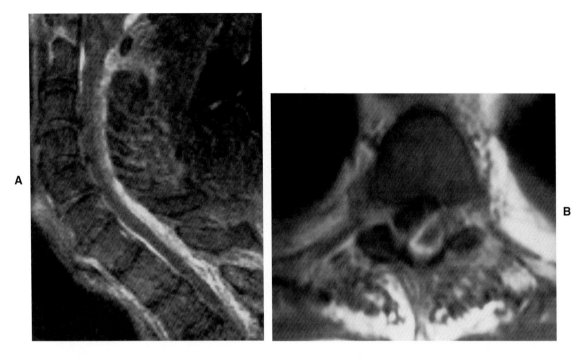

Fig. 5-27. Epidural abscess. **A,** Sagittal post-contrast, fat-suppressed image demonstrates extensive enhancement of the dorsal epidural space in the cervicothoracic region. **B,** Axial post-contrast, T1-weighted image shows an ovoid ring-like enhancement dorsally and on the left side with compression of the thoracic spinal cord.

venous drug use in the younger age group, the mean age is likely to decrease.

The most common causative organism is *Staphylococcus aureus* (62%). Tuberculous epidural abscesses are usually associated with tuberculous spondylitis (Fig. 5-28), but cases do occur where tuberculous spondylitis is not initially noted. MRI is superior to CT for the evaluation of epidural abscess. Myelography and CT-myelography may show blockage of the subarachnoid space or spinal cord compression by an epidural mass at the level of the abscess. MRI usually demonstrates epidural abscesses to be isointense to slightly hyperintense to CSF on both T1-weighted and T2-weighted sequences. Contrast-enhanced images may exhibit peripheral enhancement and diffuse homogeneous enhancement.[121,134]

Osseous Lesions

Metastasis. Metastatic disease is the most common malignant tumor of bone. Spinal metastatic disease most frequently involves the vertebral bodies, followed by the pedicles and neural arch.[2] Metastases to the spine are most frequently observed in the thoracic spine, followed by the lumbar spine.[1] The primary sites include breast, lung, prostate, kidney, lymphoma, and melanoma.[24,71,119]

Most metastases are osteolytic. Osteoblastic lesions occur with metastatic prostatic carcinoma, and less frequently with breast carcinoma. Spinal metastases begin with the replacement of fatty trabeculae.

MRI is more sensitive than plain radiographs, CT, or radionuclide bone scan for detecting early bony involvement in the spine. Metastases show hypointensity on T1-weighted images, as compared to the hyperintensity of normal bone marrow, and hyperintensity on T2-weighted images. Variable degrees of contrast enhancement are seen in bony metastases. Contrast enhancement may masquerade the lesion, making it isointense with normal bone marrow.[66] Metastatic disease is the most common epidural neoplasm.

Myeloma. Myeloma is a malignant tumor of bone marrow plasma cells.[105] The male to female ratio is 3:1 and the age of onset is usually at the fifth or sixth decade. The thoracic and lumbar spine are more frequently affected than the cervical spine and sacrum.[126] Multiple vertebral body involvement is commonly seen. Epidural disease is common. On imaging studies, multiple myeloma resembles metastatic disease.[88,126]

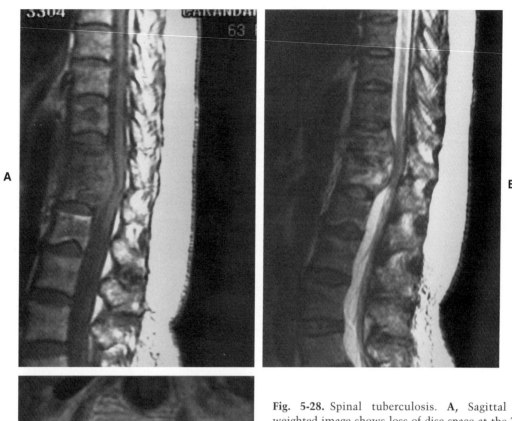

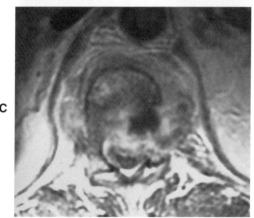

Fig. 5-28. Spinal tuberculosis. **A,** Sagittal T1-weighted image shows loss of disc space at the T11-12 level with abnormal tissue involving these two vertebral bodies, as well as ventral and dorsal tissue. The ventral epidural mass is compressing the spinal cord and displacing it dorsally. **B,** Sagittal T2-weighted image demonstrates the abnormal tissue to be of mixed high signal intensity. Loss of disc space and spinal cord compression are similar to *A.* **C,** Axial post-gadolinium, T1-weighted image shows abnormal enhancement of the paraspinal mass and a ventral epidural mass with bony destruction of the vertebral body.

Lymphoma. Osseous lymphoma may involve the bone marrow of the spine without significant epidural mass. Epidural lymphoma may result from osseous lymphoma or nonosseous lymphoma (from retroperitoneal lymph nodes). Intradural lymphoma probably results from hematogenous spread or spread via perineural lymphatics.

Hemangioma. Two histological types of hemangioma are described, cavernous and capillary. Cavernous hemangiomas are commonly found in the vertebrae. These lesions are composed of mature thin-walled vessels and large blood-filled, endothelial-lined spaces.[80,167]

The incidence of spinal hemangioma is about 10% at autopsy. Usually a single vertebral body is involved, but two or more vertebral bodies may be involved. Usually the body of the vertebra is involved, but dorsal arch involvement may also be seen. Vertical striped orientation of the bone is seen on plain radiographs or CT. The vertebral body may be enlarged.[40] High signal intensity is seen within the marrow on T1-weighted MRI due to the presence of fat and/or hemorrhage.[40,80] The cortical margin is usually intact. Occasionally, an aggressive hemangioma may be associated with cortical destruction and associated epidural mass. The differential diagnosis of an enlarged vertebral body on plain radiographs includes myeloma, lymphoma, Paget's disease, metastasis, and hemangioma.

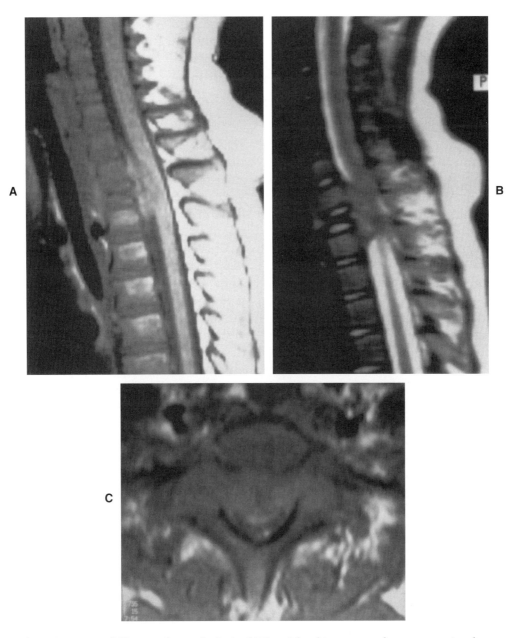

Fig. 5-29. Eosinophilic granuloma. **A,** Sagittal T1-weighted image reveals a compression fracture of the T2 vertebral body with a ventral epidural mass extending from T1 to T3. The spinal cord is compressed and displaced dorsally. **B,** Sagittal T2-weighted image demonstrates a compression fracture of the T2 vertebral body (vertebra plana) with a large ventral epidural mass. Compression of the thoracic spinal cord and obliteration of the subarachnoid space are obvious. **C,** Axial T1-weighted image shows an epidural and paraspinal mass at the ventral aspect of the spinal canal.

Langerhan's Histiocytosis. In Langerhan's histiocytosis, or eosinophilic granuloma, spinal lesions occur most commonly between the ages of 5 and 10 years. Destructive changes involve the vertebral body or pedicle without bony sclerosis. Collapse of the vertebral body results in vertebra plana. Associated paraspinal masses, which show intermediate signal on both T1-weighted and T2-weighted images may be seen (Fig. 5-29). Contrast enhancement is observed following the intravenous injection of gadolinium.[34] The differential diagnosis includes fracture, hemangioma, metastasis, myeloma, fracture secondary to steroid therapy, and Ewing's sarcoma.

Sickle Cell Disease. Loss of bone density and a coarsening of the trabecular pattern are observed on plain radiographs and CT. The spine exhibits a uniform biconcave contour of all the vertebral bodies (fish mouth vertebrae). The differential diagnosis includes Cushing's syndrome and steroid therapy. The spine in sickle cell patients is prone to salmonella osteomyelitis.

Osteoid Osteoma. Osteoid osteoma is an uncommon neoplasm of the spine and occurs in patients under the age of 30. Osteoid osteoma has a central nidus of interlacing osteoid and woven bone mixed with loose fibrovascular stroma.[70] The classical radiographic appearance is that of a small radiolucent intracortical nidus surrounded by a large sclerotic area of cortical thickening.[74] Approximately 10% of osteoid osteomas occur in the spine. In spinal osteoid osteoma the neural arch, spinous process, and transverse processes may be involved. The nidus of osteoid osteoma is low to intermediate in signal intensity on both T1-weighted and T2-weighted MRI.[165]

Osteoblastoma. Osteoblastoma is rare, accounting for about 1% of primary bone neoplasms. Patient age ranges from 5 to 50 years.[110] Approximately 40% of osteoblastomas occur in the spine. The most common location is the vertebral arch, mainly in the transverse and spinous processes. About 50% of cases have associated vertebral body involvement as well. A well-circumscribed, expansile bone lesion arising from the neural arch is observed. About one half of spinal osteoblastomas are predominantly lucent and the other half show varying degrees of matrix mineralization. MRI shows intermediate signal on T1-weighted images and mixed high signal on T2-weighted images.[139]

Aneurysmal Bone Cyst. Approximately 20% of these cysts are found in the spine, with a predilection for the cervical and thoracic spine. The bone lesion is characterized by a blown-out cortical appearance that typically involves the vertebral body, vertebral arch, or the spinous or transverse processes of the spine.[31,106] Vertebral involvement exhibits an expanding trabeculated lesion that may extend along the spine to involve several adjacent vertebral bodies with a large soft tissue mass. CT is better for demonstrating the thin shell of expanded bone. CT and MRI can both demonstrate the soft tissue mass, which is usually of mixed hypo- and hyperintensity on both T1-weighted and T2-weighted images. Fluid levels and blood degradation products may be seen.[106]

Giant Cell Tumor. Giant cell tumors of the spine are rare (3%). Approximately half of spinal giant cell tumors occur in the sacrum. Spinal giant cell tumors tend to occur earlier than those at other sites and have a peak incidence in the second and third decades. The female to male ratio for spinal lesions is 2:1. Involvement of the spine occurs at the vertebral body and the neural arch. A paravertebral mass may be observed. Radiographically they can mimic aneurysmal bone cysts.[5]

Chordoma. Chordomas can occur at any age, but the peak incidence is in the sixth decade.[136] They are rare, slow-growing malignant bone tumors that are locally invasive. Common locations include sacrococcygeal (50%), clivus (35%), and vertebral body (15%). Bone destruction with soft tissue mass usually occurs. The intervertebral disc may or may not be involved. Amorphous calcification and residual bone are better detected by CT. Chordomas have a low signal intensity on T1-weighted images and a high signal intensity on T2-weighted images.[148] Chordomas enhance variably with gadolinium.

Ewing's Sarcoma. Ewing's sarcoma has a peak incidence in the second decade, and there is a male predominance. Ewing's sarcoma of the spine is often a metastatic disease. It is an ill-defined, permeative destructive lesion of vertebral bodies, often associated with a paraspinal mass. Collapse of the vertebral body may also be seen. Differential diagnosis includes osteomyelitis and Langerhan's histiocytosis.

Chondrosarcoma. Chondrosarcomas occur predominantly in adults over 40 years. They are osteolytic expansile lesions with amorphous calcification. The spine is only occasionally involved and the dorsal elements may become involved. Chondrosarcomas may develop in pre-existing cartilaginous lesions or in association with Paget's disease or previous radiation.

Osteogenic Sarcoma. Cortical destruction, associated with sclerotic changes and soft tissue invasion, occur with osteogenic sarcoma. The vertebral body or neural arch may also be involved. Osteogenic sarcomas may be associated with pre-existing osteochondroma, Paget's disease, and previous radiation.

REFERENCES

1. Algra PR, Bloem JL, Tissing H, et al. Detection of vertebral metastases: Comparison between MR imaging and bone scintigraphy. Radiographics 11:219-232, 1991.
2. Algra PR, Hermans JJ, Valk J, et al. Do metastases in vertebrae begin in the body or pedicles? Imaging study in 45 patients. Am J Roentgenol 158:1275-1279, 1992.
3. Anson JA, Spetzler RF. Classification of spinal arteriovenous malformations and implications for treatment. BNI Quarterly 8:2-8, 1992.
4. Anson JA, Spetzler RF. Surgical resection of intramedullary spinal cord cavernous malformations. J Neurosurg 78:446-451, 1993.
5. Aoki J, Moriya K, Yamashita K, et al. Giant cell tumors of bone containing large amounts of hemosiderin: MR pathologic correlation. J Comput Assist Tomogr 15:1024-1027, 1991.
6. Araki Y, Ishida T, Ootani M, et al. MRI of paraganglioma of the cauda equina. Neuroradiology 35:232-233, 1993.
7. Augenstein HM, Sze G, Becker R. Imaging of spinal meningiomas. In Al-Mefty O, ed. Meningiomas. New York: Raven Press, 1991, pp 603-613.
8. Austin SG, Zee CS, Waters C. The role of magnetic resonance imaging in acute transverse myelitis. Can J Neurol Sci 19:508-511, 1992.
9. Avila NA, Shawker TH, Choyke PL, et al. Cerebellar and spinal hemangioblastomas: Evaluation with intraoperative gray-scale and color Doppler flow US. Radiology 188:43-147, 1993.
10. Awwad EE, Backer R, Archer CR. The imaging of an intraspinal cervical dermoid tumor by MR, CT and sonography. Comput Radiol 11:169, 1987.
11. Barakos JA, Mark AS, Dillon WP, et al. MR imaging of acute transverse myelitis and AIDS myelopathy. J Comput Assist Tomogr 14:45, 1990.
12. Barkovich AJ, Edwards MSB, Cogen PH. MR evaluation of spinal dermal sinus tracts in children. Am J Neuroadiol 12:123-129, 1991.
13. Barkovich AJ, Naidich TP. Congenital anomalies of the spine. In Barkovich AJ, Pediatric Neuroimaging. New York: Raven Press, 1990, pp 227-271.
14. Bartels RH, deJong TR, Grotenhuis JA. Spinal subdural abscess. J Neurosurg 76:307-311, 1992.
15. Bates D, Ruggieri P. Imaging modalities for evaluation of the spine. Radiol Clin North Am 29:675-690, 1991.
16. Bates DJ. Inflammatory disease of the spine. Neuroimaging Clin N Am 1:231, 1991.
17. Berman M, Feldman S, Alter M, et al. Acute transverse myelitis: Incidence and stiologic considerations. Neurology 31:966, 1981.
18. Beuls E, Gelan J, Vandersteen M, et al. Microanatomy of the excised human spinal cord and the corticomedullary junction examined with high resolution MR imaging at 9.4 Tesla. AJNR 14:699-704, 1993.
19. Biondi A, Merland JJ, Hodes JE, et al. Aneurysms of spinal arteries associated with intramedullary arteriovenous malformations. I. Angiographic and clinical aspects. AJNR 13:913-922, 1992.
20. Blaser SI, Modic MT. Herniation of the intervertebral disc. Top Magn Reson Imaging 1:25, 1988.
21. Bradley W. Intracranial hemorrhage. In Zee CS, ed. Neuroradiology: A Study Guide. New York: McGraw-Hill (in press).
22. Brooks BS, Dural ER, El Gammal T, et al. Neuroimaging features of neurenteric cysts: Analysis of nine cases and review of the literature. AJNR 14:735-746, 1993.
23. Brophy JD, Sutton LN, Zimmerman RA, et al. Magnetic resonance imaging of lipomyelomeningocele and tethered cord. Neurosurgery 25:336-340, 1989.
24. Byrne TN. Spinal cord compression from epidural metastases. N Engl J Med 327:614-619, 1992.
25. Castaneda-Zuniga WR, Sanchez R, Amplatz K. Experimental observations on short- and long-term effects of arterial occlusion with Ivalon. Radiology 126:783-785, 1978.
26. Chamberlain MC, Sandy AS, Press GA. Spinal tumors: Gadolinium-DPTA enhanced MR imaging. Neuroradiology 33:469-474, 1991.
27. Chang KH, Han MH, Choi YW, Kim OI, et al. Tubercolous arachnoiditis of the spine: Findings on myelography, CT and MR imaging. AJNR 10:1255, 1989.
28. Chaparro MJ, Young FR, Smith M, et al. Multiple meningiomas. Neurosurgery 32:298-302, 1993.
29. Cheung Y, Fung C, Chan F, Leong L. MRI features of spinal ganglioglioma. Clin Imaging 15:109, 1991.
30. Cohen MS, Wall EG, Brown RA, et al. Cauda equina anatomy II: Extrathecal nerve roots and dorsal root ganglia. Spine 15:1248-1251, 1990.
31. Cory DA, Fritsch SA, Cohen MD, et al. Aneurysmal bone cysts: Imaging findings and embolotherapy. AJR 153:99-101, 1989.
32. Criscuolo GR, Oldfield EH, Doppman JL. Reversible acute and subacute myelopathy in patients with arteriovneous fistulas: Foix-Alajouanin syndrome reconsidered. J Neurosurg 70:354, 1989.
33. Delamater RB, Ross JS, Masaryk TJ, et al. Diagnosis of lumbar arachnoiditis by magnetic resonance imaging. Spine 15:304, 1990.
34. De Shepper AMA, Ramon F, Van Marck E. MR imaging of eosinophilic granuloma: Report of 11 cases. Skeletal Radiol 22:163-166, 1993.
35. DiChiro G, Doppman J, Ommaya AK. Selective arteriography of arteriovenous aneurysms of spinal cord. Radiology 88:1065, 1967.
36. Djindjian R. Angiography of the spinal cord. Surg Neurol 2:179-185, 1974.
37. Djindjian R. Vascular malformation. In Shapiro R, Myelography, 4th ed. Chicago: Year Book Medical Publishers, 1984, pp 318-344.
38. Doppman JL. Epidural lipomatosis. Radiology 171:581-582, 1989.
39. Dormont D, Assouline E, Gelbert F, et al. MRI study of spinal arteriovenous malformations. J Neuroradiol 14:351, 1987.
40. Dorwart RH, LaMasters DL, Watanabe TJ. Tumors. In Newton TH, Potts DG, eds. Computed Tomography of the Spine and Spinal Cord. San Anselmo, Calif.: Clavadel Press 1983, pp 115-147.
41. Edwards MK, Farlow MR, Stevens JC. Cranial MR in spinal cord MS: Diagnosing patients with isolated spinal cord symptoms. AJNR 7:1003,1986.
42. El-Khoury GY, Whitten CG. Trauma to the upper thoracic spine: Anatomy, biomechanics, and unique imaging features. AJR 160:95-102, 1993.
43. Epstein FJ, Farmer JP, Freed D. Adult intramedullary astocytomas of the spinal cord. J Neurosurg 77:355-359, 1992.
44. Fessler RG, Johnson DL, Brown FD, et al. Epidural lipomatosis in steroid treated patients. Spine 17:183-188, 1992.

45. Fontaine S, Melanson D, Cosgrove R, et al. Cavernous hemangiomas of the spinal cord: MR imaging. Radiology 166:839, 1991.

46. Fredericks RK, Elster A, Walker FO. Gadolinium enhanced MRI: A superior technique for the diagnosis of intraspinal metastases. Neurology 39:734, 1989.

47. Friedman DP. Herpes zoster myelitis: MR appearance. AJNR 13:1404, 1992.

48. Friedman DP, Flanders AE. Enhancement of gray matter in anterior spinal infarction. AJNR 13:983-985, 1992.

49. Friedman DP, Tartaglino LM, Flanders AE. Intradural schwannomas of the spine: MR findings with emphasis on contrast enhancement characteristics. AJR 158:1347-1350, 1992.

50. Gero B, Sze G, Sharit HS. MR imaging of intradural inflammatory disease of the spine. AJNR 12:1009,1991.

51. Graham DV, Tampieri D, Villemure J. Intramedullary epidermoid tumor diagnosed with the assistance of magnetic resonance imaging. Neurosurgery 23:765, 1988.

52. Gundy CR, Heithoff KB. Epidural hematoma of the lumbar spine: 18 surgically confirmed cases. Radiology 187:427, 1993.

53. Hackney DB, Asato R, Joseph PM, et al. Hemorrhage and edema in acute spinal cord injury: Demonstration by MR imaging. Radiology 161:387, 1987.

54. Hajek PC, Baker LL, Goolar JE, et al. Focal fat deposition in axial bone marrow: MR characteristics. Radiology 162:245-249, 1987.

55. Halbach VV, Higashida RT, Dowd CF, et al. Treatment of giant intradural (perimedullary) arteriovenous fistulas. Neurosurgery 33:972-980, 1993.

56. Halliday AL, Sobel, Martuza RL. Benign spinal nerve sheath tumors: Their occurrence sporadically and in neurofibromatosis types 1 and 2. J Neurosurg 74:248, 1991.

57. Haughton VM, Syverston A, Williams AL. Soft anatomy within the spinal canal as seen on computed tomography. Radiology 134:649-655, 1980.

58. Helms CA, Vogler JB III. Spinal stenosis and degenerative lesions. In Newton TH, Potts PG, eds. Modern Neuroradiology, vol 1. Computed Tomography of the Spine and Spinal Cord, 251-266, 1983.

59. Hilal SK, Marton D, Pollack E. Diastematomyelia in children: Radiographic study of 34 cases. Radiology 112:609-621, 1974.

60. Hirono H, Yamadori A, Komiyama M, et al. MRI of spontaneous spinal cord infarction: Serial changes in gadolinium-DPTA enhancement. Neuroradiology 34:95-97, 1992.

61. Ho PS, Yu S, Sether LA, et al. Ligamentum flavum: Appearance on sagittal and coronal MR images. Radiology 168:469-472, 1988.

62. Hu HP, Huang QL. Signal intensity correlation of MRI with pathological findings in spinal neurinomas. Neuroradiology 34(2):98-102, 1992.

63. Isu T, Iwasaki Y, Akino M, Abe H. Hydromyelia associated with Chiari I malformation in children and adults. Neurosurgery 26:591-597, 1990.

64. Johnson CE, Sze G. Benign lumbar arachnoiditis: MR imaging with gadopentetate dimeglumine. AJNR 11:763-770, 1990.

65. Jorgensen J, Hanson PH, Steenskov V, Ovesen N. A clinical and radiological study of lower spinal arachnoiditis. Neuroradiology 9:139, 1975.

66. Kamholtz R, Sze G. Current imaging in spinal metastatic disease. Semin Oncol 18:158-169, 1991.

67. Kattenberger DA, Shah CP, Shah CP, et al. MR imaging of spinal cord hemangioblastoma associated with syringomyelia. J Comput Assist Tomogr 12:495-498, 1988.

68. Kerslake RW, Jaspan T, Worthington BS. Magnetic resonance imaging of spinal trauma. Br J Radiol 64:386, 1991.

69. Kjos BO, Norman D. Strategies for efficient imaging of the lumbar spine. In Bratzawaski M, Norman D, eds. Magnetic Resonance Imaging of the Central Nervous System. New York: Raven Press, 1987, pp 279-287.

70. Klein MH, Shankman S. Osteoid Osteoma: Radiologic and pathologic correlation. Skeletal Radiol 21:23-31, 1991.

71. Klein SL, Sanford RA, Muhlbauer MS. Pediatric spinal epidural metastases. J Neurosurg 74:70-75, 1991.

72. Kolkarni MV, McArdle CB, Kopanicky D, et al. Acute spinal cord injury: MR imaging at 1.5 T. Radiology 164:837, 1987.

73. Kramer ED, Rafto S, Packer RJ, et al. Comparison of myelography with CT follow-up versus gadolinium MRI for subarachnoid metastatic disease in children. Neurology 41(1):46-50, 1991.

74. Kransdorf MJ, Stull MA, Gilkey FW, et al. Osteoid osteoma. Radiographics 11:671-696, 1991.

75. Krol G, Sze G, Malkin M, et al. MR of cranial and spinal meningeal carcinomatosis: Comparison with CT and myelography. AJR 151:583-588, 1988.

76. Krudy AG. MR myelography using heavily T2-weighted fast spin echo pulse sequences with fat presaturation. AJR 159:1315-1320, 1992.

77. Laakman RW. Arachnoiditis, thoracic arachnoiditis with syrinx formation. In St. Amour TE, Hodges SC, Laakman RW, et al. MRI of the Spine. New York: Raven Press, 1994, pp 263-276.

78. Labischong P, et al. Normal anatomy of the spine, spinal cord and nerve roots. In Manelfe E, ed. Imaging of the Spine and Spinal Cord. New York: Raven Press, 1992, pp 1-91.

79. LaMasters DL, deGroot J, Haughton VM, et al. Normal thoracic spine. In Newton TH, Potts DG, eds. Computed Tomography of the Spine and Spinal Cord. San Anselmo, Calif.: Clavadel Press, 1983, pp 79-91.

80. Laredo JD, Assouline E, Gelbert F, et al. Vertebral hemangiomas: Fat content as a sign of aggressiveness. Radiology 177:467-472, 1990.

81. Larsson EM, Desai P, Hardin CW, et al. Venous infarction of the spinal cord resulting from dural arteriovenous fistula: MR imaging findings. AJNR 12:739, 1991.

82. Larson TC, Houser OW, Onofrio BM, et al. Primary spinal melanoma. J Neurosurgery 66:47, 1987..

83. Larsson EM, Holtas S, Nilsson O. Gd-DPTA enhanced MR of suspected spinal multiple sclerosis. AJNR 10:1071-1076, 1989

84. Latchaw RE, Harris RD, Chou SN, et al. Combined embolization and operation in the treatment of cervical arteriovenous malformations. Neurosurgery 6:131-137,1980.

85. Lee BC, Kazam E, Newman AD. Computed tomography of the spine and spinal cord. Radiology 128:95-102, 1978.

86. Lee HJ, Bansil S, Cook SD, et al. MRI of the spine in multiple sclerosis. J Neuroimaging 2:61, 1992.

87. Levy RA. Paraganglioma of the filum terminale: MR findings. AJR 160:851-852, 1993.

88. Libshitz HI, Malthouse SR, Cunningham D, et al. Multiple myeloma: Appearance at MR imaging. Radiology 182:833-837, 1992.

89. Li MH, Holtas S, Larsson EM. MR imaging of intradural extramedullary tumors. Acta Radiol 33:207-212, 1992.

90. Lyons MK, O'Neill BP, March WR, et al. Primary spinal epidural non-Hodgkin's lymphoma: Report of eight patients and review of the literature. Neurosurgery 30:675-680, 1992.

91. Manaster BJ. Skeletal Radiology. Chicago: Year Book Medical Publishers, 1989, pp 264-279.

92. Maravilla KR, Weinrob JC, Suss RA, et al. Magnetic resonance demonstration of multiple sclerosis plaques in the cervical cord. AJNR 5:685-689, 1984.

93. Mark AS. Nondegenerative, non-neoplastic disease of the spine and spinal cord. In Atlas SW, ed. Magnetic Resonance Imaging of the Brain and Spine. New York: Raven Press, 1991, pp. 967-1011.

94. Masaryk TJ, Ross JS, Modic MT, et al. Radiculomeningeal vascular malformations of the spine: MR imaging. Radiology 164:845-849, 1987.

95. Mascalchi M, Arnetoli G, Dal Pozzo G, et al. Spinal epidural angiolipoma: MR findings. AJNR 12:744-745, 1991.

96. Matsumoto S, Hasu K, Uchino A, et al. MRI of intradural extramedullary spinal neuromas and meningiomas. Clin Imaging 17:46-52, 1993.

97. Matsumura AA, Meguro K, Tsurushima H, et al. Magnetic resonance imaging of spinal cord injury without radiologic abnormality. Surg Neurol 33:281, 1990.

98. McCormick PC, Torres R, Post KD, et al. Intramedullary ependymoma of the spinal cord. J Neurosurg 62:523-532, 1990.

99. Mendelsohn DB, Zollars L, Weatherall PT, et al. MR of cord transection. J Comput Assist Tomogr 14:909, 1990.

100. Merland JJ, Riche MC, Chiras J. Intraspinal extramedullary arteriovenous fistulae draining into the medullary veins. J Neuroradiol 7:271-320, 1980.

101. Michikawa M, Wada Y, Sano M, et al. Radiation myelopathy: Significance of gadolinium DTPA enhancement in the diagnosis. Neuroradiology 33:286-289, 1991.

102. Mikulis DJ, Ogilvy CS, McKee A, et al. Spinal cord infarction and fibrocartilagenous emboli. AJNR 13:155-160, 1992.

103. Modic MT, Steinberg PM, Ross JS, et al. Degenerative disk disease: Assessment of changes in vertebral body marrow with MR imaging. Radiology 166:193-199, 1988.

104. Moufarruj NA, Palmer JM, Hahn JF, et al. Correlation between magnetic resonance imaging and surgical findings in the tethered spinal cord. Neurosurgery 25:341-346, 1989.

105. Moulopoulos LA, Varma DGK, Dimopoulos MA, et al. Multiple myeloma: Spinal MR imaging in patients with untreated newly diagnosed disease. Radiology 185:833-840, 1992.

106. Munk PL, Helms CA, Holt RG, et al. MR imaging of aneurysmal bone cyst. AJR 153:99-101, 1989.

107. Murota T, Symon L. Surgical management of hemangioblastomas of the spinal cord: A report of 18 cases. Neurosurgery 25:699-708, 1989.

108. Nabors MW, Pait TG, Byrd EB, et al. Updated assessment and current classification of spinal meningeal cysts. J Neurosurg 68:366, 1988.

109. Naidich TP, McLane DG, Harwood-Nash DC. Arachnoid cysts, paravertebral meningoceles and perineurial cysts. In Newton TH, Potts DG, eds. Modern Neuroradiology, vol 1. Computed Tomography of the Spine and Spinal Cord. San Anselmo, Calif.: Clavadel Press, 1983, pp 383-396.

110. Nemoto O, Moser RP Jr, Van Dam DE, et al. Osteoblastoma of the spine: A review of 75 cases. Spine 15:1272-1280, 1990.

111. Nichols DA, Rufenacht DA, Jack CR Jr, et al. Embolization of spinal dural arteriovenous fistula with polyvinyl alcohol particles: Experience in 14 patients. AJNR 13:933-940, 1992.

112. Ogilvy CS, Louis DN, Ojemann RG. Intramedullary cavernous angiomas of the spinal cord: Clinical presentation, patholoica features, and surgical management. J Neurosurg 31:219-230, 1992.

113. Okumra R, Minami S, Asato R, Konishi J. Fatty filum terminale: Assessment with MR imaging. J Comput Assist Tomogr 14:571-573, 1990.

114. Oller DW, Boone S. Blunt cervical spine Brown-Sequard injury. A report of three cases. Am Surg 57(6):361, 1991.

115. Osborn AG. Diagnostic Neuroradiology. St. Louis: Mosby Yearbook, 1994.

116. Osborn AG, Harnsberger HR, Smoker WRK, et al. Multiple sclerosis in adolescents: CT and MR findings. AJNR 12:521-524, 1990.

117. Pagni C, Canavero S. Spinal epidural lipoma: Rare or unreported? Neurosurgery 31:758-764, 1992.

118. Pang D, Dias MS, Ahab-Barmada M. Split cord malformation. I. A unified theory of embryogenesis for double spinal cord malformations. Neurosurgery 31:451-480, 1992.

119. Perry JR, Deodhare SS, Bilbao JM, et al. The significance of spinal cord compression as the initial manifestation of lymphoma. Neurosurgery 32:157-162, 1993.

120. Post MJ, et al. The value of computed tomography in spinal trauma. Spine 7:417-431, 1982.

121. Post MJD, Sze G, Quencher RM, et al. Gadolinium enhanced MR in spinal infection. J Comput Assist Tomogr 14:721, 1990.

122. Pratt ES, Green DA, Spengler DM. Herniated intervertebral disks associated with unstable spine injuries. Spine 15:662, 1990.

123. Preul MC, Leblanc R, Tampieri D. Spinal angiolipomas: Report of three cases. J Neurosurg 78:280-286, 1993.

124. Quint DJ, Boulos RS, Sanders WP, et al. Epidural lipomatosis. Radiology 169:485-492, 1988.

125. Raghavan N, Barkovich AJ, Edwards M, Norman D. MR imaging in the tethered spinal cord syndrome. AJR 152:843-852, 1989.

126. Rahmouni A, Divine M, Mathieu D, et al. Detection of multiple myeloma involving the spine: Efficiency of fat-suppression and contrast enhanced MR imaging. AJR 160:1049-1052, 1993.

127. Raub LW, Drayer BP. Spinal computed tomography: Limitation and application. AJR 133:267-273, 1979.

128. Resjo IM, Fitz CR, Chuang S, et al. Normal cord in infants examined with computed tomographic metrizamide myelography. Radiology 130:691-696, 1979.

129. Rosenbloom S. Thoracic disc disease and stenosis. Radiol Clin North Am 29:765-775, 1991.

130. Rosenblum B, Oldfield EH, Doppman JL, et al. Spinal arteriovenous malformation: A comparison of dural arteriovenous fistulas and intradural AVMs in 81 patients. J Neurosurg 67:795-802, 1987.

131. Ross JS, Perez-Reyes N, Masaryk TJ, et al. Thoracic disk herniation: MR imaging. Radiology 165:511-515, 1987.

132. Rothfus WE, Chedid, MK, Deeb ZL, et al. MR imaging in the diagnosis of spontaneous spinal epidural hematomas. J Comput Assist Tomogr 11:851, 1987.

133. Roux A, Mercier C, Labrisseau A, et al. Intramedullary epidermoid cysts of the spinal cord. J Neurosurg 76:528, 1992.

134. Sandhu FS, Dillon WP. Spinal epidural abscess: Evaluation with contrast enhanced MR imaging. AJNR 12:1087-1093, 1991.

135. Scotti G, Righi C, Campi A. Myelitis and myelopathies. Riv di Neuroradiol 5 (Suppl 2):49-52, 1992.

136. Sebag G, Dubois J, Beniaminovitz A, et al. Extraosseous spinal chordoma: Radiographic appearance. AJNR 14:204-207, 1993.

137. Sharif HS. Role of MR imaging in the management of spinal infections. AJR 158:1333-1345, 1992.

138. Sherman JL, Barkovich AJ, Citrin CM. The MR appearance of syringomyelia: New observations. AJNR 7:985-995, 1986.

139. Skylawer R, Osborn RE, Kerber CW, et al. Magnetic resonance imaging of vertebral osteoblastoma: A report of two cases. Surg Neurol 34:421-426, 1990.

140. Slasky BS, Bydder GM, Niendorf HP, Young IR. MR imaging with gadolinium-DTPA in the differentiation of tumor, syrinx, and cyst in the spinal cord. J Comput Assist Tomogr 11:845-850, 1987.

141. Sloof JL, Kernohan JW, MacCarty CS. Primary Intramedullary Tumors of the Spinal Cord and Filum Terminale. Philadelphia: WB Saunders, 1964.

142. Solero CL, Fornari M, Giombini S, et al. Spinal meningiomas: Review of 174 operated cases. Neurosurgery 25:153-160, 1989.

143. Solsberg MD, Lemaire C, Resch L, Potts DG. High resolution MR imaging of the cadaveric human spinal cord: Normal anatomy. AJNR 11:3-77, 1990.

144. Suh TH, Alexander L. Vascular system of the human spinal cord. Arch Neurol Psychol 41:659-677, 1939.

145. Symon L, Kuyama H, Kendall B. Dural ateriorvenous malformations of the spine: clinical features and surgical results in 55 cases. J Neurosurg 60:238, 1984.

146. Sze G. MR imaging of the spinal cord: Current status and future advances, AJR 159:149-159,1992.

147. Sze G, Stimac GK, Bartlett C, et al. Multicenter study of gadopentetate dimeglumine as an MR contrast agent: Evaluation in patients with spinal tumors. AJNR 11:967, 1990.

148. Sze G, Vichanxo LS II, Brant-Zawadski MN, et al. Chordomas: MR imaging. Radiology 166:187-191, 1988.

149. Takahashi M, Shimomura O, Sakal T. Comparison of magnetic resonance imaging with myelography and computed tomography—myelography in the diagnosis of lumbar disk herniation. NICNA (3):487-498, 1993.

150. Takahashi S, Yamada T, Ishii K, et al. MRI of anterior spinal artery syndrome of the cervical spinal cord. Neuroradiology 35:25-29, 1992.

151. Tamas DE. Trauma. In Amour TE, Hodges SC, Laakman RW, Tamas, eds. MRI of the Spine. New York: Raven Press, 1994, pp 543-592.

152. Tan RW, et al. MR imaging of recent spinal trauma. J Comput Assist Tomogr 11:412-417, 1987.

153. Taylor AJ, Haughton VM, Doust BD. CT imaging of the thoracic lumbar spinal cord without intrathecal contrast medium. J Comput Assist Tomogr 4:223-224, 1980.

154. Teal J. Lesions involving the spinal cord and nerve roots. In Zee CS, ed. Neuroradiology: A Study Guide. New York: McGraw-Hill (in press).

155. Theron J, Cosgrove R, Melanson D, Ethier R. Spinal arteriovenous malformations: Advances in therapeutic embolization. Radiology 158:163-169, 1986.

156. Truex RC, Carpenter MB. Human Neuroanatomy, 6th ed. Baltimore: Williams and Wilkins, 1969.

157. Varma DGK, Moulopoulos A, Sarat, et al. MR imaging of extracranial nerve sheath tumors. J Comput Assist Tomogr 16:448-453, 1992.

158. Viraponse C, Kier EL. Trauma to the spinal cord and nerve roots. In Shapiro R. Myelography, 4th ed. Chicago: Year Book Medical Publishers, 1984, pp 247-281.

159. Wall EJ, Cohen MS, Massie JB, et al. Cauda equina anatomy. I. Intrathecal nerve root organization. Spine 15:1244-1247, 1990.

160. Wang AM, Morris JH, Fischer EG, et al. Cavernous hemangioma of the thoracic spinal cord. Neuroradiology 30:261, 1988.

161. Wang PY, Shen WC, Jan JS. MR imaging in radiation myelopathy. AJNR 13:1049-1055, 1992.

162. Weisz GM, Lamond TS, Kitchener PN. Spinal imaging: Will MRI replace myelography? Spine 13:65-68, 1988.

163. Wolpert SM. Appropriate window settings for CT anatomic measurements. Radiology 132:775, 1980.

164. Wood BP, Harwood-Nash DC, Berger P, et al. Intradural spinal lipoma of the cervical cord. AJNR 6:452, 1985.

165. Wood ER, Martel W, Mandell SH, et al. Reactive soft tissue mass associated with osteoid osteoma: Correlation of MR imaging features with pathologic findings. Radiology 186:221-225, 1993.

166. Yamaski T, Kikuchi H, Yamashita J, et al. Primary spinal intramedullary malignant melanoma: Case report. Neurosurgery 25:117, 1989.

167. Yochum TR, Lile RL, Schultz GD, et al. Acquired spinal stenosis secondary to an expanding thoracic vertebral hemangioma. Spine 18:299-305, 1993.

168. Yoshizumi K, Sakamoto Y, Korogi Y, et al. Comparison of MRI, CT and myelography in the diagnosis of lumbar disc disease. Neuroradiology 33:337-339, 1991.

169. Yu S, Haughton VM, Lynch KL, et al. Fibrous structure in the intervertebral disk: Correlation of MR appearance with anatomic sections. AJNR 10:1105-1110, 1989.

170. Yuh WTC, March EE, Wang AK, et al. MR imaging of spinal cord and vertebral body infarction. AJNR 13:145-154, 1992.

171. Zatz LM. Basic principle of computed tomography scanning. In Newton TH, Potts DG, eds. Radiology of the Skull and Brain: Technical Aspects of Computed Tomography, vol 5. St. Louis: CV Mosby, 1981, pp 3853-3876.

172. Zawin JK, Jaramillo D. Conversion of bone marrow in the humerus, sternum, and clavicle: Changes with age on MR images. Radiology 188:159-164, 1993.

173. Zee CS, Segall HD, Terk MR, et al. J. SPIR MRI of spine diseases. J Comput Assist Tomogr 16:356-360, 1992.

174. Zweig G, Russell EJ. Radiation myelopathy of the cervical spinal cord: MR Findings. AJNR 11:1188-1190.

Intraoperative and Perioperative Management

Anesthetic Management

Steven Haddy, M.D., Stephen N. Steen, Sc.D., M.D.
and Vladimir Zelman, M.D., Ph.D.

When the elephants fight, the grass suffers.
—Old African proverb

Successful anesthesia for thoracic spine surgery requires a working knowledge of both cardiothoracic- and neurophysiology. While neurosurgeons frequently engage thoracic surgeons to expose the ventral spine, one anesthesiologist usually must perform both thoracic- and neuroanesthesia functions. In addition, the problems involved in managing unstable cervical spines require facility with specialized airway techniques. In the final analysis, close cooperation between the surgical and anesthesia staffs is the path to assure a successful outcome in these complex and challenging patients. If this harmony is not achieved only the patient suffers, as does the grass under the elephants' feet.

Various methods of treating spinal pathology have been in practice since the time of Hippocrates. During the past 30 years the surgical management of these conditions was via the dorsal approach. Since the 1970s, the ventral approach to the thoracic spine has gained wide acceptance.

PREOPERATIVE EVALUATION

Diagnostic evaluation of the stability of the spine itself and the corrective measures necessary is beyond the scope of this chapter. Obviously, close cooperation and communication with the surgeon(s) involved is critical for the success of the surgery and the safety of the patient. Specific factors that need to be considered include:

1. The position of the patient (prone vs. lateral)
2. The side that the thoracic approach will traverse
3. The stability of the spine (especially important in cases of combined cervical and thoracic pathology) that may require special techniques of airway management
4. The specific cause of the pathology (congenital, malignant, infectious, degenerative, or traumatic)
5. The cardiorespiratory system (the increased degree of curvature may warrant a transthoracic approach, necessitating one-lung ventilation [OLV]; such anesthetized patients with scoliosis are at greater risk for cardiopulmonary complications)

NEURODIAGNOSTIC PROCEDURES

Difficulties may arise during neurodiagnostic procedures due to space and equipment limitations. However, these constraints do not alter the standard of care. Monitoring for sedation and general anesthesia must be equal to that provided in other areas of the hospital.

Magnetic Resonance Imaging

The strong magnetic field generated by magnetic resonance imaging (MRI) presents special problems for the anesthesiologist. Equipment made of ferromagnetic materials may operate improperly or interfere with the imaging technique. The magnetic field may take several minutes to dissipate after the machine is turned off; should the patient require urgent attention (e.g., resuscitation) ". . . beepers, hemostats, and laryngoscopes may become unwieldy or ballistic."[129] Non-MRI-specific equipment must be at least 5 meters from the magnet.[150] There is currently no MRI-compatible anesthesia ventilator, although some of the standard ventilators may be acceptable. The use of spontaneous, assisted, or controlled ventilation using a bag and circuit is an acceptable approach should general anesthesia be required.

The Ohmeda Excel MRI anesthesia machine has been specifically designed for use in this environment. Vaporizers have little ferromagnetic material and are generally safe and accurate. Total intravenous anesthesia (TIVA) is another option if an MRI-compatible anesthesia machine is not available. Monitoring of ventilation must take into account the increased volume of compression caused by using long breathing hoses. This can be minimized by using low-compression tubing. Some aspects of ventilation can be monitored by capnography, but the long sampling tube necessary may distort the waveform if a side-stream analyzer is used.

Pulse oximeters can cause interference with the image and the magnetic field can render it inaccurate, but special units are MRI-compatible. The ECG may be distorted by the field, causing peaked T waves.[110]

Computed Tomography

Computed tomography (CT) presents fewer monitoring and equipment problems, but poses a radiation hazard to medical personnel who must remain in the immediate area. Although monitoring standards are supposed to be equivalent to those practiced in the operating room, studies indicate that this may not be the case.[79] Numerous sedative cocktails are used by radiology personnel, especially for pediatric patients. When sedation sufficient to obtund the patient's protective reflexes is required, the use of anesthesia personnel is strongly advised.

AIRWAY
Anatomy

The airway is divided into upper and lower portions by the vocal cords, which constitute the narrowest part of the adult airway and limit the size of the endotracheal tube (ETT). The trachea has an internal diameter of approximately 20 mm and is 10 to 12 cm in length, dividing at the carina into a right main stem bronchus (2.5 cm in length) with a 25 to 30-degree take-off angle and a left main stem-bronchus (5 cm long) with a 45-degree take-off angle. In the child, these angles approximate 25 degrees.

Pathology

A variety of pathological states may impact negatively on airway management. Arthritis may result in limited neck movement and in cervical instability, especially in the upper cervical spine. This is most frequently observed with rheumatoid arthritis. Temporomandibular joint disease, infection of the upper airway, and scleroderma may limit mouth opening.

Trauma and congenital syndromes (e.g., acromegaly, micrognathia, Pierre Robin, Treacher Collins, trisomy 21) may be associated with atlantoaxial instability.

Patients should be able to open their mouth 3 finger breadths or more and the thyromental distance should be about the same, otherwise visualization of the glottic chink may be difficult. Subglottic stenosis may be present if there is/was a tracheostomy. Additional studies (e.g., laryngoscopy, radiographs of trachea/cervical spine, pulmonary function tests [PFTs], and arterial blood gasses) may be helpful in airway evaluation.

Management

Anesthesia usually begins with preoxygenation of the patient. To maintain patency of the airway, an oro- or nasopharyngeal airway may be needed. Maneuvers commonly used to manage the airway (including use of an oropharyngeal airway and jaw thrust) may be associated with flexion or extension of the cervical spine. Therefore, care must be exercised if the possibility of cervical instability exists. The laryngeal mask airway (LMA) is a form of airway introduced into the hypopharynx to form a seal around the larynx so that spontaneous, assisted, or

---

THE TEN POSITIONAL STATEMENTS

Precautions (Primary)

1. The O.R. table goes into the Trendelenburg position and you know how to instruct someone to so do (in the event that you are occupied with another patient function).
2. You have a functioning suction apparatus and tubing connects (without leaks) to all catheters.
3. A functioning fiberoptic scope is in the O.R. suite. and
4. All required medications and fluids are available.

Precautions (Secondary)

5. You are familiar with the functioning of the O.R. table for all of its possible positioning.
6. You are knowledgeable in safely positioning the patient.
7. You are aware of the ready availability of back-up equipment.
8. You are knowledgeable in interfacing the back-up equipment.
9. You have, of course, followed the ASA preoperation guidelines.
10. You plan on being, at the best of times, on your own . . . all the time!

---

controlled ventilation can occur without the need for tracheal intubation. LMA should not be used when the patient's head is not easily accessible to the anesthesiologist.

Intubation with an ETT is generally required for surgeries of the spine. Nasotracheal intubation may be preferable in a patient with an unstable cervical spine because less manipulation may be required. A flexible fiberoptic scope should be available in operating room suites and considered as a first option in an anticipated difficult intubation (see accompanying box). Retrograde tracheal intubation or establishment of a surgical airway under local anesthesia are also viable options.

Occasionally an ETT needs to be changed. One method is to reintubate using direct or fiberoptic laryngoscopy; another is to use a tube changer (e.g., a hollow, malleable stylet that permits jet ventilation and suction) over which the ETT to be changed is removed and the new ETT is passed into the trachea. The management of the difficult airway described above may be expressed as algorithms (Figs. 6-1 and 6-2). Notwithstanding, failed intubation may occur in the best of hands.

In patients having undergone spinal surgery, dislodgment of the implanted instrumentation and interbody bone graft is to be avoided. Thus, one attempts to have an awake, cooperative patient who will not be reacting to the ETT. This goal is only attained with experience. Extubation may be performed with the patient awake or under general anesthesia. The former is usually reserved for a patient with a full stomach, difficult airway, or tracheal, mandibular, or facial surgery, and requires that the patient have a stable cardiopulmonary status. The latter is generally for asthmatic patients and procedures where coughing and straining may be undesirable (e.g., open-eye, middle-ear, herniorrhaphies).

PATIENT POSITIONING

Spine surgery patient positions are well known to most clinical anesthesiologists and the more unusual ones are familiar to anesthesiologists specializing in their use (e.g., neuroanesthesiologists). For an encyclopedic treatise on the subject of surgical posture, the reader is referred to *Positioning in Anesthesia and Surgery* by J. T. Martin.[97] The prone and lateral decubitus positions routinely used in spine surgery are emphasized here.

The Prone Position

Numerous frames, bolsters, and other apparatus that support the patient in the prone position have been described. No matter which system is used, the goals are similar:

1. *Avoidance of abdominal compression.* Increased abdominal pressure is transmitted to the epidural veins, which become engorged. This may lead to increased blood loss. If the abdominal contents are compressed or if the diaphragm is restricted by abdominal pressure, increased inspiratory pressures result. Increased intrathoracic pressures can decrease venous return and lower cardiac output (CO) and blood pressure (BP). There may be a higher incidence of thromboembolic complications because of venous stasis after caval compression.
2. *Avoidance of thoracic compression.* In addition to increased epidural venous pressure, peak inspiratory pressures are increased by improper positioning that allows unnecessary pressure on the thorax. The surgeon may flex

Difficult airway algorithm

I. Assess the likelihood and clinical impact of basic management problems

   A. Difficult intubation

   B. Difficult ventilation

   C. Difficulty with patient cooperation or consent

II. Consider the relative merits and feasibility of basic management choices

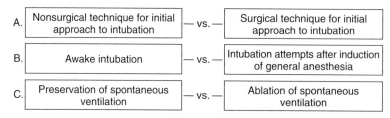

III. Develop primary and alternative strategies

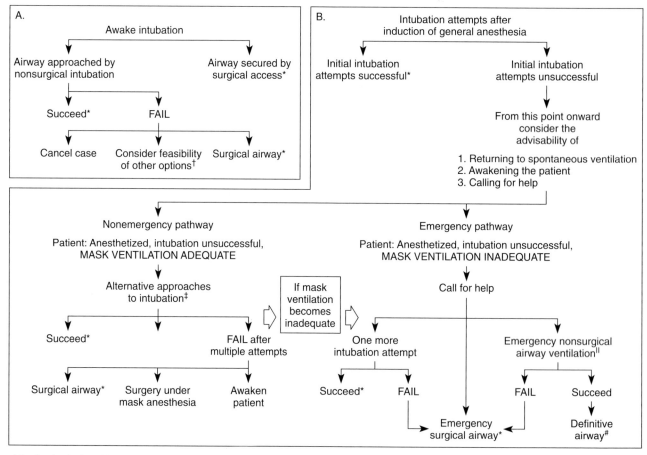

* Confirm intubation with exhaled CO_2

† Other options include (but are not limited to) surgery under mask anesthesia, surgery under local anesthesia infiltration or regional nerve blockade, or intubation attempts after induction of general anesthesia.

‡ Alternative approaches to difficult intubation include (but are not limited to) use of different laryngoscope blades, awake intubation, blind oral or nasal intubation, fiberoptic intubation, intubating stylet or tube changer, light wand, retrograde intubation, and surgical airway access.

§ See awake intubation.

‖ Options for emergency non-surgical airway ventilation include (but are not limited to): transtracheal jet ventilation, laryngeal mask ventilation, or esophageal-tracheal combitube ventilation.

Fig. 6-1. Difficult airway algorithm. (From American Society of Anesthesiologists Task Force on management of the difficult airway. Practice guidelines for management of the difficult airway. Anesthesiology 78:597-602, 1993.)

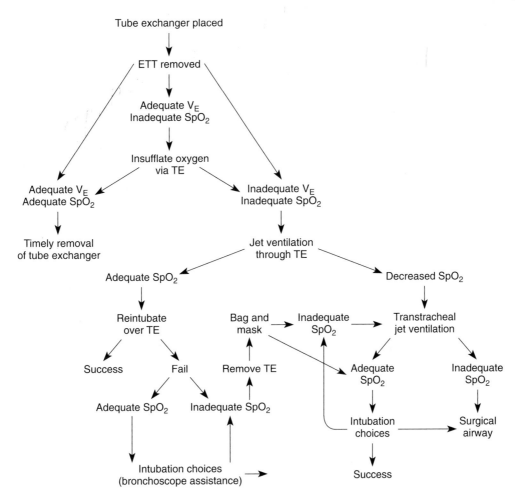

Fig. 6-2. An algorithm for extubation of the difficult airway. After placement of a tube exchanger (TE) the ETT is removed. Oxygenation and ventilation are then assessed. Hypoxemia is treated first via insufflation of oxygen via the TE if ventilation appears adequate or by jet ventilation through the TE if ventilation is inadequate. If hypoxemia resolves, reintubation over the TE should be performed (lower left arm of algorithm) after jet ventilation. If reintubation via this method fails, oxygenation should be maintained by jet ventilation through the TE while other reintubation choices are considered and performed. If jet ventilation through the TE fails to restore oxygenation (lower right arm of algorithm) transtracheal jet ventilation is recommended. If this restores oxygenation other intubation choices should be considered and performed. If transtracheal jet ventilation fails to restore adequate oxygenation, a surgical airway is necessary. This algorithm is suggested as one of several step-wise approaches to difficult airway management after extubation. Actual and optimal maneuvers may vary depending on patient conditions and skills of clinicians delivering care. (From Miller K, Harkin CP, Bailey PL. Postoperative tracheal extubation. Anesth Analg 80:149-172, 1995.)

the head upon the chest to expose the cervical vertebrae. This may compromise venous drainage, leading to swelling of the tongue and edema of the airway soft tissues as well as an increase in intracranial pressure (ICP). To avoid obstruction of the ETT due to kinking, some anesthesiologists use a wire-reinforced or "armored" tube. When forcefully compressed (e.g., by biting) the tube may not revert

to its prior configuration, leading to obstruction of the ETT. When this type of tube is used, a bite block is particularly important.[154] There is one report of coronary ischemia probably induced by compression of a coronary artery graft when the patient was placed in the prone position.[155]

3. *Avoidance of stretching of neurovascular structures.* Prime targets for injury are the

brachial plexus, ulnar nerve, and axillary artery. The arms should be placed at the sides (tucked) or extended above the patient's head on arm boards. In either event, the ulnar nerves should be padded with foam or gel pads. Care must be taken to ensure that there is no pressure from the edges of the table or arm boards.

4. *Avoidance of pressure injuries.* The soft tissues of the face (ears, nose, lips), the eyes (causing retinal blindness or corneal abrasion), and weight-bearing areas (knees, ankles, feet) are all potential sites of pressure injury and must be well padded. The authors favor the use of protective goggles (as well as lubricant and tape) to help prevent pressure on the globe.

These goals may be difficult to achieve, especially if the patient is severely deformed by his disease process or if immobility has resulted in contractures. In these instances, the frame must be adjustable or it must be modified by extra padding and supports to accommodate the needs of the patient.

Frames and Specialty Tables

Two popular systems for prone positioning are the Hall-Relton frame (Figs. 6-3 and 6-4) and the Wilson frame (Figs. 6-5 and 6-6), which have adjustable posts or radiolucent pads. This allows the abdomen to hang free (or at least be free of compression), which improves venous drainage and ventilation. One must remember to avoid compression of the female breast by placing the thoracic supports lateral to the breasts, and to avoid pressure on the brachial plexus from the lateral bolsters.

If the surgery is to include the sacral area, it is important to maintain the normal lumbar lordosis (for ambulatory patients). Extra pads may be placed under the thighs to prevent forward tilt of the lower pelvis and thus maintain the patient's lordotic posture as if he were standing.

In nonambulatory patients with marked hip flexion contractures, positioning on the Hall-Relton frame can be difficult and is modified so that the hips are flexed to a range beyond the hip flexion contracture. The lower ends of the frame or bolsters are raised so that the knees are free of pressure. The knees, lower legs, and ankles are padded.[19]

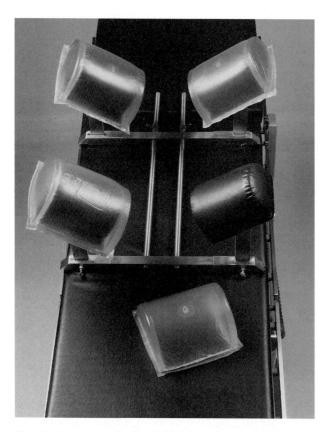

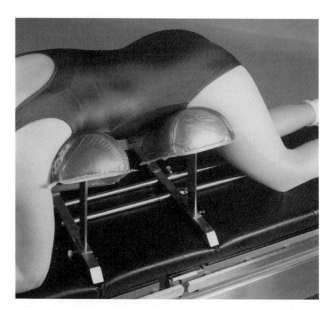

Fig. 6-3. One example of a Hall-Relton frame utilizing commercially available gel pads. Note that the positions of the supporting posts are adjustable in two planes (lateral and caudorostral) to accommodate patients of different sizes. Other frames also allow adjustment of the height of the individual posts. (Courtesy of Action Products, Inc., Hagerstown, Md.)

Fig. 6-4. The Hall-Relton frame demonstrating proper positioning of the patient. Note that the lower posts support the iliac crests. The upper posts support the thorax without compressing the axillary structures. The abdomen and lower thorax are free of compression between the two sets of posts. Under clinical conditions the elbows, knees, and ankles would receive additional padding. (Courtesy of Action Products, Inc., Hagerstown, Md.)

The Wilson frame (see Figs. 6-5 and 6-6) does not allow one to customize positioning as much as the Hall-Relton frame or bolsters, but is simple and applicable to patients without significant deformity.

Bolsters for Prone Positioning

The general guidelines and goals for using bolsters are the same as those for using a frame. Bolsters should extend from the pelvis to just below the axilla, making sure not to compress the axillary structures. The iliac crests should be well padded (Figs. 6-7 and 6-8). Although rolled sheets or blankets are commonly used, gel or foam bolsters make positioning injuries less likely. Additional padding

under the upper chest minimizes stretch on the brachial plexus and can make positioning of the head easier (especially if limited neck mobility is a problem). Females with large breasts (especially implants) require special attention to prevent traumatic compression.

If the cervical spine is involved, the head may be held in traction tongs, "a horseshoe," or pin head fixation. The head may be turned laterally (although some surgeons find that this distorts the anatomy of high thoracic lesions). Several foam pillows with cutouts for the endotracheal tube and facial structures are commercially available. Foam-lined goggles (Optigard [Dupaco, Oceanside, Calif.]) confer extra protection from pressure on the eyes.

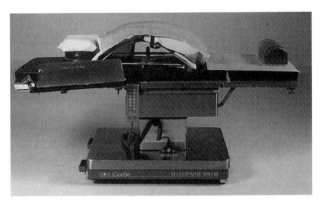

Fig. 6-5. Commercially available model of the Wilson frame with gel pads. (Courtesy of Action Products, Inc., Hagerstown, Md.)

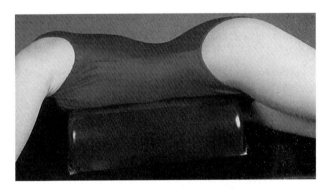

Fig. 6-7. Model demonstrating the use of bolsters to position a patient for surgery in the prone position. Note that the bolster runs from the iliac crest to the upper thorax (excluding the axilla). (Courtesy of Action Products, Inc., Hagerstown, Md.)

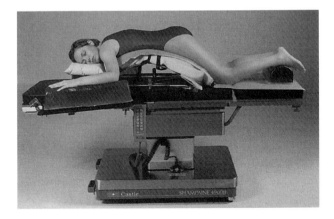

Fig. 6-6. Wilson frame with patient properly positioned. Note that the knees and ankles are padded and that the arms are placed on pads above the level of the table to decrease compression of the brachial plexus. The abdomen is free of compression between the lateral supports of the frame. (Courtesy of Action Products, Inc., Hagerstown, Md.)

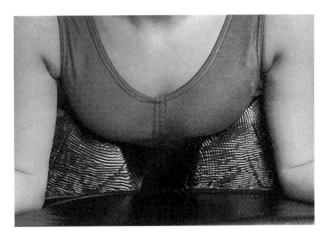

Fig. 6-8. Model on bolsters for surgery in the prone position. Note that the breasts are medial to the pads and not compressed. Under clinical conditions the elbows would receive extra padding. (Courtesy of Action Products, Inc., Hagerstown, Md.)

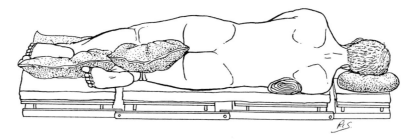

Fig. 6-9. The standard right lateral decubitus position. Note the proper padding over bony prominences, chest roll to protect axilla, and proper alignment of the cervical spine. The flexed lower leg stabilizes the torso. (From Martin JT. Positioning in Anesthesia and Surgery. Philadelphia: WB Saunders, 1988, p 1560.)

If the pathology involves the cervical spine, the surgeon may control the head during the turn. Somatosensory evoked potentials and/or a wake-up test can be used to assure that no spinal cord compromise has occurred during the intubation or turn. The surgeon may want the arms at the patient's sides and may use tape or restraints to place traction on the shoulders for better exposure. Excessive traction of the shoulders should be avoided so as not to injure the brachial plexus. If the cervical spine is not involved, the arms may be placed on well-padded arm boards above the patient's head. The elbows should be below the plane of the midaxillary line (the thorax may need to be raised on pads) to avoid stretching the brachial plexus. The arm should not be abducted more than 90 degrees. Acute flexion at the elbow may result in entrapment of the ulnar nerve and subsequent neuropathy even in the absence of pressure.

One strategy used to avoid these complications is "awake-pronation."[86] In this scenario, the patient is intubated awake using sedation and topical anesthesia of the airway. Following intubation, the patient can assist with transfer to the prone position on the operating table and assist the anesthesiologist and surgeon in finding his/her "position of comfort."

The Lateral Position

The lateral position is used if a ventral approach to the spine is indicated. Patients with scoliosis may undergo surgery on the side of the convexity. This can present problems for the anesthesiologist because the dependent lung will be on the side of the concavity. This dependent lung is already compressed by the skeletal deformity and may not be able to support the patient during OLV.

Reoperation may be performed on the same or the opposite side of a previous surgery and is based on surgical considerations. Indications to use the virgin hemithorax include avoidance of scar tissue, decreased bleeding, less chance of pulmonary compromise, and the ability to resect a rib without increasing the thoracic defect. Left-sided approaches are favored by some surgeons who feel that the aorta is easier to mobilize and less subject to accidental trauma than is the vena cava. In addition, aortic injuries may be easier to repair than caval injuries.

Following induction of anesthesia, the patient is turned so that the operative side is up. The lower leg is flexed to decrease the tendency to roll forward. The kidney rest may be elevated or the table "broken" (or both) to widen the intercostal spaces for improved surgical exposure (Fig. 6-9). At various times during surgery, the table may have to be manipulated to facilitate exposure during decompression or to "lock-in" the instrumentation or grafts in the most physiological position. An "axillary roll" is placed. In fact, this is a misnomer. The roll should be caudal to the axilla, so that the weight of the thorax is displaced from the dependent shoulder. This minimizes pressure on the neurovascular bundle of the dependent upper extremity. All other pressure points, including the ankles, dependent knee, and arm should also be protected. A pillow between the knees not only protects the underlying tissues from pressure injury, but also decreases the tendency for the patient to roll forward.

The arms may be either extended on an arm board or flexed at the elbow in the "praying position" (the potential for flexed elbows to cause ulnar nerve damage exists). A pillow or other padding should be placed between the arms. One modification of this position is to allow the nondependent arm to hang (padded by a pillow) between the dependent arm and the thorax (off the table). This has the effect of retracting the scapula rostrally and increasing the operative exposure. This is favored by some thoracic surgeons for upper lobe pulmonary surgery. An "airplane" support for the nondependent arm is another alternative. Care must be taken to assure that all of the pressure points are padded when using this device. The pulse oximeter, if placed on a finger of the dependent arm, can act as an indicator of arterial compression, as can a radial artery catheter.

Care should be taken to position the head and neck in a neutral position to avoid stretching of the nondependent cervical nerves and compression of the dependent neck vessels. Adequate protection from pressure injury of the dependent facial soft tissues is also important in this position.

A "bean bag" is frequently used to stabilize the patient in the lateral position. This is a plastic bag filled with small beads. Following positioning of the patient, the bag is molded to the patient's dependent side and suction is applied to the bag. This causes the beads to form a "solid" mass conforming to the shape of the dependent side. While this is quite efficient in stabilizing the patient in situ, the bag can be very hard and pressure injuries may occur. One approach to avoid this potential complication is the placement of a gel pad between the patient and the bag to provide padding for the dependent structures. This may make the bag less efficient in stabilizing the patient, but it usually provides satisfactory positioning and less chance of pressure injuries. Strips of adhesive tape help to stabilize the patient in the lateral position. If tape is used, avoid creating any pressure on the sciatic and peroneal nerves.

Thoracic and Thoracoabdominal Incisions

This approach to the ventral spine may require one-lung anesthesia. Many pulmonary resections have been carried out without endobronchial intubation using packs to keep the lung out of the operative field. Should endobronchial intubation and one-lung anesthesia be requested, a left-sided endobronchial tube should be acceptable in the vast majority of cases. Any time an endobronchial tube is used, a fiberoptic bronchoscope of appropriate diameter must be available to confirm proper place-

ment and to "troubleshoot" problems that may arise intraoperatively. If the region involved includes the low thoracic or high lumbar, part of the diaphragm may need to be detached and the viscera mobilized by retroperitoneal dissection. The postoperative pulmonary implications of this are discussed elsewhere.

To check for an air leak at the end of a ventral thoracic spinal procedure, the anesthesiologist may be asked to provide a period of sustained positive pressure (Valsalva maneuver). Any remaining pneumothorax can possibly be evacuated with this maneuver. However, if an otherwise unexplainable occurs, a pneumothorax should be suspected and a needle aspiration or tube thoracostomy performed.

HEMODYNAMIC CONSIDERATIONS
The Prone Position

As previously noted, it is important to keep the abdomen free of external pressure so that respiration is not hindered. If there is an increase in peak inspiratory pressure (PIP), the carbon monoxide may decrease because of obstruction to the venous return in the inferior vena cava. As a result, blood is shunted through alternate routes (e.g., the epidural veins).

Compression of the great vessels of the head must be avoided. Carotid obstruction may lead to cerebral ischemia. Venous obstruction may increase ICP and thus decrease cerebral perfusion pressure (CPP). This is even more likely to have a detrimental effect in the setting of hypotension (intentional or otherwise). Venous obstruction may also lead to the development of airway edema (as well as edema of other facial structures, such as the eyelids and conjunctivae), which may complicate extubation.

Pneumothorax is a complication of thoracic surgery in the prone position. Because access to the lung fields for auscultation is difficult, a high index of suspicion must be maintained with regard to the possibility of pneumothorax, especially in the setting of increasing PIPs, hypotension, desaturation, and a decrease in the end-tidal carbon dioxide partial pressure ($P_{ET}CO_2$). Pneumothorax may not become apparent until closure of the wound, when it may rapidly expand due to positive pressure ventilation and/or the use of nitrous oxide. Emergency treatment with a needle aspiration or tube thoracostomy may be lifesaving.

Gas (air) embolus is a potential complication any time the surgical site is higher than the right atrium. This is especially true when venous sinuses are open (as is the case when bone is resected). Hemodynamic deterioration, a falling $P_{ET}CO_2$, and desaturation should raise suspicion. The esophageal stethoscope may reveal the presence of a "millwheel" murmur associated with gas in the right atrium and ventricle. Treatment is supportive. The operative field should be flooded with saline to prevent further air entrainment. Increasing pressure on the abdomen raises the pressure in Batson's plexus of the epidural veins. This pressure is transmitted to the venous sinusoids and thus decreases air entrainment. Nitrous oxide should be discontinued. If a central venous catheter is in place, it should be aspirated in an effort to remove air, although this procedure has not been reported to be uniformly successful. Dopamine, norepinephrine, or epinephrine may be necessary for the support of circulation. Turning the patient with the right side up in an effort to confine the air to the right atrium and superior vena cava, preventing its movement through the heart, has been advocated but usually is neither practical nor efficacious.

The Lateral Position

Pulmonary artery catheters passed from the right internal jugular vein or left subclavian vein enter the right lung about 80% of the time unless directed using fluoroscopy. If the patient is placed with the right lung rostral, there is a chance that the tip will be positioned in a zone of the lung where there may not be a continuous column of blood from the pulmonary artery to the left atrium (zone 1 or 2). Without a continuous column of blood, pulmonary capillary wedge pressure (PCWP) will not accurately reflect the left atrial pressure (LAP). Measurements of the pulmonary artery diastolic pressure (PADP) and PCWP should be taken before turning to define the relationship between these two values. PADP may be the more reliable measurement once the patient is turned.

A more serious complication of pulmonary artery catheterization is pulmonary artery perforation. This can occur if the tip migrates distally. Migration is made more likely by any maneuver that decreases either right ventricular size or blood flow to the lung that has been catheterized. Deflation of the nondependent lung for one-lung anesthesia is one such risk factor. Patients with an elevated pulmonary artery pressure (PAP) are at increased risk for perforation. The pressure tracing of the pulmonary artery catheter must be observed frequently for signs of migration (e.g., loss of the PAP wave form with the balloon deflated, or a falsely elevated PAP). Any suspicion that the catheter is impinging upon the arterial wall is cause to withdraw the catheter into the main arterial tree.

Mediastinal shift can be caused by compression by the heart, by pressure from a collapsed nonventilated lung, or by placement of surgical retractors. This shift can torque the great vessels (especially the venae cavae), which may decrease venous return, cardiac output, and blood pressure.

Pulmonary artery hypertension and acute cor pulmonale is not usually a problem with the patient in the lateral position even when one-lung anesthesia is used. The increased blood flow due to gravity and to hypoxic pulmonary vasoconstriction in the nondependent lung is compensated for by recruitment of pulmonary vasculature, provided the dependent lung is relatively normal. However, in the presence of preexisting pulmonary artery (PA) hypertension (which may be present in patients with severe scoliosis), this compensatory mechanism may not be available. Acute cor pulmonale may result, requiring aggressive treatment. Such patients may not tolerate one-lung anesthesia.

RESPIRATORY CONSIDERATIONS
The Prone Position

The effects of gravity on pulmonary artery flow are similar in the supine and prone position. Therefore, the effects of anesthesia and mechanical ventilation on ventilation/perfusion ($\dot{V}/\dot{Q}$) matching in the prone position are similar to those observed in the supine position. There is some change in $\dot{V}/\dot{Q}$ matching because the ventral portion of the diaphragm tends to move less freely than the dorsal aspect. However, this is not usually clinically significant. There may actually be some improvement in $\dot{V}/\dot{Q}$ matching if the patient has been properly positioned.[121] The need to guard against airway edema and ETT kinking have already been described. When the dorsum is rostral (i.e., in the prone position) $\dot{V}/\dot{Q}$ mismatching may be increased because gravity now favors the ventral portion of the lungs.

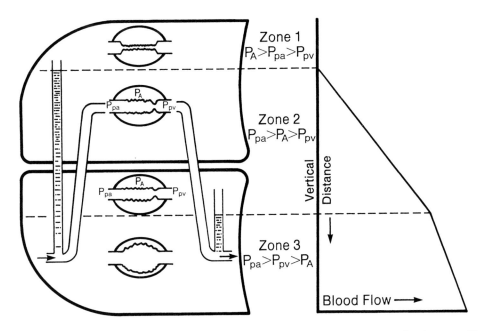

Fig. 6-10. Schematic representation of the effects of gravity on the distribution of pulmonary blood flow in the lateral decubitus position. The vertical gradient in the lateral decubitus position is less than that in the upright position. Consequently, there is less zone 1 and more zone 2 and zone 3 blood flow in the lateral decubitus position compared with the upright position. Nevertheless, pulmonary blood flow increases with lung dependency and is greater in the dependent lung compared with the nondependent lung. P_A = alveolar pressure; P_{pa} = pulmonary artery pressure; P_{pv} = pulmonary venous pressure. (Modified with permission from Benumof JL. Physiology of the open chest and one-lung ventilation. In Kaplan JA, ed. Thoracic Anesthesia. New York: Churchill Livingston, 1983.)

The insertion of an LMA is not an acceptable substitute for airway control in lieu of ETT intubation in the prone position.

The Lateral Position

Gravity plays a much greater role in the lateral position because the vertical distances between the nondependent and dependent lung zones are greater than in the supine or prone position. Therefore gravitational effects cause a gradient in distribution of pulmonary artery blood flow to a much greater degree than in the supine position (Fig. 6-10).

Under normal conditions, the right and left lungs receive approximately 55% and 45% of the blood flow, respectively. Flow to either lung is reduced about 10% when that lung is made nondependent in the lateral position. This flow is redistributed to the dependent lung (Fig. 6-11).

In the awake patient ventilation is also redistributed to the dependent lung because it is on a more favorable part of the pressure-volume curve. When anesthetized and/or mechanically ventilated, the majority of ventilation goes to the nondependent lung (about 55% of each tidal volume). General anesthesia causes a reduction in the functional residual capacity (FRC) of both lungs, changing their relative positions on the pressure-volume (compliance) curve such that the nondependent lung is better ventilated while being less well perfused. Opening the nondependent hemithorax further increases the compliance of the nondependent lung and leads to even greater redistribution of ventilation. Pressure from the mediastinum and the nondependent lung also limits ventilation to the dependent lung, as does pressure from the abdominal contents on the dependent hemidiaphragm (Fig. 6-12).

Application of positive end-expiratory pressure (PEEP) to both lungs restores most of the ventilation to the dependent lung, probably by increasing FRC and restoring it to a steeper part of the compliance curve (see Fig. 6-12). Application of PEEP only to the dependent lung has much the same effect, but can divert some blood flow to the nondependent lung. Therefore care must be used if the nondependent lung is not being ventilated, because shunt

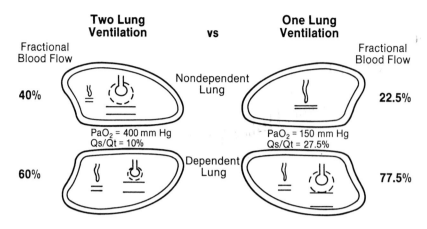

Fig. 6-11. Schematic representation of two-lung ventilation vs. one-lung ventilation. Typical values for fractional blood flow to the nondependent and dependent lungs as well as $P_{a_{O_2}}$ and $\dot{Q}s/\dot{Q}t$ for the two conditions are shown. The $\dot{Q}s/\dot{Q}t$ during two-lung ventilation is assumed to be distributed equally between the two lungs (5% to each lung). The essential difference between two-lung and one-lung ventilation is that during one-lung ventilation the nonventilated lung has some blood flow and, therefore, an obligatory shunt, which is not present during two-lung ventilation. The 35% of total flow perfusing the nondependent lung, which is not shunt flow, is assumed to be able to reduce its blood flow by 50% by hyposix pulmonary vasoconstriction. The increase in $\dot{Q}s/\dot{Q}t$ from two-lung to one-lung ventilation is assumed to be solely due to the increase in blood flow through the nonventilated, nondependent lung during one-lung ventilation. (From Benumof J. Anesthesia for Thoracic Surgery, 2nd ed. Philadelphia: WB Saunders, 1995, p 131.)

DISTRIBUTION OF VENTILATION
Closed chest, lateral decubitus position

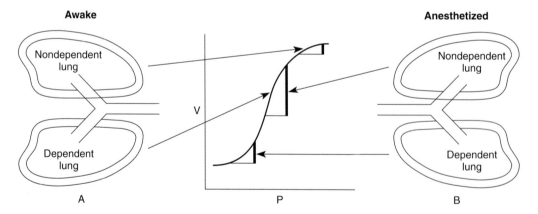

Fig. 6-12. This schematic diagram shows the distribution of ventilation in the awake patient in the lateral decubitus position (*A*) and the distribution of ventilation in the anesthetized patient in the lateral decubitus position (*B*). The induction of anesthesia has caused a loss in lung volume in both lungs, with the nondependent lung moving from a flat, noncompliant portion to a steep, compliant portion of the pressure-volume curve and the dependent lung moving from a steep, compliant part to a flat, noncompliant part of the pressure-volume curve. Thus, the anesthetized patient in a lateral decubitus position has the majority of the tidal ventilation in the nondependent lung (where there is the least perfusion) and the minority of the tidal ventilation in the dependent lung (where there is the most perfusion). Applications of PEEP to both lungs under anesthesia restores them to positions on the compliance curve that more closely resemble the awake state. (V = alveolar volume; P = transpumonary pressure. Modified with permission from Benumof JL. Physiology of the open chest and one-lung ventilation. In Kaplan JA, ed. Thoracic Anesthesia. New York: Churchill Livingston, 1983.)

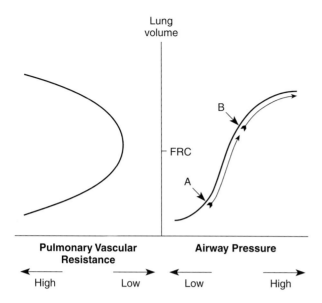

Fig. 6-13. Juxtaposition of the pulmonary compliance and composite pulmonary vascular resistance curves explains why dependent lung PEEP does not always improve arterial oxygenation during one-lung ventilation. **A,** If the initial dependent lung volume is small, PEEP brings the lung to a point on the pulmonary compliance curve where PVR is low and the beneficial effects of PEEP are realized. **B,** If the initial dependent lung volume is normal or large, PEEP increases volume to a point where the PVR is high and blood flow diversion to the up-lung occurs. (From Capan LM, Turndorf H, Miller S. Maximizing oxygenation during one-lung anesthesia. In Brodsky JB, ed. Problems in Anesthesia. Philadelphia: JB Lippincott, 1990, p 296.)

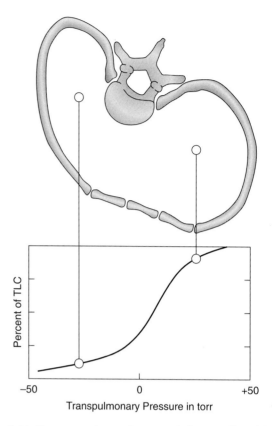

Fig. 6-14. Pressure-volume diagram of chest wall and lung and approximate position at end-expiratory lung volume of the hyperinflated (convex) and hypoinflated (concave) hemithorax. Notice that both hemithoraces are on flattened (less compliant) portions of the pressure-volume curve. (Reproduced with permission from Barash PG, Cullen BF, Stoelting RK. Clinical Anesthesia. Philadelphia: JB Lippincott, 1989, p 1179.)

may be increased by dependent lung PEEP (Fig. 6-13). This concept of different lung units behaving differently because of their relative positions on the pressure-volume (pulmonary compliance) curve takes on particular significance in the case of scoliosis. In Fig. 6-14, it can be seen that the lung on the concave side is compressed while that on the convex side is operating near total lung capacity (TLC). However, both lungs are on noncompliant portions of the pressure-volume curve. If a ventral approach is needed, it will usually be from the side of the convexity. This leaves the compressed lung to provide ventilatory function for the entire body.

ONE-LUNG VENTILATION

One-lung ventilation (single-lung ventilation [SLV]) is used when collapse of the nondependent lung is desirable to increase surgical exposure.

Because the nondependent lung is not ventilated, flow through it creates an obligatory right to left intrapulmonary shunt. Therefore for a given F_iO_2 there will be a larger $P(A-a)O_2$ and a lower PaO_2. In addition, the dependent (ventilated) lung may develop a shunt as well due to absorption atelectasis, compression by the mediastinum, compression by the abdominal contents, or by rolls used for positioning. The benefits of a high F_iO_2 outweigh the potential detrimental effects of oxygen toxicity, and the use of large tidal volumes prevents atelectasis and shunting.

With a constant minute ventilation (MV), carbon dioxide elimination is less affected than oxygen uptake. This is due to the differences in the dissociation curves for oxygen and carbon dioxide that make it possible for the ventilated lung to nearly compensate for the nonventilated lung for carbon dioxide elimination. However, because of the nature of the oxyhemoglobin dissociation curve (i.e., the flatness of the curve at high Pa_{O_2}), enough oxygen cannot be taken up in the ventilated lung to overcome the effects of the shunt. Another way of stating this is that the $P_{ET}CO_2$ to Pa_{CO_2} gradient is small while the PA_{O_2} to Pa_{O_2} gradient is large.

The immediate effect of one-lung ventilation is hyperventilation of the ventilated lung (if MV is held constant), which leads to an increased $\dot{V}/\dot{Q}$. Within 5 minutes, hypoxic pulmonary vasoconstriction (HPV) shifts flow from the nonventilated lung to the ventilated lung, shifting $\dot{V}/\dot{Q}$ back toward normal.[72] This increased blood flow through the ventilated lung (due to gravity and HPV) is usually tolerated without significant increases in pulmonary artery pressures. However, if preexisting PA hypertension is present, this increased flow may not be well tolerated.

Blood flow is distributed to the dependent lung due to gravity, surgical compression of the nondependent lung, and HPV. Mechanical stimulation of the nondependent lung may cause the release of prostaglandins that may increase nondependent lung blood flow by causing vasodilatation.[123]

HPV is an active vasoconstrictor process that increases the pulmonary vascular resistance in hypoxic areas of the lung. Hypoxia causes constriction of the small arteries of the lung. On the systemic side, hypoxia causes vasodilation. This may be related to the fact that in the fetal lung, a high pulmonary vascular resistance (PVR) shunts blood through the ductus arteriosis to maintain normal fetal circulation. The increased PVR is likely related to the pulmonary vascular smooth muscle, leading to vasoconstriction.[156] HPV is a normal response to atelectasis from whatever cause and may affect an entire lung or a small portion thereof. Its purpose is to decrease shunt flow by diverting blood from hypoxic to normoxic lung units. When HPV is fully active, there is about a 50% reduction in flow to a hypoxic lung unit.[94] The shunt through the nonventilated lung is only 20% to 30% of the cardiac output rather than the 40% to 50% that would be expected if HPV were not active.[49,81,91] If the hypoxic lung is re-expanded with nitrogen, HPV remains, indicating that active vasoconstriction rather than compression of the vessels by lung parenchyma is the mechanism of action.[10,17]

HPV can be inhibited by various drugs. Almost all vasodilators have been shown to inhibit HPV to a greater or lesser degree. Those tested and shown to be inhibitory include: sodium nitroprusside, nitroglycerin, ß-agonists (e.g.: ritodrine and salbutamol), calcium channel blockers, adenosine, prostaglandins, and nitric oxide. There is some evidence that the vasodilating prostaglandins and calcium channel blockers may affect HPV less than some of the other vasodilators.

The intravenous anesthetic agents (propofol, narcotics, and ketamine), do not inhibit HPV. The inhalation agents (at minimum alveolar concentration [MAC] levels used clinically) do not inhibit HPV to a clinically significant degree although some increase in shunt fraction is demonstrable.[126]

The beneficial effect of HPV can be overcome if high PAPs are present. The thinner muscular layers in the pulmonary circulation cannot constrict with sufficient force to overcome high PAPs.[13,51,95] Increased airway pressures due to high tidal volumes or PEEP can also reverse HPV by compressing the pulmonary vascular bed in the dependent lung thereby shunting blood to the nondependent (collapsed) lung. The acid-base status of the patient is also important. Alkalosis (respiratory or metabolic) inhibits HPV while acidosis (respiratory or metabolic) enhances HPV.

Ability to Tolerate One-Lung Anesthesia

There is little data available to predict with certainty which patients will tolerate one-lung anesthesia (OLA) and which patients will not. The ventral approach to the spine for correction of scoliosis is usually used in patients with severe curvatures because release is necessary to gain mobility prior to stabilization. The magnitude of elevation of the PAPs is related to the Pa_{O_2} rather than to the degree of curvature.[134] However, patients with the degree of curvature requiring ventral release might be expected to have hypoxemia, hypercarbia, and compression of the lung on the side of the concavity. All of these factors may lead to PA hypertension. There are some data to indicate that the hypertension is fixed (at least partially) because it fails to correct with elevation of the Pa_{O_2}.[134] In the case of scoliosis, the surgical approach may be from the side of the convexity (unless technical factors dictate otherwise, e.g., reoperation). This places the more compressed lung (the lung on the side of the concavity) dependent. It is the dependent lung that must bear the entire burden of oxygenation and increased pulmonary blood flow. Therefore the potential exists for development of hypoxemia, acute right ventricular failure, and inability to tolerate an OLA technique.

Right ventricular failure is treated with fluids and pressors (dopamine, dobutamine, norepinephrine, etc.). Vasodilators (prostaglandins, amrinone, sodium nitroprusside [SNP], nitroglycerine [NTG], and others) may be necessary to unload the right ventricle, but their potential to induce hypoxemia by inhibition of HPV must be remembered. Systemic hypotension may limit their usefulness. Because this dependent lung will be compressed by the scoliosis, smaller than usual tidal volumes may be necessary to avoid compressing the vasculature and increasing PA pressures.

For the above reasons, those patients most in need of a ventral approach for their spinal deformity may be the least able to tolerate it. Fortunately, early intervention prevents patients from reaching the severe degrees of curvature associated with significant pulmonary impairment. Ventral approaches for thoracic disc herniation, tumor, trauma, etc., should be well tolerated in the absence of preexisting cardiopulmonary disease from other causes.

Management of One-Lung Ventilation

1. Maintain two-lung ventilation as long as possible, and revert to two-lung ventilation whenever OLA is not needed for surgical exposure.

2. Ventilate with a high F_iO_2. This maximizes O_2 uptake and may dilate dependent lung vasculature, making redistribution from the nondependent lung more efficient. There is some theoretic advantage for using an F_iO_2 of 0.8 to 0.9 since the addition of a small amount of nitrogen may prevent absorption atelectasis in the dependent lung. In practice, the same results can be achieved by using liberal tidal volumes and, perhaps, low levels of dependent lung PEEP.

3. Tidal volumes of 8 to 15 ml/kg have been advocated to prevent atelectasis. Start with about 10 ml/kg, because larger volumes may shunt blood to the nondependent lung. As noted above, this may have to be adjusted downward if

the dependent lung is on the concavity of a severe scoliosis.

4. Respiratory rate is adjusted to achieve normocarbia. Hypocapnia may inhibit HPV in the nondependent lung and increase the shunt.

5. Initially PEEP should be avoided or kept under 5 cm of water. Because the effects of PEEP may be unpredictable (it may decrease oxygenation by increasing blood flow to the nonventilated lung) wait to see if it is needed. In addition, intrinsic PEEP may be present (not detectable on the anesthesia machine's manometer) and additional PEEP may worsen the situation.[138] Although external PEEP has been advocated to improve ventilation in patients with significant intrinsic PEEP, the effects of this external PEEP are variable and require graded application with close observation of ventilatory mechanics, hemodynamics, and oxygenation.

6. Differential lung management may be necessary if hypoxemia develops in spite of the above maneuvers. It is assumed that the anesthesiologist will confirm the proper placement of the endobronchial tube (or bronchial blocker) and that other technical factors are ruled out.

   a. Intermittent inflation of the nondependent lung is helpful in correcting hypoxemia for several minutes, but may require the surgeon to stop operating briefly.

   b. Nondependent lung continuous positive airway pressure (CPAP) is applied at the end of a full breath to the nondependent lung. Low levels (5 to 10 cm) of water help restore FRC and keep the airways open allowing oxygen to be entrained and some gas exchange to take place in the nondependent lung. Low levels have minimal effects on the pulmonary vasculature and do not interfere significantly with most surgeries.[12,44,139] The use of differential lung ventilation using a clamp or other device to partially obstruct the nonventilated limb of the endobronchial tube has been described.[7] This technique essentially results in CPAP (or at best minimal ventilation) of the nondependent lung. It has the advantage of not requiring a second oxygen source (as does CPAP), and is simple to set up. In addition, the resistance on the nondependent limb can be adjusted to allow as much or as little "ventilation" of the nondependent lung as is compatible with satisfactory oxygen saturation. Insufflation of the nondependent lung with oxygen at zero endexpiratory pressure (ZEEP) is of no benefit.

c. If the above does not restore oxygen saturation to an acceptable level, the addition of or increase in the level of dependent lung PEEP is a logical next step. Levels of PEEP and CPAP may be increased in stepwise alternating fashion trying to keep the level of CPAP (on the nondependent lung) higher than the level of PEEP. Jet ventilation of the nondependent lung is unlikely to be helpful if CPAP/PEEP has failed.

d. Consideration should be given to modification of the anesthetic technique to raise the Pao_2. As an example, the use of direct acting vasodilators for controlled hypotension may have to be discontinued because they may be reversing HPV.

SPINAL CORD PHYSIOLOGY
Blood Flow

The physiology of the spinal cord generally mimics that of the brain.[96] Spinal cord blood flow (SCBF) is consistent with flow to the brain.[82,130,131] As with the brain, flow is metabolically linked to the level of neuronal activity. Flow is autoregulated between approximately 50 and 150 mm Hg.[64,128]

The spinal cord also mimics the brain in its response to metabolic and respiratory conditions. Hypocapnia may constrict vessels and cause a "reverse steal." However, this does not reliably occur. Under these circumstances, it seems most prudent to maintain normo- or modest hypocapnia. If the reverse steal phenomenon is present, it has its greatest effect on the penumbral area of cord damage. Spinal cord damage is made worse by hyperglycemia, as is the case with brain injury.

SCBF decreases with hypothermia (vide: section on SSEP monitoring), as does spinal cord metabolic rate. This may be of benefit to limit progression of cord injury in the acute phase. However, SCBF may be adversely affected by temperature because a decrease of 20% to 40% is observed after exposure of the dura mater. This decreased flow is thought to be due to temperature induced vasoconstriction.

The effects of anesthetics on the spinal cord are much the same as their effects on the brain: ". . .

limited data are available concerning SCBF and metabolism. However, there is no reason to suspect that they would differ from those of the brain."[128] Injury to the spinal cord produces a decrease in blood flow and a disturbance in autoregulation just as is seen in the brain.

All inhalational anesthetics can be considered cerebral vasodilators (to a greater or lesser degree) and can therefore increase intracranial pressure. Intravenous anesthetics decrease cerebral oxygen consumption ($CMRO_2$) and thereby decrease cerebral blood flow (CBF). The exception is ketamine, which produces increased CBF and $CMRO_2$. Sodium thiopental, in doses sufficient to induce burst suppression, decreases SCBF by 50% and may therefore be of value in cord protection,[69] assuming a corresponding decrease in spinal cord metabolic rate. Coupling of metabolic rate and $CMRO_2$ is maintained with most intravenous anesthetics. Propofol also induces burst suppression and decreases $CMRO_2$. It may also act as a brain protectant.

To summarize, coupling of spinal cord metabolic rate ($SCMRO_2$) and SCBF is maintained with most of the intravenous anesthetics, but lost or at least altered with the inhalation agents. Uncoupling is more pronounced at MAC multiples. The effects of the inhalational agents are somewhat mitigated by hypocarbia.

Spinal Cord Ischemia

The spinal cord receives its blood supply from the aorta via the vertebral and segmental or radicular arteries. The main arteries of the spinal cord consist of a single anterior spinal artery and the two posterior spinal arteries. These are augmented by multiple segmental radicular and medullary arteries. The anterior spinal artery supplies the anterior two thirds of the cord. The most consistent of these is the artery of Adamkiewicz, which arises between T8 and L2 on the left side of the aorta 60% to 85% of the time. The posterior arteries supply the dorsal third of the spinal cord. The segmental radicular arteries are at risk if the lateral extracavitary approach is used. These are terminal end-arteries, and some feel that preoperative angiography is advisable to determine the arterial anatomy if this approach is planned.[25]

Most data on spinal cord protection are derived from studies on patients undergoing resection of thoracic or thoracoabdominal aneurysms. In these studies, the duration of the ischemia is the most important variable affecting the incidence of paraplegia, especially if aortic perfusion pressure is not maintained above 60 mm Hg.[34] Sixty minutes of ischemia is associated with paraplegia 90% of the time. This ischemic time can be extended by several methods.[144] Measures used to decrease the effects of ischemia include drainage of CSF to increase the spinal cord perfusion gradient. This gradient should be kept above 15 mm Hg (CSF pressure of 14 to 30 mm H_2O).[106] The midthoracic region is most susceptible to ischemia[40] because the anterior spinal artery is not functionally continuous. This can leave sections of the spinal cord as "watershed areas" that are particularly vulnerable to ischemia. Unfortunately, many of the techniques used to prevent ischemic injury in thoracic aneurysm surgery (CSF drainage, spinal cord cooling, intrathecal agents, etc.) are not suitable for use in thoracic spine surgery because the ischemia induced by instrumentation and/or distraction is not short-lived, nor is the ischemia induced by aortic cross-clamping. Indeed, the combined effects of traction (which decreases blood supply) and hypotension appear to be additive.[39,59,60]

High-dose steroids are often used in spinal surgery to mitigate the effects of surgical manipulation and ischemia, especially if the spinal cord has been previously traumatized. Their use in elective surgery is extrapolated from their demonstrated efficacy in spinal cord trauma in the National Acute Spinal Chord Injury Study (NASCIS). This multicenter, placebo-controlled study is well reviewed by Young.[163] The regimen consists of methylprednisolone, 30 mg/kg, followed by 5.4 mg/kg/h for 23 hours. This was shown to improve outcome after spinal cord injury if started within 8 hours of injury even if no function was present below the level of the lesion on admission.[18] At these doses, the steroids are probably acting as free-radical scavengers and inhibiting lipid peroxidation. Their use may be associated with an increased incidence of wound infections and gastrointestinal complications.[37]

Early reports of the beneficial effects of high dose naloxone in preventing posttraumatic spinal cord damage (based upon animal experiments) were encouraging. Unfortunately, more rigidly controlled studies (including one arm of the NASCIS study) failed to confirm their efficacy.

The *N*-methyl-D-aspartate (NMDA) antagonists show promise primarily in the patient with focal CNS lesions. They are thought to affect the penumbral area, thereby salvaging ischemic but not yet infarcted tissue. While outcome studies are lacking in humans, they might be incorporated into an overall anesthetic plan with little down-side potential. Agents shown to inhibit NMDA include MK-801, dextrorphan, dextromethorphan, levorphanol, and ketamine.[26,93]

Intrathecal papaverine[145] and magnesium sulfate have been shown to be protective in a dog model of aortic clamping. Intravenous magnesium sulfate has been protective in a rabbit model, but the dose used caused hypotension.[137]

Hypothermia, either total body or via perfusion of the intrathecal or epidural space, has been shown to be protective in animal models of aortic cross-clamping.[15] This is not surprising since even small decreases in brain temperature are neuroprotective.[22,23] The application of this technique to spine surgery remains to be determined. Mannitol may have a role in preventing injury by decreasing edema or by acting as a free-radical scavenger. Urea has also been used.

Maintenance of normothermia is important but may be difficult to achieve. Extensive dorsal spine procedures leave much of the body exposed. Intrathoracic or thoracoabdominal procedures also expose much of the body surface to ambient temperatures, and, in addition, a large incision may expose much of the viscera as well. One must also avoid hyperthermia, as small increases in temperature can increase $CMRO_2$ and precipitate or worsen ischemic damage.

Active rewarming using forced-air warming blankets (Bair Hugger [Augustine Medical Inc., Minneapolis, Minn.] and other brands) is the most efficient way to maintain or even raise temperature. However, the surface area available may be small due to the position and incision. Warming mattresses are used, but are not efficient. Blood and other fluids should be warmed. The inspired gases should be humidified and warmed because the major heat loss from the respiratory system results from the body's efforts to humidify the gases. Within pediatric patients the room should be warmed. Unfortunately, most surgeons are made uncomfortable by this maneuver.

Ischemia occurring during surgery will usually manifest as paraplegia when the patient emerges from anesthesia. However, ischemia and neurological deterioration can develop during the first 8 to 12 hours postoperatively. This has been reported as long as 72 hours following spinal surgery.

As mentioned, some groups favor preoperative angiography to evaluate the arterial supply to the spinal cord. The site of the approach or even the type of approach can then be modified depending on the origin of the spinal end-arterial feeders (especially if the lateral extracavitary approach is being contemplated).[25]

SPECIAL PROCEDURES
Chemonucleolysis

Chemonucleolysis involves injection of chymopapain into a herniated disc in an effort to dissolve it and thereby avoid surgery. The major complication of this procedure is anaphylactic response to the papain, which can be severe or even fatal. It is this complication (along with the outcome data) that have cooled enthusiasm for this procedure.

Chemonucleolysis can be performed under general, regional, or local anesthesia. Some favor regional or local in the belief that the ability to communicate with the patient allows more rapid detection of allergic reaction.

Thoracoscopic Surgery

Ventral spinal structures may be approached thoracoscopically.[70,89,127] Experience with this technique is limited, but reports describe its use to drain spinal abscesses, biopsy vertebral bodies, perform discectomy for herniated nucleus pulposus, and for ventral release in kyphoscoliosis.

It is too soon to determine the place of thoracoscopic spinal surgery. However, demonstrated advantages in pulmonary surgery include smaller incisions with less postoperative pain, less effect on respiratory function, and earlier patient discharge from the hospital. Disadvantages include increased surgical time (variable) and less control over exposure and bleeding. One still must be ready to proceed with thoracotomy in the case of failure or as a result of complications.

One-lung anesthesia is necessary for this procedure because the nondependent lung cannot be packed out of the way as it can during an open thoracotomy. This necessitates the use of a double lumen tube or bronchial blocker. Placing these tubes in a patient with a difficult airway or unstable cervical spine may be difficult and is discussed elsewhere.

Once the lungs are separated and the dependent lung ventilated, pneumothorax occurs when the chest trocar is placed. Adhesions may prevent the nondependent lung from falling away from the chest wall and may need to be lysed. The insufflation of carbon dioxide into the pleural space to produce a pneumothorax has been described.[151]

Because pressure is now atmospheric in the nondependent hemithorax, the hemodynamic and respiratory changes are similar to those described for open procedures. Use of suction by the surgeon may decrease intrathoracic pressure enough to re-expand the nondependent lung. If this occurs, placement of another trocar as a "vent" will correct this situation.

Intraoperative Position Changes

Combined ventral and dorsal approaches may require changing the patient's position from supine or lateral to prone. There is little information in the literature concerning the best way to manage these patients. If the cervical spine is involved, the authors favor the use of a Stryker or similar frame to effect the supine to prone change. This allows the patient to be turned with minimal movement of the spine, and cervical traction can be maintained if necessary.

Having enough people to manage all parts of the body cannot be overemphasized. One person (usually the surgeon) should coordinate the turn and move the most vulnerable part. Somatosensory monitoring or a wake-up test may be used following the turn to make sure no damage was done.

SCOLIOSIS

Scoliosis is defined as one or more lateral rotary curvatures in the spine. Its severity is described by the Cobb method for determining the degree of spinal curvature (Cobb angle). Eighty percent of the cases are idiopathic. Neuromuscular conditions associated with scoliosis include upper and lower motor neuron lesion, myopathic conditions such as Friedreich's ataxia and muscular dystrophy, neurofibromatosis, and mesenchymal disorders including Marfan's syndrome. Trauma, tumors, infection, and metabolic problems (e.g., rickets) also have the potential to cause kyphoscoliosis.

Patients with scoliosis may have an increased incidence of malignant hyperthermia (MH).[75] Succinylcholine (SUX) is contraindicated in muscular dystrophy, having been associated with hyperthermia, hyperkalemia, and rhabdomyolysis. Other drugs, including the inhalational agents, may trigger this response.[133] Neuropathic patients are susceptible to hyperkalemia from SUX.[29,57] Denervation of muscle causes a proliferation of extrajunctional cholinergic receptors. These muscles show resistance to the effects of nondepolarizing agents and are the cause of the hyperkalemia following SUX.

SUX produces prolonged contractions in patients with myotonia dystrophica. Shivering, percussion, and surgical manipulation may also cause spasm. Quinidine and procainamide are sometimes helpful, as is infiltration of the muscle with local anesthetics. Administration of nondepolarizing relaxants is of no benefit.

Respiratory Consequences

Respiratory complications are a major cause of morbidity in the perioperative period, and postoperative mechanical ventilation may be necessary. Curves of less than 65 degrees are not usually associated with respiratory impairment.[20] A direct relationship exists between the severity of the curvature and the decrease in vital capacity (VC).[14] The pulmonary complications are consistent with a restrictive defect. A VC less than 60% of predicted (when appropriately corrected for decreased height) is associated with increased postoperative complications including right heart failure.[75] In the scoliotic patient, one may consider armspan rather than height in predicting PFTs. Thoracic lordosis decreases the anterior-posterior diameter of the chest and therefore lung capacity.

Scoliosis associated with neuromuscular disease may cause respiratory compromise at a lesser degree of curvature than that of other etiologies. In addition, patients with neuromuscular disease may have abnormal central respiratory control, poor cough and laryngeal function, and delayed gastric emptying, leading to increased risk of aspiration. Because scoliosis due to neuromuscular disease may give lower pulmonary function tests for a given degree of curvature, the maximum voluntary ventilation (MVV) may be a better predictor of pulmonary complications.

The PFTs in scoliosis are consistent with a primary restrictive defect (normal flows with a reduced VC). As mentioned, when evaluating these tests, arm span rather than height should be used to normalize the results, since scoliosis results in decreased height and therefore the predicted values will be incorrect.[65] Compliance is reduced in the chest wall and total respiratory system and both are related to the angle of curvature.[113] Both static and dynamic compliances are reduced. In addition, a decreased maximum inspiratory force with normal expiratory pressures suggests defective mechanical coupling of the diaphragm and the thoracic cage. Therefore inspiratory impairment is a potential cause of respiratory failure in scoliosis.

The VC, TLC, FRC, and residual volume (RV) are all reduced in scoliosis. Vital capacity is reduced more than residual volume. Therefore vital capacity is a better overall test than total lung capacity. Patients with a VC test less than 30% of predicted usually need postoperative ventilation.[135]

Analysis of arterial blood gases shows progressive hypoxemia due to $\dot{V}/\dot{Q}$ imbalance. Hypercarbia is a later finding and its presence is a harbinger of respiratory failure.[140] Patients with a Pa_{O_2} less than 50 mm Hg or a Pa_{CO_2} greater than 50 mm Hg may not be able to tolerate surgery.[135] Hypoxemia may lead to increased pulmonary vascular resistance and pulmonary hypertension.

Hemodynamic Consequences

There is an increased incidence of mitral valve prolapse (MVP) in patients with scoliosis. Pulmonary artery hypertension (mentioned earlier) and cor pulmonale are especially common if the scoliosis begins in childhood, and may be out of proportion to the degree of curvature. Arrhythmias may be caused by the MVP; sudden death and cardiomyopathies are more common in scoliosis. Congenital heart disease is common in children with congenital scoliosis, cyanotic disorders being more common than acyanotic conditions.

Patients with scoliosis frequently have hypertension. This may shift the autoregulatory curve to the right, making controlled hypotension more difficult and potentially more dangerous. With time, controlled hypertensives may normalize their autoregulatory function, but this phenomenon is not consistent.

Adults with scoliosis may have atherosclerotic disease. Stress tests may be difficult or impossible due to musculoskeletal abnormalities. Dobutamine thallium testing or dobutamine stress echocardiographs are alternate methods of evaluating for coronary artery disease. Myocardial infarction within 6 months of operative intervention and congestive heart failure are consistent risk factors for perioperative cardiac events.[92] The suspicion of coronary artery disease might impact the decision to use controlled hypotension.

SPINAL CORD TRAUMA

The most common causes of traumatic spinal cord injuries are motor vehicle accidents and diving injuries. It has been estimated that between 1.5% to 3% of all major trauma victims have associated cervical spine injury.[142] Multiple trauma patients who are hypotensive, hypovolemic, and yet bradycardac should be suspected of having spinal shock.[160]

Absence of neck pain or tenderness in an alert, unmedicated patient essentially eliminates the presence of significant cervical spine injury. Often, the patient is too unstable to undergo CT or MRI and plane radiographs of the neck must be used to initially evaluate for cervical injury. Rheumatoid arthritis may lead to dislocation of C1 upon C2. This has been reported to occur spontaneously or with minimal trauma, leading to quadriparesis.

Physiology

In those patients with complete physiological spinal cord transection, there is initially flaccid paralysis below the level of the injury (spinal shock). This phase may last 1 to 3 weeks and is associated with loss of temperature regulation. Lack of sympathetic tone below the level of injury leads to hypotension, vascular dilatation with pooling of blood, and bradycardia. ECG findings include bradycardia and multiple ST segment abnormalities. Respiratory impairment due to poor cough, viscous mucus, and poor inspiratory function is seen. Gastrointestinal atony, bladder distention, and electrolyte abnormalities (especially hyponatremia) are potential complications. SUX is unlikely to provoke hyperkalemia during the first 24 hours but one might still wish to avoid it unless other techniques are unacceptable.

Neurogenic pulmonary edema was originally reported following head injury. However, it is a potential complication of spinal cord injury, stroke, increased ICP, and a variety of CNS disease. There is an initial transient increase in pulmonary and systemic vascular resistances with development of pulmonary edema. Resistances quickly return to normal, but pulmonary gas exchange (as measured by arterial blood gasses [ABGs]) is slower to improve.

The acute spinal cord lesion develops over time. The destructive process may be arrested if appropriate interventions are begun within the first several hours after injury.

The patient with chronic spinal cord injury shows altered pharmacokinetics with some medications.[132] This is probably due to increased extravascular albumin pools, decreased total body water, and increased fat content. Impaired gastric emptying and impaired motility may make oral medications unreliable. Metaclopramide may aid gastric emptying.

With time, spinal cord reflexes return. Overactivity of the sympathetic nervous system (autonomic hyperreflexia [AH]) may develop in response to visceral or cutaneous stimulation. This stimulation produces reflex vasoconstriction below the injury, which persists because the spinal cord is isolated from central modulation. If the area above the injury is too small to mitigate the blood pressure response, hypertension, bradycardia, nasal stuffiness, and flushing above the level of injury occurs. The higher the injury, the more likely the occurrence of AH. About 85% of patients with an injury above T6 will have at least one episode of AH. Peripherally acting vasodilators are used to treat AH. Prevention consists of assuring adequate anesthesia (general or regional) to prevent the sympathetic response to surgical stimulation.

As noted previously, denervated muscle undergoes proliferation at and beyond the extrajunctional cholinergic receptors. SUX can cause hyperkalemia due to massive potassium release from the extrajunctional cholinergic receptors. This is not reliably prevented by pretreatment with a nondepolarizing agent. Some authors have suggested that this response decreases over time and that SUX may be safely used after 6 months. It seems more prudent to avoid it in any spinal cord injured patient unless there is an overriding need.

Table 6-1. Effects of Some Agents Commonly Used in Anesthesia

Agent	ICP	CBF	SVR	HR	Depression (Myocardial or Respiratory)	Fluoride Ion
Halothane	+	++	o	o	++	o
Isoflurane	+	+	− −	+	+	+
Low concentration	o,+					
High concentration	−					
Enflurane	+	+	+	− +	++	+
Desflurane	o,+	*	− −	+	+	o
Sevoflurane	−	*	− −	+	+	+
N₂O	o	+	+	+	+	o
Midazolam	−	−				
Low dose	+,o,α					
High dose	−,α					
Thiopental	−	−				
Low dose	+,o,α					
High dose	−					
Etomidate	−	−				
Low dose	o					
High dose	−					
Ketamine	+	+				
Propofol	o	−				

+ = Increase
− = Decrease
o = No change
* = Not well studied
α = Dependent on use

Because these patients lack compensatory sympathetic response to hypovolemia they are more sensitive to vasodilating agents. In addition, they may need more liberal fluids. Position changes should be undertaken slowly to avoid hypotension.

DRUGS

Drugs are classified here according to their predominant effects in clinical anesthesia as follows: anxiolytic (including sedatives/hypnotics), anesthetic, analgetic, neuromuscular blocking agents, and hypotensive agents (Tables 6-1 and 6-2). All dosages should be reduced (up to 50%) for debilitated, hypovolemic, elderly, or ASA class III and IV patients. Anxiolytic drugs presently used are the benzodiazepines and droperidol—all frequently used as induction/maintenance agents. Anesthetics are those agents administered by inhalational or intravenous routes. The former include nitrous oxide (N₂O) and the volatile anesthetics; the latter are comprised of the barbiturates, propofol, etomi-date, and ketamine. Analgesics may be opioid or nonopioid (nonsteroidal anti-inflammatory drugs (NSAIDs); (e.g., ketorolac) will not be discussed here. Hypotensive agents commonly in use are discussed later.

Table 6-2. Hypotensive Agents (Commonly Used IV Dosages)

Vasodilators

Hydralazine	10-20 mg
Nitroglycerin	5-20 ug/min
Nitroprusside	0.25-8.0 ug/kg/min
Trimethaphan	0.5-5.0 ug/min

Ca⁺⁺ Channel Blocker

Nicardipine	0.10-0.25 mg
maintenance	5 mg/hr

β-Blockers

Esmolol	10-20 mg
maintenance	50-500 ug/kg/min
Labetolol	5-10 mg
Propranolol	0.5-1.5 mg

Anxiolytics

Midazolam (Versed) is probably the most frequently used benzodiazepine, because it is water-soluble and may be administered intravenously without pain. The drug has little effect on ICP and cardiopulmonary hemodynamics. The introduction of midazolam has replaced, to a great degree, the use of diazepam (Valium) and of the opioids as premedicants. For sedation, incremental intravenous (IV) doses are 0.5 to 1.0 mg; the intramuscular (IM) dosage is 0.05 to 0.1 mg/kg. IV induction dosage is about 3 times the IM sedative doses. In case of overdosage, flumazenil (Romazicon) may be administered at an initial dose of 0.2 mg IV, with additional doses as needed to reach a maximum total dose of 1.0 mg. More recently interest has turned to the potential anxiolytic effects of 5-HT$_2$ antagonists and 5-HT$_{1A}$ agonists.[143]

Droperidol (Inapsine), a butyrophenone, is presently used more for its antiemetic (approximately 1.25 mg IV) than its sedative (2.5 to 5.0 mg IV) properties and appears to have little effect on the cerebrovascular system, though anxiety, restlessness, and extrapyramidal reactions have been reported even at the lower doses.[101] A recent report based on angio-oedema with droperidol, stresses that care should be taken when butyrophenones are used in patients with known hypersensitivity to phenothiazines.[30] When the drug is added in a low dose to morphine for patient-controlled analgesia (PCA), there is a reduction in postoperative nausea and vomiting (PONV).[158] Two cases of anaphylaxis from droperidol have been reported.[112]

Inhalational Anesthetics

Because N$_2$O is about 30 times more soluble than N$_2$ in blood, the N$_2$ is replaced rapidly by N$_2$O. In a closed cavity (e.g., bowel (especially if obstructed), pneumothorax, cranium (following pneumocephalography, or traumatic or surgical pneumocephalus), the increased volume may result in increased pressure—a potentially unwelcome adverse effect.

A common practice is to administer 70% N$_2$O in oxygen, combined with a reduced concentration of other inhalational agents. The inhalational anesthetics presently in use are the halogenated hydrocarbon halothane (Fluothane) and the halogenated ethers: enflurane (Ethrane), isoflurane (Forane), and desflurane (Suprane). These are liquids that may be volatilized by vaporizers or by direct injection of the liquid into the anesthetic circuit where they vaporize (because their boiling points are below conventional ambient temperatures).

Hypocapnia induced by hyperventilation usually eliminates the increase in ICP due to cerebral vasodilatation. Some clinicians believe this to be most reliably produced during isoflurane anesthesia. Patients with intracranial lesions should not receive halothane until hypocapnia has been established. Enflurane should be used with care in these patients because it may produce seizures in the presence of hypocapnia; convulsions are less likely if concentrations are maintained below 1.5% to 2%.

Intravenous Anesthetics

Thiopental and thiamylal are generally administered IV as 2.5% solutions following a 50 mg (2 ml) test dose (because anaphylaxis, though very rare, has been reported[17]). The dose is titrated slowly to the desired effect—usually up to 5 mg/kg, but doses may reach 15 mg/kg even for induction alone (as in the UK and by one of the authors (S.N.S.) in which case other agents (volatile or narcotics) should be reduced, particularly before the end of the procedure, so that emergence is not delayed. The elimination half-life of ca 12 hours is doubled in marked obesity and halved in pediatric patients.[42]

Methohexital is usually administered in the same manner as thiopental and thiamylal, as a 1% solution. The dose used is ca 1 to 2 mg/kg. Barbiturates may impart a limited degree of brain protection.[43,103]

Propofol (Diprivan) can be given by bolus or continuous infusion. Injection through a free-running solution in a large vein minimizes the pain of administration. The use of 1% lidocaine (5 to 10 ml) prior to or with the propofol usually prevents this pain. The drug is generally administered 1 to 2 mg/kg IV. It has a rapid onset and recovery[77] with little nausea and emesis, benefits that outweigh the potential for pain on injection. It has been used in the high-risk patient[32] and for sedation (e.g., in the pediatric MRI[87] and in the ICU), but disinhibition does occur in some patients during conscious sedation.[107] Propofol appears to be a nontriggering agent in malignant hyperthermia (MH).[80] Anaphylactoid reactions to propofol have been reported.[84,99]

Etomidate (Amidate) administered IV, 0.2 mg/kg, for induction appears to have less of a respiratory depressant effect than the barbiturates or propofol and has been used as a sedative[124] in the ICU.

Ketamine (Ketalar) produces marked increases in ICP in patients with normal or elevated ICP, suggesting it not be used in the latter group. Because the drug may increase arterial pressure (up to 25%), it is contraindicated when a significant elevation of blood pressure could constitute a serious hazard (in patients with aneurysm, cerebral trauma, etc.). In burn patients (where IV access may be difficult) it is useful, because it may be given intramuscularly at 2 mg/kg (ca the same dose as intravenously).

Analgesics

Analgesics may be either opioid or nonopioid (Table 6-3). With the above in mind, we will briefly review several opioids (morphine, meperidine and members of the *Familia fentanalia*).

With morphine the onset of respiratory depression occurs after the onset of analgesic effects with peaks occurring at 30 to 60 minutes and 15 to 30 minutes, respectively. This difference between onsets and peaks may result in the not uncommon occurrence of postoperative oversedation with potential respiratory depression leading to apnea, etc. Meperidine (Demerol, Pethidine) has both a shorter onset time and duration of analgetic effects than morphine.

Fentanyl (Phentanyl, Sublimaze) has a rapid onset of action with peak analgetic and respiratory depressant effects occurring in a few minutes. Because the drug (usually given in doses of 50 to 100 µg IV and/or by infusion) has a long elimination half-life (Table 6-4), cumulative effects may occur. High blood levels are attained when the portal circulation is bypassed (i.e., when the buccal, intranasal, or transdermal routes are used). Sufentanil (Sufenta) is a derivative of fentanyl and is more potent than fentanyl. Alfentanil (Alfenta), another derivative, is less potent than fentanyl.

Muscle rigidity is most often noted at the induction of general anesthesia when a large bolus of opioid is administered intravenously. Doses as low as 50 µg fentanyl may produce this effect with inability to ventilate the patient. This complication may be treated by a small dose of muscle relaxant, such as SUX, if not contraindicated.

Small doses of opioids produce pupillary constriction (which may be reversed with opioid antagonists or ganglionic blockers [e.g., atropine]), a sign

Table 6-3. Some Properties of the Commonly Used Opioid Analgestics

Agent	Equivalent Dose (mg, IV)	Duration (hr, post-first single injection)
Morphine	1.00	3-4
Meperidine	10.00	2-3
Fentanyl	0.10	0.5-1.0
Sufentanil	0.01	0.5-1.0
Alfentanil	0.75	0.2-0.3

Table 6-4. Half-Life of Some Commonly Used Anesthetic Agents

Agent	Hours
Midazolam	2-2.5
Diazepam	20-40
Flumazenil	1
Etomidate	2-7
Ketamine	2.5
Propofol	4
Thiopental	11.5
Methohexital	2.5-4.0
Morphine	2
Demerol	3-4
Fentanyl	3-4
Sufentanil	2.5
Alfentanil	1.5
Droperidol	2

that may be important in the neurological evaluation of the patient.

Cardiovascular effects are generally of no consequence when the usual clinical analgetic doses are used. Bradycardia can occur when large doses are administered rapidly but may be reversed by vagolytic drugs. Hypotension is often observed with analgetic doses, and is frequently orthostatic in nature. This generally responds to the usual measures (positional changes, fluids, and vasopressor).

Allergic responses are rare and are generally due to a nonimmunological release of histamine; if a response is anaphylactic in nature, standard treatment should be initiated promptly. Accordingly, because opioids may precipitate bronchospasm they should be used cautiously in asthmatic patients.

It appears that all equianalgetic doses of opioids result in the same amount of respiratory depression. When respiratory depression is reversed, there is also some reversal of analgesia. When opioids are

Table 6-5. Half-Life of Some Commonly Used Anesthetic Agents

Agent	mg/kg	Time (min) to Intubation	Time (min) to 25% $T_{baseline}$
Succinylcholine	1.0	1	10
Rocuronium	0.8	1	30-60
Mivacurium	0.2	2	
Pancuronium	0.1	3	90
Atracurium	0.5	3	30
Vecronium	0.1	3	30
d-Tubocurare	0.5	3	90
Pipecuronium	0.8	5	50-100
Doxacurium	0.8	5	100-150

Maintenance doses are usually about one third of intubation dose when first twitch (T_1) = 25% $T_{baseline}$.

used alone intraoperative awareness may occur; other agents are generally added to avoid this potential complication.

Naloxone is the only available pure parenteral opioid antagonist. Reversal of opioids should be undertaken with care, as hemodynamic changes[6,102,146] and pulmonary edema[48,117] may occur and even death has been reported.[5]

Nausea and vomiting are common effects of the opioids. The most useful clinically available antiemetic appears to be ondansetron (Zofran), a serotonin receptor blocker, although other drugs (droperidol [Inapsine], metoclopramide [Reglan], prochlorperazine [Compazine], domperidone) are also effective and less expensive.

Neuromuscular Blocking Agents

Neuromuscular blocking (NMB) agents may be divided into nondepolarizing blocking drugs (Table 6-5), which compete with acetylcholine for cholinergic receptor sites, and the depolarizing drug succinylcholine dichloride (SUX, Anectine).

The duration of action of an NMB drug is of some importance. The NMBs are administered to effect, and this titration is aided measurably by the use of a peripheral neuromuscular stimulation device.

NMBs are used for skeletal muscle relaxation, to facilitate ventilation and endotracheal intubation, to relieve laryngospasm, and to maintain a lighter level of general anesthesia (but not to compensate for inadequate anesthesia).

The dosage requirements of all NMB drugs are decreased by about one third to one half when inhalation agents are used compared to N_2O/O_2 used alone. Increase in the duration of neuromuscular

block from the NMB agents may occur with most antibiotics, particularly the aminoglycosides.

Reversal of neuromuscular blocking effect, if desirable, may be undertaken when there is a muscle response of at least one or more twitches to peripheral nerve stimulation using the train of four technique. While some evidence exists that deeper levels of blockade are reversible, caution is advised, especially in cases involving a difficult airway.

An advantage of SUX is its short duration of action due to its rapid metabolism to succinyl monocholine (which is ca 0.05 times as potent) in about 95% of patients; the remaining patients have prolonged blockade.[157] SUX action may be prolonged and onset delayed with lithium. Some antibiotics, insecticides, and echothiopate eyedrops are a few of the agents known to inhibit plasma cholinesterase and thus cause prolonged responses to SUX. Prolonged apnea has been reported in patients receiving the chemotherapeutic agent cyclophosphamide (Cytoxan). This is due to inhibition of blood cholinesterase. Approximately 10 days are required to restore cholinesterase activity following the administration of cyclophosphamide.

SUX usually results in a slight increase (up to 0.5 mEq/L) in serum K^+, which is of little consequence in the normal individual. Certain pathological conditions may result in a large increase in K^+ that can produce cardiac arrhythmias and arrest. These include: burns, massive tissue trauma, upper motor neuron lesions, spinal cord and/or head trauma, amyotrophic lateral sclerosis, Friedreich's ataxia, Guillain-Barre disease, and cerebrovascular accidents. As a general rule, SUX should be avoided in any neurological condition that produces muscle wasting.

In myotonia congenita and myotonia dystrophica (myotonia atrophica, Steinert's disease, Hoffman's disease) the drug may not produce muscle relaxation, but rather contractions that are not inhibited by NMBs[2] and thus can prevent ventilation and intubation. Fortunately, these are generally self-limited. Even when the airway is secure, adequate ventilation may not be possible because of contracture of the muscles of respiration.[27,105,148]

Adverse Drug Reactions

An adverse drug reaction is any drug response that is not of therapeutic, prophylactic, or diagnostic benefit to the patient. Allergy is a hypersensitive reaction caused by exposure to a specific antigen, re-exposure to which may produce an anaphylactic reaction. Anaphylactic reactions are immunologically mediated, usually by immune globulin E (IgE) (type I hypersensitivity). Though they are uncommon intraoperatively, they may be devastating. Anaphylactoid reactions may be produced by direct release of vasoactive substances without prior exposure to an antigen. Complement activation may follow immunological or nonimmunological pathways.

There is an increased incidence of adverse drug reactions in AIDS patients, possibly due to altered patterns of drug metabolism.[85]

In the practice of anesthesia, drugs are commonly administered IV, thus bypassing the body's natural defenses to deliver an antigenic load directly to the basophils (stores of the main mediators of anaphylaxis). As a result, such reactions would be expected to be more frequent in the specialty of anesthesia. However, the incidence is difficult to assess, probably because of variations in reporting and of different patterns of drug use. For example, the incidence has been reported to be 1 in 1250 (New Zealand), 1 in 3500 (France) and 1 in 10,000 to 20,000 (Australia).

Anaphylaxis may occur late, for example, outside the operating room,[141] especially in "at risk" patients. Because ca 10% of such individuals require a second injection of epinephrine following apparent stabilization,[47] all should be observed for 6 hours, as late deterioration may occur.

Anaphylaxis to natural latex products (e.g., the anesthetic breathing bags, catheters, compression bandages, balloons, condoms, diaphragms, dental cofferdams, medication stoppers, etc.,[64] has been reported both outside of and inside the operating room.

Children with spina bifida and/or congenital urologic abnormalities are frequently exposed to latex materials and may be at increased risk for serious allergic reactions when exposed to latex intraoperatively.[54] Available data suggest that up to 50% of patients with myelodysplasia may be allergic to latex.[68]

Approximately 5% of administrations of IV iodinated contrast media result in reactions ranging from mild nausea and vomiting to anaphylaxis.[56] Seizures are possible after intrathecal contrast studies, but fortunately, MRI and CT have supplanted these tests to a large degree.

Prevention is aimed at blocking the allergic reaction and resultant histamine effects. One recommendation calls for prednisone, 50 mg orally (3 doses, 6 hours apart) and IV diphenhydramine, 50 mg, prior to exposure. In another regimen, both H_1 and H_2 blockers are used with steroids the night prior to the test as well as immediately before exposure.

Treatment of reactions is symptomatic and supportive. Discontinuation of the infusion and monitoring of vital signs are essential. Additional antihistamines and steroids (up to 1.0 gm methylprednisone) should be given as well as bronchodilators (beta sympathomimetics and/or aminophylline) if bronchospasm occurs. Epinephrine, 3 to 5 µg IV boluses followed by an infusion to support the blood pressure, may be necessary. The airway should be secured early because edema of the mucous membranes may make control of the airway difficult or impossible later.

Malignant hyperthermia (MH) is observed most commonly in fit, healthy individuals in the second and third decades of life and is a condition with which all anesthetists must be familiar. The incidence of MH is higher in North America (1 in 20,000 to 40,000 anesthetics) than in the United Kingdom (1 in 190,000).[147]

Abortive ("mild") forms of MH have an incidence of 1 in 4500 when SUX is used and may be even more frequent in children.[55] This is generally noted as masseter muscle rigidity and may be a precursor of MH, although not all masseter spasms are true MH.

The most common precipitating agents are SUX and the volatile inhalational anesthetics. Those agents considered safe comprise the anxiolytics, opioid analgetics, droperidol, ketamine, N_2O, and the nondepolarizing NMBs. Ester and amide local anesthetics are also considered nontriggering agents.

The primary signs of MH are tachycardia, tachypnea, elevated temperature, rigidity, increased $P_{ET}CO_2$, and acidosis (metabolic and respiratory). Elevated $PaCO_2$, manifested as an increased $P_{ET}CO_2$ may be the first sign.

Dantrolene is the definitive treatment, starting with 2.5 mg/kg IV and repeating as necessary up to a total dose of 10 to 20 mg/kg or until all vital signs normalize. When stable, one may convert to oral dantrolene 1 mg/kg PO every 6 hours for 24 to 48 hours. Because MH may recur following initial control with dantrolene, close observation is necessary. Supportive therapy consists of hyperventilation with 100% oxygen using a new circuit and soda lime, cooling, and treatment of metabolic acidosis (HCO_3 1 to 2 mg/kg), of hyperkalemia (glucose 0.5 to 1.0 gm and regular insulin 5 to 10 U), of arrhythmias (procainamide [Pronestyl, Procan] 3 mg/kg to a maximum of 15 mg/kg), and maintenance of urinary output (>1 ml/kg/hr using volume and diuretics). Family counseling, Medic-Alert identification, and muscle biopsy (later) are advised.

Adverse Events Related to Equipment

Equipment failure is not uncommon. Valves may malfunction in either the open or closed position. Problems may also arise due to inadequate fresh gas supply, vaporizer malfunction, or obstruction of the anesthesia circuit.[50]

ANESTHETIC TECHNIQUE
General Anesthesia
Premedication

Premedication follows the general principles of good anesthetic practice. Little or no sedation is used in patients weakened by neuromuscular disease. While the primary purpose is anxiolysis, analgesics may be needed for patients for whom moving is painful. Premedication should include maintenance of antihypertensive, cardiopulmonary medications and others as indicated. Metoclopramide and an H_2 antagonist may be added for patients at increased risk of aspiration. Antisialogogues are of particular benefit if the patient is to be intubated awake, since a dry airway accepts topical anesthesia better and secretions obstruct the view through a fiberscope. Oxygen (begun the night before surgery) may prevent desaturation during sleep, which may

lead to increased pulmonary artery pressure. Care must be used if the patient retains CO_2 or is otherwise dependent on his hypoxic drive.

Induction

Security of the airway is of primary importance, especially if the cervical spine is unstable or immobile. Once this is accomplished, any of the short-acting hypnotic induction agents may be satisfactory. SUX (if not contraindicated) allows rapid return of neuromuscular function so that response to nerve stimulation can be assessed to determine if somatosensory evoked potential (SSEP) electrodes are properly positioned.[100] A stable level of relaxation can be achieved with an infusion of a nondepolarizing relaxant. This helps eliminate background "noise" and makes it easier to obtain SSEPs and motor evoked responses. Use of a peripheral nerve stimulator may help avoid overparalysis and ensure that the block can be reversed if a wake-up test is needed. The use of a nerve stimulator is mandatory in virtually all patients receiving NMB drugs.

Maintenance

A stable level of anesthesia makes interpretation of the SSEP easier. Because all anesthetics affect the SSEP, establishing a stable level early in the procedure allows each patient to act as his own control and makes subsequent changes easier to identify. For this reason, an infusion of narcotics may be preferable to intermittent boluses.[119] Similarly, propofol/narcotic infusions (with or without nitrous oxide) are gaining popularity because they allow evaluation of the SSEP and rapid awakening at the end of surgery or for a wake-up test.[76] Etomidate may be useful in that it decreases the ICP with minimal effects upon blood pressure, therefore preserving spinal cord perfusion pressure.[36]

Benzodiazepines are useful in preventing awareness and recall during the light anesthesia that may be necessary for SSEP monitoring. In addition, they decrease the CBF, ICP, and $CMRO_2$. If necessary, they can be rapidly antagonized with flumazenil.

Isoflurane may be the potent inhalational agent of choice. It shows little change in CBF with a decrease in $CMRO_2$. Any increase in ICP can be mitigated by hypocapnia or barbiturates, which are effective even after institution of isoflurane.

In short, any technique that affects SSEP minimally (i.e., light levels of general anesthesia) and allows rapid awakening is satisfactory. The use of vasoactive drugs or beta blockers may be necessary to control hemodynamics in patients without deepening the anesthesia. Because light levels of general anesthesia are helpful in neurological monitoring, the risk of intraoperative awareness is increased. The use of ear plugs, soothing music, or prerecorded tapes of positive postoperative suggestions (through head phones) may have some value. The literature shows that intraoperative awareness is a real phenomenon. In this setting, it would appear to be a viable consideration, especially in light of its minimal down-side potential.

Emergence

Awakening from anesthesia should be smooth and safe. Coughing on the ETT has been known to dislodge a repair or instrumentation. Instillation of a topical anesthetic down the ETT before reversal of the relaxant may allow a lighter level of anesthesia without "bucking" (i.e., reacting on the ETT). Alternatively, the LITA Tube (Sheridan Catheter) may be used to instill local anesthetic into the posterior pharynx and trachea through multiple perforations in a separate channel of the ETT.

One reason for having the patient awake at the end of the surgery is to test voluntary motor function. If the patient is not awake enough to follow verbal commands, application of a peripheral nerve stimulator may elicit withdrawal of the lower extremity. Ankle clonus occurs during emergence and its presence implies intact spinal reflexes and at least some action of the upper motor neurons upon the lower spinal cord.[111]

In the patient with a normal airway, deep extubation avoids many of the problems associated with awake extubation (bucking, hemodynamic instability, arrhythmias, etc.).

Regional Anesthesia

As mentioned previously, regional anesthesia has been used for diagnostic and some therapeutic procedures (e.g., chemonucleolysis). There is a growing experience with its use as the sole anesthetic agent for lumbar spinal surgery (with appropriate sedation). Proponents cite shorter hospital stays and less postoperative pain as two of the main advantages;

ease of patient positioning is another. Unfortunately, the level required for thoracic spinal surgery makes regional anesthesia impractical for these procedures. Its use is generally restricted to postoperative pain control (discussed later in this chapter).

SPECIALIZED TECHNIQUES FOR AIRWAY CONTROL OF THE UNSTABLE CERVICAL SPINE/IMMOBILE NECK

A familiarity with fiberoptic techniques is extremely important for the anesthesiologist dealing with the unstable cervical spine or when intrathoracic procedures are undertaken. The article by Keenan, Stiles, and Kaufman[78] describing triplanar deviation of the larynx and protrusion of the odontoid process through the foramen magnum in rheumatic patients is invaluable, as are the texts by Ovassapian,[114] Roberts,[125] and Benumof.[11]

Patients with suspected cervical spine injuries are frequently immobilized in the field using a rigid (e.g., Philadelphia) collar. Additional stabilization with sand bags at the sides of the head and tape across the forehead is considered necessary to provide true immobilization. An equally effective method that allows better visualization for direct laryngoscopy is manual in-line immobilization.[33] This method permits the rigid collar and other restraints to be removed (limitation of mouth opening is a major impediment to direct laryngoscopy with the patient in a collar), which improves visualization without compromising spine immobilization.[63] Note that this differs from prior recommendations that advocated in-line traction. Application of traction has the potential to further destabilize and/or traumatize the injured cervical spine.

Awake intubation using topical anesthesia and sedation is the most conservative approach and should be considered the primary technique in patients who may be difficult to intubate, either because of anatomy or instability of the cervical spine. Not all authors agree with this approach, and indeed there is a large clinical experience suggesting that it is safe to perform direct laryngoscopy provided appropriate stabilization measures are taken. Appropriate sedation with narcotics and benzodiazepines makes this approach more acceptable to the patient. Antisialogogues improve the effect of anesthetics by drying the secretions and also permit better visualization for the same reason.

The oropharynx is sprayed with lidocaine or benzocaine. Two to four percent lidocaine is administered through a small-volume nebulizer. The patient is encouraged to inhale deeply through his mouth. This technique is simple, avoids any injections and provides excellent anesthesia to the entire airway from the pharynx to below the level of the carina. The most common cause of failure is rushing the procedure. At least 10 minutes of inhalation is necessary to achieve good results. If a nasal intubation is planned, the mucosa is topicalized with 4% cocaine or 4% lidocaine to which phenyleprine has been added. One may use a dropper to instill the solution, and follow with pledgets or applicator sticks. The pledgets or applicators must be allowed to remain in contact with the nasal mucosa for several minutes. An alternative technique is to advance a small bore catheter through the naris, spraying topical anesthetic in advance of the catheter. The sphenopalatine ganglion may be sprayed with 2 to 3 ml of 2% lidocaine using a syringe attached to a small IV catheter. It is helpful to have several syringes with local anesthetic ready for use through the suction channel of the bronchoscope. This method helps to topicalize any areas that have been missed. Prior to beginning this or any other technique, identification and marking of the cricothyroid membrane is helpful. If emergency transtracheal jet ventilation (TTJV) or cricothyroidotomy is necessary, it is helpful to have the appropriate location identified beforehand. Benumof has gone so far as to advocate prophylactic placement of a 14-ga angiocath through the membrane in selected cases.

Techniques for blocking the sphenopalatine ganglion, glossopharyngeal nerve, superior laryngeal nerve, and the recurrent laryngeal nerves are described in most standard anesthesia texts, as is transcricothyroid instillation of topical anesthetic agents. The authors have not found these techniques necessary when adequate topicalization is used as described above.

Intubation after induction of general anesthesia is rarely indicated in the patient with an unstable cervical spine. With proper use of sedation, even pediatric or mentally retarded patients can be intubated "awake." This might more appropriately be described as intubation under heavy sedation with spontaneous ventilation.

Another alternative method for the pediatric patient (if a pediatric scope is unavailable) consists of intubating the trachea with a guide wire threaded through the suction channel of a fiberoptic bronchoscope. The scope is removed after the guide wire is in place and the appropriate-sized ETT is passed over the guide wire into the trachea.

Blind nasal intubation should only be attempted if no fiberscope is available. Bleeding from attempted passage of the tube may make later use of the fiberscope (a decidedly better technique) difficult, if not impossible. In addition, some of the recommended maneuvers for nasal intubation require manipulation of the head and/or neck, which is not desirable for a patient with an unstable cervicle spine.

Some have advocated passage of increasing sizes of nasopharyngeal airways in an effort to dilate the nasal passages. Most often this is not necessary when adequate topicalization has been achieved using an anesthetic containing a vasoconstrictor. A nasopharyngeal airway, split longitudinally (split nasal trumpet), may expedite passage of the fiberoptic scope because it decreases trauma to the nasal mucosa.

Opinions differ as to whether the tube or fiberscope should be passed first through the nasal passage. Placing the tube in the nasopharynx first allows it to be used as a guide for the fiberscope. In addition, it avoids the situation where the trachea has been intubated with the fiberscope and the ETT is too large to pass through the nasal passage. The risk is that the tube will cause bleeding that may make fiberoptic visualization more difficult. Therefore some clinicians favor passing the scope first. In the unusual circumstance where one must intubate nasally and there is a suspicion of skull fracture, the scope must be passed so that the nasal passage can be traversed under visual control. This will decrease the chance of injuring intracranial structures with the ETT.

Numerous specialized blades are available for direct laryngoscopy, and some are useful in this setting. The Bullard and Upsher blades provide fiberoptic viewing through a rigid blade. The Bullard laryngoscope appears to be useful in the care of patients in whom cervical spine movement is limited or undesirable, since median values for external head extension of 2 degrees (compared to 10 degrees and 11 degrees for the Miller and Macintosh blades, respectively) have been reported.[28] The Augustine system is a blind oral technique using a special device to pass a stylet into the trachea over which an ETT is passed. The Sheridan Combitube has been

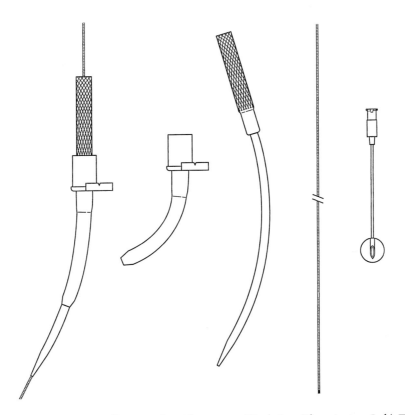

Fig. 6-15. Components of the Melker cricothyroidotomy set (Cook, Inc., Bloomington, Ind.). The needle is used to puncture the cricothyroid membrane and introduce the guide wire. An incision is then made through the skin and cricothyroid membrane. The tube and dilator are then advanced as a unit over the wire into the trachea. The wire and dilator are removed, leaving the cricothyroidotomy tube in place, which is then secured with tracheostomy tapes. The tube accepts a standard connection to an anesthesia circuit or self-inflating bag. Models with an adaptor to allow TTJV through the cricothyroidotomy tube are also available.

used as an emergency airway for patients with cervical problems. It is usually considered a "bail-out" technique if intubation is unsuccessful; however, patients have been managed on mechanical ventilation and given general anesthesia using the Combitube. The LMA has been used to "buy time" if intubation attempts fail, or as a method of administering general anesthesia while a definitive airway is being established either by endotracheal intubation or surgical means. The LMA can also be used as a guide for fiberoptic tube placement.

A retrograde technique using either an epidural catheter or a specialized retrograde intubation set (Cook Inc., Bloomington, Ind.) is an excellent choice for the patient with an unstable neck and a traumatized upper airway because bleeding may make fiberoptic endoscopy particularly difficult. If a guide wire is used rather than an epidural catheter, the wire can be threaded up the suction channel of a fiberoptic bronchoscope, allowing the scope to be passed blindly through the glottic opening. Once in the trachea the scope can be used to confirm endotracheal positioning and as a guide for passage of the ETT. Intubation using transtracheal illumination has its advocates, although this may be difficult (e.g., in the obese patient).

At times, the expeditious approach is a surgical airway (a tracheostomy or cricothyroidotomy under local anesthesia). Several emergency cricothyroidotomy sets are commercially available (Cook Melker set, Nu-Trach, and others) (Fig. 6-15). These are simple, convenient methods for establishing an emergency surgical airway. Their main drawback is that there is no cuff on the cricothyroidotomy tube. The Melker wire-dilator combination has been used to introduce a cuffed tracheotomy tube through the cricothyroid membrane, but rupture of the cuff during passage is an inherent drawback. A percutaneous tracheotomy set (e.g., Ciaglia set [Cook, Inc., Bloomington, Ind.]) can be used to introduce a cuffed tube through the cricothyroid membrane, but experience with this technique is limited. In emergency situations where a cuffed tube is immediately necessary, a surgical cricothyroidotomy using a No. 6 ETT is an alternative. Formal training and practice is necessary to perform this technique safely. The Advanced Trauma Life Support (ATLS) course offered by the American College of Surgeons is excellent training for this technique and is highly recommended for those caring for trauma victims.

If the patient becomes hypoxemic or develops laryngospasm while a definitive airway is being established, TTJV can be lifesaving. A 14-gauge catheter or one of several commercially available specialized catheters (Melker, Aldt, Patil, or TTJV catheters, [Cook, Inc., Bloomington, Ind.]) may be used to provide oxygen while fiberoptic or other techniques are being attempted. One person should be assigned to maintain the catheter in proper position. Later, if a retrograde technique is elected, the cricothyroid catheter can be used as the insertion site for the wire.

Several commercially available products are available to fix the tube in the patient's airway. This is especially important in patients in the prone position. If the cervical spine is not involved, umbilical tapes or adhesive tape can be used in a circumferential fashion. Otherwise, Mastisol, benzoin, or other skin preparatory solutions used with waterproof tape may be used to secure the tube and protect against the effects of secretions.

Extubation of the Difficult Airway

As mentioned earlier, a controlled extubation with the patient able to manage his/her own airway is the objective from both a surgical and anesthetic view. This is especially true for the patient with a difficult airway due to an unstable or immobile cervical spine.

The use of a laryngeal tracheal anesthesia (LTA) kit facilitates a smooth extubation by allowing the patient to tolerate the stimulus of the ETT at lighter levels of anesthesia. Clinically, the obtundation of tracheal reflexes seems to outlast the known duration of action of lidocaine. Spraying lidocaine down the ETT (before reversal of paralysis) can have much the same effect. Recently, the LITA Tube (Sheridan Catheter Co.), which has perforations that

allow pharyngeal and tracheal instillation of local anesthetic, has been introduced. This could facilitate smooth emergence and intubation in much the same way as an LTA kit.

Patients with a difficult airway should be extubated over a ventilating tube changer (stylet). Stylets are hollow plastic tubes with ventilation side holes, and are available from several companies (e.g., Cook Catheter, Inc., Sheridan Catheter, Co., and others) (Fig. 6-16). They are an improvement

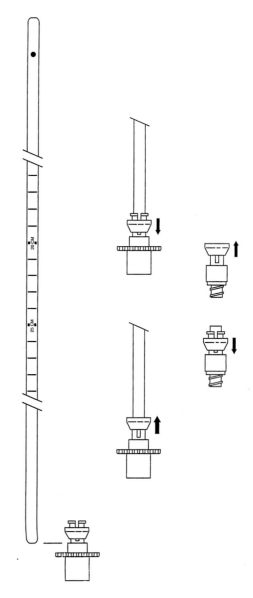

Fig. 6-16. The Cook ventilating/tube exchanging catheter (Cook, Inc., Bloomington, Ind.). Note the rapid-fit adapters for both conventional and jet ventilation. The catheter should not be advanced further than the carina. Markings on the catheter allow measurement of the length of insertion.

over such devices as gum rubber bougies, nasogastric tubes, etc., in that they have adapters that allow jet ventilation through the catheter, thus providing for ventilation and oxygenation. Stylets are well tolerated by the patient even when awake and responsive. Oxygen can be insufflated through the catheter or it can be connected to a side stream capnograph to monitor ventilation.

ASA TASK FORCE RECOMMENDATIONS FOR POSTOPERATIVE EXTUBATIDAL (ADAPTED FROM MILLER, HARKIN, AND BAILEY[104])

1. Consider the relative merits of awake extubation vs. extubation before the return of consciousness.
2. Evaluate the clinical factors that may produce an adverse impact on ventilation after the patient has been extubated.
3. Formulate an airway management plan that can be implemented if the patient is not able to maintain adequate ventilation or oxygenation after extubation.
4. Consider the short-term use of a device that can serve as a guide for expedited reintubation. The device may be rigid to facilitate reintubation and/or hollow to facilitate ventilation.

A "difficult airway" cart with the above equipment should be available for use outside the OR. This is especially important when patients are extubated in the ICU. Suggestions for the contents of such a cart are described in the ASA Practice Guidelines for Management of the Difficult Airway[24] (see Fig. 6-2).

Endobronchial Intubation

This technique of isolating the lungs for differential ventilation is desirable for any transthoracic approach to the spinal cord. It is mandatory for any thoracoscopic procedure because the lung cannot be packed away from the operative site as it can be during an open thoracotomy. The objective is to isolate the lungs, usually at the level of the mainstem bronchi, so that the dependent lung is ventilated and the nondependent lung collapses.

Several types of double-lumen tubes (DLTs), which permit intubation of either bronchus, are available (e.g., Robertshaw, Carlens and White tubes). The differences in design among these tubes

are small, but some anesthesiologists express definite preferences. Unfortunately, these are marketed, in some cases, as "endobronchial catheters, left or right bronchus," which are confusing terms, since they are not strictly single lumen endobronchial tubes per se, but DLTs.

Advantages of endobronchial tubes include ease of placement (usually), the ability to isolate both lungs to avoid soiling of one lung with contents of the other (e.g., blood), and the ability to suction down both dependent and nondependent lumina. Disadvantages include potential difficulties in placement (especially if the patient has a difficult airway), small internal lumina, carinal irritation, and the potential need to change the tube if the patient will be on mechanical ventilation postoperatively. The left mainstem bronchus is longer than the right, giving a larger margin for error when placing a left-sided tube. Most, if not all, thoracic spinal surgery can be performed using a left-sided tube. Tube placement should be checked using a standard algorithm (Fig. 6-17).

All endobronchial intubations should be confirmed using a fiberoptic bronchoscope to ensure proper positioning (Fig. 6-18). The position of the tube within the bronchus may shift when the patient's position changes, especially were the neck to be flexed or extended. The potential for distorted anatomy in scoliotic patients may require bronchoscopy for directing the tube into the endobronchial lumen of the appropriate side.[11]

Bronchial Blockers

The Univent tube (Fuji Systems Corporation, Tokyo, Japan) is a single lumen tube with a built-in bronchial blocker. The blocker can be retracted into the ETT when not needed. Advantages include the "ease of insertion" (per the manufacturer). There is no need to change the tube at the end of the surgery if mechanical ventilation is elected. The Univent may occasionally fit into the small patient whose trachea will not accept a DLT. It is easier to place in patients with a difficult airway than a DLT, especially if an awake fiberoptic intubation is planned. Because the blocker can be advanced down the mainstem bronchus, the upper or upper and middle lobes may be isolated from the lower lobe, making it possible to collapse less than a full lung. Disadvantages include the thickness of

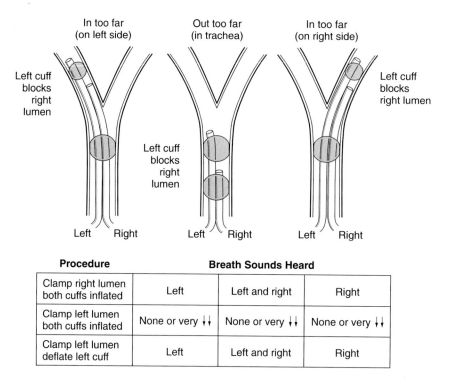

Procedure	Breath Sounds Heard		
Clamp right lumen both cuffs inflated	Left	Left and right	Right
Clamp left lumen both cuffs inflated	None or very ↓↓	None or very ↓↓	None or very ↓↓
Clamp left lumen deflate left cuff	Left	Left and right	Right

Fig. 6-17. There are three major (involving a whole lung) malpositions of a left-sided double-lumen endobronchial tube. The tube can be in too far on the left (both lumens are in the left mainstem bronchus), out too far (both lumens are in the trachea), or down the right main-stem bronchus (at least the left lumen is in the right main-stem bronchus). In each of these three malpositions, the left cuff, when fully inflated, can completely block the right lumen. Inflation and deflation of the left cuff while the left lumen is clamped creates a breath sound differential diagnosis of tube malposition. (From Benumof J. Separation of the two lungs [double-lumen tube and bronchial blocker intubation]. In Anesthesia for Thoracic Surgery, 2nd ed. Philadelphia: WB Saunders, 1995, p 347.)

the wall making the outer diameter relatively large (e.g., the 7.5 mm tube has an outer diameter of 11 mm). The authors have not found it to be as easy to place as others have reported, especially "blind." We frequently need a bronchoscope to aid in the correct placement of the blocker. Complete obstruction of the trachea is a potential problem, if the blocker slips from the bronchus to the trachea or if the blocker is accidentally inflated within the trachea by someone unfamiliar with the system. The blocker has a small lumen that allows emptying of the nondependent lung and application of CPAP, but it is too small to allow suctioning of the nondependent lung (Fig. 6-19).

If a Univent tube is unavailable, or if the patient is too small to accept it, a separate bronchial blocker is used. This is usually a Fogarty or similar catheter. It may be introduced along the side of the ETT at the time of laryngoscopy or through the lumen of the ETT (using a bronchoscope adapter to connect the ETT to the anesthetic circuit). The catheter is guided into the appropriate mainstem bronchus under fiberoptic control. It has a wire stylet, and the authors find it helpful to place a slight bend ("hockey stick") in the distal 2 to 3 cm to aid in placement of the blocker. Although useful, this technique has the following disadvantages: difficulty in placement of the blocker, inability to suction the collapsed lung or apply CPAP, and no lumen through which the gas in the nonventilated lung can escape. Nonetheless, the technique of using a Fogarty catheter may be quite useful in that the safe restoration of OLV following needle perforation of the endotracheal blocker balloon of the Univent tube has been reported.[52]

A single-lumen ETT may be positioned in the mainstem bronchus of the lung to be ventilated

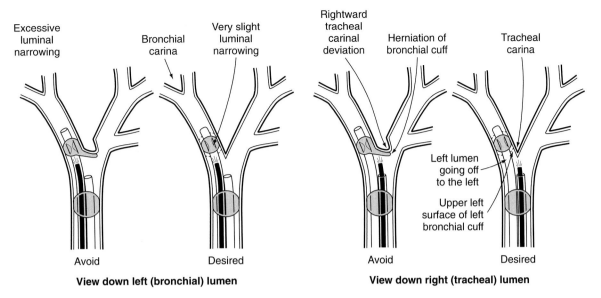

Fig. 6-18. This schematic diagram depicts the complete fiberoptic bronchoscopy picture of the left-sided double-lumen tubes (both the desired view and the view to be avoided from both of the lumens). When the bronchoscope is passed down the right lumen of the left-sided tube, the endoscopist should see a clear straight-ahead view of the tracheal carina and the upper surface of the blue left endobronchial cuff just below the tracheal carina. Excessive pressure in the endobronchial cuff, as manifested by tracheal carinal deviation to the right and herniation of the endobronchial cuff over the carina, should be avoided. When the bronchoscope is passed down the left lumen of the left-sided tube, the endoscopist should see a very slight left luminal narrowing and a clear straight-ahead view of the bronchial carina off in the distance. Excessive left luminal narrowing should be avoided. (From Benumof J. Separation of the two lungs [double-lumen tube and bronchial blocker intubation]. In Anesthesia for Thoracic Surgery, 2nd ed. Philadelphia: WB Saunders, 1995, p 352.)

using fiberoptic control. This may be a good alternative to an external bronchial blocker and it is easier to perform. It has the same disadvantages as an external blocker. One must be careful not to traumatize the mainstem bronchi.

Tube Changes

If an endobronchial tube is in place, some recommend changing to a single lumen tube before the position of the patient is changed from lateral to prone. Although a patient may be ventilated prone with an endobronchial tube in place, the size of the DLT may promote edema formation in the airway. Difficulty in changing the tube usually increases with the duration of surgery and it may be easier to change the tube before the start of the dorsal approach than at the end of surgery. Single lumen tubes (SLTs) are better tolerated; endobronchial tubes may irritate the carina and the patient may require more sedation than when SLTs are used.

Notwithstanding, if there is a question about the ability of the anesthesiologist to safely change the DLT, it should be left in place.

If one elects to change a DLT to an SLT, facilities for TTJV and emergency cricothyroidotomy should be immediately available. The DLT should be removed after the anesthesiologist has again visualized the vocal cords with the DLT in place. It is then removed over a ventilating tube changer, an SLT is passed over the tube changer, and the anesthesiologist passes this tube through the vocal cords under direct vision. If the initial intubation was difficult or required fiberoptic bronchoscopy (e.g., unstable cervical spine) the procedure will have to be undertaken "blind" over a tube changer. However, a bronchoscope may be passed into the posterior pharynx either orally or nasally to allow some visualization. If this is done, an ETT should be loaded onto the bronchoscope so that it can be used to intubate the patient were the tube changer to be displaced from between the cords. One may wish to

Insertion and Positioning of
Univent Bronchial Blocker (BB) System

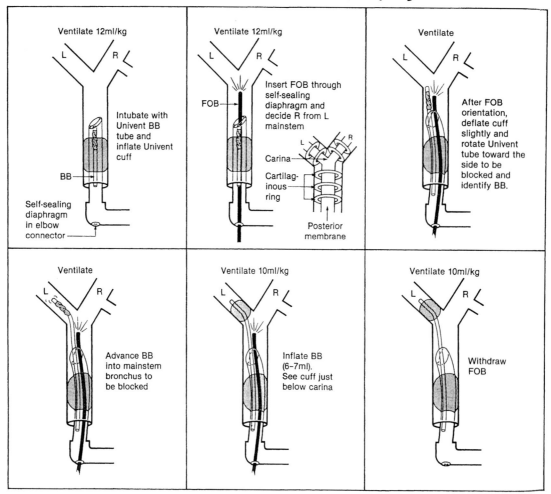

Fig. 6-19. The sequential steps of the fiberoptic-aided method of inserting and positioning the Univent bronchial blocker (BB) in the left main-stem bronchus. One- and two-lung ventilation is achieved by simply inflating and deflating, respectively, the bronchial blocker balloon. FOB = fiberoptic bronchoscope. (From Benumof J. Separation of the two lungs [double-lumen tube and bronchial blocker intubation]. In Anesthesia for Thoracic Surgery, 2nd ed. Philadelphia: WB Saunders, 1995, p 372.)

reconsider the decision to change the tube if the above procedure appears to be unduly difficult.

BLOOD CONSERVATION

Concern about transmission of disease via blood transfusion has been present almost since its introduction. However, it was not until the specter of infection with the HIV appeared that patients and physicians alike became so concerned with decreasing homologous blood transfusion. The risk of acquiring HIV infection from blood that has been tested negative is approximately 1:225,000 units transfused. The risk of acquiring hepatitis C is about 1% per unit transfused[38] (Table 6-6).

This desire to minimize the potential for acquiring transfusion related disease has led to a number of techniques designed to decrease the need for autologous transfusions. Among these are: acceptance of a low hematocrit, acute isovolemic hemodilution, autologous blood transfusion, blood scavenging techniques controlled hypotension to minimize blood loss, and pharmacologic intervention to decrease blood loss.

Table 6-6. Risks of Blood Transfusion

	Specific Adverse Outcomes	Number of Transfusions That Must Be Administered Before a Specific Adverse Outcome Is Observed
Infections:	Fatal septic reaction	$> 1 \times 10^6$
	Parasitic	$> 1 \times 10^6$
	Hepatitis A	$> 1 \times 10^6$
	Hepatitis B	$\leq 200 \times 10^3$
	Hepatitis C	5×10^3
	HIV	$\leq 250 \times 10^3$
	HTLV	50×10^3
Transfusions:	ABO incompatible RBC	33×10^3
	Fatal incompatible RBC	600×10^3
Alloimmunization:	To RBCs	100
	To platelets	?

The need for transfusion is not uncommon. Extensive surgeries with significant dissection are growing more common. Accidental injury to the great vessels with the patient in the prone position may go unrecognized until a significant volume has been sequestered in the chest or abdomen. Intrathoracic approaches place the aorta, vena cava, heart, pulmonary arteries and veins, and other vital structures in jeopardy.

Accepting a Low Hematocrit

Several studies have shown that low hematocrits are well tolerated as long as the patient is kept euvolemic and the cardiovascular system is able to increase its output to meet the metabolic oxygen requirements. Indeed, the oxygen transport and uptake may actually improve due to improved blood rheology if carbon monoxide can be maintained. Most authors now advise tolerating hematocrits in the low 30s for patients with suspected heart disease, the low 20s for otherwise healthy patients.[109,152] Signs of ischemia or cardiovascular deterioration would be signals to maintain a higher hematocrit, and at least one study suggests that prevention of early postoperative anemia (by transfusing all autologous blood on the day of surgery) leads to earlier ambulation and improved outcomes.[4]

Acute Isovolemic Hemodilution

During acute isovolemic hemodilution, 1 to 2 U of the patient's blood are withdrawn at the time of surgery (usually after induction) and replaced with an appropriate volume of crystalloid and/or colloid. This allows the patient to lose blood with a lower hematocrit during surgery. The withdrawn blood is reinfused after homeostasis is achieved. In some cases where blood loss is marked, the autologous units must be infused earlier, and thus some of the value of the technique may be lost. Isovolemic hemodilution to Hct_s of 15% or less have been shown to affect SSEPs.

The volume to be removed is calculated using a standard formula for allowable blood loss:

$$ABL = EBV \frac{(Hct_s - Hct_f)}{\frac{1}{2}(Hct_s + Hct_f)}$$

Where: ABL = Allowable blood loss
  EBV = Estimated blood volume
  Hct_s = Hematocrit at the start of the donation
  Hct_f = Hematocrit at the conclusion of the donation

The blood should be collected into standard ACD or CPD blood bags and gently agitated to assure mixing of the anticoagulant. If used within 6 hours, it may be stored at room temperature. Storage at standard blood bank refrigeration temperatures will extend this to 24 hours. It is easiest to connect the collection bag to the side arm of our central venous catheter. Placing the collection bag below the table allows the blood to drain by gravity.

Autologous Blood Transfusion

In this technique the patient predonates his own blood for intraoperative use. Blood should be withdrawn over a 3- to 4-week period to allow maximal harvesting and time for replacement. Supplementation with iron and folate is helpful in restoring red cell mass. Recently the introduction of synthetic erythropoietin has been used to speed up the red cell recovery process. Patients who have donated autologous units also benefit from having a stimulated bone marrow that will more quickly normalize the hemoglobin (Hgb) concentration in the postoperative period. If blood must be stored for more than the usual shelf life, the red cells may be frozen and stored, which increases their shelf life to over one year. However, this is quite expensive.

Blood Scavenging Techniques

With cell saver techniques, a suction device is used to collect, anticoagulate, and store blood from the operative field. In some systems, the blood is washed in normal saline and centrifuged before being returned to the patient; in others, the anticoagulated blood is filtered and returned. This lack of washing may allow fat, bone chips, etc., to be infused. Therefore only a cell saver technique that employs washing is usually considered for extensive spinal procedures. This requires a technician to operate the cell saver, which, along with the cost of the disposables, makes it impractical if less than two units are potentially salvageable.

Because the cells are washed and resuspended in saline prior to reinfusion, the plasma and clotting factors are lost. After several units, this may introduce a coagulation defect. Fresh, frozen plasma and platelets may have to be administered after multiple units are reinfused. This should not often be necessary, as only 20% to 30% of the usual factor levels are necessary for normal coagulation.

The anticoagulant used in cell savers is heparin. Washing and centrifugation processes supposedly remove the heparin from the cells to be reinfused. However, the effectiveness of this process may vary depending on the brand of machine and the volume of wash solution used by the technician. If abnormal bleeding seems to be present following transfusion of several "cell-saved" units, one may perform an activated clotting time (ACT) or similar test to look for the presence of residual heparin. Because a prolonged ACT in this setting could be due to either heparin or dilution of coagulation factors, other tests may be necessary. An automated platelet count

should be available within 30 min. An automated thrombin time and heparin-neutralized thrombin time tests are available from several companies (e.g., Hemochron [International Technidyne, Inc., Edison, N.J.] and others). These tests allow the differentiation of residual heparin from coagulation factor dilution and can be quite helpful in this setting.

Techniques to Reduce Bleeding

The techniques mentioned above are used primarily to salvage or store the patient's own blood so that homologous transfusions are not necessary. Physical techniques that have been shown to reduce bleeding itself, and therefore blood loss, are also of importance.

Infiltration

Epinephrine (1:200,000 to 1:500,000 concentration has been used to infiltrate the surgical site to decrease bleeding from the skin and subcutaneous tissues. The more dilute solutions allow for more liberal volumes to be injected. Concentrations greater than 1:200,000 do not result in more vasoconstriction.

Deliberate Hypotension

This is probably the most widely practiced technique to decrease bleeding from the surgical site. Most authors believe that the spinal cord, like the brain, autoregulates to mean blood pressure of about 50 to 60 mm Hg in the normotensive patient. Patients with hypertension shift their autoregulatory curve to the right. It has been suggested that in these patients, the pressure should only be decreased 50 mm Hg below their baseline pressure. Others have suggested reducing the systolic pressure by 25%. If the ICP is elevated because of patient position, or other factors, a higher pressure will be necessary to achieve the same CPP, and this must be taken into account when deciding on the degree of hypotension to tolerate. While the potential benefits of limiting transfusion and facilitating the surgical dissection using deliberate hypotension are substantial, one may wish to err on the more conservative side in chronic hypertensive patients, especially if they are poorly controlled. Hypotension is best achieved with vasodilators rather than negative inotropes since it has been shown that the reduction in pressure rather than reduction in cardiac output is the beneficial hemodynamic change.[136]

Potential benefits of deliberate hypotension include: a drier surgical field, which promotes faster surgery and easier dissection, and less blood loss, which decreases the need for homologous transfusions with their attendant risks. "The benefits of induced hypotension for minimizing blood loss have been demonstrated most dramatically in procedures such as total hip arthroplasty and complex spinal surgery."[152]

While not absolutely contraindicated in patients with atherosclerotic disease, the authors are more conservative when dealing with these patients. The maintenance of higher pressures and the limitation of the duration of hypotension to the period when surgical bleeding is expected to be greatest is prudent.

Invasive monitoring of the systemic BP is required for all patients undergoing deliberate hypotension. All but the most fit patients also require some monitoring of their filling pressures. If there is no suggestion of pulmonary artery hypertension, the central venous pressure (CVP) is adequate for measuring ventricular filling. Were pulmonary artery hypertension to be suspected, a pulmonary artery catheter is recommended. As noted previously, one must take care that the pulmonary artery catheter lies in zone 3 so that pressure readings are meaningful representations of filling pressure.[153] A pulmonary artery catheter capable of measuring SvO_2 or samples of mixed venous blood can be useful in assessing the adequacy of global oxygen delivery to the tissues.

Beta blockers (propranolol, metoprolol, labetalol, and others) have all been used to treat or prevent reflex tachycardia associated with the use of vasodilators for inducing hypotension. In addition, the negative inotropic state decreases the dose required to produce a given degree of hypotension. Because tachycardia is not a consistent finding, hypotension with vasodilators may be induced, and tachycardia treated if present. In this setting, a continuous infusion of esmolol has the advantages of rapid onset and offset.

Nitroglycerin, nitroprusside, and nicardipine are currently the agents most frequently used to induce hypotension. They have the advantages of rapid onset and short duration of action. The choice is usually a case of personal preference, although one group has reported better outcomes using nitroprus-side.[161] Rebound hypertension following discontinuation of nitroprusside is reported to be more common than after nitroglycerin.[31] Calcium channel blockers, angiotensin-converting enzyme (ACE) inhibitors, and beta blockers have been used to decrease the dose of nitroprusside used (and thereby limit its potential for cyanide toxicity), but the authors have not found them to be necessary, and their long duration of action is a disadvantage. Suspected cyanide toxicity (metabolic acidosis in the face of an adequate oxygen delivery) is treated with sodium thiosulfate 150 ug/kg; if preexisting B_{12} deficiency is suspected, hydroxycobalamin should be considered.[9] In emergency situations sodium nitrate 5 mg/kg precedes the administration of the thiosulfate. The sodium nitrate causes the formation of methemoglobin that binds with the cyanide (forming cyanomethemoglobin) more avidly than does the cytochrome oxidase.

Trimethaphan camsylate (Arfonad), once frequently used for controlled hypotension, has fallen into disfavor. Its ganglionic blocking properties can cause fixed pupillary dilatation (via blockade of the ciliary ganglion) that can be confusing in the perioperative setting. In addition, it may potentiate neuromuscular blockade and cause decreases in the amplitude of the EEG traces.[149]

All of the direct vasodilators inhibit hypoxic pulmonary vasoconstriction. Because of this and their blood pressure lowering effect, they increase shunting through the lung (increased zone 1) and/or dead space ventilation. Therefore, a lower PaO_2 is to be expected (especially during OLV). Nitroprusside may have a direct effect on platelet aggregation that may be reversible once it is discontinued.[62,67]

Isoflurane is a potentially useful agent for induced hypotension. The concentrations should be kept low to permit SSEP monitoring if needed. This agent may have less effect on pulmonary shunting and dead space ventilation.[83] In addition, it may have neuroprotective effects because it decreases $CMRO_2$ without decreasing CBF.[90]

Induction and control of hypotension is made easier by appropriate choices of the anesthetic technique. One should avoid agents known to cause hypertension and tachycardia, as well as those known to precipitate marked histamine release or myocardial depression. An adequate depth of anesthesia makes the blood pressure easier to control and reduces the amount of vasoactive and sympatholytic agents needed. This need for depth must be balanced against the need to monitor spinal cord function (as discussed later).

Bernstein and Rosenberg[16] believe that lowering the pressure slowly (over about 15 min) provides the spinal cord time to accommodate to the lower pressure and prevent ischemia. In addition, they believe that the pressure should be allowed to normalize during distraction and the passage of sublaminar wires or cables to prevent ischemia. Hypotension and distraction are thought to be additive in producing spinal cord ischemia.[21,61] Hypotension is capable of producing changes in the SSEP, but the effect is variable.[60] Normocarbia is recommended to prevent hypocarbic constriction of arteries supplying the spinal cord.[71] CSF drainage has been advocated to increase spinal cord perfusion pressure (SCPP) in patients undergoing thoracic aortic aneurysm resection. On this basis, some authors advocate CSF drainage as a means of spinal cord protection, especially in cases of syringomyelia.

When hypotension is no longer required, the vasoactive agents are discontinued. Blood pressure should be normalized prior to closure. This assures hemostasis and thus avoids "reactionary hemorrhage." The necessity to maintain an adequate blood volume cannot be overemphasized. Serial hematocrits, hemodynamic readings, and attention to the blood loss and urine output as well as the insensible water loss should be carefully monitored. The aim is to produce hypotension without causing the end-organ complications associated with hypovolemic shock.

Pharmacologic Techniques

Drugs known to affect platelet function should be avoided for 2 weeks prior to elective surgery.[108] Acetaminophen can be substituted for aspirin or other NSAIDs. Salsalate (Disalcid) can be used in place of aspirin since it has no acetyl group to interfere with platelet function. A short course of steroid and/or oral narcotics should control most patients' pain. Acquired platelet defects and causes of thrombocytopenia should be sought.[108]

Aprotinin has been used to reduce blood loss during a variety of operations. It currently finds its greatest use during open heart surgery where it may prevent the platelet lesion induced by cardiopulmonary bypass. However, it has also been used with success during total hip replacement and radical prostatectomies. Tranexamic acid (Cyclokapron) and epsilon aminocaproic acid (Amicar) are synthetic inhibitors of fibrinolysis and work by inhibiting conversion of plasminogen to plasmin. They too have been used during open heart surgery. Little experience is available describing their use for spinal surgery.

Desmopressin is thought to reverse the platelet lesion induced by uremia. Experience with it outside of the setting of open heart surgery or inherited factor deficiencies is limited.

INTRAOPERATIVE NEUROLOGICAL MONITORING

As previously described, the blood supply to the thoracic spinal cord is tenuous. The spinal cord is at risk for ischemic injury from surgical dissection that may interrupt blood supply or from mechanical forces acting on the spinal cord. This can result in the patient emerging from anesthesia with new neurological deficits that may be severe and permanent. While the incidence of new neurological lesions is only about 1%, their occurrence can be devastating.[98] Methods to monitor the neurological function of the cord while the patient is under anesthesia have evolved in an effort to minimize the risk of neurological injury. Additionally, the "wakeup" test may be an aid to monitoring the functional status of the spinal cord.

Evoked Potential Monitoring

Evoked potential monitoring may take one of four forms:

1. *Cortical somatosensory–evoked potentials (cortical SSEPs).* A peripheral nerve is stimulated and the resultant potential is recorded from the cerebral cortex, usually with scalp electrodes.
2. *Spinal somatosensory–evoked potentials (spinal SSEPs).* A peripheral nerve is stimulated and the evoked potential is recorded from the spinal cord, usually via electrode(s) placed within the epidural space rostral to the area of surgery.
3. *Spinal-evoked potentials (SEPs).* The spinal cord is stimulated caudal to the level of surgery, and the potential is recorded from the cord rostral to the level of surgery.

4. *Motor–evoked potentials (MEPs).* The motor cortex is stimulated either electrically or magnetically and potentials are recorded from nerves caudal to the level of surgery.

While the SSEPs do allow continuous monitoring of the functional status of the spinal cord, there are both anatomical and technical limitations that must be considered.

The primary structures monitored with SSEPs are the dorsal columns of the spinal cord, although there may be some contribution from other tracts. This leaves the ventral motor tracts unmonitored unless spinal cord ischemia is so generalized that the posterior columns are affected. Numerous reports exist detailing patients awakening from anesthesia with new motor defects that were undetected by SSEP. In one study, SSEP failed to detect 28% of new postoperative neurological deficits.[35]

During thoracic spinal surgery, the common peroneal nerves and the posterior tibial nerves are stimulated. The nerves of the upper extremities may also be monitored as a control. Changes in latency or amplitude that are reflected in both the upper and lower extremities are likely the result of anesthesia or some other metabolic factor.

Effects of Anesthesia on Evoked Potentials

In general, all volatile anesthetics decrease the amplitude of the potential and increase its latency. The exceptions are etomidate and ketamine. Etomidate increases the amplitude of the potential and may be useful in accentuating signals that are weak or difficult to detect. If technical difficulties are encountered, potentials can be recorded from the epidural space as these are less affected by anesthetics than are cortical potentials.[58,74]

A nitrous oxide/opioid anesthetic is frequently cited as the technique of choice when SSEPs are monitored. However, even N_2O and opioids can affect the signals. The combination of an infusion of propofol and a narcotic infusion provides signals with a higher amplitude than a nitrousoxide–narcotic technique. Therefore it is desirable to establish a stable level of anesthesia early so that patients can act as their own controls and changes in amplitude or latency can be more easily detected. Infusions of opioids rather than intermittent boluses have been recommended for this reason.[120]

The inhalational agents cause a dose-dependent decrease in amplitude and increase in latency.[118,122,159] The effects of N_2O are additive to those of the potent agents. Elimination of N_2O may increase the amplitude of the evoked potential. The effects of introducing inhalational agents may be difficult to differentiate from those of ischemia. This underscores the desirability of establishing a stable anesthetic level prior to maneuvers that might cause ischemia. Most authors believe that low concentrations of inhalational agents (0.5 MAC or less) are compatible with SSEP monitoring.

Multiple other factors can affect the SSEP signal. There is an inherent variability in the intensity of the signal. A 7% to 15% change in latency and/or 45% to 50% change in amplitude may occur without neurological deficit.[88,162] In addition, ischemia, hypoxemia (including that caused by a low hematocrit), hypothermia, and hypercarbia may affect the SSEP.

In the event of a change in the SSEP that might indicate cord ischemia, the following should be quickly evaluated: the integrity of the stimulating electrodes, unintentional increase in the depth of anesthesia, adequacy of ventilation and oxygenation, and hypothermia (including local hypothermia induced by irrigation with cold solution). If these evaluative tests are negative, the surgeon should be informed. The blood pressure should be normalized (if hypotension has been induced). At this point, some spinal surgeons have the anesthesiologist begin preparing the patient for a "wake-up" test.[116] If the changes persist or if the wake-up test is positive, the surgeon may consider removing spinal instrumentation and looking for other possibly reversible structural causes (e.g., blood clot, retrodisplaced bone fragment or disc, etc.).

MEPs can also be used to assess the ventral columns, which may be missed by SSEP monitoring.[115] MEPs are also sensitive to the effects of anesthetics. Transcranial MEPs of electrical or magnetic origin are even more sensitive to the effects of anesthetics than are SSEPs. A stable level of muscle relaxation allows recording of the compound muscle action potential without permitting patient movement that might interfere with surgery.

MEPs can be detected when up to 90% of the twitch is abolished by NMBs. MEPs are best recorded following stimulation of the cord using epidural, subarachnoid, or intraspinous electrodes.[3]

The motor tract can be stimulated using the same electrode used for recording spinal SSEPs. MEPs and SSEPs recorded after epidural or spinal stimulation have the advantage of being relatively insensitive to the effects of anesthesia. Transient changes associated with bolus administration of narcotics and/or barbiturates are noted, but resolve within minutes.[46]

Wake-Up Test

While SSEPs or MEPs can be used to monitor the spinal cord throughout the procedure, the wake-up test may be used at one or more points during the operation to assess the functional status of the spinal cord. It can be performed following distraction and/or placement of instrumentation or any time the SSEPs change suggesting ischemia. The wake-up test assesses primarily the ventral columns although dorsal column deficits following negative wake-up tests have been reported.[8]

If a wake-up test is planned, prior discussion with the patient may be helpful. However, most patients have little or no recall of the event.

Most anesthetic techniques acceptable for SSEP monitoring can be adapted to allow a wake-up test. The essential elements are[1]:

1. There is rapid and controlled return to consciousness.
2. There is rapid and safe reinduction following completion of the test.
3. Agents are discontinued 10 to 15 min before the anticipated time of the test. One may wish to leave some residual paralysis so that the patient cannot become too active as consciousness returns.
4. The ability of the patient to hear and follow commands should be assessed with hand grip prior to testing the lower extremities. This should help to decrease the incidence of false positive tests.
5. If short-acting narcotics and hypnotics are used, the wake-up test may be repeated as necessary.
6. This maneuver is not without risks, including: unintended extubation, dislodgment of implanted bone grafts and instrumentation, and venous air embolism.[45]

POSTOPERATIVE PAIN CONTROL
Epidural Analgesia

Epidural analgesia is frequently used for treatment of postoperative pain following many types of surgery. Unfortunately, the technique is not well suited for thoracic spinal surgery if a dorsal approach is used. If the approach is solely ventral, epidural analgesia may provide good relief from the pain of the thoracotomy. If the epidural space has been disrupted because of surgery, spread of the agent may be uneven and may lead to suboptimal analgesia, especially if local anesthetics are used.

If epidural analgesia is used, one may wish to avoid local anesthetics and rely on opioids. "Transient paraplegia" due to local anesthetic migration from an intercostal nerve block led one group to recommend against the technique following ventral approaches to the spine.[53] Similar confusion could follow an epidural technique that included the use of local anesthetics.

Citing a higher incidence of complications and studies demonstrating equivalent efficacy, Benumof[11] recommends lumbar rather than thoracic catheter placement for postthoracotomy pain. If one elects lumbar placement, appropriate adjustments of dose and volume must be made to assure adequate analgesia. If epidural narcotics are used, level of consciousness and respiratory status should be assessed at 30- to 60-minute intervals. Supplemental oxygen is also recommended.

Intrathecal Analgesia

Intrathecal injection of morphine can provide pain relief for 18 to 24 hours. It is well suited to combined ventral/dorsal approaches. This single-shot technique does not require a catheter and there is no interference in the surgical fields. The injection can be placed before induction and may provide some analgesia during the surgery. Because the authors are unable to locate studies defining the SSEP changes (if any) associated with its use, we suggest placing it following instrumentation, prior to wound closure. It would seem natural to have the surgeon inject it at the operative site; however, some surgeons fear development of a pseudomeningocele in that the tissues that usually tamponade a CSF leak have been removed during the dissection. Therefore the injection may be placed percutaneously at a lower level. Late respiratory depression is more common with intrathecal than with epidural injection and can be particularly dangerous in the patient with an immobile cervical spine because the management of the airway is more difficult. Other risk factors for late respiratory depression include advanced age, position of the patient after injection, and use of systemic narcotics. For these reasons, careful monitoring of ventilation and level of consciousness at frequent intervals is mandatory, and supplemental oxygen is strongly recommended.

Another approach to preventing late respiratory depression from spinal narcotics is the infusion of naloxone or nalbuphine. If titrated appropriately (e.g., nalbuphine 0.2 mg/kg bolus followed by 0.5 mg/kg/hr), these techniques may prevent significant respiratory depression with little effect on the analgesia.[41]

Intravenous Patient-Controlled Analgesia

Patient-controlled analgesia (PCA) is a technique familiar to most anesthesiologists. Several studies have shown its efficacy to be equivalent to epidural narcotics.[73] Most of the available narcotics have been used with little to recommend one over the others. Continuous background infusions, when added to intermittent boluses, increase patient comfort but also increase the risk of respiratory depression. If background infusions are used, monitoring similar to that recommended for spinal narcotic administration is indicated. PCA has partly replaced intermittent intramuscular injections for the relief of postoperative pain. Not only is pain relief superior to intramuscular administration, but the total dose of narcotics used is decreased.

Nonsteroidal Anti-inflammatory Drugs

Rectal indomethacin or intramuscular ketorolac (Toradol) have both been shown to improve analgesia following thoracotomy. They do not affect the carbon dioxide response curve and therefore can be safely combined with parenteral or neuraxial narcotics. Their potential for inhibiting platelet function must be kept in mind.

Intercostal Nerve Blocks

As noted above, intercostal blocks with local anesthetics have been cited as a potential cause of postoperative difficulties by mimicking ischemic cord damage. Intercostal nerve block using a cryoprobe under direct vision has been advocated as a means of providing long-lasting pain relief following thoracotomy. It should not have the same potential for problems seen with local anesthetics.

Intravenous Infusion

Ventral thoracic spinal surgery may be associated with thoracoabdominal incisions that are both extensive and painful. The authors have had favorable experience with infusions of ketamine and midazolam. Ketamine 500 mg and midazolam 25 mg are diluted in 250 ml of intravenous solution that is titrated to produce adequate analgesia (usually 5 to 15 ml/hr). Similarly, fentanyl 1250 µg can be combined with ketamine 500 mg and titrated to similar effects. End points are not only adequate analgesia, but also adequate spontaneous ventilation. These infusions can be combined with N_2O to form a general anesthesia technique that can be titrated to sedation and analgesia at the end of surgery, allowing extubation.

There are no facts, only perspectives of facts.
—Friedrich Wilhelm Nietzsche (1844-1900)

REFERENCES

1. Abbott TR, Bentley G. Intraoperative awakening during scoliosis surgery. Anaesthesia 35:298-302, 1980.
2. Abdul-Rasool IH, Sears DH, Katz RL. The effect of a second dose of succinylcholine on cardiac rate and rhythm following induction of anesthesia with etomidate or midazolam. Anesthesiology 67:795-797, 1987.
3. Adams DC, Emerson RG, Heyer EJ, McCormick PC, Carmel PW, Stein BM, Farcy JP, Gallo EJ. Monitoring of intraoperative motor-evoked potentials under conditions of controlled neuromuscular blockade. Anesth Analg 77:913-918, 1993.
4. Albert TJ, Desai D, McIntosh T, Lamb D, Balderston RA. Early versus late replacement of autotransfused blood in elective spinal surgery: A prospective randomized study. Spine 18:1071-1078, 1993.
5. Andree RA. Sudden death following naloxone administration. Anesth Analg 59:782-784, 1980.

6. Azar I, Turndorf H. Severe hypertension and multiple atrial premature contractions following naloxone administration. Anesth Analg 58:524-525, 1979.

7. Baraka A. Differential lung ventilation as an alternative to one-lung ventilation during thoracotomy. Anaesthesia 49:881-882; 1994.

8. Ben-David BT, PD, Haller GS. Posterior spinal fusion complicated by posterior column injury: A case report of a false negative wake-up test. Spine 12:540-543, 1987.

9. Bendo A, Kass IS, Hartunt JH, Cottrell JE. Neuroanatomy and neurophysiology. In Barash P, Coullen BF, Stoelting RH, eds. Clinical Anesthesia, 2nd ed. Philadelphia: JB Lippincott, 1992, p 903.

10. Benumof JL. Mechanism of decreased blood flow to atelectic lung. J Appl Physiol 46:1047-1048, 1978.

11. Benumof JL. Anesthesia for Thoracic Surgery, 2nd ed. Philadelphia: WB Saunders, 1995.

12. Benumof JL, Ghaughan S, Ozaki GT. Operative lung constant positive airway pressure with the Univent bronchial blocker tube. Anesth Analg 74:406-410, 1984.

13. Benumof JL, Wahrenbrock EA. Blunted hypoxic pulmonary vasoconstriction by increased lung vascular pressures. J Appl Physiol 38:846-850, 1975.

14. Bergofsky EH, Turingo GM, Fishman AP. Cardiorespiratory failure in kyphoscoliosis. Medicine 38:263-317, 1959.

15. Berguer R, Porto J, Fedoronko B, Dragovic L. Selective deep hypothermia of the spinal cord prevents paraplegia after aortic cross-clamping in the dog model. J Vasc Surg 15: 62-72, 1992.

16. Bernstein RL, Rosenberg AD. Manual of Orthopedic Anesthesia and Related Pain Syndromes. New York: Churchill Livingston, 1993, p 538.

17. Bjertnaes LJ, Mundal R, Hauge A, Nicolaysen A. Vascular resistance in atelectatic lungs: Effect of inhalation anesthetics. Acta Anaesthesiol Scand 24:109-118, 1980.

18. Bracken MB, Shepard MJ, Collins WF, Holford TR, Young W, Baskin DS, Eisenberg HM, Flamm E, Leo-Summers L, Maroon J. A randomized controlled trial of methylprednisolone or naloxone in the treatment of acute spinal cord injury. N Engl J Med 322:1405-1411, 1990.

19. Bradford DS. Moe's Textbook of Scoliosis and Other Spinal Deformities, 3rd ed. Philadelphia: WB Saunders, 1994.

20. Bradford DS, Moe JH, Winter RB. Scoliosis and kyphosis. In Rothman RH, Sineone FA, eds. The Spine. Philadelphia: WB Saunders, 1980, pp 316-439.

21. Brodkey JS, Richards DE, Blasingame JP, Nulsen FE. Reversible spinal cord trauma in cats: Additive effects of direct pressure and ischemia. J Neurosug 37:591-593, 1972.

22. Busto R, Dietrich WD, Globus MY, Ginsberg MD. The importance of brain temperature in cerebral ischemic injury. Stroke 20:1113-1114, 1989.

23. Busto RD, Dietrich WD, Globus MY, Vales I, Scheinberg P, Ginsberg MD. Small differences in intraischemic brain temperature critically determine the extent of ischemic neuronal injury. J Cereb Blood Flow Metab 7:729-738, 1987.

24. Caplan RA, Benumof JL, Berry FA. Practice guidelines for management of the difficult airway. A report by the American Society of Anesthesiologists Task Force on management of the difficult airway. Anesthesiology 78:597-602, 1993.

25. Champlin AM, Rael J, Benzel EC, Kesterson L, King JN, Orrison WW, Mirfakhraee M. Preoperative spinal angiography for lateral extracavity approach to the thoracic and lumbar spine. Am J Neuroradiology 15:73-77. 1994.

26. Choi DW, Maulucci-Gedde MA, Kriegstein AR. Glutamate neurotoxicity in cortical cell culture. J Neurosci 7:357-368, 1987.

27. Cody JR. Muscle rigidity following administration of succinlycholine. Anesthesiology 29(1):159-612, 1968.

28. Cohn AL, McGraw SR, King WH. Awake intubation of the adult trachea using the Bullard Laryngoscope. Can J Anaesth 42:246-248, 1995.

29. Cooperman LH, Strobel GE, Kennell EM. Massive hyperkalemia after administration of succinylcholine. Anesthesiology 32:161, 1988.

30. Corke PJ, Murray G. Angio-oedema with droperidol. Anaesth Intensive Care 21:375, 1993.

31. Cottrell J, Illner P, Kittary MJ, Steel TM Jr, Lowenstein T, Turndorf H. Rebound hypertension after sodium nitroprusside-induced hypotension. Clin Pharmacol Ther 27:32, 1980.

32. Crawford M, Pollock J, Anderson K, Glavin RJ. Comparison of midazolam with propofol for sedation in outpatient bronchoscopy. Br J Anaesth 70:419-422, 1993.

33. Criswell JC, Parr JA. Forum: Emergency airway management in patients with cervical spine injuries. Anaesthesia 49:900-903; 1994.

34. Cunningham NJ, Laschinger JC, Spencer FC. Monitoring of somatosensory evoked potentials during surgical procedures on the thoracoabdominal aorta. IV. Clinical observations and results. J Thorac Cardiovasc Surg 94:275-285, 1987.

35. Dawson EG, Sherman JE, Kanim LEA, Nuwer M. Spinal cord monitoring: Results of the Scoliosis Research Society and European Spinal Deformity Society Meeting, Scoliosis Research Society. Honolulu, Hawaii, 1990.

36. Dearden NM, McDowall DG. Comparison of etomidate and althesin in the reduction of increased intracranial pressure after head injury. Br J Anaesth 57:361-368, 1985.

37. Demaria EJ, Richman W, Kenney PR, Armitage JM, Gann DS. Septic complications of corticosteroid administration after severe nervous system trauma. Ann Surg 202:248-252, 1985.

38. Dodd RY. The risk of transfusion transmitted infection. N Engl J Med 327:14-19, 1992.

39. Dolan EJ, Transfeldt EE, Tator CH, Simmons EH, Hughes KI. The effect of spinal distraction on regional spinal cord blood flow in cats. J Neurosurg 53:756-764, 1980.

40. Domisse GF. The blood supply of the spinal cord: A critical vascular zone in spinal surgery. J Bone Joint Surg 56B: 225-235, 1974.

41. Doran R, Baxter, AD, Sampson B, Penning J, Dube LM. Prevention of respiratory depression from epidural morphine in post-thoracotomy patients with nalbuphine hydrochloride. Anesthesiology 36(5):503-9, 1989.

42. Drug Evaluations Annual 1993. Department of Drugs, Division of Drugs and Toxicology; American Medical Association, pp 165, 166.

43. Drummond T. Do barbiturates really protect the brain? Anesthesiology 78:611-613, 1993.

44. Eisenkraft JB, Thys DM, Cohen E, Kaplan JA. Hemodynamic effects of CPAP and PEEP during one-lung anesthesia with isoflurane. Anesthesiology 61:A520, 1984.

45. Engler GL, Spielholz NI, Bernard WN, Bernhard WM, Danziger F, Merkin H, Wolff T. Somatosensory evoked potentials during Harrington instrumentation for scoliosis. J Bone Joint Surg 60A:528-532, 1978.

46. Erwin CW, Erwin AC. Up and down the spinal cord: Intraoperative monitoring of sensory and motor spinal cord pathways. J Clin Neurophysiol 10:425-436, 1993.

47. Fisher MM. Clinical observations on the pathophysiology and treatment of anaphylactic cardiovascular collapse. Anaesth Intens Care 14:17-21, 1986.

48. Flacke JW, Flacke WE, Williams CD. Acute pulmonary edema following naloxone reversal of high-dose morphine anesthesia. Anesthesiology 47:376-378, 1977.

49. Friedlander M, Sandler AN, Kavanagh B, Winton T, Benumof J. Hypoxic pulmonary vasoconstriction in single lung anesthesia in the lateral position in adults. Anesth Analg 74:S100, 1992.

50. Gaba DM, Fish KJ, Howard SK. Crisis Management in Anesthesiology. New York: Churchill Livingstone, 1994, pp 195-200.

51. Gardaz J, Mc Farlane PA, Madgwick RG, Ryder WA, Sykes MK. Effect of dopamine, increased cardiac output and increased pulmonary artery pressure on hypoxic pulmonary vasoconstriction. Br J Anaesth 55:238P-239P, 1983.

52. Gayes J. Management of univent bronchial blocking balloon perforation during one-lung ventilation. Anesth Analg 79:1215, 1994.

53. Ghanayem AJ, Bohlman HH. Transient paraplegia from intraoperative intercostal nerve block after transthoracic discectomy. Spine 19:1294-1296, 1994.

54. Gold M, Swartz JS, Braude BM, Dolovich J, Shandling B, Gilmour RF. Intraoperative anaphylaxis: An association with latex sensitivity. J Allergy Clin Immunol 87:662-666, 1991.

55. Gravenstein N, ed. Manual of Complications During Anesthesia. Philadelphia: JB Lippincott, 1991, pp 108, 134-135.

56. Greenberger P, Patterson R, Lelly J. Administration of radiographic contrast media in high-risk patients. Invest Radiol 15:540-543, 1980.

57. Gronert GA, Theye RA. Pathophysiology of hyperkalemia induced by succinylcholine. Anesthesiology 43:89, 1975.

58. Grossi EA, Laschinger JC, Krieger KH, Nathan IM, Colvin SB, Weiss MR, Bauman FG. Epidural-evoked potentials: A more specific indicator of spinal cord ischemia. J Surg Res 44:224-228, 1988.

59. Grundy BL, Nash CL, Brown RH. Anterior pressure manipulation alters spinal cord function during correction of scoliosis. Anesthesiology 54:249-253, 1981.

60. Grundy BL, Nash CL, Brown RH. Deliberate hypotension for spinal fusion: Prospective randomized study with evoked potential monitoring. Can Anaesth Soc J 29:452-462, 1982.

61. Hardy RW, Nash CL, Brodkey JS. Follow-up report: Experimental and clinical studies in spinal cord monitoring. The effect of anoxia and ischemia on spinal cord function. J Bone Joint Surg 55A:435, 1973.

62. Harris S, Escobar A, Rinder C, Hines R. Nitroprusside-induced platelet dysfunction: A reversible phenomenon? Anesthesiology 77:3A:145, 1992.

63. Heath KJ. The effect on laryngoscopy of different cervical spine immobilization techniques. Anaesthesia 49:843-845, 1994.

64. Heese A, Hintzenstern J, Peters K-P, Koch HM. Horenstein OP. Allergic and irritant reactions to rubber gloves in medical health services. J Am Acad Dermatol 25:831-839, 1991.

65. Hepper NGG, Black LE, Fowler WA. Relationships of lung volume to height and arm span in normal subjects and in patients with spinal deformity. Am Rev Respir Dis 91:356-362, 1965.

66. Hickey R, Albin MS, Bunegin L, Ritter RR, Sloan T. Autoregulation of spinal cord blood flow; is the cord a microcosm of the brain? Stroke 17:1183-1189, 1986.

67. Hines R, Barash PG. Infusion of sodium nitroprusside induces platelet dysfunction in vitro. Anesthesiology 70:611, 1989.

68. Hirschman CA. Latex anaphylaxis. Anesthesiology 77:223-225, 1992.

69. Hitchon P, Kassell N, Hill T, et al. The response of spinal cord blood flow to high-dose barbiturates. Spine 7:41, 1982.

70. Horowitz MB, Moossy JJ, Julian T, Ferson PF, Huneke K. Thoracic disscectomy using video assisted thoracoscopy. Spine 19:1082-1086, 1994.

71. Jacobs HJ, Lieponis JV, Bunch WH, Barber MJ, Salem MR. The influence of halothane and nitroprusside on canine spinal cord hemodynamics. Spine 7:35, 1982.

72. Johnson D, Chang P, Hurst T, Reynolds B, Lang S, Mayers I. Changes in $P_{ET}CO_2$ and pulmonary blood flow after bronchial occlusion in dogs. Can J Anaesth 39:184-191, 1992.

73. Johnson RG, Miller M. Intraspinal narcotic analgesia. A comparison of two methods of pain relief after lumbar laminectomy. Spine 14:363-366, 1989.

74. Jones SS, Edgar MA, Ransford AO. Sensory nerve conduction in the human spinal cord: Epidural recodings made during scoliosis surgery. J Neurol Neurosurg Psychiatry 45:446, 1982.

75. Kafer ER. Respiratory and cardiovascular functions in scoliosis and the principles of anesthetic management. Anesthesiology 52:339-351, 1980.

76. Kalkman CJ, ten Brink SA, Been HD, Bovill JG. Variability of somatosensory cortical evoked potentials during spinal surgery: Effects of anesthetic technique and high-pass digital filtering. Spine 16:924-929, 1991.

77. Kearse LA, Fahmy NR. The electroencephalographic effects of propofol anesthesia in humans: A comparison with thiopental/enflurane anesthesia. Anesthesiology 71:A121, 1989.

78. Keenan MA, Stiles CM, Kaufman RL. Acquired laryngeal deviation associated with cervical spine erosive, polyarticular arthritis. Use of the fiberoptic bronchoscope in rheumatoid arthritis. Anesthesiology 58:441-449, 1983.

79. Keeter S, Benator RM, Weinberg SM, Hartenberg MA. Sedation in pediatric CT: National survey of current practice. Radiology 175:745-752, 1990.

80. Khan KJ, Cooper GM. Propofol and malignant hyperthermia: A case for day-case anesthesia? Anaesthesia 48:455-456, 1993.

81. Khanom T, Braithwaite MA. Arterial oxygenation during one-lung anesthesia (1): A study in man. Anesthesiology 38:132-138, 1973.

82. Kobrine A, Doyle T, Rizzoli H. Spinal cord blood flow as affected by changes in systemic arterial blood pressure. J Neurosurg 44:12, 1976.

83. Lam A, Gelb AW. Cardiovascular effects of isoflurane-induced hypotension for cerebral aneurysm surgery. Anesth Analg 62:742, 1983.

84. Laxenaire MC, Gueant JL, Monerek-Vautrim DA, Sullam PM. Chocs anaphylactiques an propofol lors de la premiäre utilization. Ann Fr Anesth Reanim 9(Suppl):R125, 1990.

85. Lee BL, Wong D, Benowitz NL, Sullam PM. Altered patterns of drug metabolism in patients with acquired immunodeficiency syndrome. Clin Pharmacol Ther 53:529-535, 1993.

86. Lee C, Barnes A, Nagel EL. Neuroleptanalgesia for awake pronation of surgical patients. Anesth Analg 56:276-278, 1977.

87. Lefever EB, Potter PS, Seeley NR. Propofol sedation for pediatric MRI. Anesth Analg 76:919-920, 1993.

88. Lubicky J, Spadaro JA, Yuan HA, Fredrickson BE, Henderson N. Variability of somatosensory cortical evoked potential monitoring during spinal surgery. Spine 14:790-798, 1989.

89. Mack MJ, Regan JJ, Bobenchko WP, Acuff TE. Application of thoracoscopy for disease of the spine. Ann Thorac Surg 56:736-738, 1993.

90. Madsen J, Cold GE, Hansen ES. Cerebral blood flow and metabolism during isoflurane-induced hypotension in patients subjected to surgery for cerebral aneurysms. Br J Anaesth 59:1204, 1987.

91. Malmkvist G, Fletcher R, Nortstrom L, Werner O. Effects of lung surgery and one-lung ventilation on pulmonary arterial pressure, venous admixture and immediate postoperative lung function. Br J Anaesth 63:696-701, 1989.

92. Mangano DT. Perioperative cardiac morbidity. Anesthesiology 72:153-184, 1990.

93. Marcaux FW, Goodrich JE, Dominick MA. Ketamine prevents ischemic neuronal injury. Brain Res 452:329-335, 1988.

94. Marshall B, Marshall C. Continuity of response to hypoxic pulmonary vasoconstriction. J Appl Physiol 59:189-196, 1980.

95. Marshall C, Kim SD, Marshall BE. The influence of vascular pressure on hypoxic vasoconstriction. Anesthesiology 73:A1139, 1990.

96. Marshall WV, Mostrom JL. Neurosurgical diseases of the spine and spinal cord: Anesthetics. In Cottrell JE, Smith DS, eds. Anesthesia and Neurosurgery, 3rd ed. St. Louis: CV Mosby, 1994, pp 575-576.

97. Martin JT. Positioning in Anesthesia and Surgery. Philadelphia: WB Saunders, 1988.

97. McEwen GD, Bunnell WP, Krishnaswami S. Acute neurological complications in the treatment of scoliosis. J Bone Joint Surg 57A:404-408, 1975.

99. McHale S, Konieczko K. Anaphylactoid reaction to propofol. Anaesthesia 48:446, 1993.

100. McPherson RW. Neurophysiologic brain monitoring: Evoked potentials. In Cottrell JE, Smith DS, eds. Anesthesia and Neurosurgery, 3rd ed. St. Louis: CV Mosby, 1994, p 213.

101. Melnick B, Sawyer R, Karambelkar D, Phitayakorn P, Uy L, Pater R. Delayed side effects of droperidol after ambulatory general anesthesia. Anesth Analg 69:748-751, 1989.

102. Michaelis LL, Hickey PR, Clark TA, Dixon MD. Ventricular irritability associated with the use of naloxone. Ann Thorac Surg 18:608-614, 1974.

103. Michenfelder JD. Heresy? Anesthesiology 78:613, 1993.

104. Miller K, Harkin CP, Bailey PL. Postoperative tracheal extubation. Anesth Analg 80:143-148, 1995.

105. Mitchell MM, Ali HH, Savarese JJ. Mytonia and neuromuscular blocking agents. Anesthesiology 49:44-48, 1978.

106. Miyamoto K, Ueno A, Wada T, Kimoto S. A new and simple method of preventing spinal cord damage following temporary occlusion of the thoracic aorta by draining cerebrospinal fluid. J Cardiovasc Surg 1:188-197, 1960.

107. Moore-Jeffries E, Steen SN. Efficacy of propofol for conscious sedation under regional anesthesia. Revista Espanola de Anestesiologica y Reanimacion 39:9, 1992; Anestesia 92, Barcelona, Spain: 7-12 June 1992.

108. Nanfro JJ. Anticoagulants in critical care medicine. In Chenois J, ed. The Pharmacologic Approach to the Critically Ill Patient. Baltimore: Williams & Wilkins, 1994, p 672.

109. Nelson AH, Fleisher LA, Rosenbaum SH. Relationship of postoperative anemia and cardiac morbidity in high risk vascular patients in the intensive care unit. Crit Care Med 21:860-866, 1993.

110. Nixon C, Hirsch NP, Ormerod IEC, Johnson G. Nuclear magnetic resonance. Its implications for the anesthetist. Anaesthesia 41:131-137, 1986.

111. Nolan K. Anesthetic concerns for scoliosis surgery. In Lui CP, Crosby ET, eds. Anesthesia and Musculoskeletal Disorders. Philadelphia: JB Lippincott, 1989, p 1179.

112. Occelli G, Saban Y, Pruneta RM, et al. Two cases of anaphylaxis from droperidol. Ann Fr Anesth Reanim 3:440-442, 1984.

113. Olgiati R, Levine D, Smith JP, Briscoe WA, King TK. Diffusing capacity in idiopathic scoliosis and its interpretation regarding alveolar development. Am Rev Resp Dis 126:229, 1982.

114. Ovassapian A. Fiberoptic Airway Endoscopy in Anesthesia and Critical Care. New York: Raven Press, 1990.

115. Owen JH. Motor evoked potentials. Neural monitoring. In Saltzman S, ed. The Prevention of Intraoperative Injury. New Jersey: Humana Press, 1990, pp 219-241.

116. Owen JH. Evoked potential monitoring during spinal surgery. In Bridwell KH, DeWald RL, eds. The Textbook of Spinal Surgery. Philadelphia: JB Lippincott, 1991, p 31.

117. Partridge BC, Ward CF. Pulmonary edema following low-dose naloxone administration. Anesthesiology 65:709-710, 1986.

118. Pathak KS, Ammadio M, Kalamachi A, Scoles PV, Schaffer JW, Mackay W. Effects of halothane, enflurane, isoflurane on somatosensory evoked potentials during nitrous oxide anesthesia. Anesthesiology 66:753-757, 1987.

119. Pathak KS, Brown RH, Nash CL, Cascorbi HF. Continuous opioid infusion for scoliosis surgery. Anesth Analg 62:841-845, 1983.

120. Pathak KS, Brown RH, Nash CL, Cascorbi HF. Continuous opioid infusion for scoliosis fusion surgery. Anesth Analg 73:739-759, 1983.

121. Pelosi P, Croci M, Calappi E, Cerisara M, Mulazzi D, Vicardi P, Gattinoni L. The prone positioning during general anesthesia minimally affects respiratory mechanics while improving functional residual capacity and increasing oxygen tension. Anesth Analg 80:955-960, 1995.

122. Peterson DO, Drummond JC, Todd MM. Effects of halothane, enflurane, isoflurane and nitrous oxide on somatosensory evoked potentials in humans. Anesthesiology 65:35-40, 1986.

123. Pipeer P, Vane J. The release of prostaglandins from lung and other tissues. Ann NY Acad Sci 180:363-385, 1971.

124. Prior JGL, Hinds CJ, Williams J. The use of etomidate in the management of severe head injury. Intensive Care Med 9:313-320, 1983.

125. Roberts JT. Clinical Management of the Airway. Philadelphia: WB Saunders, 1994.

126. Rogers SN, Benumof JL. Halothane and isoflurane do not decrease PaO2 during one-lung ventilation in intravenously anesthetized patients. Anesth Analg 64:946-954, 1985.

127. Rosenthal D, Rosenthal R, De Simone A. Removal of a protruded thoracic disc using microsurgical endoscopy: A new technique. Spine 19:1087-1091, 1994.

128. Sakabe T, Nakakimura K. Cerebral and spinal cord blood flow. In Cottrell JE, Smith DS, eds. Anesthesia and Neurosurgery. St. Louis: CV Mosby, 1994, p 152.

129. Sanders EG, Martin TW. Anesthesia for magnetic resonance imaging procedures. Probl Anesth 6:430-442, 1992.

130. Sandler AN, Tator CH. Effects of acute spinal cord compression injury on regional spinal cord blood flow in primates. J Neurosurg 45:660-676, 1976.

131. Sato M, Pawlik G, Heiss W. Comparative studies of regional CNS blood flow autoregulation and responses to CO_2 in the cat: Effects of altering arterial blood pressure and $PaCO_2$ or rCBF of cerebrum, cerebellum, and spinal cord. Stroke 15:91, 1984.

132. Segal JL, Brunnemann SR. Clinical pharmacokinetics in patients with spinal cord injuries. Clin Pharmacokinet 17:109-129, 1989.

133. Sethna NF, Rockoff MA, Worthen M. Anesthesia related complications in children with Duchenne muscular dystrophy. Anesthesiology 68:462-465, 1988.

134. Shneerson JM, Venco A, Prime FJ. A study of the pulmonary artery pressure, electrocardiography and mechnocardiography in thoracic scoliosis. Thorax 32:700, 1977.

135. Shook JE, Lubicky JP. Paralytic spinal deformity. In Bridwell KH, Dewald RL, eds. The Textbook of Spinal Surgery. Philadelphia: JB Lippincott, 1991, pp 279-321.

136. Silvarjam M, Armory DW, Everett GB, Duffington C. Blood pressure, not cardiac output determines blood loss during induced hypotension. Anesth Analg 59:203-206, 1980.

137. Simpson JI, Eide TR, Schiff GA, Clagnaz JF, Hossain I, Trerskoy A, Koski G. Intrathecal magnesium sulfate protects the spinal cord from ischemic injury during thoracic aortic cross-clamping. Anesthesiology 81:1493-1499, 1994.

138. Slinger PD, Hickey DR, Gottfried SB. Intrinsic PEEP during one-lung ventilation. Anesth Analg 68:S269, 1989.

139. Slinger PD, Triolet W, Wilson J. Improving arterial oxygenation during one-lung ventilation. Anesthesiology 68:291-295, 1988.

140. Smyth RJ, Chapman KR, Wright TA, Crawford JS, Rebuck AS. Pulmonary function in adolescents with mild idiopathic scoliosis. Thorax 39:901, 1984.

141. Soreide EM, Buxrud T, Harboe S. Severe anaphylactic reactions outside hospital. Aetiology, symptoms and treatment. Acta Anaesthesiol Scand 32:339-342, 1988.

142. Stoelting RK, Diefdorf SF. Anesthesia and Co-Existing Disease. New York: Churchill Livingston, 1993, p 226.

143. Strange PG. Brain biochemistry and brain disorders. Reviewed by Middlemiss DN, TiPS, 14:77, 1993.

144. Svensson LG, Loop FD. Prevention of spinal cord ischemia in aortic surgery. In Bergan JJ, Yao JST, eds. Arterial Surgery: New Diagnostic and Operative Techniques. New York: Grune and Stratton, 1988, pp 273-285.

145. Svensson LG, Stewart RW, Cosgrove DM. Intrathecal papaverine for the prevention of paraplegia after operation on the thoracic or thoracoabdominal aorta. J Thorac Cardiovasc Surg 96:38-47, 1988.

146. Tanaka GY. Hypertensive reaction to naloxone. JAMA 228:25-26, 1974.

147. Taylor TH, Major E, eds. Hazards and Complications of Anaesthesia. New York: Churchill Livingstone, 1987, pp 260-261.

148. Thiel RE. The myotonic response to suxamethonium. Br J Anaesth 39:815-821, 1967.

149. Thomas W, Cole PV, Etherington NJ, Prior PF, Stefanson SB. Electrical activity of the cerebral cortex during induced hypotension in man. A comparison of sodium nitroprusside and trimethaphan. Br J Anaesth 57:134-141, 1985.

150. Tobias M, Smith DS. Anesthesia for diagnostic neuroradiology. In Cottrell JE, Smith DS, eds. Anesthesia and Neurosurgery, 3rd ed. St. Louis: CV Mosby, 1994, p 440.

151. Tremper KK. Thoracoscopy: Anesthetic management. In Kaplan JA, ed. Cardiothoracic and Vascular Anesthesia Update. Philadelphia: WB Saunders, 1993, pp 1-5.

152. Tremper KK. Techniques and solutions to avoid homologous blood transfusions. In Barash PG, ed. Refresher Courses in Anesthesiology. Philadelphia: JB Lippincott, 1994, pp 251-262.

153. Truman KJ, Carroll GC, Ivankovich AD. Pitfalls in interpretation of pulmonary artery catheter data. J Cardiothorac Vasc Anesth 3:625-641, 1989.

154. Webb CA. Hazard of reinforced tracheal tubes. Anaesthesia 49:918-919, 1994.

155. Weinlander CM, Coombs DW, Plume SK. Myocardial ischemia due to obstruction of an aortocoronary bypass graft by intraoperative positioning. Anesth Analg 64:933-936, 1985.

156. Weir EK, Archer SL. The mechanism of acute hypoxic pulmonary vasoconstriction: The tale of two channels. FASEBJ 9:183-189, 1995.

157. Whittaker M. Plasma cholinesterase variants and the anesthetist. Anaesthesia 35:174-194, 1980.

158. Williams OA, Clarke FL, Harris RW, Smith P, Peacock TE. Addition of droperidol to patient-controlled analgesia, effect on nausea and vomiting. Br J Anaesth 70:479P, 1993.

159. Wolfe D, Drummond JC. Differential effects of isoflurane/nitrous oxide on posterior tibial somatosensory evoked response of cortical and subcortical origin. Anesth Analg 67:852-859, 1988.

160. Yashon D. Surgical management of trauma to the spine. In Schmidek HH, Sweet WH, eds. Operative Neurosurgical Techniques: Indications, Methods and Results. Philadelphia: WB Saunders, 1988, pp 1451-1452.

161. Yaster M, Simmons RS, Tolo VT, Pepple JM, Wetzel RC, Rogers MC. A comparison of nitroglycerin and nitroprusside for inducing hypotension in children: A double blind study. Anesthesiology 65:174, 1986.

162. York D, Chabot RJ, Gaines RW. Response variability of somatosensory evoked potentials during scoliosis surgery. Spine 12:864-876, 1987.

163. Young W. Neuroprotective therapy for brain and spinal cord injury. In Chernow B, ed. The Pharmacologic Approach to the Critically Ill Patient. Baltimore: Williams & Wilkins, 1994, pp 863-874.

SUGGESTED READING

Benumof JL. Anesthesia for Thoracic Surgery, 2nd ed. Philadelphia: WB Saunders, 1995.

Bernstein RL, Rosenberg AD. Manual of Orthopedic Anesthesia and Related Pain Syndromes. New York: Churchill Livingstone, 1993.

Bradford DS. Moe's Textbook of Scoliosis and Other Spinal Deformities, 3rd ed. Philadelphia: WB Saunders, 1994.

Chernow B. The Pharmacologic Approach to the Critically Ill Patient. Baltimore: Williams and Wilkins, 1994.

Cottrell JE, Smith DS. Anesthesia and Neurosurgery, 3rd ed. St. Louis: CV Mosby, 1994.

Gaba DM, Fish KJ, Howard SK. Crisis Management in Anesthesiology. New York: Churchill Livingstone, 1994, pp 195-200.

Martin JT. Positioning in Anesthesia and Surgery. Philadelphia: WB Saunders, 1988.

Ovassapian A. Fiberoptic Airway Endoscopy in Anesthesia and Critical Care. New York: Raven Press, 1990.

Roberts JT. Clinical Management of the Airway. Philadelphia: WB Saunders, 1994.

Appendix A: Abbreviations and Acronyms

hr hour(s)
min minute(s)
sec second(s)
wk week(s)
yr year(s)
ca circa
IV intravenous

po by mouth
OD outer diameter
cm centimeter(s)
mm millimeter(s)
kg kilogram(s)
mg milligram(s)
ml milliliter(s)

ga gauge
μg microgram(s)
° degree
U unit(s)

A-a alveolar arterial
ABG arterial blood gas
ABL allowable blood loss
ACE angiotensin converting enzyme
ACT activated clotting time
AH autonomic blood loss
AID antonomic hyperreflexia
ASA American Society of Anesthesiologists
ATLS Advanced Trauma Life Support
BAER brainstem auditory evoked response
BP blood pressure
CAT computed axial tomography
CBF cerebral blood flow
CMRO$_2$ cerebral O$_2$ consumption
CNS central nervous system
CO cardiac output
CO$_2$ carbon dioxide
CPAP continuous positive airway pressure
CPP cerebral perfusion pressure
CPR cardiopulmonary resuscitation
CSF cerebrospinal fluid
CT computed tomography
CVP central venous pressure
DBP diastolic blood pressure
DLT double lumen tube
EBV estimated blood volume
ECG electrocardiogram
ETT endotracheal tube
F$_i$O$_2$ fraction of inspired oxygen
FOB fiberoptic bronchoscopy
FOL fiberoptic laryngoscopy
FRC functional residual capacity
GA general anesthesia
Hgb hemoglobin
Hgb/Hct hemoglobin/hematocrit

HIV human immuno deficiency virus
H$_2$O water
HPV hypoxic pulmonary vasoconstriction
ICP intracranial pressure
ICU intensive care unit
IgE immune globulin E
IM intramuscular(ly)
IV intravenous(ly)
K potassium
LAP left arterial pressure
LMA laryngeal mask airway
LTA laryngeal tracheal anesthesia
MAC minimum alveolar concentration
MAP mean arterial pressure
MEP motor-evoked potential
mEq millequivalent
MH malignant hperthermia
MRI magnetic resonance imaging
MV minute ventilation
MVP mitral valve prolapse
MVV maximal voluntary ventilation
NASCIS National Acute Spinal Cord Injury Study
NMB(s) Neuromuscular blocker(s)
NMDA *N*-methyl-D-aspartate
NSAID(s) nonsteroidal anti-inflammatory drug(s)
NTG nitroglycerin
NTP nitroprusside
N$_2$O nitrous oxide
OLA one-lung anesthesia
OLT orthotopic liver transplant
OLV one-lung ventilation
OR operating room
O$_2$ oxygen

PA pulmonary artery
P(A-a)o$_2$ alveolar-arterial oxygen gradient
Paco$_2$ arterial CO$_2$ pressure
PADP pulmonary artery diastolic pressure
PAo$_2$ pulmonary alveolar oxygen
Pao$_2$ pulmonary arterial oxygen
PAP pulmonary artery pressure
PAR post-anesthesia room
PCA patient controlled analgesia
PCWP pulmonary capillary wedge pressure
PEEP positive end-expiratory pressure
P$_{ET}$co$_2$ end-tidal CO$_2$ partial pressure
PFTs pulmonary function test(s)
PIP peak inspiratory pressure
PO per os
PONV postoperative nausea and vomiting
PVR pulmonary vascular resistance
RV residual volume
SCBF spinal cord blood flow
SCMRO$_2$ spinal cord metabolic rate
SCPP spinal cord perfusion pressure
SLV single-lung ventilation
SNP sodium nitroprusside
SSEP somatosensory-evoked potential
SUX succinylcholine
TIVA total intravenous anesthesia
TLC total lung capacity
TTJV transtracheal jet ventilation
VC vital capacity
V̇/Q̇ ventilation-perfusion
ZEEP zero end-expiratory pressure

Management of Anemia

Srinath Samudrala, M.D.

Spine surgeons are frequently confronted with the issues of perioperative anemia and the use of blood products to manage this problem. Just as the well equipped spine surgeon is facile with various instrumentation systems and modifications of these systems, it behooves the surgeon to be well versed in transfusion technology and anemia management. While the spine surgeon can easily relate to blood transfusion technology as one would an instrumentation system, it has been considered by some authors with a pharmacological tendency as a dangerous medication. Immunologists have considered blood transfusion similar to an organ transplant due to its ability to create graft-vs.-host disease. Philosophers and Jehovah's Witnesses consider it to be the sacred carrier of life.

Many contemporary complex spinal operations would not be possible without advances in transfusion technology. Recent advances in testing of blood products, screening of blood donors, and viral inactivation of noncellular blood products have made the blood supply safer than ever before.[20] Modern surgical techniques, improved hemostatic agents, and improved anesthetic monitoring techniques and care have decreased the amount of blood loss during surgical procedures. There are now many more alternatives to allogenic transfusion than are readily available, decreasing the likelihood of allogenic exposure.

Despite these advances, the decision of who to transfuse, when to transfuse, and which blood conservation techniques to utilize seems more complex than ever. The heightened public awareness of the risks of transfusion, along with the explosion of alternatives to transfusion, has made the management of perioperative anemia more challenging and complex. In addition, society and insurers expect management of this problem to be cost-conscious. Only by meeting the challenge of perioperative anemia with a sound understanding of the issues involved and the resources available will the modern spine surgeon be able to practice effective anemia management and achieve optimal utilization of available resources.

Proper perioperative anemia management is based on four intuitively obvious goals:

1. Optimization of preoperative blood component levels
2. Minimization of operative and postoperative blood loss
3. Cost-effective and efficient use of resources to minimize the need of allogenic blood exposure
4. Proper and judicious use of allogenic products when indicated

Each intervention available to the surgeon can be used to help achieve these goals in either the pre-, intra-, or postoperative period. The effective combination of the available tools applied at the proper time during the hospital course, in the appropriate patient, should yield an effective strategy that achieves the desired goals. The surgeon should develop a strategy by understanding and becoming familiar with the issues involved, reviewing effectiveness of the strategy in his practice, and modifying the strategy as needed. Haphazard or sporadic use of some or all of these techniques may only serve to increase the cost of transfusion-related services and show no net decrease in allogenic blood exposure.

CURRENT DATA ON TRANSFUSION OF ALLOGENIC BLOOD PRODUCTS

Appropriate use of allogenic blood products is a key component of the therapy for perioperative anemia. The current status of allogenic transfusion has been molded by society's demand for blood products and technology's development of alternatives. The indications for transfusion have changed as the knowledge of anemia physiology has increased. An understanding of the forces behind these changes is helpful regarding the understanding of the evolution of transfusion technology to its current state.

History of Transfusion Medicine

Routine collection, anticoagulation, and transfusion has been commonplace in the United States since the 1940s. Transfusion services increased steadily from that time until the utilization of blood products doubled from the 1970s to the 1980s.[9] The demand for blood stabilized in the early 1990s as physician and public awareness of transfusion risks increased. In 1992 the American Red Cross reported that 5.8 million units of packed red blood cells (PRBCs) were "produced" in the United States.[9]

The indications for blood transfusion (BT) have changed during this time course as well. In 1942 Adams and Lundy[1] reported that at a hemoglobin level of less than 10g/dl, the red blood cell (RBC) mass was insufficient to provide adequate oxygen to the tissues. They suggested that a patient be transfused blood when the hemoglobin concentration fell below this level. This opinion gained widespread following and for many years this "10/30 rule" was followed as dogma. As experience with managing profoundly anemic patients without

transfusion grew, physicians realized that the transfusion trigger was not the same for all patients, and that indeed many patients could safely tolerate more severe levels of anemia than allowed by the 10/30 rule. Awareness of HIV contamination of the blood supply occurred simultaneously with a more advanced knowledge of anemia physiology and the realization that greater levels of anemia could be tolerated. Physicians sought to review the indications for blood transfusion in an attempt to decrease the public's exposure to allogenic blood products.

The National Institutes of Health Consensus Conference in 1988 was organized to evaluate the modern indications for perioperative allogenic blood transfusion. It concluded that the 10/30 rule was not valid and that no single factor could be used as an indicator of the need for blood transfusion.[7] The conference thought that moderate anemia had no proven detrimental effect in the postoperative period and that good clinical judgment and analysis of overall clinical status was essential and irreplaceable in determining the transfusion trigger for an individual patient. It was thought that while most patients with hemoglobin <7 g/dl would require transfusion, many between the levels of 7 to 10 g/dl could function without adverse sequelae.

Current Transfusion Guidelines

While it is intuitively obvious to most clinicians that transfusion of blood is indicated when the level of anemia exceeds the body's ability to maintain adequate oxygen delivery (DO_2) to the end organs, the accurate determination of this state is problematic. Normal blood hemoglobin levels insure that DO_2 far exceeds normally required levels. As hemoglobin levels fall, the body initiates a number of compensatory mechanisms to maintain adequate DO_2. (see box). The adequacy of these compensatory mechanisms, along with the patient's particular clinical situation, determines when hemoglobin levels have reached a critical stage in which ischemia of tissues is likely. In a review of perioperative Jehovah's Witnesses with moderate to severe anemia (hemoglobin <8mg/dl), mortality was found only in those with a hemoglobin <5mg/dl.[37] Other studies have confirmed that it is safe to allow a patient's hemoglobin to decrease to levels much lower than previously thought if their overall medical condition allows them to compensate. In an effort

<table>
<tr><td colspan="2">**COMPENSATORY MECHANISMS FOR ACUTE ANEMIA WITH MAINTAINED INTRAVASCULAR VOLUME***</td></tr>
</table>

Reduction in blood viscosity
Reduction in SVR
Increase in venous return
Increase in cardiac output
Redistribution of flow
Increase in oxygen extraction
Enhanced release of oxygen in tissue

*Normovolemic hemodilution.

SUGGESTED TRANSFUSION GUIDELINES: RED BLOOD CELLS

Hemoglobin ≤8 g/dl or acute blood loss in an otherwise healthy patient with signs and symptoms of decreased oxygen delivery with two or more of the following:
  Estimated or anticipated acute blood loss of $15%
    of total blood volume (750 ml in 70 kg male)
  Diastolic blood pressure ≤60 mm Hg
  Systolic blood pressure drop ≥30 mm Hg from base
    line
  Tachycardia >100 beats per minute)
  Oliguria/anuria
  Mental status changes
Hemoglobin ≤10 gl/dl in patients with known increased risk of coronary artery disease or pulmonary insufficiency who have sustained or are expected to sustain significant blood loss
Symptomatic anemia with any of the following:
  Tachycardia (>100 beats per minute)
  Mental status changes
  Evidence of myocardial ischemia including angina
  Shortness of breath or dizziness with mild exertion
  Orthostatic hypotension
Unfounded/questionable indications:
  To increase wound healing
  To improve the patient's sense of well-being
  Hemoglobin ≤10 g/dl (females ≤7) or hematocrit
    ≤30% (females ≤21%) in otherwise stable, asymptomatic patient
  Mere availability of predonated autologous blood
    without medical indication

From Fakhry SM, Sheldon GF. Blood administration, risks and substitutes. Adv Surg 28:71-92, 1995.

---

to standardize transfusion practices across geographic and physician differences, guidelines have been developed to aid physicians in determining when transfusion of allogenic blood is indicated. These guidelines should be used along with clinical and physiological indicators that could help physicians determine the proper transfusion trigger. These guidelines should supplant any dogmatic rule, such as the 10/30 rule, and should increase the appropriateness of blood transfusion (see box).

Adverse Effects Associated with Allogenic Blood Transfusion

The risk of complication from allogenic blood transfusion is lower today than it has ever been in the past. While recent technological advances have decreased the risk of transfusion, the public perception of this risk has increased. This is contrary to the past when the risks of transfusion were relatively high yet the lay person had little knowledge or concern of the potential risks. Some of the adverse effects of allogenic blood transfusion may occur immediately, while others may take years to develop (Table 7-1).

Viral Transmission

HIV infection is perhaps the most feared infectious complication associated with transfusion. While the current risk of HIV transmission is low and is estimated at 1:500,000, patients often are more concerned about this complication than any other.[26] This is undoubtedly due to an increased public awareness, the stigmata associated with the disease,

Table 7-1. Estimated Risks of Transfusion per Unit in the United States (1995)

Minor allergic reactions	1:100
Bacterial infection (platelets)	1:2500
Viral hepatitis	1:5000
Hemolytic transfusion reaction	1:6000
HTLV/II infection	1:200,000
HIV infection	1:420,000
Acute lung injury	1:500,000
Anaphylactic shock	1:500,000
Fatal hemolytic reaction	1:600,00
Graft-vs.-host disease	Rare
Immunosuppression	Unknown

HTLV = human T-cell leukemia-lymphoma virus;
HIV = human immunodeficiency virus
From: Klein, HG. Allogeneic transfusion risks in the surgical patient. Am J Surg 170:22S, 1995.

and the devastating nature of the disease. Most cases of transfusion-acquired HIV infection occurred prior to the routine serological testing of all donor blood. Since 1985, when such screening became mandatory, there have been only 33 cases of documented HIV transmission from the transfusion of blood. While the risk of acquiring HIV infection from blood transfusion is likely to remain low in the future, new mutant types of HIV that may escape current testing may pose a future threat.

Posttransfusion hepatitis has been a much more common complication of transfusion and was reported to occur as frequently as 1:3000 transfusions. Recent advances in screening have decreased the rate of infection to 1:80,000, and with the addition of a new generation of screening tests for hepatitis C, the overall risk of posttransfusion hepatitis is likely to decrease to 1:100,000.[26] Most (>90%) cases of viral hepatitis associated with transfusion are caused by the hepatitis C virus. Approximately 2% of cases are caused by the hepatitis B virus and the remainder are caused by other viruses such as cytomegalovirus (CMV), Epstein Barr virus, and hepatitis A. While posttransfusion hepatitis may be asymptomatic or have only mild symptoms in the early stages, as many as 20% of patients may go on to develop cirrhosis. Hepatitis B is also associated with the development of hepatocellular carcinoma in the later stages of the disease.

Human T-cell lymphotrophic virus 1 and 2 are retroviruses endemic in Japan and the Caribbean. HTLV 1 infection, causing tropical spastic paraparesis, has been reported in a small number of cases.[4]

Transfusion Reaction

Mild transfusion reactions may cause fever, urticaria, and chills and occur up to 1:100 transfusions. These problems are seldom difficult to manage and are caused by antibodies against white blood cells (WBCs) or plasma proteins. Febrile reactions may be prevented by premedicating the patient with acetaminophen and diphenhydramine.

Hemolytic reactions are more severe and may occur hours to days after a transfusion. The risk of a hemolytic reaction is 1:6000.[21] Patients may lose RBC mass because of the hemolysis and should be followed for anemia. More severe reactions present with immediate symptoms such as chest tightness, shortness of breath, hypotension, chills, and fever.

Fluid resuscitation, diuresis, and supportive care is essential. If a significant hemolytic reaction does occur, the blood products and new samples of the patient's blood should be sent to the blood bank for evaluation. Most fatal hemolytic reactions are due to incompatible ABO transfusions. Many of these are clerical errors and are more likely to occur in the operating room or emergency room under pressing situations.

Immunomodulatory Effects of Blood Transfusion

The immunomodulatory effects of blood transfusions in enhancing allograft survival in renal transplant patients have been known for 20 years. It has also been known that women with a history of spontaneous abortions are more likely to carry through delivery if they have been transfused allograft blood.[3] These immunosuppressive effects of allogenic transfusion are currently being studied to determine whether they increase surgical morbidity.

Gantt[10] in 1981 postulated that allogenic blood transfusion (BT) may affect the recurrence or progression of cancer. Recent concern over the impairment of the natural immunosurveilance mechanisms by allogenic blood transfusion has prompted researchers to review whether perioperative blood transfusion may affect cancer progression or patient survival. In a review of 70 studies comparing the prognosis of patients with various types of cancer who were or were not given blood, a definite causal relationship could not be found, although a detrimental association seemed to exist.[18]

PREOPERATIVE DONATION OF AUTOLOGOUS BLOOD

Preoperative autologous donation (PAD) has been increasingly used over the past several years and now accounts for 5 to 10% of transfusions in this country.[33] The demand for a low-risk transfusion alternative has led clinicians to increase the use of PAD and successfully eliminate the need for allogenic transfusion in certain subsets of patients. While PAD is considered standard of care treatment for certain procedures, such as radical prostatectomy and elective hip replacement, the efficacy and practicality in other procedures is not completely determined.[29]

PAD has many benefits. It eliminates the viral and immunological risks associated with allogenic transfusion. Physicians are likely to tolerate greater levels of anemia in PAD patients and thus the overall quantity of allogenic blood administered is less. Patient satisfaction and sense of well-being are immeasurable benefits of PAD.

While autologous blood is the safest blood product available, the process of PAD does have documented risks. Adverse events related to phlebotomy, such as vasovagal syncope, occur in 5% of patients. Cardiac or cerebral ischemia may occur in high-risk patients, although careful selection may minimize this risk.[14] Accidental administration of incompatible units is possible and, therefore, autologous units should be checked as carefully as allogenic products. Because the risk of autologous blood is perceived as extremely low, the threshold for transfusing may be lower and signs of hypervolemia or hyperviscosity may occur if administered in a susceptible patient.

The challenge of having a practical, safe, and effective autologous program involves properly managing several logistical details: (1) collecting enough blood to meet the transfusion needs without overcollecting; (2) timing the donation process with the surgical schedule to prevent blood expiration; and (3) maximizing the cost-benefit ratio. Inadequate management of these factors increases the cost of PAD and prevents the overall reduction of allogenic exposure.

PAD is not an available option for all patients, and potential candidates must meet specific donation criteria. Current protocols currently allow the donation of one unit of blood per week and patients who require more blood must be able to manage without surgery until the time necessary to collect sufficient units. Patients with anemia (hematocrit <30) are obviously not candidates and require treatment of their anemia with a resultant rise in hematocrit prior to donation. The blood donation sites must be accessible to the patients who use PAD. Because blood collected for PAD can only be preserved for 35 days, the scheduling of an operation must be reliable or the patient may lose outdated autologous units, which may increase allogenic exposure. Patients must have sufficient RBC regenerative capabilities in the time from donation to surgery, or a significant portion of the benefit of PAD may be lost.

Recent studies have documented concern over the high cost of PAD.[2] Investigators have found a 30% to 50% discard rate for unused autologous blood. This increases the cost of the PAD process.[15] While a certain degree of overcollection is important to insure the avoidance of allogenic exposure, a balance must be attempted to maintain cost-effectiveness. Given the very low risk of allogenic transfusion, the authors have questioned whether society as a whole is benefiting from the PAD process.

STANDARD PREOPERATIVE PREPARATION

Preoperative evaluation and risk assessment is the first step toward the optimization of blood use. The key aspects of the standard preoperative history and physical examination illuminate foreseeable causes of perioperative anemia. As in other aspects of surgery, the preemptive identification and treatment are the hallmarks of excellent care (see boxes).

Use of agents known to inhibit the coagulation pathway, such as heparin, Coumadin, aspirin, or nonsteroidal medications, should be discontinued preoperatively. Common causes of anemia should be evaluated and treated prior to initiation of any blood conservation strategies. Anemia due to nutritional deficiency may be corrected by simple oral supplementation. In patients requiring urgent surgery, more aggressive measures of anemia correction can be considered. These include parenteral iron, vitamin B_{12}, and folate supplementation. Anemia of chronic disease and anemia secondary to renal failure respond well to Epogen administration. Workup of blood loss from occult gastrointestinal sources should be part of the standard preoperative medical workup in elective patients. Patients who have undergone recent chemotherapy should have anemia and thrombocytopenia corrected if possible. Importantly, patients who wish to perform PAD may also develop anemia prior to their scheduled procedure. Preventing or correcting this insures that the PAD process achieves its goal of minimizing allogenic exposure. Recent use of antibiotics that may deplete vitamin K dependent co-factors for clotting should be evaluated. This commonly occurs in the setting of a critically ill patient who may have been hospitalized prior to the spinal procedure. A family history of bleeding tendencies or prior history of excessive bleeding during surgical procedures should

---

CHARACTERISTICS OF PATIENTS AT HIGH RISK FOR REQUIRING TRANSFUSION

Greater than 1000 ml blood loss expected
Preoperative anemia
Small body weight
Vascular tumor, infection
Coronary artery disease, cerebral vascular disease
Malnutrition
Prior recent surgery

PREOPERATIVE MEASURES TO MINIMIZE ALLOGENIC BLOOD EXPOSURE

Diagnose, treat, correct anemia
Obtain bleeding history
Mentally rehearse planned procedure
Schedule appropriate instruments, medical devices to
  minimize operating time
Stop use of aspirin, NSAIDs
Offer possibility of preoperative autologous donation
Lab tests:
  CBC, PT/ATT (standard)
  Vitamin B_{12}, iron, folate, factor levels (optional)
  Bleeding time (optional)
Consider erythropoietin treatment
Consider embolization, staging
Determine transfusion trigger

---

serve as a red flag that requires input from a hematological consult.

Preoperative determination of the proper transfusion trigger for each patient is likely to make subsequent transfusion decisions easier. A proper history, medical evaluation, and laboratory tests determine if the patient has any medical conditions that decrease compensatory mechanisms. Will he or she be able to tolerate a moderate anemia of hematocrit 25? Does he or she have a history of transient ischemic attacks or angina? Does his or her EKG suggest prior silent ischemic episodes? These issues are more calmly analyzed during a preoperative office visit than in the postoperative ICU setting. The individualized transfusion trigger that is likely to ensue based on this knowledge, is the ideal of anemia management. Moreover, it allows for discussion with the patient and the family, which is part of informed consent.

Optional Preoperative Measures
Embolization

Endovascular techniques have been increasingly used to decrease the amount of blood loss in spinal surgery patients. Most reports are anecdotal and conclusive studies documenting a decreased overall risk are lacking. The risks of spinal angiography and possible injury to vessels supplying the spinal cord should be weighed against the likelihood of blood loss. Because the overall risks of allogenic transfusion are quite low, (1:3000 to 6000 of a serious reaction) a prudent physician might require that embolization be extremely safe to justify its use. It is reasonable that vascular lesions, such as metastatic renal cell carcinoma and melanoma, may have blood loss risks that exceed that of transfusion. However, this requires further investigation.

Staging

Spinal surgery frequently can be staged into ventral and dorsal procedures. While one-anesthetic procedures may decrease the time to mobilization of the patient, a decreased length of stay in the hospital, decreased anesthetic length and possible risk, the risk of anemia, and the treatment of such must be considered. In the hands of some physicians and with some anemia management protocols, transfusion risks may be lessened with one-anesthetic management. Patient and surgeon preference, along with the surgical condition, often dictate whether or not this is an appropriate option.

INTRAOPERATIVE TECHNIQUES

Minimizing blood loss has long been considered an indicator of a good surgeon. This notion arose in the early days of surgery when blood transfusion was not an option. In those days, the preservation of blood during any operation was an essential aspect of patient survival. Patients with moderate anemia had no alternative but to wait for the time when the body regenerated blood lost during surgery. It is possible that the increased access to transfusion services has made surgeons more indifferent to the time-honored skill of intraoperative blood preservation. Recent public concern over the risks of transfusion have forced all physicians to reacquaint themselves with this aspect of surgery. Besides avoiding the hazards of anemia and allogenic transfusion, good hemostasis skills also allow improved visualization and decreased operative time (see box).

Because most (60% to 70%) allogenic blood is transfused during the 48 hours following the initiation of a surgical procedure, the surgeon would do well to consciously recall this fact prior to the induction of anesthesia and realize that his/her actions in the ensuing moments will be the major determinant of the necessity for allogenic blood products. Mental rehearsal of the procedure may eliminate some delay in preparing drills, instrumentation trays, and other surgical devices necessary for the procedure.[30] Reviewing the procedure with the assistant promotes efficiency. Assuring that the anesthesiologist, cell-saver technician, and circulating nurse are satisfactorily prepared goes a long way to minimize wasted time that leads to increased blood loss.

Positioning

Proper positioning should be used as a tool for minimizing intraoperative blood loss. Increased venous pressure in the epidural veins, the vertebral bodies, and paraspinal tissues can be a direct result of increased pressure in the thoracic vena cava and right heart, and the abdominal vena cava. Mechanical factors affecting the thoracic and abdominal cavities should be addressed independently during positioning.

The thoracic cage must be assessed for mechanical factors that cause compression or limit the movement necessary for ventilation. Adequate support must be provided by rolls to allow unimpeded chest excursion during ventilation. Airway pressure necessary to ventilate is also dependent on body habitus, pulmonary compliance, and dynamic airway resistance. Increased airway pressure or peak airway pressure from any number of factors may lead to increased right heart and vena caval pressures, which causes increased bleeding when the pressure is transmitted to the spinal venous system. The anesthesiologist can follow and modify such factors as inspiratory/expiratory ratio (I/E ratio), tidal volume, and ventilator rate to minimize mean intrathoracic pressure and venous pressure. The abdominal cavity should be routinely assessed in a similar fashion to the chest cage. Increased abdominal tension from improperly positioned rolls can lead to increased venous pressure transmitted from the vena cava. Inadequately sized rolls may move during the procedure, causing the patient to be supported by his abdominal wall. Properly securing the positioning devices to the bed, and securing these to the patient, is especially important for lengthy procedures. Nasogastric suctioning in patients with an ileus may help to decrease the intra-abdominal pressure that contributes to increased venous pressures.

Surgical Technique

Meticulous surgical technique could be defined as a combination of technical maneuvers that are difficult to describe but easy to identify when present. The attainment of good technique is related to proper training and experience but is also dependent upon the desire and will of each surgeon. Good surgical technique and familiarity with regional anatomy are essential in minimizing intraoperative blood loss. Knowledge of the proper use of bipolar and monopolar cautery, as well as knowing when it is prudent to pack a source of bleeding, can be gained with an earnest desire for "bloodless" surgery. Candid self-evaluation of blood loss and a desire for improvement are essential in improving technique.

Autotransfusion Devices

Salvage of intraoperative blood loss is frequently used in today's operating room. Several methods have shown a decrease in the need for allogenic blood transfusion.

Washed autotransfusion systems are most commonly used. Blood lost during a surgical procedure is scavenged using a standard sucker connected to specialized suction tubing. This tubing has two lumens: one in which the blood is aspirated into the collection canister, and another smaller channel in which heparinized saline flows at a controlled rate, insuring that the scavenged blood is quickly anticoagulated. The blood is then filtered and centrifuged. Centrifugation separates and removes waste products such as free hemoglobin, cell debris, fat globules, and surgical contaminants such as bone and metal particles. The separated RBCs are then washed with normal saline and collected. The final concentration of blood may achieve a hematocrit of 70%.[24] This blood may be reinfused at the termination of the procedure.

Autotransfusion devices such as the cell-saver have been documented to decrease the likelihood of allogenic exposure. The costs of this intervention are relatively small. The disposable costs average $100 to $400, and the technician time and overhead must be considered.[24] Autotransfusion systems are associated with a very low risk of complications. A theoretical risk of air embolus can be avoided by proper technician training and transfusion. Bacterial contamination is low. Contraindications to autotransfusion are bacterial infection in the surgical wound and malignancy. The issue of safety in cases of malignancy has not been fully evaluated. One study reported no increased risk of metastatic disease in patients with transitional cell cancer. However, the theoretical risk has precluded most surgeons from using autotransfusion in these cases.[17]

Several precautions should be taken when autotransfusion devices are used in the operating room. Bacitracin and neomycin in the irrigation solutions should be omitted with cell-saver systems because these antibiotics are not completely washed from the scavenged blood, and the intravenous administration of these drugs could be detrimental. Hemostatic agents made with microfibrillar collagen should be avoided because they may pass through the filtration system and the risk of embolization is possible.[24]

Normovolemic Hemodilution

Normovolemic hemodilution has been used successfully in series of patients undergoing scoliosis surgery. The technique involves withdrawing blood from a patient during the beginning of the procedure and reinfusing the blood at a later time, generally during the closure after most expected blood loss has occurred. During the initial phase of blood withdrawal the patient is maintained isovolemic by the infusion of colloid or crystalloid. Blood may be withdrawn until the patient's hematocrit has reached 28% (hemodilution) or 20% (profound hemodilution). The amount of blood withdrawn is dependent upon the expected blood loss, the length of the procedure, and the ability of the patient to withstand anemia. The blood is stored at room temperature in citrate preserved bags and may be stored for 6 hours. After the portion of surgery where the major expected blood loss has occurred, the blood is reinfused. Hemodilution decreases the RBC content of lost blood during the surgery because any blood loss has a lesser hematocrit than would be otherwise. The reinfused blood also returns the patient's platelets and clotting factors. The amount of blood that can be saved from this technique is variable and depends upon several factors. A 70 kg male with normal cardiopulmonary status and a preoperative hematocrit of 45 could have 5 units of blood removed to have a hematocrit of 25%.[35] Blood loss could be allowed to drop the hematocrit to 18 to 21 prior to reinfusion of the stored blood.

While extreme hemodilution should be reserved for young patients who are able to compensate for this degree of anemia, moderate hemodilution has been shown to be safe, even in patients over the age of 60. Several studies in the spine population have shown the effectiveness of this technique in blood conservation. Kafer et al.[19] showed an 85% decrease in allogenic blood utilization in pediatric patients undergoing spinal instrumentation. Martin et al[36] used extreme hemodilution to a hematocrit of 15% for adolescent scoliosis patients and obtained a reduction in mean allogenic transfusion requirements from 4370 to 750 ml.

Despite these positive results there is still underutilization of this technique. Some surgeons may perceive the procedure as dangerous or technically difficult. Others may not have adequate support from their anesthesia staff. Further studies documenting the safety of normovolemic hemodilution in routine spinal surgery may be needed to increase the popularity of this technique.

Decision of When to Transfuse

Proper determination of the intraoperative transfusion trigger can help minimize anemia associated complications and optimize use of allogenic blood. Mild to moderate anemia may be tolerated quite well by the patient if normovolemia is maintained. Many of the effects of anemia, such as decreased tissue perfusion, may be prevented if normovolemia is maintained. Infusion of volume expanders, such as colloid, should be employed to bring intravascular volume back to normal prior to the transfusion of blood.

Hypothermia

Several studies have shown the effect of hypothermia on decreasing coagulation function. Hypothermia has been shown to cause a reversible platelet dysfunction both in vivo and in vitro.[31] Other studies have shown an important prolongation of prothrombin time and activated partial thromboplastin time, which was inversely correlated to temperature.[32] The maintenance of normothermia should be attempted by minimizing exposure, maintaining warm room temperature, and the use of warming blankets as necessary.

Causes of Sudden Increased Bleeding

Intraoperative bleeding that changes suddenly should be promptly recognized. The evaluation should begin with the anesthesiologist, who can seek causes such as dislodgment of the endotracheal tube, bronchospasm, allergic reaction to medication, and hypothermia. The position should be evaluated to insure that the chest or abdominal cavity has not slipped off of the supporting devices. If blood loss has been significant, a review of the transfused products and the possible need for platelets, fresh frozen plasma, and cryoprecipitate should be considered. Also, the presence of disseminated intravascular coagulation should be considered.

Hypotensive Anesthesia

Hypotensive anesthesia has been used extensively in orthopaedic procedures and has proven to significantly decrease blood loss in patients undergoing hip replacement surgery.[30] Its use in spinal surgery has been mainly limited to scoliosis patients and

has provided conflicting results. In separate studies McNeil[28] and Knight[22] found a significant decrease in blood loss in patients who underwent hypotensive anesthesia for scoliosis surgery. Mandel et al. safely used hypotensive anesthesia with hemodilution and autologous donation in 24 patients, and clearly showed a decrease in blood loss. They were, however, unable to document a decrease in allogenic blood exposure as a result of this technique. A more recent study by Lennon et al.[25] reported no reduction in blood loss during scoliosis correction.

Despite some positive data, protocols for deliberate hypotensive anesthesia in a general spinal surgery population have not been created. As with all interventions, a risk-benefit analysis correlating specifics of anesthesia techniques and patient characteristics is needed. Variations in age, cardiopulmonary function, and anesthetic abilities are likely to make this procedure feasible and optimal for only select patients.

Jehovah's Witness patients and children who are unable to perform significant volumes of PAD may benefit from hypotensive anesthesia because it is one of the few options available to them. Consideration of this technique in other patients remains to be determined.

Pharmacological Adjuvants

Desmopressin (DDAVP) is a synthetic analog of the normal hormone vasopressin, which has been reported to decrease bleeding in spinal surgery patients. Vasopressin acts on endothelial cells to increase the release of von Willebrand factor, tissue-type plasminogen activator, and certain prostaglandins. Through these effects, DDAVP causes improved platelet aggregation and clotting in patients with uremia and chronic liver disease. The presence of impaired platelet aggregation in patients with scoliosis has led clinicians to try DDAVP as a method to reduce blood loss in patients undergoing scoliosis surgery. A randomized, double-blind trial by Kobrinsky et al.[23] in 35 patients with idiopathic or neuromuscular scoliosis related to cerebral palsy showed a 32% decrease in operative blood loss. This effect was most pronounced in patients with neuromuscular scoliosis. A study by Guay et al.,[16] however, showed no benefit from DDAVP when only patients with normal coagulation history and function were included. They suggested that DDAVP has a role in selected patients with neuromuscular scoliosis and those with proven platelet disorders, but that it does not provide benefit in the majority of patients with idiopathic scoliosis.

The current lack of data on the use of DDAVP in the general spinal surgery population indicates that further studies are required to determine which patients are likely to benefit from this drug.

POSTOPERATIVE STRATEGIES

Unwashed blood salvage systems have the greatest potential use in spinal surgery patients as a means of reducing blood loss in the postoperative anemia. These devices are currently used in cardiac surgery to collect and reinfuse shed mediastinal blood and in joint replacement surgery. In a study of patients undergoing total knee arthroplasty, postoperative autotransfusion was the only method of blood salvage necessary for 90% of patients.[6] The use of these devices in spinal surgery patients is an area for future study. Other more routine measures of blood conservation are listed in the accompanying box.

Erythropoietin

Human recombinant erythropoietin (EPO) is currently approved for use in patients with anemia secondary to chronic disease, chronic renal failure, and malignancy, and in zidovudine-treated patients with HIV. Recent studies have evaluated its use in the surgical setting, where it has shown a promising role in the management of perioperative anemia. EPO is a glycoprotein hormone produced predominantly by the kidney and by the liver to a lesser degree that serves to stimulate RBC production in the marrow. Hypoxia in the kidney and liver is the chief stimulus for EPO production and EPO is reduced to basal levels when a corrected RBC mass provides normal oxygen delivery. EPO normally circulates at basal rates and increases very little secondary to small blood losses, such as the donation of one unit of autologous blood. Only after a major blood loss does the amount of EPO increase sharply.[11] Adequate Vitamin B_{12}, folic acid, and iron stores are essential to allow the marrow to produce increased RBCs in response to this EPO rise. RBC production will not occur with inadequate nutritional stores, even if EPO has reached high levels.

Recent studies have attempted various strategies to determine the best potential use of this product. One of these strategies involves use of EPO preoperatively for a number of days to increase RBC mass and decrease the need for transfusion. This was shown in a recent study of patients undergoing hip surgery to reduce the need for transfusion by 50%.[5] EPO, in combination with PAD protocols, has been recently attempted in several series. Goodnough[13] demonstrated that EPO therapy accelerated erythropoiesis in PAD patients and allowed patients to donate 41% more blood preoperatively. The proper dosage, route, and interval of administration for perioperative EPO is still under investigation.

BLOOD SUBSTITUTES

Nonblood alternatives have been investigated as a solution to the myriad problems associated with the management of perioperative anemia. Much of the research in this field was initiated in the mid 1980s in response to the HIV contamination of the allogenic blood supply. There are two categories of products currently under investigation.

The largest category consists of modified hemoglobin molecules. Researchers are attempting to alter characteristics of the molecule, such as the affinity for oxygen, the antigenicity, and the clearance rate from the blood.[38] These drugs are currently undergoing clinical trials and may demonstrate clinical utility in the years to come.

Another category of blood substitutes are the perfluorocarbons. These are halogenated molecules that dissolve a large amount of gases, including oxygen. Spence at al.[34] performed a study using Fluosol DA in 36 Jehovah's Witness patients who had refused transfusion in the presence of significant anemia (hemoglobin 4.3/dl). They concluded that while Fluosol had no clinical benefit, it could be administered safely.

POSTOPERATIVE MEASURES TO MINIMIZE ALLOGENIC BLOOD EXPOSURE

Maintain normovolemia
Identify and correct coagulopathy
Maintain good nutrition
Utilize nonwashed autotransfusion systems

JEHOVAH'S WITNESSES AND LEGAL CONSIDERATIONS OF BLOOD TRANSFUSION

The legal aspect of allogenic transfusion in a competent adult should be considered by a surgeon as falling under two classes of laws: informed consent law and medical malpractice law. Most surgeons are familiar with the principles of these two types of laws from their surgical experience and training. Blood shield laws hold liability for the process of collection and administration of blood. This is generally not under the purview of the surgeon.[12] The increased options and variability of transfusion techniques oblige the surgeon to become well versed in the issues of blood preservation and transfusion so that discussion with the patient and proper practice of transfusion principles is carried out.

While there may be regional differences in documentation, the principles of informed consent are well known to all surgeons. Patients must be competent and have a potential procedure (in this case blood transfusion) explained to them in language that they are able to understand. They must have a discussion of the possible risks, reasonably expected benefits, and the likely course of undergoing the procedure. Importantly, the alternatives to allogenic transfusion must be explained to the patient in ample time for them to utilize these options. The patient must be able to consider these issues and ask questions as they see fit.

Medical malpractice laws find a physician liable when the standard of care has not been met by the treating physician. The standard of care is determined to be the actions a reasonable, prudent medical practitioner would take in a given circumstance. In the case of blood transfusion, malpractice could perhaps be alleged if the indications for blood transfusion were not sound or if alternatives to transfusion were not provided.

The legal issues of transfusion in Jehovah's Witness patients are actually fairly straightforward and well established by many court decisions.[8] If a Witness has given an appropriate written advance medical directive/release indicating his/her refusal to accept blood or blood product transfusion, transfusion against his/her will is battery for which the transfusing physician is liable.

The issues become more complex when an advanced medical directive is not available or when a patient is not competent to make a decision. This may occur in young patients and trauma patients. In these conditions surgeons are advised to seek assistance from their risk-management teams and members of their Hospital Liaison Committee for Jehovah's Witnesses.

While Jehovah's Witnesses do not accept transfusion of blood products, there are a number of techniques that they may accept, which can make surgery feasible and safe. Spinal surgery has been successfully performed on Jehovah's Witnesses with the use of appropriate blood salvage techniques and nonblood alternatives. Institutions where surgery with these techniques is routinely done may be useful as referral centers.

CONCLUSION

The explosion of technology in transfusion medicine has made the risks of allogenic blood transfusion less than ever before. Surgeons are now able to safely carry out operations with a reliable and safe blood supply. The risks of transfusion will never reach zero. However, patients demand an active role in determining the preferred management of their perioperative anemia. Customizing the management of perioperative anemia and utilizing transfusion alternatives are likely to be more common as current research develops. The challenge to the spine surgeon will be in assuring the least overall risk from management of this problem while maintaining the practical and cost-effective features of transfusion services.

REFERENCES

1. Adams RC, Lundy JS. Anesthesia in cases of poor surgical risk. Surg Gynecol Obstet 74:1011-1019, 1942.
2. AuBuchon JP. Cost-effectiveness of preoperative autologous blood donation for orthopedic and cardiac surgeries. Am J Med 101:38S-42S, 1996.
3. Bordin JO, Blajchman MA. Immunosuppressive effects of allogeneic blood transfusions: Implications for the patient with a malignancy. Hematol Oncol Clin North Amer 9:205-218, 1995.
4. Bove JR, Sanler SG. HTLV-1 and blood transfusion. Transfusion 28:93-94, 1988.
5. Canadian Orthopedic Perioperative Erythropoietin Study Group. Effectiveness of perioperative recombinant human erythropoietin in elective hip replacement. Lancet 341:1227-1232, 1993.
6. Carstens VL, Earnshaw PH. Postoperative orthopedic autotransfusion. Successful management for the total knee arthroplasty patient. AORN J 56:272-280, 1992.
7. Consensus Development Panel. Perioperative red blood cell transfusion. JAMA 260:2700-2703, 1988.

8. Dixon JL, Smalley MG. Jehovah's witnesses: The surgical/ethical challenge. JAMA 246:2471-2472, 1981.

9. Fakhry SM, Sheldon GF. Blood administration, risks and substitutes. Ad in Surg 28:71-92, 1995.

10. Gantt CL. Red blood cells for cancer patients. Lancet 363, 1981.

11. Goldberg MA. Erythropoiesis, erythropoietin, and iron metabolism in elective surgery: Preoperative strategies for avoiding allogeneic blood exposure. Am J Surg 170:37S-43S, 1995.

12. Goldman, EB. Legal considerations for allogeneic blood transfusion. Am J Surg 170:27S-31S, 1995.

13. Goodnough LT. Clinical application of recombinant erythropoietin in the perioperative period. Hematol Oncol Clin North Am 8:1011-1020, 1994.

14. Goodnough LT, Monk TG. Evolving concepts in autologous blood procurement and transfusion: Case report of perisurgical anemia complicated by myocardial infraction. Am J Med 101:33S-37S, 1996.

15. Goodnough LT, Rudnick S, Price TH, et al. Increased preoperative collection of autologous blood with recombinant human erythropoietin therapy. N Engl J Med 321:1163-1168, 1989.

16. Guay J, Reinberg C, Poitras B, et al. A trial of Desmopressin to reduce blood loss in patients undergoing spinal fusion for idiopathic scoliosis. Anesth Analg 75:405-410, 1992.

17. Hart OJ III, Limberg IW, Wajsman Z, et al. Intraoperative autotransfusion in radical cystectomy for carcinoma of the bladder. Surg Gynecol Obstet 168:302-306, 1989.

18. Houbiers JGA, Busch ORC, Van de Watering LMG, et al. Blood transfusion in cancer surgery: A consensus statement. Eur J Surg 161:307-314, 1995.

19. Kafer ER, Isley MR, Hansen T, et al. Automated acute normovolemic hemodilution reduces blood transfusion requirements for spinal fusion (abstract). Anesth Analg 65:S76, 1986.

20. Klein HG. Allogenic transfusion risks in the surgical patient. Am J Surg 170:21S-26S, 1995.

21. Klein HG. New insights into the management of anemia in the surgical patient. Am J Med 101:12S-15S, 1996.

22. Knight PR, Lane GA, Nichols MG, et al. Hormonal and hemodynamic changes induced by pentolinium and propranolol during surgical correction of scoliosis. Anesthesiology 53:127-134, 1980.

23. Kobrinsky NL, Letts M, Patel LR, et al. 1-Desamino-8-D-argininge Vasopressin (Desmopressin) decreases operative blood loss in patients having Harrington rod spinal fusion surgery. Ann Intern Med 107:446-450, 1987.

24. Laub GW, Riebman JB. Autotransfusion: Methods and complications. In Lake CL, Moore RA, eds. Blood: Hemostatsis, Transfusion, and Alternatives in the Perioperative Period. New York: Raven Press, 1995, pp. 381-394.

25. Lennon RL, Hosking MP, Gray JR, et al. The effects of intraoperative blood salvage and induced hypotension on transfusion requirements during spinal surgical procedures. Mayo Clin Proc 62:1090-1094, 1987.

26. Loussert-Ajaka I, Ly TD, Chaix M, et al. HIV-1/HIV-2 seronegativity in HIV-1 subtype O infected patients. Lancet 343, 1393-1394, 1994.

27. Mandel RJ, Brown MD, McCollough NC, et al. Hypotensive anesthesia and autotransfusion in spinal surgery. Clin Orthol 154:27-33, 1981.

28. McNeil TW, DeWald RL, Kuo KN, et al. Controlled hypotensive anesthesia in scoliosis surgery. J Bone Joint Surg 56A:1167, 1974.

29. Monk TG, Goodnough LT. Blood conservation strategies to minimize allogenic blood use in urologic surgery. Am J Surg 170:69S-73S, 1995.

30. Nelson CL, Fontenot HJ. Ten strategies to reduce blood loss in orthopedic surgery. Am J Surg 170:64S-68S, 1995.

31. Reed RL III, Johnston TD, Hudson JD, et al. The disparity between hyperthermic coagulopathy and clotting studies. J Trauma 33:465-470, 1992.

32. Rohrer MJ, Natale AM. Effect of hypothermia on the coagulation cascade. Crit Car Med 20:1402-1405, 1992.

33. Sculco TP. Blood management in orthopedic surgery. Am J Surg 170: 605-635, 1995.

34. Spence RK, McCoy S, Costabile J, et al. Fluosol DA-20 in the treatment of severe anemia: Randomized, controlled study of 46 patients. Crit Care Med 18:1227-1230, 1990.

35. Stehling L, Zauder HL. Acute normovolemic hemodilution. Transfusion 31:857-868, 1991.

36. Valeri CR, Khabbaz K, Khuri SF, et al. Effect of skin temperature on platelet function in patients undergoing extracorporeal bypass. J Thorac Cardiovasc Surg 104:108-116, 1992.

37. Viele MK, Weiskopf RB. What can we learn about the need for transfusion from patients who refuse blood? The experience with Jehovah's Witnesses. Transfusion 34:396-401, 1994.

38. Winslow RM. Blood Substitutes. Science and Medicine March/April: 54-63, 1997.

Monitoring

Vincent C. Traynelis, M.D., Kenneth A. Follett, M.D., Ph.D.,
and Richard K. Osenbach, M.D.

Serious spinal cord injury is the most devastating complication of thoracic spinal surgery. Over the past dozen years, intraoperative monitoring has been recommended as a means of preventing or limiting neurological injury during spinal procedures for decompression (including discectomy), deformity correction, stabilization, tumor excision (especially intradural and intramedullary neoplasms), and resection of vascular lesions.[17,79] The rationale for performing intraoperative monitoring is based on the premise that early, reversible neural dysfunction can be detected by clinical examination or evoked potentials. The surgeon, once informed of such changes, would act appropriately to limit the potential for permanent injury. Additionally, in some situations the ability to maintain stable recordings might occasionally allow for a more aggressive surgical intervention than would otherwise be possible or justified.

Generally, any patient undergoing thoracic spinal surgery may benefit from intraoperative monitoring. However, several criteria must be met to make electrophysiological monitoring worthwhile: it must be technically possible to monitor the neural pathway at risk; appropriate stimulation and recording sites must be available during the procedure; proper equipment for obtaining technically adequate recordings must be utilized; personnel skilled in the technical acquisition and interpretation of the responses must be available; and finally, if response deterioration occurs, meaningful intervention must be possible.[27]

The basic principles, advantages, and disadvantages of monitoring both ascending and descending pathways during surgery are discussed in this chapter. Current electrophysiological techniques include recording somatosensory-evoked potentials (SSEPs) at cortical levels (somatosensory cortical–evoked potentials [SSCEPs]) or spinal levels (somatosensory spinal–evoked potentials [SSSpEPs]), spinal-evoked potentials recorded as spinal levels (SpEPs), dermatomal-evoked potentials (DEPs), and motor-evoked potentials (MEPs). The wake-up test, a clinical means of assessing descending tract function, will also be reviewed. Recently, a method to evaluate nerve root function intraoperatively following pedicle screw placement has been developed, and this will also be discussed. It is emphasized that this chapter presents a basic overview, and the interested reader should consult the references for more detailed information on specific monitoring procedures.

SOMATOSENSORY-EVOKED POTENTIALS

SSEPs primarily monitor the dorsal columns. Review of the anatomical pathways involved in somatosensory perception is pertinent to understanding SSEP.

Anatomical Basis of Somatosensory-Evoked Potentials

The somatosensory system interfaces with the external environment via receptors in the skin, muscles, and joints. These receptors primarily convert mechanical stimuli into action potentials. Appropriate electrical stimulation of a peripheral nerve such as the median or posterior tibial nerve also activate the somatosensory system. Regardless of the method of stimulation, the action potential is conducted centrally through first-order neurons whose cell bodies reside in the dorsal root ganglia. First-order neuronal processes enter the spinal cord via the dorsal root entry zone and ascend in the ipsilateral dorsal column. Somatotopic order is preserved with lower extremity fibers traveling in the more medial fasciculus gracilis while axons from the upper extremity ascend via the fasciculus cuneatus. These fibers terminate and synapse in the nuclei gracilis and cuneatus, respectively, at the level of the cervicomedullary junction.

Axons from second-order neurons leave the dorsal column nuclei, decussate via the arcuate fascilulus, and continue rostrally through the brain stem as the medial lemniscus. Ultimately, they terminate in the ventral posterior lateral nucleus of the thalamus. Third-order fibers leave the thalamus, traverse the medullary center and internal capsule, and eventually terminate in the primary somatosensory cortex.

The concept that the dorsal columns and medial lemnisci serve as the conduction paths for SSEP is partially based on observations that clinical impairment of touch, vibration, proprioception, and stereognosis are associated with abnormalities in the SSEP. Furthermore, it has been noted that conditions that result in selective loss of pain and temperature loss (i.e., dissociated sensory) do not alter the SSEP.[24,27,29]

Despite classical dogma and clinical observations, the precise anatomical pathways responsible for SSEP transmission have been a topic of debate. This controversy is fueled by experimentally derived data indicating that electrical signals traveling through routes that are separate from the dorsal columns may contribute to or influence the conduction of the SSEP.[16,20,62,66] Clinically, arguments concerning the specific contribution of a given tract to the SSEP are somewhat moot. This is because intraoperative spinal cord injury causing significant neurological deficit often affects the entire spinal cord, thereby permitting the SSEP to be used as a fairly reliable monitoring tool.[11] SSEP monitoring for scoliosis correction and spinal cord tumor resection appears to be associated with a false negative rate of less than 2% and a false positive rate of about 3%.[18,32,79] Falsely positive SSEPs are usually related to anesthetic effects or technical difficulties. False negative SSEPs are almost universally the result of disproportionate damage to the descending and ascending tracts.

Detection of SSEP may be performed at the spinal and/or cortical level(s). It is preferable to record from multiple sites.[11,27,57] Recording electrodes are usually placed proximally over the peripheral nerve being stimulated, over the spine proximal to the level of surgical interest, and over the region of the somatosensory cortex that corresponds to the site of peripheral stimulation.[27,57] Scalp electrodes are usually positioned at C'3, C'4, and C'z and referenced to Fpz (according to the International Ten Twenty System).[31]

Recording from the afferent pathway distal to the surgical site (e.g., nerve or distal spinal level) will verify that successful peripheral stimulation has occurred. Monitoring should also be performed at two or more sites proximal to the surgical field. Recording from multiple locations is useful for distinguishing changes caused by surgical manipulation from those caused by technical problems. For example, loss of all potentials or one proximal potential implies a technical problem whereas loss of both proximal potentials suggests cord dysfunction secondary to surgical manipulation. Cortical and/or spinal sites may be used for proximal monitoring. If proximal recording is performed at only a single location, then a spinal site is recommended because cortical potentials are relatively more vulnerable to anesthetic or physiological alterations.

In addition to proximal spinal recording, monitoring several cortical regions will provide added assurance that the evoked responses have arrived at the cortex. Furthermore, multisite cortical monitoring allows one to "customize" the procedure. For example, the posterior tibial nerve cortical evoked-response is usually recorded from the C'z-Fpz electrode derivation, but occasionally better responses are obtained from a more lateral position (C'3 or C'4).[57]

Somatosensory Cortical–Evoked Potentials

SSCEPs are probably the most widely used responses for intraoperative spinal cord monitoring. Because they are quite sensitive, alterations in cortical activity secondary to anesthetic and/or intraoperative physiological changes may interfere with proper monitoring. Halogenated inhalational anesthetics in particular can have a profoundly detrimental effect on SSCEP recording. Excellent anesthesia and stable evoked responses can usually be achieved using a nitrous/narcotic technique. Physiological changes that can alter responses include hypotension, hypocarbia, and hypothermia.[27] These factors must be considered when evaluating intraoperative changes of the SSCEP and, as mentioned previously, simultaneous monitoring of SSSpEPs improves monitoring reliability.[17]

Preoperative SSCEP evaluation may be useful if there is an anticipated need for postoperative testing. Recordings obtained shortly after the induction of anesthesia, however, represent the true baseline against which subsequent intraoperative monitoring is compared. One reason for using the postinduction baseline is that anesthesia may attenuate responses. On the other hand, postinduction responses may actually be better than preoperative records. For example, peripheral neuropathy may limit preoperative testing because the high stimulus intensity required to evoke a response is painful. This is not a problem once the patient is anesthetized. In some institutions, it is more convenient to place electrodes and test the monitoring setup prior to anesthesia, but generally, monitoring need not begin before administering anesthetics. Exceptions to this rule occur when there is risk of spinal cord injury during induction and positioning (e.g., spinal instability).

The American Electroencephalographic Society has published specific recommendations for stimulation and recording techniques.[3] According to these recommendations, stimulating and recording electrodes may be placed before or after positioning. If they are placed prior to positioning, they must be rechecked once the patient is in the final position. This is important because there may not be clear access to the electrodes after draping, and the ability to monitor is often impaired when an electrode detaches or loses good electrical contact. Cup electrodes may be used, but they are more prone to detachment then needle electrodes. Additionally, the cup electrolyte may dry during long cases, resulting in higher impedances that can potentially alter stimulation requirements and recording effectiveness. Subdermal needle electrodes are less likely to be displaced than cup electrodes, and their interelectrode impedances are relatively low. Changes in electrode impedance are less likely to occur with needle electrodes than with cup electrodes. The disadvantages of needle electrodes relate to their invasiveness: they may break beneath the skin, promote an infection, or conceivably produce a subdermal injury if the stimulation intensity is excessive.[57]

The stimulation sites must be appropriate for the location of the surgical procedure. For most thoracic procedures, posterior tibial or common peroneal nerve activation provides an adequate stimulus for monitoring but will not permit monitoring of conus function. Caudal spinal cord monitoring may be accomplished by stimulation of the pudendal nerve or the bladder (via indwelling electrodes).[4,28,65]

Stimulation may be unilateral or bilateral. The quality and sensitivity of the SSEP may be increased with bilateral stimulation, but such a technique can hinder detection of unilateral changes.[15] Multichannel recording of individual extremities, including intermittent bilateral stimulation, is probably the most sensitive means of detecting intraoperative changes.

Stimulation is performed holding either current or voltage constant. Neuronal elements are stimulated by current flow, not voltage; therefore the effectiveness of constant voltage stimulation will vary with changes in tissue or electrode resistance (impedance). This is a potential problem in intraoperative monitoring. For example, long operative times may lead to increases in electrode impedance, especially with cup electrodes (e.g., the electrolyte may dry). This results in a decrease in the current delivered by a constant voltage stimulator. In turn, stimulation effectiveness is diminished, which can lead to loss of the evoked response being monitored (a false positive result). Changes in current delivery that are inherent with constant voltage stimulation can be averted by using a constant current stimulator, which automatically adjusts stimulus voltage to compensate for changes in resistance at the stimulation site.

The rate and number of stimulus repetitions should be such that good quality responses are produced in as little time as possible, thereby allowing rapid detection of acute intraoperative changes. Generally, the rate of stimulus repetition is four to five per second. Slower stimulation rates require an unacceptably long acquisition time for the averaged response. Increasing the frequency of stimulation allows more rapid data accumulation but attenuates the cortical response. It is important to avoid stimulation rates that might be multiples of intermittent nonbiological activity as this may produce a sinusoidal artifact. Time-locking of the stimuli and evoked responses to periodic noise artifact can usually be avoided by using noninteger stimulus frequencies.[57] The number of repetitions ranges from 100 to 2000 depending on the quality of the recorded signal. Lower extremity stimulation frequently requires a relatively higher number of repetitions.

Peripheral nerve dysfunction (e.g., neuropathy) may interfere with the ability to obtain satisfactory evoked potentials from stimulation of nerves in the extremities. Increasing the pulse duration (normally 200 to 250 microseconds) may improve both the morphology and the amplitude of the response in those patients with peripheral neuropathy. If adequate responses cannot be achieved using these maneuvers in patients with peripheral nerve disease, stimulation of the spinal cord may be necessary (see SpEP below).[26]

The equipment needed for recording SSEPs includes recording electrodes, differential amplifiers, band-pass filters, and a signal averaging computer. The microvolt amplitude of an evoked potential is significantly smaller than the ongoing baseline electroencephalographic or electromyographic activity. Without reduction of this undesirable electrical "noise," SSEP responses are uninterpretable. The processes of amplification, filtering, and averaging act to improve the signal-to-noise ratio and the definition of the evoked response.[11,57]

Recording is usually performed using differential amplifiers. These amplifiers process input from both active and reference electrodes such that activity common at both electrodes is cancelled while unique signals are amplified. Thus, extraneous electrical "noise" recorded by both electrodes (e.g., EKG activity) is eliminated from the final output of the amplifier.

Following amplification, band-pass filters are used to optimize the SSEP signal. These filters advantageously exploit the differences between axonal and dendritic potentials. Axonal potentials are usually succinct whereas dendritic responses have relatively broader configurations and longer durations.[57] Additionally, the frequency range of axonal activity is significantly wider than that of dendritic responses. Therefore band-pass filters set to record a wide range of frequencies are best for recording axonal activity. In contrast, a relatively narrow, lower frequency band-pass filter is optimal for detecting energy associated with cortical responses.[36] Despite these observations, intraoperative SSEPs have been successfully recorded using a variety of band-pass filter settings.[11,19,27,57] Brown and Nash[11] recommend a low filter setting of 0.3 Hz and a high filter setting of 250 Hz. Owens[57] has successfully recorded cortical-dendritic and subcortical axonal responses using high and low bandwidths of 10 to 250 Hz and 10 to 2000 Hz, respectively. Filter settings should be established prior to surgical manipulation because once monitoring has commenced, changing the setting will alter the configuration of the SSEP. It is difficult to discern which recording variations are due to changes in filter settings and which are due to surgical manipulation.

After the signal is filtered, it is processed by a signal-averaging computer. This computer adds each consecutive response to the preceding responses and averages them. "Noise" (random electrical activity that is not evoked by the stimulus) is gradually cancelled out while the time-locked SSEP is preserved. Reliable, reproducible recordings usually can be obtained by averaging 125 to 300 responses.[11,27,57] Fig. 8-1 illustrates a typical SSCEP and shows the advantage of signal averaging.[22]

The final recording parameter to consider is the time base or sweep duration of the recording. Selection of the sweep duration depends on numerous factors including which nerve is stimulated and whether short or long latency potentials are of primary interest. Clinically important intraoperative posterior tibial SSEP peaks usually can be recorded using a 75 msec period.[11]

One should always strive to obtain the clearest, most reproducible recordings and, to this end, the general guidelines presented in this chapter should be modified when appropriate. Techniques that can be used to improve the signal-to-noise ratio include altering the number of repetitions, increasing muscle relaxation, changing filter settings, and improving the effectiveness of stimulation (by altering stimulus intensity and/or location).[46]

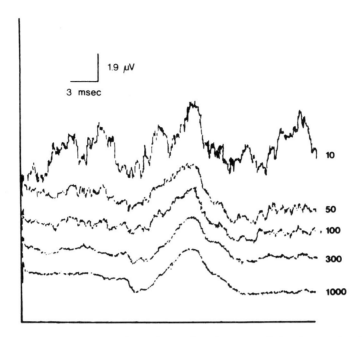

Fig. 8-1. A typical set of SSCEP recordings shows the advantage of signal averaging. The number of evoked responses collected for each averaged response is indicated on the right. The improvement in evoked response definition that occurs as the number of collected SSEPs increases is notable. (From Follett KA. Intraoperative electrophysiologic spinal cord monitoring. In Loftus CM, Traynelis VC, eds. Intraoperative Monitoring Techniques in Neurosurgery. New York: McGraw-Hill, 1994, pp 231-238.)

Somatosensory Spinal–Evoked Potentials

Depth of anesthesia, temperature, blood pressure, and changes in arterial carbon dioxide concentration all influence SSCEPs; however, these factors are much less likely to affect SSSpEPs.[27] Fast repetition rates do not attenuate SSSpEPs; thus averaged responses can be rapidly acquired.[48] Additionally, the relatively higher amplitudes of SSSpEPs provide a better quality signal than SSCEPs; therefore fewer repetitions are required to obtain a good averaged response. For these reasons, the reliability of intraoperative SSEP monitoring increases when SSSpEP responses are obtained simultaneously with SSCEP responses.[17,57]

The recording methods for SSSpEPs are more invasive than those used for SSCEPs. SSSpEP electrodes may be placed in the subarachnoid or epidural space, in the spinous processes, or in the interspinous ligament using either percutaneous or direct techniques. Midline placement is important to avoid recording a unilateral response.

Percutaneous subarachnoid electrode placement is usually accomplished with a Touhy needle.[70,71] Although Tamaki et al.[70,71] monitored 229 patients with percutaneously placed subarachnoid electrodes and reported no complications, the invasiveness and potential for injury related to this technique have been a matter of concern.[17,19] Placement under direct vision is safer, but the electrodes are necessarily within the surgical field. This makes them more susceptible to movement during surgical manipulation, and such movement can alter responses.

Epidural electrodes are less invasive than subarachnoid electrodes, and recording spinal-evoked potentials from this site has proven useful for a number of surgeons.[17,47,50,75] Epidural electrodes provide good signal amplitudes (although not as high as subarachnoid electrodes) and may be placed using one of several techniques. Directly placed electrodes should be inserted as far rostrally and caudally as possible and secured with sutures to minimize the potential for movement during the operation.[8,48,64] Despite all precautions, epidural electrodes positioned within the surgical wound are prone to displacement, which can alter evoked potential configuration. Percutaneous epidural placement carries greater risk, but there is less chance of movement (and subsequent recording error) because the electrodes are remote from the surgical field.[75]

SSSpEPs can also be monitored using electrodes (e.g., Kirschner wires) placed in the spinous processes.[9,33,38,55] Although spinous process electrodes may be displaced occasionally, they generally provide stable, consistent signals.[33,38] These electrodes are relatively safe and easy to insert in the mid- and lower thoracic regions and in the lumbar spine. A disadvantage of this technique lies in the fact that response amplitudes recorded from electrodes embedded in spinous processes are substantially less than those obtained with epidural or subarachnoid electrodes. This lowers the signal-to-noise ratio and makes obtaining good quality recordings more difficult. Furthermore, amplitude can vary greatly with this recording technique.[47] Another drawback of spinous process monitoring is that placement of the wires into the high thoracic and cervical spinous processes can be difficult and time-consuming. Furthermore, the response amplitude at these levels is frequently too small to permit reliable monitoring. McNeal et al.[52] could only obtain good quality responses above T9 in 20% of their cases. For these reasons, spinous process electrodes are not widely used.

Finally, electrodes placed into the interspinous ligament both rostral and caudal to the operative field can be used to record SSSpEPs.[18,32,37,44] Interspinous ligament responses are less variable than cortical responses, and the amplitudes are higher than those obtained with spinous process wire electrodes, possibly because the electrodes are closer to the dura. Interspinous monitoring can be particularly useful at high thoracic levels where the relatively fragile spinous processes may not support use of a spinous process electrode.[44] Care must be taken to avoid violation of the spinal canal when using this technique. Interspinous ligament electrodes may shift with surgical manipulation because they are near the surgical site, and they may have to be moved for closure.

The stimulation parameters used to elicit SSSpEPs are similar to those used for SSCEPs. Fewer stimulus repetitions are needed for good averaged SSSpEPs because spinal responses are more consistent than cortical responses. When used without cortical monitoring, the stimulation rate may be increased to 25 Hz. A higher repetition rate combined with a lower number of repetitions improves the efficiency of spinal cord monitoring; thus SSSpEPs allow for rapid assessment of spinal cord

integrity. The electrical activity evoked in spinal cord axons is much faster than in the cerebral cortex; therefore SSSpEP amplifiers are usually set to record frequencies from approximately 100 to 3000 Hz. As with SSCEPs, the filter settings should be adjusted to obtain the best evoked response with the least background noise. All filter adjustments should be made prior to surgical manipulation.

Somatosensory–Cortical Evoked Potential and Somatosensory–Evoked Potential Interpretation

The utility of SSCEP and SSSpEP monitoring is based upon detection of changes in amplitude and/ or latency of the peaks being studied. Unfortunately, clear criteria for determining the significance of intraoperative evoked response changes are not available. Generally, response amplitude seems to be the most dependable parameter for data interpretation, and a 50% to 60% decrement from baseline value should be cause for alarm.[10,11,19,27,32,79] If the signal remains stable, without further decline, permanent spinal cord damage may not occur; however, if anesthetic and technical problems have been excluded and amplitude continues to fall, one should search for a surgically related cause that can be altered to restore the SSEP. In addition to the absolute reduction, the time period of amplitude degradation also appears to be important. Specifically, loss of responses for greater than 15 minutes has been associated with new neurological deficits.[10] Latency is not as important a predictor of spinal cord dysfunction as amplitude diminution. This does not mean that latency has no significance, and latency prolongation of greater than 10% may prewarn of spinal cord injury.

Decreases in SSSpEP amplitude may be a more sensitive predictor of spinal cord injury than a drop in SSCEP amplitude. SSSpEP amplitude decreases of 40% have been associated with postoperative dysfunction. SSSpEP latency changes are of minor importance.[11,32]

Although controversial, some data suggest that preservation of the waveform components may be more meaningful than maintenance of baseline amplitude. Whittle, Johnston, and Besser[78] reported a series of patients in which persistent loss of greater than 50% of amplitude (compared to the intraoperative baseline) occurred with preservation of waveform subcomponents. These patients did not suffer postoperative neurological deficits. The speed of signal conduction across the operative site is another potential means of assessing spinal cord function.[49,50] This technique is not generally used for intraoperative monitoring, however, because it is difficult to quantify.

Significant intraoperative changes are acted upon in a systematic fashion. First, purely technical problems are excluded. Signal alterations secondary to physiological effects related to hypotension, systemic hypothermia, and cold irrigation solutions as well as anesthetic effects should be considered and handled appropriately. Once technical, physiological, and anesthetic causes have been excluded, there are several management options. One can wait for a few minutes to see if the signal improves (some of this time will have been spent excluding the potential causes previously listed). Surgical manipulations that may be utilized to reverse response changes should be considered next.[68,79] Relaxing pial retraction sutures and returning spinal alignment more toward its preoperative state by releasing any inserted instrumentation are two examples of these types of surgical maneuvers. If signal deterioration occurs during resection of intrinsic spinal cord tumors, cessation of tumor resection may be considered, particularly if the dissection plane is not readily apparent. Another course of action would be to perform a wake-up test. The above listed strategies are all reasonable depending on the given circumstances. Ignoring a degradation in response and proceeding with surgery implies that one has little confidence in the recordings, in which case it probably is preferable not to perform intraoperative recordings.

SPINAL SPINAL–EVOKED POTENTIALS

Peripheral nerve disease (e.g., peripheral neuropathy) can be so severe that the affected nerves are refractory to stimulation. This situation will preclude monitoring of SSCEPs and SSSpEPs.[32,45,48] Furthermore, recordings of SSCEPs and SSSpEPs may also be foiled by low baseline response amplitudes and, for SSCEPs, the need for low repetition rates. These problems can be circumvented by direct stimulation of the spinal cord. This is a more invasive means of monitoring in which electrodes are placed proximal and distal to the surgical site—one set for stimulation, the other for recording. SpEP monitor-

ing can be performed with either epidural or subarachnoid electrodes.[45,48,71,75] Electrodes for SpEP monitoring may be placed under direct vision or percutaneously. The risks and benefits of these two electrode placement techniques have been previously discussed. Although SpEP monitoring is not widely employed, it does offer several advantages. SpEP responses are relatively unaffected by anesthetics and general physiological changes. The relatively high SpEP response amplitudes result in favorable signal-to-noise ratios and good quality recordings. Reliable averaged evoked responses can be obtained with as few as 32 stimulus repetitions, although typically 50 to 100 are used.[71,75] SpEP repetition rates are relatively high (20 to 50 Hz). This combination of fast stimulus rate and lower number of repetitions permits assessment of spinal cord integrity in as little as 1 to 2 seconds, providing almost real-time monitoring. One disadvantage of direct spinal cord stimulation is that response interpretation is complicated by the mixture of sensory and motor fiber activity evoked by the stimulus. The problem of mixed responses can be minimized by recording from the sciatic nerve after stimulation of the spinal cord proximal to the operative site (see following section on MEPs)[57]

DERMATOMAL-EVOKED POTENTIALS

SSEPs (spinal or cortical) do not provide information about individual root function. This is because the input from each peripheral nerve is dispersed over several levels of the spinal cord so that an abnormality at one level is obscured by maintenance of normal overall activity.[15] Dermatomal monitoring has been developed in an effort to overcome the problems of mixed-nerve SSEPs. Decompressive lumbar operations constitute the primary use of DEPs. Improvement of DEP latencies following decompression of lateral recess stenosis correlates well with postoperative outcome if the patient's symptoms have not been longstanding.[11,27,30] The problem of overlapping dermatomes particularly hinders the utility of this technique in the thoracic region. Although DEPs may be only rarely helpful when decompressing thoracic roots, the authors present the technique for the sake of completeness.

Cutaneous stimulation is accomplished using electrodes placed several centimeters apart within a single dermatome. The specificity of the DEP depends on precise stimulation of the appropriate autonomous receptive field of each root to be monitored. As previously mentioned, this is especially difficult at the thoracic levels. Abnormal baseline recordings can be very helpful for determining the proper field of stimulation. Stimulation intensities should be submaximal (2 to 3 times sensory threshold) to prevent stimulation of underlying tissues (e.g., muscle and connective tissue) that would contaminate the recording. Stimuli are delivered at a rate of 3 to 7 Hz, and the recording technique is similar to that used for SSCEPs.[35] Ideally, bilateral monitoring is performed. DEPs are affected by the same factors that affect other cortical SSEP responses (anesthetics, temperature, hypotension, etc.). Unlike other SSEPs, however, the DEP latency, rather than amplitude, is the primary parameter to follow. Abnormal preoperative latencies tend to improve as the operative decompression is accomplished. Lower extremity limb latencies are generally within 3 to 6 msec of each other, and normally latency does not vary more than 3 msec from one level to the next.[57] Small latency shifts (4% or greater) may indicate root dysfunction even when amplitude changes are minor (20%), although the postoperative neurological deficits seen in patients with such response alterations are not permanent.[15]

MOTOR-EVOKED POTENTIALS

SSEPs assess afferent pathway integrity, which is primarily transmitted via the dorsal columns. SSEPs are incapable of specifically monitoring ventral or lateral spinal pathways. For this reason, patients may rarely awaken with a neurological deficit following spinal operations despite stable intraoperative SSEP recordings.[18,25,39,58] Because of this shortcoming of SSEP monitoring techniques, there has been considerable interest in developing and implementing methods for monitoring spinal motor pathways. Current MEP monitoring techniques entail activation of the motor pathways proximal to the surgical site and monitoring the motor response distally. Spinal motor pathways may be stimulated by electrical excitation of the cerebral cortex or brain stem[7,40,53,63] or the spinal cord[42,48,58], or by magnetic stimulation of the cerebral cortex.[5,67] Distal MEP responses may be recorded below the surgical site at spinal levels or more peripherally from somatic nerves or muscles. Currently, MEP monitoring is

somewhat limited by technical difficulties, but intraoperative physiological assessment of the motor pathways will undoubtedly gain prominence as equipment and procedural refinements occur.

Transcranial electrical stimulation (TES) of the motor cortex may be accomplished using EEG scalp electrodes[7,53] or electrode plates placed adjacent to the scalp and hard palate.[40] Stimulation rates vary from 0.2 to 17 Hz.[7,40] Hypertension and tachycardia limit the frequency of stimulation in some patients. Acceptable evoked response averages can usually be obtained with 30 to 250 repetitions.[40] TES is very uncomfortable due to high current densities in the scalp and extracranial tissues. The degree of pain is so intense that baseline studies cannot be obtained without anesthesia. TES is not recommended for use in patients with epilepsy or EEG evidence of seizure tendency. Additional contraindications include implanted metallic devices, skull fractures or defects, and drugs that may lower the seizure threshold.[2] TES rarely produces false negative recordings, but false positives may be common.[40,80]

Transcranial magnetic stimulation (TMS) utilizes a rapidly changing magnetic field to induce intracranial electrical currents. TMS is performed using a magnetic stimulator that consists of a high voltage power source, a storage capacitor, and electromagnetic coil. The power source charges the storage capacitor, which is connected to the magnetic coil through a low resistance circuit. A time-varying magnetic field is produced as the capacitor discharges current into the coil. Skin, fat, and bone are poor conductors (relative to neurons, blood, and cerebrospinal fluid) so the magnetic field passes through the scalp and skull without significant attenuation and induces an electrical current in underlying cerebral tissues.[12] When the induced current is of sufficient amplitude and/or duration, neuronal depolarization occurs.[12,23] Unlike TES, TMS of the motor cerebral cortex is not painful because the current flow in the scalp and extracranial tissues is negligible.[6] Pre- and postoperative assessment with TMS may therefore be easily performed.

The usefulness of intraoperative monitoring with TMS is currently limited by technical and anesthetic problems.[67] Difficulties in positioning and securing the stimulating coil have been somewhat decreased by improvements in coil design.[41,43] The use of volatile anesthetic agents, barbiturates, and droperidol should be minimized to prevent depression of cortical responsiveness.[34]

The disadvantages of magnetic stimulation include the size and expense of the required equipment, low stimulus repetition rate, and lack of specific stimulation sites in the cortex.[6] TMS is not recommended for use on a continuous basis, as the long-term effects of magnetic stimulation are unknown. Similar to TES, TMS should be avoided in patients with epilepsy or EEG evidence of seizure tendency, although the theoretical risk of inducing a seizure appears to be small.[56] TMS is contraindicated in patients with implanted metallic devices and skull defects.[2]

Direct or epidural spinal cord stimulation can also activate the motor system.[1,42,48,58,61] The stimulating electrodes must be placed in the midline to avoid unilateral stimulation.[48] The relatively high direct or epidural stimulation repetition rates (4 to 6 Hz) allow for rapid acquisition of good averaged responses.[48,58] The usefulness of this technique is adversely affected by the variability of evoked responses following spinal cord stimulation. Spinal activation of MEPs is compromised by the same anesthetic and technical factors that affect transcranial stimulation motor responses. Migration of the stimulating electrode(s) can produce response changes that suggest spinal cord injury. Likewise, current can be shunted away from the spinal cord if there is excessive fluid around the stimulating electrode or if the electrode contacts metallic instrumentation.[58] Despite these potential problems, some investigators have reported excellent results using this technique.[58,59]

Motor-evoked responses may be recorded at spinal levels, from peripheral nerves, or from muscles.[7,40,42,57,58] The more distal the recording electrode, the less the amplitude. Consistent responses to cortical stimulation can be recorded at spinal levels.[7] Spinal stimulation activates motor and sensory pathways, making interpretation of spinal responses difficult. The problem is compounded when the distance between the stimulating and recording electrodes is small. Reliable recordings can usually be obtained by averaging 100 to 500 repetitions.[48]

Peripheral nerve responses (e.g., sciatic nerve recordings) evoked by spinal cord stimulation may be more sensitive indicators of spinal cord dysfunction than spinal responses.[40,57] These peripheral nerve potentials consist of a mixture of orthodromic motor activity and antidromic sensory activity. The difference in nerve conduction velocities can be used to distinguish between sensory and motor responses. Such a technique requires that the distance between the stimulating and recording electrodes be great enough that the faster conducting motor responses are able to be cleanly separated from the sensory potentials. Peripheral nerve recordings of spinal and cortical motor-evoked responses circumvent some of the difficulties associated with studies of myogenic responses (such as effects of muscle relaxants).

Myogenic-evoked potentials are pure motor responses. Patients cannot be fully paralyzed, and the degree of muscle paralysis should be monitored because these responses will vary with the state of muscle relaxation (either voluntary or pharmacological).[73] It is preferable to maintain 75% to 90% relaxation when trying to detect magnetically stimulated MEPs, although lower extremity responses can be obtained with >95% blockade of hand muscles (which are frequently monitored by the anesthesiologists.[67] The state of muscle relaxation is more likely to vary when pharmacological relaxants are administered in boluses as compared to a continuous infusion.[40] Because of the variability associated with changes in relaxation, muscle action potential recordings may be less reliable indicators of spinal injury than MEPs recorded from peripheral nerves.[40]

Similar to SSEPs, the major criterion for assessing spinal cord integrity with MEPs is amplitude. Unlike SSEPs, however, the continued presence of a neurogenic motor potential indicates an intact motor tract even when there is some amplitude degradation.[60] No intervention is required until 50% to 60% amplitude decreases are realized. Latency changes are of lesser concern, although increases greater than 10% should be noted.[40,57]

WAKE-UP TEST

The wake-up test predates the advent of electrophysiological monitoring techniques.[76] The wake-up test represents a clinical means of assessing the descending motor pathways, and although this test may be useful, it has significant limitations. The wake-up test can only be used in cooperative, understanding patients. The surgical procedure is interrupted for each static examination; therefore continuous monitoring of spinal cord function is not accomplished.[54] Thus insults may occur prior to or after performing the wake-up test. Optimally, the need to perform a wake-up test is recognized preoperatively. This will allow the patient to be forewarned and an appropriate anesthetic technique to be performed.[74] One advantage of the wake-up test is that it does not require sophisticated, expensive equipment.

ROOT MONITORING

The development of pedicle screw fixation represents an advance in the ability to stabilize both the lumbar and thoracic spines. The excellent fixation achieved with this technique does not come without risk. In the laboratory, under controlled conditions, improper pedicle screw placement is not rare.[77] The incidence of neural dysfunction secondary to incorrectly positioned pedicle screws has been reported to be as high as 6% (although in experienced hands it is probably significantly less).[51,69,72] The relatively small size of the mid- and upper thoracic pedicles increases the risk of neural compromise. It should be noted that root deficits secondary to improper pedicle screw placement may not be apparent in the immediate postoperative period.[21] Although injury or compression of the thoracic roots does not result in significant motor deficits, painful radiculopathy may ensue. Additionally, there may be diminished fixation strength from screw penetration of the cortex of the pedicle. Monitoring may be useful for decreasing the occurrence of both immediate and delayed screw-related radiculopathy. Although not directly related to the thoracic spine, individual nerve root stimulation and monitoring may also be useful when surgically treating cauda equina lesions.

A technique for evaluating lumbar pedicle screw placement using intraoperative evoked electromyographic (EMG) monitoring has been developed at the University of Miami.[13,14] These investigators directly stimulated pedicle screws and recorded EMG potentials in segmentally appropriate muscles. Based on laboratory and intraoperative studies, they demonstrated that violation of the pedicle resulted in a significant decrease in the amount of stimulation necessary to evoke an EMG response.

Clinically, square-wave constant current stimuli of 7 mA (200 μsec pulses) administered to either the screw or a probe placed within the screw hole should not evoke EMG activity as long as the cortical pedicular bone remains intact. If stimulation of the instrumentation does not result in detectable EMG activity, the screw should be removed and the hole closely inspected. If there is only a small perforation or if the perforation cannot be found, the screw may be replaced. Screws cannot safely be placed in holes with large defects or when there is some direct evidence that the screw may compromise the nerve root. This technique is already useful, and the authors anticipate it will become more so with increasing experience.

REFERENCES

1. Adams DC, Emerson RG, Heyer EJ, McCormick PC, Carmel PW, Stein BM, Farcy JP, Gallo EJ. Monitoring of intraoperative motor-evoked potentials under conditions of controlled neuromuscular blockade. Anesth Analg 77:913-918, 1993.
2. Agnew WF, McCreery DB. Considerations for safety in the use of extracranial stimulation for motor evoked potentials. Neurosurgery 20:143-147, 1987.
3. American Electroencephalographic Society Evoked Potentials Committee. American Electroencephalographic Society guidelines for intraoperative monitoring of sensory evoked potentials. J Clin Neurophysiol 4:397-416, 1987.
4. Badr G, Carlsson C-A, Fall M, Friberg S, Lindstrom L, Ohlsson B. Cortical evoked potentials following stimulation of the urinary bladder in man. Electroencephalogr Clin Neurophysiol 54:494-498, 1982.
5. Barker AT, Freeston IL, Jalinous R, Merton PA, Morton HB. Magnetic stimulation of the human brain. J Physiol 369:3P, 1985.
6. Barker AT, Freeston IL, Jarratt JA, Jalinous R. Magnetic stimulation of the human nervous system: an introduction and basic principles. In Chokroverty S, ed. Magnetic Stimulation in Clinical Neurophysiology. Boston: Butterworths, 1990, pp. 55-72.
7. Boyd SG, Rothwell JC, Cowan JMA, Webb PJ, Morley T, Asselman P, Marsden CD. A method of monitoring function in corticospinal pathways during scoliosis surgery with a note on motor conduction velocities. J Neurol Neurosurg Psychiatry 49:251-257, 1986.
8. Britt RH, Ryan TP. Use of a flexible epidural stimulating electrode for intraoperative monitoring of spinal somatosensory evoked potentials. Spine 11:348-351, 1986.
9. Brown JC, Axelgaard J, Rowe DE. Monitoring of the human spinal cord. Orthop Trans 3:123, 1979.
10. Brown RH, Nash CL Jr. The "grey zone" in intraoperative S.C.E.P. monitoring. In Schramm J, Jones SJ, eds. Spinal Cord Monitoring. Berlin: Springer-Verlag, 1985, pp. 179-185.
11. Brown RH, Nash CL Jr. Intra-operative spinal cord monitoring. In Frymoyer JW, ed. The Adult Spine: Principles and Practice. New York: Raven Press, 1991, pp. 549-564.
12. Cadwell J. Principles of magnetoelectric stimulation. In Chokroverty S, ed. Magnetic Stimulation in Clinical Neurophysiology. Boston: Butterworths, 1990, pp 13-32.
13. Calancie B, Lebwohl N, Madsen P, Klose KJ. Intraoperative evoked EMG monitoring in an animal model. A new technique for evaluating pedicle screw placement. Spine 17:1229-1235, 1992.

14. Calancie B, Madsen P, Lebwohl N. Stimulus-evoked EMG monitoring during transpedicular lumbosacral spine instrumentation. Spine 19:2780-2786, 1994.

15. Cohen BA, Huizenga BA. Dermatomal monitoring for surgical correction of spondylolisthesis. A case report. Spine 13:1125-1128, 1988.

16. Cusick JF, Myklebust J, Larson SJ, Sances A Jr. Spinal evoked potentials in the primate: Neural substrate. J Neurosurg 49:551-557, 1978.

17. Dinner DS, Luders H, Lesser RP, Morris HH. Invasive methods of somatosensory evoked potential monitoring. J Clin Neurophysiol 3:113-130, 1986.

18. Dinner DS, Luders H, Lesser RP, Morris HH, Barnett G, Klem G. Intraoperative spinal somatosensory evoked potential monitoring. J Neurosurg 65:807-814, 1986.

19. Dinner DS, Shields RW, Leuders H. Intraoperative spinal cord monitoring. In Rothman RH, Simeone FA, eds. The Spine. Philadelphia: WB Saunders, 1992, pp 1801-1814.

20. Ducati A, Schiepatti M. Spinal pathways mediating somatosensory evoked potentials from cutaneous and muscle nerves in the cat. Acta Neurochir 52:99-104, 1980.

21. Esses SI, Sachs BL. Complications of pedicle screw fixations. Orthop Trans 16:160, 1992.

22. Follett KA. Intraoperative electrophysiologic spinal cord monitoring. In Loftus CM, Traynelis VC, eds. Intraoperative Monitoring Techniques in Neurosurgery. New York: McGraw-Hill, 1994, pp 231-238.

23. Geddes LA, Bourland JD. Fundamentals of eddy-current (magnetic) stimulation. In Chokroverty S, ed. Magnetic Stimulation in Clinical Neurophysiology. Boston: Butterworths, 1990, pp 33-44.

24. Giblin DR. Somatosensory evoked potentials in healthy subjects and in patients with lesions of the central nervous system. Ann N Y Acad Sci 112:93-142, 1964.

25. Ginsburg HH, Shetter AG, Raudzens PA. Postoperative paraplegia with preserved intraoperative somatosensory evoked potentials. Case report. J Neurosurg 63:296-300, 1985.

26. Goodridge A, Eisen A, Hoirch M. Paraspinal stimulation to elicit somatosensory evoked potentials: An approach to physiological localization of spinal lesions. Electroencephalogr Clin Neurophysiol 68:268-276, 1987.

27. Grundy BL. Monitoring of sensory evoked potentials during neurosurgical operations: Methods and applications. Neurosurgery 11:556-575, 1982.

28. Haldeman S, Bradley WE, Bhatia N. Evoked responses from the pudendal nerve. J Urol 128:974-980, 1982.

29. Halliday AM, Wakefield GS. Cerebral evoked potentials in patients with dissociated sensory loss. J Neurol Neurosurg Psychiatry 26:211-219, 1963.

30. Herron LD, Trippi AC, Gonyeau M. Intraoperative use of dermatomal somatosensory-evoked potentials in lumbar stenosis surgery. Spine 12:379-383, 1987.

31. Jasper HH. Report of committee on methods of clinical examination in EEG. Appendix: The ten-twenty electrode system of the International Federation. Electroencephalogr Clin Neurophysiol 10:371-375, 1958.

32. Jones SJ, Carter L, Edgar MA, Morley T, Ransford AO, Webb PJ. Experience of epidural spinal cord monitoring in 410 cases. In Schramm J, Jones SJ, eds. Spinal Cord Monitoring. Berlin: Springer-Verlag, 1985, pp 215-220.

33. Jones SJ, Edgar MA, Ransford AO, Thomas NP. A system for the electrophysiological monitoring of the spinal cord during operations for scoliosis. J Bone Joint Surg 65B:134-139, 1983.

34. Kalkman CJ, Drummond JC, Patel PM, Sano T, Chesnut RM. Effects of droperidol, pentobarbital, and ketamine on myogenic transcranial magnetic motor-evoked responses in humans. Neurosurgery 35:1066-1071, 1994.

35. Katifi HA, Sedgwick EM. Somatosensory evoked potentials from posterior tibial nerve and lumbosacral dermatomes. Electroencephalogr Clin Neurophysiol 65:249-259, 1986.

36. Kellway P. An orderly approach to visual analysis. Parameters of normal EEG in adults and children. In Klass D, Daley DD, eds. Current Practice of Clinical Electroencephalography. New York: Raven Press, 1979, pp 69-147.

37. Klem G, Andrish J, Gurd A, Weiker G, Lueders H. Spinal cord potentials recorded from ligamentum interspinalis. Electroencephalogr Clin Neurophysiol 50:221, 1983.

38. LaMont RL, Wasson SL, Green MA. Spinal cord monitoring during spinal surgery using somatosensory spinal evoked potentials. J Pediatr Orthop 3:31-36, 1983.

39. Lesser RP, Raudzens P, Luders H, Nuwer MR, Goldie WD, Morris HH III, Dinner DS, Klem G, Hahn JF, Shetter AG, Ginsburg HH, Gurd AR. Postoperative neurological deficits may occur despite unchanged intraoperative somatosensory evoked potentials. Ann Neurol 19:22-25, 1986.

40. Levy WJ Jr. Clinical experience with motor and cerebellar evoked potential monitoring. Neurosurgery 20:169-182, 1987.

41. Levy WJ, Kraus KH, Gugino LD, Ghaly RF, Amassian V, Cadwell J. Transcranial magnetic evoked potential monitoring. In Loftus CM, Traynelis VC, eds. Intraoperative Monitoring Techniques in Neurosurgery. New York: McGraw-Hill, 1994, pp 251-255.

42. Levy WJ Jr, York DH. Evoked potentials from the motor tracts in humans. Neurosurgery 12:422-429, 1983.

43. Linden RD, Shields CB. Comment. Neurosurgery 35:1071, 1994.

44. Lueders H. Gurd A, Hahn J, Andrish J, Weiker G, Klem G. A new technique for intraoperative monitoring of spinal cord function. Multichannel recording of spinal cord and subcortical evoked potentials. Spine 7:110-115, 1982.

45. Lueders H, Hahn J, Gurd A, Tsuji S, Dinner D, Lesser R, Klem G. Surgical monitoring of spinal cord function: Cauda equina stimulation technique. Neurosurgery 11:482-485, 1982.

46. Luders H, Lesser RP, Dinner DS, Morris HH. Optimizing stimulating and recording parameters in somatosensory evoked potential studies. J Clin Neurophysiol 2:383-396, 1985.

47. Maccabee P, Levine DB, Kahanovitz N, Pinkhasov E. Monitoring of spinal and subcortical somatosensory evoked potentials during Harrington rod instrumentation. Orthop Trans 6:19, 1982.

48. Machida M, Weinstein SL, Yamada T, Kimura J. Spinal cord monitoring: Electrophysiological measures of sensory and motor function during spinal surgery. Spine 10:407-413, 1985.

49. Macon JB, Poletti CE. Conducted somatosensory evoked potentials during spinal surgery. I. Control conduction velocity measurements. J Neurosurg 57:349-353, 1982.

50. Macon JB, Poletti CE, Sweet WH, Ojemann RG, Zervas NT. Conducted somatosensory evoked potentials during spinal surgery. II. Clinical applications. J Neurosurg 57:354-359, 1982.

51. Matsuzaki H, Tokuhashi Y, Matsumoto F, Hoshino M, Kiuchi T. Toriyama S. Problems and solutions of pedicle screw plat fixation of the lumbar spine. Spine 15:1159-1165, 1990.

52. McNeal D, Passoff T, Swank S, Satomi K. Spinal cord monitoring using epidural electrodes for stimulation and recording. Orthop Trans 6:19, 1982.

53. Merton PA, Morton HB. Stimulation of the cerebral cortex in the intact human subject. Nature 285:227, 1980.

54. Mostegl A, Bauer R, Eichenauer M. Intraoperative somatosensory potential monitoring. A clinical analysis of 127 surgical procedures. Spine 13:396-400, 1988.

55. Nordwall A, Axelgaard J, Harada Y, Valencia P, McNeal DR, Brown JC. Spinal cord monitoring using evoking potentials recorded from feline vertebral bone. Spine 4:486-494, 1979.

56. Osenbach RK, Yamada T, Traynelis VC. Transcranial magnetic stimulation of the motor cortex. In Loftus CM, Traynelis VC, eds. Intraoperative Monitoring Techniques in Neurosurgery. New York: McGraw-Hill, 1994, pp 239-250.

57. Owen JH. Evoked potential monitoring during spinal surgery. In Bridwell KH, DeWald J, eds. Textbook of Spinal Surgery. Philadelphia: JB Lippincott, 1991, pp 31-64.

58. Owen JH. Intraoperative stimulation of the spinal cord for prevention of spinal cord injury. In Devinsky O, Beric A, Dogali M, eds. Electrical and Magnetic Stimulation of the Brain and Spinal Cord. New York: Raven Press, 1993, pp 271-288.

59. Owen JH, Bridwell KH, Grubb R, Jenny A, Allen B, Padberg AM, Shimon SM. The clinical application of neurogenic motor evoked potentials to monitor spinal cord function during surgery. Spine 16:S385-390, 1991.

60. Owen JH, Jenny AB, Naito M, Weber K, Bridwell KH, McGhee R. Effects of spinal cord lesioning on somatosensory and neurogenic-motor evoked potentials. Spine 14:673-682, 1989.

61. Owen JH, Laschinger J, Bridwell K, Shimon S, Nielsen C, Dunlap J, Kain C. Sensitivity and specificity of somatosensory and neurogenic-motor evoked potentials in animals and humans. Spine 13:1111-1118, 1988.

62. Powers SK, Bolger CA, Edwards MS. Spinal cord pathways mediating somatosensory evoked potentials. J Neurosurg 57:472-482, 1982.

63. Rossini PM, Gigli GL, Marciani MG, Zarola F, Caramia M. Non-invasive evaluation of input-output characteristics of sensorimotor cerebral areas in healthy humans. Electroencephalogr Clin Neurophysiol 68:88-100, 1987.

64. Ryan TP, Britt RH. Spinal and cortical somatosensory evoked potential monitoring during corrective spinal surgery with 108 patients. Spine 11:352-361, 1986.

65. Ryken TC, Menezes AM. Intraoperative electrical and manometric monitoring in lumbosacral surgery. In Loftus CM, Traynelis VC, eds. Intraoperative Monitoring Technique in Neurosurgery. New York: McGraw-Hill, 1994, pp 257-268.

66. Schiepatti M, Ducati A. Effects of stimulus intensity, cervical cord tractotomies, and cerebellectomy on somatosensory evoked potentials from skin and muscle afferents in the cat hind limb. Electroencephalogr Clin Neurophysiol 51:363-372, 1981.

67. Shields CB, Paloheimo MPJ, Backman MH, Edmonds HL Jr. Johnson JR. Intraoperative use of transcranial magnetic motor evoked potentials. In Chokroverty S, ed. Magnetic Stimulation in Clinical Neurophysiology. Boston: Butterworths, 1990, pp 173-184.

68. Spielholz NI. Intraoperative monitoring using somatosensory evoked potentials: A brief overview. Electromyogr Clin Neurophysiol 34:29-34, 1994.

69. Steinmann JC, Herdowitz HN, El-Kommos H, Wesolowski P. Spinal pedicle fixation. Confirmation of an image-based technique for screw placement. Spine 18:1856-1861, 1993.

70. Tamaki T, Noguchi T, Takano H, Tsuji H, Nakagawa T, Imai K, Inoue S. Spinal cord monitoring as a clinical utilization of the spinal evoked potential. Clin Orthop 184:58-64, 1984.

71. Tamaki T, Tsuji H, Inoue S, Kobayashi H. The prevention of iatrogenic spinal cord injury utilizing the evoked spinal cord potential. Int Orthop 4:313-317, 1981.

72. Thalgott JS, LaRocca H, Aebi M, Dwyer AP, Razza BE. Reconstruction of the lumbar spine using AO DCP plate internal fixation. Spine 14:91-95, 1989.

73. Thompson PD, Rothwell JC, Day BL, Dressler D, Maertens de Noordhout A, Marsden CD. Mechanisms of electrical and magnetic stimulation of human motor cortex. In Chokroverty S, ed. Magnetic Stimulation in Clinical Neurophysiology. Boston: Butterworths, 1990, pp 121-143.

74. Todd MM. Anesthetic techniques for evaluation of spinal surgery patients ("wake-up test"). In Loftus CM, Traynelis VC, eds. Intraoperative Monitoring Techniques in Neurosurgery. New York: McGraw-Hill, 1994, pp 239-250.

75. Tsuyama N, Tsuzuki N, Kurokawa T, Imai T. Clinical application of spinal cord action potential movement. Int Orthop 2:39-46, 1978.

76. Vauzelle C, Stagnara P, Jouvinroux P. Functional monitoring of spinal cord activity during spinal surgery. Clin Orthop 93:173-178, 1973.

77. Weinstein JN, Spratt KF, Spendler D, Brick C, Reid S. Spinal pedicle fixation: Reliability and validity of roentgenogram-based assessment and surgical factors on successful screw placement. Spine 13:1012-1018, 1988.

78. Whittle IR, Johnston IH, Besser M. Recording of spinal somatosensory evoked potentials for intraoperative spinal cord monitoring. J Neurosurg 64:601-612, 1986.

79. Williamson JB, Galasko CSB. Spinal cord monitoring during operative correction of neuromuscular scoliosis. J Bone Joint Surg 74B:870-872, 1992.

80. Zentner J. Noninvasive motor evoked potential monitoring during neurosurgical operations on the spinal cord. Neurosurgery 24:709-712, 1989.

Surgical Principles and Techniques

Surgical Exposures of the Cervicothoracic and Upper Thoracic Spine

David Greenwald, M.D., Richard G. Fessler, M.D., Ph.D., and David Peace, M.S.

The surgical management of the cervicothoracic spine remains a difficult endeavor secondary to anatomical considerations that limit safe access. Traditional procedures approach the spinal column ventrally, ventrolaterally, dorsally, or dorsolaterally. The continual evolution of surgical technique has been, and is guided by, a desire to improve both safety and exposure of the cervicothoracic junction.

Pathological processes involving the cervicothoracic junction are infrequent, but comprise up to 10% of spinal metastases. Other pathological processes found in the cervicothoracic junction include bacterial and tuberculous infections, primary tumors of bone, vascular malformations, disc herniations, and traumatic and pathological fractures, as well as intradural intramedullary and extramedullary tumors (see accompanying box).

Dorsal approaches, including laminectomy and pediculectomy, are safe and easy to perform but provide limited access to the vertebral bodies. Thus they may exacerbate instability caused by ventral and middle column disease.

Ventrolateral approaches were first described by Gask[10] in 1933 and Hodgson and Stock[11] in 1956. The ventrolateral thoracotomy approach involves resection of the third rib and necessitate trans-

---

PATHOLOGICAL PROCESSES INVOLVING THE CERVICOTHORACIC JUNCTION

Metastatic cancer
Primary tumors of the bone
Discitis
Disc herniation
Traumatic fractures
Pathological fractures
Vascular malformations
Intramedullary tumors
Extramedullary tumors

---

pleural mobilization of the lung. It provides good exposure of T3 to T4, but access to T1 to T2 and the lower cervical spine is limited by the thoracic inlet.

The initially described dorsolateral approach was the costotransversectomy. This approach provides adequate access to the middle and lower aspects of the thoracic spine but is limited in the upper thoracic spine secondary to the scapula and parascapular musculature. In addition, it provides poor exposure of the ventral vertebral elements. The lateral rachiotomy, initially described by Capener[4] in 1954, and modified by Larson et al.[12] in 1976 as the lateral extracavitary approach, improved exposure of the middle and lower thoracic spine but continued to be inadequate in the upper thoracic region for the same reasons described above. A modification of the lateral extracavitary approach, the lateral parascapular extrapleural approach,[6-8] effectively deals with the anatomical limitations imposed by the scapula and parascapular musculature while providing excellent exposure of the upper thoracic spine up to the inferior end plate of the C7 vertebral body.

Presently, three approaches to the cervicothoracic junction are utilized at the primary author's (RGF) institution. These are the ventral transmanubrial-transclavicular approach, the lateral parascapular extrapleural approach, and the ventrolateral thoracotomy approach. Each of these procedures has advantages and disadvantages. This chapter discusses the clinical presentation of disease at the cervicothoracic junction, as well as preoperative and operative considerations necessary to make decisions regarding which of the three procedures to perform.

CLINICAL FEATURES

Patients with pathological processes involving the cervicothoracic junction may present with back and/or neck pain, with or without neurological deficits. These deficits may be radiculopathic and/or myelopathic. The most common symptoms, in decreasing order of frequency observed in the author's (RGF) series, with pathological processes from C7 to T4 are myelopathy (64%), back pain (57%), leg pain (50%), arm pain/paresthesias (29%), sensory ataxia (25%), urinary incontinence (21%), and kyphotic deformity (7%) (Table 9-1).

PREOPERATIVE EVALUATION
Radiological Evaluation

Accurate radiological assessment of pathological processes involving the cervicothoracic junction begins with ventrodorsal and lateral radiographic studies. These may reveal vertebral body and/or pedicle involvement/destruction in metastatic disease (Fig. 9-1), and disc space narrowing with involvement of the rostral and caudal end plates of the adjacent vertebral bodies in discitis, as well as traumatic or pathological fractures with or without associated malalignment (Fig. 9-2).

Radionuclide bone scintiography,[5,9,15,16] although relatively nonspecific, is very sensitive at detecting

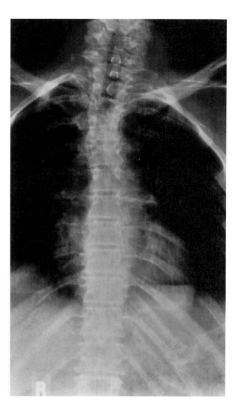

Fig. 9-1. Pedicle destruction with structural instability.

Table 9-1. Common Presenting Symptoms

Myelopathy	64%
Back pain	57%
Leg pain	50%
Arm pain/paresthesias	29%
Sensory ataxia	25%
Urinary incontinence	21%
Kyphotic deformity	7%

infections, fractures, or metastatic disease of the spine (Fig. 9-3).

Myelography and post-myelography computed tomography (CT) can be used to demonstrate pathological processes that compromise the subarachnoid space. These include thoracic disc herniations, extradural or intradural (extramedullary or intramedullary) neoplastic disease, epidural abscesses, vascular malformations, and retropulsed bone or disc fragments from traumatic or pathological fractures. In addition, two-dimensional coronal and sagittal images, as well as three-dimensional images may be reconstructed from axial CT data, providing accurate geometric configurations of frac-

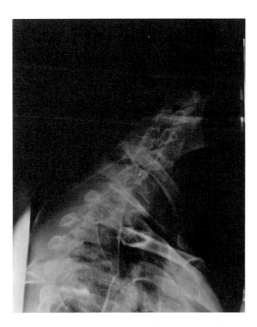

Fig. 9-2. Pathological compressive fracture of the T2 vertebral body secondary to metastatic adenocarcinoma.

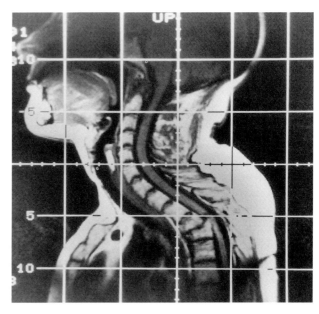

Fig. 9-4. MRI scan revealing pathological fractures of T3 and T4 with kyphotic angulation and spinal cord compression.

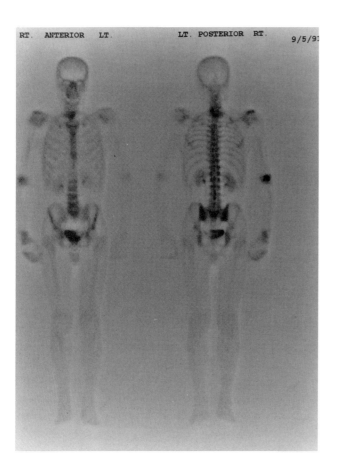

Fig. 9-3. Radionuclide bone scintiography revealing increased signal activity in the cervicothoracic vertebral bodies in a patient with metastatic spread.

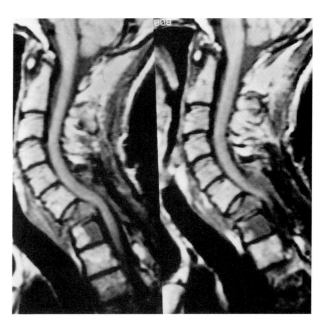

Fig. 9-5. Traumatic fracture of the body of C7 with kyphotic angulation and spinal cord compression.

tures and/or associated malalignment. This may help guide further definitive management.

MRI, although poor at imaging bone, provides a superior evaluation of neoplastic processes, infection, and spinal cord pathology[2,3,9,13] (Figs. 9-4 and 9-5). In particular, discitis, with or without epidural spread, may be accurately defined.[14] Vascular malformations can be identified by observation of characteristic dural or parenchymal flow voids.

Metabolic Evaluation

Routine preoperative evaluation should include a complete blood count (to evaluate for anemia, thrombocytopenia, leukocytosis, etc.) and a renal disease battery. In cases of suspected infection, an erythrocyte sedimentation rate (ESR) should be obtained as well. The identification of specific antigen markers may help define the site of origin of metastatic disease. In particular, carcinoembryonic antigen may help identify a gastrointestinal primary tumor, while prostate-specific antigen and serum acid phosphatase should be obtained to evaluate for prostate carcinoma. Workup for a collagen vascular disease should include ESR, antinuclear antibodies, and/or rheumatoid factor analysis. Finally, bone marrow aspiration should be performed in the evaluation of suspected hematological malignancy or blood dyscrasias.

ANESTHETIC CONSIDERATIONS

All patients undergoing surgical management of the cervicothoracic spine require general anesthesia. After induction of general anesthesia, central venous and arterial lines are placed and the bladder is catheterized. Three types of intubation may be performed: (1) routine single-lumen endotracheal intubation, (2) double-lumen endotracheal intubation, and (3) single-lumen endotracheal intubation with high-frequency ventilation. Double-lumen intubation is the most time-consuming and difficult to initiate, but allows for temporary deflation of the ipsilateral lung when indicated. Single-lumen intubation with high-frequency ventilation allows for both retraction and simultaneous ventilation of the ipsilateral lung, and as such is ideally suited for the lateral parascapular extrapleural and ventrolateral thoracotomy approaches. Routine single-lumen intubation is adequate for transmanubrial-transclavicular approaches. In cases not involving neoplastic or infectious disease the cell saver is used to minimize the need for blood transfusions.

SURGICAL TECHNIQUES
Lateral Parascapular Extrapleural Approach

This dorsolateral approach provides excellent exposure of the upper four thoracic vertebral bodies including the caudal end plate of C7. Together with the lateral extracavitary approach, this enables access to the entire thoracic spine.

The patient is placed in the prone position on chest rolls. Care is taken to position the ipsilateral chest roll somewhat medially. This allows the shoulder to fall ventrolaterally to pull the scapula out of the field. The back is prepped from the nuchal line to the sacrum. The midline incision begins at least three spinous process segments above the upper extent of the pathology and extends to three spinous processes below the lower extent. Exposure of T1 to T2 requires an incision up to C3 to C4. The caudal aspect of the incision is gently curved to the surgical side of approach (Fig. 9-6). The incision is carried caudally through the trapezius and rhomboid muscles to the plane of loose areolar tissue between the rhomboid and paraspinal musculature. This myocutaneous flap is reflected laterally, containing within it the medial border of the scapula (Fig. 9-7). Reflection of this flap requires division of the caudal fibers of the trapezius muscle. Care must be taken to ensure that an adequate cuff of muscle for suture reapproximation remains. Exposure of the caudal end plate of C7 requires the extension of the incision to C2, as well as aggressive mobilization of the levator scapulae muscle.

Deep cervical and thoracolumbar fascia cover the paraspinal muscles (erector spinae and splenius muscles). Dissection of the paraspinal muscles from the spinous processes and dorsal elements enables medial retraction of this muscle mass, thus exposing the spinous processes, laminae, pedicles, facet complexes, transverse processes, and the dorsal rib cage.

Subperiosteal dissection of the ribs allows for their removal, with care taken not to injure the neurovascular complex lying beneath the ventral surface of each rib. In general, the intercostal vein is most rostral, followed by the artery, with the nerve situated most caudally. Removal of the ribs is facilitated by incision of the costotransverse and costovertebral ligaments. Ribs are removed from the costovertebral tip to the dorsal axillary line. The intercostal neurovascular bundle is then separated from the intercostal muscle, and the intercostal artery and vein are coagulated and divided. The intercostal nerve in the neurovascular bundle can be used to trace back to the neural foramen. The sympathetic chain is then identified on the lateral surface of the vertebral bodies. The rami communicantes are divided and the

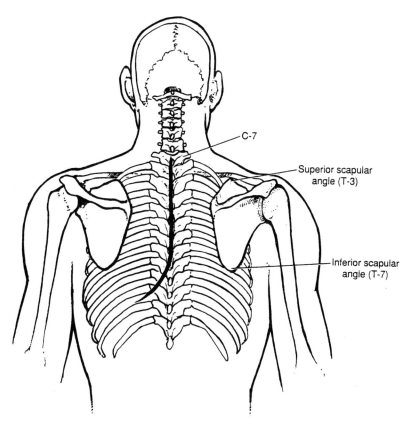

Fig. 9-6. Incision utilized for exposure of the cervicothoracic junction via the lateral parascapular extrapleural approach.

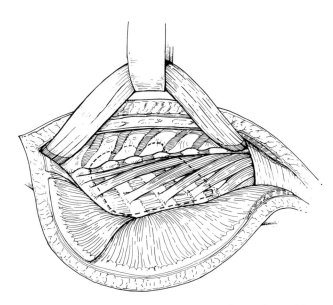

Fig. 9-7. Medial elevation of the paraspinal muscles and lateral elevation of the parascapular musculature and scapula provides exposure of the dorsal elements of the cervicothoracic region, including the dorsal rib cage.

sympathetic chain is mobilized ventrolaterally. Isolated discectomy does not require division of the intercostal nerves. Unfortunately, adequate exposure for corpectomy requires division of one or more intercostal nerves. Care must be taken not to injure or divide the eighth cervical or first thoracic intercostal nerve. This will lead to unacceptable postoperative intrinsic hand weakness. Intercostal nerves below T1 may be sacrificed and ligated proximal to the dorsal root ganglion prior to closure. Removal of the lamina, transverse process, and pedicle exposes the underlying thecal sac. Removal of ventral structures, including the vertebral body and pedicles, can be safely performed with a combination of high-speed drilling and curettage, while directly visualizing the thecal sac. Preservation of the posterior longitudinal ligament during corpectomy helps to provide a protective barrier against inadvertent injury to the thecal sac and spinal cord during drilling (Fig. 9-8). Strut graft placement and instrumentation

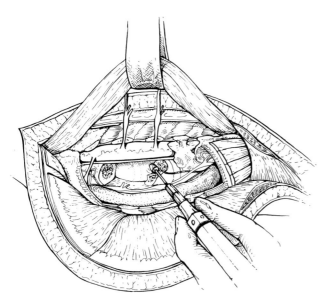

Fig. 9-8. A corpectomy performed with high-speed drilling ventral to the posterior longitudinal ligament. The latter provides a barrier for protection of the thecal sac during bone removal.

can both be accomplished through this approach. Prior to closure, the wound is filled with saline to assess for air leak. The presence of an air leak requires either primary pleural repair or the placement of a tube thoracostomy (22 Fr-24 Fr), which is brought out through a separate stab incision caudal to the main incision. Two hemovac drains are placed prior to a layered closure of the fascial planes. The skin is closed with staples.

Ventrolateral Transthoracic Approach

The patient is placed in the lateral decubitus position with the appropriate side up. The ipsilateral arm is secured above the head while the dependent axilla is well padded to protect against inadvertent neurovascular compression (Fig. 9-9).

The skin incision begins in the paraspinal region adjacent to T3. It is carried ventrolaterally along the caudal surface of the third rib to the ventral axillary line. Division of the trapezius, rhomboid major, and rhomboid minor muscles allows for rostral and lateral mobilization of the scapula. The latissimus dorsi muscle is then identified, bluntly mobilized from the underlying serratus anterior muscle, and sharply divided. This provides exposure of the free dorsal margin of the serratus anterior muscle, which is attached to the underlying rib. Division of

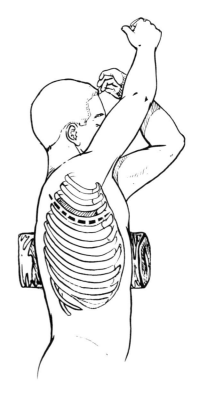

Fig. 9-9. The lateral decubitus position and skin incision used with the ventrolateral transthoracic approach.

these muscle fibers provides exposure of the third rib. Radiological confirmation of the appropriate level is undertaken prior to rib removal. Additional verification of the third rib can be accomplished by palpation of the anterior and medial scalenus muscle insertions onto the second rib above.

Once the third rib is accurately identified, the periosteum overlying the rib is sharply divided and the underlying rib is circumferentially freed from the periosteum with a combination of curved and straight periosteal elevators. Care is taken not to injure the neurovascular complex lying in a groove along the ventral and caudal surface of the rib. The rib is then resected from the costochondral junction ventrally to the dorsal angle behind. The underlying parietal pleura is then sharply divided and the second and fourth ribs are spread using a self-retaining thoracotomy retractor. The lung is manually deflated and retracted ventrally, providing visualization of the parietal pleura on the dorsal wall overlying the ventral aspects of the dorsal rib cage and thoracic vertebral bodies (T2 to T4). Sharp division of the dorsal parietal pleura over the appropriate thoracic vertebral bodies is followed by blunt dissection of the pleura, with

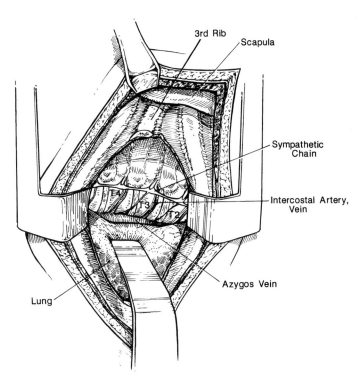

Fig. 9-10. Exposure of the T2, T3, and T4 vertebral bodies provided by the ventrolateral transthoracic approach. Note that the lung has been deflated and retracted ventrolaterally and that care has been taken not to injure the sympathetic chain.

care taken not to injure the sympathetic trunk and neurovascular bundle overlying the thoracic vertebral body (Fig. 9-10).

Structures ventral to the vertebral body (from dorsal to ventral) include the descending aorta, esophagus, and thoracic duct, the trachea, and the superior vena cava. Usually, the rostral aspect of the aortic arch extends to the T4 level and is not at risk during this approach. Structures of concern that are located ventral to the T1 to T4 vertebral bodies are the esophagus, thoracic duct, and subclavian artery. Intercostal arteries may be taken if necessary, but should be spared if possible to minimize the risk of spinal cord ischemia.

The ventrolateral transthoracic approach allows for a generous exposure of the ventrolateral upper thoracic vertebral bodies. Access to the lower cervical spine, the first thoracic vertebral body, and perhaps the second thoracic vertebral body is impeded by the narrow thoracic inlet. The third and fourth thoracic vertebral bodies and corresponding discs can be safely resected under direct vision (Fig. 9-11). Placement of strut grafts and ventral instrumentation can be accomplished as well.

Closure requires placement of two tube thoracostomies. One is placed rostrally to manage pneumothorax. The other is placed caudally in the dorsal corner to collect blood. The tubes are tunneled subcutaneously, and exit caudal to the incision line. They are secured in place with purse-string sutures. The parietal pleura in the bed of the resected third rib is closed with a running absorbable suture. The rib is reapproximated with wire ventrally to the sternum and dorsally to the remaining rib. The overlying periosteum and attached intercostal muscle are closed in a watertight fashion with a running absorbable suture. A layered closure of the serratus anterior, latissimus dorsi, rhomboid major and minor, and trapezius muscles is performed. The subcutaneous tissue is closed with 3-0 interrupted inverted Vicryl sutures, and the skin is closed with staples.

Transmanubrial-Transclavicular Approach

The transmanubrial-transclavicular approach, described by Sundaresan et al.[17,18] provides the best access to the lower cervical vertebrae of the three approaches described above.[1] It is particularly

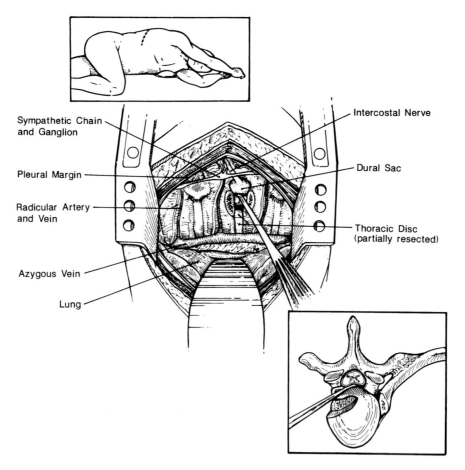

Sympathetic Chain and Ganglion

Pleural Margin

Radicular Artery and Vein

Azygous Vein

Lung

Intercostal Nerve

Dural Sac

Thoracic Disc (partially resected)

Fig. 9-11. The ventrolateral transthoracic approach provides good exposure of the third and fourth thoracic vertebral bodies and corresponding discs, allowing for their safe removal. Note that the thecal sac is approached from a ventrolateral direction.

useful for pathology involving C6 to T2. Below T2 the mediastinal great vessels limit access. In addition, occasionally severe thoracic kyphosis can obscure access to these vertebrae from this ventral approach.

The patient is positioned supine with the head turned slightly away from the side of the approach. A T-shaped incision is made with the supraclavicular transverse limb extending from the contralateral sternocleidomastoid muscle to a point 3 cm lateral to the ipsilateral sternocleidomastoid muscle. The vertical limb is made in the midline, extending to the midpoint of the sternum (Fig. 9-12). The platysma muscle is then mobilized and divided in-line with the incision. The external jugular vein overlying the sternocleidomastoid muscle is identified and divided, as are the medial branches of the supraclavicular nerves.

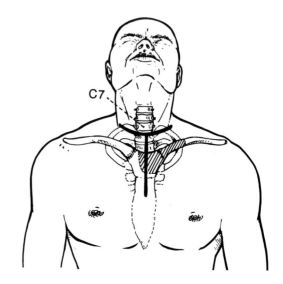

C7

Fig. 9-12. Body position with slight neck extension and proposed skin incision utilized with the transmanubrial-transclavicular approach.

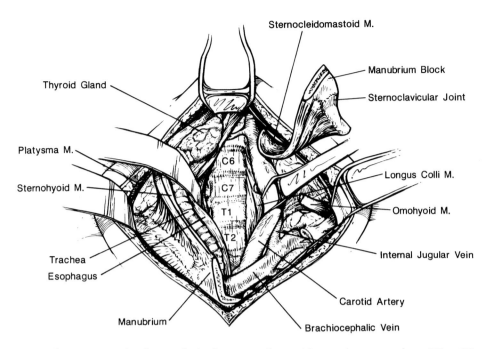

Fig. 9-13. The transmanubrial-transclavicular approach provides good exposure from C6 to T2 ventrally after retraction of the strap muscles, trachea, and esophagus medially, as well as the carotid sheath laterally. The caudal exposure is limited by the brachiocephalic vein. Note the improved caudal exposure provided by the rostral and lateral elevation of the divided manubrio-clavicular sternocleidomastoid pedicle.

The sternocleidomastoid muscle is then identified and the pectoralis major muscle is subperiosteally dissected from the medial half of the clavicle and the manubrium. Careful dissection of the superficial and middle layers of the deep cervical fascia allows for safe reflection of the sternocleidomastoid, sternohyoid, and sternothyroid muscles from the manubrium and clavicle, while protecting their neurovascular supply. Subsequently, subperiosteal dissection of the manubrium is undertaken, providing protection of the underlying brachiocephalic veins since the dorsal manubrial periosteum is a continuation of the ventral transthoracic fascia. The omohyoid muscle is divided at its midpoint and retracted, thus providing exposure of the underlying internal jugular vein and common carotid artery.

The ipsilateral two thirds of the manubrium, the midpoint of the clavicle, and the first costal cartilage are divided with a high-speed drill. The clavicle is cut in an interlocking configuration to facilitate later reconstruction. The manubrial-clavicular complex is then elevated and reflected on its sternocleidomastoid pedicle, providing exposure of the underlying trachea, esophagus, brachiocephalic veins, brachiocephalic artery, subclavian artery, and common carotid artery.

Blunt dissection medial to the carotid sheath helps to define the alar and mediastinal fascia. This prevertebral fascia is divided sharply, allowing for placement of self-retaining retractors within the wound edges and providing exposure of the carotid sheath structures laterally, as well as the tracheaesophageal structures medially (Fig. 9-13). Removal of pathological processes can be performed under direct vision with curettage, suctioning, and/or high-speed drilling.

Following decompression, reconstruction with either autologous or allograft bone may be undertaken. Stabilization of the construct can be accomplished with ventral plating techniques.

Closure requires wiring of the manubrium and wiring or screwplate fixation of the clavicle. The wound is closed in layers. Postoperatively, the ipsilateral arm is supported in an arm sling for 6 weeks.

CONCLUSION

The surgical management of pathological processes involving the cervicothoracic junction is usually challenging, secondary to limitations of exposure and maneuverability imposed by the ribs, scapula, medial parascapular musculature, lungs, great vessels, and thoracic inlet. Three approaches have been specifically developed to help overcome these obstacles to safe access to this region.

The lateral parascapular extrapleural approach is ideally suited for disease involving the upper thoracic vertebrae because it provides access from the lower end plate of C7 to the T4 vertebra. Advantages of this approach include the ability to perform the procedure with one surgical team, a short working length, direct visualization of the thecal sac during corpectomy, and the ability to remain extrapleural. In addition, bone grafting and placement of both ventral and dorsal instrumentation may be undertaken through the same incision. The main disadvantages of this approach are limited access to the lower cervical vertebrae, increased risk of lower brachial plexus nerve root injury, longer operative time, and blood loss (Table 9-2).

The ventrolateral transthoracic approach provides excellent access to the third and fourth thoracic vertebral bodies, while allowing for direct visualization and control of mediastinal vasculature. Disadvantages include poor access to the upper two thoracic vertebral bodies secondary to narrowing of the thoracic inlet, the need for transpleural mobilization of the lung, a relatively long depth of field, and potential neurovascular injury to the shoulder musculature secondary to the need for rostral and medial retraction of the scapula.

The transmanubrial-transclavicular approach provides the best simultaneous access to lower cervical and upper thoracic vertebrae. Access caudal to T2 is limited by the anatomical positions of the left brachiocephalic vein, aortic arch, and subclavian vein. Disadvantages may include the need to perform corpectomies blindly and potential risk to the carotid sheath and underlying structures, as well as potential injury to the medially retracted trachea and esophagus. Furthermore, there may be a need for a second procedure if dorsal stabilization is required.

Decision making with regard to which procedure to perform should depend upon the location of pathology, the need for thecal sac decompression and/or dorsal stabilization, as well as the extent of the spinal deformity. Exposure of the pathology above the caudal end plate of C7 is best accomplished with the transmanubrial-transclavicular approach. In the face of thecal sac compression, the lateral parascapular extrapleural approach allows for direct visualization of the thecal sac during corpectomy. The ventrolateral transthoracic approach is an alternative used in situations in which the pathology is below T2 and located ventrally.

Table 9-2. Approach-Specific Advantages and Disadvantages

Approach	Advantages	Disadvantages
Lateral parascapular extrapleural	Ventral and dorsal instrumentation may be placed through the same incision Short working length Direct visualization of the thecal sac during decompression	Limited access to the lower cervical vertebrae Increased risk of lower brachial plexus nerve root injury Longer operative time
Ventrolateral transthoracic	Direct visualization and control of mediastinal vasculature Excellent access to the third and fourth thoracic vertebral bodies	Poor access to the upper two thoracic vertebral bodies Need for transpleural mobilization of the lung Relatively long depth of field Potential neurovascular injury to the medial shoulder musculature
Transmanubrial-transclavicular	Best simultaneous access to both lower cervical and upper thoracic vertebra	Corpectomies are preformed blindly Potential risk to carotid sheath and underlying structures

REFERENCES

1. Birch R, Bonney G, Marshall RW. A surgical approach to the cervicothoracic spine. J Bone Joint Surg 72B:904-907, 1990.
2. Bruns J, Maas R. Advantages of diagnosing bacterial spondylitis with magnetic resonance imaging. Arch Orthop Trauma Surg 108:30-35, 1989.
3. Butler EG, Dohrmann PJ, Stark RJ. Spinal subdural abscess. Clin Exp Neuro 25:67-70, 1980.
4. Capener N. The evolution of lateral rachiotomy. J Bone Joint Surg 36:173-179, 1954.
5. Edylstyn GA, Gillespie PJ, Grebbel FS. The radiological demonstration of osseous metastases. Clin Radiol 18:158, 1967.
6. Fessler RG, Dietze DD. Surgical approaches to the cervicothoracic junction. Operative Neurosurg Tech 2: 1875-1886, 1995.
7. Fessler RG, Dietze DD, MacMillan M, Peace D. Lateral parascapular extrapleural approach to the upper thoracic spine. J Neurosurg 75:349-355, 1991.
8. Fessler RG, Dietze DD, Peace D. Upper thoracic spinal exposure through a lateral parascapular extrapleural approach. Neurosurgical Operative Atlas, Vol 4. Park Ridge, Ill: American Association of Neurological Surgeons, 1995, pp 173-182.
9. Galasko CSB. Skeletal metastases. Clin Orthop 210:18, 1986.
10. Gask GE. The surgery of the sympathetic nervous system. Br J Surg 21:113-130, 1933.
11. Hodgson AR, Stock FE. Anterior spinal fusion. Br J Surg 46:266-275, 1956.
12. Larson SJ, Holst RA, Hemmy DC, Sances A. Lateral extracavitary approach to traumatic lesions of the thoracic and lumbar spine. J Neurosurg 45:628-637, 1976.
13. Pauschter DM, Modic MT, Masaryk J. Magnetic resonance imaging of the spine: Applications and limitations. Radiol Clin North Am 23:551-562, 1985.
14. Sapico BL, Montgomerie JZ. Vertebral osteomyelitis intravenous drug abusers: Report of three cases and review of the literature. Rev Infect Dis 2:196-206, 1980.
15. Schlaeffer F, Mikolick DJ, Mates SM. Technetium Tc99m diphosphonate bone scan. False normal findings in elderly patients with hematogenous vertebral osteomyelitis. Arch Intern Med 147:2024-2026, 1987.
16. Staab EV, McCartney WH. Role of gallium 67 in inflammatory disease. Semin Nucl Med 8:219-234, 1978.
17. Sundaresan N, Shah J, Foley KM, Rosen G. An anterior surgical approach to the upper thoracic vertebrae. J Neurosurg 61:686-690, 1984.
18. Sundaresan N, DiGiacinto GV, Hughes JEO, Krol G. Spondylectomy for malignant tumors of the spine. J Clin Oncol 7:1485-1491, 1989.

Surgical Exposures of the Thoracic and Thoracolumbar Spine

Eric J. Woodard, M.D.

A variety of techniques are available for exposure of the midthoracic and thoracolumbar spine that allow the surgeon maximal flexibility for achieving specific surgical goals. Although the particular approach selected for a specific patient is generally based upon the spinal level, the type and distribution of the pathology are also important factors in surgical planning. Approaches have been described for each portion of the thoracic spine that reflect the unique anatomy of this region. The rib cage, the narrow thoracic spinal canal, the limited vascular supply to the spinal cord, the vulnerability of the thoracic cord to manipulation, and the transitional anatomy at the thoracolumbar junction are all factors that have contributed to the evolution of standard surgical techniques in this area.

In selecting a surgical approach the intended extent of vertebral decompression and the need for re-establishing spinal stability by arthrodesis and reconstruction are important considerations. Requirements and methods for instrumentation, individual patient characteristics (e.g., habitus, concurrent medical issues), and individual surgical experience are key factors in choosing an appropriate exposure method. As with all regions of the spine, approaches to the midthoracic and thoracolumbar regions may be divided into ventral and/or dorsal techniques (Table 10-1). This chapter outlines these standard surgical exposures of the thoracic and thoracolumbar spine, emphasizing pertinent anatomy, important points of technique, and specific advantages and limitations of each method.

VENTRAL APPROACHES

Ventral thoracic approaches afford direct access to ventrally situated pathology, providing extensive access for decompression, interbody fusion, and/or instrumentation. Appropriate clinical indications for this method include trauma (e.g., burst fractures with compression), vertebral body tumors, osteomyelitis, and midline disc herniations.[4,9,11,12] Releasing procedures for fixed kyphoscoliotic deformities also require a direct ventral approach.[23]

Three basic ventral techniques are used to approach different levels of the thoracic spine: the transthoracic approach between T2 and T10, the throracoabdominal approach for lesions between T10 and upper lumbar levels (to approximately L4), and the retroperitoneal approach for pathology between T12 and lumbar levels. The basic technique common to all of these exposures is the transthoracic approach, which at the thoracolumbar junction must be modified to accommodate the diaphragm and the transition between pleural and peritoneal cavities.

Table 10-1. Classification of Thoracic Thoracolumbar Approaches

Approach	Spinal Levels	Advantages	Disadvantages
Ventral			
Transthoracic	T2 to T10	Direct, multilevel, ventrolateral exposure; access for ventral instrumentation	Chest wall pain, pulmonary compromise, thoracostomy tube drainage, cord lies dorsal to the pathology, second procedure for dorsal instrumentation
Retropleural thoracic	T2 to T10	Extrapleural approach, avoids pulmonary compromise and chest tube drainage; access for ventral instrumentation	Chest wall pain, exposure limited to two or three levels, cord lies dorsal to the pathology, second procedure for dorsal instrumentation
Thoracoabdominal	T10 to L4	Direct, multilevel, ventrolateral exposure across the thoracolumbar junction	Chest wall pain, pulmonary compromise, thoracostomy tube drainage, diaphragm manipulation
Retroperitoneal	T12 to L4	Direct, multilevel, ventrolateral exposure across the thoracolumbar junction, extrapleural, extraperitoneal	Exposure of T12 from peritoneal side of the diaphragm, diaphragm limits lateral instrumentation trajectory at T12
Dorsal			
Dorsal midline	T1 to L5	Technical simplicity, avoids potential morbidity of ventral approaches	Limited to dorsal exposure of dorsal elements and spinal cord
Transpedicular	T1 to L5	Technical simplicity, avoids potential morbidity of ventral approaches, preserves stability	Limited to dorsolateral disc space exposure
Transfacet	T1 to L5	Technical simplicity, avoids potential less morbidity of ventral approaches, less bone destruction than the transpedicular approach	Limited to dorsolateral disc space exposure
Dorsolateral Costotransversectomy	T1 to L5	Lateral "angle of attack" with greater access to ventral structures, simultaneous access to dorsal and ventral spine, avoids potential morbidity of ventral approaches	Large soft tissue exposure, technically demanding, dorsolateral angle precludes simultaneous ventral instrumentation
Lateral extracavitary	T1 to L5	The most lateral angle of approach of the "dorsal" approaches, simultaneous access to dorsal and ventral spine, avoids potential morbidity of ventral approaches	Large soft tissue exposure, technically demanding, dorsolateral angle precludes ventral instrumentation, potential skin flap ischemia

Transthoracic Approach

The transthoracic approach is ideally suited for a ventral exposure of midthoracic segments between T2 and T10 or T11.[6,11,12,13] Advantages include a direct ventral angle of attack for ventral pathology (Fig. 10-1), extensive bilateral ventral access for decompression, and multilevel exposure.[21] It is the only routine procedure by which ventral instrumentation is applied. Principal disadvantages are the potential pulmonary morbidity of entering the chest cavity, the need for postoperative tube thora-

costomy drainage, the necessity of decompressing neural structures that lie dorsal to the pathology, and the need for a second procedure in cases requiring dorsal instrumentation.[8,12]

Positioning

Patients are generally placed on the operating table in a full lateral decubitus position using a bean bag support and an arm sling, taking great care to generously pad the axilla and all pressure

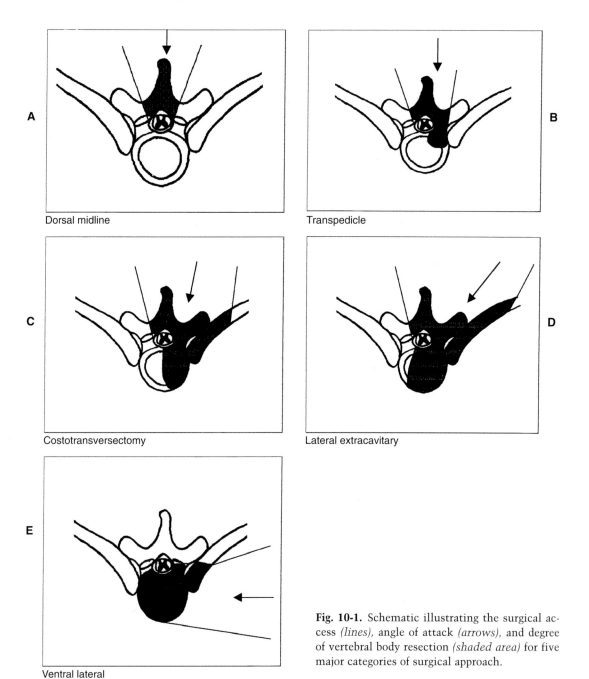

A   Dorsal midline

B   Transpedicle

C   Costotransversectomy

D   Lateral extracavitary

E   Ventral lateral

Fig. 10-1. Schematic illustrating the surgical access *(lines),* angle of attack *(arrows),* and degree of vertebral body resection *(shaded area)* for five major categories of surgical approach.

points (Fig. 10-2). Some surgeons prefer a semilateral position for more caudal, retroperitoneal exposures in which the skin incision tends to be carried more ventrally across the abdomen.[6,12] The lateral decubitus position, however, is useful for establishing a 90-degree orientation of the patient's spine to the floor. This maintains proper spatial orientation for the surgeon when approaching the thecal sac during spinal cord decompression maneuvers, and when planning the trajectories of transvertebral screws for ventral fixation.[24] The intended incision site is positioned over the break in the operating table, which is flexed to spread the rib cage and to further facilitate exposure (Fig. 10-3). By flexing the ipsilateral hip, the iliopsoas muscle is relaxed. This facilitates muscle retraction. This maneuver is especially useful for retroperitoneal exposures that extend to lumbar segments[24] (Fig. 10-4).

Incision

The side of the approach is typically the side with the greatest pathological involvement. With midline lesions, most surgeons approach mid- and

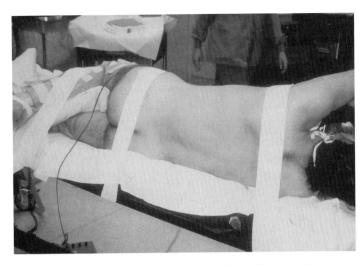

Fig. 10-2. Right lateral decubitus positioning for a left-sided transthoracic approach.

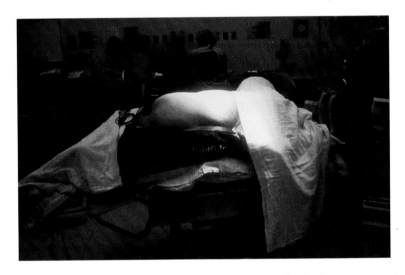

Fig. 10-3. Flexing the operating table spreads the rib cage laterally, facilitating retraction and disc space opening.

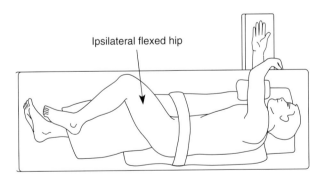

Ipsilateral flexed hip

Fig. 10-4. By securing the ipsilateral leg in a flexed position the corresponding psoas muscle group is relaxed, facilitating its retraction during ventral vertebral column exposure. (Adapted from Benzel EC, ed. Surgical Exposures of the Spine: An Extensile Approach. Park Ridge, Ill.: American Association of Neurological Surgeons, 1995.)

lower thoracic levels from the left side, because of the ease of mobilizing the heart and aorta, and the lack of obstruction from the dome of the liver. Significant controversy, however, exists regarding ischemic spinal cord injuries with left- or right-sided approaches. The major radiculomedullary artery of Adamkiewicz arises from the left side between the midthoracic to upper lumbar areas in most patients.[15] Regrettably, there is no definitive clinical or scientific evidence that adequately addresses the clinical importance of segmental vessel interruption on the spinal cord blood supply, despite well described, anecdotal reports of spinal cord ischemia after ventral procedures from the left side of the spine.[5,12] Factors thought to be important in avoiding ischemic complications, however, include preserving the anastomotic vascular arcade in the region of the proximal neural foramen, minimizing the consecutive number of segmental vessels sacrificed, and limiting the degree of spinal cord stretching, such as that which occurs during derotation maneuvers for deformity correction.[2]

For midthoracic vertebrae, an incision is made one or two rib levels above the vertebral level of interest (e.g., incise along the T7 rib to expose the T9

vertebra). This varies, depending upon the degree of rib sloping and the extent of exposure required.[21] In general, it is easier to compensate for an incision that is one level too high than one that is one level too low. Fluoroscopy or plain radiography may help incision placement in unusual cases such as spinal deformity.

A linear incision is made along the line of the chosen rib, extending from the costochondral junction to the region of the rib angle (Fig. 10-5). Dissection is carried down to the superficial layer of the thoracic musculature: the trapezius, the latissimus dorsi, the serratus anterior, and the serratus posterior muscles caudally (Fig. 10-6). In the upper thoracic spine, the inferior trapezius, the latissimus dorsi, the serratus anterior, and the underlying rhomboid muscle groups frequently require division. This is performed anatomically using electrocautery.[18,22] For the lower thoracic spine only the latissimus dorsi and serratus posterior inferior muscles typically require sectioning (Fig. 10-7). In upper thoracic approaches the tip of the scapula may be retracted laterally and dorsally with a towel clip or manually with a scapula retractor. The intended rib is exposed and its identity confirmed by either

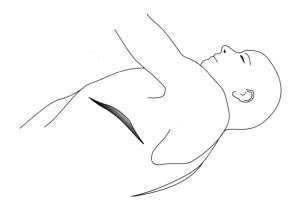

Fig. 10-5. Left transthoracic rib incision extending from the rib angle dorsally to the costochondral junction ventrally.

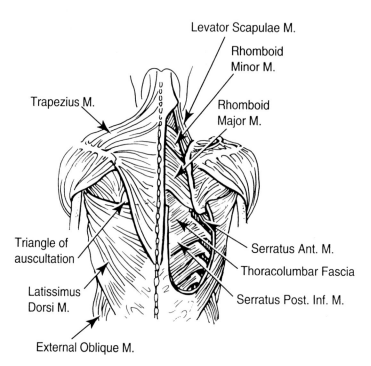

Fig. 10-6. Superficial and deep muscle layers of the thorax. (Adapted from Benzel EC, ed. Surgical Exposures of the Spine: An Extensile Approach. Park Ridge, Ill.: American Association of Neurological Surgeons, 1995.)

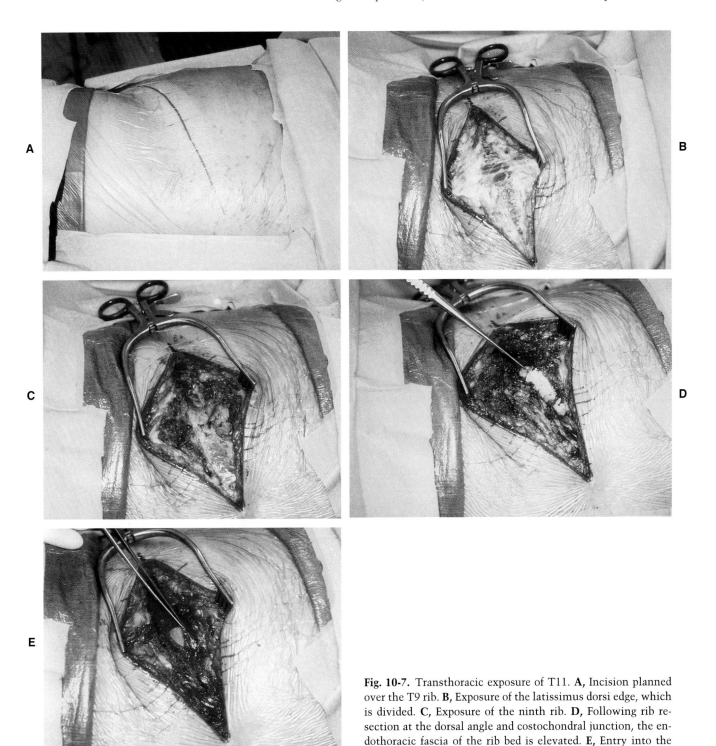

Fig. 10-7. Transthoracic exposure of T11. **A,** Incision planned over the T9 rib. **B,** Exposure of the latissimus dorsi edge, which is divided. **C,** Exposure of the ninth rib. **D,** Following rib resection at the dorsal angle and costochondral junction, the endothoracic fascia of the rib bed is elevated. **E,** Entry into the chest through the endothoracic fascia and parietal pleura.

counting down from the thoracic apex (the first rib is difficult to palpate by this method),[23] or by intraoperative radiography. The periosteum of the rib is scored with cautery and elevated with an elevator such as a Doyen, an Alexander, or a Cobb. The rib is disarticulated from the costochondral junction ventrally and cut dorsally just medial to the angle. Entry into the chest is through the rib bed periosteum and underlying endothoracic fascia and parietal pleura. The chest opening is extended the length of the rib bed. Soft, underlying pleural adhesions, if present, are easily broken with a blunt dis-

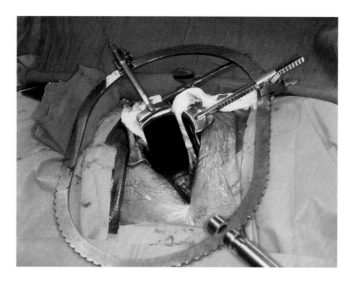

Fig. 10-8. A self-retaining, table-mounted retraction system is useful for rib cage and viscera retraction.

secting finger.[21] A rib spreading retractor, such as a Finochetto, is padded and placed, the ribs are spread, and the underlying lung is manually collapsed by packing and retraction. Use of a double-lumen endotracheal tube for unilateral ventilation facilitates lung retraction. A self-retaining, table-mounted padded retractor is also a useful means for retracting the ribs and thoracic viscera[9,18] (Fig. 10-8).

Vertebral Approach and Decompression

The ventrolateral aspect of the vertebral column is now clearly visualized; it is covered by a thin layer of parietal pleura (Fig. 10-9). The disc spaces are light in color and bulge prominently, whereas the vertebral bodies are darker and are concave on their lateral aspects.[22] Identification of the appropriate vertebral body and disc spaces is confirmed by intraoperative radiography. Placement of a smooth retractor blade between the aorta and the anterior longitudinal ligament protects the former from inadvertent trauma during the subsequent vertebral resection. The parietal pleura is incised longitudinally over the area of interest and segmental vessels are identified (Fig. 10-10). Segmental vessels are easily visualized coursing across the vertebral bodies between the aorta and the neural foramina. They should be doubly ligated at the midpoint of the vertebral body, taking care to prevent their avulsion (Fig. 10-11). Important intersegmental vascular anastomoses in the vicinity of the medial neural foramen should be preserved.[2] Only those segmental vessels that must be sacrificed,

for decompression and/or instrumentation, should be ligated. Vertebral decompression by corpectomy or discectomy is carried out as required, typically extending between normal disc spaces. Bone bleeding should be controlled with liberal use of bone wax and gelfoam sponge. Epidural venous bleeding may be problematic, because the lateral position of the patient limits access to epidural veins on the dependent side of the canal for bipolar coagulation. Gentle direct pressure with a hemostatic agent such as Gelfoam sponge, microfibrillar collagen, or powdered gelfoam mixed with bovine thrombin may be useful for this often frustrating situation.

Closure

For closure, the parietal pleura does not necessarily need to be reapproximated over the resection area. Ventral instrumentation that creates a high profile, or is in proximity to the great vessels may be covered by a Gore-Tex patch to create a protective barrier between the instrumentation and mediastinal soft tissues. The lung is then reinflated and one or two thoracostomy tubes are placed two costal levels below the incision. The ribs are compressed and reapproximated with heavy absorbable suture. The rib bed is similarly reapproximated securely to reestablish a pleural seal. Superficial muscles are repaired anatomically, and soft tissue closure is carried out in standard fashion.[12]

Extensive vertebral body resection is possible using the transthoracic approach (see Fig. 10-1).

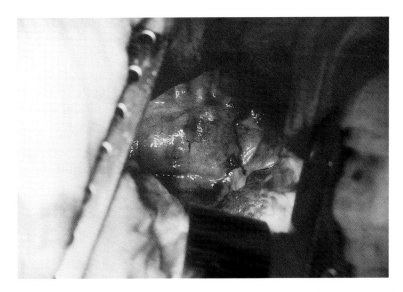

Fig. 10-9. Right lateral view of the exposed vertebral column at T6 for resection of metastatic melanoma (darkened elevation covered by parietal pleura).

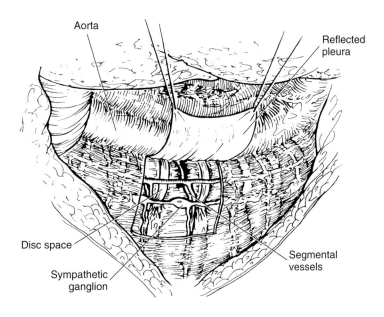

Fig. 10-10. The pleura is elevated exposing the segmental vessels and sympathetic chain. (Adapted from Benzel EC, ed. Surgical Exposures of the Spine: An Extensile Approach. Park Ridge, Ill.: American Association of Neurological Surgeons, 1995.)

Only the contralateral pedicle is not easily accessible by this technique. The ventrolateral angle of the approach also makes bone grafting for ventral interbody arthrodesis a relatively straightforward procedure. Postoperative complications of this technique are principally due to pulmonary compromise and pain from the chest wall incision.[12] Atelectasis, pneumonia, and pleural effusions should be antici-

pated. Although all patients experience some postoperative chest wall discomfort, a prolonged "post thoracotomy pain syndrome" may last longer than 6 months in up to 10% of cases.[8]

To reduce the morbidity of intrathoracic dissection, the thoracic spine can also be exposed by an extrapleural route.[16] The incision and initial technique is similar to the transthoracic approach. However, the parietal pleura is bluntly dissected and elevated from the inner chest wall and vertebral bodies. This variation avoids violation of the pleura and the subsequent need for tube thoracostomy drainage. The key to this retropleural technique is identification of a dissection plane between the endothoracic fascia of the thoracic wall and the parietal pleura.[16] Although pulmonary morbidity may be reduced with this modification, the number of possible levels that may be exposed is limited and it is technically difficult in elderly or debilitated patients to avoid inadvertent pleural tears. The retropleural approach has little effect on postoperative chest wall pain.

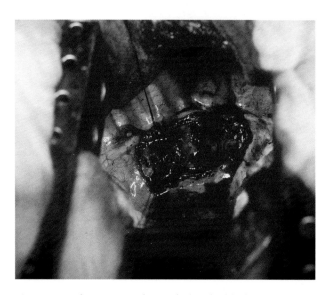

Fig. 10-11. The segmental vessels are doubly ligated and divided at the vertebral body midpoint allowing aorta retraction and vertebral body resection.

Thoracoabdominal Approach

Direct access to thoracic segments below T10 is complicated by the presence of the diaphragm.[13,21,23] This sheet of muscle originates from the dorsal aspects of the lower six ribs ventrally and inserts dorsally on the anterior longitudinal ligament of the upper lumbar vertebrae and the retroperitoneal wall via the diaphragmatic crura and the medial and lateral arcuate ligaments, respectively[18] (Fig. 10-12). Full lateral access to T11, T12, and L1 requires detachment of the dorsal-medial diaphragm from its insertion sites at L1 and L2. Further diaphragmatic detachment around its lateral periphery allows full exposure of upper- and midlumbar levels as caudal as L4. This caudal extension of the thoracoabdominal technique to the lumbar spine is used most frequently for ventral scoliosis procedures that cross the thoracolumbar junction.[13]

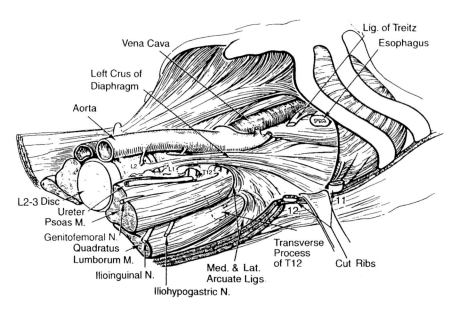

Fig. 10-12. The diaphragm arises from the lower six ribs ventrally and inserts onto the tip of the T12 rib, the lateral arcuate ligaments, the L1 transverse processes, the medial arcuate ligaments, and the ventral lumbar vertebral column via the diaphragmatic crus. (Adapted from Benzel EC, ed. Surgical Exposures of the Spine: An Extensile Approach. Park Ridge, Ill.: American Association of Neurological Surgeons, 1995.)

Thoracoabdominal approaches to the thoracolumbar junction utilize rib incisions that can vary between T7 and T12.[6,22] Most commonly, a tenth or eleventh rib incision is made in a standard transthoracic fashion. For more extensive exposures to lumbar levels the incision is fashioned more obliquely and is curved ventrally toward the abdominal midline[23] (Fig. 10-13). The tenth or eleventh rib is resected and the chest is entered. The costal cartilage of the chosen rib can be split longitudinally, allowing dissection through the costal rib bed. This maneuver takes advantage of the origin of the diaphragm from the top of the costal cartilage and the attachment of the abdominal musculature to the inferior costal cartilage.[22] Dissection at this level allows access to the properitoneal fat layer that lies caudal to the diaphragm and is continuous with the retroperitoneal space. The dissecting finger insinuated behind the diaphragm bluntly clears the peritoneum from its undersurface, thereby preventing entry into the peritoneal cavity[22,23] (Fig. 10-14). The diaphragm is then incised circumferentially along its peripheral attachment at the costal margin in a lateral to medial direction, leaving a generous cuff of muscle for later reapproximation. The lateral aspect of the lateral arcuate ligament, including its insertion at the tip of the twelfth rib, is detached along with the medial arcuate ligament at the L1 transverse process.

In this manner, the dorsal diaphragmatic attachments are freed from their medial insertions.

The retroperitoneal plane caudal to the diaphragm is then developed bluntly beneath the upper pole of the kidney and spleen. The left diaphragmatic crus should be identified and divided at its attachment to the ventrolateral margin of L1 and L2.[13] At this point, full ventrolateral exposure of the lower thoracic and upper two lumbar vertebrae has been accomplished (Fig. 10-15). After decompression and/or stabilization, great care must be taken to repair the diaphragmatic attachments accurately. The left crus is reattached to the anterior longitudinal ligament and the peritoneum, if violated, is repaired primarily. The medial arcuate ligament is reattached to the transverse process of L1, and the lateral portion of the diaphragm is reapproximated to its peripheral muscular cuff. The rib bed and thoracic musculature is closed in standard fashion.

The thoracoabdominal approach manipulates two major body cavities and creates significant soft tissue trauma. Complications may be related to visceral retraction injury (spleen, kidney, and ureter). As with any transthoracic technique, the patient is at risk for cardiopulmonary complications. This method of extensive exposure of the thoracolumbar region is usually reserved for younger, healthier patients.

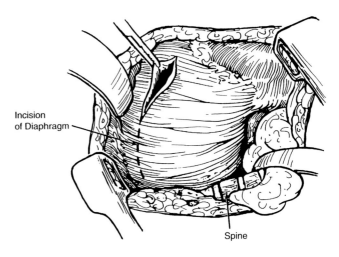

Fig. 10-14. The diaphragm incision is begun ventrally and laterally through the costal cartilage bed, which allows access to the extraperitoneal plane along the diaphragmatic undersurface. The incision is carried circumferentially to preserve the central innervation of the diaphragm. (Adapted from Benzel EC, ed. Surgical Exposures of the Spine: An Extensile Approach. Park Ridge, Ill.: American Association of Neurological Surgeons, 1995.)

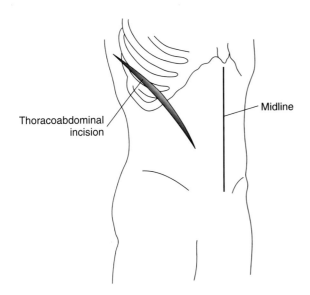

Fig. 10-13. Incision at T9 for thoracoabdominal exposure.

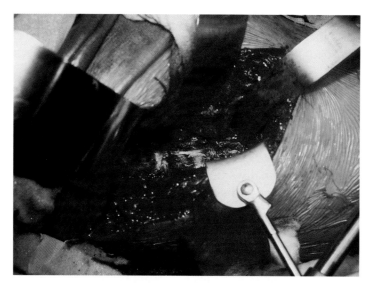

Fig. 10-15. After the medial dorsal diaphragm is free from its attachments, full ventrolateral access across multiple segments of the thoracolumbar junction is easily achieved.

Retroperitoneal Approach

The third major ventral approach to the thoracolumbar junction is through the retroperitoneal space, also known as the ventrolateral flank approach. It addresses thoracolumbar pathology from the abdominal side of the diaphragm, rather than the thoracic side. A retroperitoneal dissection does not require disruption of any major body cavity and is consequently a somewhat less morbid procedure.[24]

Like the thoracoabdominal procedure, the incision may vary depending on the particular spinal level of interest. The thoracolumbar junction is best approached by a twelfth rib incision, beginning at the lateral aspect of the paraspinous musculature and extending, as needed, obliquely downward to the lateral aspect of the rectus abdominis muscle[6,12] (Fig. 10-16).

The twelfth rib is isolated and resected, and the abdominal wall muscles are divided or split in the line of the wound. Just deep to the transversus abdominis muscle lies a layer of properitoneal fat covering the peritoneal membrane.[23] This is bluntly dissected from the undersurface of the diaphragm dorsally and medially toward the dorsal retroperitoneum. Laterally, the peritoneum becomes confluent with the transversalis fascia of the abdominal wall and the fascia behind the renal capsule (Fig. 10-17). The plane behind the kidney is developed bluntly and the peritoneum with its contents is retracted medially with a padded self-retaining retractor.[12] Care should be taken to carry this dissection ventrally toward the

ventral aspect of the vertebral bodies to avoid inadvertent dissection behind the iliopsoas muscle.[24] In this fashion, the ventral surfaces of the quadratus lumborum and psoas muscles are exposed. The genitofemoral nerve, on the ventral surface of the psoas, and the sympathetic chain between the psoas muscle and vertebral column should be identified, protected, and mobilized laterally.

This provides a relatively quick, uncomplicated exposure of the thoracolumbar and lumbar vertebrae. For simultaneous access to lower thoracic segments the arcuate ligaments can be detached from their insertions at the tip of the twelfth rib and transverse process of L1 (Fig. 10-18). This mobilizes the medial-dorsal and medial aspect of the diaphragm, allowing careful subpleural dissection for limited thoracic exposure as high as the T11-12 disc space.[13] Segmental ventral instrumentation, however, typically requires a 90-degree screw trajectory for transvertebral fixation, and may be difficult to achieve due to the overhanging rib cage and diaphragm. For this reason, when ventral instrumentation is indicated at T12, a thoracoabdominal approach should be considered. For the L1 level or below, the retroperitoneal approach is optimal.

Closure of the wound is straightforward, using simple anatomical reapproximation of diaphragmatic attachments and abdominal wall layers. A transient ileus should be anticipated. In addition to wound complications, visceral injury is a potential but infrequent problem that is often related to

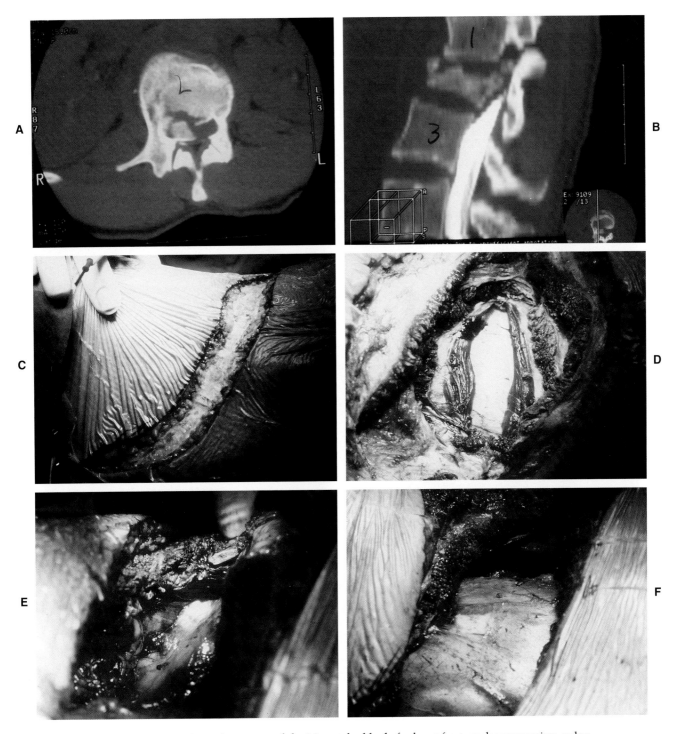

Fig. 10-16. Retroperitoneal exposure of the L2 vertebral body for burst fracture decompression, reduction, and ventral fixation. **A,** Large retropulsed bone fragment in the canal at L2. **B,** Sagittal (CT) reconstruction view. **C,** Upper right-sided flank incision along T12. **D,** Anatomical abdominal wall dissection illustrating three muscular layers: external oblique, internal oblique, transversus abdominis. **E,** The T12 rib is identified and resected to facilitate exposure. **F,** Blunt finger dissection is carried laterally around and behind the peritoneal membrane and its contents. *Continued.*

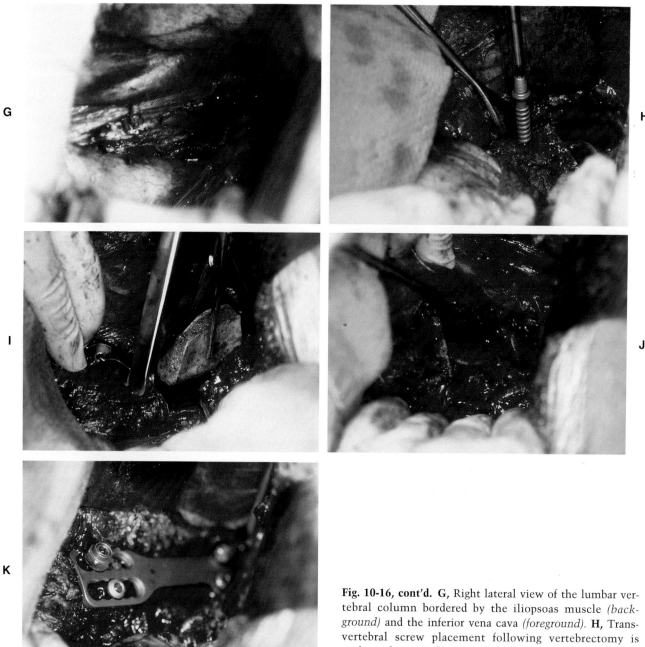

Fig. 10-16, cont'd. **G**, Right lateral view of the lumbar vertebral column bordered by the iliopsoas muscle *(background)* and the inferior vena cava *(foreground)*. **H**, Transvertebral screw placement following vertebrectomy is performed at a 90-degree angle to the long axis of the vertebral column. **I**, Iliac bone graft insertion. **J**, Properly placed interbody graft. **K**, Final plate fixation construct.

overly vigorous retraction. Dissection and retraction of the sympathetic chain may additionally result in anhidrosis and flushing of the ipsilateral lower extremity.[8]

DORSAL APPROACHES

Three standard categories of dorsal approaches are commonly described that are applicable at all thoracic and lumbar levels: dorsal midline, trans-

pedicular, and dorsolateral, which includes the costotransversectomy and lateral extracavitary techniques. Each approach provides an increasingly lateral angle to the vertebral body for improved ventral access (see Fig. 10-1).

Dorsal Midline Approach

The most common route to all levels of the spine is a standard midline dorsal approach. Well known

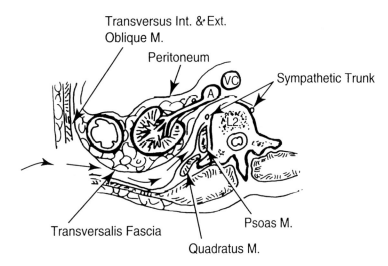

Fig. 10-17. Retroperitoneal dissection is carried behind the peritoneum and transversalis fascia over the quadratus lumborum and psoas muscles. (Adapted from Benzel EC, ed. Surgical Exposures of the Spine: An Extensile Approach. Park Ridge, Ill.: American Association of Neurological Surgeons, 1995.)

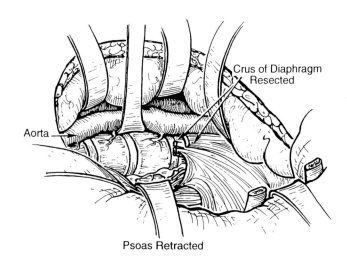

Fig. 10-18. By dividing the medial attachments of the diaphragm at the twelfth rib, the L1 transverse process, and the crus, full retropleural exposure as high as the T11-12 disc space may be achieved. (Adapted from Benzel EC, ed. Surgical Exposures of the Spine: An Extensile Approach. Park Ridge, Ill.: American Association of Neurological Surgeons, 1995.)

by most spine surgeons, it is used in a large variety of procedures ranging from simple decompressive laminectomy to dorsal fusion, with or without instrumentation. In the thoracic region, dorsal approaches are usually limited to decompressions for dorsally situated lesions (e.g., tumor, abscess, or other epidural masses), or in preparation for instrumentation.[24]

Patients are positioned prone on a chest frame, a spinal table, or laminectomy rolls, allowing the abdomen to hang freely to avoid vena cava compression. The incision is usually midline, its position being guided by the prominent spinous processes. Alternative soft tissue flaps are occasionally necessary (e.g., curved or straight paramedian) in cases with previous radiation to the area or for patients requiring future adjuvant radiation.[18] If a paramedian incision is used, it is carried down through the superficial musculature to the erector spinae muscle group. The myocutaneous flap is undermined and reflected medially to the spinous processes, allowing dorsal access to the bony elements for subperiosteal dissection.

In younger patients, a prominent cartilaginous "cap" on the tip of each spinous process can be split sharply in the midline and scraped laterally with a Cobb elevator. This maneuver leads to the appropriate plane for subperiosteal dissection along the lateral spinous processes and laminae.[24] Bilateral subperiosteal dissection is continued over the laminae with sharp elevators or electrocautery. Care should be taken to preserve facet capsules in cases not involving fusion. Blood loss may be reduced by progressive packing with epinephrine-soaked sponges and by anticipating the dorsal branches of the segmental spinal arteries that emerge lateral to the facet joints in the thoracic region and cross laterally to medially over the pars interarticularis.[1]

Meticulous attention to dissection technique and judicious muscle retraction reduces injury to the erector spinae muscle group, minimizing intraoperative blood loss, postoperative swelling, and muscle necrosis.[19] Closure simply requires anatomical reapproximation of the erector spinae muscles and the thoracodorsal fascia over the spinous processes. In the upper thoracic region, the insertions of the superficial and middle layers of the dorsal musculature (trapezius, levator scapulae, rhomboideus major and minor muscles) become confluent with the thoracodorsal fascia in the midline. Accurate closure of this layer ensures anatomical reconstruction of these important stabilizers of the scapula.[9]

Transpedicular Approach

Patterson and Arbit[18] described the transpedicular approach. It is a useful technique for herniated thoracic disc removal. The procedure is also useful for limited exposure to the ventrolateral vertebral body, such as for vertebral body biopsy or disc biopsy in suspected discitis.[7,10]

The patient is positioned prone in standard fashion on rolls or a spinal frame. A midline incision is made over the area of interest, and the paraspinal musculature and soft tissue structures are elevated subperiosteally to one side beyond the facet joint of interest. Using a high-speed drill, the entire facet joint and the associated pedicle is removed. By drilling deep into the pedicle the ventrolateral aspect of the vertebral body is accessible for limited dural decompression.[18] The disc space lies immediately above the top of the pedicle (Fig. 10-19). Disc decompression may be further facilitated by use of reverse-angled curettes. A transfacet variation of this approach that spares the pedicle has been described by Stillerman and Weiss.[20] By removing only the facet joint, the lateral aspect of the disc space is accessible for disc removal without removing the pedicle. Preserving the pedicle reportedly helps to maintain spinal stability.

The transpedicular approach is simple, easy to learn, and safe to perform. It is extremely limited,

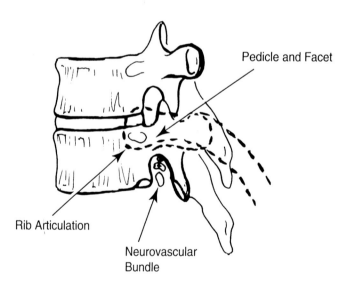

Fig. 10-19. The disc space lies immediately rostral to the top of the pedicle. The rib head articulates at the lateral disc space between the corresponding vertebral body and the next cranial vertebra. (Adapted from Benzel EC, ed. Surgical Exposures of the Spine: An Extensile Approach. Park Ridge, Ill.: American Association of Neurological Surgeons, 1995.)

however, for exposure of the ventral vertebrae. Therefore it is not generally used for extensive ventral resection, multilevel processes, or decompression of medially placed lesions.

Dorsolateral Approach

Dorsolateral techniques offer a more lateral angle of attack to vertebral pathology than dorsal approaches. They are useful for limited ventral decompression[9,10,14,19] (see Fig. 10-1). Two dorsolateral procedures are commonly described: the costotransversectomy approach and the lateral extracavitary approach.

Costotransversectomy is a dorsolateral technique that may be used throughout the spine to approach dorsal and dorsolateral structures without violating the pleural cavity. It can be considered to be an extended transpedicular procedure.[10,24] The lateral extracavitary technique is a modification of the costotransversectomy approach.[14] The major difference between the two techniques is the path each takes around the erector spinae muscle to the lateral vertebral body.

Menard[17] first described a midline costotransversectomy technique for drainage of tuberculous

abscesses. The approach uses a straight midline incision followed by a standard bilateral subperiosteal dissection. The ipsilateral dissection extends laterally beneath the erector spinae muscle to the tips of the transverse processes and proximal ribs. The appropriate rib is exposed subperiosteally and truncated medial to its angle. The costotransverse and radiate ligamentous complexes are divided and the rib is disarticulated manually. One or several ribs may be removed in this manner to provide adequate exposure. Usually only two vertebral bodies can be realistically approached by this technique. The endothoracic fascia and parietal pleura are bluntly swept from the lateral aspect of the vertebral body with a blunt dissector, creating a plane for a lateral approach to the vertebrae.

The transverse processes and corresponding pedicles are removed using rongeurs, curettes, and/or a high-speed drill, exposing the lateral aspect of the thecal sac (Fig. 10-20). Dissection of the intercostal nerve facilitates identification of the neural foramen and lateral thecal sac. This is a useful maneuver in cases of abnormal anatomy (e.g., tumor, trauma). The intercostal nerve may be sacrificed in the thoracic region by clip ligation proximal to the dorsal root ganglion. The foraminal veins and

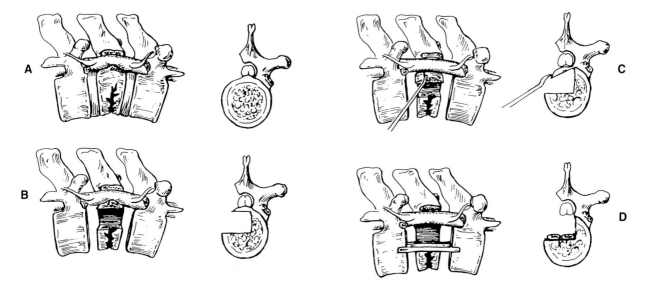

Fig. 10-20. Lateral extracavitary exposure and decompression. **A,** Simultaneous lateral view of the compressed thecal sac and ventral pathology. **B,** Initial vertebral decompression, leaving a thinned dorsal cortical shell. **C,** Impacting the cortical shell into the resection bed away from the dura mater, using a reverse-angled curette. **D,** Placement of an interbody graft following reduction. (Adapted from Benzel EC, ed. Surgical Exposures of the Spine: An Extensile Approach. Park Ridge, Ill.: American Association of Neurological Surgeons, 1995.)

medullary artery may cause troublesome bleeding and should be coagulated. Decompression is then carried out after identifying the normal disc spaces adjacent to the pathological lesion. A partial vertebrectomy is performed using a combination of rongeurs, curettes, and a high-speed drill. The plane between the thecal sac and the compressive pathology is then developed, and a down-biting curette is used to fracture the dorsal cortical shell of the vertebra ventrally into the corpectomy resection defect away from the dura mater. This maneuver fully decompresses the ventral thecal sac. A costotransversectomy provides a near-full lateral exposure of both the thecal sac and the ventral compressive lesion for controlled, direct neural decompression. The extent of decompression is only limited by the angle of approach to the ventral vertebral body.

To improve this working angle to the vertebral body, Capener[3] reported a modification of Menard's technique in which the incision is made in a parasagittal location. Dissection is carried through the superficial musculature to the lateral border of the erector spinae muscle group. This structure is elevated in a lateral to medial direction, superficial to the ribs. Alternatively, the erector spinae musculature is divided transversely and reflected. Appropriate ribs are removed approximately 8 to 10 cm lateral to the midline. The underlying parietal pleura is retracted ventrally, exposing the lateral vertebral body by a much flatter angle than that obtained by using the midline approach.

The improved angle of attack enables exposure of nearly the entire vertebral body for decompression. Decompression may be more safely performed than via direct ventral or dorsal methods, because the thecal sac and the compressive lesion are visualized simultaneously from the side. This obviates having to work around neural elements to resect the pathology or through the pathology to decompress the neural elements. Only the contralateral pedicle is not accessible using this technique. Although morbidity is thought to be less with the transthoracic approaches, the costotransversectomy techniques are technically demanding and can engender considerable blood loss due to epidural venous bleeding after decompression. Uncommon complications are neural injury, cerebrospinal fluid (CSF) leakage, segmental neuralgia, and pleural disruption.

Recently Larson, Holst, and Hemmy[14] have repopularized Capener's variation by altering the method of soft tissue approach that allows for posterior instrumentation. The classic "lateral extracavitary" approach uses a midline "hockey stick" incision with an oblique inferior limb (Fig. 10-21). After a standard midline subperiosteal dissection to the transverse processes, a plane is developed on the ipsilateral side beneath the thoracolumbar fascia. A full-thickness myocutaneous flap is retracted laterally, exposing the erector spinae muscle group to its lateral edge. A lateral to medial elevation superficial to the ribs is carried out in the same manner as the Capener procedure.

The major advantage of the lateral extracavitary technique is that it provides simultaneous access to both dorsal and ventral aspects of the spine. Following ventral decompression of the spinal cord, spinal reduction and dorsal instrumentation can be performed during the same operation. A ventral interbody arthrodesis completes the procedure (Fig. 10-22).[14]

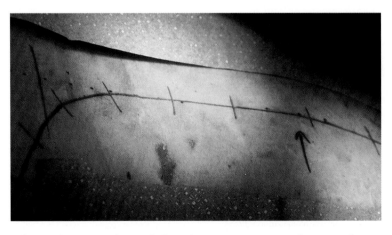

Fig. 10-21. "Hockey stick" incision for a right lateral extracavitary approach to a T10 fracture dislocation.

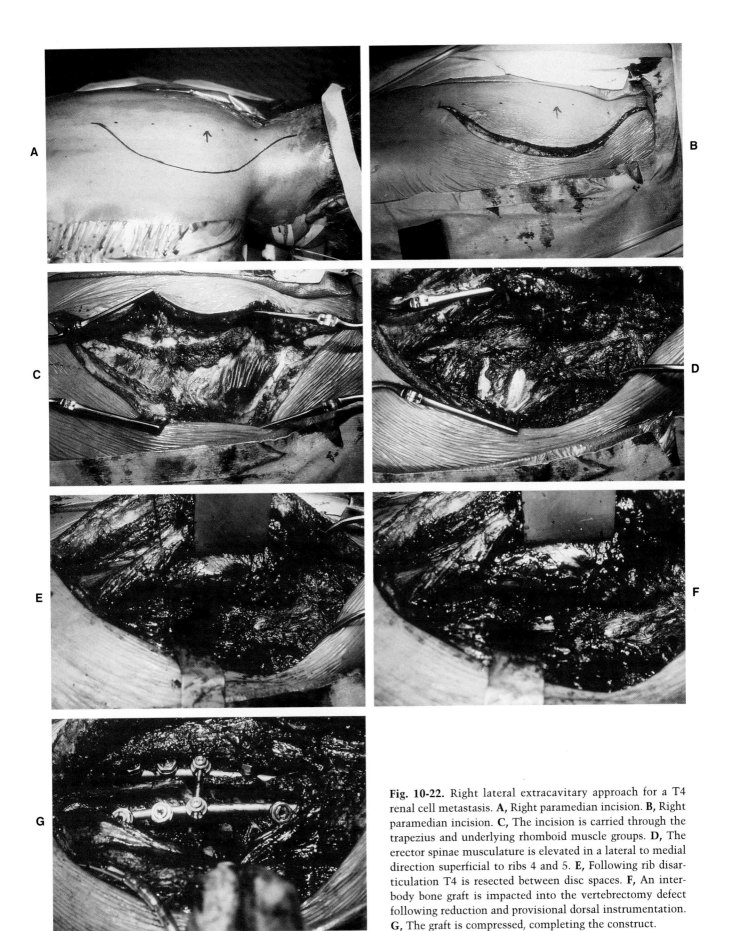

Fig. 10-22. Right lateral extracavitary approach for a T4 renal cell metastasis. **A,** Right paramedian incision. **B,** Right paramedian incision. **C,** The incision is carried through the trapezius and underlying rhomboid muscle groups. **D,** The erector spinae musculature is elevated in a lateral to medial direction superficial to ribs 4 and 5. **E,** Following rib disarticulation T4 is resected between disc spaces. **F,** An interbody bone graft is impacted into the vertebrectomy defect following reduction and provisional dorsal instrumentation. **G,** The graft is compressed, completing the construct.

Complications are similar to other costotransversectomy techniques and are principally related to the large soft tissue exposure required with secondary blood loss and postoperative pain. This procedure is technically demanding and requires an extended operating time.

CONCLUSION

There are a variety of methods for approaching the thoracic and thoracolumbar spine that reflects the unique anatomy of this region and the specific goals of a given surgical procedure. Spinal level, the degree of decompression required, the need for reconstruction, and the methods for instrumentation significantly impact the determination of the appropriateness and feasibility of the various exposure methods described.

REFERENCES

1. Amundson G, Garfin SR. Minimizing blood loss during spine surgery. In Garfin SR, ed. Complications of Spine Surgery. Baltimore: Williams & Wilkins, 1989, pp 29-52.
2. Benzel EC. Ventral exposures of the lumbar spine. In Benzel EC, ed. Surgical Exposures of the Spine: An Extensile Approach. Park Ridge, Ill.: AANS, 1995, pp 99-116.
3. Capener N. The evolution of lateral rhachotomy. J Bone Joint Surg 36B:173-179, 1954.
4. Cauchoix J, Binet JP. Anterior surgical approaches to the spine. Ann R Coll Surg Engl 21:234-243, 1957.
5. Champlin AM, Rael J, Benzel EC, et al. Preoperative spinal angiography for lateral extracavitary approach to the thoracic and lumbar spine. ANJR 15:73-74, 1994.
6. Cotler HB, Kaldis MG. Anatomy and surgical approaches of the spine. In Cotler JM, Cotler HB, eds. Spinal Fusion: Science and Technique. New York: Springer-Verlag, 1990, pp 89-124.
7. Cybulski GR. Thoracic disc herniation: Surgical management. Contemp Neurosurg 14(5):1-4, 1992.
8. Faciszewski T, Winter RB, Lonstein JE, et al. The surgical and medial perioperative complications of anterior spinal fusion surgery in the thoracic and lumbar spine in adults. Spine 20(14):1592-1599, 1995.
9. Fessler RG, Dietze DD, MacMillan M, et al. Lateral parascapular extrapleural approach to the upper thoracic spine. J Neurosurg 75:349-355, 1991.
10. Garrido E. Modified costotransversectomy: A surgical approach to ventrally placed lesions in the thoracic spinal canal. Surg Neurol 13:109-113, 1980.
11. Hodgson AR, Stock FE, Fang HSY, et al. Anterior spinal fusion: The operative approach and pathological findings in 412 patients with Pott's disease of the spine. Br J Surg 48:172-178, 1960.
12. Johnson RM, Murphy MJ, Southwick WO. Surgical approaches to the thoracic spine. In Rothman RH, Simeone FA, eds. The Spine, 3rd ed. Philadelphia: WB Saunders, 1992, pp 1696-1738.
13. Kostuik JP. Surgical approaches to the thoracic and thoracolumbar spine. In Frymoyer JW, ed. The Adult Spine: Principles and Practice, 2nd ed. New York: Raven Press, 1997, pp 1437-1470.
14. Larson SJ, Holst RA, Hemmy DC. Lateral extracavitary approach to traumatic lesions of the thoracic spine. J Neurosurg 45:628-637, 1976.
15. Leventhal MR. Spinal anatomy and surgical approaches. In Crenshaw AH, ed. Campbell's Operative Orthopedics. St. Louis: Mosby Year Book, 1992, pp 3493-3516.
16. McCormick PC. Retropleural approach to the thoracic and thoracolumbar spine. Neurosurgery 37:908-914, 1995.
17. Menard V. Causes de la paraplegie dans le mal de Pott. Rev Orthop 5:47-64, 1894.
18. Patterson RH Jr, Arbit E. A surgical approach through the pedicle to protruded thoracic discs. J Neurosurg 48:768-772, 1978.
19. Rengachary SS. Posterior and posterolateral surgical approaches to the spine. In Sudaresan N, Schmidek HH, Schiller AL, et al., eds. Tumors of the Spine: Diagnosis and Clinical Management. Philadelphia: WB Saunders, 1990, pp 488-493.
20. Stillerman CB, Weiss MH. Surgical management of thoracic disc herniation and spondylosis. In Menezes AH, Sonntag VKH, eds. Principles of Spine Surgery. New York: McGraw-Hill, 1996, pp 581-601.
21. Watkins RG. Cervical, thoracic, and lumbar complications—anterior approach. In Garfin SR, ed. Complications of Spine Surgery. Baltimore: Williams & Wilkins, 1989, pp 29-52.
22. Watkins RG. Surgical Approaches to the Spine. New York: Springer-Verlag, 1983.
23. Winter RB, Denis F. Lonstein JH, et al. Techniques of surgery. In Bradford DS, Lonstein JE, Ogilvie JW, Winter RB, eds. Moe's Textbook of Scoliosis and Other Spinal Deformities, 3rd ed. Philadelphia: WB Saunders, 1995, pp 133-217.
24. Woodard EJ. Indications, complications, and comparison of approaches. In Benzel EC, ed. Surgical Exposures of the Spine: An Extensile Approach. Park Ridge, Ill.: American Association of Neurological Surgeons, 1995, pp 157-178.

Principles and Techniques of Bone Fusion

Michael A. Morone M.D., Ph.D., Sait Naderi, M.D.,
and Edward C. Benzel, M.D.

A successful spinal fusion can be defined as solid bony union across an intervertebral space after arthrodesis. Spinal fusion and internal fixation are some of the oldest techniques used for the surgical management of the unstable spine. One of the first descriptions of spinal fusion was reported by Albee'[1] in 1911. It was performed to stabilize tuberculous infected spines (Pott's disease).[1,22,54] Spinal fusion procedures were later used to treat many other diseases associated with spinal instability.

Successful spinal fusion is associated with the elimination of motion at the arthrodesed motion segment. Failure of successful fusion results in nonunion or pseudarthrosis. Autograft and allograft bone are the most commonly used graft materials for spinal arthrodesis procedures. Although a mineralized tissue, bone is not metabolically inert. Instead, bone is continually undergoing deposition, resorption, and remodeling. These processes are influenced by different local (e.g., blood supply, hormonal) and systemic (e.g., nutritional status, presence of systemic disease, osteoporosis) factors. Understanding the principles of bone fusion requires a comprehension of the anatomy and physiology of bone, as well as its growth and healing process.

BONE ANATOMY AND HISTOLOGY

There are three main types of bone: woven bone, cortical bone, and cancellous bone. A volumetric ratio of cortical bone to cancellous bone in the human skeleton is 4:1, whereas this ratio is 1:2 in the spine.[16,33] Woven bone is found during embryonic development, during callus formation, and in some pathological situations such as hyperparathyroidism and Paget's disease. There is no discernable pattern of collagen fibers in woven bone and, incidentally, woven bone is usually remodeled to cortical or cancellous bone.

Cortical bone is remodeled from the woven bone by means of vascular channels that invade the embryonic bone from its periosteal and endosteal surfaces. Cortical bone consists of osteons, also known as Haversian systems, which are the main structural units of bone that are lined with osteogenic cells and surrounded by circular plates of bone (Figs. 11-1 and 11-2). The mechanical strength of cortical bone depends on the compact packing of the osteons. Cancellous bone (trabecular bone) contains hematopoietic elements, vascular interstices, and bone trabeculae (see Fig. 11-2). The orientation of trabeculae is perpendicular to external forces. Cancellous bone is found between

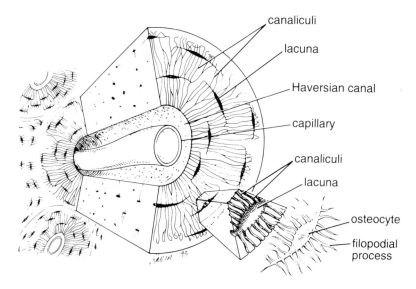

Fig. 11-1. An osteon is composed of a Haversian canal and lamellar bone.

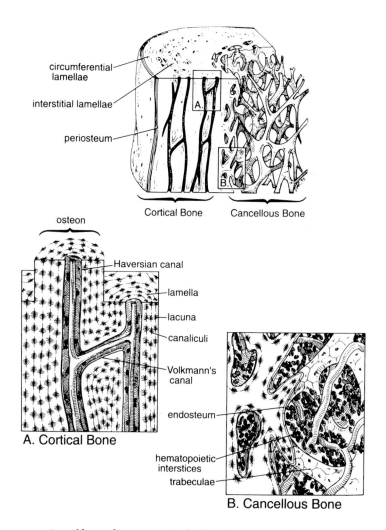

Fig. 11-2. A cross-section of bone showing cortical (*A*) and cancellous (*B*) structures of bone. Cortical bone consists of osteons and cancellous bone consists of hematopoietic elements and trabeculae.

two layers of cortical bone and undergoes remodeling at the endosteal bone surfaces.[16]

Bone Cells

The cellular elements of bone include osteoclasts, osteoblasts, osteocytes, and osteoprogenitor cells that differentiate into the bone-forming cells. Osteoprogenitor cells are small, spindled-shaped cells that are present on all nonresorptive bone surfaces. They constitute the deep layer of the periosteum that invests each bone and also the endosteum that lines the medullary cavity, Haversian canals, and other soft tissue spaces. The periosteum is a vascular and tough connective tissue membrane that covers the bone, but not its articulating surfaces. The thick outer layer of this membrane, termed its "fibrous layer," is composed of irregular, dense ordinary connective tissue. The thin, poorly defined inner region, termed the "osteogenic layer," is made up of osteogenic cells. The endosteum is a single layer of flat osteogenic cells without a fibrous layer. Its osteogenic cells are nevertheless able to participate with those of the periosteum in repairing broken bones. Osteogenic cells of the periosteum or endosteum that are stimulated to proliferate give rise to osteoblasts in regions that are well vascularized and to chondroblasts in regions that are avascular. Moreover, their capacity for self-renewal ensures that a stock of osteogenic cells persist for future need, such as for the growth and repair of bones.

Osteoblasts regulate bone remodeling and are the bone-forming cells that synthesize and secrete non-mineralized bone matrix, osteoid. Osteoid is newly synthesized, not yet calcified matrix adjacent to osteoblasts and is the organic component of bone. The cell bodies and cytoplasmic processes of osteoblasts create the lacunae and canaliculi in this matrtix. They characterize growing surfaces and can be distinguished from osteogenic cells by their large size, rounded to polygonal outline, and eccentric nucleus. Their cytoplasm is markedly basophilic, usually with a distinct negative Golgi image. In addition to lying down osteoid, osteoblasts are involved in matrix mineralization. Osteoblasts also play a role in the activation of bone resorption by osteoclasts.

Osteocytes are simply mature osteoblasts that have surrounded themselves with bone matrix. They lie in the lacunae situated between the laminae of matrix. Only one osteocyte is found in each

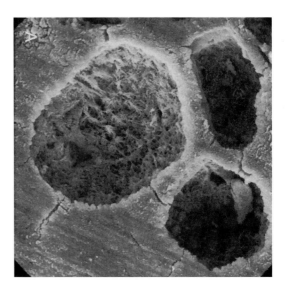

Fig. 11-3. Electron micrograph showing Howship's lacunae created by osteoclasts during bone resorption.

lacuna. The thin, cylindrical canaliculi house the osteocyte filopodial processes. Processes of adjacent cells make contact via gap junctions. This coupling provides for the intercellular flow of ions and small molecules. Osteocytes are involved in control of the extracellular concentration of calcium and phosphorus, as well as in adaptive remodeling behavior through cell-to-cell interactions in response to local environment. Death of an osteocyte results in resorption of its surrounding matrix.

Osteoclasts are multinucleated bone cells whose functions include both bone mineral and matrix absorption. Unlike osteoblasts and osteocytes, osteoclasts arise from blood monocytes. There is evidence to suggest that cells of the moncyte-macrophage line are attracted toward bare bone surfaces and that such cells can form osteoclasts by fusing with one another or by fusion with preexisting macrophage-like or osteoclast-like cells. Thus, instead of belonging to the bone cell lineage, osteoclasts represent an extension of the monocyte-macrophage-multinucleated giant cell line of differentiation. Osteoclasts reabsorb bone by attaching in groups to the bone surface where they release hydrolytic enzymes that reabsorb bone leaving small erosions known as "Howship's lacunae"[15,16] (Fig. 11-3).

Bone Matrix

The skeleton comprises 15% of the total weight and 12% of the total volume of the body. Ten percent of the skeleton changes annually because of remodeling. Cortical bone consists of inorganic components (69% by weight), organic components (22% by weight), and water (9% by weight). It imparts resilience and flexibility to the tissue.[16,37] The mineral portion of bone consists of calcium and phosphate, mainly in the form of small crystals resembling synthetic hydroxyapatite crystals.

The organic matrix of bone consists of osteoblast-secreted type I collagen (90%) and numerous noncollagenous elements, including proteins, glycoproteins, proteoglycans, peptides, carbohydrates, and lipids.[37]

THE BONE GROWTH PROCESS

Bones are formed by either membranous bone formation (intramembranous ossification) or by an intermediate step involving the formation of hyaline cartilage (endochondral ossification). The skull, face, mandible, and clavicle are formed by the former mechanism and the axial skeleton by the latter. Bone is unique in its ability for regeneration.[16] The remodeling cycle of bone is regulated by matrix deposition (by osteoblasts), matrix mineralization (by osteocytes), and matrix resorption (by osteoclasts).

REGULATORS OF BONE METABOLISM

Bone cells are modified by hormones and local factors. Three major calciotropic hormones are parathyroid hormone, vitamin D, and calcitonin. Parathyroid hormone increases the flow of calcium into the calcium pool and maintains the body's extracellular calcium concentration at a near constant level. Only osteoblasts have parathyroid hormone receptors. Parathyroid hormone causes cytoskeletal changes in osteoblasts. Vitamin D stimulates intestinal and renal calcium-binding proteins and functions in active calcium transport. Vitamin D receptors are found only in osteoblasts. Calcitonin is secreted from the parafollicular cells of the thyroid gland in response to an acutely rising plasma calcium level. Calcitonin interacts with specific receptors and inhibits calcium-dependent cellular metabolic activity.

Several polypeptide growth factors regulate bone healing. These growth factors induce mesenchymal derived cells, such as monocytes and fibroblasts that migrate, proliferate, and differentiate into bone cells. Growth factors are released from platelets, macrophages, and fibroblasts. These factors include the bone morphogenetic proteins (BMPs), insulin-like growth factor I and II, transforming growth factor beta (TGF-β), platelet derived growth factor (PDGF), and fibroblast growth factor.[25,52] The BMPs are osteoinductive, that is, they are able to induce bone growth. There are at least nine different BMPs (BMP-1 through BMP-9), all of which are members of the TGF-β superfamily of proteins except for BMP-1. In experimental studies, some of the BMPs have been shown to stimulate bone healing and promote spinal fusion healing.[10,40]

BONE GRAFTS

An ideal bone graft should (1) be biomechanically stable, (2) be osteoinductive and osteoconductive, (3) be free of disease, and (4) contain minimal antigenic features. Bone grafts are usually of two types: autograft or allograft. Autograft bone is transplanted from one part of the body (commonly from the iliac crest, fibula, spinous process, rib, or tibia). Allograft (allogenic) bone is transplanted between genetically nonidentical members of the same species, whereas a syngraft (syngenic) bone is from genetically identical members of a species, that is, twins. Xenograft (xenogenic) bone is transplanted from different species. In spinal surgery autograft bone and cadaveric allograft bone are commonly used for arthrodesis procedures.[3,4,25]

Several factors affect the strength of the graft, including the donor's age, gender, and physical characteristics, and the type of graft depending on the site from which the graft is taken (for example iliac crest vs. fibula). For all grafts, other than autograft, the manner in which the grafts are processed after harvest may affect their biomechanical strength.

Autografts

Autografts are transplanted from one part of an individual's body to another part. Autograft bone has several advantages over other types of grafts, including the fact that autograft is antigenically nonreactive, it contains osteoinductive proteins and marrow cells, and is genetically identical to the host. Disadvantages of autograft bone include the need for a separate incision for harvest, increased operating time and blood loss incurred with graft harvest, and a significant rate of persistent donor site complications.[17,51] There are different types of autografts including cortical, cancellous, cortico-cancellous, and vascularized grafts.

Cortical Bone Autograft

Cortical bone grafts are biomechanically stronger than cancellous bone grafts, in that they are more resistant to compression or shear forces. Arthrodesis with cortical bone leads to an osteoclastic (resorptive) response, while the response to cancellous bone graft is osteoblastic. This means that during the spinal fusion healing process cancellous bone grafts become stronger with time, while cortical bone grafts become weaker. During the first 6 months after arthrodesis with cortical bone, 50% of the strength is lost as the graft is resorbed. The strength is recovered within the following 1 to 2 years by ingrowth of new bone. Cortical bone graft fatigue fractures are usually seen 6 to 39 months after arthrodesis (average, 21 months).

Although cortical bone grafts are mechanically stronger than cancellous bone grafts, with regard to osteoinductive and osteoconductive properties cortical bone is less ideal than cancellous bone. In comparison to cancellous bone, cortical bone contains fewer osteocytes and osteoblasts, as well as less surface area per unit weight. The compact structure of cortical bone causes a barrier to vascular ingrowth and bone remodeling, thus requiring an osteoclastic response to the bone graft before new bone can be formed. Because of the aforementioned reasons the use of pure cortical bone graft is limited to situations requiring a strong structural support role for the graft, such as in multilevel ventral corpectomies.

Cancellous Bone Autograft

Autograft cancellous bone grafts are more cellular and become rapidly vascularized, compared with cortical bone grafts. However, cancellous bone grafts are mechanically weaker. Pure cancellous grafts are often used in dorsal spinal fusions, which do not require a structural support role for the graft. The combination of surviving marrow cells and presence of bone matrix proteins provides an ideal combination of osteogenic, osteoinductive, and osteoconductive properties for autograft cancellous bone grafts.

Corticocancellous bone grafts combine the advantages of cortical and cancellous grafts in that the corticocancellous graft can support normal axial loads under compression (similar to pure cortical grafts), while also providing the osteoinductive and osteoconductive properties of cancellous autografts.

Vascularized Bone Autograft

Vascularized bone autografts for bridging large bony defects have been used since the early 1900s. The use of such grafts has increased with time due to advances in microsurgical techniques and the use of the microscope. A vascularized graft can be used by means of either a vascular pedicle transposed to the fusion area or by a vascular microanastomosis. Vascularized bone grafts may be helpful when the recipient bed is devascularized, irradiated, or scarred.[13,22] Disadvantages of vascularized grafts include difficulty of microanastomosis and maintaining the patency of the anastomosis, as well as a longer operation time and difficulty in finding a suitable donor site.[49]

Allograft

The term graft refers to the transplantation of living tissue. It has been incorrectly used to refer to all types of grafting material. It may be more proper to use the term alloimplant instead of allograft. However, in this chapter the more commonly recognized term "allograft" is used. Because of some of the aforementioned problems with autograft use, allograft bone is often used. Autograft is not always the first choice for grafting because of (1) insufficient quantity of autograft bone, (2) poor quality of the bone, (3) postoperative donor site morbidity (e.g., pain, hemorrhage, wound problems, cosmetic problems, and infection), (4) increased operative time, (5) increased blood loss, and (6) heterotopic bone formation.

The same stages of bone healing (inflammation, repair, and remodeling) occur with the use of allograft and autograft. However, after allograft arthrodesis the healing process is slower and less extensive than with autograft.[34,44] The most common types of allograft materials include (1) fresh-frozen allograft, (2) freeze-dried allograft, (3) autolyzed, antigen-extracted allograft (AAA), and (4) demineralized bone matrix.[54,55]

Table 11-1. Spinal Fusion Rate of Frozen, Fresh-Frozen, and Freeze-Dried Allograft Bone

Author	Year	Graft Type	Bone Type	Fusion Rate (%)
Brown et al.[11]	1976	Frozen	Iliac crest	94
Aurori et al.[4]	1985	Frozen	Hip	95
Stabler et al.[43]	1985	Freeze-dried	Tibia, femur	0
McCarthy et al.[30]	1986	Frozen	Femoral head	100
Nasca and Whelchel[32]	1987	Fresh-frozen	Iliac crest	87
Knapp and Jones[24]	1988	Freeze-dried	Corticocancellous	36
Nugent and Dawson[33]	1993	Fresh-frozen	Corticocancellous	70

Transmission of infection and the lack of histocompatibility are two major problems regarding allograft. Sterilization is used to destroy infectious agents and to overcome the immune response. However, the sterilization process reduces the biomechanical, osteoconductive, and further osteoinductive properties of the graft materials.[36]

Immunogenicity decreases in the following order: fresh > frozen > freeze-dried. The immunogenicity may be further reduced by cell removal (via washing) from trabecular bone and complete soft tissue removal.[22] Today, the most important challenge is the reduction of the immunogenicity and infection rate without diminishing biomechanical strength. Freezing and freeze-drying of allografts may decrease graft immunogenicity; however, the risk of infection transmission may persist.

Deep-freezing does not appear to significantly diminish the biomechanical strength of allogenic grafts. Sedlin[41] demonstrated no change in the mechanical properties of bone after freezing to $-20°$ C, compared with fresh allograft specimens.[41] However, freeze-drying reduced the torsional and bending strength of allogenic bone.[46] Reported studies demonstrated a 4% to 100% and 0% to 92% rate of fusion using frozen and freeze-dried graft, respectively (Table 11-1).

Antigen-Extracted Allogenic Bone

Dubruc and Urist[18] developed a chemosterilized, autolyzed, antigen-extracted allogenic (AA) bone to limit the immunogenicity without loss of inductive properties. AA bone is obtained from cadaveric sources and is made of marrow-free cortical bone taken from the midshaft of long bones. AA bone is chemosterilized with 0.6 N HCl and phosphate buffers containing N-ethylmalemide. Osteocytes are removed via autolytic digestion. According to

Dubruc and Urist,[18] AA bone is more rapidly resorbed and replaced by new bone than frozen or freeze-dried whole bone. In addition, AA bone also preserves BMP activity. Dubruc and Urist[18] reported more than 80% good to excellent results with the use of AA bone compared to 70% to 80% excellent outcome with the use of autogenous bone.

Demineralized Bone Matrix

Demineralized bone matrix (DBM) is a type of allogenic bone. EDTA decalcified bone has an osteoinductive effect on fusion healing and is also resorbed faster than mineralized bone. Van de Putte and Urist[48] used HCl rather than EDTA for demineralization. Demineralization of allogenic bone diminishes allograft antigenicity. The primary active components of DBM are a series of low molecular weight osteoinductive glycoproteins, including BMPs. These BMPs comprise only 0.1% by weight of all bone protein and are most abundant in diaphyseal cortical bone. BMPs exist in the extracellular matrix and are not accessible until the bone matrix has been demineralized.[48] Many variables are involved in the preparation of DBM and the purification of BMPs, and thus the osteoinductive activity of these substances may vary considerably. DBM has a gel consistency and lacks biomechanical strength. Therefore it is often used as a supplemental inductive agent with autogenous bone.[21,48] DBM is available for clinical use under the trade name Grafton.

There are only a few uncontrolled studies that support the use of Grafton in spinal fusion. Experimental studies support the use of DBM as a graft extender (an addition to a less than ideal amount of autogenous bone) in a validated rabbit model of dorsal lumbar spinal fusion.[31,32] However, the use of Grafton in its current gel form as a graft substitute

(DBM only without the use of autograft) led to a fusion rate well below that of autograft alone.[31,32] In preliminary reports using the same rabbit model of spinal fusion new forms of DBM (Grafton putty and sheet form) have successfully been used as a graft substitute.[28] Currently there are no randomized prospective studies substantiating the beneficial use of Grafton in spinal arthrodesis procedures in humans, although trials in nonhuman primates are pending (Boden, personal correspondence).

Bone Morphogenic Proteins

In 1965 Urist[47] reported that demineralized, lyophilized bone matrix induced new bone formation in an extraskeletal intramuscular site. He demonstrated inductive substances in matrix transforming cells within muscle to follow a chondroosseous line of development.[47] There are at least nine types of BMP, of which types 2 through 9 are members of the TGF-β superfamily. The BMPs are hydrophobic, low molecular weight osteoinductive proteins isolated from insoluble bone matrix gelatin. BMPs are more abundant in cortical bone than cancellous bone. However, the mineralized matrix of cortical bone hides BMP activity until the cortical mantel is exposed, as occurs in a fracture. Other investigators confirmed the osteoinductive effects of the BMPs in animals.[25,27] Using BMP-2a, Lane et al.[25] demonstrated a dose-response ability to heal osseous defects in rats. For spinal fusions, Lovell and Dawson[27] reported the use of BMP in a canine segmental fusion model and found 2 to 3 times more bone formation with BMP. Boden, Schimandler, and Hutton[10] used a bovine derived osteoinductive protein mixture as a graft substitute and achieved 100% fusion rate in a rabbit model, compared to the use of autograft alone, which resulted in 61% fusion rate. Schimandle, Boden, and Hutton[40] used the recombinant human form of BMP-2 (rhBMP-2) added to autogenous bone graft in a rabbit model of dorsal lumbar fusion and noted a statistically significant increase in fusion rate compared to autogenous bone alone, 100% vs. 42%, respectively. In a rhesus monkey model of ventral lumbar spinal fusion using rhBMP-2 in a titanium cage, Martin et al.[29] demonstrated an increased fusion rate with rhBMP-2 use in comparison to autograft alone. This benefit of the BMPs in human spinal fusion has yet to be demonstrated. As the roles of these BMPs are elucidated,

they should become important in manipulating the complex cascade of cellular events essential to the fusion process.

Methylmethacrylate

Methylmethacrylate as an alternative to bone graft use has gained acceptance, especially for use in metastatic involvement of the spine. Methylmethacrylate provides immediate stability and facilitates early mobilization. Methylmethacrylate is truly an implant in the sense that with time there is no evidence of bone union, and the acrylic subsequently loosens. Often, the addition of Steinman pins or screws into adjacent unaffected vertebral bodies helps anchor the methylmethacrylate construct.[2] Methylmethacrylate is used most commonly for ventral vertebral column reconstruction, rather than dorsal fusions. A useful observation regarding the use of methylmethacrylate in the management of cancer of the spine is that the material properties of methylmethacrylate are unaffected by radiation and chemotherapy, both of which are known to inhibit bone healing.

Ceramics

Numerous biodegradable osteoconductive ceramic bone graft substitutes have received attention as alternatives to autogenous bone. The advantage of a biodegradable graft material is its compatibility with the new bone remodeling process required to attain optimum mechanical strength. A nonresorbable graft material may hinder remodeling and prolong the strength deficiency of new bone, as well as leave permanent stress risers in the fusion mass. Calcium phosphate ceramics, which include hydroxyapatite and tricalcium phosphate (TCP), have been the most widely used in orthopaedic surgery.

For synthetic implants to be useful in vivo, they must have certain properties: (1) compatibility with surrounding tissues, (2) chemical stability in body fluids, (3) compatibility of mechanical and physical properties, (4) ability to be fabricated into functional shapes, (5) ability to withstand the sterilization process, (6) reasonable cost of manufacturing, and (7) reliable quality control. Calcium phosphate ceramics possess these properties and have been used successfully as bone graft substitutes in dentistry and maxillofacial surgery.[20] Although biomechanical studies have demonstrated the feasibility of using ceramics in spinal surgery, there is a paucity of in vivo testing of ceramics in animal models of spinal fusion.

Hydroxyapatite and TCP ceramics are brittle materials with low fracture resistance and variability in their chemical and structural composition. Different preparative methods lead to either a compact or porous material with interconnective macropores that is the structural and spatial equivalent of cancellous bone. Commercially available hydroxyapatite is resorbed slowly, if at all, under normal physiological conditions, whereas TCP is generally resorbed by 6 weeks after implantation.

The clinical efficacy of ceramics as a graft material or as a component in a composite graft for spinal fusion has not been clearly established. In a study of 12 patients with severe scoliosis, Passuti et al.[35] used internal fixation and blocks of hydroxyapatite-TCP (3:2) alone or mixed with autogenous cancellous bone to stabilize the spine and fuse the facet joints. Clinical and radiographic assessment of the fusions were performed, and in two cases, biopsies of the graft material were obtained. At an average follow-up of 15 months, all patients exhibited complete radiographic fusions. Histological examinations of the biopsy specimens revealed the formation of new bone, which was directly bonded to the ceramic implant surface and inside the macropores.[35] Although these results are favorable, they must be interpreted with consideration for the limitations of the study. Ceramics have also been used successfully in spinal procedures such as laminoplasty procedures. Using ceramics in combination with osteoinductive agents (e.g., BMP, DBM) may make ceramics more useful.[25]

PHYSIOLOGY OF BONE REPAIR AND FUSION

The incorporation of a bone graft is the process of the envelopment and interdigitation of the old necrotic bone of the graft with new and viable bone. Bone graft properties affect the success and rate of the healing process. The properties of bone grafts that affect the rate and success of fusion healing should be discussed in terms of their osteogenic, osteoinductive, and osteoconductive properties.[37]

Osteogenesis is the ability of the graft to produce bone and is due to the presence of live bone cells within the graft. Osteogenic graft materials contain viable cells that possess the ability to form bone (determined osteoprogenitor cells) or the potential to differentiate into bone-forming cells (inducible osteogenic precursor cells). These cells participate in the early stages of the healing process to unite the graft to the host bone and must be protected during the grafting procedure to ensure viability. This potential to produce bone is characteristic only of fresh autogenous bone and bone marrow cells. Radiolabeling of graft cells has shown that very few of these transplanted cells survive.

Osteoinduction is the process by which some factor or substance stimulates an undetermined osteoprogenitor cell to differentiate into an osteogenic cell type. The BMPs and DBM are the principal osteoinductive graft materials. In addition to these materials, autogenous bone and allograft are known to possess osteoinductive properties.

Osteoconduction is the physical property of a graft material that allows the ingrowth of neovasculature and the infiltration of osteogenic precursor cells into the arthrodesed region. Osteoconduction involves the ability of the graft to act as a scaffolding to facilitate bone healing. DBM, ceramics, cancellous allografts, and autografts, are osteoconductive. Table 11-2 shows the properties of the different graft materials.

BONE HEALING PROCESS

The process of bone healing has been found to be similar in fractured long bones and spinal fusion healing.[9] There are three overlapping temporal phases of spinal fusion healing: (1) the early inflammatory phase, (2) the repair phase, and (3) the late remodeling phase (Fig. 11-4).[9,15] The inflammatory stage begins with the development of hematoma around the spinal fusion bed. Due to the arthrodesis procedure involving decortication, there is usually periosteal membrane disruption and associated muscle injury. The spinal fusion bed and hematoma are soon infiltrated by inflammatory cells, including macrophages, polymorphonuclear leucocytes, and mast cells. This infiltration is thought to be due in part to prostaglandins. Typical changes during the inflammatory phase include vasodilation, exudation of plasma, and the migration of leukocytes. Nutrient supply and oxygenation of the early spinal fusion bed is

Table 11.2 Properties of Clinical and Experimental Graft Materials

Material	Osteogenic	Osteoinductive	Osteoconductive
Autogenous cancellous bone	+	+	+
Autogenous cortical bone	+	+	+
Vascularized autograft	+	+	+
Allograft		+	+
Deproteinated xenograft			+
Bone marrow	+	?	
Demineralized Bone Matrix		+	+
Collagen			+
Ceramics			+
Bone morphogenic protein		+	

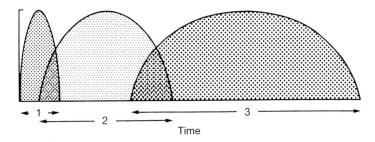

Fig. 11-4. Schematic diagram showing temporal phases of bone healing that occur during spinal fusion healing. (1)Inflammatory phase (2) Repair phase (3) Remodeling phase.

primarily via diffusion from adjacent exposed cancellous bone (after decortication) and muscle. It is during this inflammatory phase that the use of nonsteroidal anti-inflammatory drugs (NSAIDs) is thought to decrease the inflammatory response and thus decrease the chance of successful fusion.

The eventual capillary ingrowth into the spinal fusion bed increases the nutrient supply to the graft. Fibroblasts also begin to lay down a stroma that is supportive of vascular ingrowth. It is believed that nicotine inhibits capillary ingrowth into this fibrous stroma, resulting in the failure of stroma ossification, a step that requires a high oxygen tension.[14,38,39,43] A decreased union rate has been repetitively demonstrated in tobacco abusers after spinal fusion procedures.[7,8,12]

Adjacent to the exposed cancellous host bone, bone formation is rapid via intramembranous ossification. The rest of the fusion mass ossifies via endochondral ossification. Endochondral ossification requires an intermediate step in which a collagen matrix is laid down and then is resorbed while osteoid is laid down and subsequently mineralized. This period of spinal fusion healing leads to forma-tion of soft callus around the fusion bed that is very weak against movement in the first 4 to 6 weeks after the arthrodesis procedure.

In the last step of the process, the remodeling phase, bone is remodeled so that the outer part of the fusion mass consists of cortical bone, while the inner portion consists of cancellous bone. An adequate spinal fusion strength is provided in this stage. This stage may continue for months to years.

Unlike long bone fractures, spinal fusion procedures use bone graft. During the spinal fusion healing process there is replacement of the graft bone with new viable bone. This process, termed "creeping substitution," is the focal point for the incorporation of the bone graft.

Known factors that impair bony union include movement at the arthrodesis site, steroids, NSAIDs, estrogens, anemia, vitamin A and D excess, and also vitamin deficiencies associated with malabsorption, obesity, cigarette smoking, diabetes, and rheumatoid arthritis. Factors promoting the healing process include vitamins A and D, calcitonin, thyroid derivatives, and growth hormones. Radiation has an inhibitory effect on bone healing both acutely and chronically.[16]

SURGICAL TECHNIQUES

A variety of autogenous bone grafts are used in spinal surgery; these include grafts from the ventral and dorsal iliac crest, fibula, spinous processes, and ribs.

Dorsal Iliac Crest Grafts

Dorsal iliac grafts are taken from the iliac crest where the ilium is thicker. The dorsal iliac crest and the tubercle can be palpated 4 to 6 cm lateral to the midline. The graft harvesting procedure can be performed using either a separate incision or, when being performed with a lumbar spinal fusion procedure, via a subcutaneous dissection from the midline spinal exposure incision. The incision can be either vertical, just lateral to the iliac crest, or curved and parallel to the iliac crest. The dissection is performed superficially to the iliolumbar fascia and should be performed to visualize the interval between the lumbar fascia medially and the gluteus maximus laterally. Using subperiosteal dissection, the periosteum and gluteus maximus are elevated from the iliac crest. Dissection is continued to the iliac ridge between the attachments of the gluteus maximus and gluteus medius muscles. After exposure of the outer aspect of the iliac crest, a Taylor or similar retractor may be placed for retraction of the glutei muscles. Using an osteotome or an oscillating saw, a cortical or a corticocancellous bone graft can be easily taken. The first strip should be parallel to the iliac crest and removed cortical bone. A medium Cobb gouge is used to remove the cancellous bone along the inner aspect of the iliac crest. The remainder of cancellous bone can be removed by means of curettes between the two layers of the cortex. The iliac defect is filled with a large piece of gelfoam or bone wax to achieve hemostasis. The wound is copiously irrigated with antibiotic-laced normal saline and the fascial layers are closed.

Ventral Iliac Crest Grafts

Ventral iliac grafts are often used for ventral surgery and are obtained from the iliac crest lateral to the anterior superior iliac spine (ASIS) (Fig. 11-5). The ventral iliac crest is palpated while the patient is in supine position. The incision is made slightly below the ventral iliac crest. After exploration of the iliac

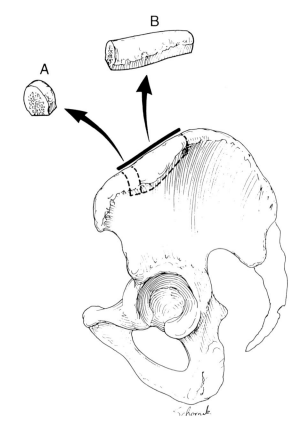

Fig. 11-5. Two different lengths of autograft that can be harvested from the anterior iliac crest. Grafts shown are for fusion after (*A*) a discectomy and (*B*) a corpectomy.

crest between oblique abdominal muscles rostrally and the tensor fascia latae and gluteus medius muscles caudally, a subperiosteal dissection is performed. Using a sponge in the depth of the incision, the external abdominal, transverse abdominal, and iliac muscles are stripped off from the iliac crest. After visualization of the outer and inner cortex of the iliac crest, a small tricortical graft is harvested. The size of the graft should be slightly larger than that required. The graft can be taken with either an osteotome or an oscillating saw.

Soft tissue around the ilium should be protected during harvesting. Two vertical ilium cuts are made and followed with a transverse cut. A small piece of the graft is enough for a disc interspace defect, whereas a larger graft is required for corpectomy. Concerning biomechanical strength, White and Hirsch[50] found horseshoe iliac crest grafts to be stronger than a dowel (Cloward) and strut (Bailey-Badgley) graft.

Fibular Grafts

Harvested fibular grafts may be used for arthrodesis procedures involving the ventral cervical and thoracic spine. Graft harvesting is performed in the supine (for cervical spine) or lateral position (for thoracic spine). The use of both a distal and a proximal tourniquet minimizes bleeding in the surgical field. An incision is made in a line joining the fibular head and lateral malleolus. The fascia of the lower leg is incised dorsal to the peroneal muscles. A sharp and careful dissection in the plane between the peroneal muscle ventrally and the flexor hallucis longus muscle dorsally exposes the dorsal crest of the fibula. The fibula graft is commonly harvested from the middle third of the fibula. Using a retractor to protect soft tissue, an oscillating saw may be used to cut the fibula. The tourniquet is released after closure of the fascia, subcutaneous tissue, and skin.

Other Autograft Materials

Other autograft materials include ribs and spinous processes. Rib and spinous process grafts are often used for dorsal spinal arthrodesis procedures. Spinous process grafts eliminate donor site problems, reduce operative time and blood loss, and produce a rate of arthrodesis equal to that of iliac crest grafts.[23] During ventral spine trauma procedures, pieces obtained from the fractured vertebral body can be used as graft material.

GRAFT PREPARATION AND PLACEMENT

A Leksell rongeur, osteotome, or high-speed drill can be used for preparation of the graft. The use of a heat-forming high-speed drill can lead to thermal injury of the graft. However, this may be reduced with continuous saline irrigation during drill use.

An adequate decortication of the fusion bed must be performed and requires exposure of cancellous bone. For this goal, osteotomes or curettes can be used. The graft should be properly fitted and placed against exposed cancellous bone to increase the chance for successful fusion. For interbody fusions improper or inadequate fitting of the bone graft to the vertebral body bed may result in inadequate

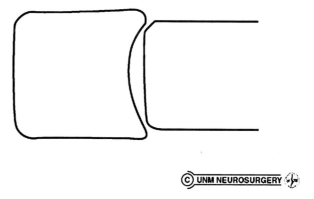

Fig. 11-6. A round vertebral body recipient bed (*left*) in which a squared-off bone graft is placed (*right*) provides very little surface area of contact between the bone graft and the recipient bed. Excessive subsidence or nonunion may ensue.

bone contact (Fig. 11-6). Cancellous bone chips may be used to fill any gaps between the graft and the fusion bed.

Ventral interbody fusion provides an optimal environment for bone growth due to the stress (compression) placed on such grafts. Ventral interbody grafts are placed in the weight-bearing region of the spine along the neutral axis. Weight bearing promotes the healing process (Wolff's law) and in turn bony fusion. The density of the graft can affect fusion. A denser graft can "knife" its way through the vertebral body; conversely, a graft that is less dense and weaker than the vertebral body may lead to failure of the graft.[5]

COMPLICATIONS OF GRAFTING

Complications of grafting include pain, neural and arterial injuries, iliac fracture, urethral injury, peritoneal perforation, hernia, infection, and sacroiliac joint injury.[6,42] Donor site pain has been reported to persist in 15% to 30% of patients 1 year after surgery.[19,26,45,53] The specific cause of persistent donor site pain is not known. However, it may be due to rich innervation and blood supply of the donor site and also to the extent of the periosteal dissection.

The vascular complications of graft harvesting include hemorrhage, bleeding due to gluteal artery injury (dorsal iliac crest grafts), radicular artery injury (rib grafts), and traumatic arteriovenous fistula formation. Hematoma formation after graft harvesting may occur in as many as 10% of cases.

Neural injuries may occur with the harvest of ventral iliac crest grafts. These include injuries of the lateral femoral cutaneous nerve and the iliogastric nerve. Superior cluneal nerve, sciatic nerve, superior gluteal nerve, and femoral nerve injuries may occur due to dorsal iliac crest graft harvests. Rib grafts may lead to injury of the segmental nerves below each rib, which results in persistent flank pain and paresthesias.

Fusion Bed Complications

Fusion bed complications include neural compression, graft breakage and collapse, malunion or nonunion, infection, and graft displacement (extrusion or intrusion).

Nonunion (pseudarthrosis) or fibrous union can be defined as the presence of ventral segmental movement at the graft site on dynamic films. Radiographically, nonunion is noted by the absence of trabecular bone 6 months (delayed union) and 12 months (nonunion) after arthrodesis. For dorsal fusion procedures, radiographically scant amounts of bone are noted or there is failure of formation of a bone bridge spanning the fused segment.

There are five types of nonunion including hypertrophic, oligotrophic, dystrophic, necrotic, and atrophic nonunion. Hypertrophic nonunion is secondary to premature weight bearing, and oligotrophic nonunion is secondary to too wide a gap for bridge formation between the bone edges. Dystrophic nonunion is a nonunion of one side of the grafted segment, and necrotic nonunion is due to vascular insufficiency. Atrophic nonunion is due to resorption of the bone graft.

Graft Failure

Graft failure can occur as a result of fracture, collapse, or resorption. The graft should be of sufficient strength to resist forces that tend to deform, displace, or fracture the strut.

Graft Displacement

Graft displacement is a serious complication after ventral spinal arthrodesis. In the cervical spine, ventral graft extrusion can result in injury to the esophagus, trachea, or carotid arteries, while dorsal extru-

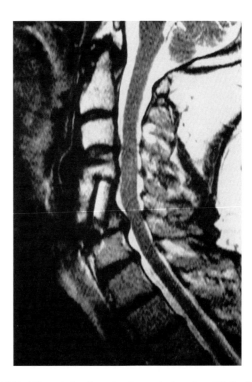

Fig. 11-7. T2-weighted sagittal cervical spine MRI of a patient in whom the fibula allograft has telescoped into the adjacent vertebral bodies. The patient had steroid-induced osteoporosis.

sion can compromise the spinal cord. Loss of graft position and deformity may necessitate a reoperation. The use of instrumentation may reduce the rate of graft displacement. A ventral spinal graft may telescope into the adjacent vertebral bodies if it is consistently denser than autogenous bone (Fig. 11-7). In such situations where bone density is decreased (osteoporosis, chronic steroid use, nutritional insufficiency, etc.), an autogenous graft may be considered.

Infection

Treatment of infection should follow surgical principles including drainage, debridement, and appropriate antibiotics. If a ventral graft becomes infected, the graft should be removed, the infected site debrided, and a new autogenous graft placed. Instrumentation removal is controversial. Several treatment methods have been proposed, including instrumentation removal and debridement vs. debridement without instrumentation removal. Such a discussion is beyond the scope of this chapter.

REFERENCES

1. Albee FH. Transplantation of a portion of the tibia into the spine for Pott's disease: A preliminary report. JAMA 57:885-886, 1911.
2. Alleyne CH Jr, Rodts GE Jr, Haid RW. Corpectomy and stabilization with methylmethacrylate in patients with metastatic disease of the spine: A technical note. J Spinal Disord 8:439, 1995.
3. An HS, Lynch K, Toth J. Prospective comparison of autograft vs. allograft for adult posterolateral lumbar spine fusion: Differences among freeze-dried, frozen, and mixed grafts. J Spinal Disord 8:131-135, 1995.
4. Aurori BF, Weierman RJ, Lowel HA, et al. Pseudarthrosis after spinal fusion for scoliosis: A comparison of autogenic and allogenic bone grafts. Clin Orthop 199:153, 1985.
5. Benzel EC: Spinal fusion. In Benzel EC, ed. Biomechanics of Spine Stabilization. Principles and Clinical Practice. New York: McGraw-Hill, 1996, pp 103-108.
6. Berchuck M, Garfin SR, Bauman T, et al. Complications of anterior intervertebral grafting. Clin Orthop 284:54-62, 1992.
7. Bishop RC, Moore KA, Hadley MN. Anterior cervical interbody fusion using autogeneic and allogeneic bone grafts substrate: A prospective comparative analysis. J Neurosurg 85:206-210, 1996.
8. Blumenthal SL, Baker J, Dossett A, et al. The role of anterior lumbar fusion for internal disk disruption. Spine 13:566-569, 1988.
9. Boden SD, Schimandle JH, Hutton WC. An experimental intertransverse process spinal fusion model. Radiographic, histologic, and biomechanical healing characteristics. Spine 20:412-420, 1995.
10. Boden SD, Schimandle JH, Hutton WC. Lumbar intertransverse-process arthrodesis with use of a bovine bone-derived osteoinductive protein. J Bone Joint Surg 77A: 1404-1417, 1995.
11. Brown MD, Malinin TI, Brown MD. A roentgenographic evaluation of frozen allografts versus autografts in anterior cervical fusions. Clin Orthop 119:231-236, 1976.
12. Brown CW, Orme TJ, Richardson HD. The rate of pseudarthroses (nonunion) in patients who are smokers and patients who are nonsmokers: A comparison study. Spine 11:942-943, 1986.
13. Buncke HJ, Furnas DW, Gordon L, et al. Free osteocutaneous flap from a rib to the tibia. Plast Reconstr Surg 59:799-804, 1977.
14. Daftari TK, Whitesides TE Jr, Heller JG, et al. Nicotine on revascularization of bone graft: An experimental study in rabbits. Spine 19:904-911, 1994.
15. Dee R. Bone healing. In Dee R, Mango E, Hurst E, eds. Principles of Orthopaedic Practice. New York: McGraw-Hill, 1988, pp 68-73.
16. Dee R, Sanders M. Bone: Structure and Function. In Dee R, Mango E, Hurst E, eds. Principles of Orthopaedic Practice. New York: McGraw-Hill, 1988, pp 53-68.
17. Depalma AF, Rothman RH, Lewinnek GE. Anterior interbody fusion for severe cervical disk degeneration. Surg Gynecol Obstet 134:755-758, 1972.
18. Dubruc F, Urist MR. The accessibility of the bone induction principle in surface-decalcified bone implants. Clin Orthop 55:217-223, 1967.
19. Fernyhough JC, Schimandle JJ, Weigel MC, et al. Chronic donor site pain complicating bone graft harvesting from the posterior iliac crest for spinal fusion. Spine 17:1474-1480, 1992.
20. Ferraro JW. Experimental evaluation of ceramic calcium phosphate ceramic as a substitute for bone grafts. Plast Reconstr Surg 63:634-640, 1979.
21. Frenkel SR, Moscovich R, Spivak J, et al. Demineralized bone matrix: Enhancement of spinal fusion. Spine 18:1634-1639, 1993.
22. Friedlaender GE, Huo M. Bone grafts and bone graft substitutes. In Frymoyer JE, ed. The Adult Spine. New York: Raven Press, 1991, pp 565-574.
23. Keene JS, McKinley NE. Iliac crest versus spinous process grafts in posttraumatic spinal fusions. Spine 17:790-794, 1992.
24. Knapp DR, Jones ET. Use of corticocancellous allograft for posterior spinal fusion. Clin Orthop 229:99, 1988.
25. Lane JM, Muschler GF, Kurz LT, et al. Spinal fusion. In Rothman RH, Simeone FA, eds. The Spine. Philadelphia: WB Saunders, 1992, pp 1739-1755.
26. Laurie SWS, Kaban LB, Mulliken JE, et al. Donor-site morbidity after harvesting rib and iliac bone. Plast Reconstr Surg 73:933-938, 1984.
27. Lovell T, Dawson EG. BMP augmentation of experimental spinal fusion. Proceedings of the Orthopaedic Research Society, 1986.
28. Martin GJ Jr, Boden SD. The use of two new forms of DBM in experimental posterolateral lumbar spine arthrodesis. Congress of Neurological Surgeons Meeting, New Orleans, La. 27 September-2 October, 1997.
29. Martin GJ Jr, Boden SD, Hutton W, et al. Laparoscopic anterior spinal arthrodesis with rhBMP-2 in a titanium interbody threaded cage. Congress of Neurological Surgeons Meeting, New Orleans, La. 27 September-2 October, 1997.
30. McCarthy RE, Peck RD, Morrissy RT, et al. Allograft bone in spinal fusion for paralytic scoliosis. J Bone Joint Surg 68A: 370-375, 1986.
31. Morone MA, Boden SD. Demineralized bone matrix (Grafton®) in experimental posterolateral lumbar spine fusion. North American Spine Society 11th Annual Meeting. Vancouver, BC: October 1996.
32. Morone MA, Boden SD. Experimental posterolateral lumbar spine fusion with a demineralized bone matrix gel. Spine 23:159-167, 1988.
33. Nasca RJ, Whelchel JD. Use of cryopreserved bone in spinal surgery. Spine 12:222-227, 1987.
34. Nugent PJ, Dawson EG. Intertransverse process lumbar arthrosis with allogenic fresh-frozen bone graft. Clin Orthop 287:107, 1993.
35. Passuti N, Daculsi G, Rogez JM, et al. Macroporous calcium phosphate ceramic performance in human spine fusion. Clin Orthop 248:169-176, 1989.
36. Pelker R, Markham T, Friedlaender G, et al. The effects of preservation on allograft strength. Trans Orthop Res Soc 7: 283, 1982.
37. Prolo DJ. Biology of bone fusion. Clin Neurosurg 36:135-146, 1988.
38. Riebel ED, Boden SD, Whitesides TE, et al. The effect of nicotine on incorporation of cancellous bone graft in an animal model. Spine 20:2198-2202, 1995.
39. Rubenstein I, Yong T, Rennard SI, et al. Cigarette smoke extract attenuates endothelium-dependent arteriolar dilation *in vivo*. Am J Physiol 261:H1913-H1918, 1991.
40. Schimandle JH, Boden SD, Hutton WC. Experimental spinal fusion with recombinant human bone morphogenic protein-2. Spine 20:1326-1337, 1995.
41. Sedlin E. A rheologic model for cortical bone. Acta Orthop Scand Suppl 36:83, 1965.

42. Shin AY, Moran ME, Wenger DR. Superior gluteal artery injury secondary to posterior iliac crest bone graft harvesting. A surgical technique to control hemorrhage. Spine 21:1371-1374, 1996.

43. Silcox DH III, Daftari T, Boden SD, et al. The effects of nicotine on spinal fusion. Spine 20:1549-1553, 1995.

44. Stabler CL, Eismont FJ, Brown MD, et al. Failure of posterior cervical fusions using cadaveric bone graft in children. J Bone Joint Surg 67A:370, 1985.

45. Tanishima T, Yoshimasu N, Ogai M. A technique for prevention of donor site pain associated with harvesting iliac bone grafts. Surg Neurol 44:131-132, 1995.

46. Triantafyllou N, Sotiropoulos E, Triantafyllou J. The mechanical properties of the lyophilized and irradiated bone grafts. Acta Orthop Belg 41:35, 1975.

47. Urist MR. Bone: Formation by autoinduction. Science 150:893, 1965.

48. Van de Putte KA, Urist MA. Osteogenesis in the interior of intramuscular implants of decalcified bone matrix. Clin Orthop 43:257, 1966.

49. Weiland AJ, Daniel RK. Microvascular anastomosis for bone grafts in the treatment of massive defects in bone. J Bone Joint Surg 61A:98-104, 1979.

50. White AA III, Hirsch C. An experimental study of the immediate load bearing capacity of some commonly used iliac bone grafts. Acta Orthop Scand 42:482-490,1971.

51. Whitecloud TS III. Complications of anterior cervical fusion. Instr Course Lect 27:223-227, 1976.

52. Wozney JM, Rosen V, Celeste AJ. Novel regulators of bone formation: Molecular clones and regulators. Science 242:1528, 1988.

53. Yonemura KS. Bone grafts: Types, harvesting and their complications. In Menezes AH, Sonntag VKH, eds. Principles of Spinal Surgery. New York: McGraw-Hill, 1996, pp 151-156.

54. Younger EM, Chapman MW. Morbidity at bone graft donor sites. J Orthop Trauma 3:192-195, 1989.

55. Zeegen N, Dawson EG. Allografts in spinal surgery. In Bridwell KH, DeWald RL, eds. The Textbook of Spinal Surgery. Philadelphia: Lippincott-Raven Publishers, 1997, pp 2347-2358.

Spinal Instrumentation: Ventral Techniques

George J. Martin, Jr., M.D., Regis W. Haid, Jr., M.D.,
and Gerald E. Rodts, Jr., M.D.

Although ventral approaches to the thoracic and thoracolumbar spine have been used since the 1930s, there is a current resurgence due to enhanced fixation techniques, lessened anesthetic morbidity, and surgeon familiarity. The correction of scoliosis in Europe and the treatment of Pott's disease in Hong Kong led the vanguard for ventral approaches. These indications have expanded to include neoplasm, trauma, and pseudarthrosis.

The goals of ventral thoracic approaches include neural decompression, arthrodesis, correction and/or prevention of deformity, short segment fixation, and early patient mobilization. Advantages of ventral approaches include direct decompression, placement of an interbody graft under compression, optimization for short segment fixation, the possibility of a single stage procedure, and the ability to reduce sagittal and/or coronal plane deformities. Potential drawbacks include lack of surgeon experience, risk of vascular and/or visceral injuries, pulmonary complications, and difficult revision surgery.

The number of ventral instrumentation techniques available to the spine surgeon has blossomed in recent years. Cable and pure distraction rod constructs have been supplanted for the most part by rod and/or plate systems that are highly versatile with improved biomechanics. There are a variety of choices of fixation devices: plate vs. rods, rigid vs. semirigid, unicortical vs. bicortical, etc. A number of factors contribute to the choice of an instrumentation system: the degree of instability, the predisposition to further deformity (e.g., thoracolumbar junction), the quality of the patient's bone, choice and/or availability of graft materials, and the surgeon's expertise. One must always remember that regardless of the rigidity of the construct, it will undoubtedly fail unless meticulous bone grafting techniques are applied.

INDICATIONS FOR THE VENTRAL APPROACH

A variety of infectious, neoplastic, congenital, and traumatic pathological conditions are suitable for ventral thoracic or thoracolumbar surgery. The initial step is to determine whether a ventral approach will truly provide the safest and most efficacious means of decompression of the neural structures, reconstruction of the ventral and middle columns, appropriate corrective forces for realignment, and an appropriate graft or spacer/implant construct. Dorsal neural compression or significant dorsal column bony/ligamentous damage are best treated by a dorsal approach. Lesions of the ventral and middle columns with associated dorsal column abnormalities, such as fracture/dislocations, may be addressed best by circumferential fusion procedures. The indications for ventral approaches, however, continue to evolve. At the present time, patients with ventral and middle column pathology and significant neural compromise are potential candidates for ventral techniques. The involvement of the dorsal column complicates matters. If there is only sagittal plane deformity with three-column involvement, strong consideration may be given to an isolated ventral reconstruction. However, if coronal deformity is also present, a dorsal fixation, either alone or in combination with a ventral procedure, should be considered.

Trauma

Trauma is the most common pathology encountered by most spine surgeons in the thoracic and thoracolumbar regions. Ventral column lesions (compression fractures) requiring operative intervention are extremely rare. Fractures that are amenable to ventral approaches include burst fractures and, occasionally, flexion-distraction injuries. It is paramount to note the presence or absence of a concomitant coronal plane deformity.

The treatment of burst fractures continues to be controversial. Historically, prolonged bed rest has been associated with significant recovery.[5] The results of nonsurgical management may be excellent in patients with limited spinal canal compromise, minimal loss of vertebral body height, and no neurological deficit.[6,11,22] Operative intervention may be warranted with thoracolumbar burst fractures with greater than 40% loss of height, greater than 50% spinal canal compromise, or a significant neurological deficit. In the thoracic region, where the spinal canal has a smaller anteroposterior (AP) diameter and the spinal cord is more susceptible to permanent neurological deficit, application of this criteria may lead to exclusion of patients best treated by surgical decompression.

Neoplasms

Neoplasms, both primary and metastatic, can involve the vertebral body. They, therefore, amend themselves to a ventral approach. Metastatic tumors are more common than primary tumors, and historically have been present in 20% to 70% of patients with malignancies.[30] With evolving improvement in the treatment of the primary disease, patients with metastatic disease will live longer. Laminectomy has been reported to offer no substantial benefit over radiotherapy for metastatic disease.[9,13,36] However, ventral decompression has been shown to be superior to laminectomy or radiation therapy, alone or in combination, in the management of metastatic tumors.[27,28,31] The type of malignancy and life expectancy, if known, before surgery or determined by frozen section, must be considered when deciding upon the optimal construct for reconstruction of the axial spine. In cases of a rapidly dividing neoplasm and short life expectancies, interbody methylmethacrylate constructs can provide immediate and short-term stability of the vertebral column.[7,8] In more indolent tumors, such as breast or prostate cancer, longer survival can be expected; and with the use of autogenous or allogenic bone as a graft substrate, one may avoid complications such as methylmethacrylate failure or migration.

Infection

Infection is another disease process that may be amenable to the ventral approach for decompression, reconstruction, and instrumentation. Severe spinal infection with deformity is an indication for operative intervention. Reconstruction with autologous or allogenic bone is feasible if a complete debridement of all necrotic tissue is accomplished. The added stability provided by instrumentation must be weighed against the low but still possible risk of persistent infection or implant failure.[18,24]

Deformity

Other conditions, such as congenital or adult deformities and posttraumatic kyphosis can be effectively treated ventrally. The treatment of scoliosis involves restoring alignment of both the thoracic and lumbar spine. Scoliotic curves with a normal lumbar lordosis may be treated with ventral instrumentation.[33] Patients with lumbar kyphosis may best be treated with a ventral release, followed by dorsal instrumentation.[20] The use of a ventral fusion in painful adult scoliosis with curves greater than 40 to 50 degrees leads to a higher rate of fusion than with a dorsal construct alone. Ventral fusion and instrumentation also play a role in the treatment of congenital kyphosis, Scheuermann's disease, and posttraumatic kyphosis where the deformities may be rigid and ventral column support is lacking.

PREOPERATIVE EVALUATION

Adequate radiographic studies before surgery can help avoid intra- or postoperative complications. Plain radiographs are essential in determining degree of instability, coronal and sagittal plane alignment, and degree of osteopenia. In cases of severe osteoporosis, poor bone density may be a relative contraindication to ventral instrumentation without a dorsal adjunct. The value of sagittal reformations of computed tomography (CT) images is often overlooked, particularly in complex lesions. The addition of myelographic dye can further pinpoint the exact location and amount of compression of the spinal cord. Axial CT is preferable over magnetic resonance imaging (MRI) for determining the amount of bony canal compromise. However, MRI often provides excellent views of the soft tissue structures (e.g., ligamentum flavum and interspinous ligaments) whose injury may commonly go unrecognized with plain radiographs and CT alone. Although MRI is the preferred imaging modality for neoplasms, it can be complemented by CT. This can aid in determining the amount of osseous destruction. MRI is also excellent in determining the exact position of the aorta. If the aorta lies directly lateral to the left side of the vertebral bodies, the placement of ventrolateral instrumentation on that side may be precluded. Although cost-effectiveness is a concern, a patient with complex spinal pathology (and for whom aggressive surgery is contemplated) may require both CT and MRI as part of their preoperative evaluation.

Although all surgical patients undergo a preoperative examination by an anesthesiologist, particular attention should be paid to the pulmonary system. Transthoracic approaches usually require retraction of the lung for adequate exposure. This is best facilitated by the placement of a double lumen endotracheal tube and complete collapse of the lung, and may be necessary for high thoracic lesions. However, for low thoracic lesions, lung deflation is much less important. Patients with severe restrictive obstructive pulmonary disease may not tolerate one-lung ventilation. Preoperative pulmonary func-

tion tests may be used to select out patients for which the ventral approach is contraindicated from a pulmonary standpoint.

Patient Positioning and Monitoring

In patient positioning, foam rubber padding is placed over pressure points on the ankles and elbows. All patients are positioned on a bean bag. The bag should not be extended to the axilla of the down arm. A softer object such as a roll (a liter bag of intravenous solution wrapped in a towel) is placed above the edge of the bag to cushion the axilla in order to prevent brachial plexus compression. The peroneal nerve in the down-side leg must also be protected with foam and/or gel padding over the fibular head. A pillow is placed between the legs, which are flexed 45 degrees at the hip and knees. The lower leg must be straight. The coronal plane of the patient's thorax should be perpendicular to the table. Wide tape may be used to secure this position. The patient will then remain secure, while allowing the rotation of the bed along its long axis ("airplaning"). Thus the surgeon can remain oriented throughout the procedure. This is crucial when confronted by complex pathology or tedious spinal canal decompression. The improved orientation of the surgeon promotes precise placement of vertebral body screws. Some tables are equipped with a level so that the desired neutral position can be recorded and reset by the anesthesiologist when appropriate. In addition, the perpendicular orientation of the coronal patient plane relative to the operating table allows for more efficient manual reduction of a kyphotic deformity by pressing on the back. The table can also be flexed at the level of the pathology to help open the disc spaces laterally and aid in the insertion of the bone graft; this is especially helpful in thoracolumbar approaches. Once the bone graft is in place, the anesthesiologist can return the table to the neutral, unflexed position. In patients of smaller stature, flexing the table promotes access to the spine by widening the space between the twelfth rib and the iliac crest.

Intraoperative monitoring or a wake-up test may be necessary when significant sagittal plane deformity correction is attempted. Although the role of somatosensory-evoked potentials (SSEP) monitoring continues to evolve, its reliability for predicting injury is fairly well-established. A decrease in SSEP amplitude of greater than 50% and limited or absent intraoperative recovery of amplitude are predictors of a postoperative neurological deficit.[10,14] Despite this reasonable sensitivity and low false negative rate, SSEP monitoring measures only dorsal column function. False positive findings are common, and are often related to anesthetic considerations that may lead to a dangerous desensitization of the surgeon to the warnings of intraoperative injury. SSEPs are most useful in severe deformity cases where a specific maneuver (typically, distraction) can be quickly reversed. In contrast, the inability to predict injury with maneuvers that are irreversible (e.g., the resection of intramedullary tissue or the coagulation of vessels) makes this method of monitoring suboptimal for this indication.

Motor-evoked potentials (MEPs) are likely a more accurate means than SSEPs for monitoring spinal cord function during surgery.[21] Some of these techniques are extremely sensitive to anesthetic agents whereas others cannot distinguish between ipsilateral and contralateral changes. Newer technologies may lessen or eliminate these disadvantages; however, they will undoubtedly be more expensive and require expertise that is not available on a widespread basis.[16]

SURGICAL APPROACHES
General Considerations

The thoracic spine can be exposed ventrally by a variety of methods. The most common approaches include the transmanubrial-transsternal approach for T2 to T4 lesion, conventional thoracotomy for T3 to T10-11 lesion, and the thoracoabdominal approach for thoracolumbar junction lesions. An intimate knowledge of the anatomy of these regions is paramount before performing these approaches. The assistance of a cardiothoracic surgeon may be necessary. Detailed preoperative and intraoperative communication with the surgical colleague, if used, ensures not only exposure of the pathological level, but also adequate exposure to allow use of instruments perpendicular to the spine for reconstructive and fixation techniques.

The localization of the desired interspace or vertebral body may be problematic, even after entering the pleural cavity. A number of methods exist. The simplest is counting the ribs. Although usually accurate, the first rib may be difficult to palpate on some patients, leading to inaccurate localization. The spine surgeon should not hesitate to obtain an intraoperative radiograph to determine the level. The level of pathology may be visible to the naked eye, but other subtle landmarks, such as vascular clips from previous surgery or distinctive osteophytes, may provide crucial information when gleaned from preoperative radiographs.

Upper Thoracic Spine

The upper thoracic spine can be exposed through a caudal extension of the ventral cervical approach down to T2 in some patients. It is usually possible to extend ventral cervical instrumentation to the T2 level. However, the sweeping thoracic kyphosis makes the placement of the caudal screws difficult below this level. One possible solution is the creation of a window in the manubrium, or a median sternotomy. However, dissection in this area may place the great vessels (particularly the brachiocephalic vein), recurrent laryngeal nerve, and thoracic duct at risk. The brachiocephalic vein may be ligated, if necessary, for optimum visualization. The caudal limit of the median sternotomy is the aortic arch, which is visible on the preoperative MRI. It cannot be retracted. The transaxillary approach can be considered for lesions affecting the upper thoracic levels. This avenue, however, offers a limited exposure at the base of a conical-shaped cavity. It is usually reserved for small, ventrolateral lesions not requiring (complete) corpectomy. The placement of instrumentation is extremely difficult due to the limited exposure.

The upper thoracic spine (T2 to T5) can also be accessed via the dorsolateral thoracotomy, in which the patient is positioned in the lateral position with the arm elevated on a rest. The left side is relatively less accessible due to the location of the aortic arch and great vessels. The straight course of the brachiocephalic artery makes the right side preferable. However, the fragility of the venous structures can complicate access as well. A curved incision is made, beginning at the dorsal axillary line, extending below the caudal angle of the scapula, and ending between the medial scapula and the spinous processes. Exposure is through the interspace above the rib. This localizes the pathology. The trapezius and latissimus dorsi muscles are divided medially to minimize denervation, and the scapula is retracted laterally. The dorsal 10 cm of the rib is resected and the segmental vessels are ligated. The pleura and upper mediastinal structures can then be bluntly dissected to allow access to the vertebral bodies. Deflation of the lung with a double lumen endotracheal tube (ETT) may be helpful. This approach requires a tube thoracostomy placement at the end of the procedure, because the parietal pleura is opened and the lung is exposed. Instrumentation can be placed via this approach. The small size of the vertebral bodies in this region, as well as the difficulty in obtaining a true perpendicular access, may also lead to difficulty regarding vertebral body screw placement in those cases where instrumentation is required.

Midthoracic Spine

Lesions involving the midthoracic region are best approached via thoracotomy. The left side is usually preferred because it is safer and easier to visualize, dissect, and mobilize the aorta and segmental vessels than the vena cava or azygous venous system. The repair of the aorta, in the event of injury, is less complicated than repair of the vena cava. If the aorta is lying very far lateral to the left on preoperative imaging studies, or if the pathology is strictly right-sided, a right-sided approach can be performed. A standard thoracotomy incision is used, beginning at the midaxillary line and extending medially and dorsally to below the angle of the scapula. One should enter the pleural cavity at the intercostal space that is directly over the level of the pathology. Usually, this corresponds to the rib that is two levels rostral to the desired vertebral body. This, however, may be altered by the obliquity of the ribs. For instance, a T9 lesion usually corresponds to the horizontal segment of the seventh rib. Resection of the rib is not necessary, unless a bone graft or an unusually lengthy exposure of the spine is needed. Once the lung is deflated via a double lumen ETT and the viscera are packed away with moist towels, the level of the pathology is then exposed.

The ligation of segmental vessels remains a controversial topic in ventral spinal surgery. A recent study[34] reviewed nearly 1200 cases in which approximately 6000 segmental arteries were ligated without any incidence of vascular related paraplegia. The authors concluded that there is virtually no risk of paraplegia provided (1) the ligation is unilat-eral, (2) performed on the convexity of a scoliosis, (3) ligated at mid–vertebral body level away from the foramen, and (4) hypotensive anesthesia is not used. These authors also thought that soft-clamping of the vessel with SSEP monitoring was not justified. However, others have reported cases of vascular paraplegia due to vessel ligation and believe that SSEP monitoring may be a useful predictor.[4,19] Some surgeons have advocated preoperative spinal angiograms in all patients to identify the artery of Adamkiewicz.[3]

The vessels are ligated at approximately the mid-body with 2-0 or 3-0 silk suture, because vascular clips may not provide enough closure strength. Sacrificing the vessels too close to the aorta risks avulsion during the procedure. Sacrificing the vessels too close to the neural foramen may interfere with the collateral circulation of the spinal cord. In anticipation of instrumentation, segmental vessels should be ligated at the levels above and below the pathology. This also allows further mobilization of the aorta, which may be at risk for vascular erosion from higher profile fixation devices.

Thoracolumbar Junction

For lesions affecting T10 through the upper lumbar spine (L1), a combined thoracoabdominal approach is most often used. As with a standard thoracotomy, the patient is positioned in the right lateral decubitus position, with a bend in the table at the level of the pathology to facilitate exposure. The incision is commonly made over the tenth or eleventh rib from the dorsal axillary line to the ventral axillary line and extended toward the anterior superior iliac spine as needed. The oblique and transversus abdominis muscles are incised, but care should be taken not to violate the peritoneal cavity. The thoracic cavity is entered and the diaphragm is immediately identified. The parietal pleura and peritoneal sac are bluntly mobilized using finger and sponge-on-a-forcep dissection. Avoiding monopolar cautery for most of this stage can prevent inadvertently entering the peritoneal cavity, lung, or abdominal viscera. If access to L1 or lower is needed to place instrumentation, the diaphragm should be mobilized. This is initiated by removing its peripheral attachment to the eleventh rib. A 2 to 3 cm cuff of diaphragmatic tissue is left to allow for reapproximation during closure. The spinal attachments of the diaphragm are taken down sharply or with monopolar cautery. The medial attachment of the lateral arcuate ligament and the lateral attachment of the medial arcuate ligament are divided close to the tip of the transverse process of L1. The crus of the diaphragm is divided 2 to 3 cm away from the vertebral body and should be tagged. At this point, large self-retaining chest retractors can be placed to displace the peritoneal contents and diaphragm. Vessel sacrifice should be performed as described above. The psoas muscle can be sharply dissected with periosteal elevators or monopolar cautery back to the attachments to the pedicle to maximize exposure of the lumbar vertebral bodies. Gentle retraction can provide exposure from T9 through L3.

Decompression

In preparation for decompression, the boundaries of the spinal canal must be established to prevent inadvertent canal entry and to promote ideal screw placement. The end plates and disc spaces above and below the pathological levels must be clearly and completely visualized. The dorsal 2 to 3 cm of the rib at the levels involved must be removed to expose the pedicle. This can be easily performed with a ¼ inch osteotome, but a rongeur or a drill may be used. Once the heads of the ribs are disarticulated, the pedicles at each level are exposed and the dorsolateral edge of the vertebral body is confirmed by palpation with a Penfield elevator. Frequently, there is a large mass of soft tissue including the ligated ends of the segmental vessels that has been swept into the area of the foramen. The bipolar rather than a monopolar should be used to cauterize any bleeding.

Before the actual decompression, the spine is "gardened." That is, the bone is well exposed from the ventral vertebral body to the dorsal wall. The lateral aspect of the vertebral bodies must be entirely exposed rostral to caudal over all levels to be instrumented. All segmental vessels are ligated. A rongeur is used to remove the "humps" or vertebral end plates to fashion a flat bone junction. It is essential to contour the plate and/or the bone to promote a strong junction. Thus the spine is fully prepared to accept a plate before any decompression.

For a vertebrectomy, the discs above and below are incised with a knife blade, or a straight osteotome can be used to separate the bulk of the disc from the end plates. One must keep in mind the concave curvature of the dorsal vertebral body in the thoracic spine in order to avoid the ventral spinal canal. Large curettes and rongeurs are used to remove disc material. A 1- to 2-inch osteotome can be used to remove a large portion of the vertebral body. The first cut is 5 to 8 mm dorsal to the ventral-most cortex of the vertebral body in the plane perpendicular to the disc space and is approximately 15 to 20 mm deep (toward the opposite side). The second cut is similarly perpendicular to the disc space and is approximately 8 mm ventral to the dorsal cortex of the vertebral body. A curved osteotome or large curette can then remove a large block of bone leaving a barrier between the decompression site and the aorta ventrally and the spinal canal dorsally. This removed bone may be used as a graft supplement. A high-speed drill is less traumatic compared with the osteotome, but at the sacrifice of increased blood loss and operative time. The remainder of bone is then removed either piecemeal with smaller curettes, or with a drill. The bone ventral to the spinal canal is thinned to "eggshell" width and is removed with a curette into the decompression site. Once the dorsal cortex and posterior longitudinal ligament have been removed, the dura mater can be inspected by direct visualization to ensure adequate decompression. The ventral and far lateral cortex of the vertebral body are preserved as much as possible to maintain stability and help secure the bone graft.

Bone Graft

The selection of bone graft depends on the distance the graft needs to span. It must take into account the location in the spine as well as the patient's underlying pathology. Factors such as the presence of osteopenia, tumor, diabetes, rheumatoid arthritis, and tobacco use are important. Autogenous tricortical iliac crest bone has been used as a graft substrate in ventral thoracic and thoracolumbar fusion. The advantage of autogenous bone is the superior healing environment of a substance that is osteoconductive, osteoinductive, and possibly osteogenic.[23] The disadvantages include the 10% to 20% complication rate associated with harvest[32] and the decreased weight-bearing ability of iliac crest grafts compared to grafts with a higher percentage of cortical bone, such as the fibula.[35] Although autogenous fibula has a high compressive strength, it is also associated with harvest complications (e.g., peroneal nerve injury and ankle joint instability). Ribs are readily available, but have less than 10% of the compressive strength of a fibula.[35] Allogenic bone has no harvest complications and is available in a variety of diameters (fibula, humerus, tibia, or femur) that can be tailored to the number and location of spinal levels to be spanned. The marrow cavity can be packed with autologous cancellous bone harvested during the vertebrectomy, autogenous cancellous iliac crest, or demineralized bone matrix. The disadvantages of allogenic bone include the possibility, though extremely remote, of infection[29] and the increased incorporation time.[12]

If autologous bone is used, all soft tissue (muscular or tendinous attachments, cartilage, fascia, etc.) must be cleanly stripped off before implantation to maximize bone surface area for fusion. Meticulous preparation of the fusion bed is paramount. The entire cartilaginous end plate should be removed. The bony end plate is decorticated in a crosshatched fashion to expose cancellous bone, but significant amounts of cortical bone must be spared in order to prevent impaction of the graft through the end plates during compression of the construct. Overaggressive end plate removal may lead to graft subsidence and subsequent pseudarthrosis. This problem is more prevalent with the use of rigid allografts such as tibia, fibula, or femur. End plates should be prepared in even, parallel fashion to ensure good fit. The wooden base of a cotton-tipped applicator (Q-Tip) makes an excellent device for determining the exact length of graft that is needed; calipers provided in many instrument sets can also be used. A graft that is too short may fall out. A graft that is too long may angle and parallelogram out, possibly into the canal. The placement of the graft can be aided by having a flexion "break" in the table to help open the space. This can also be accomplished with the use of an interspace spreader or by applying manual pressure to the dorsal spine. Once the graft is impacted, the table is returned to the neutral position to help lock in the graft.

INSTRUMENTATION
General Principles

Ventral spinal implants provide immediate rigidity, allow for compression of bone graft, and help main-

tain correction of the deformity. The three basic types of implants are rod, plate, and cable systems. With the exception of ventral cervical plates extending to the upper thoracic vertebrae, most implants in the thoracic and thoracolumbar region are placed on the lateral aspect of the vertebral body. To avoid unequal strain and stress on the metallic implant, great care must be taken to maximize the total surface area of metal-to-bone contact. This "gardening" of the spine is particularly important with plates, whose implant-to-bone surface ratio is high.

The placement of vertebral body screws should occur only after the surgeon is certain of the exact location of the spinal canal. Disorientation can be caused by a poorly positioned patient or an inadequate exposure. This may lead to perforation of the dorsal cortex by a vertebral body screw, with resultant devastating consequences. An awl or drill should be used to start screw or bolt holes to prevent instruments from skating into the spinal canal, large vessels, or viscera. Bicortical screw penetration is often preferable to provide the strongest purchase of the vertebral body, but care must be taken not to penetrate beyond 2 to 3 mm of the distal cortex of the vertebral body. Severe osteoporosis is a contraindication for vertebral body screw placement without concomitant stabilization.

Although many fixation systems are currently in use, this chapter focuses on the major categories of instrumentation. The Anterior Thoracolumbar Locking Plate System is a rigid, cantilever beam that uses unicortical screws. The Kaneda system is a rigid, cantilever beam rod system that uses bicortical screws. It can be used to correct deformities as well as to perform compression and distraction maneuvers. The Z-Plate is a rigid/semirigid cantilever beam plate that uses bicortical screw purchase and allows for graft compression and distraction. All three of these systems are available as a titanium alloy for superior postoperative imaging. They also use triangulated screws for greater pullout strength.

Anterior Thoracolumbar Locking Plate System

The Anterior Thoracolumbar Locking Plate System (ATLPS) (Synthes Spine, Paoli, Pa.) was designed for use from T10 to L5. It has a low profile. The screw heads lock to the plate, obviating the need for bicortical purchase (although this remains an

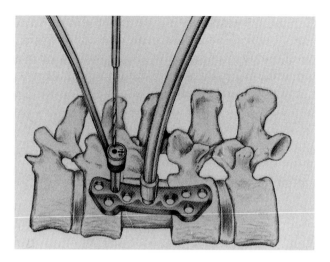

Fig. 12-1. ATLP—Plate is held in the center with a threaded drill guide applicator.

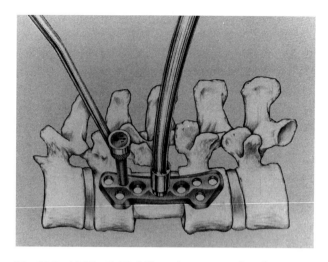

Fig. 12-2. ATLP—DCP drill guide is oriented with arrow toward the graft for drilling of temporary fixation hole.

option with longer screws). Plates are available in a variety of lengths, from 57 to 103 mm with 7.5 mm diameter vertebral body screws, ranging from 30 to 55 mm in length (in 5 mm increments). The measurement of the screws quoted by Synthes is the total screw length (the thickness of plate + length in bone); this differs from most systems, which measure only the length in bone. The use of unicortical locking screws makes the ATLPS in all likelihood the most technically straightforward device for ventral fixation. Disadvantages of this system include the fixed interval size of the plates, making them less versatile compared with other systems. Distraction cannot be applied to the screws, but only to the vertebral bodies via a spreader. This can be accomplished with the plate in position, but can be cumbersome. The screws are fixed angle, thus simplifying the system but decreasing surgeon versatility. Temporary screws allow for only 2 to 3 mm compression of the graft. Even the smallest plate may be too large for fixation above T10.

Technique

The appropriate size plate is selected so that the vertebral screws are 5 mm to 10 mm away from the end plates. The trapezoidal-shaped plate is positioned with the long end dorsally on the lateral aspect of the dorsal quarter of the vertebral body. A lateral radiograph may be obtained to confirm the position of the plate, although this is rarely necessary. It may be held in place through the center hole

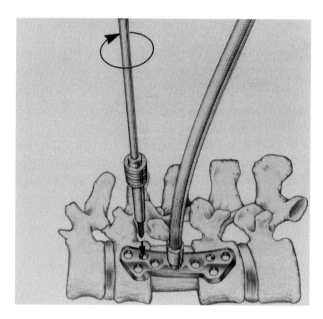

Fig. 12-3. ATLP—A hexagonal screwdriver is used to place the temporary DCP cancellous screw. After initial placement of both DCP screws, they are sequentially tightened to achieve compression.

with a threaded drill guide applicator acting as a plate holder (Fig. 12-1). The directional drill guide is placed in the first of two dynamic compression plate (DCP) holes on the plate, with the arrow on the drill barrel pointed toward the graft (Fig. 12-2); this promotes graft compression with screw placement. A 2.5 mm bit, with an automatic stop at 30 mm, is used to make the hole and the guide is removed. A 4.0 mm temporary cancellous bone screw of corresponding length is placed (Fig. 12-3) but not

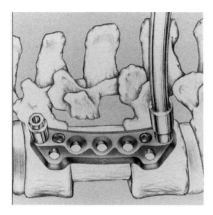

Fig. 12-4. ATLP—Threaded drill guides are placed in outer dorsal holes to ensure perpendicular placement of the drill.

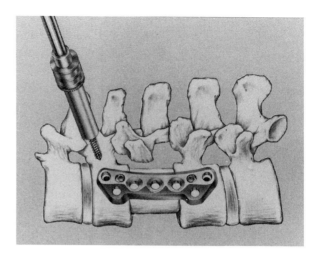

Fig. 12-6. ATLP—After removal of the drill guides, 7.5 mm locking screws are inserted and tightened until the heads are flush with the plate.

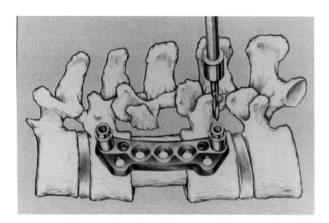

Fig. 12-5. ATLP—Dorsal holes are made with a 5.0 mm bit equipped with an automatic stop.

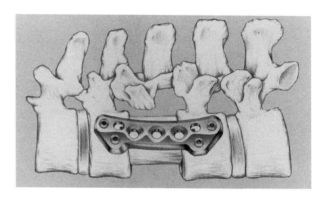

Fig. 12-7. ATLP—After the temporary screws are removed, the ventral screws are placed, completing the construct.

fully tightened until the temporary screw on the other end of the plate is inserted. These two screws are then sequentially tightened to place the graft under compression and fix the plate to the spine for permanent screw placement. The plate holder is removed and threaded drill guides, which ensure perpendicular drilling, are inserted in the outer dorsal holes of the plate (Fig. 12-4). A 5.0 mm bit, with an automatic stop at 30 mm, is inserted into the guides and used to make the holes (Fig. 12-5). A 7.5 mm locking screw is inserted perpendicular to the plate and tightened completely (Fig. 12-6). The screw heads should be flush with the plate to ensure the locking mechanism is engaged. The length of the screw is determined by the preoperative imaging studies (axial CT or MRI). Unicortical or bicortical

purchase may be obtained. The temporary screws are removed because they will obstruct proper placement of the ventral screws. The hole preparation and screw placement for the ventral screws is identical to the procedure for the dorsal screws. Sufficient retraction of the viscera will prevent soft tissue impingement on the plate holes and promote the proper perpendicular trajectory. It is paramount to seat the screws completely and to lock into the plate (Fig. 12-7) and establish the triangular geometry. This increases pull-out resistance. Postoperatively, patients should be braced with a thoracic or lumbosacral orthosis (TLSO) (Fig. 12-8). The Synthes ATLP is an excellent choice for straightforward, single level pathology not requiring extensive deformity correction.

A   B   C

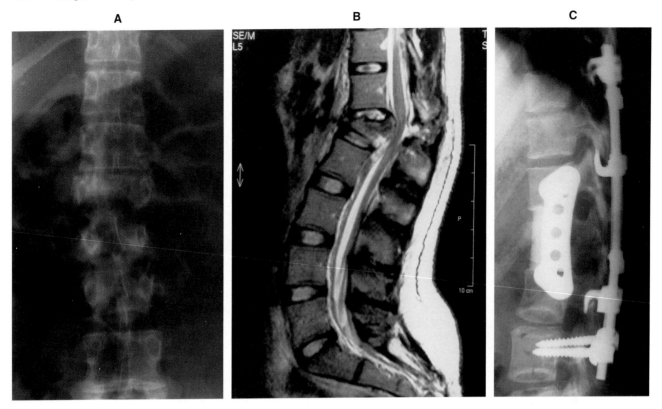

Fig. 12-8. ATLP—Case example L1 fracture/dislocation. **A,** AP thoracolumbar spine radiograph revealing increased interpedicular distance and loss of height at L1. **B,** T2-weighted sagittal MRI demonstrating retropulsed bone compressing conus medullaris and dorsal ligamentous disruption. **C,** Lateral thoracolumbar spine radiograph showing the ATLP from T12 to L2 with femoral strut allograft. Dorsal instrumentation was added due to three-column instability.

Kaneda Ventral Spinal System

The Kaneda Ventral Spinal System (AcroMed, Cleveland, Ohio) is designed for fixation from T9 to L4. It can span up to four motion segments. Advantages of this system include the ability to actively correct deformities by supplying forces via the vertebral body screws, and to perform meaningful graft compression. As a rod system, the Kaneda has the disadvantages of a higher profile as well as more cumbersome assembly compared with plating systems. A unique aspect of this system is the tetra-spiked plate that is placed on the lateral aspect of the vertebral body to act as a guide for screw placement and to decrease toggle. Fixation above T9 is difficult due to the size of the smallest spiked plate (15 × 26 mm).

The threaded rod that made this system difficult to assemble in the past has been replaced by a smooth rod, which is anchored by top tightening, open or closed head vertebral body screws. Both screw types are 6.25 mm in diameter, with lengths from 30 to 60 mm in 5 mm increments. Screw lengths are measured by length in bone only. Multisegmental constructs can be made with the placement of open head screws in the intervening vertebral bodies. Bicortical purchase is recommended for maximum pull-out strength as is the use of transverse rod couplers to increase construct stability. The system has a well proven track record for biomechanical rigidity and clinical effectiveness.[1,2,15,17,25,26,37]

Technique

After decompression and preparation of the graft site, the lateral aspect of the vertebral bodies must be "gardened" to ensure flush contact between the staple plate and the bone. The tetra-spiked plates are designed in pairs, rostral and caudal, with each side individually marked (Fig. 12-9). Proper plate placement produces a trapezoidal construct with the ventral rod greater in length than the dorsal rod. Three sizes—small, medium, or large—are

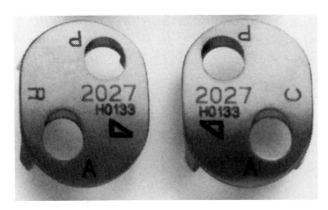

Fig. 12-9. Kaneda—Tetra-spiked plates are marked for correct orientation. A = anterior; P = posterior; R = rostral; C = caudal

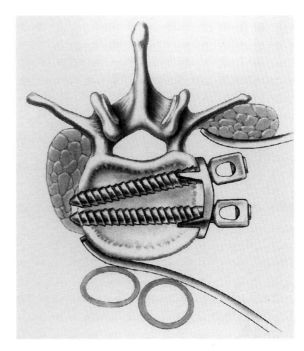

Fig. 12-11. Kaneda—Ventral screws parallel the dorsal cortex of the vertebral body while dorsal screws are directed 10 degrees away. Bicortical purchase and triangulation increase the pull-out resistance.

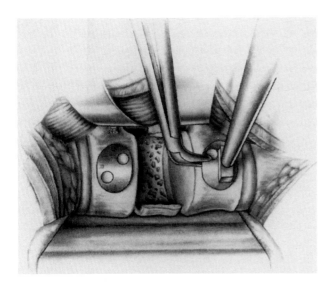

Fig. 12-10. Kaneda—Tetra-spiked plates are placed with the aid of the plate holder and plate impactor.

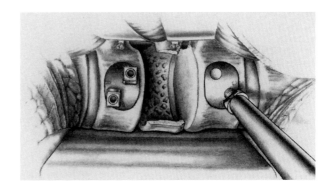

Fig. 12-12. Kaneda—Screws should be driven until the heads engage the plate and are aligned to facilitate rod placement.

available. The largest plate that fits the lateral surface of the body should be placed (Fig. 12-10). Screw length is determined from preoperative imaging studies or by direct measurement across the vertebral body. Kaneda recommends bicortical purchase be obtained with screws protruding no more than 2 mm beyond the cortex. This can be confirmed by radiography or by direct palpation after dissection of the contralateral vascular and/or visceral structures from the vertebral body. An awl is used to penetrate the cortex. The dorsal screw is placed at a 10-degree angle away from the canal, parallel to the end plate. The ventral screw is directed parallel to both the dorsal cortex of the vertebral body and the end plate (Fig. 12-11). The second set of screws is placed in the same fashion (Fig. 12-12). Open-headed screws

can be inserted into intervening vertebral bodies for multisegmental fixation. These screws must be placed through the spiked plates, precisely in line with the proposed path of the rod because Kaneda rods should not be bent. A distractor placed between the ventral screw heads is used to correct kyphotic deformities, as well as to separate the vertebral bodies for graft placement (Fig. 12-13). The bone graft should be countersunk at least 3 mm to allow for proper placement of the transverse couplers before closure. A gauge is provided to measure

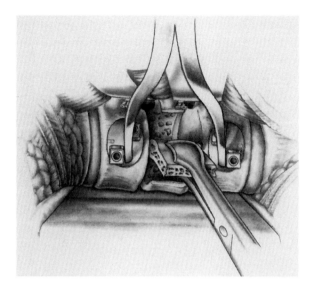

Fig. 12-13. Kaneda—The distractor is used to correct deformities and ensure proper graft placement.

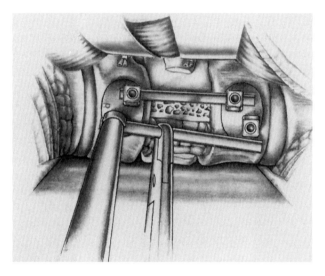

Fig. 12-14. Kaneda—Temporary rotation of one screw head by a small amount eases insertion of the rod.

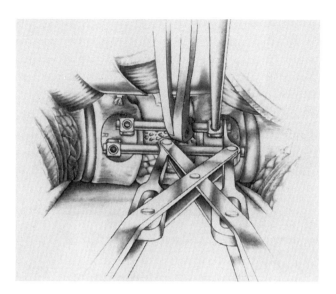

Fig. 12-15. Kaneda—Compression of the graft is accomplished over the rod holder and unsecured screw.

rod length; an overhang of 2 to 3 mm on each end should be sufficient to allow for placement of the compressor. It is helpful to have a screwdriver in place to rotate one of the screws, making rod insertion easier (Fig. 12-14). The dorsal rod can be fixated first to act as a fulcrum for further reduction of a kyphos. One set screw is completely tightened with the hex screwdriver, and a rod holder is placed approximately 2 cm from the other screw. The rod holder acts as an anchor for the compressor, which is placed across it and the unsecured screw (Fig. 12-15). Compression is applied and the hex set screw is

tightened. Further distraction can be used across the ventral screw heads if needed, but not to the degree of loosening the bone graft. If this occurs, a separate vertebral body spreader can be used temporarily, while the dorsal rod is removed and an appropriate size graft is inserted. Grafts that are poorly sized or not under compression may lead to construct failure. The ventral rod is secured in the same manner as the dorsal rod. If space permits, two transverse couplers should be placed, one close to each end of the construct. A template is provided to determine the proper coupler size. The coupler is loaded on a self-retaining wrench via the loosened bolt. The bottom portion of the coupler is positioned perpendicular to the top one to allow it to slip between the rods (Fig. 12-16). The lower portion is then maneuvered into final position by rotating the wrench followed by gentle upward tension to engage the rods. A torque wrench to 60 inch pounds is used for final tightening of all connectors (Figs. 12-17 and 12-18).

Z-Plate

The Z-Plate system (Sofamor-Danek, Memphis, Tenn.) combines the low-profile advantage of plates with the distraction and compression capabilities of vertebral body screws. The Z-Plate uses both rigid fixation bolts (fixed moment arm cantilevers) that are secured to the plate with nuts, and semirigid fixation via screws not secured to the plate (nonfixed moment arm cantilevers). Separate thoracic and

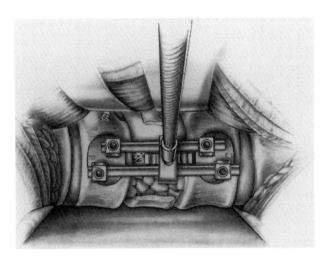

Fig. 12-16. Kaneda—The bottom portion of the transverse coupler is placed between the rods and then rotated into its final position.

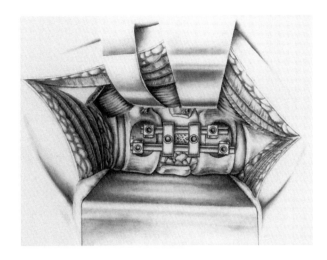

Fig. 12-17. Kaneda—The placement of two transverse couplers increases the stability of the construct. All screws should be torqued to 60 inch pounds.

lumbar plate sets exist, with the length of the plates ranging from 5 to 13 cm in 1 cm increments; thus making fixation as high as T3 and as low as L4 very feasible. The bolts are 7 mm in diameter, with lengths of 25 to 55 mm; the screws are 6.5 mm in diameter with lengths 30 to 60 mm, both in 5 mm increments. Distractive forces can be applied via the bolts, allowing for active reduction of deformities and graft placement. Compression of the graft can be accomplished as a result of the slots in the rostral end of the plate, which allow the bolts to slide before their fixation to the plate. The top tightening hardware and lack of rods and cross fixators promotes smooth assembly.

Technique

Z-Plates are shaped to accommodate the natural curvature of the lateral aspect of the vertebral bodies. All soft tissue and osteophytes must be removed to allow optimum contact of the plate to the vertebral bodies. The bolts and screws are designed for bicortical purchase. Their lengths should be determined accordingly. If no reduction is needed, a template can be used to aid in the determination of bolt entry points and plate size. The ideal entry point for the bolts is 8 to 10 mm caudal and ventral to the rostral, dorsal corner of the rostral vertebrae, and 8 to 10 mm rostral and ventral to the inferior, dorsal corner of the caudal vertebrae. An awl is used to perforate the cortex through a bolt positioning guide, which

maintains the desired 10 degree angulation away from the spinal canal (Fig. 12-19). The first bolt is inserted in this trajectory and parallel to the inferior end plate; the bolt should be driven so the head lies approximately halfway into the cortex (Fig. 12-20). The second bolt is inserted in an identical fashion with care taken to avoid dorsal cortex or end plate perforation. Deformity correction can be achieved by manual pressure maneuvers over the dorsal spine or via a lamina spreader placed in the corpectomy defect. A distractor, which is placed against the head of the bolts, is then used to maintain distraction for deformity reduction and graft placement (Fig. 12-21). When the graft is in place, the distractor is removed and interval between the bolts is measured with a template for plate sizing. The shortest plate possible is placed. Any tissues impeding full contact of the plate with the vertebral body should be removed. The nuts are placed on the nut starter shaft, with the collar of the nut toward the handle. Securing the nuts on the shaft by only one-half turn will speed their removal. The hex end of the starter shaft is inserted into the caudal bolt and the socket is advanced to engage the nut (Fig. 12-22). While maintaining counter torque on the bolt, the nut is tightened to finger tight. This process is repeated on the rostral bolt, with the nut tightened only enough to secure it on the bolt. The starter shafts are left in place and the compressor is placed around the base of the shafts (Fig. 12-23). While compression is performed, the shafts should be held

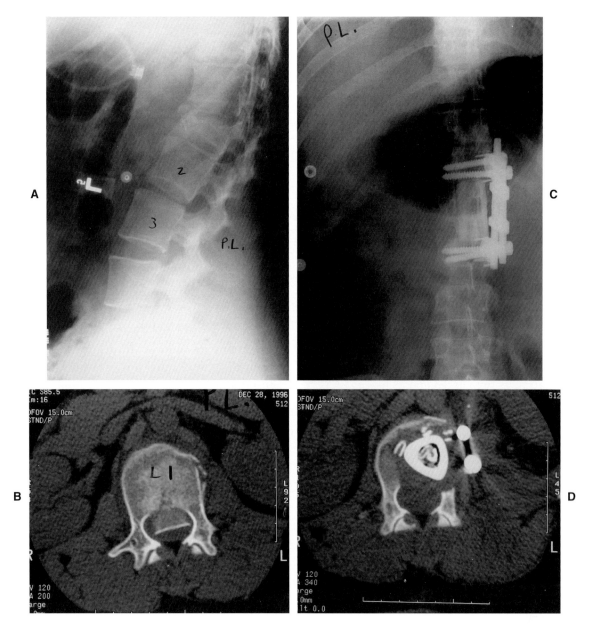

Fig. 12-18. Kaneda—Case example L1 burst fracture. **A,** Lateral thoracolumbar spine radiograph demonstrating loss of height of ventral and middle columns at L1. **B,** Axial CT of L1 revealing retropulsed bone and greater than 50% canal compromise. **C,** AP thoracolumbar spine radiograph of Kaneda device fixation at T12 to L2. **D,** Axial CT of L1 demonstrating decompressed spinal canal; femoral strut allograft is filled with morsellated vertebral bone.

parallel by an assistant to maintain even forces. The nuts are then tightened with a starter wrench while both compression on the shafts and counter torque on the bolts are maintained (Fig. 12-24). Compression is released and the nuts are tightened to 80 inch pounds with the torque wrench. The shafts are removed after placement of the bolts is completed. Preparation for ventral screw placement is initiated by perforating the cortex through the plate

with an awl. The rostral screws should be placed as close as possible but not into the inferior end plate. The length of screws needs to be 5 mm longer than the bolts to achieve bicortical purchase. Screws may be directed parallel to or up to 10 degrees toward the dorsal cortex, and are driven in with the screwdriver without tapping (Fig. 12-25). An intraoperative radiograph is obtained to ensure adequate placement before the crimping of the nut collars, which will help

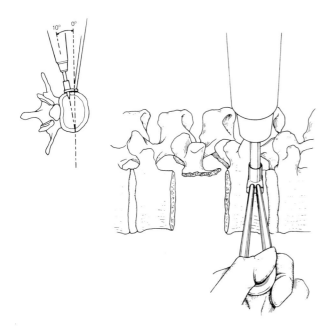

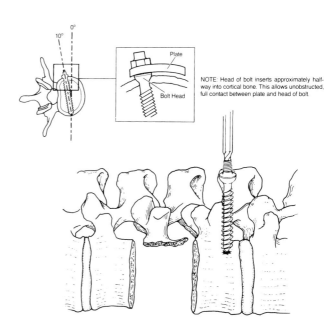

Fig. 12-19. Z-Plate—Initial cortex perforation is performed with an awl through a bolt positioning guide. The desired trajectory is 10 degrees away from the parallel of the dorsal cortex.

Fig. 12-20. Z-Plate—The 7 mm bolt is driven in this trajectory until the head seats halfway into the cortex.

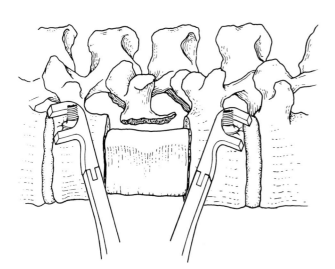

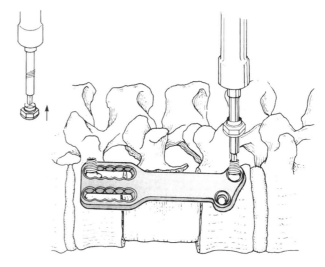

Fig. 12-21. Z-Plate—The reduced spine is held in position by the distractor, allowing for proper measurement and placement of the graft.

Fig. 12-22. Z-Plate—After placement of the nut on the starter shaft, the hex end is inserted into the bolt and the socket is advanced to engage the nut.

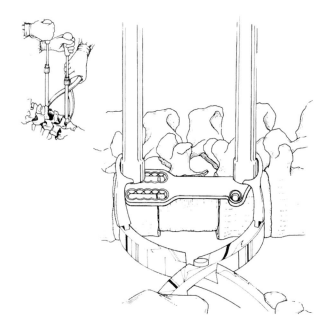

Fig. 12-23. Z-Plate—The starter shafts are held parallel while compression is applied to the graft.

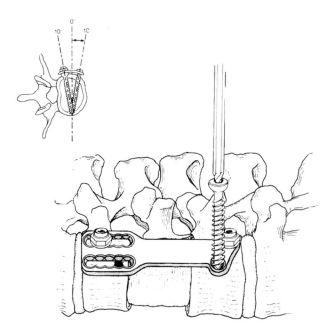

Fig. 12-25. Z-Plate—The 6.5 mm screws are driven at an angle parallel or up to 10 degrees toward the dorsal cortex.

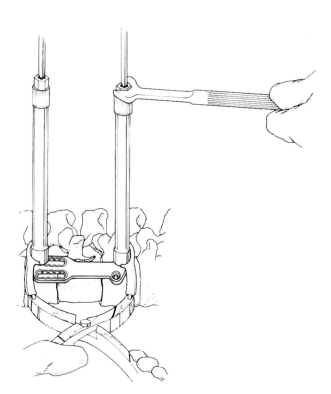

Fig. 12-24. Z-Plate—The nuts are tightened during compression while counter torque is maintained on the bolts with the hex-head screwdrivers.

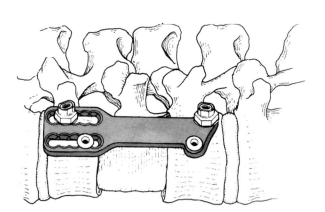

Fig. 12-26. Z-Plate—The nut collars are crimped to prevent postoperative loosening.

prevent postoperative loosening of the nuts (Fig. 12-26). Standard postoperative care should be performed, including standing anteroposterior and lateral radiographs to rule out progressive deformity and construct failure with weight bearing (Fig. 12-27).

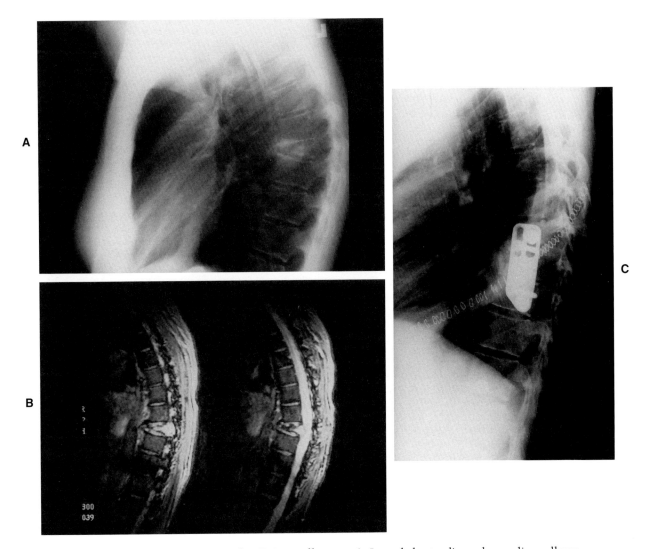

Fig. 12-27. Z-Plate—Case example T7 giant cell tumor. **A,** Lateral chest radiograph revealing collapse of T7 vertebral body. **B,** T2-weighted sagittal MRI demonstrating increased intensity in T7 body with canal compromise. **C,** Lateral chest radiograph showing thoracic Z-Plate fixation of T6 to T8 with humerus strut allograft.

CONCLUSION

The ventral approach to the thoracic spine is a powerful method for addressing pathological conditions that affect the ventral and middle columns. Instrumentation provides immediate rigidity to promote solid arthrodesis. Indications include neoplasm, trauma, infection, and deformity. Proper preoperative radiographic evaluation includes plain radiographs, which aid in quantifying instability and osteopenia; CT for evaluating bony anatomy and degree of canal compromise; and MRI to evaluate the soft tissues. Both CT and MRI can be used to determine vertebral body screw lengths. Proper patient positioning is the foundation for successful surgery and should aid surgeon orientation for optimum instrument placement.

A number of approaches exist for access to the ventral thoracic spine. The method chosen must provide adequate access to the levels that will be instrumented, as well as the level of the pathology. Before decompression, it is essential to "garden" all levels of the spine that will be instrumented to optimize implant-to-bone surface contact. The choice of bone graft, as well as its preparation (and that of the fusion bed) are paramount to the success of the procedure. Even the most rigid of implants will fail without bony union.

A number of instrumentation systems exist to fixate the ventral thoracic spine. The Synthes Anterior Thoracolumbar Locking Plate System is a rigid, cantilever beam plate that uses unicortical screws and is excellent for cases with minimal deformity. The Kaneda system is a rigid, cantilever beam rod system that uses bicortical screws and can be used to actively correct deformities as well as provide multisegmental fixation in long constructs. The Z-Plate is a rigid/semirigid cantilever beam plate that uses bicortical screw purchase. It can be applied to nearly every level of the thoracic spine.

REFERENCES

1. Abumi K, Panjabi MM, Duranceau J. Biomechanical fixation of spinal fixation devices. III. Stability provided by six spinal fixation devices and interbody bone graft. Spine 14: 1249-1255, 1989.
2. An HS, Lim TH, You JW, Hong JH, Eck J, McGrady L. Biomechanical evaluation of anterior thoracolumbar spinal instrumentation. Spine 20:1979-1983, 1995.
3. Anderson TM, Mansour KA, Miller JI. Thoracic approaches to anterior spinal operations: Anterior thoracic approaches. Ann Thorac Surg 55:1447-1452, 1993.
4. Apel A, Marrero G, King J, Tolo V, Bassett G. Avoiding paraplegia during anterior spinal surgery: The role of SSEP monitoring with temporary occlusion of segmental spinal arteries. Spine 16:S365-S370, 1991.
5. Bedbrook GM. Treatment of thoracolumbar dislocations and fractures with paraplegia. Clin Orthop 112:27-43, 1975.
6. Cantor JB, Lebwohl NH, Garvey T, Eismont FJ. Nonoperative management of stable thoracolumbar burst fractures with early ambulation and bracing. Spine 18:971-976, 1993.
7. Cooper PR, Errico TJ, Martin R, Crawford B, DiBartolo T. A systematic approach to spinal reconstruction after anterior decompression for neoplastic disease of the thoracic and lumbar spine. Neurosurgery 32:1-8, 1993.
8. Errico TJ, Cooper PR. A new method of thoracic and lumbar body replacement for spinal tumors. Technical note. Neurosurgery 32:678-680, 1993.
9. Findlay GF. Adverse effects of the management of malignant spinal cord compression. J Neurol Neurosurg Psychiatry 47:761-768,1984.
10. Forbes HJ, Allen PW, Waller CS. Spinal cord monitoring in scoliosis surgery. J Bone Joint Surg 73B:487-491,1974.
11. Frankel HL, Hancock DO, Hyslop GM, et al. The value of postural reduction in the management of closed injuries of the spine with paraplegia and tetraplegia. Paraplegia 7:179-192,1969.
12. Friedlander GE. Bone grafts, the basic science rationale for clinical applications. J Bone Joint Surg 69A:786-790,1987.
13. Gilbert RW, Kim JH, Posner JB. Epidural spinal cord compression from metastatic tumor: Diagnosis and treatment. Ann Neurol 3:40-51, 1978.
14. Goto T, Crosby G. Anesthesia and the spinal cord. Anesth Clin North Am 10:493-519,1992.
15. Gurr KR, McAfee PC, Shih CM. Biomechanical analysis of anterior and posterior instrumentation systems after corpectomy. J Bone Joint Surg 70A:1182-1191,1988.
16. Herdmann J, Deletis V, Edmonds HL, Morota N. Spinal cord and nerve root monitoring in spine surgery and related procedures. Spine 21:879-885,1996.
17. Kaneda K, Taneichi H, Abumi K, Hashimoto T, Satoh S, Fujiya M. Anterior decompression and stabilization with the Kaneda device for thoracolumbar burst fractures associated with neurological deficits. J Bone Joint Surg 79A:69-83,1997.
18. Kostuik JP. Anterior spinal cord decompression for lesions of the thoracic and lumbar spine, techniques, new methods of internal fixation results. Spine 8:512-531, 1983.
19. Kostuik JP. Point of view. Spine 21:1233-1234, 1996.
20. Kostuik JP. Adult Scoliosis. In Frymoyer JW, ed. The Adult Spine: Principles and practice, 2nd ed. Philadelphia: Lippincott-Raven, 1997, pp 1579-1621.
21. Levy WJ, York DH. Evoked potentials from the motor tracts in humans. Neurosurgery 12:422-429, 1983.
22. Mumford J, Weinstein JN, Spratt KF, Goel VK. Thoracolumbar burst fractures: The clinical efficacy and outcome of nonoperative management. Spine 18:955-970,1993.
23. Muschler GF, Lane JM, Dawson EG. The biology of spinal fusion. In Cotler JM, Cotler HP, eds. Spinal Fusion Science and Technique. Berlin: Springer-Verlag, 1990, pp 9-21.
24. Oga M, Arizono T, Takasita M, Sugioka Y. Evaluation of the risk of instrumentation as a foreign body in spinal tuberculosis: Clinical and biologic study. Spine 18:1890-1894, 1993.
25. Shono Y, Kaneda K, Yamamoto I. A biomechanical analysis of Zielke, Kaneda, and Cotrel-Dubousset instrumentations in thoracolumbar scoliosis—A calf spine model. Spine 16:1305-1311,1991.
26. Shono Y, McAfee PC, Cunningham BW. Experimental study of thoracolumbar burst fractures—A radiographic and biomechanical analysis of anterior and posterior instrumentation systems. Spine 19:1711-1722,1994.
27. Siegal T, Siegal T. Surgical decompression of anterior and posterior malignant epidural tumors compressing the spinal cord: A prospective study. Neurosurgery 17:424-432, 1985.
28. Siegal T, Siegal T. Current considerations in the management of neoplastic spinal cord compression. Spine 14: 223-228, 1989.
29. Simonds RJ. HIV transmission by organ and tissue transplantation. AIDS 7:S35-S38, 1993.
30. Sundaresan N, Digiacinto GV, Hughes JE. Surgical treatment of spinal metastases. Clin Neurosurg 33:503-522, 1986.
31. Sundaresan N, Galicich JH, Bains MS, Martini N, Beattie EJ. Vertebral body resection in the treatment of cancer involving the spine. Cancer 53:1393-1396, 1984.
32. Whitecloud TS. Complications of anterior cervical fusion. Instr Course Lect 27:223-227, 1976.
33. Winter RB. Combined Dwyer and Harrington instrumentation and fusion in the treatment of selected patients with painful adult idiopathic scoliosis. Spine 3:135-141, 1978.
34. Winter RB, Lonstein JE, Denis F, Leonard AS, Garamella JJ. Paraplegia resulting from vessel ligation. Spine 21:1232-1233, 1996.
35. Wittenberg RH, Moeller J, Shea M, White AA, Hayes WC. Compressive strength of autologous and allogenous bone grafts for thoracolumbar and cervical spine fusion. Spine 15:1073-1078,1990.
36. Young RF, Post EM, King GA. Treatment of spinal epidural metastases. Randomized prospective comparison of laminectomy and radiotherapy. J Neurosurg 53:741-748,1980.
37. Zdeblick TA, Warden KE, Zou D, McAfee PC, Abitbol JJ. Anterior spinal fixators—A biomechanical in vitro study. Spine 18:513-517,1993.

Spinal Instrumentation: Dorsal Techniques

Seth M. Zeidman, M.D., and David Polly, M.D.

Dorsal spinal instrumentation is a well established and documented treatment modality for a variety of conditions affecting the thoracic spine. The primary advantage of dorsal spinal instrumentation is that it combines well-known techniques with a dorsal midline approach. Its development for the management of various spinal conditions (trauma, neoplasms, and infection) evolved directly from the treatment of severe, progressive spinal deformities. This chapter reviews the major concepts and instrumentation systems applicable to thoracic and thoracolumbar spinal pathology.

HISTORY

The first report of dorsal spinal instrumentation was by Wilkins[23] who treated a newborn with spinal dislocation. Following open reduction, he used silver wire to maintain spinal alignment. In 1904 Lang[17] inserted 4 mm rods along the spinous processes and sewed them in with silk sutures. However, suppuration and suture breakage soon followed. The subsequent development of nonreactive metals allowed screws and other hardware to be implanted in long bones. In 1944 King[16] passed screws through the facet joints in an effort to rigidly "fix" an articulation, and thereby enhance the fusion rate. In 1959 Boucher[3] attempted to improve the

probability of achieving a solid arthrodesis by using longer screws that were angled into the pedicle. In 1963 Roy-Camille[22] improved the pedicle screw technique by interconnecting the screws with a plate. A number of pedicle screw, rod, and plate systems have since gained wide acceptance. It was within this environment that dorsal thoracic spinal instrumentation evolved.

With each advance, surgeons encountered new complications or problems. It is important to reflect on each of these problems lest we be condemned to repeat them as we apply newer techniques.

The fundamental means of fixation to the vertebral column remains the same. The current mechanisms by which a surgeon can grip the spine is via hooks, wires (or cables), or screws. Each of these mechanisms has relative advantages and disadvantages. The anatomy occasionally dictates one choice over another (e.g., if there is no lamina, a laminar hook is not an option). Through the connection of these anchors to longitudinal members (such as rods, plates, or cables, etc.), forces can be applied to achieve the desired operative goal. A race between biology and biomechanics to achieve the desired result subsequently ensues. Will the fusion mature or will the construct fatigue and fail?

Although spine surgeons have many tools at their disposal, ultimately, these tools are founded on underlying principles. The surgeon attempts to obtain and maintain optimal alignment. In turn, the ultimate solution for maintaining alignment is the achievement of a solid fusion.

The ultimate goal is a balanced, pain-free, stable spine centered over the pelvis. This should be achieved with fusion of the minimum number of motion segments. This remains a daunting task in the face of significant deformity and instability. To attain this result, the surgeon must understand the desired surgical solution, the available technology (i.e., instrumentation), and the imposed biological limitations.

Spine surgeons are only able to decompress compromised neural structures and to fuse motion segments. Despite the level of sophistication and complexity of available instrumentation systems, this remains a rather crude solution.

INDICATIONS FOR DORSAL INSTRUMENTATION

The historical development of dorsal spinal instrumentation for the management of various spinal conditions (trauma, neoplasms, and infection) evolved directly from the strategies used for the treatment of severe progressive spinal deformities, specifically neuromuscular scoliosis resulting from polio.[15]

Spinal implants are used to stabilize involved (unstable) motion segment(s). This allows for the acquisition of immediate postoperative mechanical stability and provides an environment that encourages bone fusion. Instrumentation is nearly always performed in conjunction with arthrodesis. If bony fusion does not occur, the construct is destined to fail. The general indications for fusion and instrumentation of the spine are to provide stability to the unstable spine, decrease deformity, increase the probability of fusion, prevent neurological injury, and decrease pain.

There is an increased incidence of solid arthrodesis in patients treated with internal fixation compared with those treated without instrumentation, although the clinical relevance of this increased incidence of fusion may be contested.[11]

Ventral vs. Dorsal Spinal Instrumentation

An advantage of using dorsal spinal instrumentation is the well-known and familiar dorsal midline exposure. Additionally, the spinal hardware remains farther away from prevertebral structures (i.e., aorta, vena cava, chest and abdominal cavities) than with ventral implants. Conditions in which dorsal neural compression or significant dorsal column ligamentous insufficiency are the predominant findings are best treated by a dorsal approach.

Deformity

Historically, dorsal spinal instrumentation began with neuromuscular scoliosis and the use of Harrington instrumentation.[13,15] The treatment of scoliosis involves restoring alignment of both the thoracic and lumbar spine. The indications for surgery in an adult with an idiopathic scoliotic curvature are pain relief, neurological dysfunction, prevention of further deformity, and cosmesis. Determining the site of pain generation and predicting its surgical relief remains one of the more difficult and daunting tasks in spinal surgery.

Trauma

Trauma is one of the most common pathological diagnoses encountered by spine surgeons in the thoracic and thoracolumbar regions. Dorsal spinal instrumentation is an established and well-documented treatment modality for trauma. Dorsal surgery takes less time, causes less blood loss, and is less expensive than ventral or combined ventral and dorsal surgery for traumatic spinal injury.[5] Dorsal instrumentation provides solid internal fixation with restoration of the sagittal profile without loss of correction. Rods are contoured to approximate the normal thoracic kyphosis, as well as the lumbar lordotic curve, should instrumentation across the thoracolumbar junction be required.

Neoplasms

Neoplasms, both primary and metastatic, can affect the vertebral body as well as the dorsal elements. Primary and metastatic tumors of the spinal column cause pain, instability, deformity, and neurological deficits. Metastatic lesions are more common than primary spinal tumors and are present in 20% to 70% of patients with malignancies. The definition of instability for tumors of the spinal column usually incorporates the three-column theory of Denis.[7]

The goals of surgery are to relieve pain, decompress the neural elements, and provide immediate mechanical stability. The approach and fusion technique may be ventral, dorsal, or a combination of the two. Because the vertebral body is involved in 85% of metastases, the benefit of the ventral approach for adequate decompression and fusion is clear.

Infection

Infections of the spinal column require surgical debridement and spinal reconstruction to maximize eradication of the infection and to maintain spinal alignment. Indications for instrumentation include infection progression with bony destruction of more than 50% of the vertebral body despite adequate antibiotic therapy, progressive angulation, new or increasing neurological deficit, and surgically created spinal instability.

Traditionally, debridement and stabilization were performed as separate procedures, with a prolonged interval between the procedures to minimize the possibility of infecting the hardware or graft material. However, primary reconstruction with instrumentation can be performed in acute spinal infections without infecting the inserted graft material or hardware. Successful management depends on aggressive debridement of the infectious foci and prolonged treatment with parenteral antibiotics.[8]

PREOPERATIVE EVALUATION
Imaging

Appropriate imaging studies are essential for preoperative planning. Adequate preoperative radiographic studies can potentially help to avert intra- or postoperative catastrophes.

Plain radiographs of the area of interest are critical to the performance of any operative procedure on the thoracic spine. They provide insight into the pathology in a manner not always apparent on more complex or detailed studies such as computed tomography (CT) and magnetic resonance imaging (MRI). They also provide a straightforward means to plan out the surgical approach and to determine the instrumentation to be used at each level. It is often important to carefully measure and assess the level of involvement on multiple studies.

Operating at the wrong level is not uncommon. Intraoperatively, the pathology may not be apparent until significant bony resection is completed. Trusting the counting and marking skills of colleagues, including radiologists, can be the source for problems in identifying the proper level, particularly in the thoracic spine. Relying on others to identify the level of interest will dramatically increase the likelihood of error. One must trust no one but oneself in this regard.

Upright, preferably standing, radiographs of the entire spine are needed to measure the amount of decompensation in the frontal and sagittal planes. Supine radiographs, with a firm wedge at the apex of the deformity, permit assessment of curve flexibility. Flexion/extension films should be considered if potentially dangerous clinical instability is not a concern.

For assessment of bony elements, CT is preferred. CT also provides excellent bony detail and permits an accurate assessment of spinal canal and pedicle size. CT also provides an important window to bony anatomy and involvement that is not always apparent on MRI. CT-myelography permits the assessment of the neural elements within the spinal canal, even if hardware is in place. Occasionally, three-dimensional CT imaging is of value.

MRI is the study of choice for assessing the degree of spinal cord compression and to precisely evaluate soft tissues. If there is no hardware in the field of interest, MRI provides visualization of the soft tissue component of the spinal column. It can identify spinal cord deformation, atrophy, or syrinx. MRI is preferred over CT-myelography as the evaluation of choice for most procedures requiring decompression.

Quite frequently, such as in cases of metastatic disease to the spine, MRI and CT provide complementary information. MRI provides excellent views of the soft tissues and CT views the bony structures well.

PREOPERATIVE EVALUATION AND PERIOPERATIVE MANAGEMENT

A thorough history should be obtained, including a detailed history of the present illness. A detailed physical examination should also be performed. The history determines whether the patient's symptoms warrant surgical intervention. It is important to exclude metabolic abnormalities, which can affect patients of all ages. All surgical patients should undergo preoperative evaluation by an anesthesiologist. Preoperative pulmonary consultation is warranted in patients with significant deformities or underlying pulmonary disorders. Autologous blood donation may be considered before any significant spinal procedure that might potentially require blood transfusion. A cell saver is often used, when not contraindicated. Prophylactic antibiotics are begun before surgery and continued for 48 hours postoperatively.

SURGERY
Positioning

General endotracheal anesthesia, pneumatic sequential compression stockings, and appropriate vascular access are used before positioning. The patient is positioned on a radiolucent operative frame in the prone position. The frame allows the abdomen and thorax to be free of pressure, reducing epidural venous distention. The anterior superior iliac spine region is carefully protected, because the lateral cutaneous nerve of the thigh is vulnerable to pressure application. Postoperative meralgia paresthetica may otherwise result. Fortunately, this complication is usually temporary. The positioning of the head is determined by the anesthesiologist, but usually a head rest is preferred. An adjustable fluoroscopic image intensifier may be used to provide intraoperative anteroposterior, oblique, and lateral radiographic imaging of the spine.

Monitoring
Intraoperative Monitoring

The use of somatosensory-evoked potentials (SSEPs) and or motor-evoked potentials (MEPs) has greatly aided the surgeon in assessing neurological difficulties. SSEP monitoring of the spinal cord during thoracic spinal surgery has been the standard of electrophysiological intraoperative monitoring.

Evoked potentials may be obtained through either cortical-evoked or spinal-evoked techniques. However, there may be a latency period of up to 20 minutes following injury before they can be recorded. A survey of members of the Scoliosis Research Society and the European Spinal Deformity Society revealed that despite intraoperative SSEP monitoring, 28% of neurological deficits were undetected.[6]

MEPs have been gaining wider application in recent years. Owen, Bridwell, and Grubb[21] reported 300 cases monitored with MEPs. Motor pathways within the spinal cord are stimulated with needle electrodes inserted into the spinous processes of the two intact levels immediately rostral to the zone of surgery and are recorded by electrodes over the tibial nerve behind the knee. The true value of MEPs with regard to the integrity of the ventrolateral motor pathways remains to be definitively proven.

SURGICAL APPROACHES

Exposure of the dorsal thoracic spine is rather straightforward regardless of the level because of the superficial location of the spinous processes, laminae, and transverse processes.

Before making the skin incision, the authors infiltrate the skin and underlying paraspinal musculature with local anesthetic, typically xylocaine or bupivacane. An appropriate midline incision is made, extending 2 to 3 inches above and below the segments to be instrumented. Meticulous subperiosteal dissection is performed out to the lateral tips of the transverse processes of the segments to be fused. This maximizes the amount of bone mass available to serve as bone surface for fusion. Careful attention to the integrity of the facet joints of the levels adjacent to the segments to be fused helps to prevent future transitional instability syndromes. Before instrumentation placement, neural decompression and/or vertebral body decompression is performed as indicated.

DORSAL SPINAL INSTRUMENTATION
General Principles

Dorsal implants are indicated for the treatment of dorsal, circumferential, or torsional disruption of the spinal column. They can also be used to treat ventral instability when ventral surgery is contraindicated, such as in the elderly and patients in poor medical condition and/or poor cardiopulmonary reserve. When spinal fixation is required in patients with osteoporosis or nonsegmental deformity, a dorsal device is generally indicated because it can provide multiple segment fixation.

Modern implants allow three-column purchase and provide more rotational stability than ventral devices. When properly used, they are associated with minimal risk of neurological injury.

Dorsal spinal instrumentation is safer to apply, biomechanically superior, and easier to remove than ventral implants. The complications associated with ventral approaches (e.g., pulmonary injury, bowel injury, injury to the great vessels) are avoided. Placement dorsal to the spine and away from the great vessels minimizes the potential for vascular injury.

DORSAL INSTRUMENTATION SYSTEMS
Harrington Instrumentation

In 1953 Paul Harrington assumed the care of children with progressive neuromuscular scoliosis. He sought a means to treat this complex and difficult clinical entity. These patients' pulmonary status often precluded cast treatment and the results of noninstrumented fusion were poor. Initially, he attempted to instrument the deformed spine without arthrodesis. He achieved excellent initial correction, but was unable to maintain the correction and rod breakage frequently occurred. Once the fusion was added, his results dramatically improved.

In 1960 Harrington[13] reported his initial results with instrumentation for polio patients with neuromuscular scoliosis. Harrington rods quickly became the standard of care for the treatment of scoliosis and were widely used and modified to improve stability from the 1960s through the 1980s. Harrington rods were used not only for scoliosis but also for fractures, tumors, and degenerative conditions.

Harrington spinal instrumentation is a system of stainless steel rods and hooks designed to achieve purchase on the dorsal elements of the axial skeleton from the first thoracic vertebra to the sacrum. The system is composed of two principle elements: (1) distraction rods, which are adjusted by means of a ratchet mechanism, and (2) compression rods, which are adjusted by the threaded rod and nut principle. The Harrington system is most useful in situations in which the axial thoracolumbar spine is destabilized.

Harrington Distraction Rods (HDR)

The initial Harrington dorsal spinal instrumentation system relies on rods with a ratchet on one end

and a hub on the other. The rods are connected to the dorsal bony elements by sublaminar or intrafacet hooks. The end of the rod with the ratchet locking mechanism is placed through the rostral hook. This locking ratchet design enables axial forces to be applied to the hooks. In addition to the pure distractive forces generated, a three-point or sagittal bending force is created by the rod contacting the laminae. These two forces serve to stabilize and correct flexion deformities. Bilateral distraction may restore vertebral body height compromised by axial loading, and on occasion can reduce retrodisplaced bone and disc fragments from within the spinal canal by means of ligamentotaxis. In order to reconstruct the spinal canal, while avoiding overdistraction, the anterior and posterior longitudinal ligaments must be intact.

The Harrington distraction system is useful for the treatment of early idiopathic scoliosis. For the stabilization of the traumatized spine, distraction rods are indicated when the anterior longitudinal ligament is preserved.

Numerous advancements have evolved over time.[10,15] To improve the deficiencies in rotational support, cross wiring between the rods and sublaminar wiring was introduced. Loss of physiological lordosis led to the flat back syndrome. To avoid this, rods were prebent to conform to the normal lumbar lordosis and thoracic kyphosis. The Harrington rods are rigid and difficult to contour. Sleeves were developed to slide over the rods and contact the laminae, providing a ventrally oriented vector force that helps maintain lordosis (three-point bending fixation) without the need for excessive rod bending.[10] In an effort to reduce the high incidence of hook dislocation, square-ended rods and hooks were introduced. Moe's squaring of the end of the rod and distal hook resulted in greater rotational control.[15]

Originally, the Harrington system was used for the treatment of idiopathic scoliosis. It appeared to be quite safe in this scenario. Today, Harrington dorsal instrumentation is rarely indicated for the treatment of adult scoliosis. It has several disadvantages, including limited derotating ability and the loss of lumbar lordosis. Loss of lumbar lordosis often occurs with this distracting device, even with the use of sacroalar hooks, contouring, or square-ended rods. Currently, the use of the Harrington system is appropriate for single thoracic and thoracolumbar scoliotic curves that do not require concomitant low lumbar fusion. Harrington constructs continue to be used to treat traumatic fracture dislocations.

There are several distinct disadvantages associated with Harrington rods. The original round-ended rods did not allow sagittal contouring. The importance of sagittal contour was not appreciated in the 1950s and 1960s. By its very nature distraction instrumentation induces kyphosis, producing the flat back syndrome, especially when used in the lumbar spine.

Other disadvantages of the HDR system include the need to provide long-segment fixation, the high incidence of rod breakage in the presence of nonunion, the limited ability to derotate the spine, and the potential for significant neurological complications.

Additional disadvantages of the Harrington system include (1) the forces of the system are applied directly to the upper and lower ends of the construct, (2) limited derotating ability, (3) flat back syndrome, (4) limited usefulness in translational injuries, (5) the system is entirely hook dependent, and (6) the need to rod long and fuse short.

Harrington Compression Rods

Harrington not only developed distraction instrumentation, but also a compression system.[14] He recognized that the simple distraction rod did not provide rigid fixation. It was routine to apply a body cast after the procedure so that hook dislodgment did not occur. The Harrington compression system was designed to facilitate the application of spinal compression instrumentation. By using compression instrumentation at the same time as distraction instrumentation, better fixation and better correction was achieved. Minor modifications of the hooks and the principles of application (such as wiring together the spinous processes above and below the lower hook so that it did not dislodge) have frequently been made.

Harrington compression rods were probably the earliest form of multilevel or segmental spinal fixation. The compression rods are threaded and are smaller in diameter than those used for distraction. Hooks are used to anchor the rod to the spinal column. Above T11, down-facing hooks are placed over the transverse processes. Up-facing hooks are placed in the facet joints. Small nuts are threaded onto the rod and tightened above each hook to produce compression and three-point bending forces. The Harrington compression rod acts as a hinge, producing a tension-band effect. Harrington compression rods are used to rotate the spine around its sagittal axis into extension. The compression system provides torsional support and resists flexion better than does the distraction system. The instrumentation is most useful in counteracting tension failure due to dorsal element disruption or in providing compression across an interbody graft. In scoliosis, these rods are used to enhance fixation of the thoracic spine and help preserve the lumbar lordosis. The system tends to fail at the bone-metal juncture by fracturing the transverse process, facet, or lamina.

Harrington instrumentation gave the surgeon a significant increase in corrective capability, but at the same time created a greater risk of neurological injury. There have been several solutions to this problem. One was the development of the wake-up test, which allows intraoperative assessment of the integrity of the spinal cord. Subsequently, the development and refinement of spinal cord monitoring provides a method of continuously monitoring the integrity of the spinal cord. Both methods, however, are not foolproof. Harrington instrumentation also caused sagittal plane problems. As the three-dimensional nature of scoliosis became better understood, the concept of normal spinal balance was better appreciated. Additionally, Harrington instrumentation requires long lever arms to apply corrective forces. This led to the instrumentation and fusion of normal levels even in cases in which the system was subsequently removed. Moreover, Harrington instrumentation was often inadequate for treating many destabilizing injuries, particularly when ventral column failure was present. This would often lead to late kyphotic deformity. McAfee and Bohlman[20] reported a variety of late complications associated with Harrington instrumentation for thoracolumbar fractures. These included overdistraction, fractures, loosening of the implants, infection, and lack of reduction of the fracture with resultant neurological deficit.

Luque Instrumentation

In the 1970s Eduardo Luque of Mexico City developed a segmental fixation system using sublaminar wires for the treatment of severe progressive scoliotic deformities.[18] Although Harrington's use of compression instrumentation was segmental, Luque pioneered segmental fixation. Segmental spinal fixation, in which multiple segments of the spine were fixed by the instrumentation, allowed stabilization and correction of three-dimensional deformities. Luque rod multisegmental fixation with sublaminar wiring was designed to specifically remedy the lack of segmental fixation with the Harrington system.[19] Immobilizing each vertebral level distributes the load throughout the construct and enhances resistance to flexion, extension, and rotation at each segment.

The instrumentation was designed because of a necessity for immediate stabilization of the curves in patients who often were lost to follow-up or who would not or could not comply with postoperative bracing. An additional consideration was overall cost. Sublaminar wires permitted the sequential application of corrective forces across multiple fixation points. Because of this, adjunctive postoperative immobilization was unnecessary.

The Luque system consists of solid, smooth, stainless steel rods of 3/16 or 1/4 inch diameter that are either straight, prebent in an L shape or in the form of rectangular loops. Segmental fixation to the dorsal bony elements using sublaminar wires is the conventional method of spinal attachment. The rods are contoured to conform to the sagittal alignment of the spine. The wires are gradually tightened. Prebent L rods enable the two rods to be arranged into a closed loop system. This helps prevent rod rotation, migration, and telescoping. The Luque loop or rectangle obviates the need to wire the two rods together and offers greater resistance to axial loading and rotation.

Limitations of this system include the potential neurological complications attendant to sublaminar preparation and the passage of wires, the possibility of cerebrospinal fluid (CSF) fistulas, difficulty of removal, and the inability to provide multiple plane corrective forces (e.g., distraction and compression). Luque instrumentation was initially reported to be associated with a higher probability of neurological risk. This may have been because this technique required the passage of multiple sublaminar wires, with a concomitant risk of neurological injury. Greater attention to detail when using the technique appears to have obviated most of this risk. Also, the strength of sublaminar fixation with wire, for the

slow correction of deformity, minimized the risk of sudden, catastrophic lamina failure that was so commonly observed with prolonged hook distraction.

The Luque technique requires intact dorsal elements, rendering it inappropriate for many fractures. If dorsal element involvement is present, it often requires the incorporation of an excessive number of multiple noninjured levels. Furthermore, it is difficult to apply corrective forces or to prevent additional angulation.

Advantages of the Luque system include the relative ease of application and superior fixation compared to the Harrington system. The Luque system does not resist axial loads well and should not be used in cases in which the ventral columns are destabilized.

The use of sublaminar wires in conjunction with Harrington distraction instrumentation allowed the application of distraction (which was not possible with Luque rods) and segmental wire fixation with lateral and sagittal correction. Drummond,[9] who was concerned with the neurological risk associated with the passage of sublaminar wires, modified their use via the so-called Wisconsin wire technique. With this technique, the wires were passed through the base of the spinous processes and lateral corrective force applied through a button on the far side of the spinous processes.

A major advance in conjunction with Luque instrumentation was the development of the Galveston technique by Allen and Ferguson.[1] Although Harrington had developed a sacral bar, fixation to the pelvis for long segment fusions was challenging and unsatisfactory. The placement of smooth rods into the ilium allowed for adequate fixation to aid in the correction of pelvic obliquity, a fairly common problem in neuromuscular scoliosis.

Dorsal segmental instrumentation using sublaminar wires has been largely replaced by the use of multilevel hooks and/or pedicle screws. For the treatment of deformity, the universal spinal instrumentation (USI) systems combine the rigidity of segmental fixation with the ability to perform derotation and the ability to aggressively correct deformities.

Universal Spinal Instrumentation

USI systems are characterized by a rod that is segmentally affixed to the spine via hook or screw anchors. In 1980 Cotrel and Dubousset[4] introduced a universal dorsal spinal instrumentation system, based on the multiple anchor Cotrel-Dubousset (CD) system, that allowed multiple hook fixation as a mechanism for the correction and fusion of scoliotic deformities. The CD system was designed to restore sagittal balance while correcting the obvious coronal plane deformity.

Cotrel made a significant initial contribution before the introduction of CD instrumentation. The device for transverse traction (DTT) allowed a controlled lateral force application between Harrington distraction and compression instrumentation or between stacked Harrington rods in large scoliotic deformities. This crossfixation device provided for a much more rigid construct than could be achieved without its use.

USI allows multiple anchors (hooks, screws, and wires) to be applied. By using multiple hooks, greater correction can be achieved. Rod contouring, distraction, compression, and lordosing and kyphosing forces can all be used on the same construct. The initial premise was that the scoliotic deformity could be rotated into a kyphosis, thus providing three-dimensional correction of the deformity. Subsequently, it has been determined that the rod rotation maneuver in fact applies a lateral translation force.

Nevertheless, with the advent of greater rigid fixation, difficult cases could be approached surgically. The fixation was so good that postoperative orthoses were often unnecessary. The versatility of USI provides for a customization of the implant in terms of length, anchor types and sites, and force application modes (e.g., compression, distraction, three-point bending) for the effective management of instability and deformity in any region of the thoracic or lumbar spine.

A number of instrumentation systems have provided advantages over the original CD system. A significant disadvantage of the CD system was related to the use of blockers that required the torquing off of hex-headed screws for final tightening. Once torqued off, there was no easy way of revising the construct. This problem has been solved, via other systems, in a number of different ways.

With modern USI systems, corrective forces can be applied over shorter lengths, minimizing late pain complications from the fusion of normal motion segments. The flat back syndrome resulting from the loss of lordosis due to the use of distrac-

tion rods can also be avoided. USI permits immediate segmental stabilization of the spine. This can be accomplished, even in the absence of laminae, by using a combination of pedicle screws, pedicle hooks, and transverse process hooks. The use of a rod rather than a plate as the longitudinal member allows a larger dorsolateral surface for bony fusion.

Components
Anchors

Sublaminar wires, pedicle screws, and hooks are devices that affix the construct to the spine. Each of these anchoring devices is associated with distinct positive and negative attributes. The anchors are interconnected by a longitudinal member, which in most cases is a rod. Occasionally, plates are used.

Sublaminar Wires

The sublaminar wire concept has enjoyed widespread use. Limitations include the inability to provide multiple plane corrective forces, the need for sublaminar preparation, and the risks of sublaminar wire passage. The following rules for wire passage are recommended: (1) do not pass the wires laterally; (2) the radius of curvature of the front end of the wire should be less than the laminar width; (3) the angle of the wire tip should be no greater than 45 degrees; (4) additional removal of bony lamina is not necessary, and (5) remove spinous processes before direct midline passage.[12]

Pedicle Screw Fixation

Pedicle screw fixation allows the implant to be affixed to all three columns of the vertebral axis. This facilitates the application of corrective forces over damaged motion segments. The junction between screws and bone is biomechanically stronger than the hook-bone or wire-bone junctions. This mechanical advantage over other types of dorsal fixation devices permits a shorter construct to be designed and used, thus providing sufficient stabilization without affecting adjacent levels. Care should be taken to assess the stability of the ventral column, because the implant can fail if there is marked loss of ventral stability and no ventral strut graft is placed to assist in load sharing. Pedicle screw fixation does not require intact dorsal elements, as do laminar hooks and sublaminar wires. The mechanical advantage of pedicle screws is balanced by the potential risk involved with placement.

A thorough knowledge of pedicle anatomy and orientation is critical to the safe use of thoracic pedicle screws. The ideal entry point is located on two bisecting lines in the upper corner of the outer inferior quadrant. A horizontal line from the midpoint of the transverse process is intersected by a vertical line that passes through the center of the facet joints. A drill or awl may be inserted but should not angle more than 5 degrees medially, while angulation in the sagittal plane depends on analysis of the lateral radiograph. The pedicle is closer to the rostral aspect of the vertebral body in the thoracic spine than it is in the thoracolumbar spine.

The authors favor the use of a laminotomy to allow visualization of the medial cortex of the pedicle. Intraoperative imaging or frameless stereotaxy may assist with the placement of pedicle instrumentation.

Hooks

Hook fixation has proven to be a useful method of attachment to the dorsal bony structures of the spine. Hooks are an important component of the USI systems. Hook-rod fixation is usually the dorsal anchor of choice for the treatment of thoracic instability above the thoracolumbar junction.

The three major sites for hook placement are the pedicle, the lamina, and the transverse process. The mechanical strength of the pedicle makes it the most important anchor site in the thoracic spine. Hooks are introduced into the facet joints toward the pedicles. Following hook impaction, the blade of the hook should achieve adequate purchase upon the pedicle and the inferior articular process should abut the hook throat. The bifid hook design allows for a firm purchase of the pedicle. This is critical in deformity correction. The bifid shoe is meant to engage the caudal pedicle margin.

The transverse process is the next most widely used anchor site in the thoracic spine. Although not as strong as the pedicle, the transverse process is easy to identify and prepare for hook placement. Hook placement may not be possible in the lower thoracic spine because the transverse processes become smaller in size and more vertically oriented. Transverse process hooks are caudally directed.

The third anchor site in the thoracic spine is the lamina. Hook design is such that the hook contour should closely match that of the lamina in order to avoid hook migration into the spinal canal with subsequent spinal cord injury. Laminar hooks may be rostrally or caudally directed.

Longitudinal Members
Rods

Rods are indicated as the longitudinal member in most dorsal thoracoclumbar stabilization procedures. They provide a rigid connection between anchors and are easier to apply than plating systems. Although there are other means of connecting anchors, such as plates or cables, they do not provide an optimal balance between ease of applicability and strength. Cables may be easier to apply, but they can be very difficult to apply for multiple levels of fixation. Additionally, rods allow more dorsolateral bone surface area for ultimate bony fusion to occur.

As rod-based systems have been refined, it is now easier to contour the rod, both out of the body and in situ. Rod surface characteristics have been modified to improve attachment. The CD rods are knurled with diamond-shaped asperities, which allows set screw fixation of the hook or screw implants at any point on the rod. Enhancement of resistance to fatigue and failure by improvements in metal composition and compactness of the rod, as well as variability in diameter, increases strength while making placement easier. Many systems are now available in both stainless steel and titanium.

Transverse Connectors

Interconnecting longitudinal members increase the torsional strength of a construct. This was first widely applied clinically in the 1970s with the Luque L rod. The rods were prebent so that the two rods could be connected by placing the straight end of one rod over the bent end of the other and then wiring them together.

The CD system's DTT permits controlled lateral force application between the longitudinal members. This crossfixation device increases overall construct rigidity.

Other USI systems, such as the Texas Scottish Rite Hospital (TSRH) system, provide transverse couplers with greater rigidity for strong interconnection.[2] Their primary function is to enhance resistance to rotational forces, as well as axial loads.

Crossfixators prevent rod migration and enhance the rigidity of the system.

The transverse connectors can be placed at any point along the extent of the longitudinal members. Moreover, their strategic placement can prevent migration of an adjacent anchor.

Contraindications to USI

Contraindications to USI are relative. While implantation of any foreign body in close proximity to an active infection should be avoided, spinal implants can be safely and effectively used for stabilization in the presence of acute or grossly unstable vertebral osteomyelitis.[8]

Severe osteoporosis presents a higher than normal risk of implant-related complications and failure. The instrumentation is considerably stronger than the bone. Fixation failure commonly occurs at the anchor-bone junction. Long-segment fixation distributes forces over many segments, whereas postoperative bracing, methylmethacrylate pedicle screw supplementation, and the minimization of generated force application reduce the incidence of implant failure in osteoporotic patients.

Significant loss of ventral column stability, particularly in the axial plane, can stress dorsal USI constructs and lead to fixation failure. In cases in which ventral column instability exists, consideration should be given to ventral surgical decompression and stabilization or the supplementation of the dorsal universal instrumentation implant with a ventral interbody strut graft.

SPECIFIC ANATOMICAL CONSIDERATIONS
Upper Thoracic Spine

Fractures of the upper thoracic spine (T1 to T4) are at risk for the development of progressive kyphosis and painful compensatory cervical lordosis. Long instrumentation constructs with multilevel spinal fixation usually effectively resist kyphotic deformation. The loss of mobility is less critical in the upper thoracic spine. There is little soft tissue coverage, however. Therefore a low-profile system is preferable to avoid uncomfortable and unsightly hardware prominence, as well as skin breakdown. Most surgeons prefer to use a hook-rod system supplemented with upper thoracic and lower cervical pedicle screw fixation or

sublaminar wires. Transpedicular fixation is less commonly attempted because of the narrow diameter of the pedicles in this region. However, improved familiarity with the regional anatomy, as well as the use of frameless stereotaxy, has increased the safety and use of thoracic pedicle screws.

Midthoracic Spine

In the midthoracic region, rods in combination with hooks are commonly used. Transverse process and pedicle hooks are preferable to laminar hooks because of the risk of placing instrumentation into the narrow midthoracic spinal canal. Specially designed hooks allow for a close fit between the hook and the overlying bone.

Thoracolumbar Junction

The management of thoracolumbar fractures remains controversial, because no uniform and objective definition of instability has been universally accepted. Traditional concepts of spinal stability may be inadequate to fully define the nature of the disruption at the thoracolumbar junction. Additionally, the interval from injury to presentation may have a significant effect on surgical decision making. In the acute injury phase, a kyphosis greater than 30 degrees, polytrauma, and major neurological injury may dictate more expeditious surgical intervention. Dorsal instrumentation is often quite effective in restoring vertebral body height, sagittal contour, and spinal canal configuration when undertaken within 24 to 48 hours of injury. The authors' experience has been that restoration of alignment via dorsal approaches is further facilitated when this interval is less than 8 hours.

CONCLUSION

Appropriate therapy for thoracic instability, injuries, neoplasms, infectious processes, and other entities involving the thoracic spine begins with a thorough understanding of the involved anatomy and biomechanics. Similarly of value is an understanding of the pathophysiology of the instability and a comprehension of the vectors that produced the instability.

Surgical treatment generally requires two steps: (1) decompression and (2) stabilization. The surgical approach is determined by understanding the nature of the instability. Dorsal approaches are appropriate in some situations and inappropriate in others. Dorsal decompression (laminectomy) without stabilization is uncommonly indicated in the thoracic spine.

The advantage of dorsal spinal instrumentation is that it uses well-known techniques via a dorsal midline approach. Dorsal spinal instrumentation is generally safer to apply, biomechanically superior, and easier to remove than ventral constructs. It is an effective means to re-establish balance in both the sagittal and coronal planes and is one of the more important techniques of achieving the ultimate surgical goal. This goal is a balanced, pain-free, stable spine centered over the pelvis, with the fusion of the minimum (but optimal) number of motion segments required to achieve this result. An understanding of the variety of available techniques of dorsal spinal instrumentation, as well as the principles underlying their application, should be part of the fund of knowledge of every practicing spine surgeon.

REFERENCES

1. Allen B, Ferguson R. The Galveston technique for L-rod instrumentation of the scoliotic spine. Spine 7:276-284, 1982.
2. Ashman R, Herring JA, Johnston CE, Lowery GL, eds. TSRH Universal Spinal Instrumentation. Dallas: Hundley and Associates, 1993.
3. Boucher.
4. Cotrel YJ, Dubousset J, and Guillaumat R: New universal instrumentation in spinal surgery. Clin Orthop, 1988.
5. Danisa OA, Shaffrey CI, Jare JA: Surgical approaches for the correction of unstable thoracolumbar burst fractures: A retrospective analysis of treatment outcomes. J Neurosurg 83:977-983, 1995.
6. Dawson E, Sherman JE, Kanim LE, Nove MR. Spinal cord monitoring. Results of the Scoliosis Research Society and the European Spinal Deformity survey. Spine 16:S361-S362, 1991.
7. Denis F. The three column spine and its significance in the classification of acute thoracolumbar spinal injuries. Spine 8:817-831, 1983.
8. Dietze DJ, Fessler RG, Jacob RP. Primary reconstruction for spinal infections. J Neurosurg 86:981-989, 1997.
9. Drummond D. Harrington instrumentation with spinous process wiring for idiopathic scoliosis. Orthop Clin North Am 19:281-289, 1988.
10. Edwards C, Levine A. Early rod-sleeve stabilization of the injured thoracic and lumbar spine. Orthop Clin North Am 17:121-145, 1986.
11. Fessler RG. Decision making in spinal instrumentation. Clin Neurosurg 40:227-242, 1992.
12. Goll SR, Balderston, Stambough J. Depth of intraspinal wire penetration during passage of sublaminar wires. Spine 13:503-509, 1988.
13. Harrington P. Surgical instrumentation for management of scoliosis. J Bone Joint Surg 42A:1448, 1960.
14. Harrington P. Treatment of scoliosis. J Bone Joint Surg 26:149-154, 1962.
15. Harrington P. The history and development of Harrington instrumentation. Clin Othop 227:3, 1988.
16. King D. Internal fixation for lumbosacral fusion. Am J Surg 66:357-366, 1944.
17. Lang E. Support of the spondylolytic spine by means of varied steel bars attached to the vertebra. Am J Orthop 8:344-347, 1904.
18. Luque E. The anatomic basis and development of segmental spinal instrumentation. Spine 7:256-259, 1982.
19. Luque E. Segmental spinal instrumentation for correction of scoliosis. Clin Orthop 163:192-198, 1982.
20. McAfee PC, Bohlman HH. Complications following Harrington instrumentation for fractures of the thoracolumbar spine. J Bone Joint Surg 67A:672-686, 1985.
21. Owen JK, Bridwell KH, Grubb R. The clinical application of neurogenic motor evoked potentials to monitor spinal cord function during surgery. Spine 16:S385-S389, 1991.
22. Roy-Camille, R., 1963.
23. Wilkins.

Spinal Instrumentation: Construct Design Strategies

Sait Naderi, M.D., Marc E. Eichler, M.D., Curtis A. Dickman, M.D., Charles B. Stillerman, M.D., and Edward C. Benzel, M.D.

Construct design, the act of conceiving an operative instrumentation plan for a case-specific instability problem, includes formulating both a blueprint for the instrumentation construct to be placed and a strategy for the implementation of this blueprint.[1,3,4] The construct design process should consider how to achieve spinal stability with instrumentation and the fundamental type of instrumentation to be applied. The blueprint can either be drawn or formulated clearly in the surgeon's mind, but must be conceived with forethought.[1,3]

The proper design of a spinal construct is perhaps most important in the thoracic and lumbar spine. The complexity or simplicity of the design depends on the nature of the spinal instability and on the extent of the spinal deformity. In most thoracolumbar spine applications, construct design is very complex. The number of motion segments incorporated by the construct, the mode of implant application (the force vectors applied by the implant), the mechanism of load bearing by the construct (i.e., distraction, three-point bending, four-point bending, tension-band fixation, or cantilever beam fixation), and the wide variety of implant and implant component choices are but a few of the points to consider if an appropriately conceived and designed instrumentation construct is to be used.[1,3,4]

FUNDAMENTALS OF CONSTRUCT DESIGN

The indications for spinal instrumentation are based upon the extent and types of spinal instability. Spinal instrumentation design is based on simple physical and mechanical principles. It becomes more sophisticated as newer constructs are developed. Several spinal implants are available that can be applied with a variety of construct purchase site choices. The specific advantages and pitfalls of different fixation devices must be understood for effective clinical problem solving.

The basic elements of constructs consist of (1) the spinal segments to be instrumented, (2) the longitudinal member (e.g., rod or plate), (3) the implant component of the implant-bone junction (e.g., wire, hook, or screw), (4) the transverse member(s) (cross-fixation mechanisms), and (5) interbody spacers for load bearing and/or fusion (tricoticate bone, rib, cages, pins, methylmethacrylate, etc.).[1,2] A fixation construct includes a combination of these elements in which the spine and the implant are considered as a unit. The extent of load bearing/load sharing, the degree of deformity correction, and the relief of neural compression are critical considerations in determining the surgical placement of the implant in neutral, distraction, compression, translation, flexion, extension, or lateral bending mode. The forces that act to create the spinal disruption must be understood so that appropriate counterforces can be implemented by the construct design.

MECHANISMS OF LOAD BEARING

The six mechanisms of load application by the construct are: (1) simple distraction, (2) three-point bending and related techniques (e.g., four-point bending), (3) tension-band (compression) fixation, (4) cantilever beams with fixed moment arms, (5) cantilever beams with nonfixed moment arms, and (6) cantilever beams with applied moment arms.[3,4]

Constructs may be simple or complex in design depending upon the mechanical task required of the hardware, and may be applied via a ventral, lateral, or dorsal spinal approach. Often a variety of different forces are applied simultaneously to the spine.

Simple Distraction

Simple distraction involves the application of axially directed distraction forces to the spine. These forces are associated with varying effects, depending on the perpendicular distance from the point of force application by the construct to the instantaneous axis of rotation (IAR) (Fig. 14-1). Distraction can be applied either ventral (in line with) or dorsal to the IAR. If the distraction force is in line with the IAR (interbody region) the instrumentation can resist axial loads and no bending moment is applied. When distractive forces are applied ventral or dorsal to the IAR the spine may undergo extension or flexion. The application of pure dorsally placed distraction risks increasing an already present kyphotic deformity. Dorsally placed distraction should also be avoided in cases of retro-displaced bone fragments where there is possible loss of integrity of the posterior longitudinal ligament. Distraction in this setting may not only fail to reconstruct the spinal canal but may distract the neural elements over the intracanalicular bone fragments. Distraction is often generally employed in combination with other loads applied by the hardware.

Three-Point Bending

Three-point bending is more complex than a simple distraction construct. It refers to leverage ap-

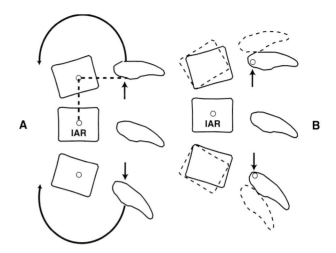

Fig. 14-1. A depiction of the forces applied to the spine by a simple dorsal distraction construct. **A,** The moment arm applied by the construct creates a bending moment *(curved arrows).* The moment arm is the perpendicular distance from the point of application of force *(straight arrows)* to the IAR. **B,** This results in an exaggeration of the flexion deformity (from solid to dashed vertebral bodies). Note that if the distraction forces were applied in closer proximity to the IAR, this bending moment would be lesser in magnitude. If they were applied in line with the IAR, the bending moment would be zero.[1,3]

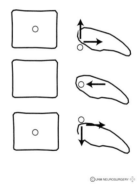

Fig. 14-2. A depiction of the forces applied to the spine by a three-point bending construct. The vertically oriented arrows depict the accompanying distraction forces. The horizontal arrows at both ends of the construct depict the dorsally directed forces, and the horizontal arrow in the middle of the construct depicts the ventrally directed force (at the fulcrum).[1,3]

plied to the spine, over three different surfaces with different vectors, to achieve bending of the spinal column at the level of the instability (as with Edwards sleeves and Harrington rods) to reduce a kyphosis. Three-point bending constructs are often applied with an accompanying distractive or compressive force. With three-point bending constructs

(Fig. 14-2), the bending moment applied to the spine is directly proportional to the length of the construct. Longer rods provide more corrective force because of greater leverage. In addition, the ability of a three-point bending construct to maintain stability once correction of the deformity has been achieved is also related to the length of the rod construct. Short segment rods over three to four spinal levels weakly resist spinal bending if a major angular deformity has been corrected.

A related concept to three-point bending force application is four-point bending, in which ventrally directed forces at two (or more) points are applied in addition to dorsally directed forces—usually both rostral and caudal to the unstable segment. Conceptually, the forces associated with three- and four-point bending are similar[1,3] (Fig. 14-3, *A*). Three- or four-point bending fixation can apply not only to midconstruct deformity reduction but can also be utilized to correct a sagittal deformity at either end of the construct terminus. In this situation, the fulcrum is located at one end of the construct (Fig. 14-3, *B*). Usually the construct is positioned so that the deformity correction occurs at the rostral end of the construct because sagittal plane deformation usually occurs with the more rostral segments translating in a ventral direction with respect to the more caudal segments.

Tension-Band Fixation

Tension-band fixation is performed by the compression of the vertebral column with forces applied at some distance either ventrally or dorsally from the IAR. This can be achieved with Luque instrumentation (rods with sublaminar wires), Harrington compression rods, universal spinal instrumentation (with claw designs), Knodt rods, Zielke instruments, Z-Plates, Kaneda plates, and a multitude of other fixation devices. Tension-band fixation applies extension (dorsal bending moment) or flexion (ventral bending moment) to the spinal segments that are compressed[1,3] (Fig. 14-4). This bending moment applied to the fracture site by the tension-band fixation device is not related to the length of the construct but instead is related to the perpendicular distance from the point of application of the force by the implant to the IAR. This is in contradistinction to the bending moment applied by three-point bending constructs, in which the length

of the implant affects the magnitude of the corrective force applied to the spine.

Cantilever Beams

A cantilever is a large projecting beam supported only at one end, usually designed to bear weight over a space where support cannot normally be placed or is not desired. There are three types of cantilever beams utilized in spinal constructs: (1) fixed moment arm cantilever beam fixation, (2) nonfixed moment arm cantilever beam fixation, and (3) applied moment arm cantilever beam fixation. Fixed moment arm cantilever beams are akin to a diving board that is rigidly affixed to the side of a swimming pool[1,3] (Fig. 14-5, *A*). The most common example of this type of construct among spinal implants is the utilization of rigid (locking) pedicle screw fixators. Such rigid fixation techniques compensate for a short moment arm by providing a fixed moment arm cantilever beam configuration for standard support. Generally a fixed moment arm cantilever construct is applied in the neutral mode. The construct must be able to withstand significant axial loads, such as when the patient assumes an upright posture. No ventrally directed force at the fulcrum is necessary because of the construct's inherent buttressing effect; this places significant stress at the point of maximum bending moment, specifically at the screw-plate or screw-rod interface. This stress may be excessive, eventually resulting in screw fracture. Nonfixed moment arm cantilever beams are akin to a board affixed via a hinge to the side of a swimming pool (analogous to a screw-through-the-plate construct; e.g., lateral mass plate, Luque ISF nonlocking pedicle plate). The toggling of the screw through the longitudinal member results in unique attributes (Fig. 14-5, *B*). These constructs do not effectively bear an axial load without assistance from other structures such as the vertebral body or a ventral strut graft. Such techniques can therefore be used only when axial load-resisting capabilities of the spine are preserved. Further, although these constructs do help the already present axial load-supporting structures to resist axial loading, the toggling of the screw on the plate allowed by this technique greatly diminishes their ability to resist screw pull-out (Fig. 14-5, *C*). Applied moment arm cantilever beams are usually rigid constructs that apply extension or flexion mo-

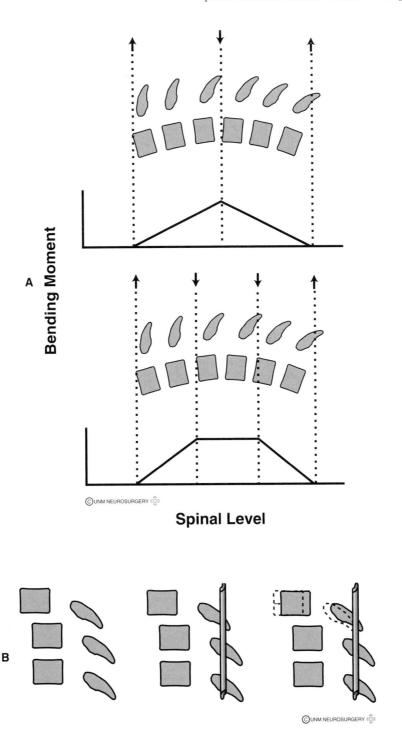

Fig. 14-3. A, A depiction of the bending moment applied to the spine by a three-point bending construct and a four-point bending construct. **B,** Terminal three-point bending constructs can be utilized to reduce a ventral translational deformity.

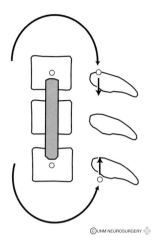

Fig. 14-4. A depiction of the forces applied to the spine by a tension-band fixation construct. The moment arm is similar in length but is associated with a bending moment *(curved arrows)* that is opposite in direction to that observed with simple distraction (see Fig. 14-1).

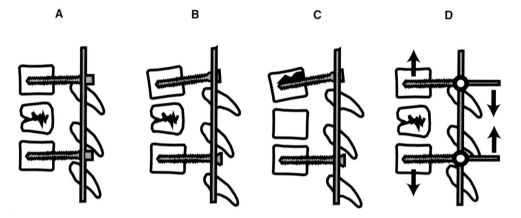

Fig. 14-5. A depiction of cantilever beam constructs. **A,** A fixed moment arm construct. Note the rigid attachment site to the longitudinal member. **B,** A nonfixed moment arm construct. Note the screw-through-the-plate configuration that allows the screw to toggle with respect to the plate. **C,** The toggling of the screw on the plate may lead to failure of the nonfixed moment arm cantilever beam construct via screw pullout. **D,** An applied moment arm construct. Note that by applying a dorsal compression via attachment sites that can be removed after screw–longitudinal member fixation and prior to wound closure (e.g., Shanz screws), extension of the spine is achieved.

ments to the spine, allowing reduction of spinal deformities (Fig 14-5, *D*). This is in contrast to the fixed and nonfixed moment arm types, in which no bending moment is applied.

MODE OF IMPLANT APPLICATION

The mode of application of the implant is critical. The placement of the implant in a distraction, compression, neutral, translation, flexion, extension, or lateral bending mode at the time of surgery affects many factors, such as (1) the extent of load bearing and load sharing by the implant, (2) the extent of deformity exaggeration or correction, and (3) the exaggeration or relief of neural compression. The first two factors directly affect the integrity of the con-

struct as a functional unit. The latter may impact on the neurological status.[1,3]

The ability to bear an axial load is an important aspect of most constructs. When axial load bearing is impaired (i.e., by vertebral body distraction or collapse), the implants may be excessively loaded if the spinal deformity is reduced. The load on the implant can be reduced by reconstructing the vertebral body with grafts, cages, or methylmethacrylate. The vertebral body prosthesis load shares with the implant to relieve stress on the hardware.

Translational force application and the resistance of translational load is important. Both may be difficult to assess unless overt structural failure occurs.

The application of distractive or compressive forces to the spine is associated with an accompa-

Table 14-1. Factors Affecting Construct Design

Construct-Related Factors

Mechanism of load bearing by the construct
Type of implant used at the implant-bone junction
Length of construct
Alloy of implant
Location of implant

Spine-Related Factors

Geometry of spine
Location of unstable spine segment
Extent of spinal instability
Bone-related factors
Axial load-bearing capacity
Orientation of instability
Presence of neural compression

nying bending moment application if the forces are applied at a distance from the IAR[4] (see Figs. 14-1 and 14-4). These bending moments play a much more significant role with shorter constructs than they do with longer constructs.[2]

DESIGNING A CONSTRUCT

The factors that affect construct design planning fall into two categories: (1) construct-related factors, and (2) spine-related factors (Table 14-1). Construct design planning in any given clinical situation relies on both of these elements.

Construct-Related Factors

Several factors influence construct design planning: (1) the mechanism of load bearing by the construct (distraction, three-point or four-point bending, tension-band fixation, cantilever beam with a fixed moment arm, cantilever beam with a nonfixed moment arm, or cantilever beam with an applied moment arm), (2) type of implant component used at the implant-bone junction (e.g., wire, hook, screw), (3) the length of the construct, (4) composition of alloy used in the construct, and (5) location of instrumentation (ventral vs. dorsal vs. lateral).

The mechanism of load bearing used by the construct dictates both the type of implant component used at the implant-bone junction (screw vs. hook vs. wire) and length of the construct used (short segment fixation vs. long segment fixation).

Spinal construct alloy selection is based on stiffness and strength. The diameter of a rod substantially affects strength (resistance to failure in flexion) and stiffness (to the third and fourth power, respectively).

Spine-Related Factors

The spine-related factors affecting construct design planning include: (1) sagittal and coronal geometry of the spine, (2) location of the unstable spinal segment, (3) extent of spinal instability, (4) bone-related factors (e.g., bone quality and bone integrity), (5) axial load-bearing capacity, (6) orientation of instability, and (7) the presence of neural compression.

Geometry of the Spine

Both sagittal and coronal geometry of the spine may affect construct design planning. An understanding of the sagittal and coronal balance is necessary. In most people the L3 vertebral body is oriented in the neutral position, and the L4 and L5 vertebral bodies are oriented ventrally. This configuration is similar to numbers on a clock (i.e., 3, 4, and 5 o'clock). A sagittal vertical axis line is the plumb line falling from C2 and passing ventral to T7, dorsal to L3, and crossing S2. Any change in the sagittal balance can affect construct design planning. The changes in the sagittal balance should be taken into account during construct design planning, as intraoperative corrective measures may be indicated.

The coronal geometry of the spine can also affect construct design planning. The coronal orientation of the spine (i.e., straight or oblique orientation of the vertebrae) may require a decompressive procedure prior to deformity correction and/or stabilization.

Location of the Unstable Spine Segment

The proximity of the construct to the rostral or caudal end of the spine (i.e., occiput or sacrum) may impact the efficacy of the instrumentation. The closer the unstable spinal segment to the termini of the spine, the shorter the lever arm applied by the affected end of the implant. This lack of an adequate length of lever arm can prevent the achievement of an appropriate bending moment. Additionally, the proximity of the construct to the apex of the thoracic kyphosis is also important. The termination of a construct at the apex of a kyphosis is a common reason of construct failure.

Extent of Spinal Instability

The extent of instrumentation should correspond to the extent of instability. A careful preoperative investigation should demonstrate the presence of overt or limited instability. In the case of limited instability, a long construct, with the accompanying advantage of a very long moment arm, may be unnecessary. The use of a compressive ventrally or dorsally placed short moment arm may be adequate in this case. On the other hand, the failure of all three columns may dictate the simultaneous use of both ventral and dorsal implants. A ventral or dorsal short segment fixation construct alone may fail in this circumstance unless it is supplemented by a concomitant construct on the opposite side of the spine.[6] The use of universal spine instrumentation, with multidirectional fixation using screws and hooks, may be the best alternative in some cases of overt thoracolumbar instability. Still, the failure to include all pathological segments of the spine in the construct may lead to failure of the instrumentation.

Instrumentation/fusion mismatch may be used with the long constructs. A long spinal fusion permanently immobilizes an excessive length of the spine, and simultaneously decreases the rate of fusion incorporation. Fusing only the unstable spinal levels, while using a long implant to gain the leverage required to achieve and maintain stabilization can cause the implant to loosen at the unfused (but instrumented) levels. The best solution is to use shorter implants, so that only the unstable spinal segments are both fused and instrumented. Technological advances and improved surgical techniques have enhanced the effectiveness of shorter constructs.[7]

Some tolerance for movement at unfused implant-bone junctions is often optimal. Hooks and wires allow some movement at this junction, whereas screws do not. Therefore when an instrumentation/ fusion mismatch is planned, screws should be avoided at the terminus of the construct.

As previously discussed, the longer the construct, the greater the moment arm applied by three-point bending. In general, an additional spinal segment above the unstable segment should be in-

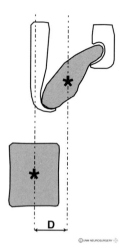

Fig. 14-6. A depiction of the point of attachment, along the long axis of the spine, of dorsally applied hooks. Note that the centroid of the site of hook attachment is at the level of the lower aspect of the vertebral body. The centroid of the vertebral body and the centroid of the hook attachment sites are thus separated by a distance (*d*) that is roughly one-half a vertebral segment in width *(vertical dashed lines)*.[1,3]

corporated by the instrumentation construct. This allows for the employment of a similar length of construct above and below the unstable segment. The point of attachment for laminar fixation is below the center of the vertebral body (Fig. 14-6). When failure of a long instrumentation system occurs, the rostral aspect usually fails. This is often due to an inadequate lever arm and to the relatively poor fixation achieved (with the often used pedicle and transverse process hooks). This may be the case when a construct is applied two spinal segments above and two spinal segments below the pathology. Therefore the extension of the construct rostrally by one segment offers a longer and more effective moment arm, which in turn strengthens this "weak" link.[1,4] Hence fusing the spine three segments above and two segments below the injury is often a logical compromise between the problems associated with long construct length and the potential for inadequate fixation achieved by short construct length (see chapter 15).

Bone-Related Factors

Relatively speaking, hooks and sublaminar wires resist pullout in bone of poor quality much better than screws. However, defects at the hook or sublaminar wire placement sites (e.g., laminectomy or fractured lamina) may dictate the use of pedicle screws despite poor bone quality. Additionally, long constructs are more effective in cases of osteoporosis, as they provide a greater moment arm.

Axial Load-Bearing Capacity

The ability to surgically reconstitute adequate axial load-bearing capacity of the spine (if lost) is an extremely important consideration regarding the choice of instrumentation constructs. If adequate axial load-bearing capacity exists or has been surgically created, the load-bearing responsibilities of the spinal implant are different than they would be if adequate axial load-bearing capacity does not exist or cannot be restored. If axial load-bearing capacity is inadequate, the instrumentation construct must provide for both prevention of translational deformity and for axial load support.

Orientation of Instability

The orientation of the instability dictates the most appropriate construct type. Translational instability often requires a four-point bending construct to reduce the deformity or "hold" the alignment. It is emphasized that the use of pedicle screws to reduce or "hold" a translational deformity dictates that the screw-bone junction resist pullout.[5] Of note is that screw-bone junctions are notoriously weak in this regard.

Presence of Neural Compression

It is worth re-emphasizing that adequate dural sac decompression, before the placement of a compression instrumentation construct, is mandatory. Both ventral and dorsal decompressive operations, however, can lead to a loss of structural stability that occasionally may be significant. Attempts at improving axial load-bearing capacity with the placement of an interbody bone graft may be beneficial but are not always successful. In most cases, destabilizing decompressive operations should be followed by a stabilization operation.

THE BLUEPRINT

A simple scheme is needed to determine (1) level of lesion or the level of the unstable segment(s), (2) the type of implant (including the implant component of the implant-bone junction, the longitudinal member, and the cross-link), (3) the mode of application at each segmental level, (4) the method of load bearing by the construct, and (5) a clear definition of the complexity of the construct. This allows, in general, for the selection of the appropriate implant components in advance and for the facilitation of intraoperative communication. This scheme is illustrated in Fig. 14-7.

Line Drawing Framework

A simple posteroanterior (PA) and lateral line drawing rendition of the spine provides a framework for the clear definition of the operative plan. Often, only a posteroanterior drawing is necessary unless the operative plan includes the reduction of a deformity in the sagittal plane—for example, a kyphotic deformity. The lateral view therefore should not depict redundant information that may potentially lead to confusion.[1]

Level of Pathology and Fusion

The level(s) of instability or pathology (designated by Xs), the level(s) to be fused (designated by cross-hatches), and the type of fusion should be clearly outlined on the line drawings (see Fig. 14-7). This becomes important when defining the number of spinal levels that a construct will span both above and below the level of pathology. The accurate delineation of the unstable motion segments is important, as the mechanical effects of immobilizing any motion segment unnecessarily may be significant. For this reason, the preoperative determination of the levels of instability is critical in the surgical decision-making process.

Type of Implant Components

The type of implant components should be clearly identified. The components utilized as spinal anchors include wires, hooks, and screws. On the PA diagram hooks are designated by a right angle arrow with the arrowhead pointing in the direction of the orientation of the hook (i.e., toward the bone purchase side of the hook). Screws may be designated by a circle with an "X." Wire may be depicted as a loop. The location of placement of each of these components is depicted by the level of the spine

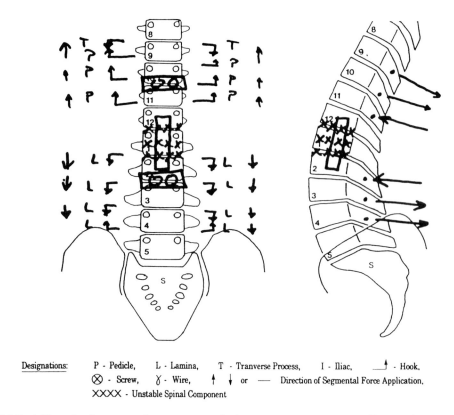

Designations: P - Pedicle, L - Lamina, T - Tranverse Process, I - Iliac, ⌐╂ - Hook,

⊗ - Screw, Υ - Wire, ↑ ↓ or — Direction of Segmental Force Application,

XXXX - Unstable Spinal Component

Fig. 14-7. A blueprint format to plan a construct design strategy. A PA view is illustrated on the left and a lateral view is illustrated on the right. Note that the diagram does not include the cervical spine. If instrumentation is planned in this region, the line drawing can be extended or the spinal segments relabeled to conform to the extent of operative plan. Space at the bottom of the page allows for other vital information, such as patient demographic data *(bottom right)* and (1) the construct type (i.e., distraction, three-point bending, tension-band fixation, cantilever beam with a fixed moment arm, cantilever beam with a nonfixed moment arm, or cantilever beam with an applied moment arm), (2) the longitudinal member type (i.e., rod or plate), and (3) a description of planned complex maneuvers (i.e., derotation maneuvers).[1,3]

that they are positioned on in the line drawing. "P" (for pedicle), "L" (for laminar or sublaminar), "T" (for transverse process), and "I" (for iliac) denotes the component type to be used.

Mode of Application at Each Segmental Level

The mode of axial load application at each level, as depicted on the PA line drawing is either that of compression (arrow facing the pathology), distraction (arrow facing away from the pathology), or neutral (horizontal line). Bending moments may be applied to the spine by the construct but are difficult to depict accurately on the line drawing and are therefore described by notations at the bottom of the line drawings. Should sagittal plane forces be necessary, such as in the correction of a scoliotic de-

formity, they are depicted in a similar fashion on the lateral line drawing (see Fig. 14-7). For long segment fixation, where cross-links may be necessary to resist torsional deformation of the rods (by creating a quadrilateral frame construct), they can be depicted by elongated rectangles with circles on the PA diagram (see Fig. 14-7).

CONCLUSION

Construct design for correction of spinal deformity and decompression of neural elements is a challenging aspect of spinal surgery. The principles of surgical correction of a spinal deformity include neural element decompression, reduction of the deformity, and stabilization. To optimize patient management, the surgeon must maintain proficiency with the wide variety of available spinal implants and understand the nuances of each particular system. Additionally, the surgeon must have an excellent comprehension of the clinical mechanics of spinal stabilization and a solid grasp of the appropriate indications for stabilization and fusion. Despite the impressive technological advances enhancing the possibilities of stabilization and deformity correction in the spine, the determining factor of success or failure is in many instances the surgeon and not the instrumentation.[7]

REFERENCES

1. Benzel EC. Biomechanics of lumbar and lumbosacral spine fractures. In Rea GL, Miller CA, eds. Spine Trauma: Current Evaluation and Management. Park Ridge, Ill.: American Association of Neurological Surgeons, 1993, pp 165-195.

2. Benzel EC. Short segment fixation. In Benzel EC, ed. Spinal Instrumentation. Park Ridge, Ill.: American Association of Neurological Surgeons, 1994, pp 111-124.

3. Benzel EC. Construct design. In Benzel EC, ed. Spinal Instrumentation. Park Ridge, Ill.: American Association of Neurological Surgeons, 1994, pp 239-256.

4. Benzel EC. Construct design. In Benzel EC, ed. Biomechanics of Spine Stabilization. Principles and Clinical Practice. New York: McGraw-Hill, 1995, pp 163-172.

5. Maiman DJ, Pintar FA, Yogananden N, et al. Pull-out strength of Caspar cervical screws. Neurosurgery 31:1097-1101, 1992.

6. McCormack T, Karaikovic C, Gaines RW. The load sharing classification of spine fractures. Spine 19:1741, 1994.

7. Stillerman CB, Gruen JP. Universal spinal instrumentation. In Benzel EC, ed. Spinal Instrumentation. Park Ridge, Ill.: American Association of Neurological Surgeons, 1994, pp 147-174.

CHAPTER

15

Deformity Correction

Edward C. Benzel, M.D., and Michael A. Morone, M.D., Ph.D.

Deformity of the thoracic spine can be acute or chronic. Acute thoracic deformities are usually of an infectious, traumatic, or neoplastic etiology. A chronic form of thoracic deformity occurs with aging. This sagittal plane deformity of aging occurs because the natural thoracic kyphosis is accentuated due to thoracic disc interspace height loss that is more extensive in the ventral aspect of the disc. This results in progression of the "natural" kyphosis as the degenerative process ensues. This progressive kyphosis is slightly offset by the rib cage, which stabilizes the thoracic spine to a significant degree.

When deformity occurs, deformity correction often requires surgical intervention. Some chronic forms of deformity may be treated with bracing (adolescent scoliosis). Acute and chronic forms of thoracic deformity are not without effects on other regions of the spinal column. The coupling phenomenon (the phenomenon whereby one movement of the spine obligates a separate movement about or along another axis) plays a significant role in the development of thoracic spinal deformities. Scoliotic deformities are nearly always accompanied by sagittal plane and rotational components of the deformity that may also involve the lumbar spine. Thus the correction of a deformity in only one plane necessitates a consideration for correction in other planes. Spinal deformity can result from unstable motion segments, or conversely, can cause them. The classification of thoracic spinal deformities can be complex.

Deformities are usually classified by their rotation or translation about the three axes of the spine as defined by the Cartesian coordinate system. There are six fundamental movements that can occur, hence there are six fundamental types of spinal deformation: (1) rotation about the long axis of the spine, (2) rotation about the coronal axis of the spine, (3) rotation about the sagittal axis of the spine, (4) translation along the long axis of the spine, (5) translation along the coronal axis of the spine, and (6) translation along the sagittal axis of the spine. Each of these movements or deformities can occur in either of two directions. Each deformity type may involve only one spinal segment or multiple segments. Spinal deformities are most often combinations of two or more of the types. They may result from either acutely or chronically applied loads.

Many factors affect the deformity correction process. A consideration of the fundamental types of force application is therefore of significance. These factors include distraction (Fig. 15-1), three-point bending (Fig. 15-2), tension-band fixation (Fig. 15-3), and cantilevered constructs (Fig. 15-4). Complications or unexpected results, however, may be observed.

Of relevance, particularly regarding long three-point bending constructs, is the location of hook placement. First, longer constructs with multiple points of spinal fixation are usually more efficacious than shorter ones. Second, the relationship between the hook attachment site and the fulcrum

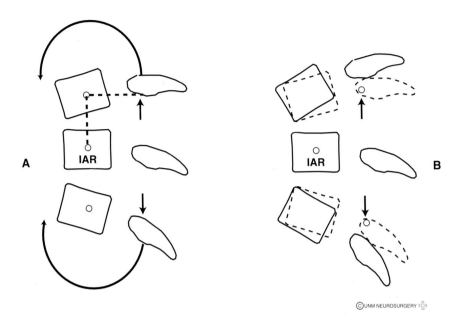

Fig. 15-1. A, A depiction of the forces applied to the spine by a simple dorsal distraction construct. Curved arrows = bending moment. Straight arrows = applied force. Instantaneous axis of rotation = IAR. **B,** A flexion deformity may result if the distraction forces are placed at a significant distance from the IAR. (From Benzel EC. Spinal Instrumentation. Park Ridge, Ill.: American Association of Neurological Surgeons, 1994.)

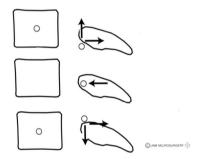

Fig. 15-2. A three-point bending construct. The vertically oriented arrows depict the accompanying distraction forces. The horizontal arrows at both termini of the construct depict the dorsally directed forces. The horizontal arrow in the middle of the construct depicts the ventrally directed force (at the fulcrum). (From Benzel EC. Spinal Instrumentation. Park Ridge, Ill.: American Association of Neurological Surgeons, 1994.)

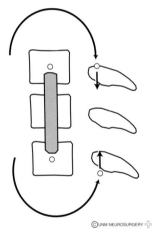

Fig. 15-3. A tension-band fixation construct. The moment arm is similar in length but is associated with a bending moment *(curved arrows)* that is opposite in direction to that observed with simple distraction (see Fig. 15-1). Applied force = straight arrows. (From Benzel EC. Spinal Instrumentation. Park Ridge, Ill.: American Association of Neurological Surgeons, 1994.)

should be carefully considered (Fig. 15-5). Finally, distraction implant efficacy is related to many factors. These include the integrity of the ligaments and the actual corrective forces applied (Fig. 15-6).

Each of these factors and their clinical applications are discussed below. Principles, rather than "cook book" procedural descriptions are emphasized.

DEFORMITY CORRECTION

Deformity correction is accomplished via the application of rotatory or translational forces to the spine along one or a combination of the three axes of the

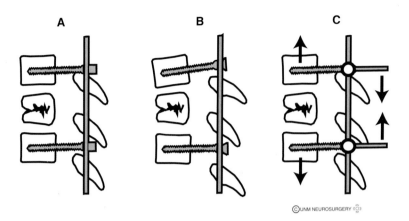

Fig. 15-4. Cantilever beam constructs. **A,** A fixed moment arm construct. Note the rigid attachment site to the longitudinal member. **B,** A nonfixed moment arm construct. Note the screw-through-the-plate configuration that allows the screw to toggle with respect to the plate. **C,** An applied moment arm construct. By applying a dorsal compression via attachment sites that can be removed after screw-longitudinal member fixation and prior to wound closure (e.g., Shanz screws), extension of the spine is achieved. (From Benzel EC. Spinal Instrumentation. Park Ridge, Ill.: American Association of Neurological Surgeons, 1994, pp 242.)

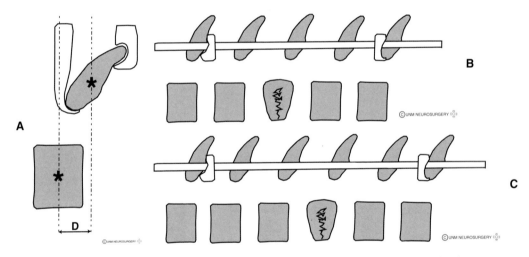

Fig. 15-5. A point of attachment, along the long axis of the spine, of dorsally applied hooks. **A,** Note that the centroid of the site of hook attachment is at the level of the lower aspect of the vertebral body ("*"). The centroid of the vertebral body and the centroid of the hook attachment sites ("*"s) are thus separated by a distance *(D)* that is roughly one-half a vertebral segment in width *(vertical dashed lines)*. **B,** A construct that is employed at the same number of segments above and below the level of pathology will apply a shorter moment arm rostrally, as is the case with a 2A-2B construct. **C,** A 3A-2B construct avoids this discrepancy. (From Benzel EC. Spinal Instrumentation. Park Ridge, Ill.: American Association of Neurological Surgeons, 1994, and Benzel EC. Biomechanics of Spine Stabilization: Principles and Clinical Practice. New York: McGraw-Hill, 1995.)

Cartesian coordinate system.[4] The clinically applicable techniques are discussed.

Distraction and Compression

Distraction may be applied to the spine to reduce coronal and sagittal plane deformations as well as compression deformations of the spine. Paraspinous soft tissue integrity is mandatory for this type of force application to be effective in these circumstances. Distraction can be effective as a method of translational deformity correction via a "ligamentotaxis mechanism" (see Fig. 15-6, *A* to *C*). It can also be used to correct scoliotic deformities (see Fig. 15-6, *D* to *F*).

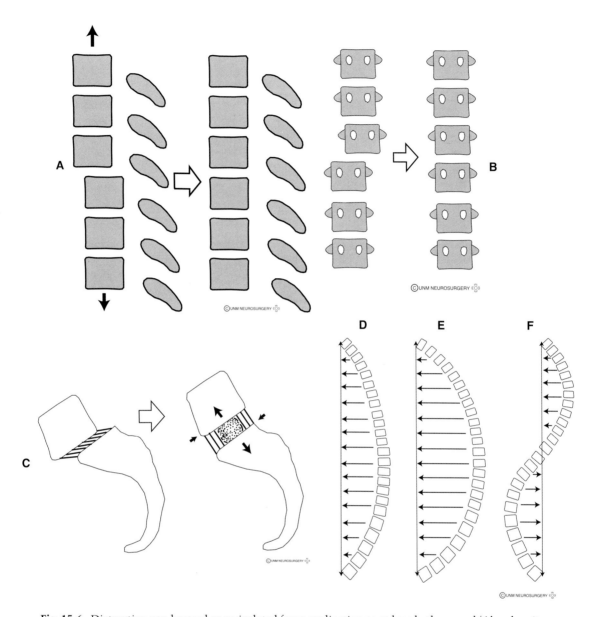

Fig. 15-6. Distraction can be used as an isolated force application to reduce both coronal (**A**) and sagittal (**B**) translational deformities. **C,** An interbody fusion technique may also be employed in this regard by acting as a "spacer" that maintains distraction of the disc interspace region. Axial distractive force application can also be employed to reduce curvatures. It is most effectively applied on the concave side of a curve; and its effectiveness *(horizontal arrows)* is proportional to the angle of the curve (**D** and **E**). **F,** Axial distraction force application can be also employed for biconcave curves. The vertical arrows depict the forces applied by the implant. The horizontal arrows depict the indirect corrective forces derived. Note that they are longest at the apex of the curve. This correlates with implant efficacy. (**C** and **F** from Benzel EC. Biomechanics of Spine Stabilization: Principles and Clinical Practice. New York: McGraw-Hill, 1995.)

Distraction of the concave side of a curve and compression of the convex side of a curve can be used to correct focal coronal plane deformities. This is a force couple that applies a coronal plane bending moment (see discussion on p. 287).[2]

Three-Point and Four-Point Bending Fixation

Three-point and four-point bending of the spine, as defined by White and Panjabi,[6] involves the loading of a long structure (i.e., the spine) with one or two transverse forces on one side and two on the other (Fig. 15-7, *A*). With a four-point bending construct, the bending moment is constant between the two intermediate points of force application. With a three-point bending construct, the bending moment peaks at the intermediate point of force application (Fig. 15-7, *B*).

Crossed-Rod Fixation

The crossed-rod technique is a complex variant of three-point bending or four-point bending fixation.[1,2] It was one of the first thoracic and lumbar deformity correction techniques employed. Recently, the sequential hook insertion (SHI) technique has been used with universal instrumentation techniques to achieve the same goal.[3] Regardless, the crossed-rod technique involves the sequential and gradual application of forces to the deformed spine (Fig. 15-7, *C* to *E*).

Applied Moment Arm Cantilever Beam Force Application

Applied moment arm cantilever beam constructs are short segment constructs that are usually used to apply sagittal plane bending moments (flexion or extension) to the spine via pedicle screw-rod implants[2,5] (Fig. 15-8, *A* and *B*). Significant force is applied to the spine. They may rarely be employed for coronal plane deformity correction. They can be utilized in combination with distraction, compression, or coronal plane bending moment force application. An accompanying ventral dural sac decompression and interbody bone graft insertion can also be simultaneously employed. This technique can be used so that a deformity is reduced and compression of the bone graft is achieved. The technique of (1) sequentially applying distraction (load bearing), (2) decompression of the dural sac, (3) interbody fusion placement, and (4) the compression of the construct, in order to share the load with the ventral spinal elements is termed "load-bearing-to-load-sharing" force application. It provides biomechanical (load-sharing) as well as clinical (shorter constructs with less stiffness) advantages[1,2] (see Fig. 15-8).

Short Segment Parallelogram Deformity Reduction

Short segment parallelogram deformity reduction is a rigid cantilever beam pedicle fixation technique. It applies a coronal plane bending moment to the spine for the reduction of lateral translational deformations.[1] This technique is most useful when short segment fixation is deemed optimal. It involves: (1) the placement of pedicle screws, (2) an appropriate dural sac decompression, (3) the attachment of the longitudinal members to the screws (i.e., rods), (4) the application of a rotatory and distraction force to the rods, (5) the maintenance of the achieved spinal reduction via rigid crossfixation, (6) the placement of a fusion (interbody and/or lateral), and finally (7) compression of the screws so that load sharing is achieved and the interbody bone graft is secured in its acceptance bed[1] (Fig. 15-9). Short segment parallelogram deformity reduction applies load-bearing forces to load-sharing forces; forces that initially bear a load by distraction intraoperatively, followed by compression of the implant and vertebral bodies onto the intervening bone graft (load sharing).

In Vivo Implant Contouring

The use of in vivo implant contouring for segmental relationship alteration is an effective method of deformity reduction. Following insertion of a spinal implant, rod contouring can be used to alter spinal curvature. Secure implant-bone interfaces are imperative. This technique may not be suitable in the presence of significant osteoporosis. Implant contouring alters the forces applied at each segmental level. Hooks may overtighten or loosen, infringe on the spinal canal, or migrate laterally or medially.[1]

Intrinsic Implant Bending Moment Application About the Long Axis of the Spine: The Derotation Maneuver

Obligatory rotatory component coexists with scoliotic deformities (coupling). Therefore they should perhaps more appropriately be termed rotatory scoliotic curvatures. This coupling phenomenon can be used to the surgeon's advantage by the application of the spinal derotation maneuver.

Fig. 15-7. **A,** Three- and four-point bending fixation consists of one or two *(left-facing dotted arrow and solid arrows)* transverse forces applied to the opposite side of the spine (intermediate forces) from the orientation of the terminal forces *(two right-facing arrows).* **B,** The bending moment associated with four-point bending fixation is constant between the two intervening points of force application and falls off to zero at the terminal points of fixation. With three-point bending fixation, the bending moment peaks at the intervening point of fixation. **C, D,** and **E,** The crossed-rod technique is a method of applying three- or four-point bending techniques to achieve deformity reduction. (**B** from Benzel EC. Biomechanics of Spine Stabilization: Principles and Clinical Practice. New York: McGraw-Hill, 1995.)

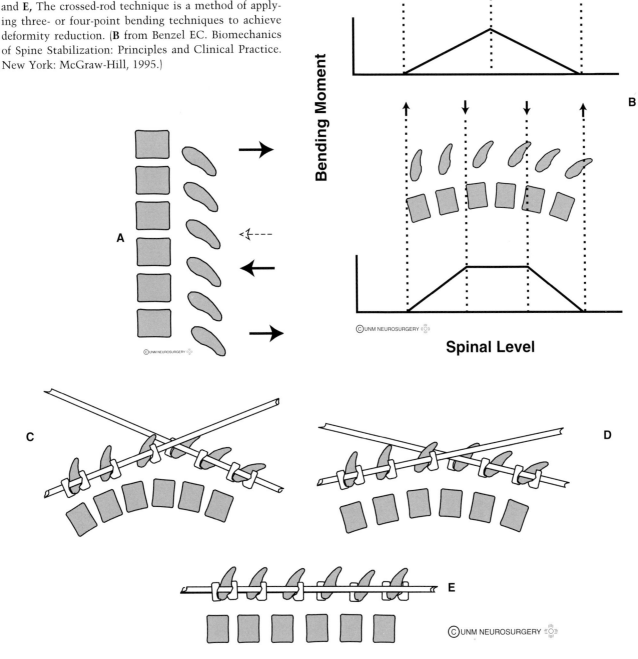

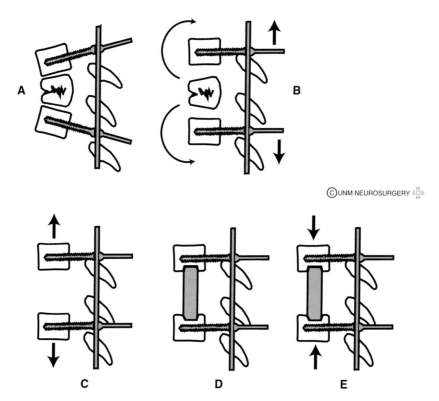

©UNM NEUROSURGERY

Fig. 15-8. A and **B,** Applied moment arm cantilever beam force application via pedicle screws. This technique can be applied in combination with other force applications to achieve a "load-bearing-to-load-sharing" force application complex. **B,** Reduction via extension force application. **C,** Distraction (the implant bears the load). **D,** Placement of an interbody bone graft. **E,** Compression provides the "load-sharing" component of the fixation complex. (From Benzel EC. Biomechanics of Spine Stabilization: Principles and Clinical Practice. New York: McGraw-Hill, 1995.)

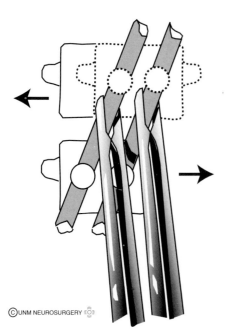

©UNM NEUROSURGERY

Fig. 15-9. Short-segment parallelogram deformity reduction. A lateral translational deformity *(dotted vertebra)* is reduced by first inserting pedicle screws into each of the pedicles located above and below the translational deformity. Next, rods are attached to each of the screws. Translational forces *(straight arrows)* are then applied to each of the vertebrae via bending moments applied by rod grippers. This reduces the deformity *(solid vertebra).* A rigid crossmember is then employed for deformity reduction maintenance and stability augmentation purposes. (From Benzel EC. Biomechanics of Spine Stabilization: Principles and Clinical Practice. New York: McGraw-Hill, 1995.)

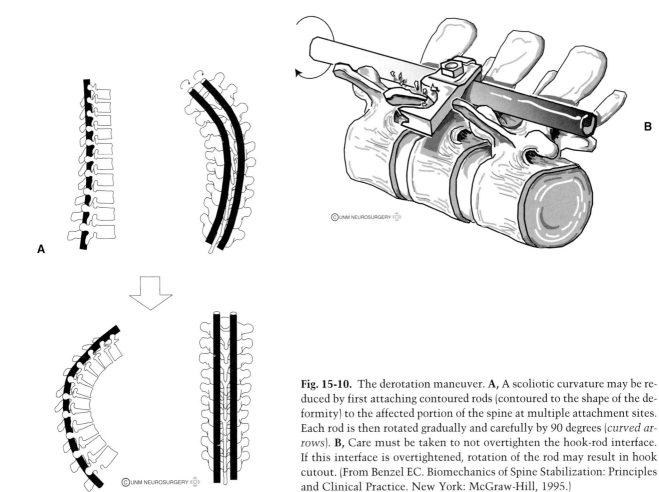

Fig. 15-10. The derotation maneuver. **A,** A scoliotic curvature may be reduced by first attaching contoured rods (contoured to the shape of the deformity) to the affected portion of the spine at multiple attachment sites. Each rod is then rotated gradually and carefully by 90 degrees (*curved arrows*). **B,** Care must be taken to not overtighten the hook-rod interface. If this interface is overtightened, rotation of the rod may result in hook cutout. (From Benzel EC. Biomechanics of Spine Stabilization: Principles and Clinical Practice. New York: McGraw-Hill, 1995.)

Although perhaps simplistic, spinal derotation is a technique that involves the conversion of a scoliotic curvature to a kyphotic curvature.[4] The derotation maneuver is accomplished by first attaching the rods to the spine (via hooks, screws, or wires). With this maneuver, the hooks, screws, or wires are relatively loosely attached to the rod (friction-glide tightness). This allows rotation of the rod at its interface with the hooks, screws, or wires. The attachment should not be so tight as to cause dislodgment at the attachment site via attachment site disruption.

The rods are then gradually and simultaneously rotated 90 degrees. This converts a scoliotic curvature to a kyphotic curvature. The rods may be contoured to eliminate an excessive kyphotic curvature, if present. Most often, however, scoliotic deformities are associated with a relatively flat back due to the coupling phenomenon. Finally, the interfaces are tightened and secured. Crossfixation is then employed to maintain the correction (Fig. 15-10, *A*). Overtightening at the hook-rod interface prior to derotation can result in hook dislodgment and hook-bone interface failure (Fig. 15-10, *B*).

Intrinsic Implant Bending Moment Application About the Axial Axes of the Spine

Intrinsic implant bending moment application can be employed in either the sagittal or coronal plane. It is most commonly used for one- or two-segment lumbar scoliotic deformities, although it could be employed in the thoracic spine.

With this technique, pedicle screws are inserted and rods are attached. The screws on the concave side of the curvature are then distracted, and the screws on the convex side of the curvature are compressed.

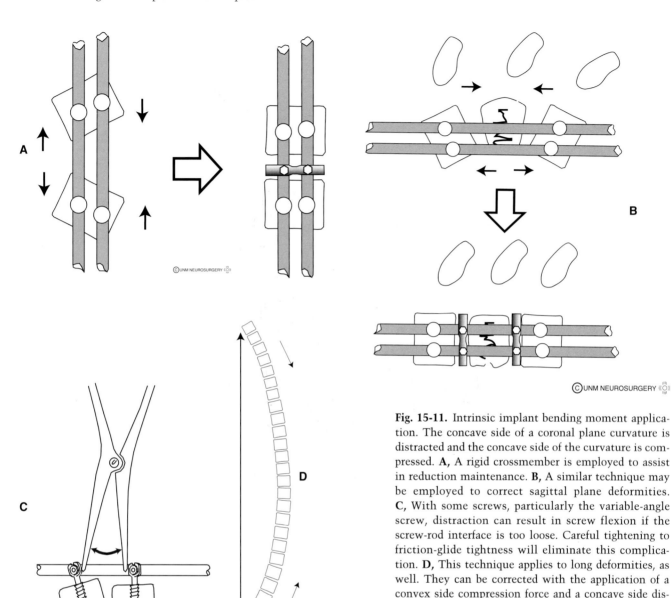

Fig. 15-11. Intrinsic implant bending moment application. The concave side of a coronal plane curvature is distracted and the concave side of the curvature is compressed. **A,** A rigid crossmember is employed to assist in reduction maintenance. **B,** A similar technique may be employed to correct sagittal plane deformities. **C,** With some screws, particularly the variable-angle screw, distraction can result in screw flexion if the screw-rod interface is too loose. Careful tightening to friction-glide tightness will eliminate this complication. **D,** This technique applies to long deformities, as well. They can be corrected with the application of a convex side compression force and a concave side distraction force. (From Benzel EC. Biomechanics of Spine Stabilization: Principles and Clinical Practice. New York: McGraw-Hill, 1995.)

Crossfixation is used to maintain the correction (Fig. 15-11, *A* and *B*). A similar technique may be used to correct sagittal plane deformities by employing rod or plate-screw systems on the lateral aspect of the spine[1] (Fig. 15-11, *C* and *D*).

The application of distraction forces to a variable-angle screw that is not adequately tightened (to a friction-glide extent) may result in screw flexion at the screw-rod interface. This undesirable event can be prevented by carefully tightening the screw to a friction-glide tightness prior to the application of the distraction forces (see Fig. 15-11, *C*). These

principles apply to longer deformities, as well (see Fig. 15-11, *D*).

THE MAINTENANCE OF CORRECTION
Crossfixation

In general, the crossfixation of short constructs is of little benefit. This excludes the fact, however, that crossfixation can be used to maintain deformity reduction in selected cases. Crossfixation provides a quadrilateral frame-like construct with longer constructs, which provides rotatory stability and implant-bone interface integrity augmentation. With long constructs, two crossmembers are better than one, yet more than two adds very little to construct integrity.[1] The crossmembers may be strategically placed behind a hook to help avoid hook backout. The crossmembers should be approximately placed at the junction of the thirds of the length of the construct.[1]

REFERENCES

1. Benzel EC. Biomechanics of Spine Stabilization: Principles and Clinical Practice. New York: McGraw-Hill, 1995.
2. Benzel EC. Spinal Instrumentation. Park Ridge, Ill.: American Association of Neurological Surgeons, 1994.
3. Benzel EC, Ball PA, Baldwin NG, Marchand EP. The sequential hook insertion technique for universal spinal instrumentation application. J Neurosurg 79:608-611, 1993.
4. Cotrel Y, Dubousset J, Guillaumat M. New universal instrumentation in spinal surgery. Clin Orthop Rel Res 227:10-23, 1988.
5. Dick W. The "fixateur interne" as a versatile implant for spine surgery. Spine 12:882-900, 1987.
6. White AA, Panjabi MM. Clinical Biomechanics of the Spine, 2nd ed. Philadelphia: JB Lippincott, 1990.

16

Thoracoscopic Approaches

Noel I. Perin, M.D.

The practice of medicine has been revolutionized in the last 10 years with the renewed interest in endoscopic surgery. Dubois et al.[2] performed the first laparoscopic cholecystectomies in 1987. The modern era of thoracoscopic surgery began in 1990 with the addition of video-to-standard endoscopic techniques. The term "video-assisted thoracic surgery" (VATS) was coined to include the broad spectrum of diagnostic and therapeutic procedures now performed thoracoscopically.

Dorsal percutaneous spinal surgery for the treatment of lumbar disc herniation has been in vogue for a long time. Starting in the 1960s with percutaneous intradiscal chymopapain injection therapy,[8] to the 1980s when Hijikata[3] and Kambin and Gellman[5] popularized manual percutaneous discectomy and automated percutaneous discectomy for contained lumbar disc herniations. Choy, Ascher, and Saddekni[1] and Mathews (unpublished abstract) in the late 1980s combined the intradiscal procedures with laser technology, and finally percutaneous endoscopic intradiscal and foraminoscopic discectomy techniques emerged in the 1990s.

Video-assisted thoracoscopic techniques to access the thoracic spine have been encouraging. Thoracoscopy affords several potential advantages over open thoracotomy for the treatment of thoracic spinal pathology. However, there is a steep learning curve with the techniques, together with the problem of interpreting three-dimensional spatial images that are projected in two dimensions on a television screen. Other drawbacks include the lack of

tactile feedback and the necessity for good hand-eye coordination. Potentially, operating time can be reduced, the length of hospital stay shortened, and patients can resume normal activities of daily living sooner. Postoperative pulmonary function is less impaired as there is less postoperative pain due to the small incisions. There is also reduced impairment of shoulder function as opposed to open thoracotomy. Scars from the thoracoscopic ports are aesthetically more pleasing than the large scar with an open procedure. Thoracoscopic spinal surgery can be used safely in a number of diagnostic and therapeutic situations affecting the thoracic spine.

THORACOSCOPIC ANATOMY

The thoracic cavity is usually entered via the fifth or sixth intercostal space in the ventral axillary line in most cases. Before starting the procedure it is well worth familiarizing oneself with the local anatomy. A thoracoscope passed through a ventrally placed port will give a panoramic view of the entire thoracic spine and dorsal chest cavity. The view and orientation on the video monitor should not be different from the view obtained in an open thoracotomy. The ventral structures appear at the top of the screen and the dorsal structures at the bottom of the screen. If the apical or basal regions of the chest cavity are to be viewed through either a rostral or caudal port, the anatomy on the video screen will change accordingly. Familiarity with the normal anatomy from different thoracoscope port positions is essential for successful surgery. Once the lung has been collapsed, the spinal column with the ribs should be well visualized. The sympathetic trunk can be seen coursing over the heads of the ribs, deep to the parietal pleura. The azygos vein runs along the ventral border of the spinal column on the right side, and the descending aorta lies in a similar position on the left side. The ribs can be counted from the apical region down to the basal areas. The diaphragm can be noted caudally and will have to be retracted caudally and laterally to access the caudal thoracic spine. The disc spaces correspond to the elevated areas of the spinal column beneath the parietal pleura. The radicular vessels lie in the troughs between the discs over the lateral surface of the vertebral bodies. The rib articulates with the adjacent end plates across a disc space and overlies the pedicle as it courses dorsally.

INDICATIONS FOR THORACOSCOPIC SPINAL SURGERY

The present indications for thoracoscopic spinal surgery will broaden with further technological advances in the field of endoscopic surgery and as physicians become more skilled.

1. *Infection.* Biopsy of disc space infection with drainage of abscess and debridement
2. *Tumor.* Biopsy of unknown tumors with tumor excision, vertebrectomy, bone grafting, and plating for stabilization
3. *Degenerative.* Excision of thoracic disc herniation[4,7]
4. *Deformity.* Ventral release in the correction of rigid scoliotic curves; ventral epiphysiodesis in skeletally immature patients at risk of developing a crankshaft with only dorsal stabilization and fusion
5. *Sympathectomy.* In hyperhidrosis and reflex sympathetic dystrophy

All patients considered for thoracoscopic spinal surgery should be evaluated for previous and present pulmonary and chest wall pathology. Patients with a history of previous thoracotomy, empyema, and pleurodesis on the ipsilateral side run a significantly higher risk of lung injury and should be excluded. Some relative contraindications are previous ipsilateral thoracoscopy, severe chronic obstructive pulmonary disease (COPD), and age under 5 years.

ANESTHETIC CONSIDERATIONS

The preoperative workup for thoracoscopic procedures is similar to open thoracotomy. Additionally, for thoracoscopic spinal surgery, the presence of lung or chest wall pathology is a contraindication. Previous history of empyema or pleurodesis again will be a contraindication for thoracoscopic spinal surgery. Single lung ventilation is necessary in thoracoscopic procedures. A knowledge of the problems associated with the use of CO_2 insufflation is essential, though CO_2 insufflation is not routinely utilized in thoracoscopic surgery. Double lumen tubes are commonly used to allow isolation of the operative lung and ventilation of the nonoperative lung. Alternatively an endobronchial tube may be used to isolate the lung. Routine insufflation is not utilized in thoracoscopic surgery unless there is difficulty with one-lung ventilation. CO_2 flow 1.5 to 2.0 L/min to a maximum pressure of 10 to 12 mm Hg is utilized when necessary to achieve maximal collapse of the ipsilateral lung. Higher pressures in the thoracic cavity may lead to mediastinal tamponade. Postoperatively epidural analgesia and intercostal nerve blocks are not necessary due to reduced levels of pain, compared to open thoracotomy.

EQUIPMENT AND INSTRUMENTATION

The basic equipment required for thoracoscopic procedures includes endoscopes (0-H and 30-degree angle), xenon light source, camera, monitors, video recorders, and CO_2 insufflators.

The most commonly used telescope is the "rigid quartz lens system" with fiber light bundles incorporated into the shaft. The most popular are the 10 mm diameter, 15-inch long, 0-degree "end viewing," and the 30-degree "angled" scopes.

Light sources are high intensity metal halide or xenon lamps. They operate in the range of 5600 to 6000 kelvin. The telescopes are connected to a camera. Three-chip camera technology now transmits truer images to the video screen. Video monitors vary from 13- to 21-inch screens. A VCR is used for recording (S-VHS). CO_2 insufflators are standard equipment in endoscopic procedures, though not usually used in thoracoscopic procedures (Fig. 16-1).

Thoracoscopic instruments (Fig. 16-2) may be divided into those required for soft tissue access and the spinal instruments. The former are instruments

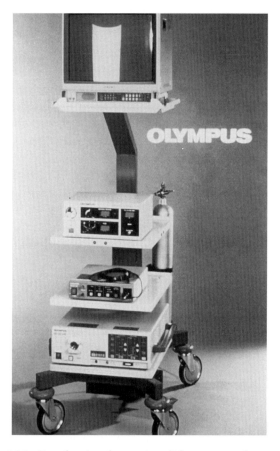

Fig. 16-1. Cart showing the monitor, light source, and camera.

used in standard endoscopic techniques, with minor modifications. "Soft" thoracic ports as opposed to the "hard" ports, were developed to reduce the postoperative intercostal neuralgic pain. Some laparoscopic instruments were shortened and, in addition, curved instruments were developed to overcome limitations placed on the straight instruments by the rigid chest cavity. In addition to the trocars for chest wall access, graspers, scissors, retractors, endoscopic staplers, and monopolar and bipolar cautery are available for use with thoracoscopic procedures.

Spinal instruments in the chest are merely extended versions of the standard spinal instruments. Any instrument, provided it is long enough, can be used, as no CO_2 insufflation is utilized with thoracoscopic spinal surgery. A standard thoracotomy set should be available in the operating room in case of emergency.

PATIENT POSITIONING AND PORT PLACEMENT

Patients are placed in the lateral decubitus position as for open thoracotomy. The patient is positioned over the break or the kidney rest so that flexion of the table can open the intercostal spaces and facilitate entry into the chest cavity. Two video monitors are placed on either side of the head when working on the mid- to upper thoracic spine, one monitor for the surgeon and one for the assistant. When the lower thoracic spine or the lumbar spine

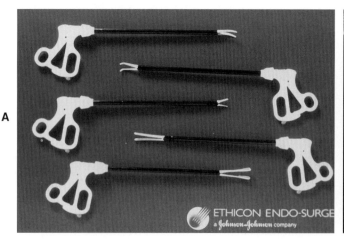

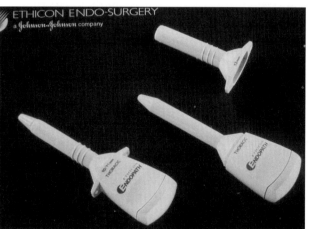

Fig. 16-2. A, Access instruments for soft tissue dissection range from graspers to scissors and bipolar forceps. **B,** Thoracoports. They are now available as soft ports.

is to be accessed, the monitors are placed at the foot end. The whole chest wall is prepared as for open thoracotomy. If the need arises, immediate thoracotomy can be performed. The anesthesiologist is asked to collapse the lung during the preparation of the patient. The initial port is placed around the sixth intercostal space in the ventral axillary line. This will of course depend on the level of the spine to be accessed. A 10 mm incision is made in the chosen space, the dissection carried down to the parietal pleura. The pleural space is entered using a kelly clamp and a finger is placed through this opening to lyse any lung adhesions before introducing the trocar. The scope is placed via this port and should provide a panoramic view of the spinal column. The subsequent port placements will be done under direct vision. The working ports should be placed dorsally in the dorsal axillary line on either side of the projected target. These ports should not be placed too close together, otherwise the instruments will tend to duel with each other. The number of ports and their locations will depend on the procedure. Typically one can start with a 0-degree scope and then switch to a 30-degree scope when working on the spine. Additional working ports can be placed as required with one directly over the site of the pathology for drilling.

THORACOSCOPIC DISCECTOMY

Large central or calcific disc herniations requiring a ventrolateral thoracotomy approach can be accessed thoracoscopically. The patient is placed in the lateral decubitus position. A right-sided approach is preferred, unless the pathology dictates otherwise. The patient's pelvis and shoulders are taped to the table. The axillary lines and sites for port placement are marked on the patient. The chest is prepared and draped as for a thoracotomy. The initial port is placed in the ventral axillary line; the intercostal space will depend on the level of the disc herniation. The rostral lung is collapsed. A 2 cm incision is made in the skin down to the intercostal muscle layer. A kelly clamp is used to separate the muscles down to the parietal pleura. The clamp is pushed gently into the pleural cavity and opened. A finger is passed into the pleural cavity and any lung adhesions lysed. A 15 mm soft thoracoport is placed in the chest and the 0-degree scope is passed into the chest cavity. A panoramic view of the chest is ob-

tained (Fig. 16-3). The remaining ports are placed under direct vision. Typically three ports are utilized, two in the ventral axillary line on either side of the target and a third caudally in the dorsal axillary line. The disc space is identified by counting the ribs from the apex, as well as placing a needle percutaneously in the disc space and obtaining a cross-table anteroposterior (AP) radiograph. Once the level is identified, the parietal pleura over the disc space and corresponding rib are opened with the Bovie. The intercostal vessels over the adjacent bodies are identified, clipped, and divided. The periosteum of the rib is scraped off, protecting the neurovascular bundle, and the rib is divided 2 to 3 cm distal to its head using an osteotome and mallet. The head of the rib is separated from its attachment to the adjacent end plates and the rib is removed in one piece. Next the soft tissue overlying the pedicle is coagulated with the bipolar, thus identifying the lateral surface of the pedicle. The Kerrison punch is used to remove the pedicle from rostral to caudal, identifying the lateral surface of the dura. At this point the dorsal, rostral margins of the end plate adjacent to the disc space are removed with the Kerrison, exposing the disc and the ventral epidural space. The disc is gently freed from the dura decompressing the cord. A drill can be used to create a trough behind the disc space to facilitate this process. A fourth port may be necessary directly

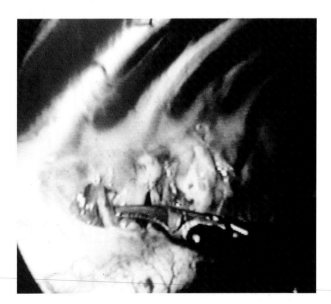

Fig. 16-3. View through the scope showing the ribs. The parietal pleura has been opened, and the radicular vessel is being dissected over the vertebral body.

over the disc space for drilling. Hemostasis is achieved with thrombin-soaked Gelfoam and bipolar coagulation. The ports are closed after achieving hemostasis with subcuticular Vicryl. A size 32 chest tube is placed adjacent to the operative site through one of the ports.

COMPLICATIONS AND COMPLICATION PREVENTION

Common problems encountered with thoracoscopic surgery include trocar site bleeding and bleeding on the endoscopic lens. These can be prevented by atraumatic placement of the ports, staying above the lower rib away from the neurovascular bundle, and adequate coagulation of the trocar site bleeding when encountered.

Fogging of the lens is a problem encountered due to the difference in the ambient and intrathoracic temperatures. The lens should be cleaned frequently with a defogger (Fred) and the scope kept in a warm saline bath, which will reduce fogging.

Dueling instruments occurs when ports are placed too close together. Careful planning and spacing of the ports using the "baseball diamond principle" will eliminate this problem.

Patients should be evaluated preoperatively for intrathoracic pathology to avoid problems during surgery.

Paralytic hemidiaphragm should be recognized prior to surgery to avoid placing the initial trocar through the diaphragm. Preoperative chest radiographs will help localize the levels of the dome of the diaphragm.

The level of the pathology should be identified by counting the ribs from the apex down with the scope and subsequently obtaining intraoperative cross-table radiographs with a percutaneously placed needle above the disc space.

Epidural bleeding when it occurs can be dealt with using bipolar coagulation and tamponaded by packing with thrombin-soaked Gelfoam and endoavitene. Dural tears are difficult to control thoracoscopically. Small tears may be packed with Gelfoam, fibrin glue, and fat graft. Larger tears however, may have to be dealt with by converting to an open thoracotomy.

Spinal cord injury is avoided by removing the head and neck of the rib and the pedicle and identifying the dural tube before embarking on disc removal.

Finally, if there is injury to large arteries or veins in the thoracic cavity, one should tamponade initially with a sponge and open the chest to obtain control. Always work with an experienced thoracic surgeon who will be available in an emergency. A standard thoracotomy set should be in the room and opened immediately when necessary.

CONCLUSION

Indications for minimally invasive spinal surgery will continue to expand with further advances in technology and refinement of current techniques. These techniques, however, will need to be cost-effective and show an improvement in the short-term and long-term outcomes.[6] The progress and outcome of such procedures will most assuredly also be closely monitored by insurers looking to cut the cost of health care delivery.

REFERENCES

1. Choy DS, Ascher PW, Saddekni S. Percutaneous laser disc decompression: A new therapeutic modality. Spine 17:949-956, 1992.
2. Dubois F, Icard P, Berthelot G, Levard H. Coelioscopic cholecystectomy: Preliminary report of 36 cases. Ann Surg 211:60-62, 1990.
3. Hijikata SA. A method of percutaneous nuclear extraction. J Toden Hosp 5:39-44, 1975.
4. Horowitz MB, Moossy JJ, Julian T. Thoracic discectomy using video assisted thoracoscopy. Spine 19:1082-1086, 1994.
5. Kambin P, Gellman H. Percutaneous lateral discectomy of the lumbar spine. A preliminary report. Clin Orthop 174:127-132, 1983.
6. Regan JJ, Mack MJ, Picetti GD. A comparison of video assisted thoracoscopic surgery (VATS) with open thoracotomy in thoracic spinal surgery. Today's Therapeutic Trends 11:203-218, 1994.
7. Rosenthal D, Rosenthal R, De Simeone A. Removal of a protruded thoracic disc using microsurgical endoscopy. Spine 19:1087-1091, 1994.
8. Smith L. Enzyme dissolution of the intervertebral disc. Nature 4887:198, 1963.

SUGGESTED READING

Friedman WA. Percutaneous discectomy: An alternative to chemonucleolysis. Neurosurgery 13:542-547, 1983.
Landreneau RJ, Hazelrigg SR, Mack MJ. Postoperative pain related morbidity. Video assisted thoracic surgery versus thoracotomy. Ann Thorac Surg 56:1285-1289, 1993.
Mack MJ, Regan JJ, Bobechko WP. Application of thoracoscopy for diseases of the spine. Ann Thorac Surg 56:736-738, 1993.
Maroon JC, Onik G, Vidovich DV. Percutaneous discectomy for lumbar disc herniation. Neurosurg Clin Am 4:125-134, 1993.
Onik G, Helms C, Ginsberg L. Percutaneous lumbar discectomy using a new aspiration probe. AJNR 6:290-293, 1985.

Thoracic Disc Herniation and Spondylosis

Thoracic Disc Disease, Spondylosis, and Stenosis

Seth M. Zeidman, M.D., Michael K. Rosner, M.D.,
and G. Jefferey Poffenbarger, M.D.

Complaints of thoracic pain are often poorly localized, vague, and enigmatic. For a small number of patients this pain is severely disabling and quite frustrating. Thoracic disc herniation is an uncommon, but clinically important cause of severe, incapacitating local and/or radicular pain and myelopathy and has long been a difficult entity to diagnose and treat. Evolution in the management of thoracic disc disease is evident in the surgical treatment of this entity, with the development of a number of operative techniques, including laminectomy, costotransversectomy, lateral extracavitary, transpedicular, transthoracic, and thoracoscopic approaches.

HISTORY

The first report of spinal cord compression resulting from a thoracic disc herniation was made by Key in 1838.[14] In 1911 Middleton and Teacher[18] described a patient with acute paraplegia from a thoracic disc herniation. The first surgical treatment of thoracic disc herniation was reported by Adson[1] in 1922, who performed a laminectomy and disc removal. Mixter and Barr[19] reported three patients who underwent thoracic laminectomy and disc excision, two of whom developed complete paraplegia.

In 1931 Antoni[3] and Elsburg[11] independently reported operative procedures performed for the treatment of thoracic disc disease. Logue's 1952 review[16] of patients undergoing laminectomy for this disorder documented the uniformly poor results with this technique.

ANATOMY AND BIOMECHANICS

The anatomy of the thoracic spinal canal predisposes it to spinal cord impingement and damage from even a small disc herniation. In the thoracic spine, the ratio of the spinal cord cross-sectional area to spinal canal area is greater than other regions of the spinal axis. The blood supply to the spinal cord in this area is often tenuous, particularly between T4 and T9. The intrathoracic spinal cord has been termed "the critical vascular zone" by Dommisse.[10] This reflects the limited direct blood supply from the radicular and intramedullary circulation, as well as the paucity of vascularization at the microcirculatory level.

Mechanical compression does not, in and of itself, necessarily result in spinal cord dysfunction. The thoracic spinal cord is immobilized by the dentate ligaments, therefore minor compression can lead to symptoms through traction. Additionally, both ischemia and venous congestion can worsen minor spinal cord compression. Angiographic studies occasionally demonstrate compression of the anterior spinal artery by a herniated thoracic disc or spondylotic disease, and distended veins can occasionally be visualized above and below the level of a herniated thoracic disc with magnetic resonance imaging (MRI).

EPIDEMIOLOGY

The incidence of clinically significant thoracic disc herniation has been estimated to be approximately one patient per million population. These represent 0.25% to 0.75% of all disc ruptures.[4] Thoracic disc surgery represents about 0.15% to 1.8% of all disc operations. However, asymptomatic disc herniations are very common. Asymptomatic disc herniation can be identified in between 11.1% and 14.5% of thoracic spines imaged with MRI.[6,25,29]

Men are affected more frequently than women. Patients often note some precipitating event including trauma, lifting heavy objects, or a fall. Trauma, particularly in younger men, is reported in up to one third of patients. The causal relationship between such events and the herniation can often be very difficult to establish with certainty.

PRESENTATION

Thoracic disc herniation does not have a characteristic clinical presentation, and misdiagnosis is common. Thoracic disc herniation typically presents with a variety of nonspecific symptoms leading to incorrect or delayed diagnoses.

Symptoms are generally progressive and of long duration, but acute presentations can and do occur. In one series of 35 patients treated with thoracoscopic spinal techniques, the mean duration of symptoms before diagnosis was 6 months.[24] Local or radicular pain is the most frequent presentation and often predates the development of neurological dysfunction or myelopathy. Diagnosis is frequently delayed until signs and symptoms of myelopathy develop. The location of maximal pain may reflect the level of disc herniation, but this is not always the case.

It is important to remember that thoracic disc herniation may mimic other disorders such as a neoplasm or demyelinating disease. However, one should also consider that identification of a herniated thoracic disc does not in and of itself constitute proof

that this is the source of the disability; exclusion of tumor and demyelinating disease must be performed before embarking upon surgical intervention.

DIAGNOSIS

Lack of accuracy of diagnostic tests is a significant problem, but CT-myelography is a major advance over myelography. MRI is now considered the standard screening examination, and has demonstrated a significantly higher incidence of thoracic disc herniation. The increased use of this noninvasive scanning technique and increased clinical awareness have resulted in the more frequent diagnosis of symptomatic thoracic disc herniation. Asymptomatic disc herniation can be identified in nearly 15% of thoracic spines imaged with MRI.[6,25,29]

Thoracic Discogenic Pain

Thoracic discogenic pain, without evidence of a true herniation, is neither well recognized nor understood. Patients typically present with a chronic thoracic pain, often without neurological complaints, secondary to a painful thoracic disc without radiologic evidence of a true or significant herniation. These patients are often refractory to conservative measures and have a serious disabling pain syndrome. As a first step, a nonoperative management program of spinal and trunk strengthening, stretching, and general conditioning is recommended. This will often eliminate or at least alleviate some of the symptomatology. If not relieved entirely, the symptoms will often be reduced to a tolerable level that enables the patient to function in a relatively normal fashion. Only when nonoperative measures have failed and debilitating pain persists is surgery considered.

The technique of thoracic discography has been well described by Skubic and Kostuik,[26] who recommend surgery by means of a ventral thoracic discectomy and fusion via a thoracotomy. With this approach, a complete discectomy is performed back to the posterior longitudinal ligament. Fixation is performed using a rib strut graft along with ventral internal fixation using the Kostuik-Harrington compression device. O'Leary et al.[20] reported two patients with nonherniated degenerated and painful thoracic intervertebral discs that were successfully treated with a transthoracic approach for the excision of the herniated disc and subsequent interbody fusion.

Thoracic Facet Arthropathy

Degenerative arthritis of the thoracic facet joints is widely accepted. Debate centers on the diagnostic criteria and treatment for this disabling condition. Thoracic facet arthropathy is more common at the cervicothoracic and thoracolumbar junctions. Isolated facet arthropathy is extremely uncommon. If facet arthropathy is suspected as being a major contributor to back pain, facet blocks and discography can serve as somewhat reliable indicators of pain generation. The presence of positive facet blocks and a negative thoracic discogram raise the possibility of dorsal thoracic fusion for this patient.

Skubic and Kostuik[26] reported three patients treated for facet arthropathy with dorsal fusion and instrumentation. Two improved. However, the efficacy of any sort of fusion in a patient with these complaints is unclear at present and awaits further study.

Thoracic Spinal Stenosis

Anatomical recognition of thoracic stenosis substantially preceded the description of its clinical symptomatology. The first clinical account of spinal cord compression due to thoracic spinal stenosis was reported by Govoni[12] in 1971. In 1979 Marzluff et al.[17] reported four patients with myelopathy due to facet hypertrophy.

Symptomatic thoracic stenosis is associated with osteophytic hypertrophy of the facet joints, hypertrophic laminae, and short, widened pedicles superimposed on a congenitally narrow spinal canal. Hypertrophic calcification of the ligamentum flavum may contribute in some cases. The process is identical to that occurring in the cervical and lumbar spine but is much less common. Spinal canal narrowing may be congenital, can occur from degenerative scoliosis, or may even represent a rare instance of thoracic spondylolisthesis. It can even result from renal osteodystrophy.

In thoracic stenosis the narrow canal is initially sufficiently large to accommodate the spinal cord. Myelopathy may occur in two ways: (1) minor trauma, resulting in small disc bulges that cannot be accommodated or (2) degenerative disc disease in the mobile lower thoracic segments, causing recurring flexion-extension stresses on the dorsal elements, hypertrophy of these structures, and dorsal encroachment on the thoracic cord. The site of spinal cord compression may be either central, in the lateral recess, within the neural foramen, or in some combination of these.

Thoracic stenosis typically presents in one of two ways. Acute thoracic disc herniation can result in acute myelopathy. This is frequently associated with acute thoracic pain, paraparesis, and sensory and sphincter disturbances. Thoracic stenosis due to degenerative changes is more common. Symptoms develop insidiously over months or years, and thoracic pain is usually absent. Sensory disturbances in the lower limbs occur first and are commonly exacerbated by prolonged standing. Spastic paraparesis develops and bladder dysfunction is usually a late manifestation. Late in the course of degenerative thoracic stenosis, symptoms persist even when supine, and the myelopathy may be so severe as to render the patient bedridden.

The neurological examination helps distinguish degenerative thoracic stenosis from pseudoclaudication due to lumbar spinal stenosis. Dorsal column dysfunction occurs early and is likely due to apophyseal impingement on the dorsal spinal cord. Increased myotactic reflexes, spasticity, and extensor plantar responses occur later. Ventral spinal cord pathways for pain and temperature are usually preserved until late in the course of the disease.

The initial treatment for symptomatic patients experiencing thoracic pain without neurological deficit includes nonsteroidal anti-inflammatory drugs (NSAIDs) and restriction of activities that aggravate the symptoms. However, aerobic conditioning, including trunk stretching, is often helpful as well. When nonoperative measures fail or a neurological deficit presents, surgical intervention should be considered.

Surgical treatment is dependent upon documenting the nature and extent of the lesion. Imaging by MRI, myelography, or computed tomography (CT) scanning is effective in depicting the morphology of the stenosis. If compression is due to only dorsal hypertrophic changes, laminectomy and partial facetectomy can restore more normal thoracic canal dimensions.

SURGICAL TREATMENT OF DISC HERNIATIONS AND SPONDYLOSIS
Indications

The ease with which thoracic disc herniation can now be identified has created a clinical dilemma, because asymptomatic disc herniation can be identified in up to 15% of thoracic spines imaged with MRI.[6,25,29]

Previously, surgery was thought to be indicated only after myelopathy developed. MRI is redefining the spectrum of symptomatic thoracic disc herniation. The decision to operate should be based on clear clinical indications that correlate with imaging findings. Asymptomatic patients with incidental thoracic disc herniation may not be suitable candidates for surgery. Intrinsic spinal cord changes should be sought, particularly changes indicative of ischemia or edema. If pain progresses and becomes incapacitating despite nonoperative treatment, operative management is indicated. These patients should be considered for operative intervention before neurological compromise occurs.

Laminectomy

The historical surgical treatment for thoracic disc herniation was a thoracic laminectomy and disc excision. This technique has largely been abandoned because addressing ventral compression via a dorsal approach in the thoracic region is associated with extremely poor outcomes, and frequently results in a greater neurological deficit. Treatments prior to 1960 (by laminectomy) resulted in a poor prognosis, and Arseni and Nash[5] reported that laminectomy failed to affect deterioration in 50% of their patients.

Skubic and Kostuik[26] reviewed a group of 12 patients who had undergone thoracic laminectomies for the treatment of thoracic disc herniation. Five patients improved, two were unchanged, and five sustained a substantial neurological injury.

The etiology of neurological injury after laminectomy for the treatment of a thoracic disc herniation is postulated to result from the excessive retraction of the thecal sac and spinal cord, which can occur during the exposure and treatment of a central disc herniation. A combination of microcontusions and alterations in microcirculation is the most likely explanation for the deterioration.

Thoracic laminectomy may be an appropriate procedure in patients with symptomatic thoracic spondylotic disease when there is significant spinal stenosis secondary to ligamentum flavum hypertrophy, facet hypertrophy, and generalized laminar thickening with a narrowed spinal canal.

Due to the substantial risk, the use of laminectomy alone is contraindicated as a decompressive procedure for thoracic disc herniation.

Transpedicular Approach

In 1978 Patterson and Arbit[21] reported the use of the transpedicular approach. They reported removal of both the entire pedicle and all of the facet to achieve decompression prior to performing a laminectomy. Many subsequent authors have reported good results with this approach. However, many practitioners do not routinely perform a laminectomy and attempt to preserve as much of the pedicle and facet as possible. After localization of the involved disc level, the facet joint dorsal to the disc space and the rostral half of the caudal pedicle are removed. The pedicle must be removed flush with the vertebral body. The disc space is entered lateral to the spinal cord, and the disc is removed by means of a cavity created ventral to the herniation. Lateral soft discs can be removed with curettes. Osteophytes and hard discs can be removed by drilling a trough in the underlying vertebral body. With the use of osteophyte impacting curettes, the mass can be delivered into the trough.

The major advantage of this approach is its minimally invasive nature. It avoids the complications and morbidity associated with thoracotomy, rib resection, and extensive muscular dissection and incision. Operating time, blood loss, and postoperative pain are less than with many of the other procedures. This approach is useful for lateral, mainly soft, lesions.

The disadvantages of this procedure are (1) limited visualization provided across the face of the thecal sac during decompression; (2) having to work "around a corner," which increases the risk of spinal cord injury when removing osteophytes and calcified discs; (3) does not allow for the removal of intradurally herniated disc fragments; (4) potential instability after pedicle removal; and (5) the inability to remove hard or central discs because the angle of approach is dorsal to the disc space. This surgery is facilitated by the use of specially designed instruments.

Lateral Extracavitary Approach

There are two main lateral approaches widely used in the treatment of thoracic spine pathology. These are the costotransversectomy and the lateral extracavitary approach. The fundamental difference between these two exposures is the extent of rib resection. The more of the rib that is removed, the better the visualization across the ventral thoracic spinal canal. In standard costotransversectomy, the extent of rib removal is limited.

The lateral extracavitary approach is a modification of the lateral rachiotomy procedure developed by Capener.[8] It was first performed for the treatment of tuberculous spondylitis by Larson et al.[15] It has been widely used for the decompression of ventral lesions. It allows decompression, stabilization and fusion to be performed circumferentially, through one incision, in a logical sequence.[28] Decompression is accomplished via ventrolateral displacement of the pleura. This is essential for adequate exposure of the lateral surface of the affected vertebral bodies.

The lateral extracavitary approach is extensive enough to guarantee a complete view of the dural sac adequate for dealing with all thoracic herniations, including calcified central ones. When compared with other lateral exposures, there is superior exposure across the ventral canal due to the extent of rib resection. This approach avoids the risks attendant with entering the pleura. Additionally, there is no need to incise the diaphragm. Placement of an interbody graft for fusion can be performed in straightforward fashion, using rib removed during the exposure.

There are several advantages to the lateral extracavitary approach to herniated thoracic discs. These include direct visualization of the dura mater immediately before and during decompression, resulting in enhanced safety during the discectomy. Removal of the rostral portion of the pedicle below the disc space further facilitates visualization. When combined with a hemilaminectomy, it allows simultaneous treatment of any stenosis of the spinal canal caused by hypertrophic spinal elements. It allows removal of intradural fragments because the spinal cord is well visualized throughout the proce-

dure. Finally, it permits application of dorsal or ventral instrumentation

Disadvantages of this technique include the risk of leaving fragments, favoring a more direct ventral approach. Additionally, it is a substantial operation. The amount of muscle dissection that must be performed to allow adequate retraction and visualization can result in substantial pain.

Transthoracic Approach

In an effort to avoid some of the complications associated with laminectomy for thoracic disc herniation, Craaford et al.[9] described a ventral approach to the thoracic spine in 1958. They described a technique utilizing fenestration of the disc. This procedure for decompressing the disc resulted in complete neurological recovery. Subsequently, Ransohoff et al.[23] and Perot and Munro[22] in 1969 reported the successful use of this procedure to remove herniated disc fragments. This technique involves the use of thoracotomy with rib resection and wide bony resection of vertebral structures to reach the ventral position of the spinal canal.

The major advantage of the transthoracic approach is the improved visualization of the thecal sac and the relationship between the dural sac and the disc herniation. It is a versatile approach that allows treatment of central and lateral disc herniations with equivalent exposure. This is particularly helpful in the management of calcified midline disc herniations, especially when they are tightly adherent to the dura mater. It is also very useful when multiple level disc herniations require surgical treatment. It is the most direct route for the attack of central disc disease, but it is somewhat demanding on the patient and is not without risk of respiratory complications.

These procedures, whether extrapleural or intrapleural, result in significant perioperative morbidity secondary to pain, difficult ventilation, shoulder girdle dysfunction, and wound healing problems. Postoperative complications include pneumothorax, pulmonary contusion, pneumonia, atelectasis, and pleural effusion. Some authors note up to a 10% loss of pulmonary function. A major contraindication to this procedure is compromised pulmonary function. Another disadvantage is the potential for substantial postoperative discomfort.

The need for bony fusion after transthoracic disc resection is controversial. Fusion has been advocated by many because of the incidence of kyphotic deformity resulting from thoracic discectomy without fusion. However, Bohlman and Zdeblick[7] advocate a transthoracic approach without fusion, contending that unless bone removal is excessive, the thoracic rib cage provides adequate stabilization.

Transsternal Approach

Transsternal procedures are rarely required. Only 6% of thoracic disc herniations occur between T2 and T6.[2] Ventral exposure of the upper thoracic spine is typically very difficult. The transsternal approach provides for a "true" ventral approach. It is critical to define the relationship between the ventral spinal column and the structures of the mediastinum, including the aortic arch, to allow for a safer procedure.

The major advantages of the transsternal approach are the improved visualization of disc lesions in the upper thoracic spine, a region difficult to manage via the other operative approaches. The major disadvantages are the formidable nature of this surgery. The substantial morbidity potentially inherent in this approach includes the risk of injury of vascular structures, the recurrent laryngeal nerve, and the thoracic duct.

Transfacet Pedicle-Sparing Approach

Stillerman et al.[27,28] developed a new approach for the microsurgical removal of thoracic disc herniations and osteophytes utilizing a transfacet pedicle-sparing procedure. This was developed to limit the amount of bone removal and muscle dissection to minimize postoperative back pain resulting from the loss of structural integrity.

Like the transpedicular approach, the transfacet pedicle-sparing approach permits thoracic disc removal from a dorsolateral trajectory. This approach is useful for the removal of calcified centrolateral, calcified lateral, and soft central discs throughout the thoracic spine. The advantages of this approach include (1) decreased operative time, (2) decreased blood loss, (3) limited bone removal, and (4) limited soft tissue disruption. Multiple levels can be approached without difficulty. Disadvantages of the procedure include (1) difficult to perform in larger patients, (2) specialized instruments may be necessary for central herniation, and (3) extent of decompression is difficult to evaluate.

Thoracoscopic Approach

The first reported application of video-assisted thoracoscopy for problems of the thoracic spine was in 1994.[13] Removal of thoracic disc herniations using thoracic endoscopes has been reported. Regan, Mack, and Picetti[24] reported results in 29 consecutive patients treated by video-assisted thoracoscopic techniques. Mean hospitalization decreased from 7 days in the first 10 patients to 3.1 days in the last 10 in the series. Overall patient satisfaction was 85%, with complete resolution of perioperative symptoms in 60% after a minimum 6-month follow-up. Improvement in overall technique, instrument design, and methods for controlling bleeding have resulted in earlier discharge from the hospital. Although intercostal dysesthesia is common after surgery, symptoms usually resolve in several weeks. No cases of neurological deterioration occurred in this series.

Advantages of this approach include a substantial reduction in surgical trauma without the need for large muscle splitting/cutting incisions. It reduces the period of confinement to bed and the postoperative hospitalization. Comparisons between thoracoscopy and open thoracotomy have demonstrated improvements in postoperative pain, shoulder girdle function, reduction in blood loss, time required in the intensive care unit, and overall hospital stay.

Disadvantages include a prolonged and steep learning curve. Additionally, many surgeons feel that the visualization provided with endoscopy is inferior to the open procedure.

CONCLUSION

Thoracic disc diseases are very difficult lesions to treat. The indirect nature of their presenting signs and symptoms generally precludes early diagnosis. Refinements and advances in neuroimaging have identified many lesions that previously would have gone undetected. However, the identification of lesions on imaging studies does not necessarily indicate surgical intervention.

The indications for operative treatment of thoracic disc herniations continue to evolve. The only absolute indication for surgery is the presence of myelopathy, particularly when it is progressive. However, radicular pain can be relieved with thoracic discectomy.

A critical review of the history of the surgical treatment of thoracic disc herniation reveals a progressive evolution of surgical technique in which successive procedures are developed that are incrementally improved over previous techniques. There is, nonetheless, a potential for further refinement.

The two major directions for future improvement in the therapy of this complex and often difficult entity will likely occur in two areas: refinement of the indications for operative intervention and the application of less invasive procedures and newer technologies. This should result in a more precise application of available technologies and less associated morbidity.

REFERENCES

1. Adson, A., 1922.
2. Alberico A, Sahni S, Hall J, Young HF. High thoracic disc herniation. Neurosurgery 19:449-451, 1986.
3. Antoni, 1931.
4. Arce C, Dohrmann G. Thoracic disc herniation: The improved diagnosis with computerized tomographic scanning and a review of the language. Surg Neurol 23:356-361, 1985.
5. Arseni C, Nash F. Thoracic intervertebral disc protrusion: A clinical study. J Neurosurg 17:418-430, 1960.
6. Awwad EE, Martin DS, Snutas, KR Jr., Baker BK. Asymptomatic versus symptomatic herniated thoracic discs: Their frequency and characteristics as detected by computed tomography after myelography. Neurosurgery 28:180-186, 1991.
7. Bohlman HH, Zdeblick TA. Anterior excision of herniated thoracic discs. J Bone Joint Surg 70A:1038-1047, 1988.
8. Capener N. The evolution of lateral rachiotomy. J Bone Joint Surg 36B:173-179, 1954.
9. Craaford T, Heirtonn, T, Lindblom K, Olson SE. Spinal cord compression caused by an intervertebral disc: Report of a case treated with anterolateral fenestration of the disc. Acta Orthop Scand 1958:103-107, 1958.
10. Dommisse G. The blood supply of the spinal cord. J Bone Joint Surg 56B:225-295, 1974.
11. Elsburg C. The extradural ventral chordomas (ecchondroses), their favorite sites, the spinal cord and root symptoms they produce, and their surgical treatment. Bull Neurol Inst NY 1:350-388, 1931.
12. Govoni A. Developmental stenosis of a thoracic vertebra resulting in narrowing of the spinal cord. AJR 112:401-404, 1971.
13. Horowitz MB, Moossy JJ, Julian T, Ferson PF, Huneke K. Thoracic discectomy using video assisted thoracoscopy. Spine 19:1082-1086, 1994.
14. Key C. On paraplegia depending on disease of the ligaments of the spine. Guy's Hosp Rep 3:17-34, 1838.
15. Larson S, Holst RA, Hemmy DC, Sance A. Lateral extracavitary approach to traumatic lesions of the thoracic and lumbar spine. J Neurosurg 45:628-637, 1976.
16. Logue V. Thoracic intervertebral disc prolapse with spinal cord compression. J Neurol Neurosurg Psychiatry 15:227-241, 1952.
17. Marzluff J, Hungerford GD, Kenpe LG. Thoracic myelopathy caused by osteophytes of the articular processes: Thoracic spondylosis. J Neurosurg 50:779-793, 1979.
18. Middleton G, Teacher J. Injury to the spinal cord due to rupture of an intervertebral disc during muscular effort. Glasgow Med J 76:1-6, 1911.
19. Mixter W, Barr J. Rupture of the intervertebral disc with involvement of the spinal cord. N Engl J Med 211:210-215, 1934.
20. O'Leary PF, Caming MB, Polifroni, NV, Flomen Y. Thoracic disc disease. Clinical manifestations and surgical treatment. Bull Hosp Jt Dis Orthop Inst 44:27-40, 1984.
21. Patterson RJ, Arbit E. A surgical approach through the pedicle to protruded thoracic discs. J Neurosurg 48:768-772, 1978.
22. Perot PJ, Munro DD. Transthoracic removal of midline thoracic disc protrusions causing spinal cord compression. J Neurosurg 31:452-458, 1969.
23. Ransohoff J, Spencer F, Sien F, Gage, L Jr. Transthoracic removal of thoracic disc. Report of three cases. J Neurosurg 31:459-461, 1969.
24. Regan JJ, Mack MJ, Picetti GR. A technical report on video-assisted thoracoscopy in thoracic spinal surgery. Preliminary description. Spine 20:831-837, 1995.
25. Ross JS, Perez-Reyes, N, Masary KT, Bohlnon HH, Modic MT. Thoracic disk herniation: MR imaging. Radiology 165:511-515, 1987.
26. Skubic J, Kostuik J. Thoracic pain syndromes and thoracic disc herniation. In Frymoyer J, ed. The Adult Spine. New York: Lippincott-Raven, 1991, pp 1444-1461.
27. Stillerman C, Chen TC Day JD, Couldwell NT, Veiss MH, The transfacet pedicle sparing approach for thoracic disc removal: Cadaveric morphometric analysis and preliminary clinical experience. J Neurosurg 83:971-976, 1995.
28. Stillerman C, Weiss M. Surgical management of thoracic disk herniation and spondylosis. In Menezes A, Sonntag V, eds. Principles of Spinal Surgery. New York: McGraw-Hill, 1995, pp 581-602.
29. Williams MP, Cherryman GR, Husband JE. Significance of thoracic disc herniation demonstrated by MR imaging. J Comput Assist Tomogr 13:211-214, 1989.

Algorithm
for Management

Charles B. Stillerman, M.D., Thomas C. Chen, M.D., Ph.D.,
William T. Couldwell, M.D., Ph.D., Edward C. Benzel, M.D.,
and Martin H. Weiss, M.D.

Herniated thoracic discs rarely require surgery. It has been estimated that only 0.15% to 4% of all disc operations are performed in this region.* There are several reasons why the management of this disorder has been problematic. The lack of a characteristic presentation pattern and the infrequency of this disease have caused delays in diagnosis. Additionally, there are numerous surgical approaches being touted as the most effective treatment for thoracic herniations. Finally, there is no general consensus regarding indications for disc removal.

CLASSIFICATION OF SURGICAL APPROACHES

Surgeries that improved access to the ventral thoracic spine and disc space evolved because, initially, laminectomy was unsuccessful. Surgical approaches may be anatomically classified. The ventral approaches include the transsternal operation, which, because of the rarity of upper thoracic her-

niations, is seldom used.[42] The ventrolateral approaches can be divided into open transthoracic thoracotomy,[8,9,12,34,35,42-47] thoracoscopy,[13,20,22,27,36,39,48] and retropleural thoracotomy.[28] The lateral approaches include the lateral extracavitary,[23,26,46] costotransversectomy,[45-47] and parascapular operations.[14,17] These provide excellent exposure to the ventral spinal canal and have been used to achieve safe and effective disc removal. They are all formidable operations, however, and may require (1) the performance of extensive muscle dissection or thoracotomy, (2) the removal of a rib, (3) working with the disc interposed between the surgeon and the spinal cord, (4) the need to detach part of the diaphragm at the thoracolumbar junction, (5) tube thoracostomy, or (6) the treatment of significant perioperative pain.

The dorsolateral surgeries include the transfacet pedicle-sparing approach[42-44] and the transpedicular approaches.[16,24,31-33] They are considered to be simpler operations that carry less physiological cost to the patient than the ventrolateral and lateral approaches.[42]

There is a potential for a unique set of complications with all surgical approaches. The surgeon must be aware of these complications so that they can be avoided. Comprehensive discussions about

---

*References 1-5, 7, 10, 11, 15, 18, 19, 21, 26, 33, 37, 38, 40, 42.

these approaches with their attendant complications have been published.*

SURGICAL APPROACH SELECTION

There is no universally accepted selection criteria to choose the best operation for each particular case. Additionally, no single surgical approach is ideally suited for all situations. As surgeons become familiar with the variety of surgical approaches, they are better able to individualize treatment, which reduces patient morbidity. Finally, there is a lack of consensus regarding the indications for disc removal. This is in large part because the natural history of this disease is as of yet unknown. Prophylactic surgery for these lesions is generally avoided. However, this preference is not based on controlled, prospective studies. Magnetic resonance imaging (MRI) may be used to facilitate longitudinal studies of both symptomatic and asymptomatic thoracic disc herniations. Certainly, if the 15% to 20% occurrence of incidental thoracic herniations is accurate, most of these patients will not require surgery for their disorder.

ALGORITHM

The surgical selection guidelines presented here have been developed from (1) experience with the surgical management of 82 symptomatic herniated thoracic discs (Fig. 18-1);[42] (2) the well-documented successes of others using the dorsolateral transpedicular approach;[16,24,32,33] (3) preliminary reports of new ventrolateral techniques, including the retropleural thoracotomy[28] and thoracoscopic operations;[13,20,22,27,36,39,48] (4) preliminary experience with the transfacet pedicle-sparing approach;[43,44] and (5) a comprehensive literature review of 13 large contemporary disc series (Tables 18-1 and 18-2).[42] Factors that influence this algorithm include the presenting signs and symptoms, the medical condition of the patient, disc size and location, the extent of calcification, degree of spinal cord deformation, and the presence of dura mater surrounding (sagging over) the dorsolateral margins of the disc (Fig. 18-2).

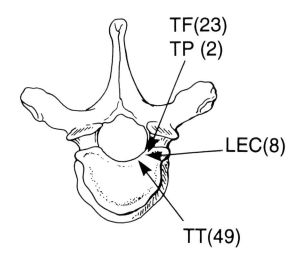

Fig. 18-1. A depiction of the four general approaches to thoracic discectomy and their respective trajectories. The two dorsolateral operations provide identical exposure to the disc. These are the transfacet (TF) pedicle-sparing approach and transpedicular (TP) approach. A true lateral exposure is achieved using the lateral extracavitary (LEC) approach. A ventrolateral trajectory is achieved with the transthoracic (TT) approach. The numbers in parentheses indicate the number of discs that were removed using each approach.[42]

The dorsolateral approaches are recommended for all soft symptomatic disc herniations, lateral calcified herniations, and selected calcified centrolateral herniations. The ventrolateral and lateral approaches, including the transthoracic, thoracoscopic, and retropleural exposures, as well as the lateral extracavitary approach, are generally reserved for densely and partially calcified centrolateral discs.[42]

Patients having only localized thoracic pain are generally not treated surgically. Conservative treatment includes the use of anti-inflammatory agents, bracing, activity modification, physical therapy, and steroid injections.

Patients with radiculopathy alone are treated nonoperatively, unless the radiculopathy proves to be refractory to treatment. On occasion, intercostal nerve injections are given. Those patients who require surgery can often be managed using a dorsolateral approach.

Patients with myelopathy are treated conservatively if the myelopathy is associated with no functional impairment or an intolerable pain syndrome is present. When the myelopathy is severe and/or progressive, patients are then entered into a high- or

Table 18-1. Thoracic Disc Series, 1986-1997

Name	Year	Surgical Approach		No. of Patients/ Discs	Pain		Motor Deficit (pre/post)	Bowel/Bladder Dysfunction (pre/post)	Complications
					Back (pre/post)	Radicular (pre/post)			
Lesoin et al.[25]	1986	Lam MTP TT	3 16 2	21/22	NR	5/5	16/10	NR	**Major 1** (4.5%) paraparesis permanent **Major 1** (4.5%) paraparesis transient Total (9%)
Bohlman and Zdeblick[8]	1988	Costo TT	11 8	19/22	13/10	4/1+NR	14/12	8/2+NR	**Major 2** (9%) 1 paraparesis permanent 1 wrong lev. → redo surgery **Minor 1** (4.5%) paraparesis transient Total (13.6%)
Blumenkopf[7]	1988	TT TP	4 3	9/*	7/7	4/4	3/2	1/1	NR
Otani et al.[30]	1988	MCos	23	23/23	NR	NR	23/23	23/18	NR
El-Kalliny et al.[15]	1991	TP TT Costo	8 8 5	21/23	15/11	13/11	10/8	6/NR	**Major 3** (13%) 1 paraparesis permanent-TT 1 pleural effusion → Surgery for CSF leak → TT 1 CVA **Minor 1** (4.3%) pleural effusion Total (17.4%)
Singounas et al.[41]	1992	Costo MCos	14 4	14/14	NR	NR	NR	NR	**Major 3** (21.4%) 1 paraparesis 1 discitis 1 comp. fx. from discitis
Le Roux, Haglund, and Harris[24]	1993	TP	20	20/23	17/14	17/16	3/3	1/1	NR
Dietze and Fessler[14]	1993	LEC	17	17/22	15/10		7/5	8/8	**Minor 2** (9%) 1 anesthesia dolorosa 1 pneumonia
Ridenour et al.[37]	1993	Lam TP Costo	4 12 15	31/33	11/7	12/5	18/9	13/8	**Major 3** (9%) 1 increased myelopathy 1 wrong level → additional surgery 1 incomplete disc removal → redo surgery **Minor 3** (9%) 3 superficial wound infection Total (18.2%)
Simpson et al.[40]	1993	MCos TP	16 5	21/23	19/19		6/4	4/3	NR
Oppenheim, Rothman, and Sachdey[29]	1993	Costo	8	12/†	7/6		NR	1/1	**Major 1** (12.5%) 1 wrong diagnosis progressive weakness. avm found 3 levels caudal operated level

Currier, Eismont, and Green[12]	1994	TT	19	19/22	15/10		11/7	6/NR	**Major 3** (13.6%)
									1 nonfatal PE
									1 intraop hemodynamic
									   instability → v. tack.+ hypotension
									1 spinal instability → kyphosis after lam
									   + TT
									Minor 9 (41%)
									1 incisional hernia
									1 dural tear → intraop repair
									   + drain
									2 transient urinary retention
									2 UTIs
									4 chronic thoracotomy pain
									Total (54.5%)

Bilsky and Patterson[6]	1998	TP	20	20/20	7/5	6/4	11/11	6/5	**Minor 3** (15%) 1 pseudomening. 1 deep wound infection 1 transient increase in myelopathy

Pre/post = preoperative signs + symptoms/postoperative patients with resolution or improvement; NR = not reported; Lam = laminectomy; TP = transpedicular; Costo = costotransversectomy; TT = transthoracic; MTP = modified transpedicular; MCos = modified costotransversectomy; LEC = lateral extracavitary.
*Seven discs operated (two treated conservatively)
†Eight discs operated (four treated conservatively)

Table 18-2. Comparative Data

	Contemporary Series[14] 1986-1997	Stillerman et al. [42]
Demographics and Disc Characteristics		
Patients/Discs	247/263	71/82
Sex (f/m)	112/95 (1.18:1)	37/34 (1.09:1)
Age	18-79	19-75
Trauma	37% (59/161)	37% (26/71)
Levels	T1-L1 (total 244)	T4-L1 (total 82)
Frequency	T8-9: 17% (41)	T9-10: 26% (21)
	T11-12: 16% (39)	T8-9: 23% (19)
	T10-11: 11% (26)	T10-11: 17% (14)
Calcified	22% (33/151)	65% (53/82)
Intradural	6% (5/90)	7% (6/82)
Canal location		
Central/centrolateral	77% (113/146)	94% (77/82)
Lateral	23% (33/146)	6% (5/82)
Multiple discs	8% (20/242)	14% (10/71)
Presenting Signs and Symptoms		
Localized/axial pain	56% (111/199)	61% (43/71)
Radicular pain	51% (94/185)	16% (11/71)
Sensory deficit	64% (145/226)	61% (43/71)
Bowel/bladder deficit	35% (72/208)	24% (17/71)
Motor impairment	55% (114/208)	61% (43/71)
Results (No. Resolved or Improved/ Total No. of Patients in Groups Reporting This Result)		
Pain: total	76% (106/140)	87% (47/54)
Localized/axial	80% (39/49)	86% (37/43)
Radicular	74% (29/39)	91% (10/11)
Sensory deficit	NR	36/43 (84%)
Bowel/bladder deficit	80% (47/59)	77% (13/17)
Motor impairment	69% (65/94)	58% (25/43)

low-risk category. Patients who are a low medical risk are divided, based on the position of their disc in the spinal canal. All patients with lateral herniations undergo dorsolateral surgery. Patients with centrolateral herniations are then stratified, based upon the degree and location of the calcification within the herniation. Those patients with soft herniations can be operated on safely and effectively using one of the dorsolateral approaches.

Densely calcified discs are likely to have dural adherence. Therefore ventrolateral approaches are appropriate when a densely calcified centrolateral herniation is more centrally located within the spinal canal. In the rare instance in which a densely calcified disc herniation occurs in the upper thoracic spine, a ventral approach may be considered. Densely calcified centrolateral discs that are more

laterally positioned may be treated with either a ventrolateral or lateral approach.

Mildly or partially calcified centrolateral herniations can be approached by using either dorsolateral, lateral, or ventrolateral operations. Factors that influence surgical selection include (1) the presence of the major bulk of the disc in the middle of the spinal canal; (2) the extent of calcification involving the dorsal aspect of the disc, which is thought to influence the likelihood of dural adherence; (3) the point of contact between the disc and the spinal cord; and (4) the extent of the spinal cord that is draped around the disc.

High-risk medical patients who have disc herniations that are not densely calcified and centrolateral in location are treated using dorsolateral decompression. Those patients with densely calcified

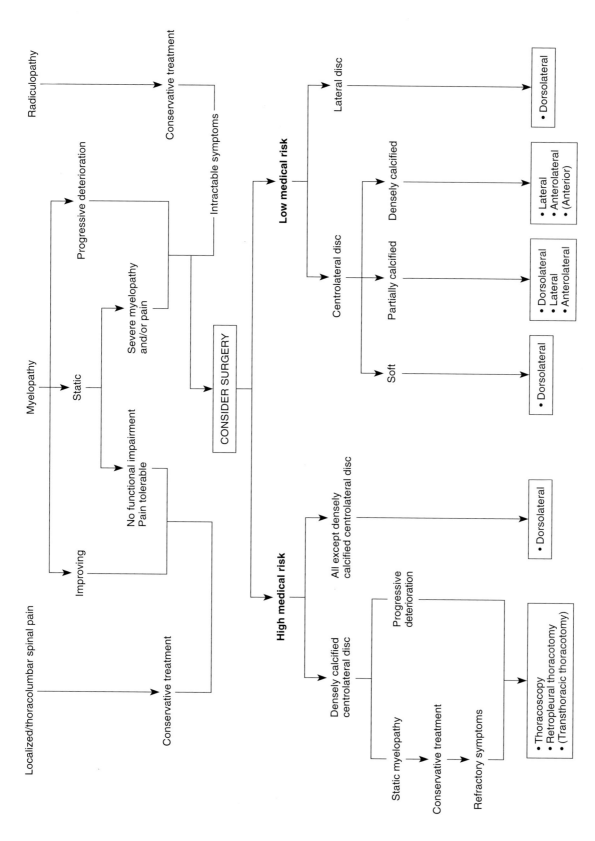

Fig. 18-2. An algorithm for the management of symptomatic thoracic disc herniations. It should be noted that the surgeon's familiarity with each particular approach influences which procedure is ultimately selected.[42]

centrolateral discs are initially treated conservatively. If the symptoms are progressive or do not improve, either a retropleural, thoracoscopic, or, if necessary, an open transthoracic thoracotomy is performed.

CONCLUSION

The surgical treatment of the thoracic herniated disc remains problematic. Although complications have dramatically been reduced since the earlier series, there still is a need to refine treatment. Fundamental questions, including which patients require surgery, as well as what the optimum surgical approach is for each particular disc herniation, remain to be answered. It seems clear that the appropriate treatment strategy should be based on the presentation pattern, medical condition of the patient, and the characteristics of the disc herniation. All of the ventral, ventrolateral, and lateral surgical approaches have the potential for significant patient morbidity. As such, continued efforts regarding the refinement of minimally invasive techniques are necessary. No single surgical approach is optimal in all situations and, as such, the treating clinician must maintain proficiency regarding the use of all, or the majority of, surgical options. The following chapters are intended to provide insights into these options.

REFERENCES

1. Arce CA, Dohrmann GJ. Herniated thoracic discs. Symposium on Neurosurgery. Neurol Clin 3:383-392, 1985.
2. Arce CA, Dohrmann GJ. Thoracic disc herniation. Improved diagnosis with computed tomographic scanning and a review of the literature. Surg Neurol 23:356-361, 1985.
3. Arseni C, Nash F. Thoracic intervertebral disc protrusions. A clinical study. J Neurosurg 17:418-430, 1960.
4. Awwad EE, Martin DS, Smith DR Jr, et al. Asymptomatic versus symptomatic herniated thoracic disc: Their frequency and characteristics as detected by computed tomography after myelography. Neurosurgery 28:180-186, 1991.
5. Benjamin V. Diagnosis and management of thoracic disc disease. Clin Neurosurg 30:577-605, 1983.
6. Bilsky MH, Patterson RH. The transpedicular approach for thoracic disc herniations. In Benzel EC, Stillerman CB, eds. The Thoracic Spine. St. Louis: Quality Medical Publishing, 1998.
7. Blumenkopf B. Thoracic intervertebral disc herniations: Diagnostic value of magnetic resonance imaging. Neurosurgery 23:36-40, 1988.
8. Bohlman HH, Zdeblick TA. Anterior excision of herniated thoracic discs. J Bone Joint Surg 70A:1038-1047, 1988.
9. Borges LF. Thoracic disc disease and spondylosis. In Tindall FT, Cooper PR, Barrow DL, eds. The Practice of Neurosurgery. Baltimore: Williams & Wilkins, 1996, pp 2461-2471.
10. Boriani S, De Lure F, Rocella P, et al. Two-level thoracic disc herniation. Spine 19:2461-2466, 1994.
11. Chowdhary UM. Intradural thoracic disc protrusion. Spine 12:718-719, 1987.
12. Currier BL, Eismont FJ, Green BA. Transthoracic disc excision and fusion for herniated thoracic discs. Spine 19:323-328, 1994.
13. Dickman CA, Rosenthal D, Karahalios DG, et al. Thoracic vertebrectomy and reconstruction using a microsurgical thoracoscopic approach. Neurosurgery 38:201-219, 1996.
14. Dietze DD Jr, Fessler RG. Thoracic disc herniations. Neurosurg Clin Am 4:75-90, 1993.
15. El-Kalliny M, Tew JM Jr, van Loveren H, et al. Surgical approaches to thoracic disc herniations. Acta Neurochir (Wien) 111:22-32, 1991.
16. Epstein JA: Thoracic disc herniation: Operative approaches and results. Comment. Neurosurgery 12:305, 1983.
17. Fessler RG, Dietze DD Jr, MacMillan M, et al. Lateral parascapular extrapleural approach to the upper thoracic spine. J Neurosurg 75:349-355, 1991.
18. Fidler MW, Godehart ZD. Excision of prolapse of thoracic intervertebral disc. A transthoracic technique. J Bone Joint Surg 66B:518-522, 1984.
19. Garrido E. Modified costotransversectomy: A surgical approach to ventrally placed lesions in the thoracic spine canal. Surg Neurol 13:109-113, 1979.
20. Horwitz MB, Moossy JJ, Julian T, et al. Thoracic discectomy using video assisted thoracoscopy. Spine 9:1082-1086, 1994.
21. Hulme A. The surgical approach to thoracic intervertebral disc protrusions. J Neurol Neurosurg Psychiatry 23:133-137, 1960.
22. Krasna MJ, Mack MJ. Atlas of Thoracoscopic Surgery. St. Louis: Quality Medical Publishing, 1994, pp 206-211.
23. Larson SJ, Holst RA, Hemmy DC, et al. Lateral extracavitary approach to traumatic lesions of the thoracic and lumbar spine. J Neurosurg 45:628-637, 1976.
24. Le Roux PD, Haglund MM, Harris AB. Thoracic disc disease: Experience with the transpedicular approach in twenty consecutive patients. Neurosurgery 33:58-66, 1993.
25. Lesoin F, Rousseaux M, Autrieque A, et al. Thoracic disc herniations: Evolution in the approach and indications. Acta Neurochir (Wien) 80:30-34, 1986.
26. Maiman DJ, Larson SJ, Luck E, et al. Lateral extracavitary approach to the spine for thoracic disc herniations: Report of 23 cases. Neurosurgery 14:178-182, 1984.
27. McAfee PC, Regan JR, Zdeblick TA, et al. The incidence of complications in endoscopic anterior thoracolumbar spinal reconstructive surgery. Spine 20:1624-1632, 1995.
28. McCormick PC. Retropleural approach to the thoracic and thoracolumbar spine. Neurosurgery 37:1-7, 1995.
29. Oppenheim JS, Rothman AS, Sachdey YP. Thoracic herniated discs: Review of the literature and 12 cases. Mt Sinai J Med 60:321-326, 1993.
30. Otani K, Yoshida M, Fujii E, et al. Thoracic disc herniation. Surgical treatment in 23 patients. Spine 13:1262-1267, 1988.
31. Patterson RH. Thoracic disc herniation: Operative approaches and results. Comment. Neurosurgery 12:305, 1983.
32. Patterson RH. Thoracic disc disease: Experience with the transpedicular approach in twenty consecutive patients. Comment. Neurosurgery 33:66, 1993.
33. Patterson RH Jr, Arbit E. A surgical approach through the pedicle to protruded thoracic discs. J Neurosurg 48:768-772, 1978.

34. Perot PL, Munro DD. Transthoracic removal of midline thoracic disc protrusions causing spinal cord compression. J Neurosurg 31:452-458, 1969.

35. Ransohoff J, Spencer F, Siew F, et al. Transthoracic removal of thoracic disc. Report of three cases. J Neurosurg 31:459-461, 1969.

36. Regan JJ, Mack MJ, Picetti GD. A technical report on video-assisted thoracoscopy in thoracic spinal surgery. Spine 20:831-837, 1995.

37. Ridenour TR, Haddad SF, Hitchon PW, et al. Herniated thoracic discs: Treatment and outcome. J Spinal Disord 6:218-224, 1993.

38. Rosenbloom SA. Thoracic disc disease and stenosis. Radiol Clin North Am 29:765-775, 1991.

39. Rosenthal D, Rosenthal R, De Simone A. Removal of a protruded thoracic disc using microsurgical endoscopy. A new technique. Spine 19:1087-1091, 1994.

40. Simpson JM, Silveri CP, Simeone FA, et al. Thoracic disc herniation. Re-evaluation of the posterior approach using a modified costotransversectomy. Spine 18:1872-1877, 1993.

41. Singounas EG, Kypriades EM, Kellerman AJ, et al. Thoracic disc herniation. Analysis of 14 cases and review of the literature. Acta Neurochir (Wien) 16:49-52, 1992.

42. Stillerman CB, Chen TC, Couldwell WT, et al. Experience in the surgical management of 82 symptomatic herniated discs and review of the literature. J Neurosurg 88:623-633, 1998.

43. Stillerman CB, Chen TC, Day JD, et al. The transfacet pedicle-sparing approach for thoracic disc removal: Cadaveric morphometric analysis and preliminary clinical experience. J Neurosurg 83:971-976, 1995.

44. Stillerman CB, Couldwell WT, Chen TC, et al. Thoracic disc (invited response). Neurosurgical forum. J Neurosurg 85:187-190, 1996.

45. Stillerman CB, Weiss MH. Principles of surgical approaches to the thoracic spine. In Tarlov EC, ed. Neurosurgical Topics: Neurosurgical Treatment of Disorders of the Thoracic Spine. Park Ridge, Ill.: American Association of Neurological Surgeons, 1991, pp 1-19.

46. Stillerman CB, Weiss MH. Management of thoracic disc disease. Clin Neurosurg 38:325-352, 1992.

47. Stillerman CB, Weiss MH. Surgical management of thoracic disc herniation and spondylosis. In Menezes AH, Sonntag VKH, eds. Principles of Spinal Surgery. New York: McGraw-Hill, 1996, pp 581-601.

48. Theodore N, Dickman CA. Current management of thoracic disc herniation. Contemp Neurosurg 18:1-6, 199.

19

Transpedicular Approaches

Mark H. Bilsky, M.D., and Russell H. Patterson, M.D.

Thoracic disc herniations have traditionally been difficult to diagnose and treat. Prior to the 1960s, the mainstay of treatment for thoracic disc herniations was laminectomy. The devastating neurological sequelae associated with laminectomy led surgeons to employ surgical strategies that decreased spinal cord manipulation and improved visualization ventral to the spinal cord by performing disc extirpation from a more lateral and/or ventral approach. These approaches include costotransversectomy, transthoracic, and transpedicular approaches. These three approaches have advantages and disadvantages, but all have resulted in a marked improvement in surgical morbidity when compared to laminectomy.

The choice of procedure is often dependent on the operating surgeon's familiarity with the particular approach. The transpedicular approach has been used exclusively at the authors' institution for the treatment of thoracic disc herniations over the last 10 years. Neurological outcome is comparable to that observed with the other approaches and is possibly associated with less overall medical morbidity.

HISTORY

Laminectomy was the first surgical procedure used to treat thoracic disc herniation. Logue[14] reviewed the 10 cases previously reported in the literature by Mueller,[18] Hawk,[11] and Mixter and Barr.[17] Six patients had complete spinal cord transection and four patients showed no improvement. In reviewing his own series of 11 patients, laminectomy resulted in three patients with functional spinal cord transections and two patients with significant neurological deterioration. The other six patients made significant recoveries, but only after suffering severe transient neurological worsening. The majority of patients who experienced poor neurological outcomes had a significant degree of spinal cord compression as evidenced by a complete block to the flow of intrathecal contrast material. Additional risk factors included calcified lesions, severe preoperative deficits, and focal degeneration of the spinal cord noted on intradural exploration.[21] The surgical procedure performed for single-level thoracic disc herniation was an extensive three- to four-level laminectomy with resection of the pedicle and facet as necessary. Disc extirpation was performed via either a transdural or extradural approach, but exposure was often poor. The poor outcomes in these patients were in part due to the difficulty encountered removing a ventral mass from a dorsal approach. A postoperative kyphotic deformity from the decompressive laminectomy combined with a residual disc or osteophyte may have been responsible for late neurological decompensation in some cases.[15] However, laminectomy performed without disc exploration also resulted in a high incidence of paraplegia.[21] Manipulation of the spinal cord over the fixed ventral mass caused mechanical damage and interfered with the already tenuous blood supply to the spinal cord.[12]

The devastating neurological sequelae associated with laminectomy led investigators to employ surgical strategies that decreased spinal cord manipulation and improved visualization ventral to the spinal cord by performing disc extirpation from a more lateral and/or ventral approach.

Costotransversectomy was initially developed for the treatment of tuberculous spondylitis. It was described by Menard (1900 Menard) and further refined by Seddon.[25] Hulme[12] was the first to apply the costotransversectomy technique to the treatment of thoracic disc herniations. He treated six patients with severe myelopathy. Four patients had good neurological recoveries. One patient with a poor outcome had undergone a previous laminectomy with a resultant functional cord transection prior to the technically successful costotransversectomy. The remaining patient had a preoperative fixed kyphotic deformity at the level of the disc herniation.

Transthoracic, transpleural thoracic disc excision was described by Crafoord et al.[8] Following this single case report, Perot and Munro[21] and Ransohoff et al.,[22] in sequential articles in the *Journal of Neurosurgery*, reported successful neurological outcomes in two and three patients, respectively. Neither article credited Crafoord with the original application of this technique to treat thoracic disc herniation, perhaps unaware that this had been previously described. All five patients in these two series presented with significant myelopathies and made excellent postoperative recoveries.

Subsequent to the application of the costotransversectomy and transthoracic approach to thoracic disc herniations, the transpedicular approach was described in a small series of patients by Patterson and Arbit.[20] All patients presented with myelopathic syndromes and made good postoperative neurological recovery. One patient had an intradural fragment that was successfully extirpated via a transdural approach. Since the original description of the transpedicular approach, the authors have used this approach exclusively for single-level thoracic disc excisions.

THE PROCEDURE

Patients are placed prone on the operating room table. For mid- to lower thoracic disc herniations, the knee-chest position is used, while for upper thoracic disc herniation, the patient is placed with the upper trunk supported and the head resting on a horseshoe. One of the major problems of thoracic disc surgery is identifying the proper level. If the thoracic disc is low in the thoracic spine, the problem is readily solved. It is then possible to take a lateral radiograph and count from L5 upwards. If the radiograph is not large enough to encompass L5 through the level of the surgery, then two or three spinal needles can be placed as points of reference and two roentgenograms taken to cover the length of spine that is necessary.

Thoracic disc herniations in the upper thoracic spine are more difficult. In this case, a PA roentgenogram is usually taken in the operating room. It is then possible to count down from the T1 level, since the T1 vertebra is distinctive in the PA projection because the transverse processes angle rostrally. The line of the roentgenographic tube may need to be angled somewhat rostrally so that the spine is thrown into a true PA projection and the levels are not overlapped. After the incision is opened, it may be advantageous to have a needle at the proper level and inject perhaps 0.25 ml of blue dye to identify the level.

A linear skin incision is made over the spinous processes of the two appropriate vertebral bodies. The paraspinous muscles are reflected off the spinous processes and laminae via a subperiosteal dissection using periosteal elevators. The dissection is carried out to expose the facet on the side of the approach. For lateral and dorsolateral disc herniations, the approach is made from the side from which the disc is most accessible. For central disc herniations, the approach is generally made from the patient's left side for a right-handed surgeon. The rostral facet and pedicle of the vertebra caudal to the disc herniation are removed. For example, intervertebral disc herniation between the eighth and ninth thoracic vertebrae would require resection of the T9 rostral facet and the T9 pedicle. Anatomically, this can be identified intraoperatively just rostral to the transverse process of T9 at the pars interarticularis. The rostral aspect of the pedicle generally lies over the disc space. The pedicle is drilled with a cutting

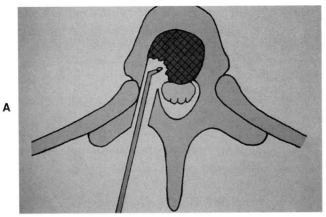

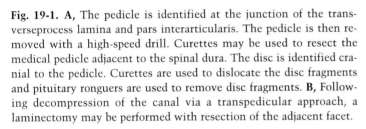

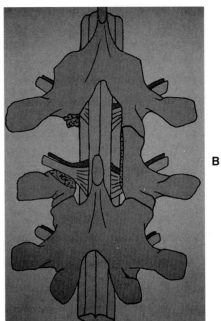

Fig. 19-1. A, The pedicle is identified at the junction of the transverseprocess lamina and pars interarticularis. The pedicle is then removed with a high-speed drill. Curettes may be used to resect the medical pedicle adjacent to the spinal dura. The disc is identified cranial to the pedicle. Curettes are used to dislocate the disc fragments and pituitary ronguers are used to remove disc fragments. **B,** Following decompression of the canal via a transpedicular approach, a laminectomy may be performed with resection of the adjacent facet.

burr, but as the dura mater is approached medially, the drill bit may then be switched to a diamond burr. The cavity created by resection of the pedicle seems surprisingly deep even though it is only 1.5 to 2.0 cm. The transition between the cancellous bone of the pedicle to the cortical bone of the vertebral body signifies the end of the pedicle dissection (Fig. 19-1).

The intervertebral disc space is incised with a No. 15 blade. It is necessary to obtain a very substantial opening into the disc interspace and remove the disc widely. When in doubt, one should remove more bone of the vertebra above and below to allow collapsing disc fragments and annulus fibrosus into the interspace for removal. Intravertebral disc is removed from the center of the disc, progressing from lateral, under the nerve root, to medial, under the spinal cord dura mater. A downbiting curette is used to force disc fragments laterally into the disc space. The pituitary rongeur is used to remove the fragments, although long downbiting curettes can be used. Generally, the fragments are removed easily and are rather distinctive because of their calcification and firmness. Sometimes the fragment will deeply penetrate the dura mater, and when teased out, a rush of spinal fluid occurs. The authors have not attempted to repair the dura mater in this case but have simply placed a sheet of Gelfoam under the dura. So far, in the authors' experience, there

have been no cases of cerebrospinal fluid (CSF) fistula into the chest or transcutaneously.

In one patient, the fragment was so adherent to the dura mater that it could not be teased from the disc interspace. In this case, the dura was opened laterally and a piece of dura that included the fragment was excised. This left a rather large defect in the dura mater ventrally. To prevent herniation of the spinal cord into the interspace, a Steinmann pin was passed into the vertebral body above and then pushed into the vertebral body below. The defect in the interspace was then filled with methylmethacrylate. The idea was to support the spinal cord and prevent herniation through the large dural defect. In general, the spinous processes and interspinous ligaments are left intact.

NEW YORK HOSPITAL EXPERIENCE

The transpedicular approach has been used exclusively at the authors' institution for patients with thoracic disc herniation since its description in 1978. From 1982 to 1992, 20 operations were performed using the transpedicular approach. Patient analysis was accomplished by hospital and clinic chart review, radiographic review, and follow-up phone calls (Table 19-1). The mean age at diagnosis was 47 years (25 to 79 years age range) with an equal sex distribution.

Table 19-1. Data From Case Review Using the Transpedicular Approach

PT NO.	Age/Sex	Level	Consistency/Location	Precipitating Event	Duration of Symptoms (Months)	Presenting Symptoms	Exam	Ambulatory Status Pre/Post	Bowel/Bladder Pre/Post	Outcome	Complication
1	38/F	T6-7	H/L Intradural	Fall	9	RLE weakness	Myelopathy (right Brown-Sequard)	NL/NL	Incontinent/NL	Improved	Pseudomeningocele/asymptomatic
2	57/F	T11-12	H/CL	Fall	12	Back and hip pain, bilateral lower extremity weakness	Radiculopathy	NL/NL	NL/NL	Asymptomatic	None
3	65/M	T1-2	S/L	NK	3.5	Neck and left arm pain, head weakness	Radiculopathy	NL/NL	NL/NL	Asymptomatic	None
4	47/F	T6-7	H/L	Spinal anesthesia, lithotomy position	1.5	Bil. lower extremity numbness	Myelopathy (right Brown-Sequard)	NL/NL	NL/NL	Improved	Transient neurological worsening
5	50/M	T8-9	S/L	Sports	1	Chest tightness	Myelopathy (left Brown-Sequard)	NI/NL	NL/NL	Asymptomatic	None
6	33/F	T7-8	H/L	MVA/thoracic compression fracture	6	Back pain, radiating pain	Radiculopathy	NL/NL	NL/NL	Improved	None
7	49/F	T2-3	S/L	NK	12	Right chest and shoulder pain	Radiculopathy	NL/NL	NL/NL	Improved	None
8	63/M	T6-7	H/CL	NK	84	Left lower quadrant pain	Myelopathy (ventral cord)	Spastic/NL	NL/NL	Improved	None
9	33/M	T9-10	S/CL	Twisting motion	4.5	Paraparesis	Myelopathy (transverse cord)	With assistance/NL	Incontinent/NL	Asymptomatic	None
10	79/M	T11-12	S/CL	NK	2	Back pain and left extremity weakness	Myelopathy (right Brown-Sequard)	Nonamb/Improved	Incontinent/NL	Improved	None

#	Age/Sex	Level	Type	Etiology	Duration	Presentation	Diagnosis	Motor/Sensory	Bladder/Bowel	Outcome	Complications
11	57/M	T11-12	S/CL	NK	4	Left extremity weakness, incontinent	Myelopathy (conus medullaris)	Nonamb/NL	Incontinent/mild dysfunction	Improved	None
12	40/M	T8-9	H/CL	MVA	4	Intermittent left extremity dysesthesias, incontinent	Myelopathy (right Brown-Sequad)	Spastic/NL	Dysfunction/NL	Asymptomatic	None
13	34/F	T7-8	H/L	Sports	3.6	Right lower extremity weakness, numbness	Myelopathy	NL/NL	NL/NL	Improved	None
14	25/F	T11-12	S/L	Lifting	6	Back pain, right lower extremity pain, bowel/bladder dysfunction	Myelopathy (conus medullaris)	NL/NL	Dysfunction/NL	Improved	None
15	35/M	T8-9	H/CL	Lifting	6	Back pain, left shoulder pain	Radiculopathy	NL/NL	Nl/NL	No Improvement	None
16	54/F	T9-10	H/CL	Fall	3.5	Back and leg pain, radiculopathy	Myelopathy (transverse cord)	With assistance/NL	Incontinent/NL	Improved	None
17	65/F	T10-11	H/CL	Hyperreflexic on pre-op testing for hip surgery	1 day	None	Myelopathy	NL/NL	NL/NL	Asymptomatic	None
18	36/M	T8-9	S/CL	NK	17	Right lower extremity numbness	Myelopathy	NL/NL	NL/NL	Improved	None
19	72/M	T9-10	S/CL	Acute deterioration postmyelogram	1	Right lower extremity weakness, numbness	Myelopathy (right Brown-Sequard)	Nonamb/ambulates w/cane	Incontinent/Continent	Improved	Wound infection (staphylococcus)
20	24/F	T8-9	S/L	MVA	48	Back and radicular pain	Radiculopathy	NL/NL	NL/NL	Unchanged	None

H = Hard; S = Soft; CL = Centrolateral; L = Lateral; NL = normal.

Presentation

A precipitating event was identified in 13 of the 20 patients. A fall, sports participation, or heavy lifting was the precipitating event in each of three patients. A twisting motion and/or spinal anesthesia in the lithotomy position was identified as the precipitating event in the remaining patients.

Predominant symptoms at the time of diagnosis included: back pain (six patients), weakness (nine patients), and paresthesias (eight patients). The mean duration of symptoms prior to diagnosis was 14.8 months (range, 1 day to 72 months). Of the 20 patients, 14 presented with myelopathy and six presented with radiculopathy. The myelopathic syndromes were characterized as Brown-Sequard (six patients), transverse cord (two patients), anterior cord (one patient), and conus medullaris (one patient). Three patients were non ambulatory and two were ambulatory with assistance only. Six patients had bladder and/or bowel incontinence or dysfunction.

Imaging

Preoperative evaluation consisted of myelogram and post myelogram computerized tomography (CT) scan (six patients), magnetic resonance imaging (MRI) (10 patients), and both myelogram, post myelogram CT, and MRI (four patients). Spinal angiography was not performed on any patient. Five of six patients who underwent myelogram demonstrated either complete or high-grade blocks to the flow of intrathecal contrast (Fig. 19-2). One patient with a complete myelographic block acutely deteriorated following myelogram, progressing from spastic paraparesis to paraplegia with loss of bowel and bladder function.

The most common level for disc herniation was T8-9 (five patients) followed by T11-12 (four patients). The majority of disc herniations occurred below the T8-9 level (13 patients). Two herniated discs were found in the upper thoracic spine at T1-2 and T2-3.

Surgical Findings

At surgery, 10 discs were found to be calcified. This was confirmed by the pathology reports. Two patients had intradural fragments removed. One of these patients had a transdural extirpation and one

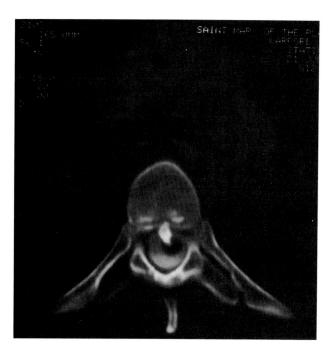

Fig. 19-2. A postmyelogram CT showing a calcified central disc herniation resected via a transpedicular approach.

patient had an extradural removal in which the dura mater was excised around the fragment. Two other patients underwent negative intradural explorations for suspected intrathoracic disc components.

Results

All 14 patients with myelopathy improved. All patients who were either nonambulatory or ambulatory with assistance preoperatively were independent ambulators postoperatively. Of the six patients who were incontinent of bowel and/or bladder preoperatively, all but one regained continence postoperatively. Hydrodynamic testing in this patient revealed a persistent neurogenic bladder.

The six patients treated for radiculopathy did not improve to the same degree as those with myelopathy. Four patients improved postoperatively; two had complete resolution of their symptoms and the other two patients showed significant improvement. The remaining two patients had no change in their preoperative status. One of these patients underwent reimaging, showing incomplete disc removal. This patient refused further surgical intervention.

Table 19-2. Presenting Symptoms of Thoracic Disc Herniation*

Presenting Symptom	Mean Percentage of Patients (%)	Range for Individual Series (%)
Back pain	57	30–80
Sensory loss	56	40–87
Leg weakness	55	21–87
Radiculopathy	44	20–80
Gait disturbances	40	15–80
Leg paresthesias	27	4–45
Bowel and/or bladder incontinence	25	5–43

*Pooled data from 238 patients.[3,4,9,10,13,15,26-28]

No patients developed signs or symptoms of postoperative instability. One patient was fused with methylmethacrylate and Steinmann pins because of the potential for the spinal cord to herniate into the large defect that had been created by the resection and not because of a perceived risk of spinal instability (i.e., progressive kyphosis or vertebral body collapse).

Complications

Three complications occurred in this series. After removal of an intradural fragment, one patient developed an asymptomatic pseudomeningocele for which no further therapy was required. The second patient developed a Staphylococcus wound infection. This patient had a number of medical risk factors, including insulin-dependent diabetes mellitus, hypertension, congestive heart failure, and chronic obstructive pulmonary disease. The third patient had transient neurological worsening from an attempted dorsal interbody fusion. The patient had a full neurological recovery.

PRESENTATION

Presenting symptoms of patients operated on for thoracic disc herniation are presented in Table 19-2. This table represents pooled data from 238 patients.[3,4,9,10,13,15,26-28] The predominant complaints were back pain, sensory loss, and leg weakness. Gait disturbance and radiculopathy were present in 40% and 44%, respectively. Lower extremity paresthesias and bowel and bladder symptoms were least likely to be presenting symptoms.

The differential diagnosis of thoracic disc herniation includes a number of intra- and extramedullary processes, including arteriovenous malformations, spinal cord tumors, syringomyelia, and primary or metastatic vertebral body tumors. Additional, multiple sclerosis (MS) and amyotrophic lateral sclerosis (ALS) should be included in the differential diagnosis, even if a herniated thoracic disc is found on imaging studies. In the two series that included patients operated on for thoracic disc herniation who either had or were subsequently diagnosed with these diseases, the surgical outcomes were significantly worse than in those patients who did not have these neurological diseases.[4,9]

The etiology of back pain may be considered a consequence of the disc herniation causing a stretch of the posterior longitudinal ligament and annulus fibrosis. Additionally, segmental spinal instability may play a role in producing back pain, particularly in cases where there is a preexisting thoracic deformity, such as from a posttraumatic kyphosis at the level of the disc herniation. Concomitant spinal deformities (e.g., Scheurmann's kyphosis) may manifest as back pain in the presence of a herniated thoracic disc. Focal back pain may be of localizing value for identifying the symptomatic disc herniation.

Myelopathy results from a combination of direct mechanical compression, venous congestion, spinal cord ischemia, and spinal cord contusion (i.e., posttraumatic). The predominant symptoms suggestive of myelopathy are leg weakness and sensory loss, followed by gait spasticity, lower extremity paresthesias, and bowel and bladder dysfunction. Brown-Sequard syndrome was the most frequently presenting myelopathic syndrome in the author's series. Paraplegia is extremely uncommon; however, it continues to be reported in series in which patients were initially approached via a laminectomy, followed by a more ventral approach.[15]

Radicular symptoms result from a direct compression or stretching of spinal roots. Thoracic radiculopathic symptoms may mimic a number of cardiac, pulmonary, intra-abdominal, or retroperitoneal diseases. Examples include myocardial infarction, abdominal aortic aneurysm, parecreatitis, renal colic, or ulcer disease. Two patients in this series underwent extensive examinations for other causes before the etiology of their symptoms was discovered to be from thoracic disc herniation. In both cases, the patients presented with radicular findings suggestive of other disease processes and subsequently developed myelopathy, which led to the correct diagnosis of thoracic disc herniation.

The first patient presented with severe left chest pain during a tennis match. An extensive cardiac workup was unrevealing. Over the subsequent 5 weeks, the patient developed progressive difficulties with ambulation, as well as urinary incontinence. Physical examination revealed a Brown-Sequard myelopathy with spastic paraparesis, loss of left-sided proprioception, and loss of right-sided pain and temperature below the T9 dermatome. The development of the myelopathy led to the diagnosis of a left centrolateral T8 to T9 soft disc herniation. Following extirpation of the disc via a unilateral transpedicular approach, the patient made a full neurological recovery.

The second patient presented with a 7-year history of left lower quadrant pain and underwent exploratory laparotomy and bowel resection without relief of his symptoms. He subsequently developed a progressive transverse myelopathy with a spastic gait, in addition to his continued radicular complaints. MRI revealed a left T6 to T7 central calcified disc herniation with significant spinal cord compression. Following the transpedicular removal of the disc herniation, the patient's myelopathy and radiculopathy resolved.

Bowel and bladder incontinence or dysfunction may result from compression of the spinal cord, conus medullaris, or cauda equina. Disc herniations at lower levels of the thoracic spine (T10-11, T11-12) have a higher incidence of urinary and/or bowel incontinence.[4,15,27] This high incidence reflects compression of the conus medullaris or sacral roots, and possibly, the increased severity of myelopathy produced by disc herniations at lower thoracic spinal cord levels.[15] Two of four patients with lesions at T11-12 presented with urinary incontinence.[15]

IMAGING

MRI provides images in both the sagittal and axial planes that are useful as a screening modality for other processes that should be considered in the differential diagnosis of thoracic disc herniation. Thoracic disc herniations are best visualized on T-1 weighted images, appearing either isointense or hypointense to the adjacent intradiscal space.[6] T-2 weighted images appear hypointense to the adjacent intradiscal space. Calcified lesions appear hypointense on both T-1 and T-2 weighted images. CT may be more definitive regarding the presence of a calcified disc. Gadolinium enhancement may increase the sensitivity of MRI for small disc herniations.[19] Images may be obscured by motion artifact caused by cardiac contractility, respiratory excursion, blood flow through the great vessels, or pulsatile CSF flow.[19,24] While less invasive than myelogram, some patients tolerate MRI less well due to the claustrophobic sensation produced in the MRI apparatus.

Myelogram with postmyelographic CT scan is as sensitive as MRI in the detection of thoracic disc herniations.[3] Prior to the advent of MRI, myelography was the gold standard for the diagnosis of thoracic disc herniation. The advantage provided by myelography, compared to MRI, is its superior delineation of the bone anatomy, including calcified discs or osteophytes. Myelography may be used as an imaging correlate for accurate intraoperative localization. The disadvantages include exposure to ionized radiation, potential for spinal headaches, and the potential for progression of symptoms in patients harboring high-grade blocks.

Plain radiographs have low sensitivity and specificity for the diagnosis of thoracic disc herniation. The most common finding is calcification of the intervertebral disc space or calcification dorsal to the disc space.[16] Other findings include disc space narrowing, osteophyte formation, segmental kyphosis, or straightening of the physiological kyphosis. Plain radiographs may be useful in identifying associated conditions, such as Scheurmann's kyphosis.

SURGICAL INDICATIONS

In a review of nine surgical series (238 patients), the most common indication for surgical intervention was myelopathy (70%), followed by intractable radiculopathy (24%), and back pain (6%)

Table 19-3. Surgical Indications*

Surgical Indications	Cumulative Series (%)	Range from Individual Series (%)
Myelopathy	70	25–96
Radiculopathy	24	0–66
Back Pain	6	0–30

*Pooled data from 238 patients.[3,4,9,10,13,15,26-28]

(Table 19-3). This was reflected in the authors' series as well, in which 70% of patients had surgery for myelopathy and 30% of patients for radiculopathy. In all series reported, myelopathy was a strong indication for surgical intervention. However, conservative management appears to have a role in patients presenting with radiculopathy.

Brown et al.[5] reviewed a series of 55 patients who presented with thoracic disc herniations. Fifteen patients presenting with myelopathy underwent surgery without a trial of conservative management. The remaining 40 patients underwent a course of conservative therapy consisting of bed rest, nonsteroidal anti-inflammatory drugs, and physical therapy (hyperextension back-strengthening exercises, postural training, and body mechanics education). Of the 40 patients treated conservatively, 77% returned to their previous level of activity without restrictions or with only slight modifications. Twenty-three percent were able to return to work. Prior to beginning physical therapy, one patient in the nonoperated group became acutely paraplegic and showed no improvement following emergency decompressive surgery.

ASYMPTOMATIC THORACIC DISC HERNIATIONS

Based on postmortem and radiographic studies, the incidence of patients with an asymptomatic thoracic disc herniation varies from 10% to 15%.[19] The use of MRI for diagnosis of spinal diseases has increased the diagnosis of thoracic disc herniation. A retrospective review of 433 myelograms performed to evaluate cervical or lumbar disc disease with incidental inclusion of the thoracic region revealed an estimated 11% to 13% incidence of thoracic disc herniation.[2] Of these patients, 88% showed dorsal displacement of the spinal cord. In 28% of those patients with dorsal displacement of the spinal cord, the deformation was greater than one half the width

of the spinal canal. The natural history of these asymptomatic disc herniations is unknown, but the percentage of patients who develop neurological deficits is clearly small. However, there have been no longitudinal prospective studies to follow these asymptomatic patients long-term.

Patients with asymptomatic disc herniations generally do not undergo prophylactic surgery, regardless of the size of the disc or degree of spinal cord compression.[23,29] However, a thorough neurological examination to ensure that there are no subtle signs of myelopathy is recommended. Additionally, patients, particularly those with central or centrolateral discs, should be counseled about the risk of progressive symptoms and should subsequently be monitored for the development of neurological signs or symptoms. Although the identification of patients who will progress is difficult, a subsegment of this asymptomatic population will develop symptoms.

USE OF THE TRANSPEDICULAR APPROACH

The transpedicular approach is effective in treating the neurological sequelae of thoracic disc herniation. While the transthoracic and lateral approaches (lateral extracavitary, lateral rachiotomy, and costotransversectomy) are better for more extensive procedures requiring vertebrectomy, such as for burst fractures or tumor, the transpedicular approach appears to be well suited for thoracic disc herniations. Review of multiple series reveals good neurological outcomes using all of these approaches. Only two previously reported series have employed the transpedicular approach for all thoracic disc herniations.[13,20] Reasons given for avoiding the transpedicular approach include the following: (1) difficulty removing midline or calcified discs,[26,28] (2) the potential for creating spinal segmental instability,[28] and (3) the inability to remove intradural disc herniations or deal with CSF fistulas created by intradural disc removal.[28] In a number of series, the transpedicular approach has been used selectively by surgeons for either lateral, noncalcified disc herniations or for patients in whom the morbidity from other approaches was prohibitive due to the patient's preexisting medical conditions.[3,10,26]

Of the 11 central or centrolateral disc herniations in the authors' series, six were calcified lesions. These midline, calcified disc herniations were safely removed using the transpedicular approach exclusively. The transpedicular approach does provide a more limited visualization of the ventral spinal cord than other procedures. Operative techniques designed to improve midline visualization when using the transpedicular approach include the use of dental mirrors and a modified arthroscope, as described by LeRoux et al.[13] Rotation of the table 15 to 20 degrees away from the operating surgeon may also improve visualization of the ventral spinal cord. Adverse neurological sequelae seen with laminectomy were not encountered using the transpedicular approach. In the authors' series, there was a transient increased neurological deficit in one patient in whom a dorsal interbody stabilization procedure was attempted (methylmethacrylate and Steinmann pins). This patient subsequently made a complete neurological recovery.

Overt spinal instability has not been reported in any series employing the transpedicular approach.[3,13,26] The thoracic spine has an inherent stability created by the costovertebral articulations and the entire thoracic rib cage structure. Delayed kyphotic deformities have not been observed with the transpedicular approach in the authors' series. Three patients developed persistent postoperative back pain, although no radiographic instability could be identified. Patients undergoing the transthoracic approach or costotransversectomy may undergo intraoperative dorsal and/or ventral fusion and are routinely placed in an external orthosis for 3 months (e.g., thoracolumbosacral orthosis [TLSO] brace) following surgery. The authors have found it unnecessary to use an external orthosis, but patients with persistent back pain may be candidates for postoperative bracing. Should dorsal spinal instrumentation become necessary, this could be readily accomplished by extending the standard dorsal midline approach used for the transpedicular approach. Patients who require a

ventral intervertebral body fusion are best approached via a transthoracic approach.

While intradural fragments are rare,[7,30] 10% incidence[28] has been reported. Intradural fragment removal and intradural exploration were readily accomplished via the transpedicular approach without adverse neurological sequelae. The transthoracic approach also allows for intradural disc removal with access to the ventral dura for repair. Costotransversectomy provides the least access of the three approaches for repair of the dural and intradural disc extirpation.

General medical complications were low in all reported series using the various approaches. Medical complications ranged from 0% to 10%. They consisted primarily of superficial wound infections,[15,26,28] deep venous thrombosis, and pulmonary embolism.[26,28] However, of the three approaches, the transpedicular approach has the least inherent morbidity. Outcomes and complications using the various approaches are listed in Table 19-4.

Thoracatomy, which is required for the transthoracic approach, may be associated with a 10% decline in pulmonary function. Additionally, it is associated with a higher incidence of atelectasis, pneumonia, and pleural effusions. Thoracostomy tube drainage is generally required for 1 to 2 days postoperatively.

Costotransversectomy requires a rib resection and has been associated with up to a 10% incidence of pleural tears, which also may require thoracostomy tube drainage. This expected intrathoracic morbidity was not encountered using the transpedicular approach.

Spinal cord vascular complications have not been reported in any series, but there is a theoretical risk of spinal cord infarction by sacrificing the neurovascular bundle at the level of the intervertebral foramen. In the series by Maiman et al.,[15] the approach had to be altered in six of 23 cases because of the presence of major radicular feeding arteries identified on preoperative angiograms. Sacrifice of radicular feeding arteries is generally performed for disc extirpation via the transthoracic approach as well, but it is performed at the ventral midvertebral body level, as opposed to the intervertebral foramen, and has not been associated with spinal cord infarction. The transpedicular approach has not been associated with sacrifice of radicular feeding arteries.

Table 19-4. Outcomes and Complications Using Various Approaches to Thoracic Disc Excision

Study	Year	Approach	No. of Cases	Neurological Outcome			Complications
				Excellent	Fair	Poor	
Logue[14]	1952	Laminectomy	11	6	0	5	NR
Arseni and Nash[1]	1960	Laminectomy	13	6	4	3	NR
Hulme[12]	1960	Costotransver.	6	4	1	1	NR
Perot and Munro[21]	1969	Transthoracic	2	2	0	0	NR
Ransohoff et al.[22]	1969	Transthoracic	3	3	0	0	NR
Patterson and Arbit[20]	1978	Transpedicular	3	3	0	0	NR
Sekhar and Janetta[26]	1983	Laminectomy Postduratomy Transthoracic Transpedicular	12	10	1	1	Wound infection (1) Bowel obstruction (1) Pulmonary embolism (1) Pleural effusion (1)
Maiman et al.[15]	1984	Lat. extracavitary	23	20	0	3	Pleural tear (3) Wound infection (2) Anesthesia dolorosa (1)
Bohlman and Zdeblick[4]	1988	Transthoracic Costotransver.	19	10	6	2	Wrong level
Blumenkopf[3]	1988	Transthoracic Transpedicular	7	6	1	0	NR
el-Kalliny et al.[10]	1991	Transpedicular Transthoracic Costotransver.	8 8 5	17	3	1	Pleural effusion (2) CVA (1)
Stillerman and Weiss[28]	1990	Transthoracic	48	37/38 (myelopathy)	1	0	Wound infection (2) Bowel obstruction (1) Pulmonary embolism (1) Pleural effusion (1)
		Lat. extracavitary	3	33/35 (pain)	2	0	
LeRoux et al.[13]	1993	Transpedicular	20	20			NR
Currier et al.[9]	1994	Transthoracic	18	12	3	3	Kyphosis after prior laminectomy

Excellent: No residual symptoms; Fair: Improved; Poor: Worse

CONCLUSION

The transpedicular approach is a safe and effective method for removing thoracic disc herniations. A number of surgeons have reserved this approach for noncalcified lateral disc herniations, preferring costotransversectomy or a transthoracic approach for central calcified lesions. In this series and the series reported by LeRoux et al.[13] the transpedicular approach was effectively employed to remove these lesions. The morbidity from this procedure is less than that associated with the other types of approaches and it does not require postoperative bracing.

REFERENCES

1. Arseni C, Nash F. Thoracic intervertebral disc protrusion. A clinical study. J Neurosurg 17:418-430-430, 1960.
2. Awwad EE, Martin DS, Smith KR, Baker BK. Asymptomatic versus symptomatic herniated thoracic disc. Their frequency and characteristics as detected by computed tomography after myelography. Neurosurgery 28:180-186, 1991.
3. Blumenkopf B. Thoracic intervertebral disc herniations: Diagnostic value of magnetic resonance imaging. Neurosurgery 23:36-40, 1988.
4. Bohlman HH, Zdeblick TA. Anterior excision of herniated thoracic discs. J Bone Joint Surg 70:1038-1047, 1988.
5. Brown CW, Deffer PA, Akmakjian J, Donaldson DH, Brugman JL. The natural history of thoracic disc herniation. Spine 17 (Suppl 6):S97-S102, 1992.

6. Chambers AA. Thoracic disc herniation. Semin Roentgenol 23:111-117, 1988.

7. Chowdhary UM. Intradural thoracic disc protrusion. Spine 12:718-719, 1987.

8. Crafoord C, Hiertonn T, Lindblom K, Olsson SE. Spinal cord compression caused by a protruded thoracic disc. Report of a case treated with antero-lateral fenestration of the disc. Acta Orthop Scand 28:103-107, 1958.

9. Currier BL, Eismont FJ, Green BA. Transthoracic disc excision and fusion for herniated thoracic discs. Spine 19:323-328, 1994.

10. el-Kalliny M, Tew JM, van Loveren H, Dunsker S. Surgical approaches to thoracic disc herniations. Acta Neurochir (Wien) 111:23-32, 1991.

11. Hawk WA. Spinal compression caused by ecchondrosis of the intervertebral fibrocartilage—With a review of the recent literature. Brain 59:204-224, 1936.

12. Hulme A. The surgical approach to thoracic intervertebral disc protrusion. J Neurol Neurosurg Psychiatry 23:133-137, 1960.

13. LeRoux PD, Haglund MM, Harris AB. Thoracic disc disease: Experience with the transpedicular approach in twenty consecutive patients. Neurosurgery 33:58-66, 1993.

14. Logue V. Thoracic intervertebral disc prolapse with spinal cord compression. J Neurol Neurosurg Psychiatry 15:227-241, 1952.

15. Maiman DJ, Larson SJ, Luck E, El-Ghatit A. Lateral extracavitary approach to the spine for thoracic disc herniation: Report of 23 cases. Neurosurgery 14:178-182, 1984.

16. McAllister C, Nash F. Protrusion of thoracic intervertebral discs. Acta Neurochirwein 11:3-33, 1963.

17. Mixter WJ, Barr JS. Rupture of the intervertebral disc with involvement of the spinal canal. New Engl J Med 211:210-214, 1934.

18. Mueller R. Protrusion of thoracic intervertebral discs with compression of the spinal cord. Acta Med Scand 139:99-104, 1951.

19. Parizel PM, Rodesch G, Baleriaux D, et al. Gd-DTPA-enhanced MR in thoracic disc herniations. Neuroradiology 31:75-79, 1989.

20. Patterson RH, Arbit E. A surgical approach through the pedicle to protruded thoracic discs. J Neurosurg 48:768-772, 1978.

21. Perot PL, Munro DD. Transthoracic removal of midline thoracic disc protrusions causing spinal cord compression. J Neurosurg 31:452-458, 1969.

22. Ransohoff JR, Spencer F, Siew F, Gage L. Case reports and technical notes. Transthoracic removal of thoracic disc. Report of three cases. J Neurosurg 31:459-461, 1969.

23. Rosenbloom SA. Thoracic disc disease and stenosis. Radiol Clin North Am 29:765-775, 1991.

24. Ross JS, Perez-Reyes N, Masaryk TJ, Bohlman H, Modic MT. Thoracic disc herniation: MR imaging. Radiology 165:511-515, 1987.

25. Seddon HJ. Pott's paraplegia—Prognosis and treatment. Br J Surgery 22:769-799, 1935.

26. Sekhar LN, Janetta PJ. Thoracic disc herniation: Operative approaches and results. Neurosurgery 12:303-305, 1983.

27. Simpson JM, Simeone FA, Balderston RA, An HS. Thoracic disc herniation. Re-evaluation of the posterior approach using a modified costotransversectomy. Spine 18:1872-1877, 1993.

28. Stillerman CB, Weiss MH. Management of thoracic disc herniation. Clin Neurosurg 38:325-352, 1990.

29. Willliams MP, Cherryman GR, Husband JE. Significance of thoracic disc herniation demonstrated by MR imaging. J Comput Assist Tomogr 13:211-214, 1989.

30. Yildizhan A, Pasoglu A, Okten T, Ekinci N, Aycan K, Aral O. Intradural disc herniations. Pathogenesis, clinical picture, diagnosis and treatment. Acta Neurochir (Wien) 110:160-165, 1991.

Transthoracic
Approach

Brian G. Cuddy, M.D., and Phanor L. Perot, Jr., M.D., Ph.D.

Until the 1960s most patients with thoracic disc herniations were treated with a standard laminectomy and removal of the protruding discs. Patients with the best results had only radicular symptoms that were caused by lateral disc herniations. Using the technique of a wide laminectomy, nearly half of these patients did not improve or worsened after the procedure.[10] Approximately 70% of the patients with a central disc herniation above the T10 to T11 level, with signs and symptoms of myelopathy, showed no improvement with a standard laminectomy approach. Furthermore, it was noted that there was a high risk of paraplegia when laminectomy was carried out in patients who had spinal cord compression with a severe preoperative neurological deficit from a central disc protrusion.

Poor surgical outcomes from a standard laminectomy precipitated a search for safer and more effective operative approaches to the thoracic spine. Carson, Gumpert, and Jefferson[3] described the technique of a far lateral laminectomy and partial facetectomy. This technique demonstrated improved results compared to those previously obtained by a standard laminectomy alone.

Patterson and Arbit[10] introduced a dorsolateral approach through the facet joint and pedicle. This was also a technical improvement compared with the standard laminectomy. Hulme[5] developed a lateral costotransversectomy approach that allowed a more lateral view of the thecal sac and dorsal disc herniation than that provided by lateral extension of a standard laminectomy alone. Although the lateral costotransversectomy improved the surgical view of the thoracic disc herniation, it still did not allow a true ventral view of the compression of the thecal sac.

In 1976 Larson et al.[6] described the lateral extracavitary approach to traumatic lesions of the thoracic spine. The approach provided access to the vertebral body and allowed resection of disc material past the midline and as far as the contralateral pedicle.

This technique has been applied specifically for thoracic disc herniations with good results.[8] The lateral extracavitary approach has improved the access to midline disc herniations, but carries the risk of interrupting significant radicular arteries at the level of the neural foramen. The artery of Adamkiewicz can arise from T5 to L2. This approach can lead to injury to this potentially important vascular supply to the spinal cord. It has been recommended that a preoperative angiogram be performed to identify the artery of Adamkiewicz before the ventral extracavitary approach. If visualized, an alteration of the surgical approach may be necessary to avoid injury, thus complicating the planned surgery if the disc herniation is at the same level. The lateral extracavitary approach provides excellent exposure of the thoracic spine, but is technically demanding.

The transthoracic approach described by Perot and Munro[13] in 1969 provides similar favorable results for thoracic disc disease. This technique is useful for central thoracic disc protrusions, especially in those causing spinal cord compression. It has the advantage of a relatively simple and direct approach to the vertebral column, with an improved visualization of the thecal sac. A major disadvantage of this technique exists with lesions above T4 or below the T12 level, because these lesions are difficult to access within the thoracic cavity. Lesions above T4 can be technically demanding because of the reversal of the thoracic kyphosis in this region, thus limiting surgical access. Thoracotomy above the level of the third rib is impractical because the first and second ribs limit the exposure. The region at the T11 to T12 level is limited by the diaphragm. To adequately visualize this region, a transdiaphragmatic-thoracoabdominal approach is required.

Since its original description, numerous reports utilizing the transthoracic approach have experienced similarly favorable clinical results, particularly when total removal of a central thoracic intervertebral disc protrusion is necessary.[1,7,11,12,14,15]

PREOPERATIVE PLANNING
Imaging Studies

The planning of a surgical approach of the thoracic spine must be done precisely, particularly with respect to the identification of the appropriate intervertebral disc space. Magnetic resonance imaging (MRI) is an excellent screening test that eliminates other spinal lesions that mimic thoracic disc disease, including tumor and demyelinating disease. Computed tomography (CT) is also useful to confirm the disc space level and to further define the surgical anatomy. CT is very helpful in delineating the size of the osteophyte (or hard disc) that is compressing the thecal sac. This can be occasionally difficult to delineate by MRI alone. CT-myelography may be used to further delineate the lesion and its anatomical relationship to the spinal cord, and is also useful for localization of the level of the lesion. Calcification within the disc space is found in 30% to 70% of symptomatic thoracic disc protrusions. This is a typical diagnostic feature on plain radiographs and CT.[9] It is also important to determine on preoperative diagnostic radiographs the number of rib-bearing vertebrae so the intraoperative radiographs correlate cor-

rectly to the level of the thoracic disc protrusion. This is a very important technical point that cannot be emphasized enough. Improper identification of the disc space level may otherwise occur. Sagittal MRI may be used to count from the C2 vertebra, down to the level of the thoracic lesion. This can be correlated with the CT scan and plain radiographs. This further lowers the chance of error regarding identification of the correct thoracic disc protrusion level.

The transthoracic approach allows entrance into the disc space at a safe distance from the dorsal intercostal arteries, crossing at the mid region of the vertebral body. Additionally, the radicular branches are also avoided because they enter at the rostral end of the intervertebral foramen. Thus with the routine transthoracic approach the use of preoperative arteriography is seldom needed.

Pulmonary Function and Evaluation

Careful preoperative preparation and evaluation reduces the risk of pulmonary complications with the transthoracic approach. During the procedure a double lumen endotracheal tube is placed so that the patient can be ventilated using the dependent lung only, while the upper lung is deflated and packed off to allow maximal surgical view of the disc space level.

Preoperative evaluation typically includes an assessment of pulmonary function, as measured by spirometry and arterial blood gases. These basic measurements permit the classification of patients (as acceptable or not acceptable). Forced vital capacity (FVC) and forced expiratory volume at one second (FEV-1) are useful regarding risks of patients undergoing lung resection, in contrast to those undergoing exposure for spinal disease. A preoperative consultation with the anesthesiologist to discuss (1) the length of the procedure, (2) the surgical exposure, and (3) the preoperative pulmonary function tests can minimize ventilatory problems during and after the procedure. If necessary during the operation, the dissection can be temporarily ceased so the collapsed lung can be ventilated. This simple maneuver can decrease intraoperative ventilation difficulties.

PATIENT POSITIONING

Lateral lesions can be approached from the side that provides the easiest access. For central thoracic disc protrusions, in the middle and upper thoracic

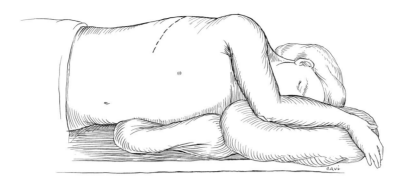

Fig. 20-1. Right-side-up thoracotomy position. The upper arm is brought in a rostral direction to allow operative exposure and intraoperative radiograph positioning.

segments, an approach from the patient's right side may be prudent because the heart and aorta are less obstructive to the surgical view. The radicular vessels that are important to spinal cord perfusion enter on the left side more often than the right. Nevertheless, in the thoracolumbar region a left-sided approach is preferred because the liver can be difficult to retract adequately.

For a right-sided approach the patient is positioned in a standard right-side-up thoracotomy position. The upper and lower extremities are carefully padded and the upper arm supported away from the operative field (Fig. 20-1). An axillary roll is used for the inferior shoulder and axillary region to prevent injury to the brachial plexus. The lower legs are flexed and pillows placed between them. The patient's position is maintained with a "bean bag" vacuum support (VAC-PAC, [Olympic Medical, Seattle, WA]). A double lumen endotracheal tube is placed so that the right lung can be deflated during the operation, thus exposing the thoracic spine. The surgeon faces the ventral side of the patient, with the assistant standing on the dorsal side. The operative microscope is readied so that it can easily be brought into the operative field when necessary. At this point, an intraoperative radiograph is obtained to confirm the appropriate location of the thoracotomy incision, as well as to ensure that the arms are not interfering with the proper placement of the radiograph during the operation so that the correct disc space can be easily verified.

SURGICAL TECHNIQUE

The ribs are attached to the vertebral bodies at the body's rostral aspect. Therefore, the thoracotomy is typically performed at one interspace above the in-

tended disc space. For example, the approach to the T6-7 disc space should be between the fifth and sixth ribs. The correct disc space level is identified from an intraoperative radiograph before preparing the surgical site. Correlation with preoperative radiographs and confirmation of the correct number of ribs are required to correctly identify the appropriate disc space at the time of the operation.

The incision is made in a curvilinear fashion from the ventral axillary line to the border of the paraspinal muscles over the rib and space selected (see Fig. 20-1). Rib resection is not usually required. The latissimus dorsi muscle is mobilized by blunt dissection and transected. The serratus anterior muscle is then mobilized, and the space between this muscle and the underlying rib is opened. The appropriate rib interspace is entered by cutting the intercostal muscles. The parietal pleura is then dissected with scissors and a self-retaining retractor inserted.

Once the thoracotomy is performed, rib spreaders are positioned and the lung deflated and packed off. The parietal pleura is opened over the appropriate disc space, exposing the articulating rib head and its radiate ligament (Figs. 20-2 and 20-3).

Great care is taken to avoid dissection over the mid portions of the vertebral bodies rostral and caudal to the disc space to avoid injuring the segmental artery (Fig. 20-4). A marker is placed into the disc space and an intraoperative radiograph is obtained to confirm the level. Next, attention is directed toward removal of the rib head. The disc space is entered with a No. 11 blade scalpel and disc material is removed so that a trough into the disc space is created. Following this, a high-speed burr is used to remove the proximal 2 to 3 cm of the rib as it articulates with the vertebral bodies above and below the disc space (Fig. 20-5).

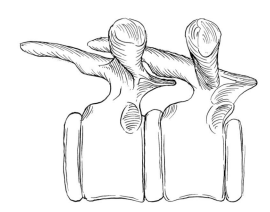

Fig. 20-2. Relationship of the vertebral body pedicle, facet, and disc space structures without the overlying rib. Note the articulation of the rib with the vertebral body is above and below the disc space. Additionally, the intravertebral disc lies at the caudal end of the intravertebral foramen.

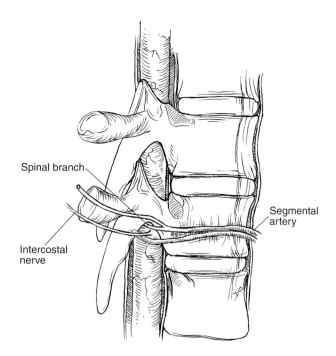

Fig. 20-4. Relationship of the exiting thoracic intercostal nerve and spinal/radicular artery. Note the exiting nerve root is located at the rostral end of the intervertebral foramen and the segmental artery is in the midsection of the vertebral body.

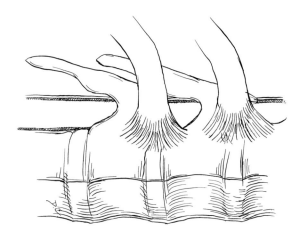

Fig. 20-3. The rib head with the radiate ligament covers the intervertebral foramen and is attached above and below the disc space in the mid- to upper thoracic spine.

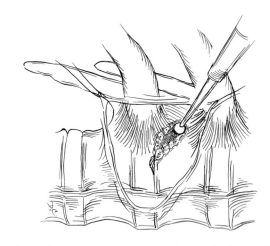

Fig. 20-5. After opening the parietal pleura, a high-speed burr is used to remove the rib head articulation as well as the dorsal aspect of the vertebral body adjacent to the intervertebral disc.

The fibrocartilaginous attachment of the rib to the vertebral bodies is removed and more disc is curetted away as the disc space is entered. The high-speed burr can also be used to thin the pedicle of the caudal vertebra. Great care is taken not to dissect into the pedicle of the rostral vertebral body. This is the location of the exiting nerve root and radicular artery.

Once enough vertebral body edge has been removed so that the disc space is fully visualized, a trough has been made into the disc itself, and the rib head has been removed, the posterior longitudinal ligament can be identified (Fig. 20-6). The fibrocartilaginous attachments of the rib head should be

completely removed. The dense fibers of the posterior longitudinal ligament are observed running in a transverse direction over the exposed field, covering the epidural space. With the removal of the proximal rib and ventral portion of the caudal pedicle, access to the spinal canal and the dura mater is "unlocked" or opened. Using a blunt nerve hook, the

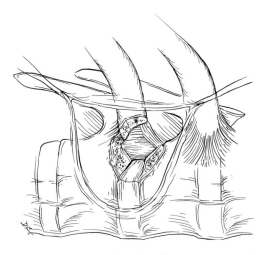

Fig. 20-6. After the rib head and its ligamentous attachment have been removed, the posterior longitudinal ligament can be identified.

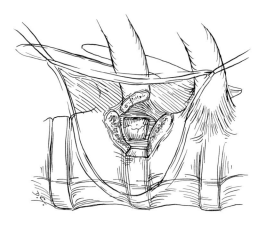

Fig. 20-8. Adjacent vertebral body surfaces have been removed as well as the ligamentous structures overlying the dura mater. At this point, the outline of the disc protrusion and thecal sac compression can be identified.

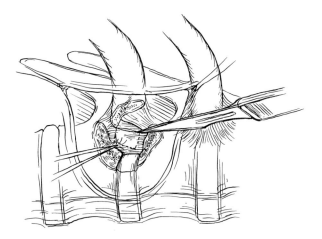

Fig. 20-7. The posterior longitudinal ligament is carefully elevated with sharp dissection and a series of curettes.

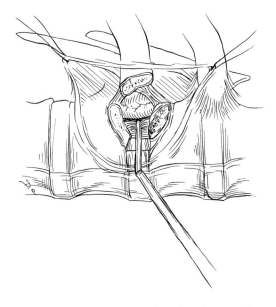

Fig. 20-9. Disc tissue is removed with a downward-cutting curette. The disc material is removed into the trough developed by removal of the intervertebral disc so that the surgeon is always working away from the dura and overlying spinal cord.

posterior longitudinal ligament can be elevated and then cut with either a No. 11 blade scalpel or a small Kerrison punch (Fig. 20-7). It is not uncommon to encounter bleeding from the epidural venous plexus at this point. Gentle bipolar coagulation, as well as small amounts of absorbable Gelfoam sponge (Upjohn Co., Kalamazoo, Mich.) can be used to obtain hemostasis.

The ligament is excised from the most rostral to the most caudal extent of the exposure (Fig. 20-8). Once the dura mater is identified, the rest of the dissection is carried out with the aid of an operative microscope. This allows the outline of the disc protrusion indenting the dura mater to be identified.

There are times when this may be completely covered by the dura mater laterally as it caps the protrusion. It is very important not to manipulate the dura mater and thus compress the spinal cord in this situation. Great care is taken to place curettes in a downward fashion, pushing the disc material into the trough previously created (Fig. 20-9). A series of curettes that use backward-angled cutting are now commercially available in various sizes. These

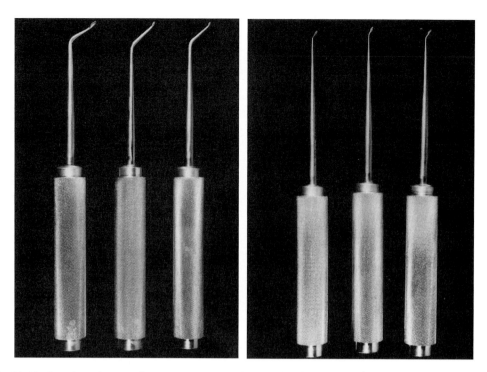

Fig. 20-10. Set of six thoracic discectomy curettes designed to facilitate removal of disc material away from the thecal sac. The curettes vary in size of cup and angle.

backward-angled curettes allow disc material to be pulled away from the ventral surface of the thecal sac without manipulation of the spinal cord (Fig. 20-10). The disc material is curetted away from the spinal cord into the trough created by the bone and disc removal ventrally (Fig. 20-11). In the situation where the disc is "hard" and composed of dorsally projecting osteophytes, the use of a high-speed burr may be necessary to thin the osteophytes adequately so that a curette can break them away from the dura mater without traumatizing the spinal cord. Under the microscope those rare situations where disc material has actually penetrated the dura mater and is adherent to the spinal cord can be visualized. This is a very difficult technical situation and extreme care must be taken. Cerebrospinal fluid (CSF) leakage is a rare event, especially with soft disc protrusions. However, with larger calcified lesions with rigid osteophytes, the dura mater can be quite thin over the dorsally projecting bone spurs. In this circumstance, a CSF leak can occur. Careful control using Gelfoam should be taken to avoid the complication of CSF leakage into the pleural space.

If a fusion is thought to be necessary (in the authors' experience this is very rare), it can be accom-

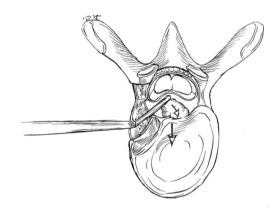

Fig. 20-11. Axial illustration of the curette entering the disc space and removal of the disc herniation against the thecal sac.

plished once the discectomy and decompression are completed. Three centimeters of rib head can be taken from its articulation with the vertebral body. Using elevators, as well as a high-speed burr, the rib head is removed in a single piece. This allows the harvested end of the distal rib to be used as a strut graft. Removal of bone along the rostral and caudal edge of the vertebral body closest to the dura mater, disc removal, and the creation of a trough in the midsection of the vertebral body permits the rib head to be tapped into the trough at the conclusion of the operation. This provides a much more rigorous removal of the disc material and the curetting of the end plates to assist in achieving an arthrodesis. Typically, an external orthosis is not used because the vertebral bodies and dorsal elements are essentially intact. Thus there is no inherent instability and the fusion can take place without the need of an external orthosis. The biomechanical effects of transthoracic microdiscectomy have been studied by Broc et al.[2] in cadaveric thoracic spines. There were minimal effects on the immediate mechanics and kinematics of the thoracic spine, which did not overtly destabilize the motion segment.

The literature contains reports of patients that were symptomatic from disc herniations at multiple levels, but this is uncommon.[4] In the unusual situation where several large disc herniations are identified, spinal excision of all of them can be accomplished in the same setting. The transthoracic technique allows exposure of more than three consecutive levels, if necessary.

POSTOPERATIVE CARE

At the time of wound closure, thoracostomy tubes are inserted to evacuate any postoperative collection of blood and air. One tube is placed toward the apex of the lung and the other curved along the dorsal gutter. Typically, these are placed one or two intercostal spaces above and below the incision, and the tubes are tunneled beneath the skin to create an air seal around the tube. A pursestring suture is placed to hold the tube in place to protect it from accidental removal during patient transfers. The ribs are reapproximated and held in place with large absorbable sutures placed around the ribs above and below the thoracotomy site. Some surgeons do not reapproximate the ribs for fear of ensnaring the intercostal nerves. In addition, a local injection of marcaine is placed along the intercostal nerves to assist in postoperative pain management. This is especially important in preventing atelectasis. The serratus anterior, trapezius, latissimus dorsi, and rhomboid muscle groups are then closed in separate layers. Scarpa's fascia is closed, the skin is closed with a subcuticular suture, and Steri-strips 3M Healthcare, St. Paul, Minn. are applied. The thoracostomy tubes are attached to a water-sealed container under constant wall suction. Most patients are extubated before leaving the operating room. The thoracostomy tubes are typically removed within 36 hours, when follow-up chest radiographs are performed to rule out pneumothorax, and drainage is less than 100 to 150 ml/24 hours.

Perioperative antibiotics are administered generally for a period of 48 hours. The authors encourage early mobilization on the first postsurgical day. Postthoracotomy pain should be controlled aggressively to assist in mobilization and avoid atelectasis. The authors typically use patient-controlled analgesia (PCA). This is switched to oral oxycodone before discharge.

SURGICAL RESULTS AND COMPLICATIONS

Patients with lateral or centrolateral protrusions with only radicular symptoms or very mild signs of a thoracic myelopathy experience the most favorable results after discectomy. Dorsolateral and lateral approaches are typically adequate for many of these lesions. The ventral transthoracic approach, however, offers a significant advantage in dealing with centrally placed intervertebral disc herniations with significant cord compression and thoracic myelopathy. Certainly patients who have severe preoperative deficits are expected to have the poorest overall results. Many of these patients, however, demonstrate significant improvement in their preoperative deficits. Patients with long-standing symptoms and a significant thoracic myelopathy should not be excluded for consideration for this surgical approach. Many of these patients may enjoy a significant recovery. Although they may remain impaired by their lower extremity spasticity, improvement in their coordination and lower extremity strength and endurance can have a significant impact upon their quality of life.

Because the incidence of thoracic disc pathology is still relatively rare in comparison to other levels of the spine, few surgeons have extensive experience with the ventral approach. However, the basic philosophy and surgical techniques for decompression of the thoracic spine share many fundamental characteristics with ventral approaches to the cervical spine, with which most spine surgeons are much more familiar. Careful preoperative evaluation, determination of soft vs. hard disc protrusions, and a careful study of the important anatomy regarding the relationship of the rib head articulation and intercostal arteries can make this surgical approach much more straightforward and comfortable for the surgeon. Allowing the dura mater to be visualized well, as well as visualizing the outline of the compression by the offending disc herniation, can allow effective and safe decompression of the spinal cord, and at the same time enable a careful inspection of the dura afterward. This confirms that the spinal cord is adequately decompressed. This visual inspection is very similar to inspecting a ventral cervical decompression for cervical stenosis and cervical myelopathy, ensuring that there is adequate decompression of the spinal cord. Having appropriate surgical instruments necessary for the extended reach, as well as a set of angled curettes allowing for disc material to be adequately removed in a downward fashion, can make this technique much safer and more straightforward.

With thoracoscopic techniques, it is critical for the surgeon to be well versed with the open procedure. Thoracoscopic disc procedures may require an open thoracotomy in an urgent fashion if the anatomy cannot be adequately dissected via thoracoscopy.

The authors have a combined experience of over 60 transthoracic procedures for thoracic disc herniations and have observed no deterioration in the neurological status nor CSF leaks. One reoperation at the original level was performed because of recurrent disc herniation 6 months postoperatively, after the patient had a traumatic injury. There was one postoperative complication of persistent pleural effusion and an eventual infection that required a reopening of the thoracotomy and debridement of the infected site.

Often when the transthoracic approach is discussed in the literature concerns regarding tube thoracostomy, pulmonary complications, and possible partial take down of the diaphragm are commonly mentioned. These disadvantages have been few in the experience of the authors and other reported series utilizing this approach.[1,14,15]

The transthoracic approach to significant protrusions of thoracic intervertebral discs offers a safe and effective alternative to previously described dorsal approaches. This effective alternative is especially important for centrally located disc hernia-tions in the midthoracic spine with significant thoracic myelopathy and spinal cord compression. It provides an optimal exposure of these ventral midline lesions, but does not require the removal of the pedicle to facilitate the exposure. Thus the risk of destabilizing the spinal column is lowered. The exposure also allows placement of a ventral interbody bone graft, if so desired by the surgeon. An additional advantage is the ability to deal with diffuse disc disease over several levels, if thought to be clinically important.

REFERENCES

1. Bohlman HH, Zdeblick TA. Anterior excision of herniated thoracic disc. J Bone Joint Surg 70A:1038-1047, 1988.
2. Broc GG, Crawford NR, Sonntag VK, Dickman, CA. Biomechanical effects of transthoracic microdiscectomy. Spine 22:605-612, 1997.
3. Carson J, Gumpert J, Jefferson A. Diagnosis and treatment of thoracic intervertebral disc protrusions. J Neurosurg Psychiatry 34:68-77, 1971.
4. Chin LS, Black KL, Hoff JT. Multiple disc herniations. J Neurosurg 66:290-292, 1987.
5. Hulme A. The surgical approach to thoracic intervertebral disc protrusions. J Neurol Neurosurg Psychiatry 23:133-137, 1960.
6. Larson SJ, Holst RA, Hemmy DC, Sances A. Lateral extracavitary approach to traumatic lesions of the thoracic and lumbar spine. J Neurosurg 45:628-637, 1976.
7. Lobosky JM, Hitchon PW, McDonnell, DE. Transthoracic anterolateral decompression for thoracic spinal lesions. Neurosurgery 14:26-30, 1984.
8. Maiman DJ, Larson SJ, Lucky E, El-Ghatit A. Lateral extracavitary approach to the spine for thoracic disc herniation. Report of 23 cases. Neurosurgery 14:178-182, 1984.
9. McAllister VL, Sage MR. The radiology of thoracic disc protrusion. Clin Radiol 27:291-299, 1976.
10. Patterson RH, Arbit E. A surgical approach through the pedicle to protruded thoracic discs. Neurosurg 48:768-772, 1978.
11. Perot PL Jr. Transthoracic removal of thoracic disc protrusions. In Symon L, Thomas DGT, Clark K, eds. Neurosurgery, 4th ed. Rob & Smith's Operative Surgery series. London: Butterworths, 1989, pp 398-404.
12. Perot PL Jr. Thoracic disc disease. In Wilkins RH, Rengachary SS, eds. Neurosurgery, vol 3, 2nd ed. New York: McGraw-Hill, 1996, pp 3795-3800.
13. Perot PL Jr, Munro DD. Transthoracic removal of midline thoracic disc protrusions causing spinal cord compression. J Neurosurg 31:452-458, 1969.
14. Ransohoff J, Spencer F, Siew F, et al. Transthoracic removal of thoracic discs. Report of three cases. J Neurosurg 31:459-461, 1969.
15. Sekhar, LN, Jannetta, PJ. Thoracic disc herniation: Operative approaches and results. Neurosurgery 12:303-305, 1983.

Lateral Extracavitary Approach

Leslie A. Sebring, M.D., Ph.D., Dennis J. Maiman, M.D., Ph.D.,
and Sanford J. Larson, M.D., Ph.D.

Thoracic disc herniations are identified in as many as 15% of autopsy specimens and magnetic resonance imaging (MRI) scans of asymptomatic individuals. Symptomatic thoracic herniations, however, are quite rare, accounting for only 0.2% to 0.8% of all disc operations.[8] The majority of symptomatic thoracic discs or osteophytes produce pain that may be localized to the midline thoracic region, or may radiate ventrally around the trunk, into the groin, or into the lower extremities. The initial pain of a herniated disc in this region is often incorrectly attributed to an intrathoracic or intraabdominal process, and thus the diagnosis is frequently delayed until the patient presents with the neurological findings of myelopathy, such as lower extremity weakness, spasticity, ataxia, or bowel/bladder disturbances.

In the absence of neurological deficit, nonoperative treatment can be expected to result in a resolution of symptoms in the majority of cases.[2] When myelopathy is present, or when conservative therapy fails to improve radicular pain, surgical treatment should be considered. The removal of a thoracic disc herniation or osteophyte, however, presents a particular challenge. The anatomy of the thoracic spine is such that the cross-sectional area of the bony spinal canal barely exceeds that of the spinal cord. Hence spinal cord impingement may result from even a relatively small disc herniation in this region. Moreover, thoracic disc herniations are commonly central or paracentral in location and thus present as poorly-accessible ventral mass lesions. Many thoracic discs are calcified and some 10% to 15% are intradural, further complicating their removal.[10] Additionally, the tenuous blood supply to the thoracic region of the spinal cord results in a relative intolerance to surgical manipulation during disc removal.

As might be expected, laminectomy for thoracic disc removal has historically been associated with dismal results.[11] Special surgical approaches have therefore evolved to allow a safer ventral access to the thoracic spine. An ideal approach for the removal of a ventral thoracic disc herniation or osteophyte should include the following: (1) access to the entire width of the ventral spinal canal without spinal cord retraction, (2) direct visualization of the dura mater during separation of the disc/osteophyte from the thecal sac, (3) an ability to open and repair the dura mater in the event of intradural migration, (4) adequate exposure for access to multiple levels and placement of a bone graft, and (5) minimization of associated risks, including spinal destabilization, damage to the great vessels and intrathoracic organs, or sacrifice of the radicular arteries. The technique that best accomplishes these goals is the lateral extracavitary approach.

INDICATIONS

The lateral extracavitary approach was initially designed for the treatment of tuberculous spondylitis, which typically presents with an extradural, ventral, or ventrolateral mass lesion.[3] Later adaptation proved useful for thoracolumbar trauma, tumor, inflammatory diseases, and disc herniations.[5-7] Currently accepted indications for this technique in the setting of a thoracic disc herniation include a symptomatic lesion, located between T3 and T12, with signs of myelopathy and/or lack of response to nonoperative management for radicular pain. Access to disc herniations at the level of T2 and above may be difficult because of the presence of the scapula.[4] Multiple adjacent herniations may be treated via this approach, but if more than three levels are involved, transthoracic methods may be advisable. In the presence of spinal instability or deformity, spinal instrumentation with fusion or laminectomy can easily be incorporated in the surgery. The procedure may be performed bilaterally in the rare instance that complete decompression cannot be accomplished through a unilateral access.

PREOPERATIVE EVALUATION AND PREPARATION

Preoperative evaluation should include adequate radiographic studies to precisely establish the level of disc herniation. An anteroposterior (AP) chest radiograph of good quality is essential to confirm the presence of twelve ribs; the lowest rib may serve as the landmark for determining the correct spinal level once the patient is positioned during surgery. The preoperative MRI or computed tomography (CT) study of the involved disc should include lateral "scout" radiographs encompassing the lesion and either the odontoid process, in the case of an upper thoracic disc herniation, or the sacrum, when a lower thoracic herniation is present. A preoperative skin marking may be helpful, but should be confirmed intraoperatively. Spinal angiography is commonly obtained for lesions between T6 and L2 to identify the radiculomedullary artery of Adamkiewicz. This artery arises between T10 and L1

85% of the time and provides a significant blood supply to the middle and lower thoracic cord.[1] If the artery is found at the level of the lesion or immediately proximal or distal, the authors recommend the contralateral approach.

Preoperative preparation is minimal. Informed consent should include a discussion of the risks of worsened neurological status, pneumothorax, extensive hemorrhage, superficial or deep wound infections, nonunion of bone grafts, and lack of relief or worsening of radicular pain. A general history, physical examination, and screening blood work should be performed. Preoperative autologous blood donations can be obtained; in addition, cell savers (autotransfusion devices) are used routinely and are strongly recommended.

SURGICAL TECHNIQUE

The operation is conducted under general anesthesia, combining both narcotic and inhalation agents. Antiembolism stockings with intermittent pneumatic compression and a foley catheter are placed. Large-bore peripheral and central catheters are essential given the possibility of rapid blood loss intraoperatively. Direct arterial pressures and oxygenation status are carefully monitored. The authors do not use intraoperative evoked potential monitoring because the results of such neurophysiological monitoring have been inconsistent and the disc removal is performed under direct visualization.

The patient is positioned prone on padded chest rolls or on a spinal frame, but supported so that a lateral tilt away from the operator may safely be applied. Arms are carefully tucked at the sides or above the head, with pressure points padded. In the case of morbid obesity, a lateral decubitus position provides adequate exposure.

The skin is incised in the midline with a curved "hockey-stick" shape (Fig. 21-1, *A*). When used for trauma, the vertical portion generally extends three vertebral levels above and three vertebral levels below the lesion; for disc herniation a much smaller incision is possible. Two vertebral levels above and below a single-level lesion is generally adequate. The curved portion of the incision is angled laterally 8 cm to allow adequate soft tissue retraction. The approach may be from either side, and the choice will depend on the presence of lateralizing features and the results of the preoperative spinal angiogram. The incision is then carried through the subcutaneous tissue and thoracodorsal fascia. The fascia is elevated off the underlying musculature by blunt and sharp dissection, working from the midline. When the fascia has been freed over the entire extent of the vertical incision, it is incised along the angled portion. The thin muscles dorsal to the fascia remain attached to it. The skin, subcutaneous tissue, and fascia are then retracted laterally, exposing the lateral border of the erector spinae muscles. The paravertebral muscles are then elevated as a group off the ribs and reflected medially. This exposes the dorsal aspects of the ribs, medial to their angles as well as the tips of the transverse processes (Fig. 21-1, *B*). Muscular branches of the dorsal intercostal arteries require cautery and division during this process.

Alternatively, the incision may be paramedian, corresponding to the outer border of the paravertebral muscle mass and centered at the level of the lesion. In this case, the muscle layers are divided in the line of the incision until the outer border of the paravertebral muscles is exposed. The tissues are then reflected as above.

The appropriate spinal level is now confirmed by radiograph and by palpation of the ribs. For the spinal levels T3 to T10, a single rib articulates at the disc space and requires detachment. The seventh rib, for instance, adjoins the T6-7 interspace and attaches to the T7 transverse process, thus necessitating removal for full exposure of a T6-7 disc herniation. At T11 and T12, however, the ribs articulate directly with the vertebral body so that detachment of the ribs immediately above and below

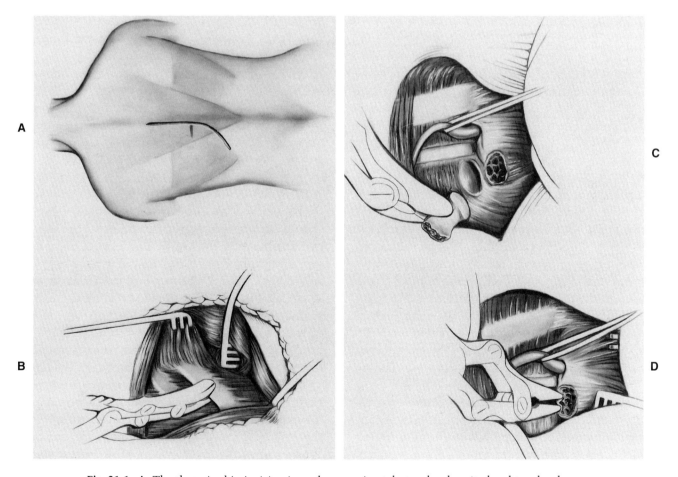

Fig. 21-1. A, The thoracic skin incision is made approximately two levels rostral and two levels caudal to the lesion, with a gently curved lateral portion. **B,** Paraspinous muscles are elevated from lateral to medial to expose the ribs. **C,** Tips of the transverse processes adjacent to the lesion are resected. **D,** A portion of rib 7 to 10 cm lateral to the costovertebral junction is removed.   *Continued.*

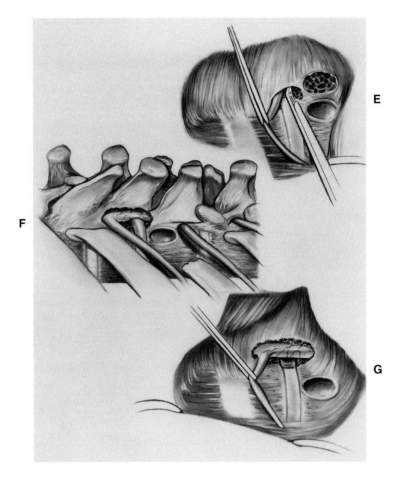

Fig. 21-1, cont'd. **E** and **F,** Bone and disc are removed from the dorsal aspect of the vertebral bodies, **G,** Annulus is excised and removed.

the disc space may be required for adequate exposure at these levels.

To assist with rib removal, the pleura, muscles, and attached ligaments are stripped from the rib circumferentially, taking care to protect the intercostal vessels. The rib is then transected 7 to 10 cm lateral to the costovertebral junction (Fig. 21-1, *C*). The joint of the capsule is excised with a scalpel, elevating the rib away from the pleura (Fig. 21-1, *D*). This maneuver is facilitated by first rongeuring the tip of the corresponding transverse process. The rib is saved for later use as a graft, if desired.

Following rib removal, the intercostal neurovascular bundle is identified. Historically, the intercostal nerve is isolated and divided distally to provide access to the intervertebral foramen and to prevent stretch injury to the nerve root. This helps avoid injury to the spinal cord from nerve root injury. However, this is optional and with careful dis-

section and retraction, the nerve root can be saved. If the nerve was initially sectioned distally, it should be cut and clipped proximal to the dorsal root ganglia prior to closure. The band of hypesthesia that results is rarely problematic and usually resolves over time. The intervertebral foramen and attendant disc are identified by tracing the corresponding intercostal nerve medially. A second localization radiograph is taken with a blunt spinal needle placed into the appropriate disc space. At this point, it may be advantageous to tilt the table 15 to 20 degrees away from the surgeon.

The foramen is enlarged by thinning away and removing the rostral portion of the pedicle inferior to the disc space with small Kerrison rongeurs and curettes until the lateral aspect of the thecal sac is exposed. Epidural bleeding may be encountered at this point, but is usually controlled with a cellulose hemostatic agent and packing with cottonoids.

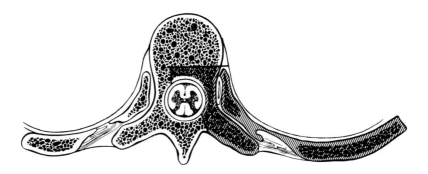

Fig. 21-2. Extent of decompression possible from the lateral extracavitary approach.

Electrocautery should be avoided adjacent to the thecal sac. The presence of a disc protrusion is confirmed by introducing a thin, flat instrument ventral to the sac. The annulus is incised below the floor of the canal, and, by curettage, the intervertebral disc and contiguous portions of bone are removed as far as the opposite side of the vertebral bodies (Fig. 21-1, *E* to *G*). This resection is facilitated by bone removal using a high-speed surgical burr. The object is to create a cavity ventral to the disc protrusion into which the disc can be withdrawn away from the dural sac, thus avoiding any distortion of the thoracic cord. The adjacent floor of the spinal canal is preserved as long as possible to avoid epidural veins. Finally, sharp curettes are introduced between the dura and the floor of the canal, and the disc material and adjacent bone are broken downward into the cavity (see Fig. 21-1, *E* and *F*). Adequacy of resection can be determined by means of a dental mirror or flexible endoscope placed ventral to the dura. The extent of ventral decompression possible from the lateral extracavitary approach is depicted in Fig. 21-2.

The amount of bone removed is usually insufficient to endanger the stability of the spinal column, particularly when the dorsal elements are not violated. The question of whether the initial disc herniation is the result of mild instability at a single motion segment, however, remains unanswered. In view of this, the authors choose to perform a ventral interbody fusion utilizing the resected rib as graft following the discectomy. Prior to placing the rib graft, slots are carved into the vertebral bodies adjacent to the decompression. The rib is prepared by trimming a length of rib that is 10% to 15% longer

than the defect to be spanned. The ends are trimmed to 45 degree angles, with the shorter length as the leading edge. At least two pieces of rib are impacted into position, at least 1 cm away from the dural sac, to prevent spinal cord compression.

At this time, the exposed pleura is examined during the respiratory cycle for the presence of an air leak after the wound is filled with saline. If the pleura has been opened, a No. 32 thoracostomy tube is placed in the pleural space and connected to water-seal suction and drainage. A large surgical drain is placed in the paravertebral region (optional) and the wound is then carefully closed in layers.

POSTOPERATIVE CARE

Aggressive pulmonary toilet is instituted, assisted by adequate doses of narcotics to prevent chest wall splinting. Surgical drains and chest tubes (necessary in less than 10% of cases) are typically removed at 48 to 72 hours. The patient is mobilized 3 days postoperatively in a custom bivalved jacket; however, the brace is optional as the body, dorsal elements, and one pedicle are left intact.

RESULTS AND COMPLICATIONS

In the authors' surgical series at the Medical College of Wisconsin, 41 patients with thoracic disc herniations and/or osteophytes underwent the lateral extracavitary approach to the thoracic spine from 1973 to 1994.[9] Each patient received CT, myelography, and/or MRI scanning preoperatively, and most patients underwent spinal angiography to determine the presence of a radiculomedullary artery in the area of the proposed operation. A ventral interbody fusion utilizing the resected rib as the graft was performed in most cases. Average length of stay has dropped from 11 to 5 days. Postoperatively, most patients were treated in bivalved jackets for 8 to 10 weeks, except when recumbent.

Presenting complaints and neurological status are summarized in Table 21-1 and the accompanying box. Most cases presented with local pain in combination with weakness and sensory loss. Approximately one half of the patients reported a radicular pain component as well. Each case was graded according to the degree of myelopathy immediately before (box and Fig. 21-3) and 3 months after the operation (Table 21-2 and box). The majority of the patients in this series were myelopathic and most improved significantly with surgery. For instance, 12 of the 13 patients with moderate myelopathy and 10 of 18 patients with severe to complete myelopathy showed substantial recovery of neurological function. Fourteen patients who could not walk before operation could do so after surgery and rehabilitation.

Local pain disappeared or regressed in all but two of the 41 patients. Anesthesia dolorosa developed at the level of the thoracic rhizotomy in one case in which the intercostal nerve had been divided distal to the dorsal root ganglion. At reoperation, the ganglion was completely resected and the pain was abated.

In four patients, intraoperative pleural tears required postoperative closed drainage for a period of

Table 21-1. Presenting Complaints

Complaint	% of Patients
Weakness	85
Sensory loss	85
Local pain	83
Bowel/bladder loss	46
Radicular pain	54

SEVERITY OF MYELOPATHY

Mild

Minimal sensory disturbance
Intact or mild impairment of motor function
Intact bowel/bladder status

Moderate

Prominent sensory level
Ambulation with external support only
Intact bowel/bladder status or mild dysfunction

Severe

Prominent sensory level
Slight movement; nonambulatory
Moderate to severe bowel/bladder dysfunction

Complete

Little or no sensation
No motor function
No bowel/bladder function

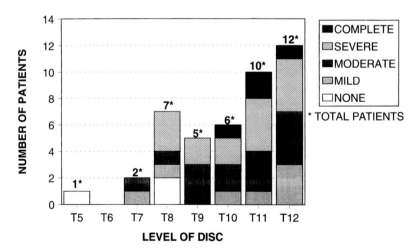

Fig. 21-3. Level of disc herniation and neurological status.

Table 21-2. Results of Operation

Initial Status	No. of Patients With Improvement in Myelopathy			
	None	Slight	Moderate	Marked
No myelopathy; pain only			2	1
Mild myelopathy		2	3	2
Moderate myelopathy		1	6	6
Severe myelopathy	1	1	3	9
Motor complete	3			1

not more than 5 days. Two superficial wounds cleared with antibiotic coverage and local care; urosepsis was treated in one patient with parenteral antibiotics. Other common complications of the procedure included pulmonary atelectasis or hypovolemia secondary to a continued low-volume blood loss. One patient with postoperative atelectasis required temporary reintubation. There were no deaths in this series.

CONCLUSION

The lateral extracavitary approach to the thoracic spine is an effective technique for the removal of herniated thoracic discs and osteophytes. It permits adequate visualization of the dural sac across the spinal canal and allows complete removal of offending lesions without cord manipulation. The morbidity is low, and the complications associated with dorsal procedures or transthoracic methods are avoided.

REFERENCES

1. Arnold PM, Hollowell JP, Bates SR, Mark LP. Role of spinal arteriography in the preoperative management of thoracolumbar pathology. AANS/CNS Joint Section on Disorders of the Spine and Peripheral Nerves. Ft. Lauderdale, Fla.: February 1994.
2. Brown CW, Deffer PA, Akmakjian J, Donaldson DH, Brugman JL. The natural history of thoracic herniation. Spine 17: S97-102, 1992.
3. Carpener N. The evolution of lateral rachatomy. J Bone Joint Surg 36A:173-179, 1954.
4. Flesser RG, Dietze DD, Millan MM, Peace D. Later parascapular extrapleural approach to the upper thoracic spine. J Neurosurg 75:349-355, 1991.
5. Larson SJ, Holst RA, Hemmy DC, Sances A Jr. Lateral extracavitary approach to traumatic lesions of the thoracic and lumbar spine. J Neurosurg 45:628-637, 1976.
6. Maiman DJ, Larson SJ. Lateral extracavitary approach to the thoracic and lumbar spine. In Rengachary SS, Wilkins RH, eds. Neurosurgical Operative Atlas. Baltimore: Williams & Wilkins, 1992, pp 153-161.
7. Maiman DJ, Larson SJ, Luck E, El-Ghatit A. Lateral extracavitary approach to the spine for thoracic disc herniation: Report of 23 cases. Neurosurgery 14:178-182, 1984.
8. Patterson RH, Arbit E. A surgical approach through the pedicle to protruded thoracic discs. J Neurosurg 48:768-772, 1978.
9. Sebring LA, Maiman DJ. Lateral extracavitary approach to the spine for thoracic disc herniation: Report of 41 cases. Abstr: Joint Section on Disorders of the Spine and Peripheral Nerves. February 1995.
10. Stone JL, Lichtor T, Banerjee S. Intradural thoracic disc herniation. Spine 19:1281-1283, 1994.
11. Terry AF, McSweeny T, Jones HWF. Paraplegia as a sequela to dorsal disc prolapse. Paraplegia 19:111-117, 1981.

Transfacet Pedicle-Sparing Approach

Charles B. Stillerman, M.D., Thomas C. Chen, M.D., Ph.D.,
William T. Couldwell, M.D., Ph.D., and Martin H. Weiss, M.D.

Several operative techniques have evolved for the management of herniated thoracic discs. These include the ventrolateral (transthoracic,[2-4,19,20,23-28] thoracoscopic,[5,9,10,14,21,22,29] and retropleural thoracotomy[15]), lateral (lateral extracavitary,[11,13] costotransversectomy,[26-28] and parascapular[6,8]), and dorsolateral (transpedicular[7,12,16-18]) approaches. It has been well documented that all of these procedures may facilitate safe removal of herniated discs, including central osteophytes and intradural fragments.[26-28] Outcomes with respect to improvement of myelopathy and radicular pain have been excellent.

The ventrolateral and lateral procedures are formidable operations, generally requiring more extensive bone removal than the transpedicular approach.[26-28] These operations are usually combined with an interbody fusion. The ventrolateral and lateral approaches have been reported to be associated with superior back pain results, compared to the transpedicular operation.[13,17,24,26,27]

The authors have developed the transfacet pedicle-sparing approach as a simpler alternative to the formidable ventrolateral and lateral procedures.[23-25] This operation enables a safe and effective microdiscectomy through a limited partial facetectomy without removal of the ipsilateral, caudal pedicle. Morphometric analysis and clinical experience has shown that the keyhole bone removal does not sacrifice the exposure achieved using the transpedicular approach, and it may diminish the potential for chronic back pain arising from disruption of the facet, pedicle, and disc.

MORPHOMETRIC INVESTIGATIONS

Prior to proceeding with the clinical investigation, a cadaveric analysis was carried out, using 180 thoracic vertebral segments.[23,25] Fifteen formalin-fixed human adult thoracic spines were used to (1) evaluate the exposure, (2) develop special thoracic microdiscectomy instrumentation, and (3) establish morphometric measurements, which would improve the orientation to the disc space.

The three key measurements that enhanced orientation between the facet joint and the underlying disc are shown in Fig. 22-1. These include the sagittal distance from the inferior articular facet to the disc space (column a). This distance remained constant over varying vertebral body levels, except at T11-12, because of the increased thickness of the facet joints at these levels. The vertical distance from the bottom of the inferior articular process to a point on the facet overlying the center of the disc space increases with descending levels (column b). The width of the disc space remained constant at all levels, until T10-11 (column c).

LEVEL	FACET TO DISC (mm)	INFERIOR ARTICULAR PROCESS TO DISC CENTER (mm)	DISC SPACE WIDTH (mm)
	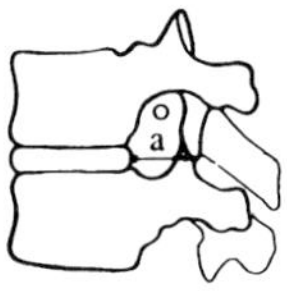	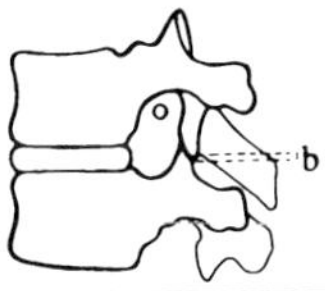	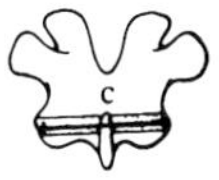
T1-2	15.2 +/- 2.1	0.3 +/- 0.8	31.6 +/- 2.1
T2-3	14.8 +/- 1.9	0.3 +/- 0.7	31.8 +/- 3.4
T3-4	14.6 +/- 1.6	0.8 +/- 1.1	30 +/- 2.4
T4-5	14.5 +/- 1.7	1.2 +/- 1.4*	28.6 +/- 3.8
T5-6	14.7 +/- 1.4	1.6 +/- 1.2*	30.8 +/- 4.8
T6-7	14.8 +/- 0.9	2.0 +/- 1.2*	33.2 +/- 5.6
T7-8	14.8 +/- 0.9	3.5 +/- 1.7*	34.6 +/- 4.6
T8-9	15.1 +/- 0.8	4.5 +/- 1.5*	35.8 +/- 5.8
T9-10	15.2 +/- 1.4	5.3 +/- 1.8*	38.4 +/- 6.0
T10-11	16.3 +/- 1.6	6.5 +/- 1.7*	40.2 +/- 6.8*
T11-12	19.2 +/- 2.6*	7.7 +/- 2.1*	42.2 +/- 7.0*
T12-L1	21.8 +/- 2.8*	10.3 +/- 3.2*	46.2 +/- 6*

Fig. 22-1. Morphometric data. Asterisk indicates significant difference between a certain level compared to the initial level at T1-2 (p <0.05) using Student's T-test. +/− represents standard deviation. **Column a,** The distance from the facet to the disc remained constant over varying vertebral body levels except at T11-12 because of increased thickness of the facet joints at these levels. **Column b,** The vertical distance from the inferior articular process to the point on the facet directly over disc center increased with descending levels. **Column c,** The width of the disc remained constant at all levels until T10-11.[23,25] (Used with permission from Stillerman CB, Chen TC, Day JD, et al. The transfacet pedicle-sparing approach for thoracic disc removal: Cadaveric morphometric analysis and preliminary clinical experience. J Neurosurg 83:971-976, 1995.)

OPERATIVE TECHNIQUE

The patient is placed in the prone position on a radiolucent spinal table. Chest rolls are used. An anteroposterior (AP) fluoroscopic image is used to identify the involved disc space. (Fig. 22-2, *A* and *B*). A 3 to 4 cm incision is centered over the disc space. The muscle on the side of the disc herniation is reflected laterally and a self-retaining retractor is placed. The rostral and caudal transverse processes are exposed. Under microscopic vision, a high-speed drill is used to perform a partial mesial facetectomy (Fig. 22-3, *A*). Intraoperative fluoroscopy guides the extent of the facetectomy. The underlying neural foramen is entered. Soft tissue is coagulated with bipolar cautery. The lateral margin of the annulus fibrosus is identified and exposed (Fig. 22-3, *B*). Incision of the lateral portion of the annulus fibrosus is made with a microknife and the disc is removed (Fig. 22-3, *C*). The Manny-Mark Stillerman Thoracic Microdiscectomy Instruments were developed to facilitate disc removal, in order to avoid injuring the medially situated spinal cord[23,25] (Fig. 22-4). Endoscopy can also be used to monitor disc removal,

as well as to evaluate the extent of the decompression. No fusion is performed.

CLINICAL RESULTS

Initial clinical results have previously been published.[23-25] The transfacet pedicle-sparing approach was initially used with success to remove eight thoracic herniations; segmental levels ranged from T7 through T11. Most of the discs were centrolateral in location. One patient's herniated disc occupied nearly the entire ventral spinal canal (Fig. 22-5). Two of the discs were densely calcified. Two patients underwent multiple level decompressions (Table 22-1).

Table 22-2 depicts the patient demographics. The initial six patients consisted of four men and two women, with ages ranging from 31 years to 63 years. There is a mean age of 46 years. All patients had severe axial pain preoperatively. Three patients had radiculopathy. Four patients were myelopathic. The initial follow-up ranged from 7 to 23 months, with a mean of 12.9 months. Postoperatively, all

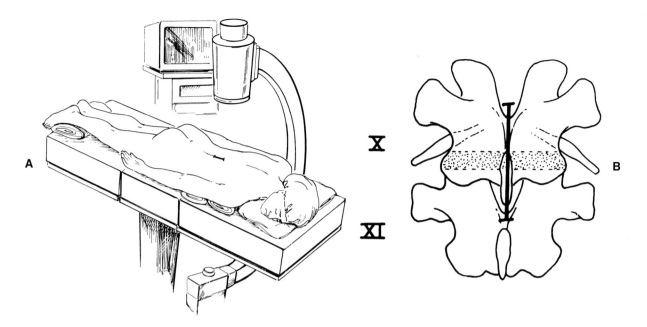

Fig. 22-2. Fluoroscopic guidance is used for localization. **A,** The patient is placed prone on radiolucent chest rolls and secured with tape so that the table may be rolled away from the surgeon to facilitate exposure during the disc removal. **B,** A 3 to 4 cm incision is centered over the appropriate disc space *(shaded region)* using fluoroscopy. Fluoroscopic guidance is desirable to plain radiographs because it can be easily repeated in planning the skin incision, determination of the portion of facet to be removed, and the postdecompression evaluation of the extent of disc removal. (Used with permission from Stillerman CB, Chen TC, Day JD, et al. The transfacet pedicle-sparing approach for thoracic disc removal: Cadaveric morphometric analysis and preliminary clinical experience. J Neurosurg 83:971-976, 1995.)

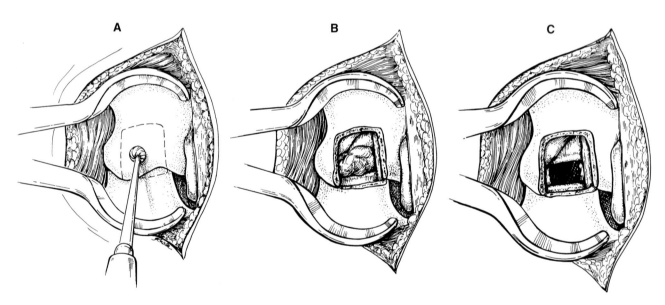

Fig. 22-3. Depiction of the transfacet pedicle-sparing approach. **A,** Under microscopic vision a partial facetectomy is performed with a high-speed drill. Fluoroscopy is used to guide the extent of facetectomy. An attempt to preserve the lateral facet margin is made. **B,** After the partial facetectomy is completed, the dorsal aspect of the neural foramen is entered. Foraminal soft tissue may be coagulated with bipolar cautery. In this case a large herniation can be seen along the lateral aspect of the dura (which is situated medially). Note, in this instance, the rostral nerve root is exposed. **C,** The lateral margin of the annulus fibrosus has been incised and the disc has been removed using specially designed instrumentation. The postdiscectomy appearance is depicted. (Used with permission from Stillerman CB, Chen TC, Day JD, et al. The transfacet pedicle-sparing approach for thoracic disc removal: Cadaveric morphometric analysis and preliminary clinical experience. J Neurosurg 83:971-976, 1995.)

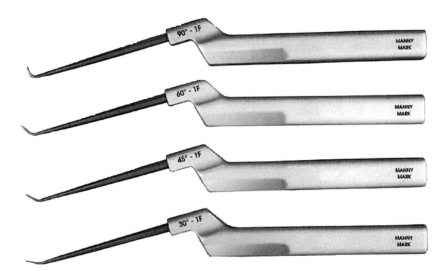

Fig. 22-4. Photograph of the Manny-Mark Stillerman microdiscectomy instruments. These instruments were designed to facilitate safe and thorough disc removal without causing injury to the medially situated spinal cord. (Used with permission from Stillerman CB, Chen TC, Day JD, et al. The transfacet pedicle-sparing approach for thoracic disc removal: Cadaveric morphometric analysis and preliminary clinical experience. J Neurosurg 83:971-976, 1995.)

Table 22-1. Thoracic Disc Characteristics in Six Patients Undergoing Operation for Herniated Discs

Case No.	Consistency	Location	Operated Levels
1	Soft	Centrolateral	T8-9/T9-10
2	Partially calcified	Centrolateral	T10-11
3	Soft	Entire ventral canal	T10-11
4	Calcified	Lateral	T9-10
5	Calcified	Centrolateral	T8-9/T10-11
6	Soft	Centrolateral	T10-11

Used with permission from Stillerman CB, Chen TC, Day JD, et al. The transfacet pedicle-sparing approach for thoracic disc removal: Cadaveric morphometric analysis and preliminary clinical experience. J Neurosurg 83:971-976, 1995.

Table 22-2. Characteristics of Six Patients Undergoing Operation for Herniated Thoracic Discs

Case No.	Age, Sex	Axial Pain		Myelopathy		Radiculopathy		Disc Recurrence
		Preop	Postop	Preop	Postop	Preop	Postop	
1	47, F	Yes	Resolved	Yes	Resolved	Yes	Resolved	None
2	53, M	Yes	Sig improved	No	NA	No	NA	None
3	62, M	Yes	Sig improved	Yes	Resolved	Yes	Resolved	None
4	31, F	Yes	Sig improved	No	NA	Yes	Resolved	None
5	36, M	Yes	Resolved	Yes	Resolved	No	NA	None
6	63, M	Yes	Resolved	Yes	Improved	No	NA	None

sig = significantly; NA = not applicable.
Used with permission from Stillerman CB, Chen TC, Day JD, et al. The transfacet pedicle-sparing approach for thoracic disc removal: Cadaveric morphometric analysis and preliminary clinical experience. J Neurosurg 83:971-976, 1995.

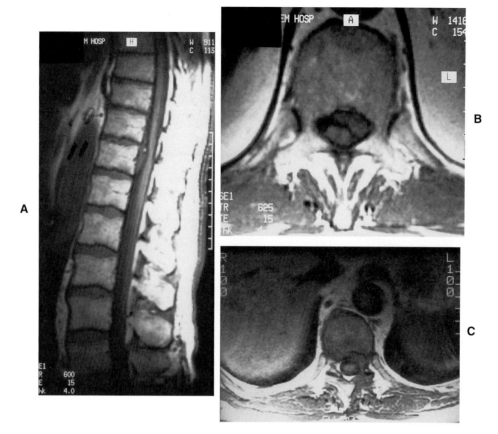

Fig. 22-5. MRI images revealing a large extruded T10-11 disc herniation. **A,** Preoperative T1-weighted sagittal MR image demonstrating a large ventral lesion with dorsal displacement of the spinal cord. **B,** Axial view demonstrating that nearly the entire ventral spinal canal is occupied by the disc fragment. **C,** The transfacet pedicle-sparing approach was used for microdiscectomy. A postoperative axial gadolinium-enhanced MR image was obtained to evaluate the extent of disc removal. There is no intracanalicular disc material present. Note that the spinal cord has returned to its normal position and is no longer being deformed. (Used with permission from Stillerman CB, Chen TC, Day JD, et al. The transfacet pedicle-sparing approach for thoracic disc removal: Cadaveric morphometric analysis and preliminary clinical experience. J Neurosurg 83:971-976, 1995.)

patients had significant improvement or resolution of myelopathy and axial pain. There were no complications.

APPROACH-SPECIFIC SURGICAL INDICATIONS

The ventral (transsternal), ventrolateral (transthoracic thoracotomy, thoracoscopy, and retropleural thoracotomy) and lateral (lateral extracavitary, costotransversectomy, and parascapular) approaches provide excellent exposure to the disc space. These procedures enable total disc removal with good results regarding improving myelopathy, radiculopa-

thy, and localized thoracic back pain. They are, however, all formidable procedures from the standpoint of operative time, perioperative pain, and physiological stress to the patient, compared to the dorsolateral operations.[23-25] The main indication for these more formidable operations is usually in lower medical risk patients, with densely calcified central or centrolateral herniations[24] (Table 22-3).

A less formidable surgery, the transpedicular approach was first described by Patterson and Arbit[18] and has been used with great success for the treatment of myelopathy and radicular pain. It has been pointed out, however, that "outcome in patients with pain alone has not been entirely satisfactory."[17]

Table 22-3. Surgical Approaches for Thoracic Discectomy

Approach	Primary Indications
Transthoracic	T4-11: densely calcified central disc
Lateral extracavitary	T6-12: calcified centrolateral disc
Transfacet pedicle-sparing	All levels: soft central disc; calcified centrolateral disc
Transpedicular	All levels: soft central disc; calcified centrolateral disc

Used with permission from Stillerman CB, Chen TC, Day JD, et al. The transfacet pedicle-sparing approach for thoracic disc removal: Cadaveric morphometric analysis and preliminary clinical experience. J Neurosurg 83:971-976, 1995.

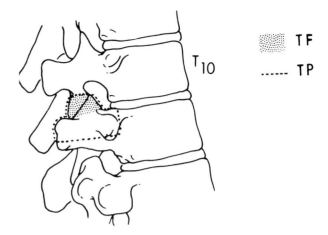

Fig. 22-6. Drawing depicting the degree of bone removal for the transfacet pedicle-sparing approach (TF) vs. the transpedicular approach (TP). In addition to removal of the pedicle, the transpedicular approach entails a more extensive facetectomy than does the transfacet approach. (Used with permission from Stillerman CB, Chen TC, Day JD, et al. The transfacet pedicle-sparing approach for thoracic disc removal: Cadaveric morphometric analysis and preliminary clinical experience. J Neurosurg 83:971-976, 1995.)

Perhaps this relates to the loss of the mechanical integrity from destruction of the facet-pedicle and disc (Fig. 22-6).

To improve localized back pain reported with the transpedicular approach and provide a low-risk surgical option, the authors developed the transfacet pedicle-sparing approach. Like the transpedicular approach, the transfacet pedicle-sparing approach allows disc removal through a dorsolateral trajectory (see Fig. 22-6). Currently, the authors use it for the removal of all soft disc herniations, as well as all densely calcified lateral herniations and selected partially calcified centrolateral discs.[23-25] Pedicle removal is not necessary. Preservation of the pedicle may, in fact, explain why preliminary results have been favorable from the standpoint of postoperative back pain. Of notable importance is the utilization of specially designed microdiscectomy instrumentation and, when necessary, the use of endoscopic visualization of the disc and ventral dura mater during disc removal.

ADVANTAGES AND DISADVANTAGES OF THE TRANSFACET PEDICLE-SPARING APPROACH

The main advantages of the transfacet pedicle-sparing approach include (1) diminished operative time, (2) decreased blood loss, (3) limited bone removal, and (4) limited soft tissue disruption. Perioperative pain reduction, decreased length of hospitalization, and reduction in the time interval to return to work compared with the ventrolateral and lateral op-

erations should be observed. Removal of the rare upper thoracic herniation can be carried out without difficulty, as can multiple disc herniations. The extent of facet removal is limited to only a portion of the facet without the need to remove the caudal pedicle.

The disadvantages of the procedure include (1) the limited skin incision makes it more difficult to perform the microdiscectomy in larger patients, (2) disc removal may be difficult without the use of specially designed instruments, and (3) the extent of decompression after microdiscectomy may be difficult to evaluate. The authors frequently use intraoperative endoscopy for this purpose.

Finally, the authors have not shared the success of others using a posterolateral operation for large, densely calcified centrolateral discs with significant central bulk. Densely calcified discs often have significant dural adherence, making centrolateral disc removal difficult using a dorsolateral approach. It is in these instances that a ventrolateral or lateral approach is selected.[23-25]

Lateral calcified discs and selected centrolateral calcified discs are generally well suited for the transfacet operation, especially in high medical risk patients.[23-25] The parameters used to determine the ease of removal of the calcified centrolateral herniations via this approach include the size of the disc, the density of the calcification, the degree of spinal cord deformity, and the presence of dura mater surrounding the dorsolateral margins of the herniated disc.[23-25]

The authors have not found soft extradural discs, regardless of size, to be difficult to remove by a dorsolateral approach (see Fig. 22-5).

COMPARISON WITH THE LAMINOFORAMINOTOMY APPROACH

There are several important features that distinguish this surgery from Spurling and Scoville's laminoforaminotomy.[25] The transfacet approach relies only on a keyhole facetectomy to expose the thoracic neural foramen, whereas the laminoforaminotomy involves a laminotomy as well as a foraminotomy.

The portion of the facet removed in the transfacet approach is varied, depending upon the position of the underlying disc space and/or disc fragment. This can be determined intraoperatively using fluoroscopy, as well as by relying on the cadaveric morphometric data (see Fig. 22-1) and preoperative imaging studies. In the cervical laminoforaminotomy a lateral laminotomy, mesial facetectomy, and lateral ligamentum flavum removal exposes the proximal and distal nerve root. The location and extent of the facet removal is fairly constant and involves the medial one third to one half of the joint.

The laminoforaminotomy exposes the cervical nerve root, but is too medial to be used in the thoracic spine without additional facet removal. The transfacet pedicle-sparing approach is a more lateral operation, facilitating entry into the lateral disc space and ventral spinal canal. This is a function of increasing vertebral body and disc space widths as the spinal axis is descended.[1]

CONCLUSION

The authors' experience suggests that the transfacet pedicle-sparing approach may become the procedure of choice for the surgical management of all soft symptomatic herniations, lateral calcified, and selected centrolateral calcified thoracic discs. It has been especially valuable when treating the high-risk patient. Patient outcomes thus far have been excellent for the treatment of myelopathy, radiculopathy, and back pain.

REFERENCES

1. Benzel, EC. Biomechanics of Spinal Stabilization: Principles and Clinical Practice. New York: McGraw-Hill, 1995, p 4.
2. Bohlman HH, Zdeblick TA. Anterior excision of herniated thoracic discs. J Bone Joint Surg 70A:1038-1047, 1988.
3. Borges LF. Thoracic disc disease and spondylosis. In Tindall GT, Cooper PR, Barrow DL, eds. The Practice of Neurosurgery. Baltimore: Williams & Wilkins, 1996, pp 2461-2471.
4. Currier BL, Eismont FJ, Green BA. Transthoracic disk excision and fusion for herniated thoracic discs. Spine 19:323-328, 1994.
5. Dickman CA, Rosenthal D, Karahalios DG, et al. Thoracic vertebrectomy and reconstruction using a microsurgical thoracoscopic approach. Neurosurgery 38:201-219, 1996.
6. Dietze DD Jr, Fessler RG. Thoracic disc herniations. Neurosurg Clin N Am 4:75-90, 1993.
7. Epstein JA. Thoracic disc herniation: Operative approaches and results. Comment. Neurosurgery 12:305, 1983.
8. Fessler RG, Dietze DD Jr, MacMillan M, et al. Lateral parascapular extrapleural approach to the upper thoracic spine. J Neurosurg 75:349-355, 1991.
9. Horwitz MB, Moossy JJ, Julian T, et al. Thoracic discectomy using video assisted thoracoscopy. Spine 9:1082-1086, 1994.
10. Krasna MJ, Mack MJ. Atlas of Thoracoscopic Surgery. St. Louis: Quality Medical Publishing, 1994, pp 206-211.
11. Larson SJ, Holst RA Hemmy DC, et al. Lateral extracavitary approach to traumatic lesions of the thoracic and lumbar spine. J Neurosurg 45:628-637, 1976.
12. Le Roux PD, Haglund MM, Harris AB. Thoracic disc disease: Experience with the transpedicular approach in twenty consecutive patients. Neurosurgery 33:58-66, 1993.
13. Maiman DJ, Larson SJ, Luck E, et al. Lateral extracavitary approach to the spine for thoracic disc herniation: Report of 23 cases. Neurosurgery 14:178-182, 1984.
14. McAfee PC, Regan JR, Zdeblick, TA, et al. The incidence of complications in endoscopic anterior thoracolumbar spinal reconstructive surgery. Spine 20:1624-1632, 1995.
15. McCormick PC. Retropleural approach to the thoracic and thoracolumbar spine. Neurosurgery 37:1-7, 1995.
16. Patterson RH. Thoracic disc herniation: Operative approaches and results. Comment. Neurosurgery 12:305, 1983.
17. Patterson RH. Thoracic disc disease: Experience with the transpedicular approach in twenty consecutive patients. Comment. Neurosurgery 33:66, 1993.
18. Patterson RH Jr, Arbit E. A surgical approach through the pedicle to protruded thoracic discs. J Neurosurg 48:768-772, 1978.
19. Perot PL, Munro DD. Transthoracic removal of midline thoracic disc protrusions causing spinal cord compression. J Neurosurg 31:452-458, 1969.
20. Ransohoff J, Spencer F, Siew F, et al. Transthoracic removal of thoracic disc. Report of three cases. J Neurosurg 31:459-461, 1969.
21. Regan JJ, Mack MJ, Picetti GD. A technical report on video-assisted thoracoscopy spinal surgery. Spine 20:831-837, 1995.

22. Rosenthal D, Rosenthal R, De Simone A. Removal of a protruded thoracic disc using microsurgical endoscopy. A new technique. Spine 19:1087-1091, 1994.

23. Stillerman CB, Chen TC, Day JD, et al. The transfacet pedicle-sparing approach for thoracic disc removal: Cadaveric morphometric analysis and preliminary clinical experience. J Neurosurg 83:971-976, 1995.

24. Stillerman CB, Chen TC, Couldwell WT, et al. Experience in the surgical management of 82 symptomatic herniated thoracic discs and review of the literature. J Neurosurg 88:623-633, 1998.

25. Stillerman CB, Couldwell WT, Chen TC, et al. Thoracic disc (invited response). Neurosurgical forum. J Neurosurg 85:187-190, 1996.

26. Stillerman CB, Weiss MH. Principles of surgical approaches to the thoracic spine. In Tarlov EC, ed. Neurosurgical Topics: Neurosurgical Treatment of Disorders of the Thoracic Spine. Park Ridge, Ill.: AANS, 1991, pp 1-19.

27. Stillerman CB, Weiss MH. Management of thoracic disc disease. Clin Neurosurg 38:325-352, 1992.

28. Stillerman CB, Weiss MH. Surgical management of thoracic disc herniation and spondylosis. In Menezes AH, Sonntag VKH, eds. Principles of Spinal Surgery. New York: McGraw-Hill, 1996, pp 581-601.

29. Theodore N, Dickman CA. Current management of thoracic disc herniation. Contemp Neurosurg 18:1-6, 1997.

Vascular Malformations and Tumors

Intramedullary and Dural Vascular Malformations

Donald W. Larsen, M.D., George P. Teitelbaum, M.D.,
Steven L. Giannotta, M.D., and John A. Anson, M.D.

Vascular malformations of the spine can be subdivided into several categories based on their anatomical location and angioarchitecture. The anatomical location, configuration, arterial supply, and venous drainage pattern determine the pathophysiology, natural history, appropriate treatment option, and therapeutic results. They may present with a wide variety of signs and symptoms that may be manifested distant to the site of vascular pathology. Recent advances in imaging, endovascular, and neurosurgical techniques have greatly improved the diagnosis and treatment of these complicated lesions.

CLASSIFICATION

Spinal vascular malformations have been previously classified according to their relation to the vertebral body, dura, pia, and spinal cord.[1,2,8,20,27,34,41] The earliest investigators recognized two types of vascular malformations: a venous type consisting of abnormally enlarged perimedullary veins, usually dorsal to the lower thoracic spinal cord, without high-flow arteriovenous (AV) shunting, and an arteriovenous type consisting of an intramedullary nidus of abnormal vessels with high-flow AV shunting and engorged draining veins.[41] The venous type originally described probably corresponds to what is now known as a spinal dural arteriovenous fistula (SDAVF) and the arteriovenous type to what is now known as a true intramedullary arteriovenous malformation (AVM).

Spinal vascular malformations with arteriovenous shunting can be further classified as arteriovenous fistulas (AVFs) or true arteriovenous malformations (AVMs). Anatomically, AVFs are recognized as a direct connection between an artery and a vein, without an intervening nidus of abnormal vessels. The AV shunting may be rapid, as with perimedullary AVFs, or relatively slow, as with SDAVFs. True AVMs demonstrate high-flow AV shunting across a tangle of abnormal vessels in a nidus between the artery and vein. The pathological distinction between these lesions is important to delineate angiographically because the natural history, pathophysiology, and treatment among these lesions differs.

VASCULAR ANATOMY

The arterial supply to the spinal cord is via three distinct arterial axes: one anterior spinal artery and two posterior spinal arteries. The anterior spinal artery is located in the anterior median sulcus, and the posterior spinal arteries are on the dorsolateral surface of the spinal cord, dorsal to the dorsal nerve root on each side. These arteries are supplied by the

349

anterior or posterior radiculomedullary arteries that accompany their corresponding nerve roots to join the spinal cord. The radiculomedullary arteries are located irregularly along the spinal cord. In the cervical region, they may arise from branches of the subclavian arteries (ascending and deep cervical branches of the thyrocervical trunk and costocervical trunks, respectively) and the vertebral arteries. The vertebral artery gives rise to a small anterior spinal artery proximal to the vertebrobasilar junction. This branch descends in front of the medulla and unites with a similar vessel on the opposite side to become one anterior spinal artery in the high cervical spinal region. It is not uncommon to observe duplication of the anterior spinal branches in the cervical area. A fairly constant radicular artery arises from the vertebral or ascending cervical artery at the C5 or C6 level and is termed the "artery of the cervical enlargement." In the thoracic and thoracolumbar regions, the radiculomedullary arteries arise from dorsospinal branches of intercostal and lumbar arteries. One of these contributors is larger than the others and is termed "arterial radicularis magna" or the "artery of Adamkiewicz." It commonly arises from the lower intercostal or lumbar artery on the left side and is responsible for the supply of most of the thoracic spinal cord and conus medullaris. Angiographically or in the anteroposterior (AP) projection, the anterior spinal artery can be recognized by its characteristic "hairpin" appearance with ascending and descending midline branches. Each posterior spinal artery arises dorsolaterally from radicular branches and has a similar, but usually smaller, hairpin appearance to the anterior spinal artery, positioned laterally instead of at the midline.

The anterior spinal artery supplies the ventral two thirds of the spinal cord, whereas the two posterior spinal arteries supply the dorsal third. The anterior and posterior spinal arteries anastomose through a pial perispinal network.

The spinal cord is drained by radical veins that reach the pial surface to form the coronal venous plexus and longitudinal spinal veins. Venous blood passes from the subarachnoid space via medullary veins that penetrate the dura mater adjacent to the penetrating nerve roots to join the systemic venous drainage of the paraspinal venous system.

INTRAMEDULLARY ARTERIOVENOUS MALFORMATIONS

Intramedullary AVMs usually present in childhood or adolescence with spinal subarachnoid hemorrhage or an acute medullary syndrome.[8,22,35] These patients usually have a poor prognosis if untreated, resulting in intermittent, progressive deterioration of spinal cord function with multiple hemorrhages. The nidus of these malformations is located partially or totally within the spinal cord parenchyma and is supplied by enlarged anterior and posterolateral spinal arteries and drains into medullary veins. Nearly half of these patients have an associated aneurysm of either the feeding arteries or the draining veins.[35] When hemorrhage involves the spinal cord substance, it can produce an abrupt neurological decline and even complete functional spinal cord transection. Less commonly, a ruptured arterial or venous aneurysm can produce subarachnoid hemorrhage without intraparenchymal hemorrhage. Fig. 23-1 shows magnetic resonance imaging (MRI) scans and selective angiograms that demonstrate an intramedullary AVM presenting with subarachnoid hemorrhage in an 18-year-old male. The onset of localized back or neck pain helps to clinically differentiate these hemorrhages from those caused by rupture of an intracranial aneurysm.

Patients suffering repeated episodes of hemorrhage usually have a less favorable prognosis.[1,2] Intramedullary AVMs may be further classified based on nidus morphology. If the nidus of the AVM is compact within the spinal cord parenchyma, it is generally referred to as a glomus type; if the nidus is diffusely infiltrating within the spinal cord parenchyma, it is referred to as a juvenile type.[35]

Radiographic Evaluation

Plain radiographic studies are generally unremarkable unless a large arteriovenous fistula has caused bone erosion.

MRI is an excellent screening modality for intramedullary AVMs because the nidus usually is associated with a signal void (decreased signal) on T1- and T2-weighted images within the spinal cord parenchyma.[6] In addition, T2-weighted spinal echo images may identify the feeding arteries and drain-

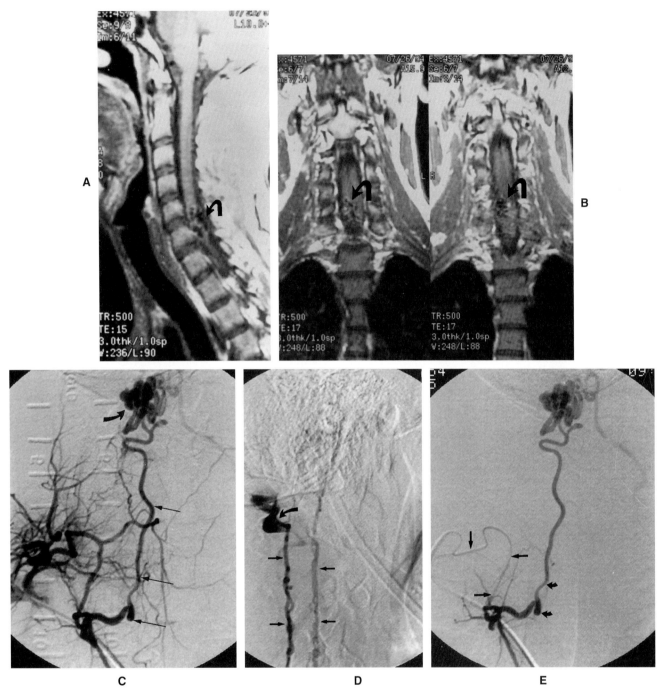

Fig. 23-1. An 18-year-old male presented with neck pain and spinal subarachnoid hemorrhage. T1-weighted MR scans of the cervical spine. Sagittal (**A**) and coronal (**B**) scans demonstrate intramedullary areas of absent signal consistent with flow voids of an intramedullary AVM *(curved arrows)* at C5 to C6. Spinal angiogram, AP view, right costocervical trunk injection (**C**), demonstrates ascending posterolateral artery *(straight arrows)* supplying the AVM nidus *(curved arrow)*. **D,** Late venous phase of spinal angiogram, lateral view, right costocervical trunk injection (**D**), demonstrates enlarged anterior and posterior draining perimedullary veins *(straight arrows)* with venous aneurysm (varix) *(curved arrow)* responsible for subarachnoid hemorrhage. Subselective spinal angiogram, AP view (**E**), subselective injection through microcatheter *(straight arrows)* in deep cervical branch of costocervical trunk providing radicular artery supply *(curved arrows)* to the AVM nidus. Polyvinyl alcohol (PVA) embolization performed through microcatheter in this location. *Continued.*

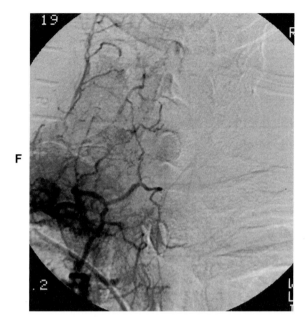

Fig. 23-1, cont'd. Late arterial phase of spinal angiogram, AP view, right costocervical trunk injection, postembolization, (**F**), demonstrates occlusion of AVM.

ing medullary veins as dark serpentine structures outlined by bright cerebrospinal fluid (CSF). Intraparenchymal hemorrhage, myelomalicia, spinal cord atrophy, and edema are more clearly discerned with MRI than with any other modality. Chronic hemorrhage, characterized by a rim of decreased signal produced by hemosiderin-laden macrophages, can best be visualized with gradient refocusing techniques and heavily T2-weighted images. Recent advances in MRI techniques, such as high-resolution fast spin-echo images, cardiac gating, and motion compensation, have markedly improved conspicuity of these lesions.

Computed tomography (CT), performed with intravenous iodinated contrast media, may demonstrate enhancement within the spinal cord at the level of the malformation. However, screening of the entire spine with CT is cumbersome, time-consuming, and exposes the patient to excessive ionizing radiation. CT, after administration of intrathecal contrast, may show abnormal spinal cord enlargement, atrophy, enlarged arteries, and draining veins. There is a report of spinal myoclonus and clinical deterioration after the intravenous administration of contrast material in a patient with a spinal cord AVM, presumably caused by a leakage of contrast into the surrounding spinal cord parenchyma through a defective spinal cord–blood

barrier.[4] CT is inferior to MRI as a screening modality in terms of both sensitivity and specificity of spinal vascular lesions.

Myelography has been used in the past to evaluate spinal cord AVMs and commonly shows focal spinal cord enlargement, enlarged feeding arteries, and dilated draining medullary veins. Like CT with intrathecal contrast, myelography may not identify intraparenchymal lesions that do not result in an abnormal spinal cord contour.

Although MRI is now the screening method of choice for spinal chord AVMs selective spinal angiography remains essential for complete evaluation.[9] Intra-arterial digital subtraction angiography has been shown to be an effective modality for the evaluation of spinal cord AVMs.[11,26,43] Occasionally, small focal spot, cut film subtraction angiography may be necessary for improved spatial resolution. To fully evaluate the entire extent of the malformation, it is important to use selective injections involving multiple spinal arteries. Oblique and lateral projections are useful to establish the relation of the vascular supply to the spinal cord and to differentiate intramedullary AVMs from other spinal vascular lesions. Rapid filming is imperative to identify feeding arterial aneurysms and draining venous aneurysms.[7] Arteriography demonstrates the AVM, usually with feeding arteries of increased diameter and tortuosity, arising from the anterior spinal artery and only rarely from the posterior spinal arteries. AVMs in the cervical spinal cord may be supplied by branches of the vertebral arteries, costocervical and thyrocervical trunks, supreme intercostal and upper thoracic intercostal arteries. Venous drainage occurs through dilated medullary veins, to radicular veins, and occasionally to the epidural plexus. Occasionally, it is difficult to distinguish hemangioblastoma from intramedullary AVM.

Treatment

Treatment of these lesions depends on their location within the spinal cord and their angiographic morphology, but generally falls into three categories: (1) surgical excision of the malformation, (2) endovascular embolization, and (3) combined therapies. The desired goal of surgical therapy is complete excision of the malformation. However, the location and extent of the lesion within the spinal cord parenchyma occasionally makes this goal unattainable.[42] Advances in microsurgical techniques have greatly facilitated the excision of these malformations. In addition, intraoperative ultrasonography to localize the nidus,[15] as well as spinal cord–evoked potentials, have been useful adjuncts during neurosurgical procedures.[33]

If the feeding arteries to the AVM are of sufficient caliber, superselective catheterization and subsequent transcatheter endovascular embolization may be performed, either as an adjunct to surgical excision[22] or as the sole treatment.[10,19,25,40] Because the supply to the malformation generally arises from spinal arteries, it is imperative that the embolic agent passes through the anterior and posterior spinal cord supply and lodges within the malformation itself without occluding medullary perforators or important draining veins. Embolization may be performed with particulate emboli, especially PVA of known particle size.[5,24] In humans, the normal anterior spinal artery diameter is in the range of 110 to 340 microns and the diameter of the normal central spinal artery varies between 60 to 72 microns.[39] Therefore calibrated PVA sponge particles, with diameters of 150 to 250 microns should pass through a normal anterior spinal artery without lodging in the central spinal arteries. In most cases the feeding anterior spinal posterior spinal arteries have hypertrophied in size to supply the AVM, allowing the use of larger particles (500 to 700 microns) that can more safely be flow-directed into the nidus if necessary. Particle embolization with PVA has the disadvantage of long-term recanalization. This may necessitate repeat embolization if endovascular treatment is the sole therapy, but would not be necessary if surgical excision is planned after embolization. Particle embolization of cervical and thoracic AVMs provides immediate clinical improvement in the majority of cases. This improvement may continue if repetitive embolization is performed. Repetitive embolizations every 6 months to a year may be necessary to maintain clinical improvement. Embolization with liquid acrylic agents, such as N-butyl cyanoacrylate (NBCA) has the advantage of achieving more permanent occlusion and is less likely to recanalize. However, it is associated with a higher risk of spinal cord infarction, especially when the anterior spinal artery is involved.

Surgical treatment of vascular malformations should be considered when endovascular therapy cannot be safely performed or when endovascular therapy is not effective in completely obliterating the lesion. Surgical techniques include ligation and/or excision of extradural fistula components and subtotal or total resection of perimedullary or intramedullary nidi. Coordination between the treating surgeon and the endovascular practitioner is of paramount importance in determining the roles. Only in those centers where both work as a coordinated team (or are one and the same) will successful and safe treatment of these complex lesions be accomplished. Specific surgical techniques are discussed in relation to each individual diagnosis. In rare instances, the microcatheter can be navigated to the malformation nidus or an associated arterial aneurysm, and platinum coils or particles deposited. The majority of these procedures may be performed in an awake patient under local anesthesia to allow continuous monitoring of neurological status. Provocative testing with sodium amobarbital (Amytal) or lidocaine can be performed to assess the functional territory to be embolized. Evoked potentials may also be obtained at this time in patients under general anesthesia.

PERIMEDULLARY ARTERIOVENOUS FISTULAS

Perimedullary AVFs are a recently recognized entity in which there are direct fistulas located on the surface of the spinal cord (see accompanying box). They are supplied by the anterior or posterior spinal arteries. The majority occur in the region of the conus medullaris. Like intramedullary AVMs, perimedullary AVFs are presumed to be congenital lesions and present with neurological dysfunction, such as progressive paraparesis secondary to venous hypertension. Less commonly, they can present with hemorrhage secondary to rupture of a feeding artery aneurysm.

Radiographic Evaluation

Visualization of small fistulas on MRI can be difficult due to artifacts of CSF pulsation that may obscure the lesion (seen as flow voids) on the surface of the cord. Cardiac gating and thin sections are essential. Intramedullary increased signal on T2-weighted images may be evident due to venous hypertension, but is nonspecific and may be misleading (Fig. 23-2, *A*). Myelography usually demonstrates dilated feeding arteries and engorged medullary veins. Selective spinal arteriography (Fig. 23-2, *B* and *C*) is essential to confirm the diagnosis and to demonstrate the

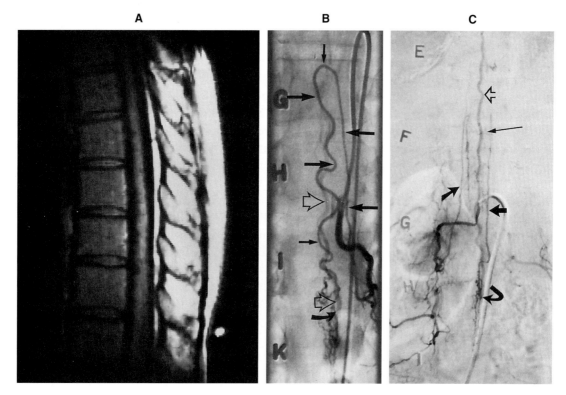

Fig. 23-2. A 31-year-old female presented with progressive lower extremity weakness. **A,** Sagittal T1-weighted MRI of the thoracic spine demonstrates perimedullary "scalloped" areas suggesting vascular flow voids. **B,** Spinal angiogram, AP projection, left T12 intercostal injection, demonstrates filling of the artery of Adamkiewicz and anterior spinal artery *(straight arrows)* with characteristic "hairpin" turn. The anterior spinal artery fills a high-flow perimedullary fistula at the L1 level *(curved arrow)* with ascending draining perimedullary veins *(open arrows)*. **C,** Spinal angiogram, AP view, right T12 intercostal injection, demonstrates filling of right posterolateral spinal artery *(oblique arrow)* and left posterolateral spinal artery (short straight arrow) via a pial collateral network *(long straight arrow)*. Recruited branches of left posterolateral spinal artery also supply the fistula *(curved arrow)*. Ascending perimedullary vein *(open arrow)*. The fistula was cured by surgical resection.

PERIMEDULLARY ARTERIOVENOUS FISTULA CLASSIFICATION[29]

Type I

Small or minimally dilated artery
Point of AVF is where the vessel changes caliber
Little dilated ascending venous drainage (dorsocervical)

Type II

Tortuous dilated artery
Point of AVF is marked by vascular ectasia
Extensive ascending dilated venous drainage
Rapid AV shunting

Type III

Multiple markedly dilated feeding arteries
Difficult to identify point of the AVF
Giant draining vein
Rapid AV shunting

exact morphology, location, and arterial supply to a perimedullary AVF, as well as to differentiate it from the other vascular malformations.

Treatment

Treatment may consist of surgical clipping of the fistula site or embolization with coils, balloons, or liquid adhesive agents. These fistulas are subdivided into three types, depending on the number and size of the feeding arteries and the degree of shunting. The degree of neurological impairment, however, does not often parallel the size of the fistula.[17] Surgery appears to be the best therapy for type I lesions that have small arterial feeders and are therefore not suitable for superselective catheterization. Type II fistulas have larger arterial feeders and more prominent arteriovenous shunting. They are more suitable for endovascular therapy. Type III lesions are giant fistulas in which the arterial feeders are very large and allow placement of detachable balloons or coils. Surgical therapy in this case usually takes the form of clip ligation of the fistula itself. In some cases, the fistula size is too large to be occluded by detachable balloons or coils. Following partial embolization therapy, the fistula itself is exposed surgically and is ligated, usually with aneurysm clips. In those large lesions where a certain amount of mass effect is contributing to symptoms, partial excision of the tangles has allowed for decompression of nerve roots or the spinal cord itself. Intraoperative angiography may be extremely helpful in cases in which it is unclear whether or not the entire fistula is obliterated. In most circumstances however, a dramatic decrease in turgidity of the lesion, as well as changes in color of the draining veins (from red to bluc), signifies satisfactory obliteration.

SPINAL-DURAL ARTERIOVENOUS FISTULAS

These recently recognized entities are mainly found in older adults (mean age, 51 years) and are thought to be acquired lesions.[35] They are found in males 85% of the time and can present with a slowly progressive myelopathy or radiculopathy.[30] If they are untreated, patients can progress to complete paraplegia or quadriparesis. For many years these lesions were classified incorrectly as retromedullary AVMs, but with the availability of superselective angiography, the abnormal arteriovenous connection has been localized to the dura mater itself (Table 23-1 and Fig. 23-3). Generally, the feeding artery is normal in caliber and flow through these lesions is exceptionally slow. The venous drainage is to a dilated radicular vein that drains retrograde into medullary veins and the coronal venous plexus surrounding the spinal cord. The pathophysiology results from spinal cord ischemia secondary to chronic venous hypertension, which results in chronic medullary ischemia. If recognized and treated, clinical symptoms

Table 23-1. Summary of Spinal Dural Arteriovenous Fistula Types

Category	Supply	Location of Nidus	Drainage	Presentation	Clinical Course
Type I	Meningeal branches of radicular artery	Nerve root sleeve	Directly into meningeal vein with arterialized and dilated dural venous plexus (venous drainage of spinal cord is not affected)	Radiculopathy	Often benign, high rate of spontaneous remission
Type II	Meningeal branches of radicular artery	Nerve root sleeve	Directly into meningeal vein with retrograde flow into subarachnoid veins	Radiculopathy and neurological deficit	Progressive neurological deficit
Type III	Meningeal branches of radicular artery	Nerve root sleeve	Dorsal spinous venous plexus through subarachnoid anastomotic vein (arterialized)	Myelopathy, neurological deficit, and subarachnoid hemorrhage	Progressive neurological deficit

From Borden JA, Wu JK, Shucart WA. A proposed classification for spinal and cranial dural arteriovenous fistulous malformations and implications for treatment. J Neurosurg 82:166-179, 1995.

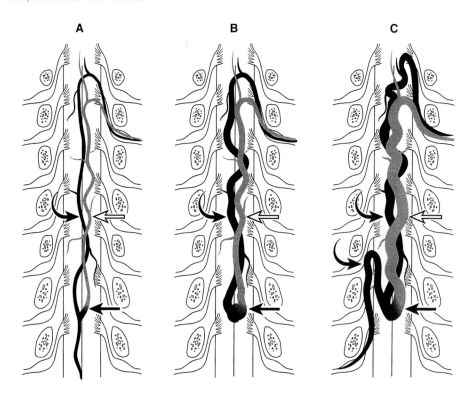

Fig. 23-3. Perimedullary arteriovenous fistula classifications.[29] Fistula site denoted by solid arrows. Feeding arteries and draining veins shown by curved and open arrows, respectively. **A,** Type I. **B,** Type II. **C,** Type III (see box on p. 354 for description).

can often improve dramatically. The chance of improvement after closure of the fistula is inversely related to the length of duration of the fistula. An abrupt clinical decline is often associated with venous infarction and has a much poorer prognosis. Rapid and severe neurological decline may also be a result of the spontaneous thrombosis in the draining veins.

Radiographic Evaluation

Although early reports suggest that MRI can be useful for the diagnosis of these fistulas,[28] these small connections can be easily missed, even with excellent quality, thin-section, cardiac gated MRI. Flow in dilated medullary veins can occasionally be seen as serpentine signal voids along the dorsal aspect of the spinal cord. The spinal cord itself may be mildly enlarged, with focal or diffuse enhancement following the administration of gadolinium contrast media, which presumably reflects venous ischemia (Fig. 23-4, *A*). A sensitive MRI finding is diffusely increased spinal cord signal on T2-weighted images, probably due to edema or ischemia secondary to venous hypertension (Fig. 23-4, *B*). Rare cases of con-

firmed spinal radicular artery dural fistulas have been entirely missed with excellent quality MRI. Therefore MRI should not be used as a screening modality for this disease, but may be useful in evaluating secondary changes, such as venous infarction, that may indicate a poor prognosis.

The screening method of choice for this disease is water-soluble contrast myelography of the entire spine, performed in both supine and prone positions. The preferential venous drainage is to the retromedullary veins, which can be imaged to best advantage in the supine position (Fig. 23-4, *C*). Myelography usually demonstrates dilated and tortuous medullary veins on the dorsum of the spinal cord. Occasionally, arterial pulsations may be observed under fluoroscopy. The spinal cord may be of normal caliber, increased caliber due to spinal cord edema, or decreased caliber due to chronic ischemic changes. If dilated medullary veins are observed on myelography, complete spinal angiography must be performed (Fig. 23-4, *D*). Angiography must be of excellent quality with filming continued into the late venous phase, because opacification of the shunts can be delayed up to several seconds after the injection. Occasionally, the AVF may be supplied by

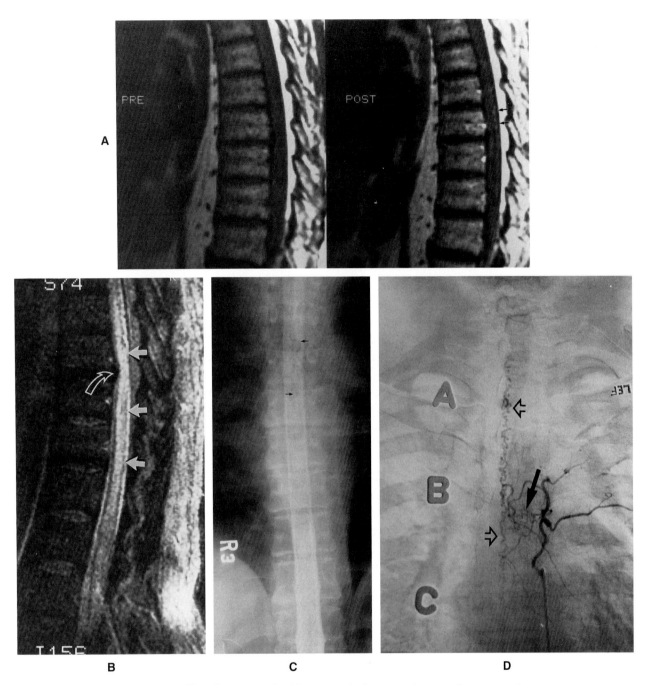

Fig. 23-4. A 62-year-old male presented with progressively worsening spastic paraparesis over a period of several years. **A,** Sagittal T1-weighted MRI of the thoracic spine. Post-gadolinium enhancement image *(right)* reveals dorsal medullary enhancement *(arrows)* probably representing dilated medullary veins. **B,** T2-weighted sagittal MRI reveals diffuse central band of abnormal high signal *(arrows)* and an inconsequential thoracic disc *(open arrow)*. **C,** Supine thoracic myelogram demonstrates serpentine filling defects representing enlarged perimedullary veins *(arrows)*. **D,** Spinal angiogram, AP view, left T5 intercostal injection, reveals filling of a SDAVF at the T5 level *(straight arrow)* with tortuous ascending and descending perimedullary veins *(open arrows)*. Subselective catheterization with a microcatheter was achieved and curative occlusion of the fistula with liquid adhesive (NBCA) was performed.

dural branches fed from more than one level. It is important to examine adjacent levels after finding the primary fistula site on angiography. Such fistulas may occasionally arise from an internal iliac arterial branch.[23] The location of the shunt is usually on the dura mater, but rarely can be on the ventral surface of the spinal cord. Rarely, spontaneous closure of the fistula may occur. Spontaneous thrombosis of the draining veins can occur (Foix-Alajouanine syndrome), which can result in a marked deterioration in neurological function. As a result of the insidiousness of the presenting symptoms of pain, radiculopathy, or myelopathy, it is not unusual for this disease to be misdiagnosed as ascending myelitis, transverse myelitis, or spondylosis.

Treatment

This disease can be effectively treated by both endovascular and surgical strategies. In the lumbar and thoracic regions, the majority of patients have supply to the fistula arising from intercostal or lumbar arteries that do not supply the spinal cord. These frequently can be cured with embolization alone using either liquid adhesive or particles. Because recanalization of SDAVFs treated with PVA has been observed, it is therefore preferable to use liquid adhesive if the anatomy is favorable.[32] A risk of liquid adhesive embolization is excessively distal occlusion on the venous side, which can exacerbate venous hypertension.

Surgical treatment is reserved for those cases where endovascular treatment fails to completely occlude the fistula. In most of these cases, the abnormal communication resides extradurally along the course of the nerve root. Surgical strategy here is to obliterate the fistula and observe the change in turgor and color of the draining vein, which is invariably intradural. Thus extradural and intradural exposure of the involved spinal segment is mandatory. In the event that obliteration of the extradural component does not obliterate the fistula, intradural sources of arterial input must be identified and obliterated. Frequently this is not necessary and may be contraindicated to remove the serpiginous series of draining veins on the surface of the spinal cord. As long as these carry venous blood at normal pressure, they may be left in situ.

EPIDURAL ARTERIOVENOUS MALFORMATIONS

These lesions are primarily extradural and may have drainage to either the epidural venous plexus or medullary veins.[12,18,21,22,36] These patients can present with spontaneous cervical epidural hemorrhage,[12] progressive radiculopathy,[36] or subarachnoid hemorrhage.[18] Significant findings may be absent on MRI (Fig. 23-5, *A*), CT, and myelography. Angiography may reveal the arterial supply from vertebral, thyrocervical, or costocervical arteries (Fig. 23-5, *B*). These lesions may be treated by complete closure of the fistula with endovascular embolization.

SPINAL HEMANGIOMAS

These are the most common benign spinal neoplasms, occurring most frequently in thoracic and lumbar vertebral bodies, with a peak incidence in the fourth to sixth decades. They are a relatively common finding at autopsy, occurring in 11% in a large series.[37] Most (60%) are asymptomatic[13] without gender preference. However, symptomatic hemangiomas are more common in females. When hemangiomas are symptomatic, they can present with local back pain, radicular pain, or spinal cord compression. Most acute symptoms occur due to compression fracture, epidural extension, hemorrhage, and sudden mass effect.

Radiographic Evaluation

On plain radiographs, hemangiomas demonstrate a coarse, striated appearance of the vertebral body, which on CT has a characteristic "polka dot" appearance. Most vertebral hemangiomas are incidental findings on MRI[13] and appear as well-delineated hyperintense vertebral body lesions on T1- and T2-weighted images (Fig. 23-6, *A*). They may expand into the arch or dorsal elements and encroach on the spinal cord by extension into the epidural space (Fig. 23-6, *B* and *C*).[14]

Treatment

Those patients presenting with neurological deficits require aggressive treatment.[16] The optimal treatment is still somewhat unclear, but basically cen-

Fig. 23-5. Elderly male presented with neck pain. **A,** Sagittal proton-density *(left)* and T2-weighted *(right)* spin-echo cervical MR images demonstrate enlarged dorsal perimedullary veins serving as drainage pathway for epidural AVF *(arrows)*. **B,** Lateral right vertebral angiogram in same patient demonstrates a dorsal cervical epidural AVF with multiple enlarged arterial feeders from right vertebral artery *(arrows)*.

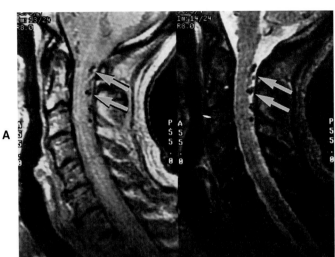

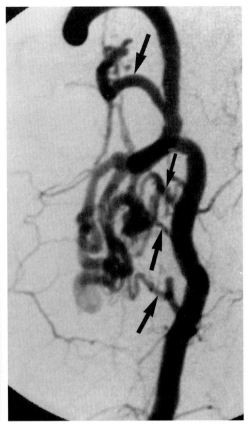

ters on surgery or radiation. The disadvantages of surgery alone are based on earlier reports of high complication rates from excessive blood loss.[38] If the blood loss can be controlled preoperatively, either by embolization therapy or possibly preoperative radiation, then the surgical risks can be greatly decreased. In general, surgery involves removing the expanded vertebral body containing the hemangioma. Once successful dural decompression is accomplished, fusion may be required.

Radiation alone represents a second form of therapy. It is usually reserved for painful lesions without acute spinal cord compression.

Isolated reports of treatment with embolization alone suggest that this markedly reduced the necessity for emergent laminectomy.[37] Others however, have not had similar results.[26,31] This is not entirely unexpected, as symptoms are usually due to mass effect in part caused by bony expansion, which is not likely to shrink acutely after embolization.

CONCLUSION

No single diagnostic imaging modality is ideal for visualization of all types of spinal vascular malformations. MRI is ideal as a screening modality for intramedullary pathology. However, it is not suitable to screen for SDAVFs or epidural AVMs. While myelography is an ideal screening modality for SDAVFs, it can miss epidural AVMs and cavernous malformations. Spinal angiography is essential for complete evaluation of high-flow AVMs, perimedullary AVFs, and SDAVFs.

Advances in microcatheter technology and the use of new embolic materials have improved the endovascular treatment of complicated vascular abnormalities. Certain anatomical locations favor surgical excision, while others can be approached by endovascular techniques. Certain lesions require a combined approach consisting of preoperative embolization followed by surgical resection.

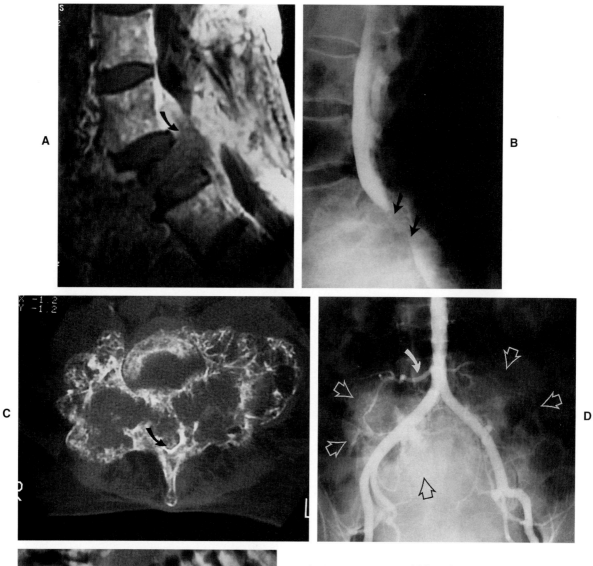

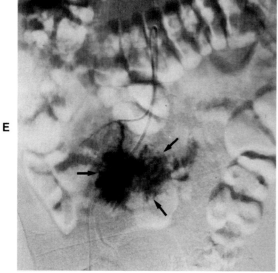

Fig. 23-6. A 56-year-old female presented with progressive paraparesis. **A,** Sagittal T1-weighted MRI of the lumbar spine demonstrates compression fracture of the L5 vertebral body with dorsal extension causing severe compromise of the spinal canal *(arrow).* The normal high signal of fatty marrow has been replaced with low signal. **B,** Lateral lumbar myelogram demonstrates almost complete block of the lumbar subarachnoid space by extradural compression *(arrows).* **C,** Axial CT scan after intrathecal contrast administration demonstrates diffuse expansion of the vertebral body and dorsal elements and severe narrowing of the contrast opacified spinal canal *(arrow)* consistent with an expansile vertebral hemangioma. **D,** AP pelvic arteriogram, late arterial phase, lower abdominal aortic injection, demonstrates diffuse intense contrast stain involving the expanded L5 vertebral body *(open arrows)* and a dilated right L4 dorsospinal artery *(curved arrow).* **E,** Selective L4 injection, AP projection, demonstrates to best advantage the abnormal hypervascularity of the hemangioma *(arrows)* without arteriovenous shunting. This arterial supply was preoperatively embolized with PVA particles prior to surgical decompression with subsequent marked improvement in symptoms.

REFERENCES

1. Aminoff MJ, Logue V. Clinical features of spinal vascular malformations. Brain 97:197-210, 1974.
2. Aminoff MJ, Logue V. The prognosis of patients with spinal vascular malformations. Brain 97:211-218, 1974.
3. Borden JA, Wu JK, Shucart WA. A proposed classification for spinal and cranial dural arteriovenous fistulous malformations and implications for treatment. J Neurosurg 82:166-179, 1995.
4. Casazza M, Bracchi M, Girotti F. Spinal myoclonus and clinical worsening after intravenous contrast medium in a patient with spinal arteriovenous malformations. AJNR 6:965-968, 1985.
5. Castaneda-Zuniga WR, Sanchez R, Amplatz K. Experimental observations on short- and long-term effects of arterial occlusion with Ivalon. Radiology 126:783-785, 1978.
6. DiChiro G, Doppman JL, Dwyer AJ, et al. Tumors and arteriovenous malformations of the spinal cord; Assessment using MR. Radiology 156:689-697, 1985.
7. DiChiro G, Doppman JL, Ommaya AK. Selective arteriography of arteriovenous aneurysms of spinal cord. Radiology 88:1065-1077, 1967.
8. Djindjian A, Djindjian M. Arteriovenous malformations of the spinal cord: Clinical, anatomical and therapeutic consideration—A series of 150 cases. Prog Neurol Surg 9:238-266, 1978.
9. Djindjian R. Angiography of the spinal cord. Surg Neurol 2:179-185, 1974.
10. Doppman JL, DiChiro G, Ommaya AK. Percutaneous embolization of spinal cord arteriovenous malformations. J Neurosurg 34:48-55, 1971.
11. Enzmann DR, Brody WR, Djang WT, et al. Intra-arterial digital subtraction spinal angiography. AJNR 4:25-26, 1983.
12. Foo D, Chang VC, Rossier AB. Spontaneous cervical epidural hemorrhage, anterior cord syndrome, and familial vascular malformation: Case report. Neurology 30:308-311, 1980.
13. Fox MW, Onofrio BM. The natural history and management of symptomatic and asymptomatic vertebral hemangiomas. J Neurosurg 78:36-45, 1993.
14. Golwyn DH, Cardenas CA, Murtagh FR, et al. MRI of a cervical extradural cavernous hemangioma. Neuroradiol 34:68-69, 1992.
15. Gooding GA, Berger MS, Linkowski GD, et al. Transducer frequency considerations in intraoperative US of the spine. Radiology 160:272-273, 1986.
16. Grahm JJ, Yang WC. Vertebral hemangioma with compression fracture and paraparesis treated with preoperative embolization and vertebral resection. Spine 9:97-101, 1984.
17. Halbach VV, Higashida RT, Dowd CF, et al. Treatment of giant intradural (perimedullary) arteriovenous fistulas. Neurosurgery 33:972-980, 1993.
18. Halbach VV, Higashida RT, Hieshima GB. Treatment of vertebral arteriovenous fistulas. AJNR 8:1121-1128, 1987.
19. Horton JA, Latchaw RE, Gold LHA, et al. Embolization of intramedullary arteriovenous malformations of the spinal cord. AJNR 7:113-118, 1986.
20. Houdart R, Rey A, Djindjian M, et al. Arteriovenous malformations of the cord (spinal angiomas). In Carrea P, ed. Neurological Surgery—International Congress Series. Oxford: Excerpta Medica Amsterdam, 1978, p 194.
21. Janda J, Mracek Z. Angioreticuloma of the brain stem. Simultaneous occurrence of an arteriovenous malformation in the epidural space of the cervical spinal cord. Cesk Neurol Neurochir 41:397-399, 1978.
22. Kendall BE, Logue V. Spinal epidural angiomatous malformations draining into intrathecal veins. Neuroradiology 13:181-189, 1977.
23. Larsen DW, Halbach VV, Teitelbaum GP, et al. Spinal dural arteriovenous fistulas supplied by branches of the internal iliac arteries. Surg Neurol 43:35-40, 1995.
24. Latchaw Re, Gold LHA. Polyvinyl foam embolization of vascular and neoplastic lesions of the head, neck, and spine. Radiology 131:669-679, 1979.
25. Latchaw RE, Harris RD, Chou SN, et al. Combined embolization and operation in the treatment of cervical arteriovenous malformations. Neurosurgery 6:131-137, 1980.
26. Levy JM, Hessel SJ, Christensen FK, et al. Digital subtraction arteriography for spinal arteriovenous malformations. AJNR 4:1217-1218, 1983.
27. Malis LI. Arteriovenous malformations of the spinal cord. In Younmans JR, ed. Neurological Surgery, vol 3, 2nd ed. Philadelphia: WB Saunders, 1982, pp 1850-1874.
28. Masaryk TJ, Ross JS, Modic MT, et al. Radiculomedullary vascular malformation of the spine: MR imaging. Radiology 164:845-849, 1987.
29. Merland JJ, Reizine D, Laurent A, et al. Embolization of spinal cord vascular lesions. In Vinuela F, Halbach VV, Dion JE, eds. Interventional Neuroradiology: Endovascular Therapy of the Central Nervous System. New York: Raven, 1992, pp 153-165.
30. Merland JJ, Riche MC, Chiras J. Intraspinal extramedullary arteriovenous fistulae draining into the medullary veins. J Neuroradiol 7:271-320, 1980.
31. Nguyen JP, Djindjian M, Gaston A, et al. Vertebral hemangiomas presenting with neurologic symptoms. Surg Neurol 27:391-397, 1987.
32. Nichols DA, Rufenacht DA, Jack CR, et al. Embolization of spinal dural arteriovenous fistula with polyvinyl alcohol particles: Experience in 14 patients. AJNR 13:933-940, 1992.
33. Owen MP, Brown RH, Spetzler RF, et al. Excision of intramedullary arteriovenous malformation using intraoperative spinal cord monitoring. Surg Neurol 12:271-276, 1979.
34. Pia HW. Diagnosis and treatment of spinal angiomas. Acta Neurochir (Wien) 28:1-2, 1973.
35. Rosenblum B, Oldfield EH, Doppman JL, et al. Spinal arteriovenous malformation: A comparison of dural arteriovenous fistulas and intradural AVMs in 81 patients. J Neurosurg 67:795-802, 1987.
36. Ross D, Olsen W, Halbach VV, et al. Cervical root compression by a traumatic pseudoaneurysm of the vertebral artery: Case report. Neurosurgery 22:414-417, 1988.
37. Schmorl G. Tumors and tumor metastases. In Bessemann EF, ed. The Human Spine in Health and Disease, 2nd ed. New York: Grune and Stratton, 1971, pp 325-327.
38. Smith TP, Koci T, Mehringer CM, et al. Transarterial embolization of vertebral hemangiomas. JVIR 4:681-685, 1993.
39. Suh TH, Alexander L. Vascular system of the human spinal cord. Arch Neurol Psychol 41:659-677, 1939.
40. Theron J, Cosgrove R, Melanson D, et al. Spinal arteriovenous malformations: Advances in therapeutic embolization. Radiology 158:163-169, 1986.
41. Wyburn-Mason R. The vascular abnormalities and tumors of the spinal cord and its membranes. London: Kimpton, 1943.
42. Yasargil MG, DeLong B, Guarnaschelli JJ. Complete microsurgical excision of cervical extramedullary and intramedullary vascular malformations. Surg Neurol 4:211-224 1975.
43. Yeates A, Drayer B, Heinz ER, et al. Intra-arterial digital subtraction angiography of the spinal cord. Radiology 155:387-390, 1985.

Intramedullary Tumors

Paul C. McCormick, M.D.

Intramedullary tumors of the spinal cord account for about 3% to 4% of central nervous system neoplasms.[11] They occur throughout the spinal cord, although most series note a cervical preponderance.[6,8] Most intramedullary tumors are benign primary glial neoplasms. Astrocytomas and ependymomas comprise greater than 80% of intramedullary neoplasms in most series.[6,11] Whereas astrocytomas predominate in childhood and adolescence, ependymomas are more common than astrocytomas in adults. Nearly all spinal ependymomas are histologically benign and noninfiltrative. Although most astrocytomas are benign, about 20% of astrocytomas in adults are malignant. This percentage rises with increasing age. By their nature, astrocytomas are infiltrative tumors but the degree of cord infiltration is variable. A small number are diffusely infiltrative without a distinct tumor mass. Others are well circumscribed, particularly in children, and may allow gross total resection. Most astrocytomas exhibit a gradual indistinct transition into the surrounding spinal cord.

Hemangioblastomas account for 5% to 10% of intramedullary tumors.[6,11] Most arise in the cervical spinal cord. Less than 25% occur in association with von Hippel-Lindau syndrome. Multiple intracranial and intraspinal tumors may occur in these cases. These are well-circumscribed vascular tumors that usually arise from a dorsal or lateral pial surface and are buried into the spinal cord substance to a variable degree from a pial attachment. Inclusion tumors and cysts are congenital lesions that result from disordered embryogenesis. Lipoma, dermoid and epidermoid, and teratoma arise within the substance of the spinal cord as a result of defective cleavage of germ cell layers. They most commonly involve the thoracic spinal cord. Most present in childhood and are often associated with sinus tracts, overlying cutaneous abnormalities, and/or spina bifida occulta. Lipomas are the exception. These lesions usually present in adults with a progressive myelopathy as tumor enlargement from increased fat deposition occurs in nonneoplastic adipose cells. A wide variety of tumorous and nontumorous pathology, such as metastatic tumors, pigmented neoplasms, neurocytomas, aberrant Schwann cell tumors, cavernous malformations, and inflammatory (e.g., abscess) conditions account for the remaining 5% of intramedullary mass lesions.[6]

EVALUATION

Most patients present with a prolonged clinical history that reflects the extremely slow growth rate of most intramedullary tumors. Diagnosis is now routinely achieved with gadolinium-enhanced magnetic resonance imaging (MRI) before the onset of significant neurological deficit. Back pain followed by spasticity and gait disturbance is the most common presentation of thoracic intramedullary mass lesions. Quite frequently, subtle or nonspecific symptoms may persist for several months or years prior to diagnosis or development of a significant objective neurological deficit.

A   B   C

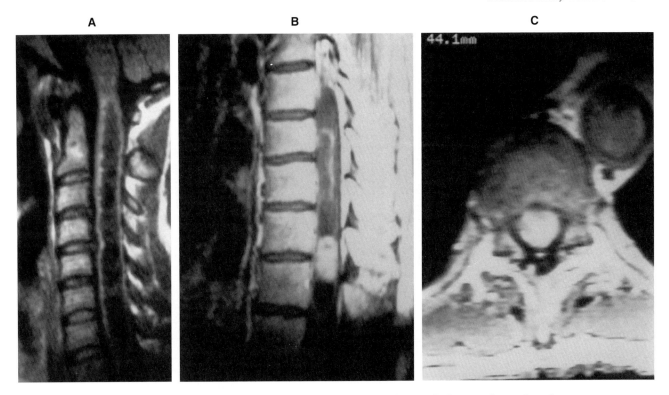

Fig. 24-1. Sagittal T1-weighted MRI (**A**) of the cervical spine shows a holocervical spinal cord syrinx extending up to the cervicomedullary junction. In the absence of a hindbrain abnormality (e.g., Chiari malformation) a thoracic spinal cord tumor should be suspected. Sagittal (**B**) and axial (**C**) gadolinium-enhanced MRI in same patient demonstrates a thoracic intramedullary tumor. Note the linear enhancement extending rostrally from the solid tumor mass that is most likely a small draining vein. At surgery, a well-circumscribed benign ependymoma was encountered and completely removed.

The gadolinium-enhanced MRI provides valuable information. Spinal cord enlargement and at least some degree of enhancement are the characteristic findings. Often, polar cysts are present and may account for much of the length of spinal cord enlargement. Ependymomas most commonly appear as a symmetrical sausage-shaped, uniformly enhancing mass with well-defined margins (Fig. 24-1). Cystic, hemorrhagic, or heterogeneous enhancement may occur, however. This precludes confident tumor type identification on the basis of MRI appearance. Astrocytomas present a more variable MRI appearance. Enhancement may be minimal, intense, or heterogeneous (Fig. 24-2). Intratumoral cysts are common. Margins may be sharply demarcated, irregular, or infiltrative. Hemangioblastomas appear as an eccentric intensely enhancing mass or nodule with a variable amount of spinal cord enlargement above and below the tumor mass (Fig. 24-3). Cavernous malformations present the only other characteristic MRI appearance. These nontumorous mass lesions demonstrate a heterogeneous core of

mixed signal intensity surrounded by a hypointense rim of hemosiderin.[5] Nonsurgical inflammatory lesions such as transverse myelitis or multiple sclerosis may also be imaged with MRI. These patients typically present with the acute or subacute onset of neurological deficit. MRI shows focal or patchy spinal cord enhancement that is often confined to the white matter. Spinal cord enlargement is minimal or absent.

MANAGEMENT

Management of intramedullary tumors is surgical removal whenever possible. Gross total removal of benign well-circumscribed and noninfiltrative neoplasms such as ependymoma, hemangioblastoma, and some astrocytomas can be performed with minimum morbidity and is the most effective method of achieving long-term tumor control with preservation of neurological function.[3,5-8,13] Although radiation therapy after subtotal resection or biopsy may provide long-term tumor control in some patients

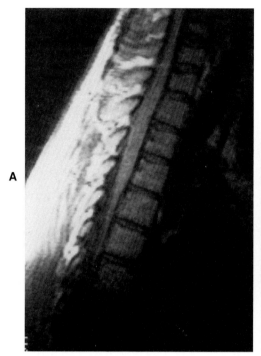

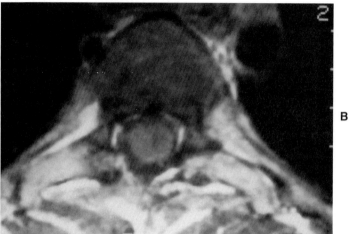

Fig. 24-2. Sagittal (**A**) and axial (**B**) gadolinium-enhanced MRI shows diffuse intramedullary spinal cord widening without significant enhancement. This patient had a diffusely infiltrative astrocytoma for which only biopsy for diagnosis could be performed.

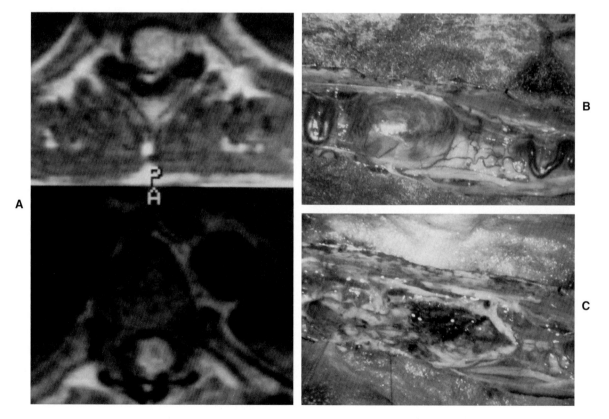

Fig. 24-3. A, Axial gadolinium-enhanced MRI demonstrates a focal, intensely enhancing eccentric tumor mass. **B,** Operative photograph after exposure demonstrates a large pial-based hemangioblastoma. **C,** Operative photograph after total removal. Note that a circumscribing pial incision is used to detach and remove the hemangioblastoma from the spinal cord.

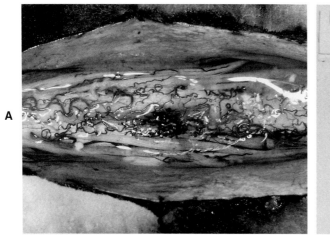
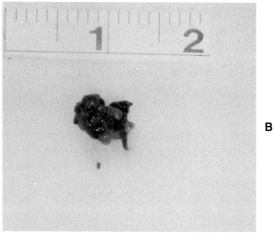

Fig. 24-4. A, Operative photograph demonstrates typical bluish discoloration of the spinal cord surface, consistent with a cavernous malformation. **B,** Photograph of a classic mulberry-appearing resected cavernous malformation.

with ependymomas, this response is inconsistent.[6,8,14] Clearly, gross total resection alone represents the treatment of choice because long-term tumor control is more consistently achieved and preservation of neurological function is routinely possible. The effectiveness of surgery in the management of infiltrative tumors such as astrocytomas is less clear.[9,10] Treatment of astrocytomas remains individualized because of heterogeneity with respect to physical characteristics in relation to the spinal cord, histology, and natural history. Gross total removal is not possible for diffusely infiltrative tumors, nor of any benefit for malignant tumors. Furthermore, the extent of removal has not been definitively correlated with clinical outcome or tumor control for most astrocytomas.[6,9,10] Even the most well-circumscribed astrocytomas that allow gross total resection demonstrate microscopic tumor infiltration into the spinal cord interface. Management of less common intramedullary lesions is determined by the nature of their interface with the spinal cord. Cavernous malformations, metastatic tumors, and certain inclusion tumors may be reasonably well circumscribed and present a clear dissection plane. Gross total removal should be accomplished in these patients (Fig. 24-4).[5] Tumors without a definable interface with the spinal cord are biopsied or subtotally decompressed, depending upon the clinical circumstance.

SURGICAL CONSIDERATIONS

Because surgery represents the most effective treatment of benign intramedullary tumors, every attempt must be made to optimize its benefits. Early diagnosis and aggressive initial treatment are particularly important because preservation of neurological function is more effectively achieved than restoration of lost neurological function. Patients with the least amount of neurological deficit benefit the most from surgical removal. Indeed, not only do significant or long-standing neurological deficits rarely improve after technically successful tumor excision, but the surgical morbidity is greater in more impaired patients. This probably reflects the tenuous nature of the surrounding spinal cord that is relatively intolerant to even gentle surgical manipulation. Therefore the surgeon should assume that each intramedullary tumor is resectable and plan the operation accordingly. Assumption of tumor type and potential resectability based on patient factors or MRI characteristics alone is often incorrect and may unfairly influence the surgical objective. The most important factor determining resectability is the nature of the tumor–spinal cord interface. Tumors that are clearly separable from the surrounding spinal cord can and should be removed. Accurate determination of the presence or absence of a definable tumor–spinal cord interface requires an adequate myelotomy that extends over the entire length of the solid tumor component.

SURGICAL TECHNIQUE

After administration of steroids and prophylactic antibiotics, routine induction and intubation are accomplished. Baseline somatosensory responses are obtained and compared to an earlier preoperative screening study. Motor potentials are generated with subarachnoid electrodes that are placed after dural opening. A nitrous/narcotic anesthetic technique with controlled neuromuscular blockade is used in most cases.[1]

In truth, however, intraoperative monitoring of motor- and somatosensory-evoked potentials is of little practical value to the surgeon. Although simultaneous monitoring of both motor and sensory information increases the reliability of the monitored data, it rarely alters the technique or surgical objective.

Exposure

A standard midline incision and subperiosteal dissection is performed. The appropriate level should be verified with a marking film or intraoperative portable radiograph. Discrepancies can exist between the MRI and intraoperative plain radiograph localization because of variability in rib number and/or rib size. A standard bilateral laminectomy that extends at least one level above and below the solid tumor component is accomplished in the adult. Although resection of the medial one fourth to one third of the facet joint is required to achieve adequate thoracic spinal cord exposure, delayed spinal instability is not a concern in adults. Laminoplasty is recommended in children and adolescents, although its effectiveness in reducing the risk of delayed kyphotic deformity has yet to be critically evaluated. A dorsal fusion that often occurs after laminoplasty in young patients (aged under 10 to 11 years), may result in a crankshaft phenomenon. The latter is the result of persistent ventral vertebral body axial growth in the face of a dorsal fusion (no dorsal growth).

Ultrasound tumor imaging is useful to assure adequate tumor exposure before dural entry. Hemostasis should be secured at this point to prevent annoying blood drainage into the dependent microsurgical operative field. Moist cottonoid wall-offs are placed over the exposed muscle and Surgicel mesh is placed around the base of the field and lateral dural gutters.

The dura mater is opened longitudinally in the midline and tented laterally to the muscle with 4-0 silk suture. Hemostats are hung on the long suture tails to compress the wall-offs against the raw muscle wall. The arachnoid is opened separately. The spinal cord is inspected for any surface abnormalities. Most glial tumors are totally intramedullary and their presence may be apparent only through focal spinal cord widening (Fig. 24-5). Occasionally, an eccentric tumor or polar cyst may be visible through the thinned spinal cord surface and intact pial layer. Hemangioblastomas usually appear as a light orange pial discoloration that may be obscured by enlarged overlying epipial draining veins (see Fig. 24-3). Their location is usually dorsal or dorsolateral. The size of the pial attachment may belie a large intramedullary component. Lipomas are usually subpial in location and are visualized as a faint yellow mass immediately below the thinned pia mater (Fig. 24-6).

Intradural Dissection

The technique of tumor exposure and removal depends upon the tumor's size, location, and relationship to the surrounding spinal cord. Most intramedullary glial tumors are exposed through a dorsal midline myelotomy (see Fig. 24-5). The dorsal midline is identified as the midpoint between corresponding dorsal root entry zones. This estimation of the dorsal midline allows the surgeon to maintain a midline orientation despite occasional spinal cord rotation. The midline epipial vessels, irrespective of size, are cauterized over the entire extent of the intended myelotomy. The pia is incised in an avascular segment at the point of maximum spinal cord widening. The midline pial incision is continued rostrally and caudally with a knife or microscissors. Crossing vessels may be recauterized more effectively by passing bipolar forceps on either side of the pia, perpendicular to the pial edges. The myelotomy is deepened with gentle blunt dissection with microforceps and dissectors. A vertical array of penetrating vessels on each side of the dorsal hemicords maintains the midline orientation.

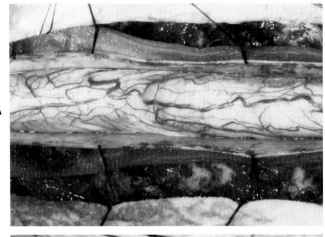

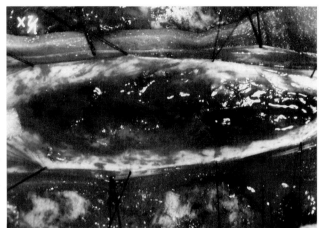

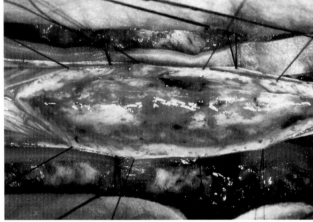

Fig. 24-5. A, Intraoperative photograph of an intramedullary ependymoma shows only spinal cord enlargement. There is no visible surface abnormality. **B,** Operative photograph after dorsal midline myelotomy that extends over the entire dorsal tumor component. Note the glistening tumor surface that is well differentiated from the surrounding spinal cord. This appearance is typical of benign intramedullary ependymomas. Note the pial traction sutures that provide gentle, constant superior spinal cord retraction. **C,** Operative photograph after gross total resection.

The dorsal tumor surface is first encountered at its widest central point. For well-circumscribed tumors, such as ependymomas and some astrocytomas, microforceps can be passed in either direction on the tumor surface, along the axis of the spinal cord, to expose the polar regions of the tumor. Firm gliosis at the polar tumor regions may not be easily separated with gentle blunt dissection and may require sharp incision with a microknife. Both tumor poles are identified and polar cysts, if present, are entered and drained before any tumor is removed. An attempt is made to further define the dorsal tumor margin by gentle blunt lateral displacement of the overlying dorsal hemicords with dissectors. A biopsy is obtained at this point for frozen section examination.

The surgeon may encounter a number of scenarios at this point. If a well-defined tumor–spinal cord interface exists, then continued surface dissection is indicated (virtually irrespective of biopsy results). The only exception is the histological identification of a malignant astrocytoma that independently signals an end to further tumor removal. Surgery has no therapeutic value in the latter group of patients.[2] Histological identification of a benign ependymoma generally corroborates the surgeon's gross impression of a well-circumscribed noninfiltrative and resectable neoplasm. In some cases, however, a distinct tumor–spinal cord interface may not be immediately apparent. This may occur with large tumors with surrounding edematous spinal cord tissue. In these cases, confident histological identification of ependymoma helps the surgeon to "see" the dissection plane.

Histological diagnosis of astrocytoma must be interpreted carefully by the surgeon in the context of the gross findings for several reasons. First, many benign astrocytomas are well circumscribed, particularly in children, and gross total resection may be possible. Second, precise histological interpretation of tiny biopsy fragments may be inaccurate. Indeed, the intraoperative frozen section diagnosis of astrocytoma is often changed to ependymoma or other neoplasm following review of the permanent sections. This can occur either because the initial biopsy of surrounding gliotic nontumorous tissue or the tiny fragments did not reveal diagnostic features of ependymomas such as cell clustering or pseudorosettes. Indeed, in the absence of these features, it can be difficult even on permanent sections to distinguish astrocytoma from ependymoma.

Tumor Resection

Once the dorsal tumor surface of a well-circumscribed tumor has been exposed, 6-0 prolene pial sutures are placed and hung on small mosquito clamps to provide constant, gentle traction on the dorsal hemicords (see Fig. 24-5). The lateral and polar tumor margins are developed with forceps traction on the tumor against pial suture and blunt dissector countertraction on the spinal cord. Fibrous adhesions and vascular attachments between the spinal cord and tumor are systematically cauterized and divided. Internal decompression with laser or ultrasonic aspirator facilitates mobilization of large tumors. Occasionally, the tumor–spinal cord interface may appear obscured or unclear in certain regions. In these cases, the surgeon should retreat to a well-defined interface and approach the unclear margin from a different direction. The ventral tumor–spinal cord interface is defined with vertical tumor forceps traction and systematic cautery and division of vascular attachments.

An "inside-out" method of tumor removal is used for neoplasms in which distinct tumor margins are not identified. After myelotomy and pial suture retraction, laser or ultrasonic aspirator tumor removal begins centrally and is continued peripherally until the surgeon can no longer clearly differentiate tumor from spinal cord tissue. This is usually the case with most benign intramedullary astrocytomas.

Hemangioblastoma removal begins by defining the margins of its pial attachment. Some of the overlying epipial draining vessels may need to be cauterized and divided for exposure. The pial margin is circumferentially divided. The tumor is delivered with gentle traction on the detached pial origin and systematic bipolar cautery on the tumor surface to shrink tumor volume.[12] Small polar myelotomies

may improve visualization of particularly large intramedullary tumor components (see Fig. 24-3).

Intramedullary lipomas are subpial in location and require only a longitudinal pial incision for exposure.[4] Aggressive subtotal internal decompression with laser or ultrasonic aspirator is the surgical objective (see Fig. 24-6). No attempt is made to define tumor margins because none exist.

After tumor removal, the pial sutures are removed. The dorsal hemicords are reapproximated without suture. All blood and debris are irrigated out of the subarachnoid space with warm saline solution. The dura mater is closed primarily with a running lock 4-0 silk suture. An autologous thoracodorsal facial graft is preferred in reoperative cases that require a dural patch graft. The remainder of the wound is closed meticulously in layers to prevent a postoperative cerebrospinal fluid (CSF) fistula. No drains are used.

POSTOPERATIVE MANAGEMENT
Routine Considerations

Most patients report subjective sensory loss in the immediate postoperative period. This probably reflects dorsal column dysfunction from the midline myelotomy. These complaints tend to persist despite surprisingly little, if any, subjective sensory complaints. Preexisting motor deficits are often worse in the early postoperative period but tend to improve over several weeks to months postoperatively. The new onset of significant neurological deficit should occur uncommonly. This complication most often accompanies radical resection of malignant glial neoplasms.

Early mobilization is encouraged to prevent the complications of recumbency. Orthostatic hypotension may temporarily exist following upper thoracic tumor removal. CSF leaks are aggressively managed with wound revision and/or a spinal drain to prevent meningitis. Early physical therapy is instituted for mobilization and gait training which are often impaired significantly in the immediate postoperative period despite minimal objective deficit.

Long-term intensive rehabilitation is critical for patients with significant neurological deficit. A follow-up MRI is obtained six weeks postoperatively to determine the extent of tumor resection. Long-term clinical and radiographic follow-up is

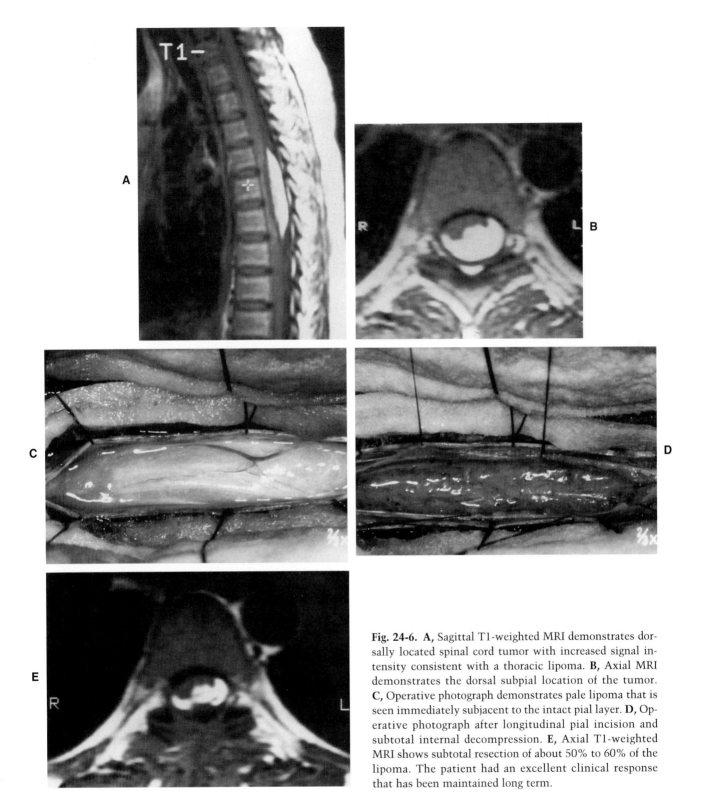

Fig. 24-6. A, Sagittal T1-weighted MRI demonstrates dorsally located spinal cord tumor with increased signal intensity consistent with a thoracic lipoma. **B,** Axial MRI demonstrates the dorsal subpial location of the tumor. **C,** Operative photograph demonstrates pale lipoma that is seen immediately subjacent to the intact pial layer. **D,** Operative photograph after longitudinal pial incision and subtotal internal decompression. **E,** Axial T1-weighted MRI shows subtotal resection of about 50% to 60% of the lipoma. The patient had an excellent clinical response that has been maintained long term.

recommended because of the continued risk of tumor recurrence. Management of tumor recurrence is based on the patient's age and clinical condition, size and growth of the recurrent tumor, previous response to tumor excision, and tumor histology. Whereas small asymptomatic recurrences may be followed in older or higher-risk surgical patients, elective resection of a progressively enlarging recurrent ependymoma may be appropriate in asymptomatic younger patients with minimal surgical risk. In general, whereas surgical excision of asymptomatic recurrent ependymomas is recommended in low-risk patients, repeat surgery for astrocytomas is contemplated only for clinically symptomatic tumor recurrence in patients who have demonstrated a reasonable response to previous surgery.

Radiation Therapy

The role of radiation therapy is unclear. Some studies demonstrate improved long-term tumor control after subtotal resection of benign ependymomas.[14] The response, however, is inconsistent and long-term results are not comparable to patients treated with gross total microsurgical resection alone.[6,8] Furthermore, radiation therapy complicates the prospect of further surgery by increasing the risk of CSF fistula and possibly obscuring tissue planes, secondary to radiation-induced gliosis. No convincing data are available to suggest any efficacy of radiation therapy for tumor control of benign astrocytomas. Radiation therapy is appropriate in patients with malignant astrocytic neoplasms and may improve tumor control after resection of malignant metastatic tumors.

CONCLUSION

Surgery represents the most effective treatment of benign well-circumscribed intramedullary tumors. Long-term tumor control or cure with preservation of neurological function can be achieved in most cases. Early clinical diagnosis, definitive initial treatment if possible, and meticulous microsurgical technique will maximize the benefit of surgery in these patients. The precise role of surgery for benign infiltrative tumors has not been established. Aggressive tumor removal until loss of clear demarcation between tumor and spinal cord is advocated. Although surgery may be effective in selective cases of metastatic spinal cord involvement, no therapeutic role for surgery exists for malignant primary glial neoplasms. Radiation therapy may confer partial tumor control in some patients with benign intramedullary tumors, but this response is inconsistent. Gross total removal whenever possible is the preferred method of treatment.

REFERENCES

1. Adams DC, Emerson RG, Heyer EJ, et al. Intraoperative evoked potential monitoring with controlled neuromuscular blockade. Anesth Analg 77:913-918, 1993.
2. Cohen AR, Wisoff JH, Allen JC, et al. Malignant astrocytomas of the spinal cord. J Neurosurg 70:50-54, 1989.
3. McCormick PC. Spinal ependymoma. Neurosurg Q 3:178-191, 1993.
4. McCormick PC. Anatomic principles of the intradural spinal surgery. Clin Neurosurg 41:204-223, 1994.
5. McCormick PC, Michelson WJ, Post KD, et al. Cavernous malformations of the spinal cord. Neurosurgery 23:459-463, 1988.
6. McCormick PC, Stein BM. Intramedullary tumors in adults. Neurosurg Clin N Am 1:609-630, 1990.
7. McCormick PC, Stein BM. Spinal cord tumors in adults. In Youmans JR, ed. Neurological Surgery, 4th ed. Philadelphia: WB Saunders, 1996, pp 3102-3122.
8. McCormick PC, Torres R, Post KD, et al. Intramedullary ependymoma of the spinal cord. J Neurosurg 72:523-533, 1990.
9. Rossitch E, Zeidman S, Burger PC, et al. Clinical and pathological analysis of spinal and astrocytomas in children. Neurosurgery 27:193-196, 1990.
10. Sandler HM, Papadopoulos SM, Thuntan AF, et al. Spinal cord astrocytoma: Results of therapy. Neurosurgery 30:490-493, 1992.
11. Sloof JL, Kernohan JW, MacCarthy CS. Primary Intramedullary Tumors of the Spinal Cord and Filum Terminale. Philadelphia: WB Saunders, 1964.
12. Solomon RA, Stein BM. Unusual spinal cord enlargement related to intramedullary hemangioblastoma. J Neurosurg 68:550-553, 1988.
13. Stein BM, McCormick PC. Intramedullary neoplasms and vascular malformations. Clin Neurosurg 39:361-387, 1992.
14. Whitaker SJ, Bessell EM, Ashley SE, et al. Post-operative radiotherapy in the management of spinal cord ependymoma. J Neurosurg 74:720-728, 1991.

Extramedullary Tumors

Felipe C. Albuquerque, M.D., Michael L. Levy, M.D.,
and Michael L.J. Apuzzo, M.D.

Meningiomas and neurilemomas are the most common tumors of the thoracic spine. Indeed, their preponderance renders other lesions of this area rare.[20] Each presents with characteristic signs and symptoms, and the resection of both offers substantial potential for recovery. A discussion of the epidemiology, symptomatology, histology, and surgery of these lesions follows.

MENINGIOMAS
Epidemiology

Meningiomas represent approximately 25% of primary tumors of the spinal cord, up to 90% of which are in the thoracic region.[9,18,26,28] Typically, such lesions are found in women over 40 years of age.[5,9,18,20,25] While meningiomas of the spine do occur in men, they do so throughout the spinal cord without a predilection for the thoracic segment.[9] The theory that meningiomas rely on female sexual hormones for growth does not explain their affinity for women as most of these lesions produce symptoms after menopause.[25] Dural sac irritation in the midthoracic region may predispose to the development of meningiomas.[5,18]

Signs and Symptoms

Symptoms produced by meningiomas are secondary to their broad dural attachment and gradual im-

pingement on the spinal cord with growth.[5] The slow progression of these lesions creates an insidious clinical course that is often confused with other lesions of the spinal cord, peripheral nervous system, and thorax.[5,20,21] The duration of symptoms may span 6 to 23 months and is rarely characterized by an abrupt onset.[5,9,18] Because meningiomas do not arise from nerve roots themselves, as do neurilemomas, they typically present with myelopathic rather than radiculopathic findings. With substantial growth of the lesion, however, patients may present with signs and symptoms of both nerve root and spinal cord compression.[3] Most often, patients complain of regional back pain, or night pain, followed by sensorimotor changes and, finally, bowel and bladder dysfunction.[5,9,18,20,26] Sensory changes range from diffuse paresthesias over the lower extremities to an actual thoracic, sensory level. Motor weakness often progresses slowly to paraplegia.[5] Undoubtedly, a delay in diagnosis adversely affects outcome. A middle-aged woman complaining of diffuse back pain, presenting with a spastic myelopathy should arouse one's suspicion of a thoracic meningioma and hasten the appropriate diagnostic investigation.

Location

Meningiomas of the thoracic spine originate from clusters of arachnoid cells located at nerve root

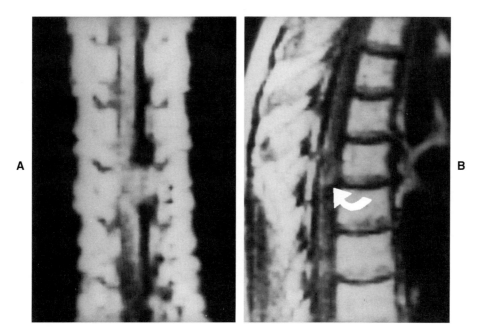

Fig. 25-1. Laterally located T9 meningioma with mass effect on the spinal cord as seen on coronal (**A**) and sagittal (**B**) CT scans.

entry zones or at the junction of the dentate ligaments and dura mater, where the spinal arteries penetrate.[3] For this reason, laterally located tumors are more common than dorsal and ventral lesions[12,18,25] (Fig. 25-1). Of the latter, dorsal tumors are more common than their ventral counterparts.[4,5] The fact that meningiomas predominate in the lateral compartment explains the eventual presentation of radicular symptoms. While the majority of thoracic meningiomas are entirely intradural, some authors report an extradural component to these lesions in 10% to 15% of cases.[3,25]

Histopathology

Spinal meningiomas differ from their intracranial counterparts by a greater proclivity to psammomatous change.[26] Generally, all histological features seen in the intracranial variety are present in spinal meningiomas. Meningotheliomatous and transitional features are also more common in spinal lesions.[26] The extent of calcification, furthermore, is more predominant than that of intracranial meningiomas.[3,26] Typically, spinal meningiomas are globoid-shaped and vary in consistency depending on the extent of calcification.[3] Multiple lesions are rare, occurring at a rate of 2% of all spinal meningiomas, and are most often associated with von Recklinghausen's neurofibromatosis. These tumors, moreover, have a higher rate of malignancy.[4] Finally, en plaque meningiomas of the thoracic spinal cord are exceedingly uncommon.[28] Such lesions can take a circumferential or hemicircumferential position, thus complicating their removal and increasing the risk of postoperative deficit.

Surgical Resection

Ease of resection varies with the location of the tumor. Optimally, the tumor should sit between the surgeon and the spinal cord. This configuration lessens the amount of traction placed on the cord and improves the surgeon's visibility of the lesion.[3] For those tumors situated dorsally or laterally, a standard thoracic laminectomy often suffices for exposure.[26] Once the bone has been removed the surgeon must resect the ligamentum flavum and coagulate branches of the overlying epidural venous plexus.[26] The dura mater is then opened over the tumor.[10] Devascularization of the mass by cautery of its overlying vessels speeds resection and minimizes blood loss.[3] Care must be taken not to sacrifice arterial branches to the spinal cord. The latter is particularly critical when operating on the left side in the lower thoracic spine, where the artery of Adamkiewicz enters the spinal canal. En bloc resection of the mass is not recommended, as this may transmit retraction forces to the spinal cord itself.[26] By gradually debulking the tumor laterally and internally, the surgeon can fold the lesion on itself and better visualize the tumor-cord interface.[19,25,26] Division of the dentate ligaments or sacrifice of a dorsal nerve root may enhance the exposure, especially with tumors lying within the lateral compartment.[19]

Having completed the debulking, the surgeon must then focus on establishing or locating the plane between the mass and the spinal cord. This step poses a considerable challenge, because growth of the lesion stretches and attenuates the arachnoid membrane lying between the mass and the pial surface of the spinal cord.[26] By identifying this membrane, the surgeon can complete the dissection in the epiarachnoid plane, dramatically reducing the likelihood of spinal cord injury. If this membrane is mistakenly judged to be tumor capsule, the surgeon may inadvertently denude the surface of the spinal cord by violating the pia mater. Once again, internal decompression of the lesion should provide enough maneuverability around the lesion to identify both the arachnoid and pial surfaces.

Ventral, and some lateral, lesions can be difficult to resect through a simple laminectomy. Ventrolateral access is limited in the thoracic region by the small size of the spinal canal, the rib cage, and the adjacent paraspinal musculature.[27] In cases where such exposure is necessary, the surgeon may choose to perform a unilateral or partial facetectomy.[26] It is believed that a portion of one pedicle may also be removed without significantly compromising spinal stability. However, this enlarged dissection exposes nerve roots and vessels in the area of the neural foramina to increased risk. A dorsolateral, or lateral extracavitary, approach to the thoracic spinal canal is another option when attempting to resect ventral and/or lateral lesions.[27] Disarticulation of the rib at the level of the tumor allows access to the entire ipsilateral spinal canal space and minimizes the amount of retraction needed to complete tumor resection. Drawbacks of this approach include a greater risk to pleural and mediastinal structures, a significantly longer operative time, and the requirement of a higher degree of technical expertise. Transthoracic resection of ventrally located tumors is a final option. This approach necessitates a vertebrectomy and carries a much higher morbidity than the operations previously discussed.[27]

Whether to resect and graft the dura mater overlying the lesion is a matter of preference and accessibility. For those meningiomas lying dorsally, complete excision of the dural segment abutting the tumor is recommended. The defect may be repaired with a cadaveric specimen, a silastic patch, or autogenous fascia, or may closed primarily.[9,19,20,27] In lesions located ventrolaterally, dural resection may not be feasible. In these cases, electrocautery of that segment of dura involved with the tumor will not raise considerably the risk of recurrence.[9,19]

Results

Rates of recovery are generally very high after resection of thoracic meningiomas.[5,9,18,25] Recurrence, furthermore, is significantly lower than that of intracranial lesions.[17,25,26] The latter may be secondary to a higher rate of complete resection, which in itself is secondary to a greater ease of resectability.[17] Factors associated with a poor outcome include: calcified tumors, ventrally located lesions, elderly patients, duration and severity of symptoms, subtotal resection, and an extradural component.[5,21,26] As mentioned previously, calcified tumors are more difficult to debulk in a piecemeal fashion and cause undue traction on the spinal cord with manipulation. In addition, they are more likely to adhere to the arachnoid surface of the spinal cord, complicating identification of the dissection plane.[26] Resection of ventral lesions is associated with a worse postoperative function because of their proximity to vital neurovascular structures, including the ventral horns and anterior spinal artery.[5] Tumors with an extradural component are more likely to invade bone and rapidly progress. Retraction and manipulation of the dural sac during resection of the extradural component can also jeopardize outcome.[3] Regardless of these deleterious factors, resection of thoracic meningiomas is associated with a remarkably high recovery rate. Even paraplegic patients have recovered the ability to ambulate.[5]

In their series of 97 cases of spinal meningiomas, 73 of which were thoracic, Levy, Bay, and Dohn[9] report a complete resection of the lesion in 82% of patients. Six months after surgery 85% of their patients were either without deficit or neurologically improved compared to preoperative function. Two of the six paraplegic patients in this study regained the ability to walk. Solero et al.[25] achieved complete tumor resection in 168 of 174 patients with spinal meningiomas. In this group, 144 patients had tumors of the thoracic spine. At late follow-up, 74% of patients were normal, 18% were partially disabled, and 8% were severely disabled. The authors also report that only 6% (nine of 150 patients) had a recurrence of their tumor on follow-up examination (average duration, 14 years). Furthermore, only two of these lesions (1.3%) recurred within the first 5 postoperative years. In two smaller studies, Namer et al.[18] and David and Washburn[5] report similarly impressive results. In the former, the authors performed a complete resection in 27 of 29 cases, 19 of which involved the thoracic spine. Total cure or significant improvement was observed in 86.5% of their patients. Davis and Washburn resected 45 meningiomas, 35 of which were located in the thoracic segment and 26 of which were between T3 and T8. The authors report a "highly satisfactory" recovery in 36 patients.

NEURILEMOMAS
Epidemiology

Like meningiomas, neurilemomas account for nearly 25% of primary spinal cord tumors.[10] Several authors believe that these lesions are more common than meningiomas, though statistically, their incidence is similar.[2,3,15] Unlike meningiomas, men and women are affected equally by neurilemomas.[3,10] The vast majority of cases represent single lesions, with multiple tumors occurring usually in cases of von Recklinghausen's neurofibromatosis.[1,10] Typically, patients present with insidious symptoms starting in the fifth decade.[12,20]

Signs and Symptoms

Given that these lesions arise from nerve roots, patients typically first manifest radicular complaints.[3,10] In the thoracic region this consists of pain and paresthesias in a dermatomal distribution. With growth, neurilemomas produce both radiculopathic and myelopathic findings.[3,10,20] Symptoms develop insidiously over several months and are frequently disregarded by the patient.[3,10,20,21] Pain is typically the most frequent complaint and can be seen in more than 80% of patients.[10] In comparison to meningiomas, bowel and bladder dysfunction and weakness are less common, occurring in 25% and 30% of patients, respectively.[10]

Location

Unlike meningiomas, neurilemomas have no predilection for the thoracic spine, occurring with nearly equal frequency throughout the spinal canal.[10,12] Lesions typically arise from a single, dorsal nerve root, and hence tend to expand in a dorsolateral direction.[3,27] The majority of neurilemomas are purely intradural.[3,10] "Dumbbell" lesions growing out of the dural sac and through the neural foramina are observed in 7% to 13% of cases.[3,10]

Histopathology

Neurofibromas originate from the endoneurium and are characterized by elongated Schwann cell cylinders intermingled with axonal elements in a mucinous matrix.[3,7,23] They occur predominantly in patients with von Recklinghausen's neurofibromatosis and are less frequently observed in a sporadic fashion.[7,23] In patients with von Recklinghausen's neurofibromatosis, these lesions have a greater proclivity toward malignant degeneration (Fig. 25-2). Schwannomas grow as extensions of the perineurium and are characterized by a combination of two histological features: Antoni type A and type B tissue.[7,23] Antoni type A tissue consists of elongated spindles of cells, compactly arranged, with darkly-staining nuclei. These features are frequently found in association with Antoni type B elements, which are typified by a looser arrangement of stellate and pleomorphic cells.[23] Schwannomas occur with greatest frequency in patients with type 2 neurofibromatosis and in sporadic cases.[7] Grossly, both lesions are globoid in shape, avascular, and soft in consistency.[3] Neurofibromas tend to be poorly defined and often merge insensibly with the nerve root, in contradiction to Schwannomas, which tend to be smooth growths blossoming from around the root.[23] Both lesions are rarely calcified.[3] Because these tumors are benign growths with similar histological features, clinicians frequently fail to distinguish between them. For the purpose of this review, these lesions will collectively be addressed as neurilemomas.

Surgical Resection and Results

As with meningiomas, results of neurilemoma resection are usually gratifying. Even patients with severe deficits can benefit from removal of their le-

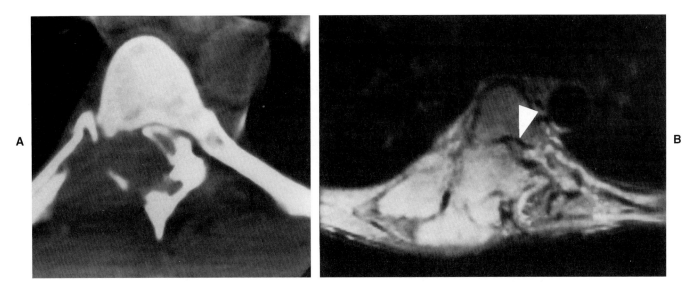

Fig. 25-2. Malignant T6 neurilemoma in a patient with von Recklinghausen's neurofibromatosis. **A,** CT demonstrates bony erosion of the canal. **B,** MRI reveals significant displacement of the cord in a ventrolateral trajectory *(arrowhead)*.

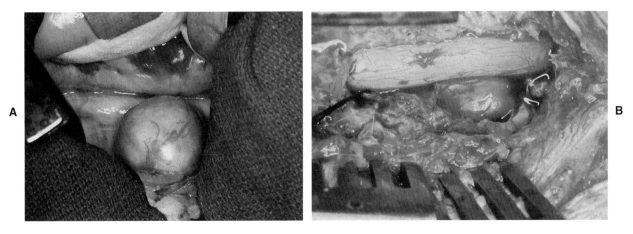

Fig. 25-3. A, Massive neurilemoma with significant canal expansion as seen after laminectomy. **B,** The stitch *(lower left corner)* demarcates the dural edge.

sions.[3,10] Resection arrests the progression of disease, generally relieves associated pain, and often enhances recovery of function.[3] The same technical points apply in approaching these tumors via a standard laminectomy (Fig. 25-3). The dura mater is incised either lateral or medial to the lesion.[10] Critical to completing the resection is early identification of the nerve root of origin.[3] The nerve root itself can be used to retract the mass from the spinal cord, and must be sacrificed to ensure total excision of the lesion.[3] In those cases with an extradural component, the lesion may be divided and that part outside the neural foramen addressed after removal of the in-

tradural component.[3] This technique lessens traction forces placed on the spinal cord by manipulation of the lesion en masse.[3] Dural repair is usually primary and is considerably simplified by the lack of the dural attachment commonly observed with meningiomas.[20]

RESULTS

In the sister study to their analysis of spinal meningiomas, Levy et al.[10] report similar surgical results with the resection of neurilemomas. Of the 66 neurilemomas resected, 42% of which were in the

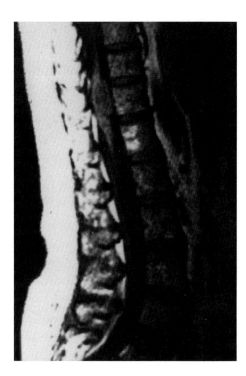

Fig. 25-4. T10 ventral neurilemoma as seen on contrast-enhanced MRI scan.

thoracic segment, 60% of patients made a full post-operative functional recovery. Pain was relieved in 85%, and the sensory level resolved in 88%. Three patients had worse motor function postoperatively, and one patient had recurrence of the lesion 3 years after a partial resection. Other complications specific to resection of both spinal neurilemomas and meningiomas include CSF leakage and infection.[4,10,25]

Because neurilemomas originate from the dorsal root, they usually grow in a dorsolateral trajectory. Nonetheless, in those rare cases with a significant ventral component, the lateral extracavitary approach can be employed (Fig. 25-4). In their review of six patients, four of whom had thoracic neurilemomas, Steck, Dietze, and Fessler[27] report "sustained neurological improvement" in five. Complications specific to this approach include: pneumothorax, sympathetic pleural effusion, and pneumonia.

RADIOGRAPHIC FEATURES

Magnetic resonance imaging (MRI) is the diagnostic standard for spinal meningiomas and neurilemomas.[24] With the improvement in image quality, one can often differentiate the lesions based on specific radiographic characteristics. Distinction between the

two may be seen when assessing signal intensities, lesion margins, dural attachments, extension into the neural foramina, and contrast enhancement.[14] Neurilemomas usually appear hypointense in comparison to the spinal cord on unenhanced T1-weighted images and hyperintense on T2-weighted images.[11,14,25] Typically, meningiomas appear isointense on both T1- and T2-weighted images.[14,25] Neurilemomas often have smoother margins but more irregular enhancement in comparison to meningiomas.[11,14] The latter is likely secondary to a greater propensity for neurilemomas to undergo cystic degeneration and internal necrosis.[11,14] The intensity of enhancement is higher, however, in neurilemomas—a factor with a likely histological explanation.[11,14] Neurilemomas have open, short, straight gap junctions that communicate with the extracellular spaces, while those of meningiomas are tortuous and elongated.[13,14] Presumably, gadolinium penetrates the gap junctions of neurilemomas unencumbered, resulting in more intense enhancement. Meningiomas typically demonstrate a wide dural base, while neurilemomas may lack one or have one that is very narrow.[11,14] Extension of the lesion into the neural foramen is virtually diagnostic of a neurilemoma.[14]

Plain radiographs are not a reliable means of diagnosing meningiomas and neurilemomas.[5,18,26] Despite the fact that neurilemomas more often reveal abnormal plain radiographic findings than meningiomas, these findings do not occur with enough frequency to be diagnostic, and certainly not with enough detail to differentiate between the two lesions. Abnormalities on plain radiographs may be detected in nearly 20% of cases of spinal meningiomas, and include vertebral body erosion, widening of the interpedicular space, scoliosis, and expansion of the spinal canal.[9,18] Neurilemomas may demonstrate abnormal features on plain radiographs in up to 50% of cases. These include widening of the intervertebral foramina and erosion and decalcification of the pedicle in contact with the lesion.[10,12] Unlike plain radiography, myelography nearly always reveals a lesion, but again, often will not provide enough detail to discriminate between the two types of tumor. With meningiomas, a myelogram typically reveals a complete or near-complete block, while with neurilemomas, it may show the lesion tracking into a neural foramen.[9]

The use of intraoperative ultrasonography serves as a useful tool in guiding the dissection and determining the quantity and location of residual tumor.[16] Mimatsu et al.[16] performed intraoperative ultrasonography on 17 patients with neurilemomas and nine with meningiomas. All lesions were highly echogenic. In this study neurilemomas typically had smooth surfaces and occasional cystic areas, while meningiomas were more echogenic and tightly opposed to the dura.

MISCELLANEOUS LESIONS

As mentioned previously, the overwhelming majority of intradural extramedullary tumors of the thoracic spine are meningiomas and neurilemomas. Other tumors of this region are considered rare.[20] Cases of purely extramedullary thoracic lipomas, chordomas, and metastatic lesions exist.[6,11,22] In 1992 Levy et al.[8] reported the first case of a thoracic intradural-extramedullary ganglioneuroma. Metastatic lesions to the thoracic spine include uterine cancers and malignant melanomas. Nearly all lipomas of the spinal cord have an intramedullary component, and the majority of metastatic lesions remain extradural.

CONCLUSION

Meningiomas and neurilemomas are the most common tumors of the thoracic intradural extramedullary compartment. These benign lesions generally produce an insidious clinical course characterized by myelopathic and radiculopathic symptoms, respectively. With substantial growth, the symptom complexes may merge and can leave the patient with significant deficits, including paraplegia. Even in those cases with poor preoperative function, however, resection of these lesions can be associated with excellent recovery. Surgical morbidity is low given that the majority of lesions are resectable through a simple laminectomy. In those cases with ventrolateral extension, an extracavitary approach may be warranted and is associated with a higher, but nonetheless low, morbidity. Radiographically, these tumors are best delineated by MRI. Meningiomas are characterized by a wide dural base, homogeneous enhancement, and an irregular surface. Neurilemomas are smoother and enhance heterogeneously due to a greater tendency toward cystic degeneration. Intraoperative ultrasound is a useful adjunct that can guide the surgeon toward residual tumor and can better define the tumor-cord interface. Other tumors of this region are rare, and include lipomas and metastases.

REFERENCES

1. Akeson P, Holtas S. Radiological investigation of neurofibromatosis type 2. Neuroradiology 36:107-110, 1994.
2. Ardehali MR. Relative incidence of spinal canal tumors. Clin Neurol Neurosurg 92:237-243, 1990.
3. Bloomfield SM, Carter LP. Intradural-extramedullary tumors of the thoracic spine. Curr Ther Neurol Surg 2:236-238, 1989.
4. Chaparro MJ, Young RF, Smith M, Shen V, Choi BY. Multiple spinal meningiomas: A case of 47 distinct lesions in the absence of neurofibromatosis or identified chromosomal abnormality. Neurosurgery 32:298-302, 1993.
5. Davis RA, Washburn PL. Spinal cord meningiomas. Surg Gynecol Obstet 131:15-21, 1970.
6. Dillon WP, Norman D, Newton TH, Bolla K, Mark A. Intradural spinal cord lesions: Gd-DTPA-enhanced MR imaging. Radiology 170:299-237, 1989.
7. Halliday AL, Sobel RA, Martuza RL. Benign spinal nerve sheath tumors: Their occurrence sporadically and in neurofibromatosis types 1 and 2. J Neurosurg 74:248-253, 1991.
8. Levy DI, Bucci MN, Weatherbee L, Chandler WF. Intradural extramedullary ganglioneuroma: Case report and review of the literature. Surg Neurol 37:216-218, 1992.
9. Levy WJ, Bay J, Dohn D. Spinal cord meningioma. J Neurosurg 57:804-812, 1982.
10. Levy WJ, Latchaw J. Hahn JF, Sawhny B, Bay J, Dohn DF. Spinal neurofibromas: A report of 66 cases and a comparison with meningiomas. Neurosurgery 18:331-334, 1986.
11. Li MH, Holtas S, Larsson EM. MR imaging of intradural extramedullary tumors. Acta Radiol 33:207-212, 1992.
12. Lombardi G, Passerini A. Spinal cord tumors. Radiology 76:381-391, 1961.
13. Long DM. Vascular ultrastructure in human meningiomas and schwannomas. J Neurosurg 38:409-419, 1973.
14. Matsumoto S, Hasuo K, Uchino A, Mizushima A, Furukawa T, Matsuura Y, Fukui, M, Masuda K. MRI of intradural-extramedullary spinal neurinomas and meningiomas. Clin Imaging 17:46-52, 1993.
15. McGuire RA, Brown MD, Green BA. Intradural spinal tumors and spinal stenosis. Spine 12:1062-1066, 1987.
16. Mimatsu K, Kawakami N, Kato F, Saito H, Sato K. Intraoperative ultrasonography of extramedullary spinal tumours. Neuroradiology 34:440-443, 1992.
17. Mirimanoff RO, Dosoretz DE, Linggood RM, Ojemann RG, Martuza RL. Meningioma: Analysis of recurrence and progression following neurosurgical resection. J Neurosurg 62:18-24, 1985.
18. Namer IJ, Pamir MN, Benli K, Saglam S, Erbengi A. Neurochirurgia 30:11-15, 1987.
19. Ojemann RG. Management of cranial and spinal meningiomas [honored guest presentation]. Clin Neurosurg 40:321-383, 1993.
20. Onofrio BM. Intradural extramedullary spinal cord tumors. Clin Neurosurg 25:540-555, 1978.
21. Pena M, Galasko CSB, Barrie JL. Delay in diagnosis of intradural spinal tumors. Spine 17:1110-1116, 1992.
22. Ramiro J, Ferreras B, Calvo JMP, Zafra A. Thoracic intradural chordoma. Surg Neurol 26:571-572, 1986.
23. Rubinstein LJ. Tumors of the cranial and spinal nerve roots. In Tumors of the Central Nervous System. Washington,

D.C.: Armed Forces Institute of Pathology, 1972, pp. 205-214.

24. Schroth G, Thron A, Guhl L, Voigt K, Niendorf HP, Garces LRN. Magnetic resonance imaging of spinal meningiomas and neurinomas. J Neurosurg 66:695-700, 1987.

25. Solero CL, Fornari, M, Giombini S, Lasio G, Oliveri G, Cimino C, Pluchino F. Spinal meningiomas: Review of 174 operated cases. Neurosurgery 25:153-160, 1989.

26. Souweidane MM, Benjamin V. Spinal cord meningiomas. Neurosurg Clin N Am 5:283-291, 1994.

27. Steck JC, Dietze DD, Fessler RG. Posterolateral approach to intradural extramedullary thoracic tumors. J Neurosurg 81:202-205, 1994.

28. Stetchison MT, Tasker RR, Wortzman G. Spinal meningioma *en plaque:* Report of two cases. J Neurosurg 67:452-455, 1987.

26

Primary Bone Tumors

Kevin M. Deitel, M.D., and Michael G. Fehlings, M.D., Ph.D.

Primary tumors of the spine are rare lesions that may be classified as benign (10%) or malignant (90%) neoplasms (see box). Some of the clinical features of primary bone tumors are summarized in Table 26-1. Benign tumors can be difficult to diagnose. They are rare, seldom suspected, and lack specific symptoms and signs. The most common presentation is that of unremitting back pain in a young adult. The pain may radiate in a radicular fashion; however, specific neurological deficits caused by compression of the spinal cord and nerve roots are rare. Malignant spinal tumors also commonly present with back pain, which may be constant in nature, unresponsive to analgesia, and typically present at night. The severity of the symptoms tends to progress more rapidly than with benign lesions. Spinal deformities such as scoliosis may occur with either benign or malignant lesions. Patients with benign lesions tend to be younger with an average age at presentation of 21 as compared to 49 for malignant lesions.[29] Involvement of the vertebral body occurs in 80% of malignant lesions and only 40% of benign lesions. Neurological deficits are more common with malignant lesions, presenting in 55% of patients vs. 35% in benign lesions.

Upper motor neuron findings, including paraparesis, spasticity, extensor plantar responses, sensory abnormalities, and neurogenic involvement of bowel or bladder function, are more common in malignant lesions due to direct tumor extension or pathological fractures. In contrast, symptoms and

> **PRIMARY BONE TUMORS OF THE THORACIC SPINE**
>
> **Benign**
>
> Osteoid osteoma
> Osteoblastoma
> Osteochondroma
> Giant cell tumor
> Aneurysmal bone cyst
> Hemangioma
> Eosinophilic granuloma
>
> **Malignant**
>
> Osteosarcoma
> Chondrosarcoma
> Chordoma
> Multiple myeloma
> Ewing's sarcoma

signs of radicular compression are more common in benign spinal lesions.

Malignant lesions tend to penetrate the capsule and are surrounded by a reactive zone that is outgrown by aggressive lesions. These tumors grow by direct tissue destruction and by the stimulation of osseous resorption. Reactive bone formation is often present. Bone formation by the tumor itself occurs in some osteosarcomas.

It can be difficult to differentiate between primary and secondary malignant spinal tumors. They both exhibit vertebral body involvement, bony

Table 26-1. Clinical Features of Primary Bone Tumors of the Thoracic Spine

	Benign	Malignant
Age	Young adults (mean age 21)	Middle-aged adults (mean age 49)
Back pain	Common	Common (severity progresses more rapidly than with benign lesions)
Neurological deficit	35%	55%
Scoliosis	May occur	May occur
Involvement of vertebral body	40%	80%

destruction, and collapse. Primary spinal tumors, however, are usually solitary whereas secondary lesions are usually multiple upon presentation. Bone scanning can be useful to determine the number of bony lesions.

BENIGN LESIONS
Osteoid Osteoma/Osteoblastoma

Although osteoid osteoma and osteoblastoma (Fig. 26-1) have some differences clinically, they are identical histologically. These tumors are most common in the second and third decades of life with a male preponderance of 2 to 3:1. In the spine, osteoblastomas occur more commonly than osteoid osteomas.

Patients present with localized pain that tends to be intermittent in nature, lasting weeks to months before clinical presentation. The pain tends to increase with activity, is unrelieved with rest, and may occur at night, awakening patients from sleep. Neurological findings may be present and are more common with osteoblastomas. The pain is usually relieved by aspirin or other nonsteroidal anti-inflammatory drugs (NSAIDs).

There may be local tenderness over the lesion. The lesion itself may be palpable. Scoliosis or other spinal deformities may be present with or without a neurological deficit (Fig. 26-1, *A*). Osteoid osteoma and osteoblastoma are the most common causes of painful scoliosis in adolescents.

These lesions tend to involve the dorsal elements of the spine. When they cause scoliosis, the lesions are present on the concave side within two vertebrae of the apex. Osteoid osteomas tend to be less than 1.5 cm in diameter while osteoblastomas tend to be larger. On plain radiographs and computed tomography (CT) scans, osteoid osteomas have a round or oval radiolucency or "nidus" surrounded by a sclerotic margin (Fig. 26-1, *B* and *C*). Osteoblastomas

tend to have a larger area of radiolucency with more irregular margins and less sclerosis. About half of osteoblastomas that involve the spine have epidural extension. Cortical expansion or thinning may be present within these lesions. In contrast to osteosarcoma, periosteal new bone formation is not present. Bone scanning has a high specificity for these lesions and shows intense activity that is present in the blood pool (immediate) image and persists in the delayed image. Because these are very vascular tumors, selective angiography may be helpful to define these lesions. Embolization may then be employed.

Morphologically, these lesions are well circumscribed with randomly interconnected trabeculae of woven bone surrounded by a rim of osteoblasts. The stroma surrounding the lesion consists of loose connective tissue with many dilated or congested capillaries.

Microscopically, there is an extremely active formation of osteoid and immature bone by osteoblasts in a highly vascularized stroma. High levels of prostaglandin E_2 and prostaglandin metabolites are present, explaining the relief of symptoms with NSAIDs.

The goal of treatment is early diagnosis and complete surgical excision. CT and bone scans allow accurate localization of the tumor, which aids in surgical planning. Patients with painful scoliosis who present within 15 months of symptoms onset have a decrease of or complete correction of the scoliosis with surgical excision. In contrast, patients with greater than 15 months of symptoms usually do not have a change in the scoliosis.[15] Complete resection of the lesion is invariably associated with complete elimination of osseous pain. Failure to relieve pain postoperatively has a poor prognosis for cure of the lesion and its symptoms. Indeed, persistence of pain and a positive bone scan indicate recurrence of the tumor.[10]

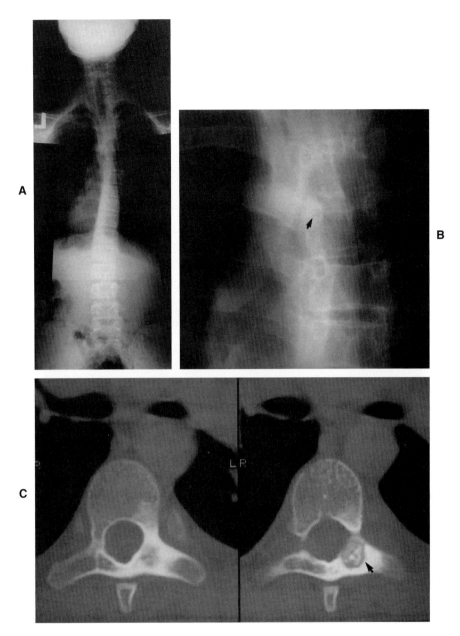

Fig. 26-1. Osteoid osteoma. **A,** This 14-year-old male presented with a painful right thoracic scoliosis of 27 degrees. **B,** Closer examination of the film shows a sclerotic left pedicle at T6 *(arrow)*, near the apex of the deformity. **C,** CT scan of the lesion at T6 shows involvement of the left pedicle and lamina. The characteristic findings of a well-defined nidus and surrounding sclerosis are present *(arrow)*. The patient is pain-free postoperatively after resection of the lesion and T5 to T7 fusion.

Osteochondroma

Osteochondromas (Fig. 26-2) likely arise from lateral displacement of aberrant growth cartilage and result in a bone-like outgrowth capped by cartilage. These lesions grow as the cartilage tip undergoes ossification. Thoracic lesions account for approximately 25% of all spinal osteochondromas. They may be solitary or multiple. Multiple lesions are known as multiple exostoses or osteochondromatosis. They can occur sporadically but usually are inherited as an autosomal dominant trait. Spinal osteochondromas show a male preponderance of 1.8:1 for multiple exostoses with an average age of 21.6 years. In contrast, solitary lesions show a greater male preponderance (3:1) and a slightly older mean age of presentation (30 years). Nine percent of patients with multiple exostoses have spinal involvement, accounting for 12% of all cases of osteochondroma. In addition, osteochondromas may be radiation-induced in children with open epiphyses and occur in 12% of cases within 8 years of treatment. The frequency increases in younger patients with higher doses of irradiation.[1]

Clinically, patients present with a painless mass. They tend to be asymptomatic unless the lesions cause compression of neurovascular structures or pathological fractures. Myelopathy occurs in 77% of patients with multiple lesions and only 34% of those with solitary lesions. The lesions usually stop growing at skeletal maturity. Pain or rapid growth may indicate malignant transformation. This occurs in less than 1% of lesions, usually to chondrosarcoma (low grade) or rarely to osteosarcoma or fibrosarcoma.

Plain radiographs show blending of the cortex of the exostosis with normal bone (see Fig. 26-2). In younger patients, the cartilage cap cannot be visualized but may be seen on CT scan. In older patients, the cap calcifies irregularly, giving a spotty appearance. Changes in the radiographic appearance, including poor definition of the lesion's margins, may indicate sarcomatous transformation. Bone scan findings correlate with the level of active ossification in relation to adjacent bone and are thus not helpful in diagnosis of this lesion. Magnetic resonance imaging (MRI) shows the cap to have a high signal density surrounded by low signal perichondrium on T2-weighted images.

Morphologically, these lesions are mushroom-shaped and may appear either sessile or pedunculated. The outer layer consists of hyaline cartilage, which by endochondral ossification forms the head and stalk. The center of the lesion is formed by mature lamellar bone.

Treatment consists of surgical excision of all symptomatic lesions. Excision may be technically difficult due to the rock-hard consistency of these lesions, and requires the use of drills or osteotomes in the vicinity of neural structures. Incomplete resection leads to recurrence that may present clinically within several months up to 14 years later. Almost all patients have a relief of symptoms postoperatively.[14,17]

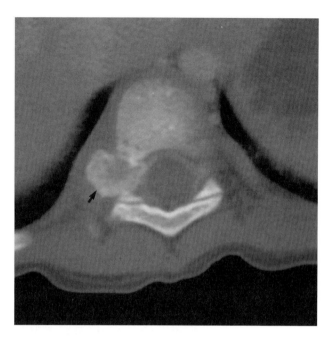

Fig. 26-2. Osteochondroma. A 4-year-old female presented with a 3-month history of severe back pain without neurological symptoms. CT scan shows a lytic, expansile lesion involving the left pedicle of T9 *(arrow)*. The patient is pain-free postoperatively after resection of the lesion and a T8 to T10 fusion.

Giant Cell Tumor

Giant cell tumors (Fig. 26-3) rarely occur in the spine. Of all recorded cases in the literature, less than 3% occur in the spine, including the sacrum. They are benign but locally aggressive lesions. Rarely, they may undergo sarcomatous transformation, usually to osteosarcoma or fibrosarcoma. A very small number of these lesions are anaplastic. This occurs more frequently with a history of irradiation. Histologically benign distant metastasis may occur, often to the lungs. Giant cell tumors present in the third to fifth decades of life with a slight female preponderance and an increased incidence in Asians. These tumors may occur in association with Paget's disease of bone, and in this setting present in the sixth decade of life.

The clinical presentation consists of local pain that is intermittent and dull in nature. There may be a tender, palpable mass. Pathological fractures may occur, resulting in more severe, acute symptoms.

On plain radiographs, these lesions are expansile, radiolucent, and may have a characteristic "soap-

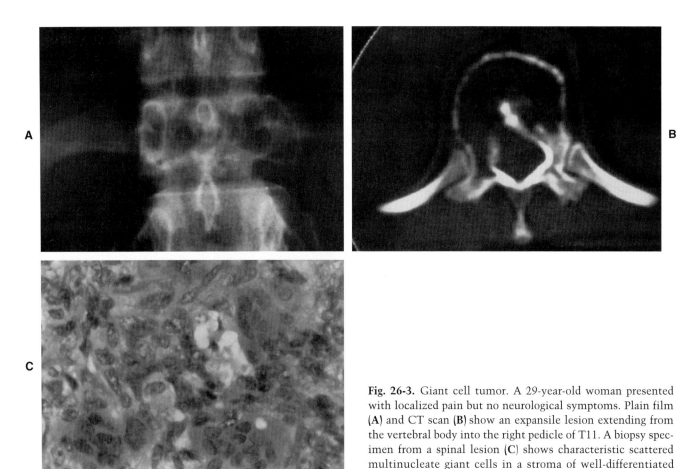

Fig. 26-3. Giant cell tumor. A 29-year-old woman presented with localized pain but no neurological symptoms. Plain film (**A**) and CT scan (**B**) show an expansile lesion extending from the vertebral body into the right pedicle of T11. A biopsy specimen from a spinal lesion (**C**) shows characteristic scattered multinucleate giant cells in a stroma of well-differentiated mononuclear cells.

bubble" appearance. The margin of osteolysis is well defined without a sclerotic rim. The periosteum is expanded and thinned; however, there is no periosteal bone formation, even with pathological fractures. There is rarely calcification within the tumor. The cortex may be broken by soft tissue invasion of the tumor. CT scans are helpful in showing bony involvement, spinal canal encroachment, and soft tissue extension. Characteristically, the cortex of the vertebra is preserved, though thinned. Angiography can be helpful because giant cell tumors are the most vascular of the benign bone tumors. MRI shows the extent of soft tissue invasion. T1-weighted images show diminished intensity while T2-weighted images may show the same or increased intensity compared to the surrounding bone. Bone scan shows intense uptake.

Morphologically, giant cell tumors are well-circumscribed, multilobular red-brown lesions with prominent areas of hemorrhage. Cyst formation may be present with foci of yellow-white necrosis. These tumors may rarely penetrate the surrounding soft tissue. They are usually solitary lesions, but may be multiple. They usually involve the vertebral body, but may involve the dorsal elements.

Histologically, these tumors are characterized by two types of cells: (1) mononuclear ovoid cells that are uniform in size with large spindle-shaped nuclei and numerous mitotic figures and (2) multinucleated giant cells that can have >100 nuclei (see Fig. 26-3).

Treatment consists of curettage and stabilization as necessary of symptomatic lesions. Angiography with embolization is useful preoperatively. Embolization may also reduce the size of these tumors. Postoperatively, angiography can be used to evaluate the efficacy of treatment and assess any revascularization of the lesion. Radiation therapy may be used postoperatively to minimize the chance of symptomatic recurrence. Patients who develop spinal cord compression may require emergent decompression. Complete resection may be possible if the lesion is well circumscribed. Even with incomplete resection, the incidence of local recurrence is less than 5%, suggesting that vertebral giant cell tumors are less aggressive than in other locations.[3,5,6,13,18]

Aneurysmal Bone Cyst

Aneurysmal bone cysts (ABCs) (Fig. 26-4) are expansile, vascular lesions with a peak occurrence in the second decade of life. ABCs occur more commonly in the dorsal elements than in the vertebral body. Half the cases involve more than one vertebra. There is a slight female preponderance.

Clinically, ABCs present with pain and swelling for a period of several months. They may grow very rapidly, often reaching an enormous size, and may rupture, causing local hemorrhage. Spinal cord or nerve root compression may occur. Pathological fractures may result from excessive replacement of normal bone.

Plain radiographs show bone resorption with cortical thinning or expansion. This is usually better visualized on CT scan (Fig. 26-4, *A*). A zone of transition between the lesion and medullary bone is poorly defined with some sclerosis. CT shows blood- or fluid-filled spaces of varying size. There may be fluid-fluid levels due to blood layering. Angiography shows the high vascularity of these lesions. MRI shows multiple septations and cysts with fluid-fluid levels with a rim of low intensity (Fig. 26-4, *B*).

Morphologically, the lesions are spongy with multiple blood-filled cysts with fibrous septae. The septae are composed of granulation tissue with multinucleated giant cells and occasional osteoid trabeculae.

Treatment of symptomatic lesions consists of surgical excision. These lesions can disappear spontaneously. Preoperatively, angiography with embolization may be used to reduce the vascularity, facilitating a more complete resection. Partial resection has a high rate of recurrence that tends to

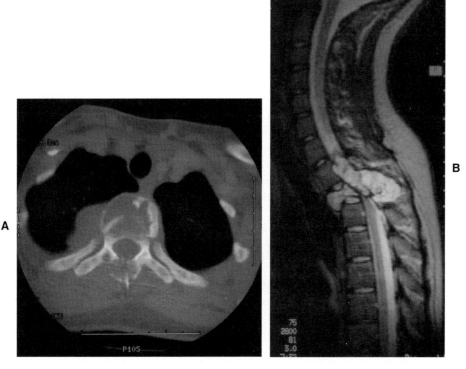

Fig. 26-4. Aneurysmal bone cyst. A 13-year-old female presented with painful scoliosis and spinal cord compression. **A,** CT scan at T2 shows expansile and lytic lesions involving the ventral and dorsal elements. **B,** Sagittal T2-weighted MRI shows vertebra planum and spinal cord compression. This patient was managed with a combined ventral (transsternal) and dorsal resection and fusion.

occur rapidly (1 to 12 months). If there is no evidence of recurrence after 1 year, then the lesion can be considered to be completely excised.[7,27]

Hemangioma

Hemangiomas (Fig. 26-5) are benign vascular tumors that are slow growing, small, and usually asymptomatic. They can involve the vertebral body or the dorsal elements. They are common, with autopsy studies showing hemangiomas in 12.5% of spines.

Although the majority of spinal hemangiomas are clinically silent, patients may present with pain or neurological deficits caused by direct extension of the tumor into the epidural space or expansion of the vertebra, causing spinal stenosis. Pathological fractures can occur, causing pain, neurological deficits, or rarely paraplegia. Rarely a palpable mass is present.

On plain radiographs, exaggerated trabeculae are seen as vertical striations. These are best visualized on lateral films and are due to bone resorption. CT myelogram or MRI show extraosseous epidural extension. MRI shows high signal intensity on T1- and T2-weighted images. Bone scan shows increased activity on the delayed phase.

The lesions are usually of the cavernous type that consist of many large vascular channels varying in size. They are separated by a scant connective

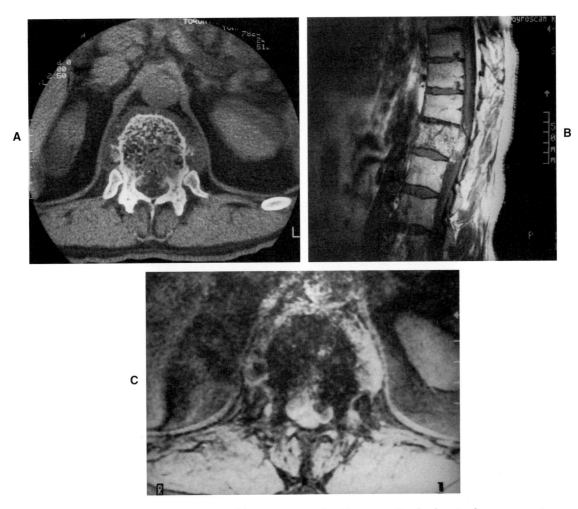

Fig. 26-5. Hemangioma. A 45-year-old man presented with progressive back pain, lower extremity weakness, and decreased sensation. **A,** CT scan shows extension of the lesion from the T12 vertebral body into the epidural space. **B** and **C,** T1-weighted MRI scans show compression of the spinal cord by the lesion. The patient underwent ventral resection, decompression, and T11 to L1 fusion. The patient's symptoms resolved postoperatively.

tissue stroma. Bone resorption is present. Occasionally, lesions are of the capillary type, which consist of closely packed aggregations of thin-walled capillaries filled with blood.

Symptomatic lesions are treated by surgical excision. Preoperatively, angiography with embolization is used to minimize the problem of excessive bleeding during the surgery. Radiotherapy has been used postoperatively to reduce recurrence.

Eosinophilic Granuloma

These are benign lesions that are usually asymptomatic but may cause pain and tenderness as the lesion erodes the bone and occasionally result in pathological fractures. They tend to occur in children between the ages of 5 and 10 years and in young adults before age 30. There is a male preponderance of 4:1. Vertebral involvement occurs in 10% to 15% of cases, affecting the vertebral body and pedicle. Multifocal disease can occur and can result in systemic syndromes: (1) Hand-Schüller-Christian disease occurs in infants and young children and consists of lytic bone lesions involving the skull, exophthalmos, and diabetes insipidus; granulomas may affect bone, orbit, hypothalamus, pleura, lung, spleen, pericardium, liver, or skin; (2) Letterer-Siwe disease is a fulminant disseminated condition of infancy that consists of skin erythema, hepatomegaly, splenomegaly, eosinophilia, and histiocytic infiltration of lymph nodes and skin.

Radiologically, three phases can be identified. First, there is the destructive phase in which spotty lucencies can be observed. Next, the collapse phase results in compression fractures. Finally, the regenerative phase occurs, resulting in residual vertebra plana. Bone scans have a lower sensitivity than plain radiographs but may be useful to detect recurrent lesions.

These lesions occur in medullary bone. They consist of expanding, erosive accumulations of histiocytes known as Langerhans' cells. They are mixed with eosinophils, lymphocytes, plasma cells, and neutrophils. Regions of necrosis may be present.

This is usually a self-limiting disease. Biopsy or curettage, followed by irradiation, frequently cause the lesion to regress. Vertebrae that have been flattened by the disease will partially regain their height. Surgical decompression is rarely indicated, as neurological deficits will resolve with conservative therapy.

MALIGNANT LESIONS
Osteosarcoma

These are high-grade, malignant tumors of mesenchymal cells. The peak incidence is between ages 10 to 20 years with a slight male preponderance. When they occur in patients over the age of 40 they are usually associated with a preexisting condition, such as Paget's disease, multiple enchondromas, multiple osteochondromas, osteomyelitis, fibrous dysplasia, or exposure to a carcinogenic influence such as irradiation. They often metastasize to lung with 30% to 40% of patients having pulmonary metastases upon presentation. They may also metastasize to bone, brain, and other distant sites. Although osteosarcomas are the second most common primary malignancy of bone, primary osteosarcomas rarely affect the spine.

Pain is the most common presenting symptom. It begins insidiously and intermittently, gradually becoming more constant in nature. Neurological symptoms are present in 70% of patients. More acute symptoms accompany pathological fractures. A firm, slightly tender soft tissue mass may be present. The serum alkaline phosphatase may be elevated. This correlates with a poorer prognosis. Neurological findings commonly occur in spinal lesions.

CT scans show the bony and soft tissue extent of the lesions that typically are expansile and lytic and/or blastic in nature. The tumors may cause pathological fractures of the vertebral body and may also involve the dorsal elements. An adjacent soft tissue mass may be ossified or have amorphous calcifications. MRI scans on T2-weighted images delineate extraosseous disease. Bone scans show increased uptake and are useful in detecting bone metastasis and multiple lesions.

The lesions are gray-white, aggressive appearing masses with focal areas of hemorrhage and cystic softening. Erosion through the cortex and periosteum is common at the time of presentation. They consist of anaplastic mesenchymal parenchyma with formation of osteoid or cartilaginous matrix. The mesenchymal cells are wildly anaplastic with atypical mitoses and hyperchromasia. In the telangiectatic type, multiple vascular channels are present.

Osteosarcomas of the spine have a very poor prognosis. Only seven of 27 patients in one study survived for greater than 1 year.[20] Chemotherapy is often used in treatment of these tumors. Angiography with embolization may also be useful. Surgical options include vertebral body resection with margins as complete as possible. These tumors usually have extracompartmental extension at presentation, thus only a limited resection may be possible. Patients with limited resection of these tumors have a poorer prognosis. Radiotherapy to the tumor bed may be of benefit postoperatively, particularly when the resection is incomplete. The response can be monitored with serial CT scans. Given the very poor prognosis for these lesions, it has been recommended to perform a biopsy and give chemotherapy to all patients. If they show evidence of response, surgical resection followed by irradiation can then be undertaken.[24]

Chondrosarcoma

Six percent of all primary chondrosarcomas occur in the spine. These lesions vary in behavior depending on the grade of tumor. Generally, they evolve slowly and metastasize late. High-grade lesions metastasize to lungs, liver, kidney, and brain. These tumors generally have a better prognosis than osteosarcomas. Seventy-five percent of the lesions arise de novo. The remainder arise from benign cartilaginous tumors, exostoses (solitary or multiple), or rarely from chondroblastomas. They occur in middle age to later in life. There is a slight male preponderance.

Due to their indolent clinical course, they present as a slowly enlarging mass for years or decades. Symptoms include back pain due to cortical expansion. Neurological symptoms are common.

Plain radiographs and CT scans show destruction of the vertebral body with possible involvement of the lamina (Fig. 26-6, *A*). The lesions are osteolytic and expansive with an irregular, well-defined margin. They progress to cortical destruction with invasion of the surrounding soft tissues. Dense, irregular, punctate calcifications are present.

Most chondrosarcomas arise centrally, but some arise subperiosteally. They consist of lobules of gray-white translucent tissue with spotty calcifications. Central necrosis leading to cyst formation may be present. The adjacent cortex is thickened or eroded. The lacunar cells show anaplasia with hyperchromatic nuclei and with two or more cells per lacuna. There are multinucleated and giant tumor cells. The lesions engulf trabeculae of normal surrounding cancellous bone. Bone formation occurs within the cartilage, in contrast to osteosarcoma (Fig. 26-6, *B*).

These tumors are resistant to radiation and chemotherapy. Surgical management consists of definitive surgical resection with wide margins. Partial or contaminated resections lead to recurrence due to spillage of neoplastic cells. Postoperative radiation is indicated when complete resection is not

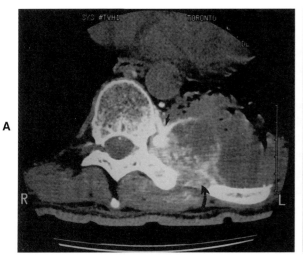
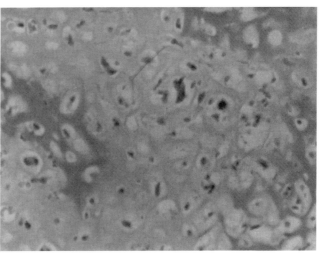

Fig. 26-6. Chondrosarcoma. A 38-year-old man presented with severe back and left thoracic radicular pain. **A,** CT scan with angiography shows the mass to the left of T9 with microcalcifications *(large arrow)* and close proximity to the artery of Adamkiewicz *(small arrow)*. **B,** Microscopic sections of this tumor show anaplastic chondrocytes. Resection of the lesion resulted in elimination of pain and did not cause any spinal cord symptoms.

possible, if there are doubts about the adequacy of the surgical margins, or if gross tumor remains. Serial CT scans are useful to detect tumor recurrence. Paraplegia often precedes death.[21,26]

Chordoma

These are rare, slow-growing malignant tumors arising from notochordal remnants in the midline, involving adjacent bone (Fig. 26-7). Chordomas are rare in the thoracic spine, with 85% involving the sacrum or skull base. They are aggressive lesions with a high rate of recurrence. They occur in patients aged 30 to 70 years. Documented metastases occur in 40% of patients to lung, lymph nodes, bone, liver, intra-abdominal viscera, or skin. Vertebral lesions tend to occur in a younger age group and they are clinically more aggressive than those found at other sites. Almost all present with epidural extension. The median survival of patients with spinal chordomas is 5 years.[23]

Clinically, patients present with pain, neurological dysfunction, and occasionally a palpable mass. These lesions occur in the midline, usually in the vertebral body, but may involve the dorsal elements. The radiographic appearance is character-ized by bony destruction and cortical expansion. A paraspinal mass may be present and calcified. Two or more vertebrae and an intervertebral disc may be involved. CT and MRI are most useful in defining the extent of the tumor.

Chordomas are infiltrative, osteodestructive, and lobulated in appearance. Microscopically, the lobules are round or oval with stomal septations. The cells are epithelial or vacuolated and are arranged in rows or cords. Malignant foci with cellular pleomorphism, hyperchromatism, and mitoses may be present.

Chemotherapy is not effective in treating chordomas. Radiation has been shown to increase the disease-free interval, prolong survival, and improve palliation.[22] The goal of surgical intervention is total resection of the tumor. Incomplete resection leads to tumor recurrence within several years. Postoperatively, high-dose radiation therapy is given. Patients succumb to the debilitating and destructive effects of locally recurring tumors rather than from widespread metastases.[4,16,28]

Multiple Myeloma

Multiple myeloma (Fig. 26-8) arises from myeloid elements in the bone marrow and is the most common primary malignant neoplasm of bone in the thoracic spine. It is twice as common in males than in females and twice as common in blacks than in whites. Seventy-five percent of cases occur in patients between the ages of 50 and 70 years. Clinical presentation before age 30 is rare. In most cases, the disease presents with disseminated lesions, commonly in extraspinal locations, but on occasion may be solitary (plasmacytoma).

Clinically, these neoplasms present with bone pain that may be severe and acute due to compression fractures. Neurological symptoms, when present, tend to appear abruptly and progress rapidly. Patients may also have anemia due to extensive marrow involvement, renal failure due to the nephrotoxicity of excessive immunoglobulins, and immunodeficiency due to the production of immunosuppressive cytokines. Myeloma neuropathy, hyperviscosity syndrome, and hypercalcemia may also be present. Diagnosis may be made by bone marrow smears and serum or urine immunoelectrophoresis. Renal failure and systemic infections are the most common causes of death.

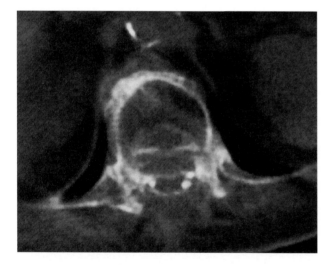

Fig. 26-7. Chordoma. A 75-year-old woman presented with lower back pain radiating to both legs. She underwent dorsal decompression and postoperative radiotherapy with relief of symptoms. Two years later her symptoms recurred. CT myelogram shows a complete block of CSF flow and tumor recurrence at T12. The patient expired intraoperatively during the fourth decompression.

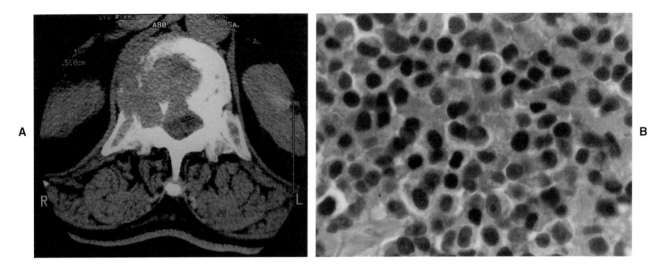

Fig. 26-8. Multiple myeloma. **A,** A 70-year-old woman with known multiple myeloma presented with severe back pain and no neurological symptoms. CT scan shows a lytic lesion involving T12. **B,** A photomicrograph of this tumor shows masses of plasma cells, most of which are mature, with some anaplastic cells.

Plain radiographs show a loss of bone density with a reduction in trabeculae and thinning of cortices. Multiple myeloma involves the vertebral bodies more than the pedicles (Fig. 26-8, *A*), due to their lack of marrow. This can help differentiate these tumors from metastatic lesions. Destruction of the dorsal elements, however, can occur. Punched-out lytic lesions with a sclerotic margin may occur but are rarer findings in the spine. Sclerosis may be of three patterns: focal, generalized, and uniform. Invasion of the soft tissues may manifest as a paraspinal extrapleural mass. MRI shows diminished signal intensity on T1-weighted images. Focal increased signal intensity on T2-weighted images indicates replacement of marrow with tumor.

Morphologically, the lesions are red, soft, and gelatinous. They consist of abnormal aggregates of plasma cells that are mostly well differentiated, but also have some anaplasia and tumor giant cells. There is destructive infiltration, invasion, and erosion of both cancellous and cortical bone. Osteolysis is mediated by the activation of osteoclasts (Fig. 26-8, *B*).

The mainstay of treatment is chemotherapy (melphalan and prednisone) and radiation. Surgical intervention is indicated for stabilization of unstable pathological fractures or when neural decompression is required despite a course of chemotherapy and radiation.[2,9,12,25]

Ewing's Sarcoma

Secondary involvement of the spine in Ewing's sarcoma is very common, particularly in patients with advanced disease (Fig. 26-9). Primary spinal lesions, excluding the sacrum, however, account for only 0.9% of all cases of Ewing's sarcoma. These tumors consist of cells of unknown cellular origin. Neoplastic transformation is associated with translocation of chromosomes 11 and 22. Ewing's sarcoma has a peak incidence in the second decade of life. There is a male preponderance of 2:1.

Clinically, patients present similarly to osteomyelitis. Findings include pain, swelling, dilated veins, fevers, neurological deficits, and a palpable mass. The erythrocyte sedimentation rate is consistently elevated.

Radiographically, a small focus of poorly-defined radiolucency is present initially. With time, large areas of bone lysis occur, eroding cancellous and cortical bone from within. Usually, periosteal new bone formation (onion skinning) is present but periosteal elevation may occur. Vertebra planum may be present. CT scan is useful in defining the soft tissue extension, bony destruction, and thecal compression (Fig. 26-9, *A*).

Morphologically, the lesions consist of soft gray-white tissue with bony expansion. The tumors may rupture into surrounding tissues. Histologically, these tumors are characterized by sheets of uniform

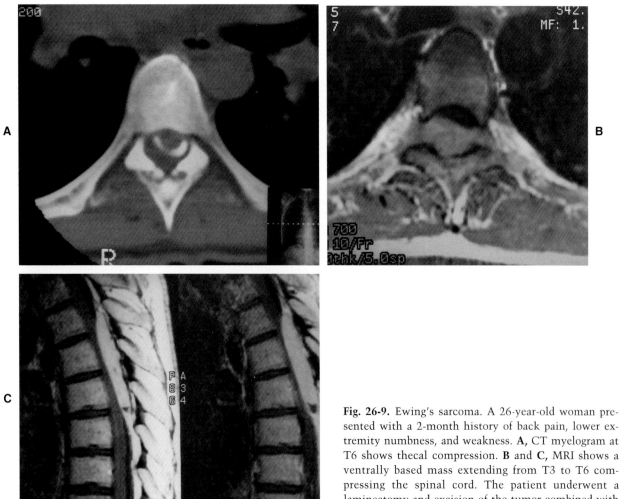

Fig. 26-9. Ewing's sarcoma. A 26-year-old woman presented with a 2-month history of back pain, lower extremity numbness, and weakness. **A,** CT myelogram at T6 shows thecal compression. **B** and **C,** MRI shows a ventrally based mass extending from T3 to T6 compressing the spinal cord. The patient underwent a laminectomy and excision of the tumor combined with postoperative chemotherapy and radiotherapy. The symptoms resolved postoperatively.

cells with rare mitotic figures that resemble lymphocytes. Lesions with greater cellular pleomorphism have a poorer prognosis. There is little intercellular stroma, and tumor necrosis may be present.

The diagnosis of Ewing's sarcoma is confirmed by biopsy. If epidural compression with rapidly progressing neurological symptoms is present, prompt surgical decompression is undertaken. If the patient is neurologically stable, chemotherapy is given. The response to chemotherapy is subsequently evaluated by clinical, radiological, and histological (if available) means. If there is a good response, further chemotherapy and radiation therapy is the definitive treatment. If, however, there is a poor response to chemotherapy, treatment consists of aggressive surgical resection in addition to chemotherapy and radiation therapy (Fig. 26-9, *B* and *C*). In pediatric patients, chemotherapy and high doses of corticosteroids with neurological monitoring is the initial therapy. Surgical resection is undertaken if there is a poor response. Surgery may also be indicated if spinal instability results from tumor resection or tumor necrosis. Prognostic factors include extent of disease, neurological symptoms, age of patient, and response to chemotherapy. Spinal lesions have a better prognosis than those occurring in sacral or pelvic sites. There is an 86% long-term survival rate and a 100% local control rate in primary spinal lesions.[8,11,19]

ACKNOWLEDGMENTS

The authors wish to thank Dr. Douglas M. Hedden, Department of Orthopaedic Surgery, Hospital for Sick Children, and Dr. Walter Montanera, Department of

Neuroradiology, The Toronto Hospital, Western Division, for contributing cases to this publication, and Dr. John Provius, Department of Pathology, The Toronto Hospital, Western Division, for help with pathology specimens.

REFERENCES

1. Albrecht S, Crutchfield JS, SeGall GK. On spinal osteochondromas. J Neurosurg 77:247-252, 1992.
2. Avrahami E, Tadmor R, Kaplinsky N. The role of T2-weighted gradient echo in MRI demonstration of spinal multiple myeloma. Spine 18:1812-1815, 1993.
3. Biagini R, De Cristofaro R, Ruggieri P, Boriani S. Giant-cell tumor of the spine. A case report. J Bone Joint Surg 72A:1102-1107, 1990.
4. Bjornsson J, Wold LE, Ebersold MJ, Laws ER. Chordoma of the mobile spine. A clinicopathologic analysis of 40 patients. Cancer 71:735-740, 1993.
5. Dahlin DC. Giant-cell tumor of vertebrae above the sacrum. A review of 31 cases. Cancer 39:1350-1356, 1977.
6. Di Lorenzo N, Spallone A, Nolletti A, Nardi P. Giant cell tumors of the spine: A clinical study of six cases, with emphasis on the radiological features, treatment and follow-up. Neurosurgery 6:29-34, 1980.
7. Dolatzas TH, Keramidas DK, Dendrinos GK. Haemothorax from aneurysmal bone cyst of the spine. J Bone Joint Surg 73B:345-346, 1991.
8. Grubb MR, Currier BL, Pritchard DJ, Ebersold MJ. Primary Ewing's sarcoma of the spine. Spine 19:309-313, 1994.
9. Jonsson B, Sjostrom L, Jonsson H, Karlstrom G. Surgery for multiple myeloma of the spine. A retrospective analysis of 12 patients. Acta Orthop Scand 63:192-194, 1992.
10. Kirwan EO, Hutton PAN, Pozo JL, Ransford AO. Osteoid osteoma and benign osteoblastoma of the spine. Clinical presentation and treatment. J Bone Joint Surg 66B:21-26, 1984.
11. Kornberg M. Primary Ewing's sarcoma of the spine. A review and case report. Spine 11:54-57, 1986.
12. Kyle RA. Multiple myeloma. Review of 869 cases. Mayo Clin Proc 50:29-39, 1975.
13. Larsson S, Lorentzon R, Boquist L. Giant-cell tumors of the spine and sacrum causing neurological symptoms. Clin Orthop Rel Res 111:201-211, 1975.
14. Marchand EP, Villemure JG, Rubin J, Robitaille Y, Ethier R. Solitary osteochondroma of the thoracic spine presenting as spinal cord compression. A case report. Spine 11:1033-1035, 1986.
15. Pettine KA, Klassen RA. Osteoid-osteoma and osteoblastoma of the spine. J Bone Joint Surg 68A:354-361, 1986.
16. Rich TA, Schiller A, Suit HD, Mankin HJ. Clinical and pathologic review of 48 cases of chordoma. Cancer 56:182-187, 1985.
17. Roblot P, Alcalay M, Cazenave-Roblot F, Levy P, Bontoux D. Osteochondroma of the thoracic spine. Report of a case and review of the literature. Spine 15:240-243, 1990.
18. Savini R, Gherlinzoni F, Morandi M, Neff JR, Picci P. Surgical treatment of giant-cell tumor of the spine. The experience at the Istituto Ortopedico Rizzoli. J Bone Joint Surg 65A:1283-1289, 1983.
19. Sharafuddin MJA, Haddad FS, Hitchon PW, Haddad SF, El-Khoury GY. Treatment options in primary Ewing's sarcoma of the spine: Report of seven cases and review of the literature. Neurosurgery 30:610-618, 1992.
20. Shives TC, Dahlin DC, Sim FH, Pritchard DJ, Earle JD. Osteosarcoma of the spine. J Bone Joint Surg 68A:660-668, 1986.
21. Shives TC, McLeod RA, Unni KK, Schray MF. Chondrosarcoma of the spine. J Bone Joint Surg 71A:1158-1165, 1989.
22. Sundaresan N. Chordomas. Clin Orthop Rel Res 204:135-142, 1986.
23. Sundaresan N, Galicich JH, Chu FC, Huvos AG. Spinal chordomas. J Neurosurg 50:312-319, 1979.
24. Sundaresan N, Rosen G, Huvos AG, Krol G. Combined treatment of osteosarcoma of the spine. Neurosurgery 23:714-719, 1988.
25. Unander-Scharin L, Waldenstrom JG, Zettervall O. Surgical treatment of myelomatosis. A review of 18 cases. Acta Med Scand 203:265-272, 1978.
26. Vanderhooft JE, Conrad EU, Anderson PA, Richardson ML, Bruckner J. Intradural recurrence with chondrosarcoma of the spine. A case report and review of the literature. Clin Orthop Rel Res 294:90-95, 1993.
27. Vandertop WP, Pruijs JEH, Snoeck IN, Van Den Hout JHW. Aneurysmal bone cyst of the thoracic spine: Radical excision with use of the Cavitron. A case report. J Bone Joint Surg 76A:608-611, 1994.
28. Walsh TM, Mayer PJ. Chordoma of the thoracic spine presenting as a second primary malignant lesion. A case report. Spine 17:1524-1528, 1992.
29. Weinstein JN, McLain RF. Primary tumors of the spine. Spine 12:843-851, 1987.

27

Metastatic Tumors

Julie E. York, M.D., David M. Wildrick, Ph.D.,
and Ziya L. Gokaslan, M.D.

According to the American Cancer Society, 1.4 million new cases of cancer are diagnosed every year. Approximately half of these patients die as a result of their illness, with the major cause of death in this patient population being complications related to metastatic disease.[10] The skeletal system is the third most common site of metastases, following lung and liver.[99] Within the skeletal system, the spinal column is the most common site of involvement.[13,14] Autopsy studies show metastatic deposits in the spinal column in up to 90% of patients with cancer. Approximately 30% of patients with neoplastic conditions present with symptomatic spinal metastases during the course of their illness, and about 20% of patients with spinal involvement have evidence of spinal cord compression at the time of their presentation.[24,118]

There is a great deal of controversy regarding the management of patients with metastatic disease of the spine. The reasons for this controversy include the lack of controlled clinical studies comparing the various treatment modalities, as well as an absence of standard criteria for evaluating the response to treatment. Early studies certainly showed no improvement in the overall outcome in patients treated with surgery relative to those treated with radiotherapy.* However, only one surgical procedure (laminectomy) was used as the basis for com-

parison with radiotherapy. Because metastatic disease involves the vertebral body in up to 80% of cases, decompression of the spinal canal by laminectomy is less than ideal. In most patients, laminectomy provides inadequate access to the part of the spinal column where the pathology is located.[44] Therefore tumor resection is usually incomplete. Furthermore, the procedure has the potential for further destabilizing the spinal column in the presence of an already existing ventral column pathology. Certainly, poor patient selection in the past may also have played a role in demonstrating no benefits from surgery.

The recent advances in cancer management are prolonging the life expectancies of patients with various types of neoplastic conditions. More effective chemotherapy regimens and, particularly, the availability of bone marrow transplantation are contributing to improvement in the survival of patients in certain disease categories. These factors are resulting in more patients surviving long enough to present with spinal involvement. With the widespread availability of computed tomography (CT) and magnetic resonance imaging (MRI), more patients are being diagnosed with spinal metastases at an earlier stage. More recently, and especially during the last decade, new surgical approaches to the spinal column have also been developed. More effective methods of spinal stabilization with both ventral and dorsal instrumentation systems have become widely available. Therefore the physicians and surgeons treating these patients have not only

---

*References 6,8,24,25,31,41,42,44,46,48,64,66,67,69,72,74, 76,78,107.

earlier and more frequent encounters with patients who have spinal metastases, but also better means of treating these patients surgically.

Aggressive surgical approaches have been shown to improve the survival and the quality of life in patients with lung, liver, and brain metastases in certain instances.[70] It is reasonable to assume that a more aggressive surgical approach to the metastatic involvement of the spinal column can potentially improve both the quality of life and survival in these patients.

The purpose of this chapter is to review the management of patients with metastatic thoracic spine disease, with particular emphasis on surgical treatment.

INCIDENCE

It has been estimated that 5% of patients with cancer will develop neoplastic spinal cord compression.[10,65,73] The annual incidence of traumatic spinal cord injury has been reported to be 3.5:100,000 patient population. Compared to this, the annual incidence of cancer-induced spinal cord injury is 8.5:100,000 patient population. Thus the calculated incidence of neoplastic paraplegia exceeds that of traumatic spinal cord injuries. Table 27-1 summarizes the incidences of spinal involvement for various tumor types seen

at The University of Texas M. D. Anderson Cancer Center between 1984 and 1994. Over this 10-year period, more than 113,000 new patients were referred with neoplastic disease. Of these, 11,884 (10.4%) were found to have metastatic disease involving the spinal column. Three major categories of primary disease—lung, breast, and prostate cancer, account for the majority of patients with metastases to the spine from solid tumors. A 30-year review of the literature published in 1988 by Brihaye[19] revealed that in 1477 patients with symptomatic metastatic disease of the spine, 16.5% of metastases arose from breast cancer, 15.6% from lung cancer, 9.2% from prostate cancer, and 6.5% from kidney cancer. The location of the primary tumor was unknown in 12.5% of these patients. In terms of disease distribution within the spinal column, many patients had multilevel involvement. However, even in those patients with multilevel disease, only one particular level was usually symptomatic.[25,44,92,107,116] The thoracic spine is the most common site for symptomatic metastases, presumably related to the relative large number of thoracic vertebrae and the small size of the thoracic spinal canal relative to the neural structures.[15,30,44,107] A published review of 1585 cases of symptomatic spinal metastasis revealed that the thoracic and thoracolumbar regions were involved in 70.3% of the cases.[19]

Table 27-1. Metastatic Disease of the Spine (The University of Texas M. D. Anderson Cancer Center* 1984-1994)

Site	Primary Tumors			Spinal Metastases	
	No. of Cases	% of Total	% With Spinal Metastases	No. of Cases	% of Total
Lung	10,568	9.3	22.8	2410	20.2
Breast	13,977	12.3	25.7	3592	30.2
Prostate	6975	6.1	16.3	1137	9.6
Colon	7107	6.2	2.6	185	1.6
Urinary tract	5692	5.0	8.4	478	4.0
Uterus	2224	2.0	0.7	16	0.1
Mouth	5174	4.5	1.4	72	0.6
Blood	12,907	11.3	9.4	1213	10.2
Pancreas	1637	1.4	0.6	10	0.1
Skin	10,844	9.5	3.4	369	3.1
Ovary	2916	2.6	0.6	17	0.1
Bone	1167	1.0	1.2	14	0.1
Unknown	4099	3.6	8.4	344	2.9
Other	28,544	25.1	7.1	2027	17.1
Total	113,831			11,884	

*Patient population identified through a search of the Tumor Registry maintained by the Department of Medical Informatics.

Metastatic tumors producing spinal cord compression in children are histologically and biologically different from those of adults.[65] Ewing's sarcoma and neuroblastoma are the most common tumors causing spinal cord compression in children. They account for greater than 50% of cases, followed by osteogenic sarcoma and rhabdomyosarcoma.[65] Most pediatric tumors invade the spinal canal through the neural foramina, rather than by extending from within the vertebral body.[99]

PATHOPHYSIOLOGY

A number of experimental models have been developed to study the pathophysiology of spinal cord compression by epidural metastases.[58,95,97,100,101,102,103] It has been demonstrated that the first step that occurs with an expanding epidural mass is obstruction of the epidural venous plexus. This leads to vasogenic edema within the white matter and myelin destruction.[58,117] A variety of insults to the central nervous system (CNS) lead to the release of arachidonic acid from membrane phospholipids and to the formation of prostaglandins.[97,98] Experimental rat models of neoplastic spinal cord compression show a significant increase in prostaglandin E_2 (PGE_2) production in the compressed segments of the spinal cord. This production appears to precede edema formation, thus implicating PGE_2 as a mediator in the formation of vasogenic edema.[95,97,98,100,101,102,103] Additional studies have suggested that certain serotonin receptors mediate some of the deleterious consequences observed in the compressed spinal cord by a mechanism not coupled to PGE_2 synthesis.[97,98] This early stage is considered to be reversible,[58] and if the spinal cord is surgically or medically decompressed at this stage it is likely that spinal cord function will return. In cases where the axons have already undergone demyelination, patients will take longer to regain their functional capacity. As the tumor mass increases, mechanical compression of the spinal cord leads to a reduction in blood flow. When the spinal cord blood flow decreases to a critical level, spinal cord ischemia ensues, leading to cytotoxic edema and cell death.[58,95,97,100,101,102,103] Thus loss of spinal cord function is probably the result of the combined effects of compression, ischemia, and myelin loss.[117] As expected, at this late stage, decompression is not effective in restoring neurological function.

Table 27-2. Symptoms in Patients Presenting with Spinal Metastases

Clinical Presentation	%
Pain	96
Weakness	76
Sensory loss	50
Autonomic dysfunction	57
Other	7

Modified from Gilbert RW, Kim JH, Posner JB. Epidural Spinal Cord Compression from Metastatic Tumor. Ann Neurol 3:40-51, 1978.

CLINICAL PRESENTATION

Patients with spinal metastases most commonly present with pain as their chief complaint.[44] By the time of diagnosis, neurological dysfunction exists in the majority of patients (Table 27-2). Rarely, a patient will present with a mass lesion. As the use of imaging studies to screen cancer patients has become more widespread, more patients are presenting with asymptomatic spinal lesions. Management of patients with asymptomatic spinal metastases, especially those who harbor chemo- or radioresistant tumors such as renal cell cancer, remains controversial.

The issue of pain deserves further attention, as it has significant clinical implications in terms of surgical treatment. In the past, surgical intervention has been directed toward the restoration of neurological function or prevention of further neurological decline, and has not been focused on alleviating pain. Prior to the use of spinal instrumentation for stabilization, pain could not be relieved as effectively and actually worsened after many of the decompressive procedures.

Three types of pain are encountered in cancer patients who have metastatic spinal involvement. The first is local pain. This pain is constant, and generally there is no worsening with movement nor any improvement with recumbency. Imaging studies usually reveal no evidence of vertebral body collapse or spinal deformity. However, enlargement of the vertebral body is often evident. The cause of this local pain has been attributed to periosteal stretching of the vertebral body from an expansile mass. In these patients, radiation therapy may be of benefit in relieving pain, particularly if the patient harbors a radiosensitive tumor. It is believed that radiation therapy causes reduction in tumor mass and therefore relief of the periosteal stretching.

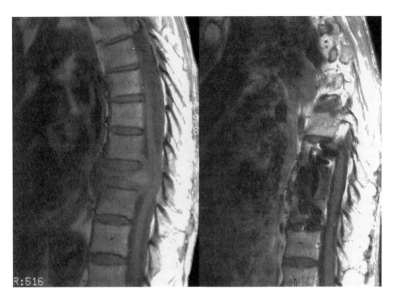

Fig. 27-1. Preoperative and postoperative sagittal MRI of a patient who underwent vertebrectomy with ventral stabilization for metastatic lung cancer invading the T9 vertebral body. This patient presented with typical axial spinal pain, which was alleviated with surgical resection and spinal stabilization. The postoperative image *(right)* illustrates the well-aligned, decompressed spinal column with minimal artifact generation from either the ventral plates and screws or the methylmethacrylate spacer.

The second type of pain seen in this patient population is axial spinal pain, which is a significant cause of morbidity (Fig. 27-1). It is a mechanical pain and is the result of structural abnormality in the spinal column. This type of pain worsens with movement and is relieved with recumbency. When the patient lies down, the pain is usually significantly improved. Imaging studies usually reveal vertebral body collapse and/or spinal deformity. Because the cause of axial spine pain is spinal instability, for obvious reasons spinal stabilization is usually very effective in relieving the pain. Radiation therapy is of no benefit in alleviating the discomfort in these patients.

The final category of pain is the radicular type, which is related to compression of a nerve root. It is usually constant, but may be worsened or relieved with movement. The pain occurs in a dermatomal distribution and is usually associated with dysesthesia. The cause of this type of pain is nerve root compression, either as a result of the tumor mass or produced by a bony fragment and/or disc from a compression fracture. Depending upon the cause, the nerve root may be decompressed either surgically or with the use of chemotherapy and/or radiation treatment. This type of pain can usually be controlled quite satisfactorily with the appropriate treatment.

Neurological dysfunction is the second most common presentation in patients with thoracic spinal metastases. Because the thoracic spinal canal is relatively small in proportion to the spinal cord inside the space, spinal compression here occurs early in the course of the illness. The patient may present with motor dysfunction leading to weakness in both lower extremities. Sensory loss can occur as a result of compression of the dorsal columns or spinothalamic tracts. Dorsal column dysfunction is manifested by loss of proprioception and vibration sense in the lower extremities. Autonomic dysfunction, including bowel, bladder, and sexual dysfunction, is present in approximately half of patients at the time of diagnosis.[22]

DIAGNOSIS/PREOPERATIVE WORKUP

Most spinal metastases are osteolytic, although those from breast and prostate tumors can cause osteoblastic or sclerotic lesions.[87] In the evaluation of patients with cancer metastatic to the spine, a variety of radiographic studies are utilized. Plain radiographs reveal vertebral metastases in about 85% of adults who have symptomatic metastatic epidural compression,[10,44,107] with the frequency of bony abnormality depending upon the tumor type. In a published series of patients with metastatic disease, plain radiographs were abnormal in 94% of patients with breast cancer and 74% of patients with lung cancer. The vertebral body, and specifically its dorsal portion, is the earliest and most commonly involved portion of the spinal column. Whereas pedicle destruction is the most common radiographic finding, loss of contours of the pedicle occurs rather late in the metastatic process and often accompanies extensive destruction of the trabecular bone within the vertebral body.[18,59,74] In fact, it has been shown that 50% to 70% of the trabecular bone must be destroyed before lysis is visible on plain radiographs.[2,32,87] An indistinct dorsal vertebral body margin is a subtle radiographic finding suggestive of epidural metastatic disease. Plain radiographs remain an important tool in assessing the alignment of the spinal column. When necessary, dynamic radiographic studies are obtained to assess stability.

The myelogram was previously the procedure of choice for identifying epidural mass lesions; however, MRI has now become the preferred imaging technique. Myelography depicts displacement and compression of the spinal cord and/or nerve roots, although the extent of disease outside of the spinal column cannot be determined. The utility of myelography can be increased by obtaining a postmyelogram CT. CT scans provide good bone detail, and the postmyelogram CT provides a more direct visualization of the compressive mass within the spinal column relative to the myelogram alone.[62] At the present time, there is little need for myelography, although it does have an added advantage of permitting cerebrospinal fluid (CSF) collection at the time of the procedure. Relevant CSF studies include cell count, determination of protein content, and cytopathological examination. Cytological studies may reveal the tumor type if it lies in the subarachnoid space and may also diagnose leptomeningeal carcinomatosis. Lumbar puncture performed below the level of a high-grade block causing rapid neurological deterioration has been reported in 14% of patients.[56] Considering the excellent results obtainable with other imaging studies and the ease with which they are obtained, the use of myelography is usually limited to cases where there is a delay in obtaining an MRI, or where the patient has a contraindication to MRI, such as claustrophobia, extreme obesity, or the presence of a pacemaker or previously placed stainless steel hardware in the area of interest.

Bone scans are very sensitive in detecting alterations in local metabolism associated with osseous metastatic lesions and serve as a practical and simple tool to screen cancer patients for skeletal involvement.[40,60,87,91] However, bone scans are nonspecific and can be abnormal in cases of trauma, infection, and degenerative disease.[85,87]

The definitive imaging study of choice in most patients is MRI, because it is even more sensitive than bone scans in detecting vertebral metastases.[45,87,105] It allows visualization of the relation of the tumor mass to the neural structures and soft tissues in multiple planes and is minimally invasive. Contrast-enhanced MRI is especially helpful in detecting leptomeningeal metastases and may also provide additional information regarding epidural lesions.[22] Benign compression fractures can usually be distinguished from pathological causes with MRI. Benign compression fractures, such as those associated with osteoporosis, have a marrow signal intensity that is isointense with normal vertebrae on all sequences. Pathological fractures show low signal on T1-weighted sequences and high signal on T2-weighted sequences relative to uninvolved vertebrae.[7] Involvement of the pedicle is more common with pathological compression fractures.[87] A radiological feature that can be helpful in distinguishing neoplastic destruction of the vertebral body from vertebral osteomyelitis is the condition of the intervertebral disc. Although the vertebral body may be destroyed by the neoplastic process, the intervertebral disc is usually maintained because it is resistant to invasion by tumor. Although MRI findings are helpful in differentiating osteoporotic fractures from pathological ones, CT-guided needle biopsy may eventually be needed to establish the diagnosis.

The CT scan has one important advantage over MRI that must be recognized. It provides excellent visualization of the bone. This becomes particularly important if one is planning to use radiation therapy as the primary treatment modality in the presence of spinal cord compression. If the compressive pathology is a tumor mass, radiotherapy may be effective in relieving the pressure. However, if the CT scan reveals a retropulsed bone or disc fragment, surgical decompression is the only treatment option (Fig. 27-2).

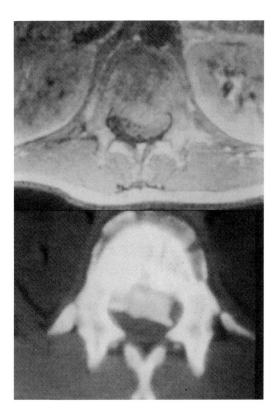

Fig. 27-2. Preoperative MRI and CT scans of a patient with multiple myeloma who presented with acute back pain. MRI *(top)* shows a ventral mass compressing the neural elements. CT *(bottom)* scan of the same patient demonstrates a burst type fracture with a retropulsed bone fragment. This patient was treated with a surgical decompression/stabilization, and would not have benefited from radiation therapy.

Preoperative spinal angiography and preoperative embolization can be invaluable in certain cases, especially with tumors that are known to be vascular, such as renal cell carcinomas, thyroid tumors, sarcomas, and myelomas[20,110] (Fig. 27-3). Several reports in the literature have demonstrated that with the use of preoperative arterial embolization, resectability of a variety of tumor types is enhanced as a result of the reduction in intraoperative blood loss.[20]

MANAGEMENT

The management of metastatic disease of the spine is controversial because there are few good controlled studies in the literature comparing the available treatment modalities. Because cure is usually beyond expectations for most patients, palliation is a reasonable goal in the management of patients with spinal metastases. Preservation or restoration of neurological function and adequate pain relief are the criteria of successful therapy. The only surgical procedure that has been used for comparison with nonsurgical treatments in the past is laminectomy, which is a very ineffective procedure for spinal cord decompression in the cancer setting.[11,21,29,50,54,79,88,90,94,106] The two main reasons for poor results following laminectomy are (1) the posterior approach rarely provides adequate exposure

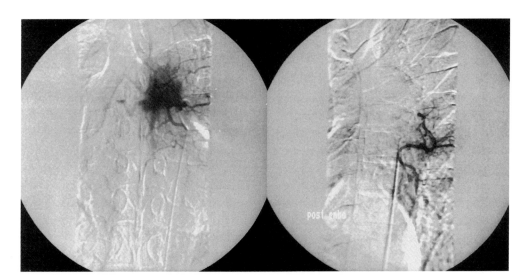

Fig. 27-3. Pre- and postembolization spinal angiogram of a patient with renal cell carcinoma metastatic to the midthoracic spine. A robust vascular blush observed with injection of corresponding segmental vessel completely resolved following embolization with Gelfoam particles.

for resection of the metastatic lesion, which is most often located in the vertebral body, and (2) laminectomy can cause or worsen spinal instability. In the majority of these patients, cancer has already destroyed a portion of the spinal column, and laminectomy further destabilizes the spine. Several reviews have shown that in patients with spinal metastases, over 80% of these lesions are located in the vertebral body.[96] Any attempt to resect this ventrally-located lesion from a dorsal approach in order to decompress the spinal cord is fraught with difficulty. Sound methods of spinal stabilization were not widely available in the past, thus limiting spine surgeons' ability to resect these tumors in a radical manner. Whether from a lack of understanding of the metastatic process or lack of available spinal instrumentation techniques, it is not surprising that these early studies showed no advantage to the use of surgical intervention over radiation therapy alone.

Certain events have taken place over the past decade that significantly impact the management of metastatic spinal disease. MRI and CT allow for the early diagnosis of spinal metastases, including asymptomatic disease. More effective chemotherapy regimens are available, resulting in longer survival from the patients' primary cancers and therefore more metastases. New surgical approaches have been developed in the past decades, along with more effective methods of spinal reconstruction and instrumentation that together have revolutionized the management of metastatic disease of the spine. In selecting the optimal therapeutic approach for patients with metastatic tumors of the spinal column, the three major categories of options are medical, radiation, and surgical treatments.

The use of steroids in the treatment of spinal cord compression is widely accepted.[15,44,96,115] The reasons for their efficacy are multiple. They provide dramatic pain relief, and in most patients, the neurological dysfunction is arrested or may be reversed.[26,95,101,102,113,115] Steroids should be instituted immediately upon the diagnosis of spinal cord compression because they may benefit the patient by relieving pain and improving neurological function. Ushio et al.[113] reported a reduction in spinal cord edema and an improvement in the neurological function of rats harboring a neoplastic spinal cord compression who were treated with 10 mg/kg dexamethasone twice daily. Clinical studies have demonstrated no difference in neurological outcome between high- and low-dose steroid protocols, but greater pain relief has been seen with high-dose steroids.[47,114] Greenberg, Kim, and Posner[47] reported a rapid and complete relief of pain in the majority of patients after the initiation of high-dose steroids (100 mg bolus followed by 24 mg every 6 hours). There are, of course, inherent complications related to the long-term use of steroids that need to be factored into the decision-making process. The authors advocate the use of high-dose steroids in the presence of significant spinal cord dysfunction.

Aside from the use of steroids, the real question is whether radiation therapy or surgery should be the front-line treatment for metastatic disease of the spine. Beginning with radiotherapy alone, Table 27-3 lists the studies published from 1966 through 1995. Over this 29-year period, results from a total of 996 patients are reported. The reported rate of neurological improvement with radiotherapy alone is 43%; however, 19% of the patients worsened neurologically during the course of radiotherapy or immediately afterward. The results are somewhat better for radiosensitive tumors, such as lymphoma, myeloma, and neuroblastoma.[9] The outlook is less favorable for tumors less sensitive to radiotherapy, including lung carcinoma, melanoma, and sarcoma.[9]

The published series for laminectomy, with or without radiotherapy, are listed in Table 27-4. As indicated previously, dorsal decompression is not an effective procedure for decompression of the spinal cord in the majority of patients. In almost 2000 patients reported in the literature, the neurological improvement rate was only 44%—not much different than the rate for radiotherapy alone. Thirteen percent of the patients treated with laminectomy worsened neurologically, with an overall mortality rate of approximately 8%. Wound infection rates as high as 35% are reported with laminectomy.[96] The results of these types of analyses are the basis for the opinion that is held by many oncologists, that surgery rarely has a role in the first-line treatment of metastatic spinal tumors.

Table 27-5 summarizes the results of laminectomy combined with dorsal stabilization for the management of spinal metastases. Again, dorsal decompression is not often the most efficacious surgical procedure for the management of spinal metastases, although with the addition of spinal stabilization, surgeons were perhaps provided the

Table 27-3. Results of Treatment for Spinal Cord Compression: Radiotherapy Alone

Authors	Year	No. of Patients	% Improved Motor	% Worse
Mones, Dozier, and Berrett[80]	1966	41	34	–
Kahn et al.[61]	1967	82	42	–
Cobb, Leavens, and Eckles[24]	1977	18	50	22
Marshall and Langfitt[76]	1977	29	41	21
Gilbert, Kim, and Posner[44]	1978	130	49	–
Greenberg, Kim, and Posner[47]	1980	83	57	7
Stark, Henson, and Evans[107]	1982	31	35	–
Constans et al.[25]	1983	108	39	26
Obbens et al.[83]	1984	83	28	23
Harrison et al.[53]	1985	33	27	36
Bach et al.[6]	1990	149	35	18
Maranzano and Latini[75]	1995	209	76	0
Mean		–	43	19
Total		996		

Updated from Siegal T, Siegal T. Surgical management of malignant epidural tumors compressing the spinal cord. In Schmidek HH, Sweet WH, eds. Operative Neurosurgical Techniques. Indications, Methods, and Results. Philadelphia: WB Saunders, 1995, pp 186-193.

Table 27-4. Results of Treatment for Spinal Cord Compression: Laminectomy With or Without Radiotherapy

Authors	Year	No. of Patients	% Improved Motor	% Worse	% Mortality
Hall and Mackay[48]	1973	129	30	–	–
Brady et al.[17]	1975	90	61	–	–
Merrin et al.[78]	1976	22	22	0	0
Cobb, Leavens, and Eckles[24]	1977	26	46	23	–
Marshall and Langfitt[76]	1977	17	29	–	–
Gianotta and Kindt[42]	1978	33	30	18	12
Gilbert, Kim, and Posner[44]	1978	65	45	–	–
Kleinman, Kiernan, and Michelsen[66]	1978	20	15	5	15
Livingston and Perrin[74]	1978	100	77	–	9
Gorter[46]	1978	31	39	–	13
Baldini et al.[8]	1979	140	30	19	0
Dunn et al.[31]	1980	104	33	23	10
Levy et al.[72]	1982	39	82	15	8
Stark, Henson, and Evans[107]	1982	84	37	–	–
Constans et al.[25]	1983	465	46	13	–
Klein, Richer, and Schafer[64]	1984	194	54	16	–
Kollmann et al.[67]	1984	103	56	–	–
Garcia-Picazo et al.[41]	1990	53	41	–	–
Bach et al.[6]	1990	91	59	11	–
Landmann, Hunig, and Gratzl[69]	1992	127	58	2	–
Mean			44	13	8
Total		1933			

Updated from Siegal T, Siegal T. Surgical management of malignant epidural tumors compressing the spinal cord. In Schmidek HH, Sweet WH, eds. Operative Neurosurgical Techniques. Indications, Methods, and Results. Philadelphia: WB Saunders, 1995, pp 186-193.

opportunity to more effectively resect the tumor and consider the issue of spinal instability. The neurological recovery rate increased to 65%, and the issue of pain relief is addressed in the majority of articles. These studies reveal a remarkable 89% improve-ment in pain. In previous studies, an assessment of pain was not routinely reported, possibly because without spinal instrumentation axial pain cannot be relieved. Morbidity and mortality rates are accept-able for those studies in which they were reported.

Table 27-5. Results of Treatment for Spinal Cord Compression: Laminectomy and Stabilization

Authors	Year	No. of Patients	% Improved Motor	% Improved Pain	% Mortality
Brunon et al.[21]	1975	20	—	100	—
Hansebout and Blomquist[50]	1980	82	84	100	—
Miles et al.[78]	1984	23	65	100	—
DeWald et al.[29]	1985	17	45	65	6
Overby and Rothman[88]	1985	12	75	—	—
Solini et al.[106]	1985	33	48	—	3
Heller et al.[54]	1986	33	70	79	—
Perrin and McBroom[90]	1987	200	82	80	8
Olerud and Jonsson[84]	1996	51	≥38	100	0
Bauer[11]	1997	67	76	—	0
Mean			65	89	3
Total		538			

Updated from Siegal T, Siegal T. Surgical management of malignant epidural tumors compressing the spinal cord. In Schmidek HH, Sweet WH, eds. Operative Neurosurgical Techniques. Indications, Methods, and Results. Philadelphia: WB Saunders, 1995, pp 186-193.

Table 27-6. Results of Treatment for Spinal Cord Compression: Vertebral Body Resection and Stabilization

Authors	Year	No. of Patients	% Improved Motor	% Improved Pain	% Mortality
Slatkin and Posner[104]	1982	29	56	60	7
Harrington[52]	1984	52	65	80	6
Siegal and Siegal[96]	1985	61	80	91	6
Sundaresan et al.[109]	1985	101	70	85	8
Onimus et al.[86]	1986	36	72	97	6
Perrin and McBroom[90]	1987	21	95	90	5
Moore and Uttley[81]	1989	26	62	71	30
Sundaresan et al.[108]	1991	54	100	90	6
Hall and Webb[49]	1991	15	86	—	20
Fidler[37]	1994	18	93	94	20
Hosono et al.[55]	1995	90	81	94	0
Mean			78	85	10
Total		503			

Updated from Siegal T, Siegal T. Surgical management of malignant epidural tumors compressing the spinal cord. In Schmidek HH, Sweet WH, eds. Operative Neurosurgical Techniques. Indications, Methods, and Results. Philadelphia: WB Saunders, 1995, pp 186-193.

Table 27-6 summarizes the results for vertebral body resection as the primary mode of decompression, followed by spinal stabilization in most cases. An impressive 78% of the patients improved neurologically, with a large proportion of the patients reporting an improvement in pain. All of this was accomplished with an acceptable morbidity and mortality rate.

In summary, the published literature supports a pathology-directed approach for the treatment of metastatic spinal disease. The addition of spinal stabilization appears to be critical in improving overall neurological recovery rate and relieving axial spinal pain.[37,49,57,81,86,90,96,104,108,109]

INDICATIONS FOR RADIOTHERAPY

Radiation therapy, the aim of which is to palliate pain and prevent irreversible neurological complications, has long been the initial therapy of choice for patients with spinal metastases. Radiotherapy has been shown to relieve pain in up to 50% of patients with spinal cord compression and to produce neurological improvement in approximately 40% of patients who have metastatic spinal cord compression (see Table 27-3). The most important prognostic factor in determining functional outcome in these patients is the level of neurological function at the initiation of radiation therapy.[71] The majority of ambulatory patients retain their ability to walk after radiation therapy, whereas the rate of ambulation recovery in patients who are paraplegic at presentation is less than 5%.[44] From the published literature, it is difficult to determine how various factors such as tumor biology, radiosensitivity, and degree of spinal column involvement impact the outcome of radiotherapy. A large prospective study demonstrated that early diagnosis of metastatic spinal cord compression was the primary predictor of outcome. Tumor histology influenced outcome only when the diagnosis of spinal involvement was delayed.[75] Tolerance of the thoracic spinal cord to radiation has been reported to be less than at other levels, but more recent reviews discount this finding.[36] Therefore at present there is no objective reason to support poorer tolerance of the thoracic spine to radiation. It is reasonable to consider that radiotherapy is indicated if the patient has a radiosensitive or moderately radiosensitive tumor, there is no evidence of spinal instability or bony compression, and the patient is in satisfactory or stable neurological condition.

After the decision is made to proceed with radiotherapy, the question of timing still remains. A number of studies have shown that radiation therapy has a deleterious effect on bone formation, fracture healing, and graft incorporation.[16,33] Bouchard et al.[16] studied the effects of the timing of radiotherapy on dorsal bone graft healing in a rabbit model. They found that grafts irradiated preoperatively or immediately postoperatively had less histological evidence of bony fusion and were biomechanically weaker. Delayed radiotherapy (day 21) did not have a significant impact on bony fusion or biomechanical strength, compared to nonradiated grafts. Ventral spinal fusions may be more resistant to the adverse effects of radiotherapy.[16,33] Emery et al.[33] used a canine model to study the effects of radiation on graft healing using a ventral strut model. Their results were similar to Bouchard's except that preoperative radiotherapy did not have a significant influence on bone healing or strength of graft for ventral spinal fusions. Reasons for the difference in results between ventral and dorsal fusion rates may relate to a better blood supply to the vertebral body and the ventral graft being under compression, rather than distraction. Additionally, the healing process in dorsal grafts is more dependent upon the status of surrounding tissue, and this tissue is dele-teriously affected by radiation.[16,33] The authors advocate 3 to 4 weeks of delay following surgical intervention prior to initiation of radiation therapy if a bone graft has been placed during surgery.

INDICATIONS FOR SURGERY

The goals of surgery are restoration or preservation of neurological function, immediate stabilization of the spine, pain relief, and a potential cure in selected patients who have a single, purely intraosseous metastatic lesion. Surgical intervention, including tumor resection and spinal reconstruction with stabilization, is indicated if (1) the patient has a radioresistant tumor, (2) there is evidence of instability or bony compression, (3) the patient is neurologically compromised, or (4) the patient has a recurrence despite previous radiotherapy. It has been suggested that curative resection may be considered when the metastasis is limited to the vertebral body.[109]

Multiple series have attempted to delineate the factors that are important in determining surgical success, but the criteria for selecting patients with metastatic spinal disease for surgery remain rather ill-defined.[9] Tokuhashi et al.[112] reported an interesting scoring system for preoperative prognostic assessment of patients with metastases to the spine. Each of six parameters were given a score of 0 (high risk) to 2 (low risk), for a possible total of 12 points. Utilizing this scoring system (outlined in Table 27-7), they found that in 113 patients studied, 92% of the patients who scored less than six points survived less than 6 months, whereas 78% of the patients who scored greater than eight points survived more than 1 year. The utility of this scoring system was recently assessed by Enkaoua et al.[34] in a retrospective study. They concluded that the Tokuhashi preoperative score was a useful prognostic indicator, although they proposed reducing the score assigned to metastases of unknown origin.

There is no consensus regarding the life expectancy required to justify surgical intervention. Requirements of 3 to 6 months expected survival have been proposed, although it is frequently difficult to accurately determine life expectancy for any given patient. Each patient needs to be assessed individually. Tatsui et al.[111] recently studied the survival of patients diagnosed with metastatic spinal tumors. Serial bone scans were performed on 2372 patients,

Table 27-7. Evaluation System for the Prognosis of Patients With Metastatic Spine Tumors

	Score
General Condition (performance status)	
Poor	0
Moderate	1
Good	2
Number of Extraspinal Bone Metastatic Foci	
≥3	0
1–2	1
0	2
Number of Metastases in the Vertebral Body	
≥3	0
2	1
1	2
Metastases to the Major Internal Organs	
Unresectable	0
Resectable	1
No metastases	2
Primary Site of the Cancer	
Lung, stomach	0
Kidney, liver, uterus, others, unidentified	1
Thyroid, prostate, breast, rectum	2
Spinal Cord Injury	
Complete	0
Incomplete	1
None	2

Modified from Tokuhashi Y, Matsuzaki H, Kawano H, Sano S. The indication of operative procedure for a metastatic spine tumor: A scoring system for the preoperative evaluation of the prognosis. Nippon Seikeigeka Gakkai Zasshi—Journal of the Japanese Orthopaedic Association 68:379-389, 1994.

beginning at the time each was initially diagnosed with a primary neoplasm. During the follow-up, 425 patients were found to have spinal metastases. The 1-year survival rate, beginning at the time of metastatic spinal disease diagnosis, ranged from 22% in lung cancer to 83% in prostate cancer.

When assessing a patient's general physical condition, hematological and nutritional status must be considered. Many patients have bone marrow suppression with leukopenia and thrombocytopenia from chemotherapy or radiation therapy.[5] Patients who are malnourished or who have previously irradiated tissues are at increased risk for infection and poor wound healing. Irradiated nonhealing wounds in the thoracic region present a difficult problem.[43]

Exposure of the underlying bone and hardware can be disastrous. Various techniques of plastic surgical closure for dorsal spinal wounds have been described.[23,43] These include latissimus dorsi and trapezius rotational flaps. In addition, a number of free flap options are available to the plastic surgeon. A paramedian, as opposed to a midline, incision has been advocated in those patients who have received radiation therapy previously.[99] The authors advocate early consultation with plastic surgeons in treating patients who have received prior radiation, to minimize the chance of wound complications associated with the dorsal approach.

Most series suggest that motor function recovery following 24 to 48 hours of complete paraplegia is very unlikely; yet, the pediatric population tends to have a better prognosis.[4,6,55] The Frankel classification has been proposed to document the ambulatory capacity of patients with spinal cord compression.[39] A visual analog pain scale is a simple method of documenting the patient's pain status and response to treatment.

INDICATIONS FOR STABILIZATION

The definition, and therefore management, of spinal instability in the setting of metastatic cancer is controversial. Although much has been written regarding the management of spinal fractures, most reports address traumatic injury as opposed to metastatic involvement. Denis's three-column spine concept is widely accepted as the biomechanical model for thoracolumbar spine fractures and has application to neoplastic involvement of the spinal column.[27,28,89] His concept evolved from a retrospective review of thoracolumbar injuries and observations on spinal instability. He defined the ventral column as the ventral one half of the vertebral body, the ventral annulus fibrosus, and the anterior longitudinal ligament; the middle column consists of the dorsal one half of the vertebral body, dorsal annulus fibrosus and posterior longitudinal ligament; the dorsal column consists of the pedicles, laminae, ligamenta flava, and interspinous and supraspinous ligaments.

Criteria for spinal instability secondary to trauma are generally accepted as (1) ≥ two-column injury, (2) >50% collapse of vertebral body height, (3) > 20 to 30 degree kyphotic angulation, or (4) involvement of the same column in two or more adjacent levels.[27,63]

Additional factors that should be considered in patients with neoplastic disease of the thoracic spine are the quality of surrounding bony and ligamentous structures and the ability of the patient's spine to heal. The thoracic rib cage and the orientation of facet joints at the level of the thoracic spine create a relatively protected spinal region. However, the thoracic spinal cord and segmental nerves are contained in a narrow canal, and any compromise of the available space may result in profound neurological deficit.[63] The cervicothoracic and thoracolumbar junctions represent high-stress regions of the spine. Normally the cervical and lumbar spine segments assume lordotic curvatures. The interposed kyphotic curvature of the thoracic spine predisposes the spine to exaggerated stresses of increased bending moments at each of the two junctional regions.[63] The relatively abrupt changes in regional mechanics between the mobile cervical, rigid thoracic, and mobile lumbar spine segments increase the risk of fracture and instability at the cervicothoracic and thoracolumbar regions.[27,28,63] These considerations have significant implications for spinal stabilization.

A systematic approach to assess spinal stability in patients with metastatic disease of the thoracic spine should include the preoperative studies outlined previously, as well as consideration of the iatrogenic spinal instability that may be unavoidably caused during the approach to, or resection of, the tumor. Performing a laminectomy in a patient who has metastatic involvement of either the ventral or middle columns will result in instability. By definition, a two-column injury (and therefore an unstable spinal injury) is created when performing a vertebrectomy, regardless of the state of the dorsal column. Both of these examples may require spinal instrumentation for stabilization, although in selected cases, vertebrectomy and reconstruction alone (without additional fixation) can provide satisfactory support, provided the rib cage is intact.

SELECTION OF SURGICAL APPROACH

The surgical approaches to the thoracic spine (see box) may be divided into those that provide access ventrally (vertebrectomy), dorsally (laminectomy), and dorsolaterally (costotransversectomy). The position and extent of the tumor with respect to the spinal column will determine which approach is

SURGICAL APPROACHES	
Laminectomy	All levels
Transpedicular	All levels
Costotransversectomy	All levels
Vertebrectomy	
Median sternotomy	T1 to T2
"Trap door" exposure	T3 to T4
Dorsolateral thoracotomy	T5 to T11
Thoracoabdominal approach	T12 to L1

most appropriate (Fig. 27-4). As metastases to the spine usually involve the dorsal portion of the vertebral body and cause spinal cord compression by extending dorsally, tumor resection most often requires a vertebrectomy. Therefore a ventral approach usually provides the best access in patients with metastatic involvement of the spinal column. The exact surgical approach taken to perform a vertebrectomy depends upon the level at which the metastasis resides (Fig. 27-5). A vertebrectomy can be performed in the high thoracic (C7 to T2) spine through a median sternotomy or a costotransversectomy. The trap door exposure, described by Nazzaro, Arbit, and Burt[82] is a ventral method for exposing lesions in the high thoracic region involving T3 and T4 levels. This exposure combines a standard ventral approach to the cervical spine along the sternocleidomastoid muscle with both a partial median sternotomy and a ventrolateral thoracotomy. In the mid- and lower thoracic spine, lesions that are primarily ventral or ventrolateral can be effectively approached through a dorsolateral thoracotomy. A thoracoabdominal approach provides exposure for decompression and stabilization in the thoracolumbar region.

A dorsolateral approach is especially effective when the tumor wraps around the spinal cord circumferentially. Tumor and/or retropulsed bone from a compression fracture can be adequately decompressed, and supplemental dorsal fixation can be performed during the same procedure (Fig. 27-6).

A dorsal approach (laminectomy) can be performed at any spinal level. A tumor confined to the lamina, which is a very uncommon finding, can be effectively removed with a laminectomy. Occasionally, a patient cannot tolerate a ventral procedure because of his or her medical condition, and it is necessary to utilize a dorsal approach even though the pathology is located ventrally.

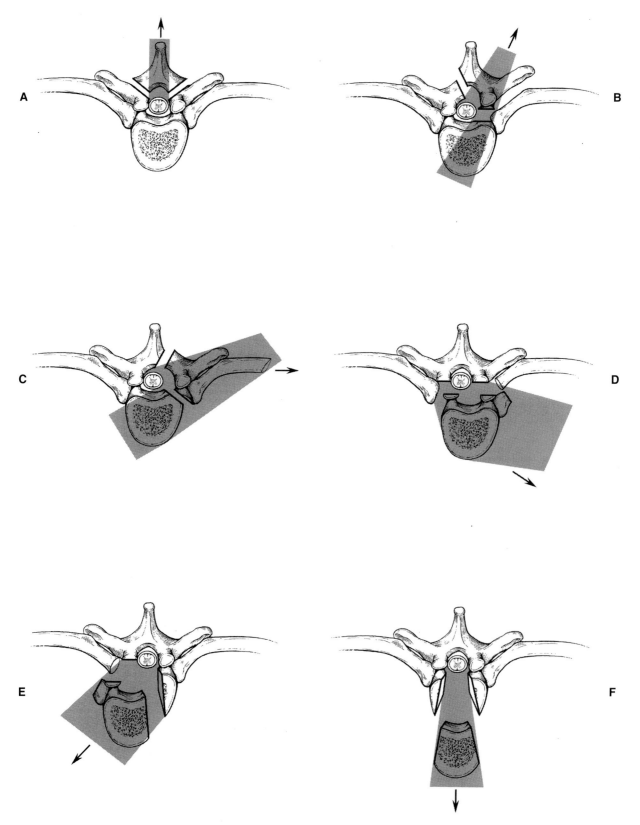

Fig. 27-4. Artist's illustrations showing various routes available to the surgeon, bone elements removed, and field of view. Optimal surgical approach is dictated by the location of pathology. **A,** Laminectomy (strictly dorsal involvement). **B,** Transpedicular (dorsolateral involvement). **C,** Costotransversectomy (dorsolateral and lateral involvement). **D,** Vertebrectomy via dorsolateral thoracotomy (T5 to T12) (strictly ventral involvement). **E,** Vertebrectomy via "trap door" exposure (T3 to T4) (strictly ventral involvement). **F,** Vertebrectomy via median sternotomy (T1 to T2) (strictly ventral involvement).

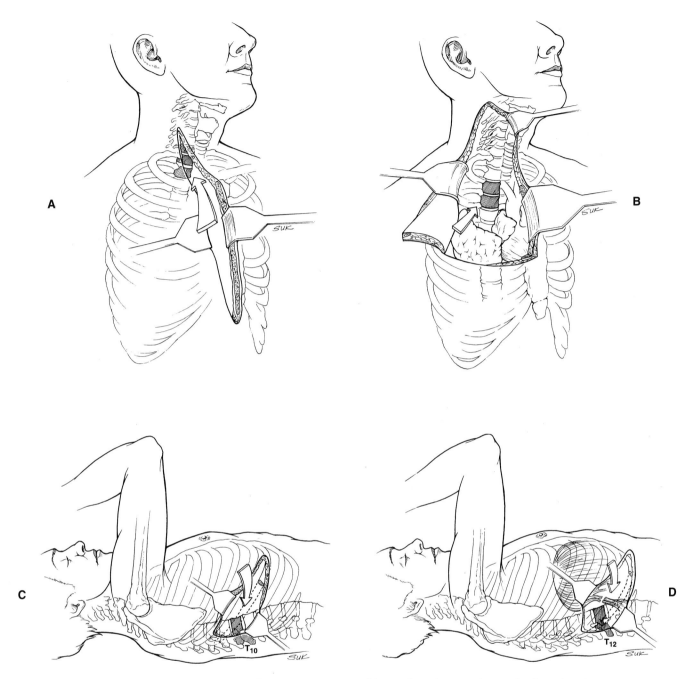

Fig. 27-5. Artist's illustrations showing various ventral/ventrolateral approaches to the thoracic spine, depending upon the level(s) involved with neoplastic process. **A,** Ventrolateral surgical approach combined with median sternotomy for lesions at C7 through T2. **B,** "Trap door" exposure (ventrolateral cervical approach combined with median sternotomy and ventrolateral thoracotomy) for tumors located at T3 through T4. **C,** Dorsolateral thoracotomy for lesions at T5 through T11. **D,** Thoracoabdominal approach for lesions located at the thoracolumbar junction. Crus of the diaphragm is taken down to expose this region.

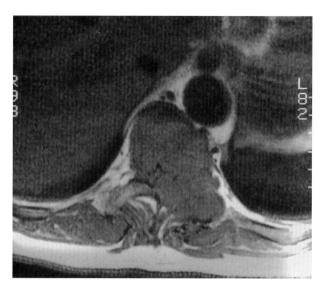

Fig. 27-6. Axial MRI demonstrating a metastatic thyroid cancer involving primarily the dorsal/dorsolateral elements in which a dorsolateral surgical approach is most appropriate.

RECONSTRUCTION/STABILIZATION OF THE THORACIC SPINAL COLUMN

As mentioned previously, the goals of surgical intervention include (1) decompression of neural structures, (2) reduction of anatomical deformity, and (3) rigid fixation. Ventrally, cervicothoracic and upper thoracic spine stabilization is performed using locking plate and screw constructs, provided that the ventral column can be reconstructed. The cervicothoracic junction is a high-stress region, and in the presence of severe kyphosis, supplemental dorsal fixation may be necessary. Several options for dorsal stabilization are available. These include hooks, rods, and Wisconsin wires, cables, or plates with lateral mass and/or pedicle screws (Fig. 27-7). The remainder of the thoracic spine can be stabilized ventrally using a ventral thoracolumbar plate and screws (Fig. 27-8). The standard dorsal method for stabilizing the midthoracic spine involves the use of hooks and rods in a claw configuration above and below the lesion (Fig. 27-9), although segmental fixation with a Luque rectangle and sublaminar wires/cables has also been used successfully.[1,77] The thoracolumbar junction, another high-stress area, can be stabilized dorsally with a combination of hooks, rods, and pedicle screws. If a significant spinal deformity exists at the thoracolumbar junction, both ventral and dorsal fixation should be used

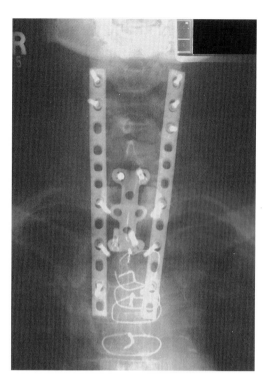

Fig. 27-7. Anteroposterior (AP) cervicothoracic radiograph of a patient who underwent ventral and dorsal tumor resection and stabilization procedures for circumferential metastatic osteogenic sarcoma of T1. Whereas cervical plate and screw constructs can be used for ventral fixation of this region, cervical lateral mass plates, combined with thoracic pedicle screws, are effective means of dorsal fixation.

to achieve a long-lasting, durable, construct for weight bearing (Fig. 27-10).

Reconstruction of the spinal column following vertebrectomy is required in order to obtain a stable construct. The vertebral body may be replaced with bone, methylmethacrylate, or spacers.[3,29,35,50,51,57] For patients in whom a long survival is expected, a bone graft is optimal, because this probably provides the greatest chance for fusion and long-term stability. Reconstruction with methylmethacrylate is often appropriate in cancer patients. Various methods of fixation have been proposed to anchor methylmethacrylate to the vertebral bodies rostral and caudal to the vertebrectomy defect. These include Steinmann pins, fixation screws, and chest tube techniques.[35,38,68,109] We believe the technique described by Errico and Cooper[35] provides the best method of reconstruction with methylmethacrylate. With this method, one can anchor the methylmethacrylate spacer to the normal vertebral bodies above and below in a solid manner. Because there is

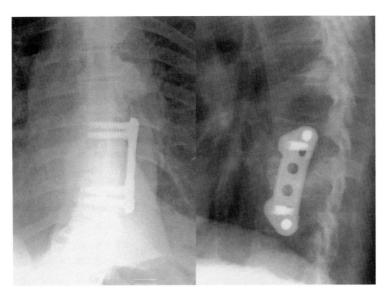

Fig. 27-8. AP and lateral radiographs of a patient with metastatic lung cancer who underwent T9 vertebrectomy, reconstruction with methylmethacrylate, and ventral fixation with a thoracolumbar locking plate and screws.

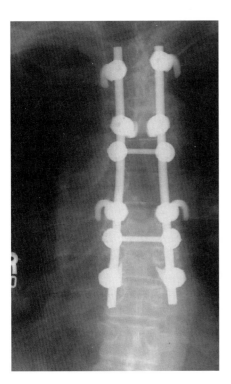

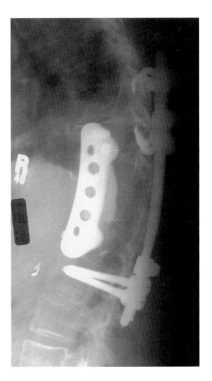

Fig. 27-9. AP radiograph of a patient with metastatic melanoma confined to the dorsal elements who underwent a T6 through T7 laminectomy and bilateral facet removal, resection of tumor, and dorsal thoracic fixation using hooks and rods in a typical claw configuration above and below the lesion.

Fig. 27-10. Lateral thoracolumbar radiograph of a patient with metastatic thyroid cancer who underwent T11 and T12 vertebrectomy, reconstruction with methylmethacrylate, and fixation with a thoracolumbar plate and screws. Because of severe preexisting kyphosis, supplemental dorsal instrumentation was carried out using pedicle screws, hooks, and rods.

no need for Steinmann pins or screws for anchorage, artifact formation on postoperative MRI is not an issue. Methylmethacrylate, when used ventrally following a vertebrectomy, is very stable in compression. However, in most cases we recommend additional ventral fixation (plate and screws inserted into rostral and caudal vertebral bodies) to prevent distraction failure.

The feasibility of ventral vertebral resection and replacement with methylmethacrylate was first reported in 1967 by Scoville.[93] There has been no convincing evidence in the literature that the presence of methylmethacrylate interferes with local radiation therapy, nor that radiation affects the compressibility, shear strength, or durability of methylmethacrylate. This reconstruction technique is ideal in the cancer setting because it achieves immediate stabilization following radical tumor resection, allowing patients to ambulate without any external orthosis and permitting the administration of radiation therapy without delay.

CONCLUSION

In conclusion, the treatment of patients with metastatic disease of the thoracic spine should be individualized depending upon many factors, including location of the pathology, radiosensitivity of the tumor, and general condition and life expectancy of the patient. Early diagnosis and intervention improve the patient's likelihood of remaining or becoming ambulatory following treatment. Management must be balanced in terms of medical, radiation, and surgical treatment options, realizing that surgical resection with spinal reconstruction and stabilization has the potential for playing a major role in improving the quality of life in certain patients with metastatic disease of the spinal column.

REFERENCES

1. Akeyson EW, McCutcheon IE. Single-stage posterior vertebrectomy and replacement combined with posterior instrumentation for spinal metastasis. J Neurosurg 85:211-220, 1996.
2. Algra PR, Heimans JJ, Valk J, Nauta JJ, Lachniet M, Van Kooten B. Do metastases in vertebrae begin in the body or the pedicles? Imaging study in 45 patients. AJR 158:1275-1279, 1992.
3. Ammirati M, Sundaresan N, Lane JM. Technique of vertebral body resection and stabilization for the treatment of spinal metastases. Surgical Rounds: 21-34, 1985.
4. Ampil FL. Epidural compression from metastatic tumor with resultant paralysis. J Neurooncol 7:129-136, 1989.
5. Asdourian PL. Metastatic disease of the spine. In Bridwell KH, DeWald RL, eds. The Textbook of Spinal Surgery, vol 2. Philadelphia: JB Lippincott, 1991, pp 1187-1241.
6. Bach F, Larsen BH, Rohde K, Borgesen SE, Gjerris F, Boge-Rasmussen T, Agerlin N, Rasmusson B, Stjernholm P, Sorensen PS. Metastatic spinal cord compression. Occurrence, symptoms, clinical presentations and prognosis in 398 patients with spinal cord compression. Acta Neurochir (Wien) 107:37-43, 1990.
7. Baker LL, Goodman SB, Perkash I, Lane B, Enzmann DR. Benign versus pathologic compression fractures of vertebral bodies: Assessment with conventional spin-echo, chemical-shift, and STIR MR imaging. Radiology 174:495-502, 1990.
8. Baldini M, Tonnarelli GP, Princi L, Vivenza C, Nizzoli V. Neurological results in spinal cord metastases. Neurochir 22:159-165, 1979.
9. Barcena A, Lobato RD, Rivas JJ, Cordobes F, de Castro S, Cabrera A, Lamas E. Spinal metastatic disease: Analysis of factors determining functional prognosis and the choice of treatment. Neurosurgery 15:820-827, 1984.
10. Barron K, Hirano A, Araki S, Tery R. Experiences with metastatic disease involving the spinal cord. Neurology 9:91-106, 1959.
11. Bauer HC. Posterior decompression and stabilization for spinal metastases. Analysis of sixty-seven consecutive patients. J Bone Joint Surg 79A:514-522, 1997.
12. Bauer HC, Wedin R. Survival after surgery for spinal and extremity metastases. Prognostication in 241 patients. Acta Orthop Scand 66:143-146, 1995.
13. Berrettoni BA, Carter JR. Mechanisms of cancer metastasis to bone. J Bone Joint Surg 68A:308-312, 1986.
14. Bhalla SK. Metastatic disease of the spine. Clin Orthop 73:52-60, 1970.
15. Black P. Spinal metastasis: Current status and recommended guidelines for management. Neurosurgery 5:726-746, 1979.
16. Bouchard JA, Koka A, Bensusan JS, Stevenson S, Emery SE. Effects of irradiation on posterior spinal fusions. A rabbit model. Spine 19:1836-1841, 1994.
17. Brady LW, Antonaides J, Prasasvinichai S, Torpie RJ, Asbell SO, Glassburn JR, Schatanoff D, Mancall EL. The treatment of metastatic disease of the nervous system by radiation therapy. In: Seydel HG, ed. Tumors of the Nervous System. New York: John Wiley and Sons, 1975:176–188.
18. Brice J, McKissock W. Surgical treatment of malignant extradural spinal tumours. Br Med J 1:1341, 1965.
19. Brihaye J, Ectors P, Lemort M, Van Houtte P. The management of spinal epidural metastases. Adv Tech Stand Neurosurg 16:121-176, 1988.
20. Broaddus WC, Grady MS, Delashaw JB, Jr, Ferguson RD, Jane JA. Preoperative superselective arteriolar embolization: A new approach to enhance resectability of spinal tumors. Neurosurgery 27:755-759, 1990.
21. Brunon J, Satreaux JL, Sinday M, Fischer G. Posterior osteosynthesis in the treatment of spinal cord tumors. Neurochirurgie 21:435-446, 1975.
22. Byrne TN. Spinal cord compression from epidural metastases. N Engl J Med 327:614-619, 1992.
23. Casas LA, Lewis VL, Jr. A reliable approach to the closure of large acquired midline defects of the back. Plast Reconstr Surg 84:632-641, 1989.
24. Cobb CAI, Leavens ME, Eckles N. Indications for nonoperative treatment of spinal cord compression due to breast cancer. J Neurosurg 47:653-658, 1977.

25. Constans JP, de Divitiis E, Donzelli R, Spaziante R, Meder JF, Haye C. Spinal metastases with neurological manifestations. Review of 600 cases. J Neurosurg 59:111-118, 1983.

26. Delattre JY, Arbit E, Thaler HT, Rosenblum MK, Posner JB. A dose-response study of dexamethasone in a model of spinal cord compression by epidural tumor. J Neurosurg 70:920-925, 1989.

27. Denis F. The three column spine and its significance in the classification of acute thoracolumbar spinal injuries. Spine 8:817-831, 1983.

28. Denis F. Spinal instability as defined by the three-column spine concept in acute spinal trauma. Clin Orthop 189:65-76, 1984.

29. DeWald RL, Bridwell KH, Prodromas C, Rodts MF. Reconstructive spinal surgery as palliation for metastatic malignancies of the spine. Spine 10:21-26, 1985.

30. Dommisse GF. The blood supply of the spinal cord. A critical vascular zone in spinal surgery. J Bone Joint Surg 56B:225-235, 1974.

31. Dunn RC, Jr, Kelly WA, Wohns RN, Howe JF. Spinal epidural neoplasia. A 15-year review of the results of surgical therapy. J Neurosurg 52:47-51, 1980.

32. Edelstyn GA, Gillespie PJ, Grebbell FS. The radiological demonstration of osseous metastases. Experimental observations. Clin Radiol 18:158-162, 1967.

33. Emery SE, Brazinski MS, Koka A, Bensusan JS, Stevenson S. The biological and biomechanical effects of irradiation on anterior spinal bone grafts in a canine model. J Bone Joint Surg 76B:540-548, 1994.

34. Enkaoua EA, Doursounian L, Chatellier G, Mabesoone F, Aimard T, Saillant G. Vertebral metastases. A critical appreciation of the preoperative prognostic Tokuhashi score in a series of 71 cases. Spine 22:2293-2298, 1997.

35. Errico TJ, Cooper PR. A new method of thoracic and lumbar body replacement for spinal tumors: Technical note. Neurosurgery 32:678-680; 680-681, 1993.

36. Faul CM, Flickinger JC. The use of radiation in the management of spinal metastases. J Neurooncol 23:149-161, 1995.

37. Fidler MW. Radical resection of vertebral body tumours. A surgical technique used in ten cases. J Bone Joint Surg 76B:765-772, 1994.

38. Fielding JW, Pyle RN, Jr, Fietti VG, Jr. Anterior cervical vertebral body resection and bone-grafting for benign and malignant tumors. A survey under the auspices of the Cervical Spine Research Society. J Bone Joint Surg 61A:251-253, 1979.

39. Frankel HL, Hancock DO, Hyslop G, Melzak J, Michaelis LS, Ungar GH, Vernon JD, Walsh JJ. The value of postural reduction in the initial management of closed injuries of the spine with paraplegia and tetraplegia. I. Paraplegia 7:179-192, 1969.

40. Galasko CS. Skeletal metastases. Clin Orthop 210:18-30, 1986.

41. Garcia-Picazo A, Capilla Ramirez P, Pulido Rivas P, Garcia de Sola R. Utility of surgery in the treatment of epidural vertebral metastases. Acta Neurochir (Wien) 103:131-138, 1990.

42. Gianotta SL, Kindt GW. Metastatic spinal cord tumors. Clin Neurosurg 25:495-503, 1978.

43. Giesswein P, Constance CG, Mackay DR, Manders EK. Supercharged latissimus dorsi muscle flap for coverage of the problem wound in the lower back. Plast Reconstr Surg 94:1060-1063, 1994.

44. Gilbert RW, Kim JH, Posner JB. Epidural spinal cord compression from metastatic tumor: Diagnosis and treatment. Ann Neurol 3:40-51, 1978.

45. Godersky JC, Smoker WR, Knutzon R. Use of magnetic resonance imaging in the evaluation of metastatic spinal disease. Neurosurgery 21:676-680, 1987.

46. Gorter K. Results of laminectomy in spinal cord compression due to tumors. Acta Neurochir (Wien) 42:177-178, 1978.

47. Greenberg HS, Kim JH, Posner JB. Epidural spinal cord compression from metastatic tumor: Results with a new treatment protocol. Ann Neurol 8:361-366, 1980.

48. Hall AJ, Mackay NNS. The results of laminectomy for compression of the cord or cauda equina by extradural malignant tumors. J Bone Joint Surg 55B:497-505, 1973.

49. Hall DJ, Webb JK. Anterior plate fixation in spine tumor surgery. Indications, technique, and results. Spine 16:S80-S83, 1991.

50. Hansebout RR, Blomquist GA. Acrylic spinal fusion. J Neurosurg 53:606-612, 1980.

51. Harrington KD. The use of methylmethacrylate for vertebral-body replacement and anterior stabilization of pathological fracture-dislocations of the spine due to metastatic malignant disease. J Bone Joint Surg 63A:36-46, 1981.

52. Harrington KD. Anterior cord decompression and spinal stabilization for patients with metastatic lesions of the spine. J Neurosurg 61:107-117, 1984.

53. Harrison KM, Muss HB, Ball MR, McWhorter M, Case D. Spinal cord compression in breast cancer. Cancer 55:2839-2844, 1985.

54. Heller M, McBroom RJ, MacNab T, Perrin R. Treatment of metastatic disease of the spine with posterolateral decompression and Luque instrumentation. Neuroorthopedics 2:70-74, 1986.

55. Helweg-Larsen S, Rasmusson B, Soelberg-Sorensen P. Recovery of gait after radiotherapy in paralytic patients with metastatic epidural spinal cord compression. Neurology 40:1234-1236, 1990.

56. Hollis PH, Malis LI, Zappulla RA. Neurological deterioration after lumbar puncture below complete spinal subarachnoid block. J Neurosurg 64:253-256, 1986.

57. Hosono N, Yonenobu K, Fuji T, Ebara S, Yamashita K, Ono K. Vertebral body replacement with a ceramic prosthesis for metastatic spinal tumors. Spine 20:2454-2462, 1995.

58. Ikeda H. Ushio Y, Hayakawa T, Mogami H. Edema and circulatory disturbance in the spinal cord compressed by epidural neoplasms in rabbits. J Neurosurg 52:203-209, 1980.

59. Jacobson JG, Poppel MH, Shapiro JH. The vertebral pedicle sign. AJR 80:817, 1958.

60. Joo KG, Parthasarathy KL, Bakshi SP, Rosner D. Bone scintigrams: Their clinical usefulness in patients with breast carcinoma. Oncology 36:94-98, 1979.

61. Kahn FR, Glicksman AS, Chu FC, Nickson JJ. Treatment by radiotherapy of spinal cord compression due to extradural metastases. Radiology 89:495-500, 1967.

62. Kamholtz R, Sze G. Current imaging in spinal metastatic disease. Semin Oncol 18:158-169, 1991.

63. Kern MB, Malone DG, Benzel EC. Evaluation and surgical management of thoracic and lumbar instability. Contemp Neurosurg 18:1-8, 1996.

64. Klein HJ, Richer HP, Schafer M. Extradural spinal metastases. A retrospective study of 197 patients. Adv Neurosurg 12:36-43, 1984.

65. Klein SL, Sanford RA, Muhlbauer MS. Pediatric spinal epidural metastases. J Neurosurg 74:70-75, 1991.

66. Kleinman WB, Kiernan HA, Michelsen WJ. Metastatic cancer of the spinal column. Clin Orthop 136:166-172, 1978.

67. Kollman H, Diemath HE, Strohecker J, Spatz H. Spinal metastases as the first manifestation. Adv Neurosurg 12:44-46, 1984.

68. Kostuik JP, Errico TJ, Gleason TF, Errico CC. Spinal stabilization of vertebral column tumors. Spine 13:250-256, 1988.

69. Landmann C, Hunig R, Gratzl O. The role of laminectomy in the combined treatment of metastatic spinal cord compression. Int J Radiat Oncol Biol Phys 24:627-631, 1992.

70. Lang FF, Sawaya R. Surgical management of cerebral metastases. Neurosurg Clin N Am 7:459-484, 1996.

71. Leviov M, Dale J, Stein M, Ben-Shahar M. Ben-Arush M, Milstein D, Goldsher D, Kuten A. The management of metastatic spinal cord compression: A radiotherapeutic success ceiling. Int J Radiat Oncol Biol Phys 27:231-234, 1993.

72. Levy WJ, Latchaw JP, Jr, Hardy RW, Hahn JP. Encouraging surgical results in walking patients with epidural metastases. Neurosurgery 11:229-233, 1982.

73. Lewis DW, Packer RJ, Raney B, Rak IW, Belasco J, Lange B. Incidence, presentation, and outcome of spinal cord disease in children with systemic cancer. Pediatrics 78:438-443, 1986.

74. Livingston KE, Perrin RG. The neurosurgical management of spinal metastases causing cord and cauda equina compression. J Neurosurg 49:839-843, 1978.

75. Maranzano E, Latini P. Effectiveness of radiation therapy without surgery in metastatic spinal cord compression: Final results from a prospective trial. Int J Radiat Oncol Biol Phys 32:959-967, 1995.

76. Marshall LF, Langfitt TW. Combined therapy for metastatic extradural tumors or the spine. Cancer 40:2067-2070, 1977.

77. McAfee PC, Bohlman HH, Ducker T, Eismont FJ. Failure of stabilization of the spine with methylmethacrylate. A retrospective analysis of twenty-four cases. J Bone Joint Surg 68A:1145-1157, 1986.

78. Merrin C, Avellanosa A, West C, Wajsman Z, Baumgartner G. The value of palliative spinal surgery in metastatic urogenital tumors. J Urol 115:712-713, 1976.

79. Miles J, Banks AJ, Dervin E, Noori Z. Stabilisation of the spine affected by malignancy. J Neurol Neurosurg Psychiatry 47:897-904, 1984.

80. Mones RJ, Dozier D, Berrett A. Analysis of medical treatment of malignant extradural spinal cord tumors. Cancer 19:1842-1853, 1966.

81. Moore AJ, Uttley D. Anterior decompression and stabilization of the spine in malignant disease. Neurosurgery 24:713-717, 1989.

82. Nazzaro JM, Arbit E, Burt M. "Trap door" exposure of the cervicothoracic junction. Technical note. J Neurosurg 80:338-341, 1994.

83. Obbens EA, Kim JH, Thaler H, Deck MD, Posner JB. Metronidazole as a radiation enhancer in the treatment of metastatic epidural spinal cord compression. J Neurooncol 2:99-104, 1984.

84. Olerud C, Jonsson B. Surgical palliation of symptomatic spinal metastases. Acta Orthop Scand 67:513-522, 1996.

85. O'Mara RE. Bone scanning in osseous metastatic disease. JAMA 229:1915-1917, 1974.

86. Onimus M. Schraub S, Bertin D, Bosset JF, Guidet M. Surgical treatment of vertebral metastasis. Spine 11:883-891, 1986.

87. Osborn AG. Diagnostic Neuroradiology. St. Louis: Mosby-Year Book, 1994, p 936.

88. Overby MC, Rothman AS. Anterolateral decompression for metastatic epidural spinal cord tumors. Results of a modified costotransversectomy approach. J Neurosurg 62:344-348, 1985.

89. Panjabi MM, Oxford TR, Kifune M, Arand M, Wen L, Chen A. Validity of the three-column theory of thoracolumbar features. A biomechanic investigation. Spine 20:1122-1127, 1995.

90. Perrin RG, McBroom RJ. Anterior versus posterior decompression for symptomatic spinal metastases. Can J Neurol Sci 14:75-80, 1987.

91. Roberts JG, Gravelle IH, Baum M, Bligh AS, Leach KG, Hughes LE. Evaluation of radiography and isotopic scintigraphy for detecting skeletal metastases in breast cancer. Lancet 1:237-239, 1976.

92. Ruff RL, Lanska DJ. Epidural metastases in prospectively evaluated veterans with cancer and back pain [published erratum appears in Cancer 66:935, 1990]. Cancer 63:2234-2241, 1989.

93. Scoville WB, Palmer AH, Sandra K, Chong G. The use of acrylic plastic for vertebral replacement or fixation in metastatic disease of the spine: Technical note. J Neurosurg 27:274-279, 1967.

94. Sherman RPM, Waddell JP. Laminectomy for metastatic epidural spinal tumors. Posterior stabilization, radiotherapy and postoperative assessment. Clin Orthop 207:55-63, 1986.

95. Siegal T, Shohami E, Shapira Y, Siegal T. Indomethacin and dexamethasone treatment in experimental neoplastic spinal cord compression. II. Effect on edema and prostaglandin synthesis. Neurosurgery 22:334-339, 1988.

96. Siegal T, Siegal T. Surgical decompression of anterior and posterior malignant epidural tumors compressing the spinal cord: A prospective study. Neurosurgery 17:424-432, 1985.

97. Siegal T, Siegal T. Participation of serotonergic mechanisms in the pathophysiology of experimental neoplastic spinal cord compression. Neurology 41:574-580, 1991.

98. Siegal T, Siegal T. Serotonergic manipulations in experimental neoplastic spinal cord compression. J Neurosurg 78:929-937, 1993.

99. Siegal T, Siegal T. Surgical management of malignant epidural tumors compressing the spinal cord. In Schmidek HH, Sweet WH, eds. Operative Neurosurgical Techniques. Indications, Methods, and Results, vol 2, 3rd ed. Philadelphia: WB Saunders, 1995, pp 1997-2025.

100. Siegal T, Siegal T, Lossos F. Experimental neoplastic spinal cord compression: Effect of anti-inflammatory agents and glutamate receptor antagonists on vascular permeability. Neurosurgery 26:967-970, 1990.

101. Siegal T, Siegal T, Shapira Y, Sandbank U, Catane R. Indomethacin and dexamethasone treatment in experimental neoplastic spinal cord compression. I. Effect on water content and specific gravity. Neurosurgery 22:328-333, 1988.

102. Siegal T, Siegal T, Shohami E, Shapira Y. Comparison of soluble dexamethasone sodium phosphate with free dexamethasone and indomethacin in treatment of experimental neoplastic spinal cord compression. Spine 13:1171-1176, 1988.

103. Siegal T, Siegal TZ, Sandbank U, Shohami E, Shapira J, Gomori GM, Ben-David E, Catane R. Experimental neoplastic spinal cord compression: Evoked potentials, edema,

prostaglandins, and light and electron microscopy. Spine 12:440-448, 1987.

104. Slatkin NE, Posner JB. Management of spinal epidural metastases. Clin Neurosurg 17:698-716, 1982.

105. Smoker WR, Godersky JC, Knutzon RK, Keyes WD, Norman D, Bergman W. The role of MR imaging in evaluating metastatic spinal disease. AJR 149:1241-1248, 1987.

106. Solini A, Paschero B, Orsini G, Guercio N. The surgical treatment of metastatic tumors of the lumbar spine. Ital J Orthop Traumatol 11:427-442, 1985.

107. Stark RJ, Henson RA, Evans SJ. Spinal metastases. A retrospective survey from a general hospital. Brain 105:189-213, 1982.

108. Sundaresan N, DiGiacinto GV, Hughes JE, Cafferty M, Vallejo A. Treatment of neoplastic spinal cord compression: results of a prospective study. Neurosurgery 29:645-650, 1991.

109. Sundaresan N, Galicich JH, Lane JM, Bains MS, McCormack P. Treatment of neoplastic epidural cord compression by vertebral body resection and stabilization. J Neurosurg 63:676-684, 1985.

110. Sundaresan N, Scher H, DiGiacinto GV, Yagoda A, Whitmore W, Choi IS. Surgical treatment of spinal cord compression in kidney cancer. J Clin Oncol 4:1851-1856, 1986.

111. Tatsui H, Onomura T, Morishita S, Oketa M, Inoue T. Survival rates of patients with metastatic spinal cancer after scintigraphic detection of abnormal radioactive accumulation. Spine 21:2143-2148, 1996.

112. Tokuhashi Y, Matsuzaki H, Kawano H, Sano S. The indication of operative procedure for a metastatic spine tumor: A scoring system for the preoperative evaluation of the prognosis. Nippon Seikeigeka Gakkai Zasshi 68:379-389, 1994.

113. Ushio Y, Posner R, Posner JB, Shapiro WR. Experimental spinal cord compression by epidural neoplasm. Neurology 27:422-429, 1977.

114. Vecht CJ, Haaxma-Reiche H, van Putten WL, de Visser M. Vries EP, Twijnstra A. Initial bolus of conventional versus high-dose dexamethasone in metastatic spinal cord compression. Neurology 39:1255-1257, 1989.

115. Weissman DE. Glucocorticoid treatment for brain metastases and epidural spinal cord compression: A Review. J Clin Oncol 6:543-551, 1988.

116. Weissman DE, Dufer D, Vogel V, Abeloff MD. Corticosteroid toxicity in neurooncology patients. J Neurooncol 5:125-128, 1987.

117. Welch WE, Jacobs JB. Surgery for metastatic spinal disease. J Neurooncol 23:163-169, 1995.

118. Wong DA, Fornasier VL, MacNab I. Spinal metastases: The obvious, the occult, and the imposters. Spine 15:1-4, 1990.

28

Radiation Therapy and Chemotherapy

Thomas A. Buchholz, M.D., Natalie S. Callander, M.D., and John H. Schneider, M.D.

For nearly 100 years, metastatic disease involvement of the thoracic spine has been a common and difficult problem for oncologists. Only 2 months after Roentgen's 1895 publication on the discovery of x-rays, radiation was used in the treatment of a patient with bony metastases.[104] Since the time of this first treatment, over a million cancer patients have undergone effective treatments for thoracic spine metastases, making this group of patients one of the most common challenges confronting radiation, medical, and spinal oncologists. The past century has seen dramatic improvements in all aspects of cancer care. Improvements in imaging have enabled radiation oncologists to better localize the extent of disease and improve radiation dose delivery. Modern linear accelerators offer dose-sparing of skin and subcutaneous tissues, greatly reducing the morbidity of radiation treatments. Improvements in surgical techniques have enabled safe and effective decompression of epidural thoracic metastases and improved stabilization of collapsed vertebral bodies. Finally, the evolution of chemotherapy and hormonal therapies over the past three decades has allowed the first effective systemic treatments of metastatic disease.

Metastatic disease involving the thoracic spine presents many unique challenges. It is important to recognize the diverse spectrum of patients with disease in this region and understand this variability in prognosis. Some patients die within weeks to months of diagnosis, while others may be cured. Metastatic spread of cancer to the thoracic spine can occur with nearly any type of malignancy. However, certain malignancies have a predilection for spread to the bone. Most studies of metastatic bone disease have found breast, lung, and prostate cancer to be the most common.[42,98,104,112] Other malignancies known to have a predilection for bony spread include lymphoma, thyroid cancer, kidney cancer, and myeloma. The majority spread via the hematogenous route, although local extension from growth of a paraspinous mass is possible, particularly in the upper thoracic spine. Tumor growth typically induces osteoclastic activity and bone reabsorption, resulting in an osteolytic radiographic appearance. However, osteosclerotic appearances resulting from osteoblastic activity are also a possibility, particularly with metastases from prostate cancer. Thoracic metastases usually cause localized pain resulting from malignant growth and invasion of the bone and periosteum. The etiology of bony pain is poorly understood, but is likely related to periosteal destruction or expansion and the release of prostaglandins and other chemical factors from the tumor and the destroyed bone.[67]

The goal of this chapter is to provide an overview of radiation and systemic treatments of metastatic disease involving the thoracic spine. To help practitioners gain a greater appreciation of the principles involved in radiotherapy treatment decisions, underlying principles of radiobiology and radiation physics are reviewed. The technical aspects of radiation delivery are explained, and the toxicity associated with thoracic spine irradiation is discussed. The general principles and toxicities of chemotherapy are also discussed. Radiotherapeutic approaches for patients with spinal cord compression are reviewed. Finally, the management of thoracic spine metastases for specific types of malignancies is covered, with an attempt to outline the general principles involved in radiation and systemic treatments decision making.

THERAPEUTIC INDICATIONS

There are few universal guidelines that govern the management of patients with thoracic spine metastatic disease. The goal of treatment in the vast majority of these patients is to provide maximal quality of life through resolution of pain and prevention of spinal cord injury. Treatments must take into account the extent of metastatic disease, the histology and site of the primary tumor, the stability of the involved vertebral bodies, the effect of the metastases on the quality of life of the patient, and the life expectancy of the patient. Table 28-1 provides estimated survival times from the onset of metastatic disease for various malignancies.[89] The spectrum of survival rates highlights the need to individualize treatment recommendations. The guidelines for treatment provided in this chapter must be interpreted within this concept.

The majority of thoracic spine metastases require some form of local therapy. In a series of 2467 patients with spinal metastases, 72% underwent local field radiation.[21] In addition, approximately 40% of patients with thoracic spine metastases receive systemic treatment. The patients in whom supportive care without intervention is appropriate include patients with life expectancies of less than a month regardless of therapy. Close clinical follow-up without treatment is also appropriate for patients with asymptomatic lesions from malignancies in which systemic treatment does not improve survival. Patients in whom no treatment is recommended

Table 28-1. Estimated Survival of Various Metastatic Malignancies[89]

Primary Tumor	Time to Metastases After Diagnosis of Primary (mo)	Mean Survival After Diagnosis of Spinal Metastases (mo)
Lung	2.2	7.7
Breast	89	116
Renal	—	6
Prostate	18.6	44.2

should have spine radiographs to assure spinal stability. Local therapy should be used for patients with pedicle erosion or marked vertebral body involvement to prevent spinal cord compression and transverse myelopathy. Plain radiographs correctly predict the presence or absence of epidural tumor over 80% of the time.[92] Patients receiving only supportive measures require periodic spine radiographs, careful clinical follow-up, and patient education concerning the signs and symptoms of spinal cord compression.

The role of surgery for treatment of spinal metastases without spinal cord compression is thought by some to be limited. More recently some authors advocate a more aggressive surgical treatment plan as the initial strategy. Bone biopsies may be required to confirm the spread of cancer. Biopsies should be performed in cases in which there is a relative uncertainty about the presence of metastatic disease. For example, a 54-year-old woman 6 years status posttreatment for localized breast cancer who develops thoracic back pain and an isolated area of increased uptake on bone scan should have biopsy confirmation of metastatic disease prior to treatment. In contrast, a 75-year-old man treated 2 years ago for lymph node positive prostate cancer who presents with back pain, a rising serum prostate-specific antigen, and multiple new areas of increased uptake on bone scan may not need pathological confirmation prior to treatment. The authors generally believe that surgical intervention beyond biopsy is appropriate only in settings of instability or in selected patients with spinal cord compression (as discussed later in this chapter).

Radiation is the most commonly employed treatment for thoracic spine metastases. However, asymptomatic lesions detected on bone scan imaging often do not require radiation. In a large series of patients with asymptomatic thoracic spine metastases from breast cancer, the subsequent

Table 28-2. Response Rates to Conventional Chemotherapy in Previously Untreated Patients With Metastatic Disease

Primary	Response Rates (%)
Lung, small cell	75-85
Lung, non-small cell	30-40[14]
Renal cell carcinoma	15-20 (slightly higher for some studies with biological response modifier therapy)
Breast, hormone receptor negative	50-70
Breast, hormone receptor positive	70-80 (hormonal agents or conventional chemotherapy given as primary therapy)
Colorectal	25-40[12]
Prostate	60-80 (hormonal agents)[25]
Melanoma	15-25 (includes biological agents)[63]
Multiple myeloma	45-65[1]
Non-Hodgkin's lymphoma, stage IV	60-80[4]
Ewing's sarcoma (pediatric)	70[85]
Neuroblastoma	60-70[85]
Rhabdomyosarcoma	75[76]

*Response rates include complete and partial responses.

development of spinal cord compression was only 5%.[21] As a general rule, radiation therapy is indicated in the majority of patients with symptomatic thoracic spine metastases. Contraindications for radiation include previous external beam radiation in the area of disease or patient life expectancy less than 1 month. Radiation treatments need to be carefully coordinated with any planned systemic treatment. For patients with structurally stable but symptomatic thoracic spine metastases from malignancies with a high likelihood of responding to a systemic regimen, radiation may be deferred until a time when the systemic regimen is considered ineffective. The most common example of such a scenario is patients with newly diagnosed metastatic prostate cancer beginning hormonal therapy.

The appropriateness of systemic therapies in metastatic disease is highly dependent on response rates and the toxicities of therapy. Table 28-2 provides response rates of various malignancies in the setting of metastatic disease.[1,4,12,14,25,63,76,85] Systemic treatment is frequently combined with local field radiation to assure that palliation of pain is achieved as soon as possible. More details concerning the success rates of radiation in achieving pain palliation and the systemic treatments of various malignancies with thoracic spine metastases are provided later in this chapter.

RADIATION THERAPY
General Principles: Radiobiology and Radiation Physics

Ionizing radiation achieves therapeutic effects through the deposition of energy within cells, which causes either single or double strand DNA injuries. The goal of selective tumor cell kill without normal tissue injury is achieved through both radiobiological means (taking advantage of intrinsic biological differences between tumor cells and normal tissue) and physical means (achieving selective delivery of the radiation to the tumor with sparing of dose to the normal tissue).

One of the most important radiobiological principles involved in achieving the optimal therapeutic ratio between tumor cell death and normal tissue complication is the concept of fractionation. Fractionation is the number of treatments into which the total dose of radiation is divided. Fractionation preferentially reduces the probability of obtaining a lethal event in a late responding normal tissue (such as the spinal cord) relative to the probability of a lethal event occurring in a tumor. This sparing of normal tissue with fractionation is a result of the following factors that occur during a course of fractionated treatment: reoxygenation of radiation-resistant hypoxic regions within tumors, redistribution of tumor cells in radioresistant cell cycle phases to more radiosensitive phases, repopulation of normal cells and tumor cells, and repair of sublethal radiation damage.[118]

Perhaps the most important reason for fractionating radiation treatments concerns the difference between normal tissues and tumors in their ability to repair damage induced by radiation. In the laboratory, the repairing ability of normal and tumor cells can be determined through cell survival curves that measure the fraction of cells surviving escalating radiation doses. It has been found that cell survival can be predicted and described by the linear-quadratic formula:

$$SF = e^{-\alpha D - \beta D^2}$$

where SF = surviving fraction, D = dose, D^2 = square of the dose, α = linear constant, β = quadratic constant.[111] Normal cells differ from one another and from tumor cells in the α and β constants of their cell survival curve, commonly described as their α/β ratio. Tissues with a high α/β ratio are late responding tissues, whereas tissues with a low α/β ratio, such as most tumors, are acutely responding tissues. Injuries to late responding tissues are more sensitive to the size of the daily radiation fraction compared to acutely responding tissue.[118] These differences in α/β ratios allow a course of radiation to be designed that maximizes the probability of tumor control while minimizing the risk of injuring late responding normal tissues.

The dose of radiation used in treatment is determined by the tolerance of normal tissue as well as the sensitivity of the tumor. In standard treatments of the thoracic spine, radiation inevitably leads to dosage of the spinal cord, skin, subcutaneous tissue, and vertebral body, and likely provides some dosage to the esophagus, stomach, heart, and lungs. Of these normal structures, the dose-limiting organ is usually the spinal cord. The spinal cord is a late responding tissue with a high α/β ratio. The α/β ratio of the spinal cord and tumors can be used in a linear-quadratic equation to predict how changes in fractionation can affect therapy. For example, a 10 cm length of thoracic spinal cord has a radiation tolerance of 4500 cGy when delivered in 25 180 cGy fractions over 5 weeks. If the dose per fraction is increased, the biologically effective dose to the tumor becomes less for an equivalent tolerance dose to the spinal cord. The linear-quadratic equation predicts that fractions of 300 cGy, 600 cGy, and 800 cGy per

day would give, respectively, 84%, 64%, and 58% of the biologically effective dose to the tumor if the tolerance dose to the spinal cord is maintained (assuming α/β ratios of 2 Gy for spinal cord and 10 Gy for tumors). This example does not take into account important parameters such as repopulation, and is only provided to show that as the dose per fraction is decreased to 180 to 200 cGy per day, the late responding tissues are tolerant of higher total radiation dosages and the tumor can receive a higher biologically effective dose. From a biological perspective, therefore, the best therapeutic ratio for the patient with metastatic disease to the thoracic spine entails a 5-week radiation course.

Safe and effective radiation treatments are not solely dependent on biological factors. Physics, which governs the delivery of radiation, also plays an important role. Normal tissue injuries are minimized by minimizing the volume of normal tissue irradiated. The simplest technique for achieving this goal is through customized contoured fields. In the treatment of thoracic spine metastases, this is usually achieved by limiting the borders of the radiation field to the region in which the metastasis is located. Because of the proximity of the disease to the spinal cord, no attempt is made to shield this structure from the treatment volume. Dose is typically given solely from a dorsal field, which limits the total radiation dose to the more ventral organs such as the heart and lungs. Under certain clinical circumstances, such as when treating patients following a dorsal decompression surgery, a decreased dose may be desired within the surgical field and a ventral field may be added to offer greater dorsal skin sparing.

Sophisticated radiation delivery techniques are available that can further improve the radiation dose delivery for patients with thoracic spine disease. Examples of such forms of treatment are proton beam irradiation and heavy ion treatment. These types of radiation require a cyclotron to accelerate charged particles into the range of energies required for therapeutic usage. The advantages of these treatments compared to conventional radiation treatment is that the dose can be contoured much more precisely around a targeted area, with a rapid falloff of dosages around critical structures such as the spinal cord.[109] This permits the treatment of malignant lesions with higher radiation doses before spinal cord tolerance is reached. For patients with nonmetastatic malignant diseases involving the thoracic spine region, proton or heavy ion therapy are appropriate considerations. However, for patients with metastatic disease of the spine the expense, difficulty of delivery, inconvenience for the patient, and lack of survival benefit in this population limit the clinical use of these treatments. Brachytherapy (the use of radioactive implants) is also rarely indicated for patients with thoracic spine metastatic disease because the tumor burden usually prohibits a more localized dose distribution compared to conventional therapy, and because of the potential for morbidity with the operative procedure required for radioactive seed placement.

Techniques and Results

The majority of patients receiving radiation for symptomatic thoracic spine metastases have limited life expectancies. The goal of treatment for most patients is to provide a short and effective therapy that achieves pain relief as quickly as possible with a minimal amount of treatment morbidity. Pretreatment workup for these patients should include a careful neurological examination. A bone scan helps localize the radiation ports, and radiographs of the thoracic spine help assess bony stability. Radiation treatments begin with a treatment planning session known as a simulation. For the majority of patients, a single dorsal field is designed that encompasses the involved vertebral bodies plus a vertebral body margin above and below the extent of disease. For patients with radiculopathy or plain radiographs that are suspicious for a paraspinous mass, further imaging, which may involve computed tomography (CT) imaging, may help define the lateral borders of the treatment field. However, CT scanning is not usually required and the lateral margins are set to include the spinous processes of the vertebral bodies, with a small margin for beam build-up and variations in day to day patient positioning. A lateral radiograph is obtained during simulation to determine the depth from the dorsal skin surface to the spinal cord. In obese patients, in whom this depth is 10 centimeters or greater, or in patients being treated after a dorsal decompression surgery, a matched ventral field can be added to minimize the dose to the dorsal skin and subcutaneous tissues. More sophisticated workup and planning of treatment fields are frequently unnecessary as they may not be cost-effective.

Fractionation and total dosages are dependent on the individual circumstances. For unfavorable patients, the usual treatment prescription is 3000 cGy total dose delivered in ten 300 cGy treatments over a 2-week period. For patients with very limited life expectancies, shorter courses of treatment are appropriate. 2000 cGy in five treatment fractions and even 800 cGy delivered in a single treatment have been reported to achieve symptomatic palliation in one half to two thirds of patients.[42,87] For patients with diffuse bony disease and a very short life expectancy, single-dose hemibody radiation can be safely delivered as an alternative to local field therapy, with efficacy in achieving temporary pain relief being reported as high as 73%.[97]

Radiation has a high success rate in achieving prolonged palliation of symptomatic bony metastases. Series that have employed fractionation schedules commonly used in practice today (3000 cGy in ten fractions) report good to excellent pain relief rates of 70% to 90%, with complete relief rates of 50% to 60%.[10,104] There are conflicting data concerning the effect of histology on palliation rates. Many authors have found a lower palliation rate in non-small cell lung cancer with good to excellent palliation achieved in only 40% to 50%.[87,104,112] Others have found and equal palliative rate among various histologies.[42] The recurrence of symptoms following complete pain relief occurs in 27% to 54% of patients, with a range of median pain-free intervals from 12 weeks to 12 months.[42,112] Local field palliation of bony metastases is unlikely to affect survival rates. In a series of 158 patients treated with palliative radiation for bony metastases, the median survival from the time of treatment was 12 months, with 24% of the patients surviving less than 3 months. Patients with lung cancer had the shortest median survival (3 months).[42]

Radiation is very successful in preventing the development of epidural spinal cord compression. In one series of 1742 breast cancer patients radiated for symptomatic spinal metastases, only seven patients subsequently developed a spinal cord compression in the area of previous radiation.[21]

There exists a subset of patients with thoracic spine metastatic disease in whom the short-term prognosis is favorable. Such patients include subsets of patients with hormone-sensitive prostate cancer, breast cancer patients with metastases limited to bone, patients with newly diagnosed multiple myeloma, patients with metastatic non-Hodgkin's lymphomas, and certain pediatric malignancies such as neuroblastoma, Ewing's sarcoma, and rhabdomyosarcoma. Effective systemic chemotherapeutic or hormonal therapies are available for these diseases. In some of these patients, symptomatic lesions without compromise of the vertebral body or epidural disease can be initially treated with systemic therapy, with radiation used for recurrence or persistence of symptoms. In patients with long life expectancies who receive radiation, a more protracted course of treatment should be considered. As mentioned earlier, decreasing the daily fraction size permits a higher radiobiologically effective tumor dose in most malignancies. This was shown to have clinical relevancy in a Radiation Therapy Oncology Group randomized multicenter trial comparing various fractionation schemes for the treatment of bony metastases. Results from this trial noted that as a group, 90% of the 759 patients experienced a partial relief of pain and 54% achieved complete pain relief.[112] In a reanalysis of the data using a multivariate logistic regression analysis, an increased number of treatment fractions was a statistical factor in achieving pain relief.[10] The reanalysis concluded that more protracted courses of radiation that deliver higher total radiation dosages improve the palliation of bone metastases.

Complications

Serious complications resulting from radiation treatments of metastatic disease in the thoracic spine are rare. Effects of radiation on normal tissues are classically divided into acute effects and late effects. Acute effects arise during or shortly after radiation treatments and affect organs with rapidly proliferating stem cells. In treatment of the thoracic spine, acute effects consist of mainly minor dermatological, gastrointestinal (esophagus, stomach), and hematological toxicities. The most common toxicity that is of consequence to patients is radiation esophagitis. Typically, esophagitis occurs toward the end of the second week of treatment and usually resolves within 1 week of completion of treatment. Symptoms consist of dyspepsia and dys-

phagia and are treated symptomatically with topical anesthetic solutions and antacids. Rarely, in patients receiving steroids, chemotherapy, and radiation, severe esophagitis may occur from fungal superinfection. In these patients, therapy should include an antifungal agent and symptomatic support with narcotics. In patients with lesions in the low thoracic spine, the exit dose of radiation passes through the upper abdomen and may lead to temporary nausea and/or diarrhea. Treatment of thoracic metastatic disease with modern linear accelerators provides adequate skin sparing, minimizing the acute dermatological toxicities of erythema, puritis, and dry desquamation of the skin within the irradiated volume. Concurrent administration of radiation and doxorubicin should be avoided due to the risk of brisk erythema and acute ulceration of the skin. Hematological toxicities in patients receiving radiation alone are rare. The thoracic spine typically contains less than 30% of the functioning bone marrow in the normal adult[94] and therefore neutropenia or thrombocytopenia is usually limited to patients with previous histories of prior radiation treatments to the bony pelvis and/or chemotherapy. A weekly complete blood count with platelets should be followed in patients with previous treatment histories.

Late toxicities of radiation of the thoracic spine are more concerning than the acute effects because, if they occur, resulting deficits can be permanent. Because radiation most often kills cells as they enter into mitosis or DNA synthesis, lethal damage to cells not actively proliferating may not be clinically apparent for months following the radiation treatments. For example, radiation damage to the spinal cord, lung, and heart are typically seen anywhere from 6 months to 3 years posttreatment, and rarely, if ever, during the actual course of therapy.

Radiation myelopathy is the most serious potential toxicity of radiation therapy to the thoracic spine. Fortunately, spinal cord injuries are rare because the dosages effective in the palliation of pain are usually below the spinal cord tolerance dose. However, sporadic injuries are possible even with the dosages used in treatment of thoracic spine metastases. Myelopathy typically occurs 9 months to 3 years following radiation treatments and leads to a spectrum of deficits.[100] Initial symptoms consist of paresthesias and sensory deficits that can progress to complete loss of neurological functioning below the level of the injury.[44,82] Risk factors for the development of radiation myelopathy include previous radiation to the area of treatment, increased length of spinal cord within the irradiated volume, hypertension, and concurrent or sequential treatment with vincristine, actinomycin D, or intrathecal methotrexate.[5,22,44,68] In addition, patients with previously irradiated thoracic spinal cords are at high risk for the development of radiation myelitis with reirradiation, as the cumulative dose typically exceeds the spinal cord tolerance. The pathophysiology of radiation myelopathy suggests the etiology of the injury can be either vascular endothelial damage or a direct neural injury with the demyelination of axons and subsequent liquefaction necrosis of white matter.[101] In patients with metastatic disease, radiographic studies need to be performed in patients with a clinical history suggestive of radiation myelopathy. It is not uncommon to find a malignant etiology of the neural deficits.[82] Unfortunately, there are no effective treatments for radiation myelopathy. Experimental therapy with hyperbaric oxygen or pentoxifylline aim at attempting to improve oxygenation within the area of involved spinal cord. Corticosteroids are often used in patients with radiation myelopathy, but their effectiveness has not been proven and their pharmacological effects do not address the underlying pathophysiology.

Radiation injury involving bone most commonly manifests as bone marrow rather than vertebral body toxicity. Dosages ranging from 1600 to 3600 cGy have been found to cause temporary adipose tissue replacement of bone marrow, with blood-forming elements recolonizing 9 months to 2 years after treatment.[81] Dosages over 4000 cGy have a high likelihood of permanent adipose tissue replacement of bone marrow.

Clinically significant radiation injury of vertebral bodies is extremely rare in most patients receiving thoracic spine radiation. However, the effect of radiation on normal bone is of clinical concern in pediatric patients and in adult patients who have undergone surgical stabilization of a vertebral body with strut graft placement. In preadolescent children, high-dose thoracic spine radiation (greater than 3500 cGy in 180 to 200 cGy fractions) causes growth plate damage resulting in abnormal growth and development leading to decreased sitting heights.[34] In addition, radiation in young children leads to soft tissue atrophy and fibrosis within the irradiated volume, which can cause significant future cosmetic and functional back problems. Without careful attention to radiation technique, differential bone growth resulting in severe scoliosis can occur.

Adult patients requiring ventral decompression for vertebral body collapse from malignant disease often require vertebral strut grafts for stabilization. Postoperative radiation in these patients has the potential of adversely affecting the healing of these grafts. Unfortunately, few clinical studies have been performed to determine the affect of radiation on bone graft healing. In a canine model, radiation delivered to a dose of 2500 cGy in 500 cGy fractions beginning on postoperative day 3 adversely affected the strength of the grafts, as defined by measurements of torsion and left lateral bending 3 months following treatments. However, in animals treated with the same radiation regimen preoperatively or on postoperative day 21, no adverse affects were observed.[37] This data suggests that postoperative radiation in patients with grafts should not begin prior to a 3-week period of healing. This period is unlikely to lead to significant tumor regrowth.

Radiation-induced carcinogenesis is often a concern of patients receiving radiation treatments. Radiation-induced second malignancies, most commonly bone or soft tissue sarcomas, occur in 1% to 2% of long-term survivors. Because the median time to the development of these tumors is 11 years after treatment, this risk for the patient with thoracic spine metastases is negligible.[58]

Spinal Cord Compression

Approximately 20% of patients with metastatic involvement of the spine develop epidural tumor extension and compression of the spinal cord.[98] The location of spinal cord compression is the thoracic spine in two thirds of patients (combined data from four series).[43,60,75,98] Acute neurological deterioration in a patient with a history of cancer necessitates immediate diagnostic and therapeutic intervention. The initial symptom of patients with spinal cord compression is back pain in 80% to 96% of the cases.[43,60] The back pain, on average, precedes the diagnosis of spinal cord compression by 6 weeks.[60] At the time of first clinical presentation, the majority of patients have motor, autonomic, and sensory dysfunction and two thirds to three fourths are non-ambulatory due to neurological deficits.[43,60]

Thoracic spinal cord compression can occur with any type of malignancy. The four most common malignancies are breast cancer, lung cancer, prostate cancer, and kidney cancer.[43,60] Thoracic spinal cord compression usually results from preexisting vertebral body metastases. Extra-axial spinal cord compression without bony metastases should raise the suspicion of a nonmetastatic etiology, such as meningioma. Bony metastasis can cause spinal cord compression, either from local tumor growth into the epidural space or by vertebral body collapse with resulting kyphotic angulation of the spinal cord.

The workup of patients with spinal cord compression should begin emergently. A complete history should ascertain the length of time neurological deficits have been present. Physical examination should document motor and sensory deficits, rectal sphincter tone, and region of spinal tenderness. Following examination, high-dose intravenous corticosteroids should be started and the patient admitted to the hospital for neurological status monitoring. The optimal dosage and administration of corticosteroids is unknown. In a small randomized trial, 10 mg of intravenous dexamethasone bolus followed by 16 mg daily was noted to be as effective as 100 mg intravenous bolus followed by 16 mg daily in improving pain and preventing progressive neurological sequelae in patients with metastatic spinal cord compression.[114] Radiographic studies should be obtained immediately to ascertain the level of the spinal cord compression and structural integrity of the involved vertebral bodies. A magnetic resonance imaging (MRI) study is preferred over a myelogram because in addition to determining the level of the spinal cord compression, MRI provides a more sensitive delineation of the vertebral and paraspinous disease extent, and perhaps a more sensitive assessment of the structural integrity of the bones. This information is vital to optimal radiation and/or surgical treatment planning.

An immediate question that arises regarding the management of patients with spinal cord compression is whether a surgical decompression of the spinal cord would benefit the patient. This question needs to be answered on an individual case basis based on the patient's overall medical condition, the degree of neurological impairment and its timing, the radiosensitivity of the malignancy, the pre-

vious treatment history, the structural integrity of the involved vertebral body, the presence of a paraspinous mass, and the location of the spinal cord compression. There has been much debate over the value of surgical decompression in metastatic cord compression. Only one randomized trial has compared surgery and postoperative radiation to radiation alone.[122] In this study, only 7% of the patients treated with surgery and postoperative radiation had an improvement in their ambulatory status compared to 16% of the patients treated with radiation alone. The certainty of this finding is limited, due to the fact that only 29 patients were enrolled in the trial. However, the results of this trial mirror the largest nonrandomized series that compared radiation alone to surgery with postoperative radiation in 130 patients. In this series, 46% of the surgery and postoperative radiation group were ambulatory following treatment compared to 49% of those treated with radiation alone.[43] In addition, an analysis of 31 series studying the treatment of spinal cord compression in over 2300 total patients noted improvement in neurological functioning in 30% of the patients treated with surgery alone, 44% in those treated with surgery and postoperative radiation, and 46% in patients treated with radiation alone.[7] Furthermore, in this analysis, the combined surgical morbidity (deterioration in neurological functioning) was 12%, and the surgical mortality was 9%. It is important to keep in mind, however, that early surgical series frequently entailed a dorsal decompression (laminectomy) alone. In many instances the major bulk of the spinal cord compression involves the ventral spinal canal. A laminectomy may not reduce the ventral forces acting on the spinal cord, and in fact may create additional problems by further destabilizing the spinal column. In these situations a lateral or ventral exposure may achieve better results when compared to dorsally decompressed patients or those undergoing radiation alone.

Surgical decompression has a role in the management of spinal cord compression. Surgery is indicated in patients in need of a tissue diagnosis, as well as patients who have a history of previous radiation to the area of the compression. In addition, for patients with compression secondary to vertebral body collapse and kyphotic angulation of the spinal cord rather than epidural tumor extension, surgery for decompression and stabilization with postoperative radiation is the treatment of choice. In a series of 52 patients with spinal instability secondary to metastatic vertebral fractures, 21 out of the 40 patients with major neurological impairment had complete recovery following ventral spinal decompression and spinal stabilization using methylmethacrylate.[47] Surgery is also indicated in patients experiencing a progressive neurological deterioration during or following radiation treatments. In a series studying the effectiveness of up-front medical therapy, two out of six patients in whom steroids, radiation, and chemotherapy were unsuccessful in halting neurological progression became ambulatory following surgical decompression.[75]

The greatest area of controversy regarding the role of surgery in patients with spinal cord compression concerns the optimal management of patients with radioresistant histologies (non-small cell lung cancer, renal cell carcinoma, sarcoma, and melanoma) and acute neurological defects. In the largest retrospective study, patients with radioresistant histologies had poorer outcomes compared to patients with radiosensitive histologies. However, despite the poorer outcome in the patients with radioresistant tumors, there was no apparent benefit in the use of surgery in this subgroup.[43] A composite study of 31 series similarly found that patients with radioresistant histologies had poorer outcomes, but again, these patients did not benefit from surgery.[7] In contrast, in a single-arm prospective study investigating spinal cord decompression in patients with radioresistant histologies, 17 ambulatory and 21 nonambulatory patients improved neurologically following surgery and 23 out of the 25 patients alive 2 years after treatment maintained their ambulation.[110] In this series, surgical morbidity was 15% and mortality 6%.

There are also conflicting data regarding the use of surgery in patients with acute neurological deterioration from spinal cord compression. In one series, none of the nine surgically treated patients who presented with weakness less than 48 hours from onset recovered from their neurological deficits. In contrast, of the 13 patients who presented with weakness less than 48 hours and were treated with radiation alone, seven had neurological improvement.[43] However, another article that combined the results of 31 series and analyzed multifactorial variables in determining outcomes concluded that surgery was appropriate in patients with severe

but not complete neurological deficits resulting from a dorsal compression of the spinal cord.[7]

Chemotherapy has been used successfully as a sole treatment modality of spinal cord compression in germ cell tumors and pediatric malignancies. One series reported complete neurological recovery in three patients with spinal cord compression from metastatic germ cell tumors treated with corticosteroids and cisplatin.[26] In 14 pediatric patients with spinal cord compression from neuroblastoma or Ewing's sarcoma, surgery led to neurological improvement in only one out of five patients, with all 14 patients recovering neurologically following chemotherapy.[48]

If radiation is to be used as the primary treatment, the setup and delivery for patients with spinal cord compression are quite similar to treatments of symptomatic metastatic disease to the vertebral bodies. Aspects unique to patients with spinal cord compression include the timing of initiation of treatment and the dose of radiation given in the first two to three fractions. The treatment of spinal cord compression should begin immediately, with a clinical setup if necessary. Subsequent simulation should be performed to ensure that the field size, and thus the amount of normal tissue being treated, is minimized. In patients presenting with neurological deficits, dose per fractions under 300 cGy should not be given for at least the first three fractions. It has been shown that the edema and the overall mass effect in the area of compression are decreased by large dose per fraction treatment compared to conventional fraction sizes.[93]

The acute prognosis for neurological recovery is dependent on several factors. As mentioned, numerous authors have described the importance of histology in neurological recovery and overall prognosis. Lung cancer has been noted to have the lowest neurological recovery rate, 17%, and shortest survival rate from treatment, 2.6 months.[7] Success rates are highest for lymphomas and myelomas, with a recovery rate of 58% and survival of 88 months.[7] Another important prognosticator of neurological recovery is ambulatory status and neurological functioning at the time of treatment. Paraparetic patients regain ambulatory function in 40% to 50% of cases compared to paraplegic patients, who recover ambulation in only 3% to 33%.[7,43,74] Recovery from paralysis may be more dependent on the interval from motor symptoms to paralysis than the interval from paralysis to treatment.[49] Furthermore, in patients treated with radiation, recovery of ambulation may not occur until 3 to 6 months following completion of therapy.[49] A final prognostic factor that may influence the success in treating spinal cord compression is the presence of paraspinal disease. One series noted that none of the 15 nonambulatory patients with paravertebral masses and histologies other than lymphoma regained ambulatory function with radiation treatments.[59] This compared to an approximately 20% recovery rate in similar patients without paravertebral disease.

In summary, patients with spinal cord compression should be treated emergently. Therapy should be decided on after multidisciplinary evaluation by a radiation oncologist and a neurosurgeon. The majority of patients should be treated with radiation alone. Surgical therapy is appropriate for patients with vertebral body collapse with kyphotic angulation of the spinal canal, the need for tissue diagnosis, progressive disease during or after radiation, and possibly in patients with good performance status who are paraplegic from a radioresistant tumor.

CHEMOTHERAPY
General Principles

The use of cytotoxic drugs as antineoplastic agents dates back to the 1940s, when nitrogen mustard, an alkylating agent used as a poisonous gas during World War I, was found to have activity treating lymphomas. In the 1960s combination chemotherapy was shown to cure Hodgkin's disease, a malignancy that was often fatal until this development. Many of the chemotherapeutic drugs in use today were discovered in the 1950s and 1960s, and as experience with pharmacokinetics and an understanding of tumor cell biology has grown, the application of these agents continues to evolve. In addition, new chemotherapy agents continue to be evaluated each year by the National Cancer Institute through its anticancer drug screening program.

Several categories of antineoplastic drugs are in use today. The first is traditional chemotherapy, in which drugs kill or suppress tumor cells through interference with critical enzymes necessary for DNA synthesis and function. Many of the side effects of these agents occur because their antireplicative effects are not selective, and rapidly growing normal cells can also be affected. A second type of systemic

therapy, biological therapy or biological response modifiers, achieves antitumor effects through the manipulation of natural host defense mechanisms, or through the administration of natural mammalian substances. Examples of biological response modifiers are the interferon and interleukin families of agents. Lastly, hormonal agents such as tamoxifen and leuprolide have been found to be highly effective in both the treatment of prostate and breast cancer.

Chemotherapy drugs can be grouped loosely through their mechanisms of action. It is important to remember that some drugs can work at multiple points during the cell cycle, especially if the route and schedule of administration is altered. Alkylating agents are highly reactive compounds that have the ability to substitute alkyl groups ($R-CH_2-CH_2^+$) for hydrogen atoms in certain compounds. These substitutions result in cross-linking of DNA strands, which interferes with cell replication. Examples of alkylating agents include nitrogen mustard derivatives (such as melphalan and chlorambucil), cytoxan, and ifosfamide, thiotepa, busulfan, dacarbazine, nitrosoureas (BCNU, CCNU), and platinum derivatives (cisplatin, carboplatin).

Antibiotic chemotherapy drugs are natural products of various strains of the soil fungus streptomyces. This group includes the anthracyclines or adriamycin (doxorubicin) and daunorubicin, and the related synthetic compounds mitoxantrone, bleomycin, dactinomycin, mitomycin, and streptozotocin. All the antibiotics are capable of binding to DNA, often between base pairs (thus the name intercalating agents). Anthracyclines, in addition, inhibit the enzyme topoisomerase II, which is critical for DNA replication.[124]

Plant derivatives are the source of the vinca alkaloids (vincristine and vinblastine), which are extracted from the common periwinkle plant. Podophyllins were originally derived from the mandrake root, and currently two semisynthetic derivatives of podophyllins are in wide use, etoposide (VP-16) and teniposide (VM-26). The antimetabolite drugs include agents such as methotrexate, which blocks dihydrofolate reductase; fluorouracil (5-FU), which inhibits thymidylate synthase; the related compound floxuridine (FuDR); cytarabine (ara-C), which inhibits DNA polymerase; and hydroxyurea (hydrea), which inhibits ribonucleotide reductase. Finally, a group of miscellaneous agents features drugs such as procarbazine, l-asparaginase, and mitotane.

The side effects and dose limiting toxicities of chemotherapy depend largely on the dose and route of administration; however, certain special side effects of each drug bear mentioning. For example, anthracyclines can cause cumulative myocardial damage, and often these agents must be discontinued to protect against the development of congestive heart failure. Bleomycin can cause pulmonary fibrosis. BCNU can also cause lung damage. Cisplatin use can be complicated by renal damage, as well as neuropathy and ototoxicity. Vincristine and vinblastine also are neurotoxins.

An evolving method of using antineoplastic drugs is high-dose therapy, often synonymous with bone marrow transplantation. The theory behind high-dose therapy is that inherent or acquired tumor resistance can be overcome by using extraordinarily large doses of agents, sometimes in combination with radiation. In an autologous bone marrow transplant, a patient's bone marrow cells, which would be seriously damaged by high-dose therapy, are first removed from the patient either by a "bone marrow harvest" or through newer techniques of apheresis. After chemoradiation is completed, the patient's stored cells are reinfused intravenously. In an allogenic transplant, the patient is furnished with a "new" or "reset" immune system provided by marrow cells from a sibling or a tissue matched unrelated donor. The donor cells are thought to provide an additional "graft against tumor" effect that an autologous transplant cannot provide. The development of high-dose therapy has enabled some patients to be cured of otherwise fatal diseases, but its application in patients with metastatic disease is still investigational.

Tumor Resistance

Resistance of tumors to chemotherapeutic agents is in part related to inherent growth cycle. In a small, young population of tumor cells, the number of dividing cells represents a large fraction of that population, as opposed to an older, larger, well-established population in which a much smaller fraction of cells are dividing. Because many drugs are cell cycle specific (i.e., effective only during periods of DNA synthesis and cellular replication), a larger tumor may be more inherently chemoresistant compared to a small one.

Another important consideration is drug resistance due to cellular defense mechanisms. Cells can inherently possess or acquire the ability to pump out chemotherapy drugs (often referred to as the multidrug resistance or MDR phenotype[27]), to change specific enzyme targets, or to change growth requirements. Such alterations probably arise spontaneously, but treatment with chemotherapy can also selectively pull out a resistant clone. Chemoresistant tumors such as renal, thyroid, pancreatic, and hepatobiliary tumors probably possess one or all of these mechanisms. Other malignancies such as germ cell tumors, Hodgkin's lymphomas, Burkitt's lymphoma, and many types of acute leukemia appear to lack these resistance traits and are curable with chemotherapy.

Chemotherapy and Surgery

In many cases, the administration of chemotherapy following surgery in patients with metastatic disease can wait until a patient has fully recovered from their operation. There is often concern that the use of chemotherapy will interfere with wound healing. Although the initial inflammatory phase of wound healing involves neutrophils and macrophages, which release cytokines and phagocytose debris, experimental studies have shown that wound healing can take place in the face of leukopenia or lymphopenia. However, if the wound is contaminated with sufficient bacteria, healing is delayed and infection may ensue.[65] Fibroblast proliferation typically begins 3 to 5 days postoperatively and lasts approximately 2 weeks. Because of cellular replication occurring during this time, this may be the most susceptible portion of wound healing to chemotherapy agents.[80] Following this proliferative phase, the maturation phase of wound healing begins about 2 to 3 weeks after the initial injury. There appears to be less of an effect of chemotherapy when given in this period, although collagen continues to be laid down for about 8 weeks.

In patients who require surgery during a course of chemotherapy, the surgery ideally should be delayed until 10 to 14 days after the last dose of chemotherapy to allow time for fibroblast recovery. However, even patients with severe pancytopenia have been taken to the operating room successfully. An additional consideration in the selection of surgical candidates is the overall condition of the patient. Often, patients with metastatic disease are less than optimal surgical candidates because of chronic poor nutrition rather than because of the chemotherapy they have received.

Some chemotherapy agents can be given immediately following surgery. For example, the steroids commonly used to lessen edema caused by a metastatic spinal cord lesion are in themselves potent agents in the treatment of lymphomas and myeloma. Women with osseous metastases secondary to breast cancer or men with metastases from prostate cancer can safely begin or continue hormonal therapy postoperatively.

Chemotherapy and Radiation

Many commonly used chemotherapy agents may potentiate side effects of radiation. Adriamycin has long been known to cause an increase in radiation therapy morbidity, especially when given very close to a course of radiation.[3,17,115] In addition, adriamycin has been implicated in the development of radiation pneumonitis when given several months after a patient has completed radiation to the thorax, and also has the possibility of causing erythema and desquamation of the skin in the areas of previous radiation. The mechanisms responsible for these effects have not been clearly identified, but it has been postulated that anthracyclines interfere with repair of sublethal radiation damage to lung parenchymal cells or capillary endothelium.[72] Other agents that have been reported to cause the same sort of recall reaction are bleomycin, actinomycin-D, vincristine, cyclophosphamide, and vinblastine.[56,79]

In certain cases, the use of chemotherapy may positively impact the therapeutic effects of radiation. For example, the halogenated pyrimidine analogs (which include 5-FU) have been shown to improve response rate and survival when given with radiation to patients with rectal, anal, esophageal, pancreatic, and laryngeal cancer.[30,40,41,64,105] Mitomycin-C and cisplatin may also act as radiosensitizers.[23,51] However, no study to date has investigated whether these agents given concurrently with radiation therapy are advantageous for the treatment of spinal metastases.

Hematological Toxicities of Chemotherapy

Many patients with spinal metastases have previously received extensive treatment with either radiation or chemotherapy and their ability to recover from chemotherapy-induced cytopenias is often impaired. This is particularly true of patients who have previously received radiation to areas of active marrow, such as the pelvis or major portions of the spine. In adults, the vertebral bodies contain about 42% of the active red marrow.[36] Patients who have received radiation therapy to the entire spine frequently show a reduction in their capacity to recover counts after receiving standard doses of chemotherapeutic agents. Additionally, patients with previous chemotherapy exposure may develop cumulative marrow toxicity. Often, these patients require dose reductions of the chemotherapy agents. Because the majority of these patients are receiving palliative chemotherapy, the potential negative impact on response because of a reduction in dose intensity may be a minor consideration.

In patients in whom dose reductions could reduce the likelihood of cure, the availability of growth factors may make the use of full-dose chemotherapy possible, despite extensive pretreatment. Clinical trials have shown that recombinant erythropoietin can reduce the need for red cell transfusion as well as improve some patients' sense of well-being.[71,86] Erythropoietin has been used in patients concomitantly receiving radiotherapy with no apparent increase in side effects or decrease in response to radiation.[66] However, not all patients respond to erythropoietin and uniform dosing recommendations and cost-effectiveness are being studied.[108] Granulocyte-colony stimulating factor (G-CSF) and granulocyte-macrophage-colony stimulating factor (GM-CSF) can ameliorate neutropenia caused by chemotherapy and allow the maintenance of dose intensity. It is unclear if the use of colony stimulating factors to support a neutrophil count is advisable during prolonged radiation therapy. In two trials of patients with lung cancer, G-CSF was given in conjunction with radiation and chemotherapy. In both studies, patients receiving the growth factor experienced significantly more thrombocytopenia.[15,78] Some have argued that colony stimulating factors may mobilize stem cells from bone marrow into circulation whereby they can be damaged as they pass through a radiation field. The 1994 consensus statement on the use of colony stimulating factors that was issued by the American Society of Clinical Oncology recommends the concomitant use of growth factors and radiotherapy be avoided.[2]

Thrombocytopenia is often a limiting side effect of chemotherapy and at this time there is no specific pharmaceutical intervention to improve platelet counts. There is some data that interleukin 6 (IL-6) can increase platelet counts in animals who have received radiation.[50,123] Recently, human thrombopoietin (TPO, mpl-ligand) has been cloned and clinical trials testing the efficacy of this agent in improving chemotherapy or radiation-induced thrombocytopenia should begin shortly.[11,31] Recently, IL-11 (oprelvekin) given as a daily subcutaneous injection has been shown to reduce the requirement for platelet transfusions in 2 separate placebo controlled blinded studies of patients receiving intensive chemotherapy.[54a,110b] This medication appears to be well tolerated and is now commercially available for this indication.

Chemotherapy for Thoracic Spine Metastases

For patients with thoracic spine metastases, the role of chemotherapy is highly dependent on the type of primary malignancy. As previously shown in Table 28-2, many of the tumors that metastasize to the thoracic spine are relatively resistant to chemotherapy. However, in patients with metastases from prostate cancer, breast cancer, small cell carcinoma of the lung, and hematological malignancies, chemotherapy or hormonal therapy can play an important and occasionally curative role. As with surgery and radiotherapy, the goals of chemotherapy for metastatic disease are recovery or preservation of function, local and systemic disease control, maintenance of stability, pain relief, and, if possible, prolongation of survival. In many cases the decision to use chemotherapy comes after definitive local treatment of the thoracic spine disease. However, in certain clinical situations chemotherapy may be the appropriate primary treatment. For example, symptomatic patients with low-grade non-Hodgkin's lymphoma with medullary cavity involvement of the thoracic spine and no evidence of instability can be effectively treated with chemotherapy alone and rarely require radiation or surgery. Similarly, pediatric patients with thoracic spine metastases often receive chemotherapy alone, because of the undesirable long-term effects of radiotherapy on bone growth. Ultimately the decision to use chemotherapy is based on the goals of treatment (curative vs. palliative), the overall physical condition of the patient, the inherent toxicity of the proposed chemotherapeutic regimen, life expectancy, and patient desires.

Monitoring the response of bone metastases to chemotherapy can be difficult. Perhaps the most sensitive indicator of response is palliation of pain. Repeat of bone scintigraphy studies is less helpful in that the expected decrease of radiopharmaceutical uptake may be masked by differences in scan techniques or differences in the amount of radiopharmaceutical administered. Additionally, 10% to 15% of breast cancer patients can experience an initial flare in pain and scan uptake resulting not from tumor progression, but rather from new nonneoplastic bone formation. Magnetic resonance imaging (MRI) offers an alternative means to track disease response,[78a] but its routine use is limited by cost and lack of specificity.

MANAGEMENT OF SPECIFIC TUMOR TYPES
Breast Cancer

Carcinoma of the breast is the most common malignancy among women in the United States, with approximately 182,000 new cases projected to be diagnosed in 1998.[65a] Breast cancer is the second leading cause of cancer death in American women, surpassed only by lung cancer. The majority of women (49% to 85%) with metastatic breast cancer will eventually develop bone metastases, and in 20% to 25% of these patients, bone will be the only site of metastatic disease.[99] Unlike other solid tumors, a number of reasonable treatment options exist for women with thoracic metastases following initial treatment. Patients with symptomatic thoracic spine metastases commonly receive both systemic therapy and local field radiation. In addition, the group of drugs known as bisphosphonates, which inhibit osteoclast activity among other effects, offer a new approach to the treatment of metastatic bone lesions. In two randomized blinded trials, pamidronate given intravenously once a month decreased the incidence of new bone fractures as well as the need for surgery and radiation in patients with lytic bone lesions secondary to breast cancer.[53a,111a] Pamidronate is very well tolerated and more potent bisphosphonates such as zoledronate are currently being tested in clinical trials.

Breast cancer chemotherapy can be divided into hormonal and nonhormonal therapy. The drug tamoxifen, a synthetic antiestrogen, was first reported to be useful in 1971,[24] and its use has grown tremendously. In postmenopausal women with metastatic breast cancer that is estrogen and progesterone receptor positive, response rates are upwards of 50% to 70%. Women with bone metastases only often respond well. Other hormonal therapies that can be used include progestins (e.g., megestrol acetate and medroxyprogesterone acetate), adrenal suppressants (aminoglutethimide, aromatase inhibitors), and luteinizing hormone-releasing hormone antagonists (leuprolide). Many nonhormonal agents are also effective against metastatic breast cancer. Combinations such as CMF (cytoxan, methotrexate, and fluorouracil), CAF (cytoxan, adriamycin, fluorouracil), and MFL (mitoxantrone, fluorouracil, leucovorin) have been observed to yield response rates of 50% to 75% in untreated women with metastatic breast cancer, though these therapies are rarely curative.[8,13,106] Taxol (paclitaxel), first isolated from the Western yew tree in 1971,[116] is another extremely active agent in metastatic disease, even in women who have progressed through anthracycline therapy.[28a,52] Finally, high-dose chemotherapy followed by autologous bone marrow or peripheral blood stem cell transplantation is also being used in women with metastatic breast cancer with some promising initial results.[83] However, data from randomized trials proving transplantation's benefit over traditional chemotherapy are still in progress, and transplantation for metastatic breast cancer is still best performed within the context of a clinical trial.[35]

Prostate Cancer

Prostate cancer is the most common cancer in American men, with 184,500 new cases projected for 1998.[110b] While many of these cases will be detected early, given the widespread use of prostate-specific antigen (PSA) screening , about 45,000 men will be diagnosed with metastatic disease and 65% of these will have osseous metastases.[29] An important discovery was made in the first part of this century when it was reported that prostate cancer is hormonally dependent.[54] Many men with metastatic prostate cancer to bone have an excellent short-term prognosis. Because 95% of circulating testosterone is synthesized in the testicles, an effective approach has been bilateral orchiectomy, and this therapy has been the gold standard of treatment for metastatic disease. Alternatives to castration include therapy with the estrogen diethyl stilbestrol (DES) or the luteinizing hormone-releasing hormone agonists (e.g., leuprolide, goserelin). Both therapies cause impotence and hot flashes, as well as other side effects, although DES is infrequently used today because of the associated cardiovascular risks.[28] An area of controversy is that of "total androgen blockade." Because the adrenal glands still make a small amount of testosterone even after castration or leuprolide, some investigators have explored the addition of an antiandrogen in combination with leuprolide. In a randomized trial supported by the National Cancer Institute, there was no overall survival difference at 6 years between the group treated with leuprolide and flutamide, and those treated with flutamide alone. However, a "good performance" subgroup appeared to do better with the combination therapy.[29] Overall, about 60% to 80% of men with metastatic disease respond favorably to hormonal therapy.[25] Some patients who have progression of metastases after orchiectomy benefit from an antiandrogen. As a rule, response to therapy of bone metastases can be monitored through reduction in pain, improvement or stabilization of bone scans, and in many patients a decline or stabilization of the prostate-specific antigen level.

Patients with symptomatic osseous metastases that no longer respond to hormonal manipulation can be treated with conventional external beam radiation, or in cases in which the disease is widespread, systemically administered strontium-89. Strontium-89 is a beta-emitting radioisotope with a half-life of approximately 50.5 days[77] that is preferentially taken up by bone, as it mimics calcium metabolism. Given intravenously, a single injection of 40 to 60 μCi/kg has been shown to significantly improve pain in 80% of patients with metastatic prostate cancer, despite previous treatment with hormonal agents.[91] Side effects appear to be quite tolerable, with the most important being a transient pain flair in 10% to 20% of patients occurring several days posttreatment (and usually predictive of a favorable outcome) and mild thrombocytopenia occurring 5 to 6 weeks after treatment in 20% to 30% of patients. It is important to note that unlike hormonal therapy, strontium is not an antitumor therapy, and therefore will not prolong survival. However, it appears to be a safe and effective therapy for painful bony metastases. It is also possible to treat patients a second time (generally 6 months later), although the response rate is often lower.

Finally, although prostate cancer is often thought of as a "chemoresistant" tumor, reports of good responses to combination chemotherapy with vinblastine given with the oral alkylating agent/estrogen derivative estramustine, or estramustine in combination with oral etoposide, have yielded responses in some hormone refractory patients.[84,102] More recently, a randomized trial showed that the combination of mitoxantrone and prednisone provided superior pain relief and quality of life compared to prednisone alone in patients with hormone resistant metastatic prostate cancer.[110a]

Renal Cell Carcinoma

About 29,900 cases of kidney cancer will be diagnosed this year in the United States.[65a] About 30% of these patients will present with metastatic disease.[73] About 20% to 40% of patients with metastatic renal cancer will develop osseous metastases. Unfortunately, patients with metastatic disease seldom respond to conventional chemotherapy, with response rates well under 10%.[88] The key behind this chemoresistance may be due to inherent abundant expression of the multidrug resistance gene in tumor cells.[62] More promising have been studies conducted using biological response modifiers such as interferon and interleukin-2, either alone or in combination or with specially manipulated patient-derived lymphocytes.[6,9,38] While responses do occur with these regimens, they are rarely seen in patients with widely metastatic disease. Therefore patients with symptomatic spinal metastases from renal cell carcinoma should be treated with radiotherapy or surgery, if indicated. Patients can subsequently be invited to participate in clinical trials.

Lung Cancer

Currently, lung cancer is the single most frequent cause of cancer death in the United States. In 1998, approximately 171,500 cases will be diagnosed and 160,000 people will die from the disease.[65a] There is

little doubt as to the link between smoking and lung cancer. It is sobering to note that in the nineteenth century lung cancer was exceedingly uncommon. About 40% of patients present with metastatic disease, and another 40% will be poor surgical candidates, and therefore likely incurable. Most patients die from complications of metastatic disease. Bone metastases are a very common finding. Radiation is the mainstay of therapy for symptomatic bone lesions in patients with non-small cell carcinoma. Although there is a modest response rate to agents such as cisplatin combined with vincristine, the routine use of chemotherapy for palliation of bone metastases is probably not warranted outside of a clinical trial.[19,55,119]

Patients with metastatic small cell carcinoma (also known as oat cell), however, generally benefit from chemotherapy. Response rates to combination chemotherapy such as cisplatin and etoposide or cytoxan/adriamycin/vincristine are in the neighborhood of 50% to 90%, although long-term survivors are rare.[61] Patients with bony metastases that are not causing neurological compromise often benefit from chemotherapy alone, provided there is no evidence of impending fracture or instability. Once a patient progresses after one combination of agents, it is sometimes possible to change therapy, either with other intravenous agents or oral etoposide, and achieve a second response. Oral etoposide can also be a first line treatment in elderly or frail patients who refuse, are refractory to, or otherwise too ill to receive chemotherapy. The median survival of patients presenting with metastatic disease who receive chemotherapy is around 9 to 12 months.[18,107]

Multiple Myeloma

Multiple myeloma is a rare malignancy of plasma cells (13,800 new cases expected in 1998) that strikes predominantly patients in their seventh and eighth decades of life.[65a,90] Approximately 70% of the patients present with bone pain, and 10% will present with cord compression. Most patients present with diffuse bony involvement, but rarely a patient can have a solitary collection of plasma cells, the so-called plasmacytoma. The spine is the most common location of plasmacytomas.[33] These patients should be assessed for systemic disease, and then are generally treated with radiation and/or surgery. Most patients with a solitary bone plasmacytoma progress to full-blown myeloma within 10 years. Patients with systemic disease often receive radiotherapy for painful osseous lesions and frequently surgical stabilization is required as well, particularly of weight-bearing bones. A number of effective chemotherapeutic regimens exist,[1] but they are palliative and median survival despite treatment remains only 3 years. Special problems of patients with multiple myeloma are the frequent occurrence of renal failure and infection. Autologous bone marrow transplantation has been shown to improve overall survival and disease free survival over conventional chemotherapy in a large randomized trial and is now considered the treatment of choice for patients with good performance status and organ function.[5a,39,113] Allogeneic transplantation is associated with a high mortality rate and probably should be limited to a very select group of patients.[8a] Finally, most patients with multiple myeloma benefit from the routine monthly use of pamidronate, which recently has been shown to decrease bone fractures and need for radiation and surgery in a large multinational placebo controlled trial.[8b]

Non-Hodgkin's Lymphoma

Bone marrow involvement with lymphoma is a frequent finding in patients with non-Hodgkin's lymphoma, particularly in those patients with small cleaved cell, either follicular or diffuse. In these patients, 50% to 100% will have marrow involvement at presentation.[20] Bone marrow involvement in the low-grade lymphomas is located in peritrabecular regions, whereas in diffuse large cell lymphomas, the involvement may be accompanied by focal or diffuse myelofibrosis. True lytic bone metastases are found in only 5% to 15% of patients, mostly those with more aggressive histologies.[69] It is rare that lymphomatous involvement produces instability or significant destruction of vertebral bodies. When osseous metastases are present, these lesions generally are quite responsive to a number of interventions. Corticosteroids are directly lymphocytic, and often patients with lymphoma respond dramatically to modest doses of dexamethasone or prednisone. Secondly, a large number of chemotherapeutic agents can be used to treat lymphomas, including alkylating agents, antimetabolites, vinca alkaloids, and other plant derivatives.[4] Finally, lym-

phomatous lesions tend to be extremely sensitive to intermediate doses of radiation. It is indeed unusual to encounter a patient with lymphoma in whom no treatment option exists, except for those with end stage refractory disease.

Carcinoma of Unknown Primary

About 5% to 10% of patients diagnosed with a malignancy will fall into the category of "occult primary malignancy" or "carcinoma of unknown primary." The definition of this syndrome is the finding of a biopsy-proven neoplasm at a metastatic site for which no primary tumor mass can be located. Most often these tumors are adenocarcinomas. Bone metastases are the only site of disease in 10% to 15% of patients with this syndrome. It is extremely important to rule treatable causes of bone metastases in a logical fashion. For example, it is recommended that men receive a prostate-specific antigen determination and women receive a mammogram or perhaps a sampling of the tumor tissue for estrogen/progesterone receptors to rule out breast cancer. In these two groups of patients, very effective therapy for metastatic disease could be recommended. However, in many cases a primary site is not located antemortem, and it is not cost-effective to pursue a long, expensive search.[46] The median survival of all patients with carcinoma of unknown primary who present with isolated bone metastases is only 8 months.[66a] The role of chemotherapy in these patients is quite limited. There is some data suggesting that combination chemotherapy with cisplatin and etoposide can produce responses in selected patients.[44a,45] The decision to offer chemotherapy in this setting should depend on the assessment of a patient's overall state of health, age, personal desires, and clinical suspicion regarding the origin of the primary and possible inherent responsiveness.

Pediatric Tumors

One of the most significant differences between pediatric and adult cancers is their general chemosensitivity and the possibility that patients can be cured even when they present with widely metastatic disease. The pediatric tumors most likely to metastasize to bone, excluding leukemia and osteogenic sarcoma, are Ewing's sarcoma, rhabdomyosarcoma, and neuroblastoma. A detailed discussion of these tumors is beyond the scope of this chapter; the following is a general outline of the tumors most commonly metastasizing to bone.

Ewing's sarcoma is the most common tumor of bone in children under 10 years, and the second most common in children older than 10, following osteogenic sarcoma.[121] These tumors are characterized by a chromosomal translocation, t(11,23) (q24; q11-12), also seen in peripheral primitive neuroectodermal tumors (PNET).[53] Ewing's sarcoma can involve the spine primarily[103] or metastasize or extend locally to vertebral bodies. Rarely Ewing's sarcoma has been reported to arise primarily in the spinal epidural space.[57] Before the routine use of adjuvant chemotherapy, long-term survivors were uncommon. Ewing's sarcoma is quite sensitive to a number of agents, including doxorubicin, actinomycin-D, ifosfamide, etoposide, vincristine, and cytoxan. Chemotherapy is generally combined with radiation therapy for maximum benefit. Every patient should be treated with curative intent, as even patients with widely metastatic disease can be cured, or at least have excellent responses to therapy that can translate to years of survival. Bone marrow transplantation is also being examined in patients with relapsed or refractory disease.[120]

About one fourth of children with rhabdomyosarcoma present with metastatic disease, and bone and bone marrow involvement is common.[95] Although combination chemotherapy, surgery, and radiation do produce some long-term survivors in patients with metastatic disease, children with marrow involvement or an alveolar histology do particularly poorly.[96] Patients with these tumors should be treated as part of the intergroup rhabdomyosarcoma studies, which were inaugurated in 1972 in order to coordinate international treatment standards for this disease.[32]

Neuroblastomas are the most common malignant tumors in infancy.[70] About 50% of patients present with bone marrow involvement, although true lytic metastases are much less common. These tumors are very sensitive to both radiation and chemotherapy, but unfortunately only 15% of patients with disseminated disease survive. Newer interventions such as bone marrow transplantation hold hope for more cures.[108a]

REFERENCES

1. Alexanian R, Dimopoulos M. The treatment of multiple myeloma. N Engl J Med 330:484-489, 1994.

2. American Society of Clinical Oncology. American Society of Clinical Oncology recommendations for the use of hematopoietic colony-stimulating factors: Evidence based, clinical practical guidelines. J Clin Oncol 12:2471-2508, 1994.

3. Aristizaba SA, Miller RC, Schlichtemeier AL, Jones SE, Boone MLM. Adriamycin-irradiation cutaneous complications. Int J Radiat Oncol Biol Phys 2:325-331, 1977.

4. Armitage JO. Treatment of non-Hodgkin's lymphoma. N Engl J Med 328:1023-1030, 1993.

5. Asscher AW, Anson SG. Arterial hypertension and irradiation damage to the nervous system. Lancet 2:1343-1346, 1962.

5a. Attal M, Harosseau JL, Stoppa AM, et al. A prospective randomized trial of autologous bone marrow transplantation and chemotherapy in multiple myeloma. N Engl J Med 335:91-97, 1996.

6. Atzpodien J, Poliwoda H, Kirchner H. Alpha interferon and interleukin-2 in renal cell carcinoma: Studies in nonhospitalized patients. Semin Oncol 18:108-112, 1991.

7. Barcena A, Lobato RD, Rivas JJ, Cordobes F, De Castro S, Cabrera A, Lamas E. Spinal metastatic disease: Analysis of factors determining functional prognosis and the choice of treatment. Neurosurgery 15:820-827, 1984.

8. Bennett JM, Muss HB, Doroshow JH, Wolff S, Krementz ET, Cartwright K, Dukart G, Reisman A, Schoch I. A randomized multicenter trial comparing mitoxantron, cyclophosphomide and fluorouracil with doxorubicin, cyclophosphomide, and fluorouracil in the therapy of metastatic breast carcinoma. J Clin Oncol 10:1611-1620, 1988.

8a. Bensinger WI, Buckner CD, Anasetti C, et al. Allogeneic marrow transplantation for multiple myeloma: An analysis of risk factors on outcome. Blood 88-2787-2793, 1996.

8b. Berenson JR, Lichtenstein A, Porter L, et al. Efficacy of pamidronate in reducing skeletal events in patients with advanced multiple myeloma. N Eng J Med 334:488-493, 1996.

9. Bergmann L, Fenchel K, Weidmann E, Enzinger HM, Jahn B, Jonas D, Mitrou PS. Daily alternating administration of high-dose alpha-2b-interferon and interleukin-2 bolus infusion in metastatic renal cell cancer. Cancer 72:1733-1742, 1993.

10. Blitzer, PH. Reanalysis of the RTOG study of the palliation of symptomatic osseous metastasis. Cancer 55:1468-1472, 1985.

11. Broudy VC, Lin NL, Kaushansky K. Thrombopoietin (c-mpl ligand) acts synergistically with erythropoietin, stem cell factor, and interleukin-11 to enhance murine megakaryocyte colony growth and increases megakaryocyte ploidy in vitro. Blood 85:1719-1726, 1995.

12. Bruckner HW, Motwani BT. Chemotherapy of advanced cancer of the colon and rectum. Semin Oncol 18:443-461,1991.

13. Bull JM, Tormey DC, Li SH, Carbone PP, Falkson G, Blom J, Perlin E, Simon R. A randomized comparative trail of adriamycin versus methotrexate in combination drug therapy. Cancer 41:1649-1657, 1978.

14. Bunn PA. Lung Cancer: Current Understanding, Staging and Treatment. Princeton: Bristol-Myers Squibb, 1992, pp 39-61.

15. Bunn PA, Crowley J, Hazuka M. The role of GM-CSF in limited stage SCLC: A randomized phase III study of the southwest oncology group [abstract]. Proc Am Soc Clin Oncol 11:292, 1992.

16. Carney DN, Grogan L, Smit EF, Harford P, Berendsen HH, Postmus PE. Single-agent oral etoposide for elderly small cell lung cancer patients. Semin Oncol 17:49-53, 1990.

17. Cassady JR, Richter MP, Piro AJ, Jaffe N. Radiation-adriamycin interactions: Preliminary clinical observations. Cancer 36:946-949, 1975.

18. Catane R, Lichter A, Lee YJ, Brereton HD, Schwade JG, Glatstein E. Small cell lung cancer: Analysis of treatment factors contributing to prolonged survival. Cancer 48:1936-1943, 1981.

19. Cellerino R, Tummarello D, Guidi F, Isidori P, Raspugli M, Biscottini B, Fatati G. A randomized trial of alternating chemotherapy versus best supportive care in advanced non-small lung cancer. J Clin Oncol 9:1453-1461, 1991.

20. Chabner BA, Fisher RI, Young RC, DeVita VT. Staging of non-Hodgkin's lymphoma. Semin Oncol 7:285-291, 1980.

21. Cobb CA, Leavens ME, Eckles N. Indications for nonoperative treatment of spinal cord compression due to breast cancer. J Neurosurg 47:653-658, 1977.

22. Cohen ME, Duffner PK, Terplan KL. Myelopathy with severe structural derangement associated with combined modality therapy. Cancer 52:1590-1596, 1983.

23. Coia L, Engstrom P, Paul A, Stafford P, Hanks G. Long term results of infusional 5-FU, mitomycin-C, and radiation as primary management of esophageal carcinoma. Int J Radiat Oncol Biol Phys 20:29-36, 1991.

24. Cole MP. A new anti-oestrogenic agent in late breast cancer. An early clinical appraisal with ICI 46474. Br J Cancer 25:270-275, 1971.

25. Cookson MS, Sarosdy MF. Hormonal therapy for metastatic prostate cancer: Issues of timing and total androgen blockage. South Med J 87:1-6, 1994.

26. Cooper K, Bajorin D, Shapiro W, Krol G, Sze G, Bosl GJ. Decompression of epidural metastases from germ cell tumors with chemotherapy. J Neurooncol 8:275-280, 1990.

27. Cordon-Cardo C, O'Brien JP. The multidrug resistance phenotype in human cancer. In DeVita VT, Hellman S, Rosenberg SA, eds. Important Advances in Oncology. Philadelphia: JB Lippincott, 1991, pp 19-39.

28. Crawford ED. Hormonal therapy of prostatic carcinoma. Cancer 66:1035-1038, 1990.

28a. D'Andrea GM, Seidman AD. Docctaxel and paclitaxel in breast cancer therapy: Present status and future prospects. Semi Oncol 24 (Suppl 3):27-44, 1997.

29. DeAntoni EP, Crawford ED. Pretreatment of metastatic disease. Prostate cancer in the older male. Cancer 74:2182-2187, 1994.

30. Department of Veterans Affairs Laryngeal Cancer Study Group. Induction chemotherapy plus radiation compared with surgery plus radiation in patients with advanced laryngeal cancer. N Engl J Med 324:1685-1690, 1991.

31. de Sauvage FJ, Hass PE, Spencer S, Malloy BE, Gurney AL, Spencer SA, Darbonne WC, Henzel WJ, Wong SC, Kuang WJ, Oles KJ, Hultgren B, Solber LA, Goeddel DV, Eaton DL. Stimulation of megakaryocytopoiesis and thrombopoiesis by the c-Mpl ligand. Nature 369:533-538, 1994.

32. Diller L. Rhabdomyosarcoma and other soft tissue sarcomas of childhood. Curr Opin Oncol 4:689-695, 1992.

33. Dimopulous MA. Solitary plasmacytoma of bone and asymptomatic multiple myeloma. Hematol Oncol Clin North Am 6:356-369, 1992.

34. Donaldson SS, Kaplan HS. Complications of treatment of Hodgkin's disease in children. Cancer Treat Rep 66:977-989, 1982.

35. Eddy DM. High-dose chemotherapy with autologous bone marrow transplantation for the treatment of metastatic breast cancer. J Clin Oncol 10:657-670, 1992.

36. Ellis RE. The distribution of active bone marrow in the adult. Phys Med Biol 5:255-258, 1961.

37. Emery SE, Brazinski MS, Koka A, Bensusan JS, Stevenson S. The biological and biomechanical effects of irradiation on anterior spinal bone grafts in a canine model. J Bone Joint Surg 76A:540-548, 1994.

38. Fisher RI, Coltman CA, Doroshow JH, Rayner AA, Hawkins MJ, Mier JW, Wiernik P, McMarins JD, Weiss GR, Margolin KA. Metastatic renal cancer treated with interleukin-2 and lymphokine activated killer cells. Ann Intern Med 108:518-523, 1988.

39. Gahrton G , Tura S, Ljungman P, Belanger C, Brandt L, Cavo M, Facon T, Granena A, Gore M, Gratworth A, Lowenber B, Nikoskelain J, Reiffers JJ, Samson D, Verdonck K, Volin L. Allogeneic bone marrow transplantation in multiple myeloma. N Engl J Med 325:1267-1273, 1991.

40. Gastrointestinal Tumor Study Group. Prolongation of disease free interval in surgically treated rectal carcinoma. N Engl J Med 312:1465-1472, 1985.

41. Gastrointestinal Tumor Study Group. Further evidence of effective adjuvant combined radiation and chemotherapy following curative resection of pancreatic cancer. Cancer 59:2006-2010, 1987.

42. Gilbert HA, Kagan AR, Nussbaum H, Rao AR, Satzman J, Chan P, Allen B, Forsythe A. Evaluation of radiation therapy for bone metastases: Pain relief and quality of life. Am J Roentgenol 129:1095-1096, 1977.

43. Gilbert RW, Kim JH, Posner JB. Epidural spinal cord compression from metastatic tumor: Diagnosis and treatment. Ann Neurol 3:40-51, 1978.

44. Goldwein JW. Radiation myelopathy: A review. Med Pediatr Oncol 15:89-95, 1987.

44a. Hainsworth JD, Erland JB, Kalman LA, et al. Carcinoma of unknown primary site: Treatment with 1-hour paclitaxel, carboplatin and extended schedule etoposide. J Clin Oncol 15:2385-2393, 1997.

45. Hainsworth JD, Johnson DH, Greco FA. The role of etoposide in the treatment of poorly differentiated carcinoma of unknown primary site. Cancer 67 (Suppl 1):310-314,1991.

46. Hamilton, CS, Langlands AO. ACUPS (adenocarcinoma of unknown primary site): A clinical and cost benefit analysis. Int J Radiat Oncol Biol Phy 13:1497-1503, 1987.

47. Harrington KD. Anterior cord decompression and spinal stabilization for patients with metastatic lesions of the spine. J Neurosurg 61:107-117, 1984.

48. Hayes FA, Thompson EI, Hvizdola E, O'Connor D, Green AA. Chemotherapy as an alternative to laminectomy and radiation in the management of epidural tumor. J Pediatr 104: 221-224, 1984.

49. Helweg-Larsen S, Rasmusson B, Sorensen PS. Recovery of gait after radiotherapy in paralytic patients with metastatic epidural spinal cord compression. Neurology 40:1234-1235, 1990.

50. Herodin F, Mestries JC, Janodet D, Martin S, Mathieu J, Gascon MP, Pernin MO, Arnaud Y. Recombinant glycosylated human interleukin-6 accelerates peripheral blood platelet count recovery in radiation induced bone marrow depression in baboons. Blood 80:688-695, 1993.

51. Herskovic A, Martz K, Al-Sarraf M. Combined chemotherapy and radiotherapy compared with radiotherapy alone in patients with cancer of the esophagus. N Engl J Med 326:1593-1598, 1992.

52. Holmes FA, Walter RS, Theriault RL, Forman AD, Newton LK, Raber MN, Buzdar AU, Frye DK, Hortobagyi GN. Phase II trial of taxol, an active drug in metastatic breast cancer. J Natl Cancer Inst 83:1797-1805, 1991.

53. Horowitz ME, Tsokos MG, DeLaney TF. Ewing's sarcoma. CA Cancer J Clin 42:300-320, 1992.

53a. Hortobagyi GN, Theriault RL, Porter L, et al. Efficacy of pamidronate in reducing skeletal complications in patients with breast cancer and lytic bone metastases. Protocol 19 Aredia Breast Cancer Study Group. N Engl J Med 335: 1985, 1996.

54. Huggins C, Stevens RE, Hodges S. Studies of prostate cancer. The effects of castration of advanced carcinoma of the prostate. Arch Surg 43:209-228, 1941.

54a. Isaacs C, Robert NJ, Bailey FA. Randomized placebo-controlled study of recombinant human interleukin-11 to prevent chemotherapy-induced thrombocytopenia in patients with breast cancer receiving dose-intensive cyclophosphamide and doxorubicin. J Clin Oncol 15:3368-3377, 1997.

55. Kass S, Lund E, Thorud E, Hatlevoll R, Host H. Symptomatic treatment versus combination chemotherapy for patients with extensive non-small cell lung cancer. Cancer 67:2443-2447, 1991.

56. Karvonen RL. An animal model of pulmonary radiation fibrosis with biochemical, physiologic, immunologic and morphologic observations. Radiat Res 111:68-80, 1987.

57. Kasper GJ, Kamphorst W, van de Graaff M, van Alphen AM, Veerman AJP. Primary spinal epidural extraosseous Ewing's sarcoma. Cancer 68:648-654, 1991.

58. Kim JH, Chu FC, Woodward HQ, Huvos A. Radiation induced sarcomas of bone following therapeutic radiation. Int J Radiat Oncol Biol Phys 9:107-110, 1983.

59. Kim RY, Smith JW, Spencer SA, Meredith RF, Salter MM. Malignant epidural spinal cord compression associated with a paravertebral mass: Its radiotherapeutic outcome on radiosensitivity. Int J Radiat Oncol Biol Phys 27:1079-1083, 1993.

60. Kim RY, Spencer SA, Meredith RF, Weppelmann B, Lee JY, Smith JW, Salter MM. Extradural spinal cord compression: Analysis of factors determining functional prognosis—Prospective study. Radiology 176:279-282, 1990.

61. Klasa RJ, Murray N, Coldman AJ. Dose-intensity meta-analysis of chemotherapy regimens in small-cell carcinoma of the lung. J Clin Oncol 9:499-508, 1991.

62. Klein EA. The multidrug resistance gene in renal cell carcinoma. Semin Urol VII:207-214, 1989.

63. Koh HK. Cutaneous melanoma. N Engl J Med 325:171-182, 1991.

64. Krook JE, Moertel CG, Gunderson LL, Wieand HS, Collins RT, Beart RW, Kubista JP, Poon MA, Meyers WC, Maillard JA. Effective surgical adjuvant therapy for high risk rectal carcinoma. N Engl J Med 324:709-715, 1991.

65. Laing EJ. Problems in wound healing asssociated with chemotherapy and radiation therapy. Probl Vet Med 2:433-441, 1990.

65a. Landis SH, Murray T, Bolden S, et al. Cancer statistics 1998. CA Cancer J Clin 45:6-39, 1998.

66. Lavey RS, Dempsey WH. Erythropoietin increases hemoglobin in cancer patients during radiation therapy. Int J Radiat Oncol Biol Phys 27:1147-1152, 1993.

66a. Lenzi R, Hess KR, Abbruzzese MC, et al. Poorly differentiated carcinoma and poorly differentiated adenocarcinoma of unknown origin: Favorable subsets of patients with unknown primary carcinoma? J Clin Oncol 15:2056-2066, 1997.

67. Levick S, Jacobs C, Loukas DF, Gordon DH, Meyskens FL, Uhm K. Naproxen sodium in treatment of bone pain due to metastatic cancer. Pain 35:253-258, 1988.

68. Littman P, Rosenstock JG, Bailey C. Radiation myelitis following craniospinal irradiation with concurrent actinomycin-D therapy. Cancer 52:1590-1596, 1983.

69. Longo DL, DeVita VT, Jaffe ES, Mauch P, Urba WJ. Lymphocytic lymphomas. In DeVita VT, Hellman S, Rosenberg SA, eds. Cancer: Principles and Practice. Philadelphia: JB Lippincott, 1993, pp 1859-1927.

70. Lopez-Ibor B, Schwart AD. Neuroblastoma. Pediatr Clin North Am 32:755-778, 1985.

71. Ludwig H, Elke F, Kotzman H, Hocker P. Gisslinger J, Barnas U. Erythropoietin treatment of anemia associated with multiple myeloma. N Engl J Med 322:1693-1699, 1990.

72. Ma LD, Taylor GA, Wharam MD, Wiley JM. Recall pneumonitis: Adriamycin potentiation of radiation pneumonitis in two children. Radiology 187:465-467, 1993.

73. Maldazys JD, derKernion JB. Prognostic factors in metastatic renal carcinoma. J Urol 136:376-379, 1986.

74. Maranzano E, Latini P, Checcaglini F, Ricci S, Panizza BM, Aristei C, Perrucci E, Beneventi S, Corgna E, Tonato M. Radiation therapy in metastatic spinal cord compression: A progressive analysis of 105 consecutive patients. Cancer 67:1311-1317, 1991.

75. Marshall LF, Langfitt TW. Combined therapy for metastatic extradural tumors of the spine. Cancer 40:2067-2070, 1977.

76. Maurer HM, Geahn EA, Beltangandy M, Crist W, Dickman PS, Donaldon SS, Fryer C, Hammond D, Hays DM, Herrmann J, Heyn R, Jones PM, Lawrence W, Newton W, Ortega J, Abdelsalam HR, Raney RB, Ruymann, FB, Soule E, Tefft M, Webber B, Wiener E, Wharam M, Vietti TJ. The intergroup rhabdomyosarcoma Study-II. Cancer 71:1904-1922, 1993.

77. Mertens WC, Stit L, Porter AT. Strontium therapy and relief of pain in patients with porstatci carcinoma metastatic to bone: A dose response relationship? Am J Clin Oncol 16:238-242, 1993.

78. Momin F, Kraut M, Lattin P. Thrombocytopenia in patients receiving chemoradiotherapy and G-CSF for locally advanced non-small cell lung cancer (NSCLC) [abstract]. Proc Am Soc Clin Oncol 11:410, 1992.

78a. Moulopoulos LA, Dimopoulos MA. Magnetic resonance imaging of the bone marrow in hematologic malignancies. Blood 90:2127-2147,1997.

79. Nemechek PM, Corder MC. Radiation recall associated with vinblastine in a patient treated for Kaposi sarcoma related to acquired immune deficiency syndrome. Cancer 70:1605-1609,1992.

80. Newcombe JF. Effect of intra-arterial nitrogen mustard infusion on wound healing in rabbits. Ann Surg 163:319-329, 1966.

81. Orlandini GE, Ruggiero C, Gulisano M, Ruggiero M, Villari N, Casamassima F. Magnetic Resonance (MR) evaluation of bone marrow in vertebral bodies. Arch Ital Anat Embriol 96: 93-100, 1991.

82. Pallis CA, Louis S, Morgan RL. Radiation myelopathy. Brain 84:460-479, 1961.

83. Peters WP, Shpall EJ, Jones RB, Olsen GA, Blast RC, Gackeman JP, Moore JD. High-dose combination alkylating agents with bone marrow support as initial treatment for metastatic breast cancer. J Clin Oncol 6:1368-1376, 1988.

84. Pienta KJ, Redman B, Hussain M, Cummings G, Esper PS, Appel C, Flaherty LE. Phase II evaluation of oral estramustine and oral etoposide in hormone-refractory adenocarcinoma of the prostate. J Clin Oncol 12:2005-2012, 1994.

85. Pizzo PA, Horowitz ME, Poplack DG, Hays DM, Kun LE. Solid tumors of childhood. In DeVita VT, Hellman S, Rosenberg SA, eds. Cancer: Principles and Practice. Philadephia: JB Lippincott, 1993, pp 1738-1761.

86. Platanais LC, Miller CB, Mick R, Hart RD, Ozer H, McEvilly JM, Jones RJ, Rataian MJ. Treatment of chemotherapy-induced anemia with recombinant human erythropoietin in cancer patients. J Clin Oncol 9:2021-2026, 1991.

87. Price P, Hoskin PJ, Eastan D, Austin D, Palmer SG, Yaynold JR. Prospective randomized trial of single and multifraction radiotherapy schedules in the treatment of painful bony metastases. Radiother Oncol 6:247-255, 1986.

88. Quesada JR. Biologic response modifiers in the therapy of metastatic renal cell carcinoma. Semin Oncol 15:396-407, 1988.

89. Rao S, Badani D, Schildauer T, Borges M. Metastatic malignancy of the cervical spine. Spine 17S:407-412, 1992.

90. Riedel DA, Pottern LM. The epidemiology of multiple myeloma. Hematol Oncol Clin North Am 6:225-247, 1992.

91. Robinson RG, Preston DF, Baxter KG, Dusing RW, Spicer JA. Clinical experience with strontium-89 in prostatic and breast cancer patients. Semin Oncol 20 (Suppl 2):44-48, 1993.

92. Rodichok LD, Harper GR, Ruckdeschel JC, Price A, Roberson G, Barron KD, Horton J. Early diagnosis of spinal epidural metastases. Am J Med 70:1181-1187, 1981.

93. Rubin P. Extradural spinal cord compression by tumor. Radiology 93:1243-1260, 1969.

94. Rubin P, Landman S, Mayer E, Keller B, Ciccio S. Bone marrow regeneration and extension after extended field irradiation in Hodgkin's disease. Cancer 32:699-771, 1973.

95. Ruymann FB, Newton WA, Ragab AH, Donaldson MH, Foulkes M. Bone marrow metastases at diagnosis in children and adolescents with rhabdomyosarcoma. A report from the Intergroup Rhabdomyosarcoma Study. Cancer 53:368-373, 1984.

96. Ruymann FB. Rhabdomyosarcoma in children and adolescents. Hematol Oncol Clin North Am 1:621-654, 1987.

97. Salazar OM, Rubin P, Hendrickson FR, Komaki R, Poulter C, Newall J, Asbell SO, Mohiuddin M, Van Ess J. Single-dose half-body irradiation for palliation of multiple bone metastases from solid tumors. Cancer 58:29-36, 1986.

98. Schaberg J, Gainor BJ. A profile of metastatic carcinoma of the spine. Spine 10:19-20, 1985.

99. Scheid V, Buzdar AU, Smith TL, Hortobagyi GN. Clinical course of breast cancer paitents with osseous metastasis treated with combination chemotherapy. Cancer 58:2589-2593, 1986.

100. Schultheiss TE, Higgins EM, El-Mahdi AM. The latent period in clinical radiation myelopathy. Int J Radiat Oncol Biol Phys 10:1109-1115, 1984.

101. Schultheiss TE, Stephens LC, Maor MH. Analysis of the histopathology of radiation myelopathy. Int J Radiat Oncol Biol Phys 14:27-32, 1988.

102. Seidman AD, Scherr HI, Petrylak D, Dershaw DD, Curley T. Estramustine and vinblastine: Use of prostate specific antigen as a clinical trial end point for hormone refractory prostatic cancer. J Urol 147:931-934, 1992.

103. Sharafuddin MJA, Haddad FS, Hitchon P, Haddad SF, El-Khoury GY. Treatment options in primary Ewing's sarcoma of the spine: Report of seven cases and review of the literature. Neurosurgery 30:610-619, 1992.

104. Shocker JD, Brady LW. Radiation therapy for bone metastasis. Clin Orthop 169:38-43, 1982.

105. Sischy B, Doggett RL, Krall JM, Taylor DG, Sause WT, Lipsett JA, Seydel HG. Definitive irradiation and chemotherapy for radiosensitization in management of anal carcinoma. J Natl Cancer Inst 81:850-856, 1989.

106. Smalley RV, Carpenter J, Bartolucci A, Vogel C, Krauss S. A comparison of cyclophosphomide, adriamycin, 5-fluorouracil (CAF) and cyclophosphomide, methotrexate, 5-fluorouracil, vincristine and prednisone (CMFVP) in patients with metastatic breast cancer. Cancer 40: 625-632, 1977.

107. Sorensen JB, Hansen HH. Recent advances in diagnosis and treatment of small cell and non-small cell lung cancer. Curr Opin Oncol 6:162-170, 1994.

108. Spivak JL. Recombinant human erythropoietin and the anemia of cancer. Blood 84:997-1004, 1994.

108a. Straum DO, Matthay KK, O'Leary M. Consolidation chemoradiotherapy and autologous bone marrow transplantation versus continued chemotherapy for metastatic neuroblastoma. A report of two concurrent children's cancer group studies. J Clin Oncol 14:2417-2426, 1996.

109. Suit H, Urie M. Protein beams in radiation therapy. J Natl Cancer Inst 84:155-164, 1992.

110. Sundaresan N, Digiacinto GV, Hughes JE, Cafferty M, Vallejo A. Treatment of neoplastic spinal cord compression: results of a prospective study. Neurosurgery 29:645-650, 1991.

110a. Tannock IF, Osoba D, Stockler MR, et al. Chemotherapy with mitoxantrone plus prednisone or prednisone alone for symptomatic hormone-resistant prostate cancer: A Canadian randomized trial with palliative end points. J Clin Oncol 14:1756-1764, 1996.

110b. Tepler I, Elias I, Smith JW, et al. A randomized placebo-controlled trial of recombinant human interleukin-11 in cancer patients with severe thrombocytopenia due to chemotherapy. Blood 87:3607-3614, 1996.

111. Thames HD, Withers HR, Peters LJ, Fletcher GH. Changes in early and late radiation responses with altered dose fractionation: Implication for dose-survival relationships. Int J Radiat Oncol Biol Phys 8:219-226, 1982.

111a. Theriault RL, Lipton A, Leff R, et al. Reduction of skeletal related complications in breast cancer patients with osteolytic bone metastases receiving hormone therapy, by monthly pamidronate sodium infusion. Proc Am Soc Clin Oncol 16:130a, 1997.

112. Tong D, Gillick L, Hendrickson FR. The palliation of symptomatic osseous metastases. Cancer 50:893-899, 1982.

113. Tricot G, Jagannath S, Vesole D, Nelson J, Tindle S, Miller L, Cheson B, Crowley J, Barlogie B. Peripheral blood stem cell transplants for multiple myeloma. Idenitification of favorable variables for rapid engraftment in 225 patients. Blood 85:588-596, 1995.

114. Vecht CJ, Haaxma-Reiche H, Van Putten WLJ, De Visser M, Vries EP, Twijnstra A. Initial bolus of conventional versus high-dose dexamethasone in metastatic spinal cord compression. Neurology 39:1255-1257, 1989.

115. Vegesna V, Withers HR, McBride WH, Holly FE. Adriamycin induced recall of radiation pneumonitis and epilation in lung and hair follicles of mouse. Int J Radiat Oncol Biol Phys 23:977-981, 1992.

116. Wani MC, Taylor HL, Wall ME, Coggon P, McPhail AT. Plant antitumor agents. VI. The isolation and structure of taxol, a novel antileukemic and antitumor agent from Taxus brevifolia. J Am Chem Soc 93:2325-2327, 1971.

117. Wingo PA, Tong T, Bolden S. Cancer statistics, 1995. CA Cancer J Clin 45:8-30, 1995.

118. Withers HR, Thames HD. Dose fractionation and volume effects in normal tissues and tumors. Am J Clin Oncol 11:313-329, 1988.

119. Woods RL, Williams CJ, Levi J, Page J, Bell D, Byrne M, Kerestes ZL. A randomised trial of cisplatin and vindesine versus supportive care only in advanced non-small cell lung cancer. Br J Cancer 61:608-611, 1990.

120. Yaniv I, Bouffet E, Irle C, Negrier S, Biron P, Favrot M, Philip I, Brunat-Mentigny M, Philip T. Autologous bone marrow transplantation in pediatric solid tumors. Pediatr Hematol Oncol 7:35-46, 1990.

121. Young JL, Miller RW. Incidence of malignant tumors in children. J Pediatr 86:254-258, 1975.

122. Young RF, Post EM, King GA. Treatment of spinal epidural metastases. J Neurosurg 53:741-748, 1980.

123. Zeidler C, Kanz L, Hurkuck F, Rittman KL, Wildfand I, Kadoya T, Mikayama T, Souza L, Welte K. In vivo effects of interleukin-6 on thrombopoiesis in healthy and irradiated primates. Blood 80:2740-2745, 1992.

124. Zwelling LA. Topoisomerase II as a target of antileukemia drugs. A review of controversial areas. Hematol Pathol 3:101-112, 1989.

Special Considerations

Orthotics

Seth M. Zeidman, M.D.

Orthotic device use is widespread and contributes a significant amount to overall expenditures on spinal health care. Correctly and appropriately used, orthoses are often highly effective, facilitating healing and deformity correction. When used incorrectly or inappropriately, they are ineffective, uncomfortable, and a costly waste of resources. Proper use and application of orthoses to clinical problems affecting the thoracic spine is dependent upon an understanding of the underlying biomechanics of the spine and the biomechanical capabilities of orthotic devices. This chapter will focus on (1) the goals of bracing, (2) the biomechanics of the spine and how this relates to orthoses, (3) an assessment of common thoracic orthoses, (4) the role of these devices for specific clinical problems affecting the thoracic spine, and (5) the limitations of orthoses.

The spine has three major functions: support, mobility, and spinal cord protection. The science of spinal orthotics alters the existing patterns of deformation and kinematics of the spine by the application of forces in an effort to control the spine by providing, in general, support, rest, immobilization, protection, deformity, and correction.

The specific aims of spinal bracing as applied to the thoracic spine and thoracolumbar junction include (1) trunk support, (2) decrease loading of the thoracic spinal column and decrease muscular activity, (3) limit intersegmental and overall trunk motion, (4) increase intra-abdominal pressure (thus stabilizing the spine), and (5) spinal realignment.

To support and rest the spine, the orthosis often must substitute for and assist the musculature. Immediately after spinal surgery or injury, protection of the spinal cord and nerve roots is paramount. In this situation, the orthosis substitutes for the spine and musculature by providing support. When certain positions or movements are painful, the orthosis limits motion. The orthosis can serve as a comforter or psychological reminder, thereby limiting undesired activity or motion. An orthosis provides a supportive role that includes heat, massage, and placebo effects. Finally, spinal orthoses can be used to correct scoliotic and kyphotic deformities.

An understanding of the reasons for bracing, along with knowledge of the properties of individual orthoses, is imperative for their successful usage. Erroneous judgment and inappropriate assumptions in orthotic selection may result in limited benefit and may even cause injury to the patient.

Although progress has been made, there is still a paucity of quality research on spinal orthotics, particularly controlled clinical trials to assess their efficacy. Thus a significant portion of our knowledge is based on inferences from objective information regarding clinical biomechanics and physical properties of the spine.

BIOMECHANICS OF BRACING

Clinical bracing is based on the application of forces to the spine. The magnitude and resultant effects of these forces ultimately depend upon the biomechanics of the orthosis and the patient. The spine is a series of linked semirigid bodies (vertebrae) separated by viscoelastic linkages (discs and ligaments), and encased in materials with multiple moduli of elasticity and viscosities. The thoracic spine is surrounded by skin, subcutaneous fat, muscles, ribs, air, and lungs. With the exception of the ribs, which are significantly stiffer, the materials adjacent to the spinal column have minimal stiffness. The ribs stiffen the thoracic spine by forming a box-like construct that increases the stiffness of the thoracic spine in bending by 200%.[1]

The biomechanical aim of any spinal orthosis is the transmission of sufficient and appropriate forces to the vertebrae via "nonstiff," viscoelastic transmitters. Force is not generally applied directly to the spine but must be transmitted via the surrounding structures (such as ribs). Whether the goal is support, immobilization, or correction, the mechanism is dependent upon the transmission of forces to the spine. Spinal bracing presents unique problems, the most significant of which is its relative lack of effectiveness in achieving success. The volume of soft tissue separating the spine and the brace minimizes effectiveness. There is an inverse relationship between the thickness of soft tissue between the spine and the inner surface of the brace and the effectiveness of the brace. External forces applied to the spine are limited by discomfort and the characteristics of the structures through which they are transmitted.

The major mechanical factor limiting the transmission of forces to the spine is the stiffness of the structures through which the force must be applied. The stiffness of these transmitters varies considerably. The ribs (although not particularly stiff) represent the stiffest available transmitter; fat, which has a much lower stiffness, is at the other end of the continuum.

The thoracic spine is unique because it is the only segment of the spine to which traditional external splinting principles can be applied. The thickness of soft tissue separating the spine and the external orthosis is relatively unimportant in this region because of the stabilizing effect of the firm rib cage. It is possible to apply forces more effectively to a thoracic scoliosis than to one in the lumbar region because the ribs are better transmitters than the muscle, fat, and viscera in the lumbar region.

Limitations to the application of forces include the pain sensitivity of the skin and the deeper tissues. The skin must be able to be cleansed of dirt, debris, and excretions, and it must be provided with adequate ventilation. These factors limit the magnitude and the duration of force that can be applied. As a result, the clinician is able to apply forces to the spine by means of orthoses but is not able to completely and continuously control motion.

All of these factors must be considered during evaluation of the forces that can be expected to be transmitted to the particular region of the spine in order to achieve the desired therapeutic goal.

Normal Kinematics of the Thoracic Spine and Appropriate Orthosis Selection

The clinician must understand the normal kinematics of the spine and their role in influencing bracing problems. The thoracic spine experiences significant motion, but is significantly less mobile than either the cervical or lumbar regions. Flexion is greater than extension and the amount of rotation in the sagittal plane progressively increases in a rostral to caudal manner. Transition to the kinematic pattern of the lumbar spine typically occurs between T9 and T12.

Selection of the optimal orthosis for controlling the spine requires consideration of regional kinematics, along with an analysis assessing the seven degrees of freedom (see box).[8] This includes evaluation of translation along each of the three Cartesian coordinates and rotation about each of the three axes. The clinician is typically most concerned with two or three of the seven degrees of freedom. However, an awareness and an analysis of all six are preferable. When orthotics are used to compensate for instability, a basic understanding of clinical instability is essential. It is necessary to consider which structures have been rendered nonfunctional so that appropriate compensatory support may be applied. Spines that are unstable as a result of the loss of the functional integrity of the ventral elements are more unstable in extension. Spinal instability due to disruption of dorsal elements is more unstable in flexion. Certain orthoses protect against ventral displacement more effectively than against dorsal displacement and vice versa. Attention is then focused on the rigidity of fixation. The orthotic device must compensate for instability and the device selected should be the most appropriate one for the particular type of instability being treated.

Bone and ligaments adapt to repetitive loading. An example of this adaptation is the change ob-

served in Scheuermann's disease with bracing.
Here, the actual configuration of the spine changes.
Alterations are more readily mediated in the growing skeleton, where Volkmann's laws can operate
through the epiphysis. Time (duration of bracing) is
an important consideration in the design and use of
spinal orthotics for these purposes.

Once a diagnosis is made, the particular therapeutic goals are set for each individual patient—
whether to support, immobilize, or correct the
spine. An analysis of the six degrees of freedom in
which the involved vertebrae can move is performed to decide which degrees of freedom are to be
controlled, as well as the manner and the extent of
control required. First the movement that must be
prevented is determined. On the basis of these determinations, the orthosis that is best able to
achieve stability is selected.[8]

Mechanical Principles of Spinal Orthoses

Spinal orthoses use some combination of five major
forces to control the spine: (1) balanced horizontal
forces, (2) fluid compression, (3) distraction, (4) sleeve
principle, and (5) skeletal fixation.[8] Horizontal
forces provide efficient bending moments for the
correction of lateral curvature, vertebral derotation,
and spinal immobilization. Most orthotic loading
situations are mediated via a three-point bending
mechanism. Three horizontal forces are applied at
points along the length of the spine. Two in one direction, and one in the opposite direction.

Because the system is in equilibrium, the sum of
forces and the sum of the resulting bending moment equals zero. Consequently, the site of application of the forces and their magnitudes are closely
interrelated.

The bending moment applied to the spine produces the angular correction. The bending moment
varies, depending upon the segmental level. It is
maximal at the site of the middle force and decreases to zero at the termini of the brace. The two
terminal forces should be positioned as far from the
middle force as is feasible. In a three-point bending
fixation system, the middle force should be located
at the site of maximum deformity or instability. By
placing the middle force at the apex of the curve,
maximal correction is possible.

Fluid compression permits soft tissues (muscles,
fat, fascia, and tendons) to support a compressive
load. Nature employs the diaphragm and abdominal
muscles to compress the viscera. Soft tissue under
pressure supports or splints the spine. Distraction
permits the application of tension to immobilize
and stabilize the spine.

The sleeve principle involves the construction of a
cage around the patient with two fixation points, one
above the other. Between the two points of fixation
there are various uprights. The uprights may be at the
sides of the patient, or they may be dorsal and/or
paraspinous. These uprights serve as a sleeve, as a
splint, as a distractor, and as a point for attachment
of various accessory devices.

Skeletal fixation provides the most effective
methods of reliably controlling spinal motion. Examples include halo fixation and halo pelvic fixation devices.[8]

CORSETS AND THORACIC BRACES

Corsets provide little spinal control. Corsets with
stiff uprights provide slightly better control. A
longer brace is more efficacious for providing spinal

stability than a shorter one. Long braces have greater leverage, which provides a mechanical advantage. The length/width ratio of the brace plays a significant role is in its efficacy in stabilizing the spine.

Mechanical devices added to braces provide additional support. Examples include devices limiting axial rotation, usually via pads and supports that apply discrete, localized loads for particular purposes. These can often be used effectively in the treatment of scoliosis or kyphosis. Spinal orthoses incorporating the thigh may be efficacious. Increased fixation can be achieved through the use of more rigid material, such as plaster.

Substantial immobilization is achieved through the use of external skeletal fixation with the halo apparatus in conjunction with a body cast. A molded plaster cast offers the best nonskeletal fixation against axial spinal rotation. The long body cast offers greater immobilization because of greater purchase and leverage. The most effective device at present for immobilizing the entire spine is the halo pelvic apparatus. For the most effective control of the degrees of freedom, the halo pelvic skeletal fixation, halo cast, halo vest, or a Minerva plaster jacket should be used.

Corsets provide some degree of immobilization, however, the support is minimal. Corsets should not be used when rigid external fixation is required. Newer corsets are fabricated with low-temperature thermoplastic polymers that can be custom molded for each patient. These form-fit plastics are then placed within Lycra envelopes and fastened with Velcro. These systems are light, fit better than off-the-shelf models, and are more affordable.

When custom fitted, some long thoracic corsets provide significant immobilization. However, they are not as effective as some of the other appliances. Their main indication is chronic, benign, thoracic pain, for which the orthosis gives good symptomatic relief. In addition to the increased warmth and massage, they may provide a distinct placebo effect.

Conformation to the Torso

Splinting devices that do not closely conform to the torso have several disadvantages. The Jewett hyperextension brace applies a dorsally directed force at the sternum and pubic region. Because the pressure applied may be significant, it frequently causes discomfort. In the case of lumbar instability, it does not place the ventrally directed force in an appropriate location (i.e., the low lumbar or lumbar spine).

Furthermore, the Jewett brace and similar techniques do not promote maintenance of the cylindrical body shell. That is, contact with the torso is made over a relatively small surface area. The Jewett brace provides a three-point bending biomechanical advantage, which has been shown to be an important factor in the stability achieved with external bracing. The maintenance of the body shell also increases the stability of the ventral and dorsal spinal columns. The trunk serves as an important stabilizer of the spine. Finally, the Jewett and similar braces do not significantly restrict lateral bending.

The conformation and fit between the ventral and dorsal halves of the brace are critical to the brace's ability to stabilize the spine. The lack of a close fit between halves allows parallelogram deformation of the bracing construct. This in turn diminishes protection. The halves of the brace should be secured so that one does not slide. They should be rigidly attached to one another.

Thoracolumbar Orthoses

Thoracic orthoses can be classified as either flexible or rigid devices. The flexible orthoses are similar to the rigid ones with regard to the overall architecture. The flexible thoracolumbosacral orthosis (TLSO) extends higher, with the upper border at the midscapular level at the xiphoid process. These garments are circumferentially adjustable by means of side, front, and back laces or hooks, or more recently with Velcro straps.

The flexible TLSO is often used for low back pain. It reportedly decreases the myoelectric activity of the paraspinal muscle groups and increases intra-abdominal pressure, thus diminishing disc loading.

Jewett Hyperextension Brace

The Jewett hyperextension brace applies a three-point bending truncal force with two ventral supports, one on the symphysis pubis and another at the sternomanubrial junction. The third point of fixation is at the thoracolumbar junction. It is designed to resist motion primarily in flexion, and attempts to extend the thoracic and upper lumbar spine. This brace shifts weight from the ventral to the dorsal elements of the thoracic vertebrae.

The primary advantage of the Jewett hyperextension brace is the ability to adjust the levels at which maximal fixation can occur. It is able to relatively immobilize a particular segment of the thoracolumbar spine. It is less effective in restricting bending in the coronal plane and offers virtually no resistance to axial rotation (y-axis). When the brace is adjusted into hyperextension, it shifts the weight-bearing axis more toward the dorsal elements of the vertebrae, diminishing stresses on the ventral elements.

Jewett hyperextension braces require some degree of bone contact. They are best used for symptomatic relief of compression fractures, where there is not significant fear or risk of further collapse. They do not provide significant resistance against flexion, but are poorly tolerated by elderly patients.

Nagel et al.[5] demonstrated that the Jewett hyperextension brace reduced intersegmental motion and flexion at the thoracolumbar junction. Because this brace has no pelvic support, however, lateral and axial rotation were not affected. Outcome studies of patients treated with Jewett braces are not available.

Patwardhan et al.[6] evaluated the effectiveness of the Jewett hyperextension brace in controlling deformity progression under gravitational and flexion loads using a finite element analysis that simulated three severities of thoracolumbar injury. They found that the Jewett brace restored stiffness to normal values in injuries simulating one- and two-column fractures. For three-column injuries, which had greater than 85% loss of segmental stiffness, the Jewett brace was ineffective.

The Knight-Taylor brace is another example of a commonly prescribed TLSO. This device is similar to a TLSO corset, but has lateral as well as dorsal uprights, with over-the-shoulder straps to limit lateral bending and flexion-extension. Adding crossed uprights makes this device more rigid. However, the rotational control, even with uprights, is poor. The Knight-Taylor TLSO is one of the standards for thoracic and thoracolumbar spine stabilization. The immobilizing efficacy of this brace is good in the lower thoracic region.

Custom-Molded Total Contact Orthoses

The total contact orthosis is the most effective orthosis for the immobilization of the patient with a midthoracic or thoracolumbar fracture. This brace is indicated for patients who have instabilities in more than one plane, in patients with impaired skin sensation, or in patients with osteoporotic compression fractures. A total contact orthosis is contraindicated for very obese or noncompliant patients.

A custom-fitted TLSO provides rotational control. An example of this is a high-temperature polyform TLSO that is custom fitted from a plaster shell taken from the patient. A TLSO provides restriction of motion up to approximately the T5 level rostrally to approximately L4 caudally. If the injury is in the upper thoracic spine a cervical extension should be added. To immobilize L4 and below, one rigid thigh extension with 15 to 30 degrees of hip flexion can be added to limit pelvic rotation and motion.

The advantages of custom-molded total contact orthoses include: distribution of forces over a large surface area, improved pelvic and thoracic fixation, better control of lateral bending and axial rotation, better patient and nursing acceptance, and an ability to obtain unobscured radiographs. Also, at least theoretically, deformity can be corrected by patient positioning during the molding process. In insensate patients, a total contact orthosis offers substantial advantages because of its ability to monitor the skin and readily adjust areas of excessive pressure.

The brace should be fabricated by a skilled orthotist. After fitting, the brace should be checked for excessive pressure, and if present, the brace should be modified. Molding for the orthosis should be delayed if patients have abdominal distention or excessive weight gain from fluid retention. Patients with spinal cord injury or multiple injuries may have significant weight gain and may require reassessment of the fit of the total contact orthosis. Occasionally, patients with significant weight change may require the fabrication of a second brace.

Protocols for brace use vary. Most authorities recommend that patients wear braces full time, including nighttime. Patients may shower and swim in the orthosis, but they must lie flat in bed until the orthosis dries and can be reapplied. Standard total contact orthoses or other braces do not immobilize below L4 or above T5 to T6, and may increase loads and range of motion at these levels. Injuries above T5 to T6 are immobilized by adding chin and occipital pads to the custom-molded orthosis.

For rigid immobilization, a custom-molded body jacket of polyvinyl chloride (or equivalent) or a custom-fitted plaster jacket is required.[2] Closed reduction and hyperextension casting affords the ability to achieve and maintain fracture reduction until consolidation. Biomechanically, a cast is more effective than any orthosis.[5] Because casting is enforced, it is not as dependent upon patient cooperation. Disadvantages of casting include cast weight, pressure sores, inability to monitor skin, neurapraxia of the lateral femoral cutaneous nerve, deep venous thrombosis secondary to groin pressure, and poor patient acceptance. Closed reduction casting is indicated in younger patients with two- and three-column injuries who have significant deformity, in patients who are likely to be noncompliant, and when reduction is required, such as patients with Chance type fractures.

SPINAL TRAUMA

Spinal orthoses have been traditionally used for the management of thoracolumbar injuries treated with or without surgical stabilization. However, the orthotic treatment modality for the management of spinal fractures remains subjective, because few objective data are available on the effectiveness of orthoses in stabilizing injured spinal segments.

Orthoses decrease intersegmental range of motion and overall trunk motion, but do not decrease axial loads across the intervertebral discs. To provide maximum effect, the center of the orthosis must be centered at the segmental level of the injury. After placement of the orthosis, serial upright radiographs are assessed for fracture alignment. During healing, isometric trunk strengthening exercises and aerobic training are performed so that the patient may achieve early ambulation.

The treatment of thoracolumbar spine burst fractures in neurologically intact patients is controversial. Reid et al.[7] reported 21 neurologically intact patients with thoracolumbar burst fractures treated with early ambulation in a custom-molded total contact orthosis. No complications occurred as a result of the brace and none of the patients required surgery for brace failure or the development of a neurological deficit. They concluded that it was possible to treat patients with burst fractures nonoperatively if they fulfill the following criteria: (1) the patient is neurologically intact; (2) the kyphosis angle is less than 35 degrees; (3) other injuries do not preclude the use of a total contact orthosis; and (4) the patient is capable of understanding and cooperating with the treatment regime. These criteria are irrespective of the computed tomography (CT) findings of dorsal

vertebral body retropulsion and spinal canal narrowing. Cantor et al.[3] and Mumford et al.[4] both reported similar good and excellent results and no complications for patients with thoracolumbar burst fractures treated with total contact orthoses. Cantor et al.[3] attributed their good results in these patients with intact dorsal elements and thoracolumbar burst fractures to the exclusion of patients with posterior column disruption.

Benzel and Larson[2] assessed the efficacy of postoperative external splinting techniques for patients with thoracic and/or lumbar spine trauma. The modified Minerva jacket offered the most efficacious immobilization and maximum patient comfort for fractures in the upper thoracic region. Thoracic and thoracolumbar injuries may be stabilized with either a Jewett hyperextension brace or a body jacket. The lack of maintenance of the cylindrical body shell, as well as excessive discomfort, make the Jewett brace and similar orthotic devices a second choice to body shell jackets for fractures in this region. The application of plastic polymer (Thermoplast) to spine splinting techniques offers the patient increased comfort and stability, as well as facilitating easy application and a more snug fit.

OSTEOPOROSIS

It is important to be aware of the limitations of a brace in protecting an osteoporotic vertebra. It should be recognized that a brace will be significantly limited in its ability to compensate for the very large loss of supporting elements in the osteoporotic vertebra. The Jewett hyperextension brace cannot be relied upon to prevent additional collapse of severely comminuted osteoporotic thoracic spine fractures. The decrease in strength of the vertebral bodies in osteoporosis is such that the orthosis is not likely to be completely effective in protecting them from collapse. If this is a major concern, a full body cast should be applied in hyperextension.

DISADVANTAGES OF BRACING

Surprisingly, the long-term effects of spinal bracing have not been investigated. Contraction of soft tissue, muscle atrophy, decreased joint range of motion, decreased bone mass, increased fatigability of postural muscles, and diminished cardiovascular endurance are potential consequences.

Spinal bracing is associated with numerous complications, the most significant of which is its relative ineffectiveness in achieving its stated goal, the minimization of spinal movement. The amount of soft tissue separating the spine and the brace minimizes the effectiveness of any brace.

Trunk strengthening and cardiovascular exercise have been shown to be of benefit in patients with other low back conditions.

CONCLUSIONS

Mechanical and psychological factors often interact and become major considerations in the prescription for an orthosis. It is important to have realistic expectations of an orthosis from a practical as well as a mechanical point of view.

With all the foregoing considerations, a clinical biomechanical approach to the use of orthotics may be taken through answers to the following questions. What are the pathological conditions that are involved? What are the therapeutic mechanical goals? In what way should the mechanics of the spine be changed? Is the goal to protect the spine, to rest it, or to correct deformity? What forces need to be applied to achieve these therapeutic aims?

The type of forces necessary can be determined by a review of the basic kinematics of the spine that are specific for the region where the forces are to be applied. Finally, it is then possible to decide which orthotic devices are able to apply the required loads. There are limitations in the extent to which forces may be applied to the spine. These involve psychological, physiological, and mechanical factors.

REFERENCES

1. Andriacchi T, Schultz A, Belytschco T, et al. A model for studies of mechanical interactions between the human spine and rib cage. J Biomech 7: 497, 1974.
2. Benzel EC, Larson SJ. Postoperative stabilization of the post-traumatic thoracic and lumbar spine: A review of concepts and orthotic techniques. J Spinal Disord 2: 47-51, 1989.
3. Cantor JB, Lebwohl, NH, Garvey, T, Eiswant FJ. Nonoperative management of stable thoracolumbar burst fractures with early ambulation and bracing. Spine 18:971-976, 1993.
4. Mumford J, Weinstein JN, Spratt KF, Goel VK. Thoracolumbar burst fractures. The clinical efficacy and outcome of nonoperative management. Spine18:955-970, 1993.
5. Nagel DA, Koogle TA, Pizialli RL, et al. Stability of the upper lumbar spine following progressive disruptions and application of individual internal and external fixation devices. J Bone Joint Surg 63A:62, 1981.
6. Patwardhan AG, Li SP, Gavin T, et al. Orthotic stabilization of thoracolumbar injuries. A biomechanical analysis of the Jewett hyperextension orthosis. Spine 15:654-661, 1990.
7. Reid DC, Hu R, Davis LA, Seboc LA. The nonoperative treatment of burst fractures of the thoracolumbar junction. J Trauma 28:1188-1194, 1988.
8. White AA, Panjabi MM. Spinal braces: Functional analysis and clinical applications. In White AA, Panjabi MM, eds. Clinical Biomechanics of the Spine, 2nd ed. Philadelphia: JB Lippincott, 1990, pp 475-510.

The Elderly Patient

Shari Miura Ling, M.D., Geoffrey Shiu-Feng Ling, M.D., Ph.D.,
and Seth M. Zeidman, M.D.

Older adults commonly complain of musculoskeletal pain and discomfort. Recent studies suggest that arthritis is the leading chronic condition in the United States that increases both in prevalence and incidence with advancing age.[1] The care of older adults with musculoskeletal symptoms challenges practitioners on several levels. In older adults, symptom reporting may differ from clinical presentation. Patients may mistakenly attribute their painful and other symptoms to old age and dismiss them without reporting them to a physician. Patients may also inaccurately attribute their musculoskeletal pain to arthritis, without the necessary medical confirmation. Clinicians are also challenged by atypical, nonclassical, and even vague presentations of rheumatic diseases in older adults.

Back pain is a common complaint that can originate from a wide variety of structural and medical conditions. Current management strategies are based upon data obtained from young adults who acquire this problem in the workplace. Because the underlying causes of back pain in older adults differ significantly, extrapolation of management strategies to this often frail patient population is inappropriate. This chapter reviews the diagnostic considerations and the evaluation of elderly patients with back pain.

CLINICAL PRESENTATION
Acute Back Pain

The causes of acute back pain (less than 7 days duration) differ significantly from the causes of persistent or chronic back pain (present for at least 3 months). Although not specific to elderly patients, Borenstein[2] provides a systematic and methodical approach to patients with low back pain. The first important step should be to exclude life- or function-threatening conditions that require emergent evaluation and treatment. Abdominal aneurysms can result in throbbing back pain that is often associated with lower extremity claudication, syncope, or physical evidence of circulatory insufficiency. Patients with acute back pain accompanied by saddle anesthesia and/or bowel or bladder incontinence may have cauda equina syndrome. These two conditions warrant emergent radiographic and surgical evaluation.

Having excluded the life-threatening conditions mentioned above, the next recommended step is to carefully review the patient's history for clues that suggest systemic medical illnesses. Surgical specialists are well acquainted with the importance of eliciting neurological deficits in patients with back pain. Radicular pain suggests nerve impingement. In the elderly population, this is most commonly due to osteoarthritis of the spine. However, other

442

causes must be sought. Many surgeons are less familiar with association of back pain that worsens at night or during recumbency. These symptoms may signal occult infection or tumor. Infectious osteomyelitis, discitis, and pyogenic sacroiliitis are usually accompanied by constitutional symptoms. A variety of malignant neoplasms that may or may not exhibit direct bony involvement are also accompanied by constitutional symptoms. Nonradiating midline back pain in the elderly patient raises the possibility of vertebral body fracture. The occurrence of a spontaneous, nontraumatic fracture in this group most commonly arises from significant osteoporosis, however, other causes (e.g., tumor and infection) may be responsible. In a series of 900 patients aged 55 years and older, referred for evaluation of their back pain, 46% were found to have underlying spinal pathology, including 11% with a malignant condition.[3] Back pain that develops in the setting of inflammatory joint disease, such as psoriatic arthritis, Reiter's syndrome, and ankylosing spondylitis, usually is worse in the early morning and also results in stiffness that extends over 1 hour beyond awakening. Seronegative spondyloarthropathies may develop in the later years, contrary to previous beliefs.

Persistent Low Back Pain

The causes of persistent low back discomfort in the elderly differ significantly from those observed in younger age groups and may represent concerning pathology in the back as well as surrounding areas. In young adults, only 10% to 15% of all patients with acute back pain fail conservative management. Similar data are not available for older adults, however, a protracted course is not uncommon. Several disease states are associated with persistent low back pain in elderly patients.

Osteoarthritis

Osteoarthritis is characterized by mechanical pain that worsens with standing and spine extension, but lessens with sitting, bending, and forward spinal flexion. Radiographic evidence of structural abnormalities of the lumbar apophyseal (facet) joints and/or degenerative disc disease are prevalent in this population. Characteristic findings include bony sclerosis, osteophyte formation, and disc space narrowing. It is necessary for the clinician to question whether the patient's clinical presentation is explained by the radiographic findings or if osteoarthritis of the spine is an incidental finding.

Spinal Stenosis

Spinal stenosis is a common cause of lower back and lower extremity pain that worsens with activity or spine extension. As with osteoarthritis, symptoms may improve with sitting and forward spine flexion. Physical findings include poor balance, a wide-based gait, and diminished strength, lower extremity reflexes, and/or sensation. The Romberg test may also be abnormal. Spinal stenosis most commonly occurs in conjunction with spinal osteoarthritis, but also can occur in the setting of Paget's disease and after previous surgery (e.g., spinal facia and decompression laminectomy leading to postoperation spinal deformity). Neurogenic claudication due to spinal stenosis must be differentiated from vascular claudication. Patients with vascular claudication will have relief with standing and lying flat, and have diminished peripheral pulses on examination. Patients with spinal stenosis have worsened pain when standing upright in the extended position and may have normal distal lower extremity pulses. Bicycle exercise testing can occasionally distinguish neurogenic from vascular claudication by reproducing vascular claudication and not reproducing neurogenic claudication.

Osteoporosis

Osteoporosis can involve the entire spine and other bones. Pain due to osteoporotic fractures is severe and can result in compromised mobility and function. Pain can persist despite radiographic evidence of healing. Retropulsed bone and/or disc fragments can impair neurological function. Elderly patients with osteoporosis should also be evaluated for hyperthyroidism, myeloma, osteomalacia, Paget's disease of the bone, and metastatic disease.

Inflammatory Diseases

Inflammatory diseases of the spine often result in back pain. As previously described, these conditions are usually accompanied by morning stiffness that persists for 1 hour or longer. Peripheral arthritis should be sought because rheumatoid arthritis, ankylosing spondylitis, and psoriatic arthritis can afflict elderly patients. Radiographs can help to identify spinal and sacroiliac pathology. Laboratory studies, including a sedimentation rate and rheumatoid factor, can be helpful, but should not be obtained as a screening test for rheumatic disease, particularly in elderly patients who have a high rate of false positive results.

Fibromyalgia Syndrome

Recent evidence suggests that older adults are not spared from fibromyalgia syndrome. Originally thought to afflict young to middle-aged women, recent studies suggest that the peak incidence of this chronic condition is in the later years. Fibromyalgia syndrome is characterized by back pain, fatigue, nonrestorative sleep, and the presence of tender points on physical examination. Management options for elderly patients are limited in that the recommended medical therapies (tricyclic antidepressants and cyclobenzaprine) are associated with side effects that may be problematic in the elderly, including anticholinergic orthostasis, constipation, confusion, drowsiness, and increased risk of falling. Low impact exercise may be a more prudent treatment option for these patients.

DIAGNOSTIC EVALUATION

Adults aged older than 55 years, having a history of malignancy, steroid use, recent trauma, or symptoms that localize to the thoracic spine should undergo radiographic evaluation of the symptomatic area to rule out a bony lesion or involvement of the adjacent areas. In addition, laboratory studies should be included in the evaluation if constitutional or infectious symptoms are present.

There are many diagnostic procedures available to the clinician. Plain radiographs of the spine are helpful in evaluating patients in whom malignancy or fracture are suspected. Lateral, anteroposterior (AP) and oblique views should be obtained. Sacroiliac views must be requested specifically if inflammatory back disease is suspected. Computed tomography (CT) provides the best resolution of cortical bone and should be requested if cortical erosions are suspected but not visualized on plain radiographs of the spine or sacroiliac joints. Magnetic resonance imaging (MRI) is the best available test when neurological impairment or encroachment is of concern. MRI also provides the best resolution of intramedullary and intraosseous processes, such as tumor or infection. MRI has largely supplanted myelography, except that myelography assists the surgeon in planning the surgical approach, precisely localizing the segmented level of pathology, and excluding other lesions that are not clinically apparent. Nuclear studies are most helpful when bony infections, tumors, occult trauma, or advance degeneration changes (e.g., facet arthropathy) are suspected.

Laboratory studies are helpful in evaluating patients with systemic or inflammatory symptoms and as part of a preoperative evaluation.

MANAGEMENT

Although less common in elderly patients than young adults, simple muscular strain can be treated nonoperatively with rest, local measures (such as gentle massage and heat), and the use of analgesics (such as acetaminophen), low doses of nonsteroidal anti-inflammatory agents, or narcotic analgesics if necessary. Recovery should occur in 2 to 4 weeks. Because of this excellent prognosis, glucocorticoid injection therapies are rarely necessary nor are they more effective than placebo in management of acute back pain due to disc herniation in young adults. Muscle relaxants have not been studied in the management of back pain in older adults. Furthermore, they place the patient at risk for anticholinergic side effects, including drowsiness and urinary retention.

The current literature is sparse in terms of systematic trials of interventions to treat persistent back pain in the older patient. Clinicians often extrapolate recommendations derived from trials using young adults, but this may not be appropriate because the causes of pain frequently differ between the two populations. The adverse consequences of immobility and deconditioning suggest that prolonged bed rest should be avoided. Recent evidence suggests that tricyclic antidepressants provide some benefit for those who are also depressed but offer little to those patients who are not depressed. Muscle relaxants, nonsteroidal anti-inflammatory agents, and local glucocorticoid injections have not been systematically studied. Neuromuscular and/or transcutaneous electrical nerve stimulation probably are more effective when used together than when either is used alone. However, this has not been studied in the elderly. Experimental therapies including epidural steroids and acupuncture are currently under investigation. Calcitonin and pamidronate have been used in the management of musculoskeletal complications of Paget's disease but have not been applied to the management of back pain due to other processes.[4]

SURGICAL EVALUATION

There are three critical components that determine whether any given patient is a suitable candidate for operative management. The first is the determination of whether surgical intervention is clearly indicated. Secondly, a detailed preoperative assessment is necessary to determine whether the patient's overall medical condition will allow surgery to proceed safely. The third component is one that is often overlooked but is believed by the authors to be important. This involves a patient-directed values history. Patients differ vastly with regard to the treatments they are willing to try in hopes of relieving painful symptoms, and also differ in the extent of pain or disability they are willing to tolerate and accept.

PERIOPERATIVE MANAGEMENT

Elderly patients are at greater risk for complications, including death, from operative procedures. Small problems that are well tolerated by young, healthy adults may be quickly compounded in geriatric patients, sometimes with catastrophic results.

Patients over 65 years of age are at risk for generalized atherosclerosis and may have poor myocardial and renal reserve. Elderly patients often develop cardiac failure if they are fluid overloaded. These patients mandate close monitoring of vital signs, intake, output, body weight, and serum electrolytes. These patients generally require smaller doses of narcotics, sedatives, and anesthetics than younger patients. Barbiturates, sedatives, and steroids may cause confusion, and narcotics can produce respiratory depression.

Finally, advanced age is a serious independent risk factor for the development of postoperative deep-venous thrombosis and pulmonary embolism, which are major causes of morbidity and mortality after surgical procedures.

CONCLUSION

Surgery for the treatment of thoracic spinal abnormalities has its own unique considerations in the elderly patient. The potential for increased perioperative risks mandates that a thoughtful and deliberate preoperative evaluation be carried out to recognize problems and optimize the overall medical condition. A multidisciplinary approach to postoperative care utilizing an internist/gerontologist along with the surgical team may be desirable.

REFERENCES

1. Amundsen T, Weber H, Lilleas F, Nordal H, Abdelnoor M, Magnaes B. Lumbar spinal stenosis: Clinical and radiologic features. Spine 20:1178-1186, 1995.
2. Borenstein DG. Low back pain. In Klippel JH, Dieppe PA, eds. Rheumatology. St. Louis: Mosby, 1994, pp 1-26.
3. Katz JN, Dalgas M, Stucki G, Katz NP, Bayley J, Fossell AH, Chang LC, Lipson SJ. Degenerative spinal stenosis diagnostic value of the history and physical examination. Arthritis Rheum 38:1236-1241, 1995.
4. Wong E, Wong J, Reid IR. Pamidronate treatment of the neurologic sequelae of pagetic spinal stenosis. Arch Intern Med 155:1813-1815, 1995.

SUGGESTED READINGS

Baumgartner E, Heitmann L, Duvoisin B. Back pain in the older patient. Ann Iheun Dis 55:600-602,1996.
Bonaiuti D, Fontanella G. The affective dimension of low back pain: Its influence on the outcome of back school. Arch Phys Med Rehabil 77:1239-1242,1996.
Borenstein DG, Burton JR. Lumbar spine disease in the elderly. J Am Geriatr Soc 41:167, 1993.
Deen HG, Zimmerman RS, Lyons MK, McPhee MC, Verheijdge JL, Lemens SM. Measurement of exercise tolerance on the treadmill in patients with symptomatic lumbar spinal stenosis: A useful indicator of functional status and surgical outcome. J Neurosurg 83:27-30, 1995.
Deyo RA. Drug therapy for back pain: Which drugs help which patients. Spine 21:2840-2849, 1996.
Deyo RA, Deihl AK. Patient satisfaction with medical care for low back pain. Spine 11:28-30, 1986.
Deyo RA, Diehl AK, Rosenthal M. How many days bed rest for acute low back pain? A randomized clinical trial. N Engl J Med 315:1064-1070, 1986.
Engle C, Von Korff M, Katon W. Back pain in primary care: Predictors of high health-care costs. Spine 65:197-204, 1996.
Frank A. Low back pain: Education and debate. BMJ 306:901-909, 1993.
Frost H, Klaber Moffett JA, Moser JS, Fairbanks JCT. Randomised controlled trial for evaluation of fitness programme for patients with chronic low back pain. BMJ 310:151-154, 1995.
Garvey TA, Marks MR, Wiesel SE. A prospective, randomized double-blind evaluation of trigger-point injection therapy for low-back pain. Spine 14:962-964, 1989.
Indahl A, Velund L, Reikeraas O. Good prognosis for low back pain when left untampered. Spine 20:473-476, 1995.

Jensen MC, Brandt AA, Zawadzki MN, Obuchowski N, Modic M, Malkasian D, Ross JS. Magnetic resonance imaging of the lumbar spine in people without back pain. N Engl J Med 331:69-73, 1994.

Klippel JH, Dieppe PA, eds. Rheumatology. St. Louis: Mosby, 1994.

Liang MH, Sturrock RD. Evaluation of musculoskeletal symptoms. In Klippel JH, Dieppe PA, eds. Rheumatology. St. Louis: Mosby, 1994, p 2:1.7-8.

Malmivaara A, Hakkinen U, Aro T, Heinrichs M-L, Koskenniemi L, Kousma E, Lappi S, Paloheimo R, Servo C, Vaaranen V, Hernberg S. The treatment of acute low back pain—Bed rest, exercise or ordinary activity? N Engl J Med 332:351-355, 1995.

Moore S, Shurman J. Combined neuromuscular electrical stimulation and transcutaneous electrical nerve stimulation for treatment of chronic back pain: A double-blind, repeated measures comparison. Arch Phys Med Rehabil 78:55-60, 1997.

Ondel D, Sari H, Donmez C. Lumbar spinal stenosis: Clinical/radiologic therapeutic evaluation in 145 patients: Conservative treatment or surgical intervention? Spine 18:291-298, 1993.

Ross PD, Davis JW, Epstein RS, Wasnich RD. Pain and disability associated with new vertebral fractures and other spinal conditions. J Clin Epidemiol 47:231-239, 1994.

Skekella PG, Adams AH, Chassan MR, Hurwitz EL, Brook RH. Spinal manipulation for low back pain. Ann Intern Med 117:590-598, 1992.

Turner JA. Educational and behavioral interventions for back pain in primary care. Spine 21:2851-2859, 1996.

VonKarff M, Barlow W, Cherkin D, Deyo RA. Effects of practice style in managing back pain. Ann Intern Med 121:187-195, 1994.

The Obese Patient

Gregory J. Przybylski, M.D., and Wade M. Mueller, M.D.

The prevalence of obesity has progressively increased during the last few decades.[40] In fact, nearly one third of adult Americans are considered obese.[33,40,64] Because an increased frequency of herniated discs, osteoarthritis, and disc degeneration is associated with obesity,[10,35,39,44,53] a large proportion of patients evaluated by the spine surgeon are overweight. Moreover, the many comorbid conditions associated with obesity can have a significant impact upon the management of the obese patient. Consequently, additional consideration must be given in the treatment of spinal diseases in the obese patient in order to optimize successful results.

A thorough understanding of the interaction of obesity in all aspects of patient management requires defining the condition of obesity and a review of its epidemiology. Secondly, the impact of the multisystem abnormalities associated with obesity is analyzed. An understanding of this background can facilitate initial patient management to improve their preoperative condition. In addition, specific operative considerations are evaluated. Finally, methods to improve postoperative management to reduce complications and enhance rapid recovery are discussed.

DEFINITION AND EPIDEMIOLOGY OF OBESITY

Although many apply the term "obesity" to describe individuals who have a higher than average proportion of adipose tissue to lean body mass,[55] the purpose of objectively defining this condition is to identify the group of people with a higher frequency of mortality related to their body mass index (BMI).[34] The BMI is the height-adjusted weight calculated by dividing the weight in kilograms by the square of the height in meters. According to the National Institutes of Health Consensus Conference in 1985, a person with a BMI greater than 28 kg/m² has increased health risks.[40] This approximates a weight 20% above ideal as described by Metropolitan Life actuarial statistics.[64]

An analysis of mortality frequency reveals a linear relationship with BMI greater than 30 kg/m² (Table 31-1).[34] [Severe and morbidly obese groups represent one third of all obese people,[19] while the morbidly obese group represents less than one tenth of obese people.[14]]

However, the distribution of weight on the body is more strongly associated with mortality than BMI.[34,44,53,54] Abdominal localization of weight, termed "central obesity," is characterized by a high waist to hip ratio. Central obesity, independent of BMI, may be as strong a risk factor for cardiovascular mortality as hyperlipidemia, smoking, and hypertension.[34]

In the late 1970s 26% of the American population was considered obese.[33] The frequency has steadily increased to a prevalence of nearly one third of the population in this decade.[40,64] Moreover, African-American and Hispanic-American women have proportionally more obese people in groups stratified by gender and race.[33,64] Although

Table 31-1. Ranges of Obesity Identifying Risk of Mortality

Obese	BMI of 30-35 kg/m²	Moderate risk
Severely obese	BMI of 35-40 kg/m²	High risk
Morbidly obese	BMI of 40 kg/m² and over	Very high risk

Adapted from Bray GA. Pathophysiology of obesity. Am J Clin Nutr 55:488S-494S, 1992.

the mortality risk of the obese is twice that of nonobese people,[54] risk increases between five- and twelvefold among obese men aged 30 to 60 years.[40,56] However, mortality risk decreases with increasing age[42] until similar risks exist for obese and nonobese people after the age of 80 years.[54]

The economic impact of obesity is staggering. Medical costs attributable to obesity are estimated at $40 billion annually, representing 5.5% of all medical expenditures.[40,53] Moreover, nearly half of the costs are associated with the severely obese.[19] Consequently, the prevalence, mortality risk, and medical cost of obesity justify selective consideration of this group.

COMORBIDITIES ASSOCIATED WITH OBESITY
Cardiovascular

The greatest proportion of mortality in the obese is related to cardiovascular abnormalities.[34,50,53,55] After accounting for other cardiovascular risk factors such as hypertension and smoking, obesity has been identified as an independent cardiovascular risk factor.[28] Most of the cardiovascular effects can be attributed to hyperlipidemia, increased portal fatty acids, and hypoxemia.

Obesity is associated with increased plasma lipids, including cholesterol and triglycerides,[11,34,40,44] but decreased high density lipoprotein.[11] This contributes to a greater frequency of occlusive coronary artery disease.[44] The risk of myocardial infarction is further aggravated by maximal coronary vasodilation.[28]

Increased portal fatty acid concentration may contribute to hypertension.[53] Nearly two thirds of obese people have hypertension,[1,34] which is linearly related to weight.[44] The increased afterload contributes to abnormal diastolic ventricular function, resulting in a subclinical cardiomyopathy.[2,66]

Finally, hypoxemia results from increased oxygen consumption with insufficient respiratory reserve. Although adipose tissue is hypovascular, it is metabolically active, requiring 3 L of blood flow per minute for every 100 kg of adipose tissue weight.[1,14] To accommodate the required blood flow and oxygen demand, blood volume must increase.[1,28] As a result, eccentric left ventricular hypertrophy develops, with proportionally greater ventricular volume than ventricular wall thickness.[1,8,28,50] Measured hemodynamic parameters reflecting these changes include increased cardiac output, pulmonary capillary wedge pressure, right ventricular stroke work, and right atrial pressure.[1,8,50] The strain of increased preload and afterload[22] eventually reduces left ventricular contractility.[50]

Despite these significant alterations in cardiac function, only 10% of obese people develop congestive heart failure, although the majority have pulmonary hypertension.[55] The most common electrocardiographic findings include T-wave flattening, low voltage, and left or right axis deviation.[1,14,42] Weight loss can reverse the majority of cardiovascular changes, although its effect on coronary artery disease is unknown.[8,28]

Pulmonary

The predominant pulmonary abnormality encountered is hypoxemia.[1,14,44,61] The severity of hypoxemia is reflected in the degree of polycythemia.[1,14] The increased oxygen consumption required by excess adipose tissue becomes difficult to accommodate as thoracoabdominal size restricts pulmonary mechanics.[14] There is a progressive decrease in lung compliance, with reduction in tidal volume, vital capacity, expiratory reserve volume, and functional reserve capacity.[30,44,50,55] The resultant small airway and alveolar closure results in ventilation-perfusion mismatch, reducing oxygen delivery in the setting of increased oxygen demand.[14,42,50,55]

Consequently, maximum voluntary ventilation occurs at rest.[42,55] Despite these changes, less than 10% of obese people develop hypoventilation syndrome.[1,2,13,42] However, the supine position significantly reduces effective ventilation and aggravates hypoxemia.[23,27,50] Although weight loss does not improve oxygenation, it can increase measured lung volumes[27] and reduce atelectasis[27] and oxygen consumption.[1]

Thromboembolic

Obesity is an independent risk factor for thromboembolism, increasing the risk of disease twofold over the risk in nonobese people.[13] Hypercoagulability results from polycythemia,[1,14] increased fibrinogen and plasminogen activator inhibitor levels,[34,42,53] and decreased antithrombin III concentration.[42] Stasis from decreased activity or spinal cord injury further aggravate the risk of thromboembolic disease.[18] Although plasma viscosity and red cell aggregation diminish with weight loss, fibrinogen levels remain elevated.[45]

Gastrointestinal

An increased gastric volume in association with increased gastric acidity and more frequent hiatal hernia compound the risk of aspiration pneumonitis.[55] Diminished gastric pH and cirrhosis affect drug metabolism.[13,42,55] Hepatomegaly from fatty liver infiltration is common in the obese patient, aggravating restricted diaphragmatic motion.[1,13,55] Although weight loss can reduce fatty infiltration, it is associated with portal fibrosis and inflammation.[3] Cholelithiasis is also frequently encountered,[44,55] and can be aggravated by weight loss.[4,43]

Endocrine

Diabetes is commonly identified, with its prevalence increasing from twofold among the mildly obese to tenfold among the severely obese.[28,40,53,55] Increased metabolism results in a greater demand for insulin.[11,34] This eventually leads to the insulin resistance and glucose intolerance observed in noninsulin-dependent diabetics.[34] Significant control of glucose can be achieved with weight loss.[40]

Musculoskeletal

Obesity has been identified as an independent risk factor in osteoarthritis,[39] increasing the incidence by two- or threefold over nonobese people.[44,53] The distribution of osteoarthritis includes both weight-bearing and non–weight-bearing joints, implying a pathogenesis independent of mobility and mechanical stress.[60] Osteophytic disc degeneration and herniated discs are both more commonly observed in the obese.[10,35] However, obesity is protective against the postmenopausal bone loss observed with idiopathic osteoporosis.[22,46] The effect of weight loss on the progression of osteoarthritis is not well elucidated.

An uncommon disease termed "idiopathic epidural lipomatosis" is also associated with obesity.[6,26,59] The disease more commonly affects the thoracic spine, causing compressive neurological symptoms.[26,59] The condition can be reversed with weight loss.[26,59]

PREOPERATIVE EVALUATION
History and Physical Examination

In addition to a musculoskeletal and neurological history, a thorough review of systems is imperative to help identify cardiovascular, pulmonary, gastrointestinal, thromboembolic, or endocrine disorders that may require preoperative management. Significant abnormalities are uncommon, despite severe obesity.[1,2,13,42,55] However, obese patients may have asymptomatic disease that will only become evident during the perioperative period.

Identification of neurological signs referable to the thoracic spine may be affected by peripheral neuropathy from undiagnosed or untreated diabetes mellitus. Osteoarthritis of the hip and knees may be the cause of lower limb pain and weakness. Hypertension may be underestimated, even with a larger blood pressure cuff, unless the width and length of the bladder cuff, are 50% and 80% of the arm circumference, respectively.[13] Thoracoabdominal adipose tissue adversely affects auscultation of the heart and lungs, causing difficulty in identifying cardiopulmonary disease on examination alone.[1,28]

Laboratory Studies

Particular attention must be given to glucose levels to identify uncontrolled hyperglycemia.[40] Preoperative arterial blood gases and hematocrit are recommended, particularly in the case of a weight to height ratio greater than 1, to identify patients at risk for intraoperative hypoxia and postoperative hypoventilation.[14] Basic liver function or coagulation tests are unlikely to reveal significant abnormalities. An electrocardiogram and chest radiograph are particularly important in the obese patient given the limitations of the physical examination and the occurrence of asymptomatic cardiopulmonary disease.[14] Although preoperative pulmonary function tests[14] and echocardiography[1,28] have been recommended by some physicians, spirometry results have poorly predicted the occurrence of perioperative pulmonary complications.[9,21] The utility of preoperative Swan-Ganz catheter pressure measures or echocardiography in improving perioperative management are unknown.[50]

Imaging

Although the standard studies of myelography, computed tomography (CT), and magnetic resonance imaging (MRI) are still utilized, the patient's size may require special arrangements or maneuvers to successfully obtain the required imaging. When a "swimmer's view" fails to demonstrate the alignment of the cervicothoracic junction, half-arc tomography may be useful.[36] Lumbar puncture for myelography can be facilitated by coaxial needle placement, with the patient in a seated position.[31] Eccentric positioning of the patient on the CT scanner can eliminate ring artifacts within the spinal canal.[20] Finally, open MRI scanners can facilitate imaging of patients weighing nearly 500 pounds.[48]

PREOPERATIVE MANAGEMENT

Preoperative weight loss is often recommended in an attempt to reduce the impact of comorbid conditions on perioperative complications for elective surgery.[1,8,21,27,28,42,45] Even a 10% to 15% weight loss may reduce the risk of cardiovascular, pulmonary, and thromboembolic diseases.[42] Because weight loss from exercise is easily overcome by caloric intake,[17] a combination of dietary management and behavioral modification is suggested as the best method to achieve long-term weight control.[4,40,43,65] Several studies have shown that commercial programs, unsupervised dietary treatment, and even monitored very low-calorie diets fail to maintain weight loss in the majority of patients without inclusion of strict behavioral management.[5,40,54] Beyond a BMI of 35 kg/m^2, drug treatment[12] and surgical techniques are recommended for reducing caloric intake.[11,32,40,54,56]

However, several studies have failed to demonstrate a reduction of postoperative complications after preoperative weight loss management.[24,41] Consequently, it may be reasonable not to delay elective surgery to achieve preoperative weight loss.[42] Moreover, weight loss fails to improve oxygenation[27] or reduce fibrinogen levels,[45] and may even contribute to hepatic inflammation[3] and cholelithiasis.[4,43]

Cessation of smoking at least 4 weeks preoperatively is particularly important in the obese patient.[42] The risk of perioperative alveolar closure and hypoxemia is significant in the setting of maximum voluntary ventilatory capacity at rest.[42,55] Elimination of smoking, learning cough and deep breathing techniques, and weight loss can contribute to reducing postoperative atelectasis.[27]

OPERATIVE MANAGEMENT
Equipment and Positioning

Preoperative planning is important to ensure that the necessary operative tables, transporting stretchers, hospital beds, and surgical equipment are available to accommodate the morbidly obese patient. Specifically designed stretchers and wheel chairs (Custom Extra-Duty Chair [Everest and Jennings, St. Louis, Mo.]) that are modified with additional bracing can support larger patients. Common operative tables such as the AMSCO 1080/2080 (American Sterilizing Co., Erie, Pa.) are narrow and can only accommodate weights less than 140 kg. Other tables, such as the AMSCO Quantum 3080 RL (American Sterilizing Co.) and the Maquet 1120 (Siemens, Englewood, Colo.) are designed to tolerate up to 180 kg. An alternative to a special larger table is bolting together a pair of standard tables.[49] Modified versions of other tables such as the Jackson JST-5928 (Orthopaedic Systems Inc., Hayward, Calif.) are available to accommodate weights up to 230 kg.

A careful choice of positioning requires not only consideration of the injury location, adequacy of visualization, and availability of long instruments, but also the need to optimize ventilation and hemodynamics, to attain intraoperative radiographs, and to access table rails for attachment of fixed retractor systems. Thoughtful preoperative planning is rewarded by fewer intraoperative difficulties. A trial of transporting and positioning the patient before the scheduled surgery date may reveal unanticipated problems that can be remedied preoperatively.[49]

Intraoperative positioning can have a large impact on pulmonary and cardiovascular dynamics. The supine position is associated with increased oxygen consumption, pulmonary arterial pressure, and reduced chest wall mechanics.[14] Significant difficulty with ventilation and consequent hypoxemia can develop with poor positioning.[50] Allowing the patient to position himself after an awake intubation can ensure an optimal prone position before anesthetic induction.[58] In contrast, the lateral decubitus position, with an axillary roll to prevent brachial neurovascular injury, reduces intra-abdominal pressure and improves diaphragmatic excursion.[14] However, elimination of chest and abdominal restrictions can result in similarly reduced abdominal pressures in the supine and prone positions.[14] Suggested alternatives to longitudinal rolls are the modified Hastings frame, Wilson frame, and vacuum pillow to reduce intra-abdominal pressure with prone positioning.[23,57] Careful attention must also be given when flexing the lower limbs in a kneeling prone position to prevent development of a compartment syndrome.

It is imperative that the patient is padded and secured properly to the table, regardless of the position chosen. Straps, wide tape, kidney rests, and vacuum mattresses (Olympic VAC-PAC [Olympic Medical, Seattle, Wash.]) can be utilized to maintain the desired position, even if rotation of the table is desired during the procedure to improve visualization. However, the security of these various devices with table rotation should be confirmed before prepping. Particular care should be given to padding joints where superficial neurovascular bundles can be injured from prolonged compression against the securing devices. Similarly, skin overlying bony prominences like the sacrum and iliac crests should be well padded to prevent skin injury. Padded arm supports are also useful adjuncts with lateral positioning. Finally, taping of abdominal skin folds can facilitate exposure of the iliac crests for harvesting bone graft.

Anesthetic Management

Although obesity itself may not be associated with greater morbidity related to anesthesia,[42,50] several factors must be considered to optimize mainte-nance of ventilation and timely recovery from anesthesia. The most common difficulties associated with the anesthetic management of the obese patient are obtaining venous access and intubation.[55] Central venous access may be necessary when peripheral veins cannot be cannulated. Limitation of cervical mobility in the obese patient contributes to problems with intubation.[55] Fiberoptic guidance[49] or application of continuous nasal positive airway pressure[47] have been used to overcome difficulties with intubation.

Moreover, adequate oxygenation and medication dosing require additional attention. Because the functional reserve capacity in the obese patient is small, there is less nitrogen available for displacement during preoxygenation for intubation or positioning.[9] In fact, oxygen saturation falls below 90% in nearly two thirds less time in the obese patient compared with a slender patient despite lengthy preoxygenation.[9,30] Consequently, rapid intubation and maintenance of ventilation during turning and positioning are recommended.[9] Continuous monitoring of oxygen saturation by pulse oximetry as well as arterial cannulation for accurately measuring blood gases and blood pressure are likewise important.[14,55] Neither large tidal volume ventilation[7,14] nor positive end expiratory pressure[14] improve oxygenation. Consequently, adequate ventilation, security of the endotracheal tube, and proper function of the pulse oximeter, venous, and arterial pressure monitors must be confirmed after positioning to minimize manipulation after draping.

Medication dosing must be adjusted not only for body weight but also for estimated body water.[13,16] At the same time, one must avoid administering excess muscle relaxants and anesthetics given the poor reliability of surface electrode stimulation and accumulation of fat-soluble drugs, respectively.[14,55] Moreover, there is a risk of hepatic toxicity from halothane and renal toxicity from some inorganic fluoride inhalational agents.[14] In contrast, short-acting sevoflurane is not associated with inorganic fluoride accumulation,[25] whereas propofol does not accumulate to the degree of other anesthetic agents.[51] Finally, the use of epidural narcotics at the end of the operation has been quite effective in controlling thoracic pain, reducing the quantity of systemic narcotics used, and allowing for more rapid postoperative ambulation.[14,15]

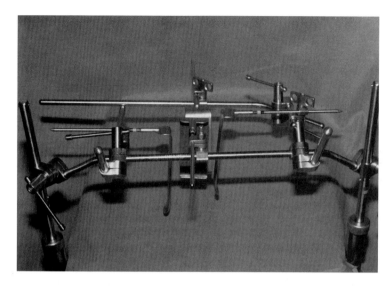

Fig. 31-1. Components of the Thompson-Farley Retractor System (Thompson Surgical Instruments, Traverse City, Mich.), which can be used to achieve exposure in ventrolateral surgical approaches.

Surgical Approaches and Retraction

The surgical approaches used for the treatment of thoracic spine abnormalities have been described in earlier chapters. The pathological process rather than the size of the patient should dictate the approach. However, the size of the surgical exposure and choice of retractor systems are very much influenced by patient size. Incisions should be longer than usual, with greater subcutaneous and fascial exposure to enhance deep visualization and to prevent progressive narrowing of the surgical field as the spine is approached.

Retractor systems fixed to the operating table can be invaluable in maintaining exposure. Intrathoracic, retropleural, and retroperitoneal approaches are facilitated with devices such as the Upper Abdominal Retractor System (Omni-Tract Surgical, Inc., St. Paul, Minn.) and the Thompson-Farley Retractor System (Fig. 31-1). Although the time required to attach the table posts and cross-links diminishes with experience, the versatility of rapidly adding additional retractors or changing their orientation is an invaluable time-saving benefit. Because the crossbars are designed for attachment to a single operating table, customized crossbars may be needed when using paired tables bolted together.[49] Similarly, customized Miskimon (Fig. 31-2) and Scoville (Fig. 31-3) retractors can provide excellent paraspinal muscle retraction in deep wounds. These are only a few examples of available retractor systems that may facilitate a deep exposure in the obese patient.

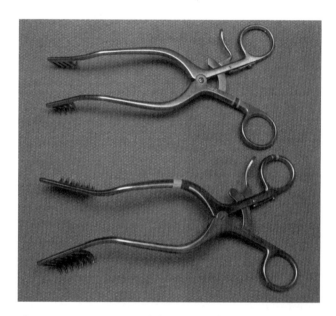

Fig. 31-2. Comparison of the standard angled Weitlanner *(above)* (Codman, Randolph, Mass.) and the customized Miskimon retractor *(below)* (Ruggles Surgical Instrumentation, Atlanta, Ga.) with longer arms and wider, more angled blades to achieve better exposure in dorsal surgical approaches.

Stabilization and Fusion

The influence of the type and extent of instrumentation on achieving temporary stability, successful bony fusion, and infrequent instrumentation failure in the obese spine-injured patient is unknown. Although patient size did not increase the frequency of implant failure after total hip replacement,[37] a

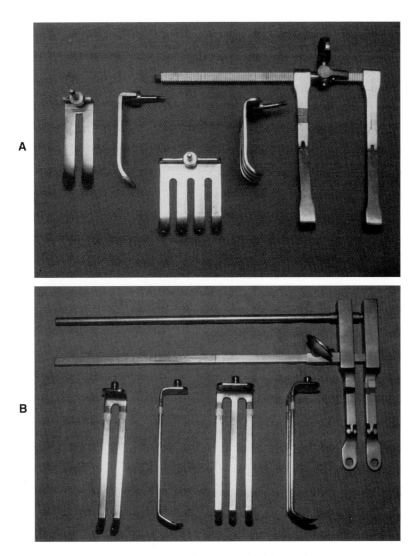

Fig. 31-3. Comparison of the standard Scoville retractor **(A)** (Aesculap Instruments Co., Burlingame, Calif.) and the customized retractor **(B)** (Adtech Medical Instrument Co., Racine, Wis.) with longer blades to achieve exposure in dorsal surgical approaches.

biomechanical analysis of the force and moment distributions would suggest that the more ventral center of gravity compounded by the greater body mass in the obese patient would accentuate the stress upon the injured spine as well as the attached instrumentation.[62] Consequently, it seems reasonable to use larger materials with more attachment points over a greater length to achieve greater dispersion of forces and reduce the chance of instrumentation failure. Conversely, the greater bone density observed in the obese[22,46] may help accommodate the greater forces and moments anticipated.

For example, inserting larger pedicle screws (both in major diameter and length) in the lower thoracic spine when feasible may reduce metal fatigue and

screw pullout.[62] Similarly, a longer hook-rod construct, with more segmental attachment points, may prevent early instrumentation failure. Likewise, the integrity of the ventral column or its adequate structural reconstruction with a bone graft may be more important if dorsal instrumentation alone is used to maintain stability.

In addition, the effectiveness of external orthoses in protecting instrumentation or maintaining stability may be reduced because of the patient's size. For example, a halo orthosis for immobilization of cervicothoracic injuries might be ineffective in the obese patient.[63] Similarly, a poorly fit thoracolumbosacral orthosis may result in cutaneous complications without offering significant immobilization.

Consequently, stress on the instrumentation may be greater in the obese patient.

Wound Closure

The postoperative complications frequently observed in the surgical treatment of obese patients are superficial wound infections and separations.[24,42,55] The thick, relatively avascular adipose layer heals slowly and may be less resistant to bacterial exposure. It may be beneficial to suture the adipose tissue in several layers, eliminate dead space, and perhaps utilize temporary drainage to prevent wound complications. Perioperative antibiotics may also be important in reducing the frequency of superficial infections.[42]

POSTOPERATIVE MANAGEMENT

Although postoperative complications unrelated to wound closure may not be more common in the obese patient,[24,37] additional attention must be given to preventing pulmonary, cardiovascular, and thromboembolic complications. Atelectasis is commonly encountered and may aggravate preoperative hypoxemia.[42,50,55] A metabolic acidosis may compound the risk of hypoventilation.[61] The degree of hypoxemia reaches a maximum on the second postoperative day.[61] In fact, supplemental oxygen may be required for as long as the first postoperative week.[14] Consequently, careful monitoring of oxygen saturation during the first few days is imperative. Moreover, a semirecumbent or seated position can significantly improve hypoxemia encountered with supine positioning.[3,14,50,55,61] Reintubation for hypoxemia and hypercapnia may be avoided by using nasal continuous positive airway pressure, particularly at night.[52]

While cardiovascular complications are less prominent, arrhythmias, myocardial infarction, and left ventricular dysfunction have been observed in the early postoperative period.[24,28] Judicious use of diuretics, nitrates, digoxin, and angiotensin-convertins enzyme (ACE) inhibitors may assist in managing hemodynamics.[1,2] Brief postoperative intensive care unit monitoring may be beneficial.

The increased risk of thromboembolic complications from hypercoagulability and stasis in the obese patient have been recognized.[13,14,18,29,42,55] The risk may be reduced with postoperative anticoagulation with heparin.[24] In addition, perioperative sequential compression devices are recommended.[18]

Rapid ambulation is very important in reducing these cardiopulmonary and thromboembolic complications. Because intramuscular narcotics for pain control are often ineffective,[13] obese patients may resist mobilization. Epidural narcotics have successfully controlled pain while reducing the time to ambulation and discharge.[14,15] Likewise, patient-controlled intravenous anesthesia with continuous pulse oximetry and apnea monitoring has been recommended for postoperative pain management.[13,38]

CONCLUSION

Management and treatment of the obese patient with thoracic spine disease requires special consideration. Awareness of the possibility of multisystem abnormalities is particularly important given the frequency of obesity in the general population. Although comorbid conditions may increase the risk of operative treatment, careful attention and planning can be effectively used to minimize perioperative complications and achieve satisfactory results.

ACKNOWLEDGMENTS

We would like to thank Mary Braun, R.N., and Lynda Rae Pearson, R.N., for their assistance in obtaining product information and in preparing the figures.

REFERENCES

1. Alexander JK. Obesity and the heart. Heart Dis Stroke 2:317-321,1993.
2. Alpert MA, Hashimi MW. Obesity and the heart. Am J Med Sci 306:117-123,1993.
3. Andersen T, Gluud C, Franzmann M, Chrisoffersen P. Hepatic effects of dietary weight loss in morbidly obese subjects. J Hepatol 12:224-229,1991.
4. Anderson JW, Brinkman VL, Hamilton CC. Weight loss and 2-year follow-up for 80 morbidly obese patients treated with intensive very-low-calorie diet and an education program. Am J Clin Nutr 56:244S-246S, 1992.
5. Atkinson RL. Massive obesity: Complications and treatment. Nutr Rev 49:49-53,1991.
6. Badami JP, Hinck VC. Symptomatic deposition of epidural fat in a morbidly obese woman. Am J Neuroradiol 3:664-665,1982.
7. Bardoczky GI, Yernault JC, Houben JJ, d'Hollander AA. Large tidal volume ventilation does not improve oxygenation in morbidly obese patients during anesthesia. Anesth Analg 81:385-388,1995.
8. Benotti PN, Bistrian B, Benotti JR, Blackburn G, Forse RA. Heart disease and hypertension in severe obesity: The benefits of weight reduction. Am J Clin Nutr 55:586S-590S,1992.

9. Berthoud MC, Peacock JE, Reilly CS. Effectiveness of pre-oxygenation in morbidly obese patients. Br J Anaesth 67:464-466,1991.

10. Bostman OM. Body mass index and height in patients requiring surgery for lumbar intervertebral disc herniation. Spine 18:851-854,1993.

11. Bray GA. Pathophysiology of obesity. Am J Clin Nutr 55:488S-494S,1992.

12. Bray GA. Drug treatment of obesity. Am J Clin Nutr 55:538S-544S,1992.

13. Brentin L, Sieh A. Caring for the morbidly obese. Am J Nurs 91:41-43,1991.

14. Brodsky JB. Anesthetic management of the morbidly obese patient. Int Anesthesiol Clin 24:93-103,1986.

15. Brodsky JB, Merrell RC. Epidural administration of morphine postoperatively for morbidly obese patients. West J Med 140:750-753,1984.

16. Caldwell JB, Nilsen AK. Intravenous ciprofloxacin dosing in the morbidly obese patient. Ann Pharmacother 28:806, 1994.

17. Calles-Escandon J, Horton ES. The thermogenic role of exercise in the treatment of morbid obesity: A critical evaluation. Am J Clin Nutr 55:533S-537S,1992.

18. Clagett GP, Anderson FA, Heit J, Levine MN, Wheeler HB. Prevention of venous thromboembolism. Chest 108:312S-334S,1995.

19. Colditz GA. Economic costs of obesity. Am J Clin Nutr 55:503S-507S,1992.

20. Coulden RAR, Dixon AK. Avoidance of ring artefacts in lumbar spine computed tomography in obese patients. Br J Radiol 60:518, 1987.

21. Crapo RO, Kelly TM, Elliott CG, Jones SB. Spirometry as a preoperative screening test in morbidly obese patients. Surgery 99:763-767,1986.

22. Dawson-Hughes B, Shipp C, Sadowski L, Dallal G. Bone density of the radius, spine and hip in relation to percent ideal body weight in postmenopausal women. Calcif Tissue Int 40:310-314,1987.

23. DiStefano VJ, Klein KS, Nixon JE, Andrews ET. Intraoperative analysis of the effects of position and body habitus on surgery of the low back. Clin Orthop Rel Res 99:51-56,1974.

24. Fasol R, Schindler M, Schumacher B, Schlaudraff K, Hannes W, Seitelberger R, Schlosser V. The influence of obesity on perioperative morbidity: Retrospective study of 502 aorto-coronary bypass operations. Thorac Cardiovasc Surg 40:126-129,1992.

25. Frink EJ, Malan TP, Brown EA, Morgan S, Brown BR. Plasma inorganic fluoride levels with sevoflurane anesthesia in morbidly obese and nonobese patients. Anesth Analg 76:1333-1337,1993.

26. Haddad SF, Hitchon PW, Godersky JC. Idiopathic and glucocorticoid-induced spinal epidural lipomatosis. J Neurosurg 74:38-42,1991.

27. Hakala K, Mustajoki P, Aittomaki J, Sovijarvi ARA. Effect of weight loss and body position on pulmonary function and gas exchange in morbid obesity. Int J Obes 19:343-346,1995.

28. Herrera MF, Deitel M. Cardiac function in massively obese patients and the effect of weight loss. Can J Surg 34:431-434,1991.

29. Holliday DM, Watling SM, Yanos J. Heparin dosing in the morbidly obese patient. Ann Pharmacother 28:1110-1111,1994.

30. Jense HG, Dubin SA, Silverstein PI, O'Leary-Escolas U. Effect of obesity on safe duration of apnea in anesthetized humans. Anesth Analg 72:89-93,1991.

31. Johnson JC, Deeb ZL. Coaxial needle technique for lumbar puncture in the morbidly obese patient. Radiology 179:874, 1991.

32. Kral JG. Overview of surgical techniques for treating obesity. Am J Clin Nutr 55:552S-555S, 1992.

33. Kuczmarski RJ. Prevalence of overweight and weight gain in the United States. Am J Clin Nutr 55:495S-502S, 1992.

34. Larsson B. Obesity, fat distribution and cardiovascular disease. Int J Obes 15:53-57,1991.

35. Lawrence JS. Hypertension in relation to musculoskeletal disorders. Ann Rheum Dis 34:451-456,1975.

36. Lee LH. Half-arc tomography of the cervical-thoracic junction. Radiology 103:462, 1972.

37. Lehman DE, Capello WN, Feinberg JR. Total hip arthroplasty without cement in obese patients. A minimum two-year clinical and radiographic follow-up study. J Bone Joint Surg 76A:854-862,1994.

38. Levin A, Klein SL, Brolin RE, Pitchford DE. Patient-controlled analgesia for morbidly obese patients: An effective modality if used correctly. Anesthesiology 76:857-858, 1992.

39. Marmor L. Surgery for osteoarthritis. Geriatrics 27:89-95, 1972.

40. Martin LF, Hunter SM, Lauve RM, O'Leary JP. Severe obesity: Expensive to society, frustrating to treat, but important to confront. South Med J 88:895-902, 1995.

41. Martin LF, Tan TL, Holmes PA, Becker DA, Horn J, Bixler EO. Can morbidly obese patients safely lose weight preoperatively? Am J Surg 169:245-253, 1995.

42. Paskula PS, Bistrian BR, Benotti PN, Blackburn GL. The risks of surgery in obese patients. Ann Intern Med 104:540-546, 1986.

43. Pi-Sunyer FX. The role of very-low-calorie diets in obesity. Am J Clin Nutr 56:240S-243S, 1992.

44. Pi-Sunyer FX. Medical hazards of obesity. Ann Intern Med 119:655-660, 1993.

45. Poggi M, Paraleti G, Biagi R, Legnani C, Parenti M, Babini AC, Baraldi L, Coccheri S. Prolonged very low calorie diet in highly obese subjects reduces plasma viscosity and red cell aggregation but not fibrinogen. Int J Obes Relat Metab Disord 18:490-496, 1994.

46. Ribot C, Tremollieres F, Pouilles JM, Bonneu M, Germain F, Louvet JP. Obesity and postmenopausal bone loss: The influence of obesity on vertebral density and bone turnover in postmenopausal women. Bone 8:327-331, 1987.

47. Rothfleisch R, Davis LL, Kuebel DA, deBoisblanc BP. Facilitation of fiberoptic nasotracheal intubation in a morbidly obese patient by simultaneous use of nasal CPAP. Chest 106:287-288, 1994.

48. Rothschild PA, Domesek JM, Eastham ME, Kaufman L. MR imaging of excessively obese patients: The use of an open permanent magnet. Magn Reson Imaging 9:151-154,1991.

49. Sarr MG, Felty CL, Hilmer DM, Urban DL, O'Connor G, Hall BA, Rooke TW, Jensen MD. Technical and practical considerations involved in operations on patients weighing more than 270 kg. Arch Surg 130:102-105, 1995.

50. Savino JA, Del Guercio LRM. Preoperative assessment of high-risk surgical patients. Surg Clin North Am 65:763-791, 1985.

51. Servin F, Farinotti R, Haberer JP, Desmonts JM. Propofol infusion for maintenance of anesthesia in morbidly obese patients receiving nitrous oxide. A clinical and pharmacokinetic study. Anesthesiology 78:657-665, 1993.

52. Shivaram U, Cash ME, Beal A. Nasal continuous positive airway pressure in decompensated hypercapnic respiratory failure as a complication of sleep apnea. Chest 104:770-774, 1993.

53. Sjostrom LV. Morbidity of severely obese subjects. Am J Clin Nutr 55:508S-515S, 1992.

54. Sjostrom LV. Mortality of severely obese patients. Am J Clin Nutr 55:516S-523S, 1992.

55. Strauss RJ, Wise L. Operative risks of obesity. Surg Gynecol Obstet 146:286-291, 1978.

56. Summers G, Hocking MP. Surgical approach to the obese patient. J Fla Med Assoc 79:396-399, 1992.

57. Sunden G, Walloe A, Wingstrand H. A new device to reduce intra-abdominal pressure during lumbar surgery. Spine 11:635-636, 1986.

58. Swerdlow BN, Brodsky JB, Butcher MD. Placement of a morbidly obese patient in the prone position. Anesthesiology 68:657-658, 1988.

59. van Rooij WJJ, Borstlap ACW, Canta LR, Tijssen CC. Lumbar epidural lipomatosis causing neurogenic claudication in two obese patients. Clin Neurol Neurosurg 96:181-184, 1994.

60. van Saase JLCM, Vandenbroucke JP, van Romunde LKJ, Valkenburg HA. Osteoarthritis and obesity in the general population. A relationship calling for an explanation. J Rheumatol 15:1152-1158, 1988.

61. Vaughan RW, Engelhardt RC, Wise L. Postoperative hypoxemia in obese patients. Ann Surg 180:877-882, 1974.

62. White AA, Panjabi MM, eds. Clinical Biomechanics of the Spine, 2nd ed. Philadelphia: JB Lippincott, 1990.

63. Whitehill R, Richman JA, Glaser JA. Failure of immobilization of the cervical spine by halo vest. A report of five cases. J Bone Joint Surg 68A:326-332, 1986.

64. Williamson DF. Descriptive epidemiology of body weight and weight change in U.S. adults. Ann Intern Med 119:646-649,1993.

65. Wing RR. Behavioral treatment of severe obesity. Am J Clin Nutr 55:545S-551S, 1992.

66. Zarich SW, Kowalchuk GJ, McGuire MP, Benotti PN, Mascioli EA, Nesto RW. Left ventricular filling abnormalities in asymptomatic morbid obesity. Am J Cardiol 68:377-381, 1991.

The Osteopenic Patient

James P. Hollowell, M.D., and Thomas C. Chen, M.D., Ph.D.

Osteoporosis is estimated to affect 25 million Americans. It is a state characterized by abnormally low bone mass and architectural changes that result in weakening of bones and ultimately in bone failure. Vertebral fractures cause significant pain, deformity, and disability, and are estimated to occur in 25% of women over 70 years of age. The surgical treatment of patients with reduced bone density necessitates special considerations, often altering usual practice. As the quantification of bone mineralization has become easier to establish, and as better understanding of bone physiology has been achieved, new techniques have emerged to help prevent or reverse the loss of bone mineralization.

BONE PHYSIOLOGY AND ANATOMY

Bone is composed of an organic and inorganic matrix, and cellular elements. Type I collagen constitutes more than 90% of the organic matrix of bone, while other noncollagenous proteins, glycoproteins, phospholipids, polysaccharides, and glycosaminoglycans constitute the remainder. An extensive complement of proteins such as bone gla protein, osteonectin, osteopontin, osteocalcin, and others are thought to participate in bone mineralization by incompletely defined mechanisms.

The inorganic or mineral component of bone consists of calcium hydroxyapatite and small amounts of other elements. The mineralization of bone depends on the availability of large amounts of calcium and phosphate.

The cellular component includes osteoblasts, osteoclasts, osteocytes, osteogenic precursors, and hematopoietic and vascular cells. Osteoblasts are bone-forming cells that synthesize the organic matrix and participate in the regulation of mineralization. Osteoblasts are derived from stromal cell precursors of the bone marrow. Differentiation is stimulated by thyroid hormone, parathyroid hormones, growth hormones, prostaglandins, transforming growth factor-β, (TGF-β), and other growth factors. Control of osteoblast function is complex and incompletely understood. It is believed that stimulating factors include thyroid hormone, insulin-like growth factors I and II, and vitamin D. Estrogen and progestins also stimulate osteoblasts in rodent models, and stimulate the production of certain cytokines including TGF-β and interleukin-1 in human bone cells. Inhibiting factors include nicotine and corticosteroids (Fig. 32-1).

Osteocytes are end stage osteoblasts that have trapped themselves in mineralized bone. They maintain interconnections with other osteocytes through slender long processes and gap junctions, though their precise role in bone metabolism is not well understood. They may function as mechanoreceptors.

Osteoclasts are syncytial giant cells that resorb bone under complex control. These cells form a "ruffled border" of contact with bone and secrete bone-digesting lysozymal enzymes such as acid phosphatase, and proteolytic enzymes to digest the organic matrix. These breakdown products of osteoclast function are released into the serum and urine

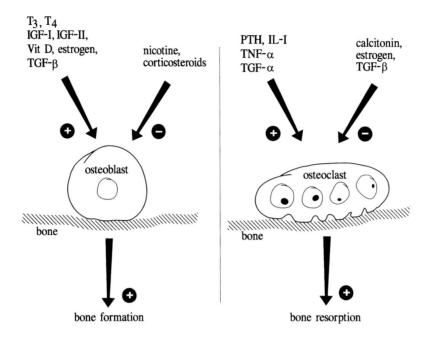

Fig. 32-1. Control of osteoblast and osteoclast function is complex and poorly understood. Stimulation of osteoblast function by thyroid hormone *(T₃,T₄)*, insulin growth factor-I *(IGF-1)*, insulin growth factor II *(IGF-II)*, vitamin D *(Vit D)*, estrogen, and transforming growth factor-β *(TGF-β)* leads to new bone formation. Nicotine and corticosteroids inhibit osteoblast function, decreasing the rate of new bone formation and increasing the likelihood of developing osteoporosis. Osteoclasts, which actively resorb bone, are stimulated by parathyroid hormone *(PTH)*, interleukin-1 *(IL-1)*, tumor necrosis factor-α *(TNF-α)*, and transforming growth factor-α *(TGF-α)*. On the other hand, estrogen, calcitonin, and TGF-β inhibit osteoclast function, resulting in decreased bone resorption.

and serve as markers of osteoclast activity. Osteoclast recruitment, differentiation, and activity are controlled by numerous agents. Calcitonin is known to inhibit osteoclast function, and estrogens are thought to inhibit osteoclast recruitment.

Mature bone is predominantly cortical or cancellous. Cortical bone makes up approximately 80% of skeletal mass and is found mostly in long bones. Cancellous bone represents only 20% of the whole skeleton and is significantly more prominent in spinal vertebrae. Cortical bone is organized in a tubular structure of concentric lamellae surrounding a central vascular canal, while cancellous bone is composed of a meshwork of trabeculae 50 to 400 μm in diameter. The trabeculae are arranged in a pattern that responds to the stress experienced by that bone. Metabolic and pathological changes affect the cortical and cancellous components differently. Therapeutic interventions similarly may affect one bone type more than the other.

Both cortical and cancellous bone are continuously remodeled in a tightly coupled process. Any subtle derangement permitting even slight imbalance in the degradation or formation of bone would

necessarily result in a net gain or loss of skeletal bone mass. A bone remodeling unit is a cylindrical structure that tunnels through cortical bone. At one end active osteoclasts initiate resorption followed by osteoblastic bone formation to fill the cavity, ultimately resulting in a new bone structural unit. In cancellous bone a similar process occurs on the surface of a trabecula forming a pit, which is subsequently filled with new bone. The process takes about 3 months in cortical bone and 6 months in cancellous bone. Exactly how the coupling of resorption and formation occurs is not well known. There is some evidence that a substance in the bone matrix is released as osteoclasts dissolve the bone. This substance may be inhibitory to osteoclasts or stimulate osteoblasts to "repair the damage" of the tunneling osteoclasts.

Maximal bone mass is reached by 25 to 30 years of age. As further aging occurs bone mass is lost. The exact mechanism of bone loss is not completely understood and appears to differ depending on the disease process and skeletal location. There are clear differences between cortical and cancellous bone. There may be a rapid increase in the number of resorption lacunae, initially resulting in a net loss of bone. As the subsequent bone formation increases, a new steady state may be achieved without a net loss of bone. This mechanism results in a transient (reversible) loss of bone. In cancellous bone irreversible bone loss may occur when each resorption pit on the surface of a trabecula is incompletely filled with new bone, resulting in the thinning of the trabecula. When two resorption pits occur directly opposite each other on both sides of a trabecula, a perforation may occur, resulting in irreversible bone loss. Cortical bone loss may occur if there is an increase in the number of bone remodeling units, causing increased porosity on a reversible or irreversible basis. The cortical shell can be thinned by active resorption at the endosteal surface at the interface with the cancellous bone.

BONE MINERALIZATION

Bone mass increases until it peaks at age 25 to 30. The peak bone mass obtained is influenced by sex, race, heredity, nutrition, and exercise. After a brief period of relative stability, there is a constant loss of bone in both men and women with aging. Women demonstrate a transient acceleration of bone loss at menopause that lasts 6 to 10 years before returning to the baseline rate of loss. The exact rate of bone loss differs between cortical and cancellous compartments and depends on the site measured. Meier, Orwall, and Jones[84] demonstrated a 0.2% to 0.34% loss of bone mineral density (BMD) per year for cortical bone of the radius as compared to a 1.2% loss per year of cancellous bone of the spine. Marked disparity between trabecular and cortical bone loss occurs with age in healthy men. The loss of cancellous bone appears to start about a decade earlier than loss of cortical bone.[108] Beyond age 40, loss of bone in females occurs at approximately 0.5% per year until menopause.[99] In males it is somewhat less at 0.3% to 0.4% per year.[60] At menopause, females may experience accelerated loss of bone (up to 6% per year) before returning to baseline rate of loss.[108] Other studies of postmenopausal bone loss have not demonstrated such a significant acceleration of loss. The Postmenopausal Estrogen/Progestin Interventions Trial (PEPI) demonstrated a mean 1.8% loss of vertebral BMD over 3 years.[13] The cumulative effect of this bone loss over a lifetime, results in women losing about 35% of their cortical bone and about 50% of their trabecular bone,

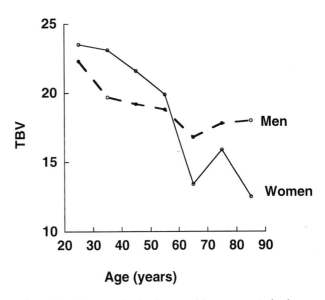

Fig. 32-2. Aging results in decreased bone mass in both men and women. Trabecular bone volume (TBV) from iliac crest biopsies may be used to assay these changes in bone mineral density. Women lose up to 50% of their trabecular bone, while men may lose only one half of this amount. (From data summarized by Mazess.[82])

while men lose about one half of this amount (Fig. 32-2).[82,109]

The maintenance of BMD requires a delicate balance of bone formation and resorption. Both processes are active throughout life and tightly coupled in young people. In osteoporosis, bone formation and resorption become uncoupled. There appear to be different abnormalities of this uncoupling process in premenopausal vs. postmenopausal bone loss. The age dependent premenopausal bone loss appears to be the failure of bone formation to keep up with a near normal rate of bone resorption. In the accelerated postmenopausal state, there appears to be an increase in bone turnover. The magnitude of the increased resorption is greater than that of the increased formation, resulting in a net loss of bone.

MEASUREMENT OF BONE MASS

As more attention is directed toward early intervention for the prevention of clinical manifestations of osteoporosis, the development of accurate, reproducible assessments of BMD has become a central focus. Several techniques to determine BMD have included plain radiogammetry, single photon absorptiometry (SPA), dual photon absorptiometry (DPA), quantitative computed tomography (QCT), and dual x-ray absorptiometry (DXA). Certain measurement techniques are more sensitive to alterations of cortical or cancellous bone. Bone loss or therapeutic interventions may selectively affect certain bone (cortical or cancellous) or certain sites (axial vs. appendicular). The measurement technique may be selected based on the specific skeletal site or bone type expected to be involved in the specific disease process or therapeutic intervention.

Standard spinal radiographs reflect clear evidence of bone loss only when the extent of bone loss is 30% to 50%. This makes routine spine radiographs inadequate to diagnose early bone loss or to follow response to interventions.

Radiogammetry was introduced in the 1960s to assess the thickness of cortical bone. This technique simply measures the cortical thickness of a long bone from the periosteal to the endosteal margins with calipers, allowing calculation of the total cross-sectional area of cortical bone. However, it does not provide for estimation of cortical bone or cancellous bone porosity, and is inadequate for most uses.

SPA, also introduced in the early 1960s, utilizes single-beam monoenergetic radiation (often [125] I) across the longitudinal axis of a long bone. The beam passes through cortical and trabecular components together and is sensitive to the surrounding soft tissues. It is typically used in appendicular bones such as the radius, and not in the spine.

DPA, developed several years later, has the advantage of reducing the effect of surrounding soft tissues to permit accurate scanning of the spine and hip. The technique uses two discrete monoenergetic radiation sources. This can be provided by a mixture of radionuclides or a dual energy emitter. Scanning patients with severe deformity, collapsed vertebral bodies, previous surgery, or certain spinal diseases such as Paget's or metastatic disease, may produce data that are difficult to interpret or reproduce. A lumbar scan is usually done in the anteroposterior (AP) direction and measures all cortical and trabecular spinal elements, including the vertebral body, spinous process, articular facets, and transverse processes. Hypertrophic facet disease in the elderly population may mask real changes of mineralization of the vertebral body. DPA has also been used to scan the femur or determine total body mineral content through whole body scans.

QCT utilizes conventional or modified CT scanners with specialized software to analyze the spine and appendicular bones. It is the only technique that provides a true BMD (gm/cm^3), in contrast to other techniques that provide only area density (gm/cm^2). This technique offers the ability to define a region of interest in the central portion of a vertebral body consisting entirely of trabecular bone. This permits elimination of areas of hypertrophic facet changes or vertebral spurring to give a more accurate measurement of the trabecular vertebral component. QCT studies necessitate a radiation exposure 10 to 60 times greater than DPA or DXA, approximately representing the exposure of a single chest radiograph. QCT is available as single-energy (SEQCT) or dual-energy (DEQCT). The SEQCT study takes about half as long (10 minutes) and has about half the radiation exposure. Unfortunately, SEQCT may underestimate BMD due to the presence of fatty marrow in the vertebral body. Fatty content varies with age and also due to disease. DEQCT has been designed to reduce the effects of fatty marrow. It is more accurate but may be less reproducible. Sometimes both determinations are used together when high accuracy and reproducibility is required in certain areas of research. Either method is considered acceptable for clinical determinations of spinal BMD.

DXA, a technique commercially introduced in 1987, is similar to DPA but uses an x-ray source (Fig. 32-3). DXA is three to four times faster than DPA with improved precision, similar accuracy, and lower radiation exposure. A DXA study typically costs about $200. The two sources of energy can be obtained from an x-ray tube switching rapidly back and forth between energies, or a constant x-ray source that is filtered into two energies. Scanning can be performed in a posteroanterior or lateral projection. Posteroanterior projections may incorporate osteophytes, aortic calcifications and sclerotic degenerative facet changes, which can significantly alter results. Lateral projections eliminate most of these problems and image a sample of nearly all cancellous bone. Determination of BMD in a lateral projection correlates much better than PA projections when compared to QCT determinations. Unfortunately, due to the iliac crest and rib

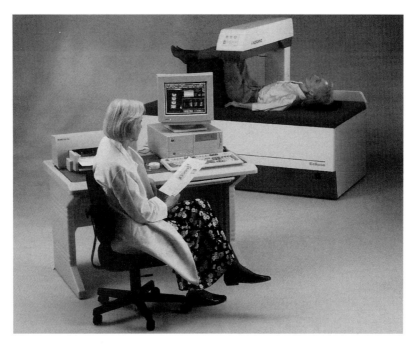

Fig. 32-3. Typical DXA device and control computer with patient positioned for AP imaging. (Permission from Norland Medical Systems, Inc, Fort Atkinson, Wis.)

Table 32-1. WHO Diagnostic Criteria for Osteoporosis

Category	Definition*
Normal	Less than 1 SD
Low bone mass (osteopenia)	Greater than 1 SD; less than 2.5 SD
Osteoporosis	Greater than 2.5 SD
Osteoporosis (severe)	Greater than 2.5 SD, with 1 or more fragility fractures

*BMD or BMC deviation from young adult reference mean

overlap, lateral projections may be restricted to L3 and L4. Scanning may be performed in both projections, and results are compared to a known reference database. The BMD is often expressed as the number of standard deviations from peak BMD of young normal individuals (T score) and the number of standard deviations from age-matched controls (Z score). A Z score of –2.0 would suggest a BMD two standard deviations below the mean for this age group (Fig. 32-4). The World Health Organization (WHO) and others are attempting to standardize the definition of osteoporosis as 2.5 standard deviations from the mean for young normal individuals (Table 32-1). DXA appears to have nearly replaced all other techniques of BMD determination in the last few years.

CELLULAR BASIS OF OSTEOPOROSIS

It has been proposed that there are two types of involutional osteoporosis.[2,107] Type I is postmenopausal due to estrogen deprivation. Type II is considered osteoporosis associated with aging. Bone loss in type I osteoporosis is due to increased activity of osteoclasts deprived of the suppressive influence of estrogen.[36,95] Type II osteoporosis appears to be due largely to a relative osteoblastic insufficiency.[35] Type I osteoporosis occurs predominantly in females, mostly involves cancellous bone, and is typified by increased osteoclastic activity and normal or near normal osteoblastic activity. In contrast, type II osteoporosis is more evenly distributed among males and females, occurs in an older age group, and is typified by near normal osteoclastic activity and reduced osteoblastic activity.

In a young mature spine a lumbar vertebral body has a load-bearing capacity of about 1000 kg.[88] Total load-bearing capacity is significantly related to the size or cross-sectional area of a vertebral body. Men have vertebral bodies that are typically 20% to 30% larger than those of women, and therefore a similarly

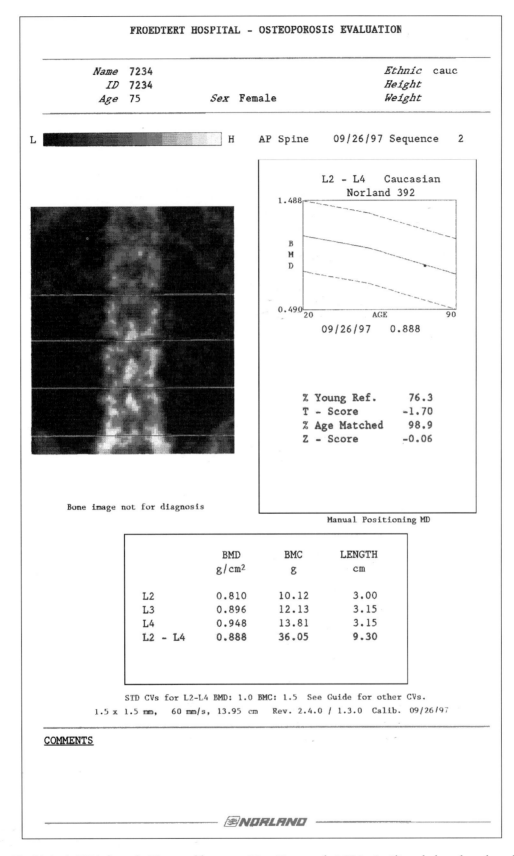

FROEDTERT HOSPITAL - OSTEOPOROSIS EVALUATION

Name	7234		*Ethnic* cauc
ID	7234		*Height*
Age	75	*Sex* Female	*Weight*

L ▮▮▮▮▮▮▮▮ H   AP Spine   09/26/97 Sequence   2

L2 - L4   Caucasian
Norland 392

09/26/97   0.888

% Young Ref.   76.3
T - Score   -1.70
% Age Matched   98.9
Z - Score   -0.06

Bone image not for diagnosis

Manual Positioning MD

	BMD g/cm²	BMC g	LENGTH cm
L2	0.810	10.12	3.00
L3	0.896	12.13	3.15
L4	0.948	13.81	3.15
L2 - L4	0.888	36.05	9.30

STD CVs for L2-L4 BMD: 1.0 BMC: 1.5 See Guide for other CVs.
1.5 x 1.5 mm,   60 mm/s, 13.95 cm   Rev. 2.4.0 / 1.3.0 Calib. 09/26/97

COMMENTS

NORLAND

Fig. 32-4. A, DXA data of a 75-year-old woman. Note T score of –1.70 is significantly less than that of a young normal individual; however, the Z score of –0.06 is quite similar to the expected age-matched control. The patient has diminished bone density typical for a female of her age.

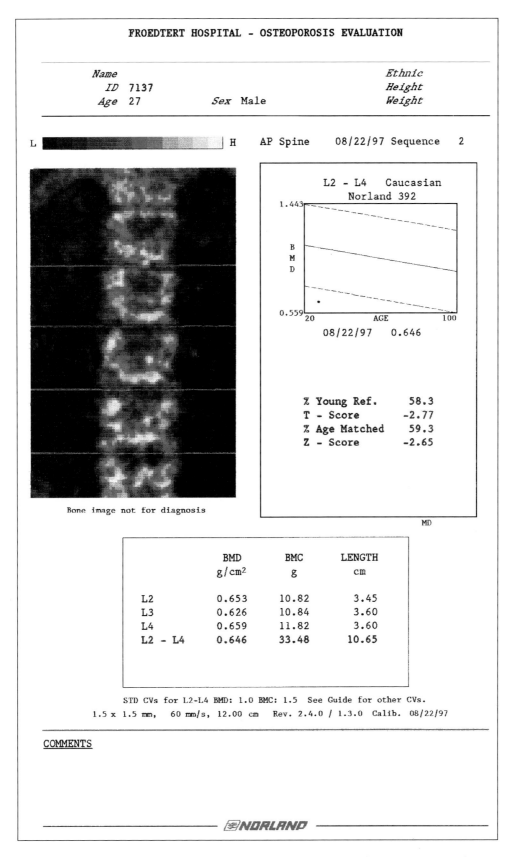

FROEDTERT HOSPITAL - OSTEOPOROSIS EVALUATION

Name   *Ethnic*
  ID   7137   *Height*
  Age   27   *Sex*   Male   *Weight*

L ▮▮▮▮▮▮▮▮ H   AP Spine   08/22/97 Sequence   2

L2 - L4   Caucasian
Norland 392

1.443

B
M
D

0.559

20   AGE   100

08/22/97   0.646

% Young Ref.	58.3
T - Score	-2.77
% Age Matched	59.3
Z - Score	-2.65

Bone image not for diagnosis

MD

	BMD g/cm²	BMC g	LENGTH cm
L2	0.653	10.82	3.45
L3	0.626	10.84	3.60
L4	0.659	11.82	3.60
L2 - L4	0.646	33.48	10.65

STD CVs for L2-L4 BMD: 1.0 BMC: 1.5   See Guide for other CVs.
1.5 x 1.5 mm,   60 mm/s, 12.00 cm   Rev. 2.4.0 / 1.3.0   Calib. 08/22/97

<u>COMMENTS</u>

🔁NORLAND

Fig. 32-4, cont'd, B, DXA data of a 27-year-old man. Note both T and Z scores are quite low, consistent with a diagnosis of osteoporosis.

greater load-carrying capacity. As men age there is a further increase in the cross-sectional area of the vertebral body that largely offsets the gradual loss of BMD, resulting in a preservation of vertebral strength. This same increase in cross-sectional area of the vertebral body does not occur in women, leaving them even more vulnerable to the effects of decreased BMD aggravated by the accelerated loss after menopause.

Cancellous bone is composed of a regular meshwork of trabeculae. There are vertical trabecular struts with a usual thickness of 200 to 220 μm supported by somewhat thinner horizontal struts (180 to 200 μm). After menopause the activation frequency of resorption increases and perforation of the trabecular struts increases. The perforations are more common in the horizontal struts, possibly due to their initial thinner width. The strength of a trabecula is proportional to its radius squared. Moderate trabecular thinning results in an even more drastic loss of strength. The compressive strength of the trabecular structure is proportional to the square of the distance between the supporting horizontal struts. As more horizontal struts are removed by perforation, the vertical struts may begin to fail by buckling.[8] In addition, the cortical end plate in osteoporosis may be thinned by 50% to 120 to 150 μm. The overall effect of these changes significantly reduces the load-carrying capacity of the vertebra. The load-carrying capacity may decline to 60 to 90 kg, making it vulnerable to failure with physiological loads.

BIOCHEMICAL MARKERS OF BONE METABOLISM

Several markers of bone turnover have been identified. Many are collagen-based and indicate either bone formation or bone degradation. Markers of bone formation include serum studies for procollagen type I C-terminal propeptide (PICP), serum procollagen type I N-terminal propeptide (PINP), osteocalcin, and total and bone-specific alkaline phosphatase. Markers of degradation often found in urine include hydroxyproline, hydroxyl glycosides, pyridinium cross-links, collagen type I cross-linked N-telopeptide, collagen type I cross-linked C-telopeptide, carboxyterminal telopeptide, and tartrate-resistant acid phosphatase. It appears that assays for pyridinium cross-links are more specific and less expensive than hydroxyproline, the first generation marker.

For several reasons, many of the markers do not necessarily provide completely accurate assessments of bone turnover. In some cases the marker of interest is not entirely specific to bone or may be affected by certain physiological or pathological states such as renal or liver failure and pregnancy. The costs of these tests range from about $16 to nearly $300. Most are some type of radioimmunoassay. Because they indicate the rate of bone turnover at one particular moment rather than bone density, they cannot be used to diagnose osteoporosis. They may be effective at determining response to treatment, but even this role is not clearly established. Markers may ultimately be used to identify patients at greater risk for osteoporosis but they are not presently used routinely for this purpose. The study of biochemical markers and their clinical utility is relatively new and it is likely that we will soon have available reliable markers and well-established indications for their usage.

FACTORS INFLUENCING BONE MINERALIZATION

Bone mineralization is influenced by hereditary, mechanical, nutritional, and hormonal factors (see box). Some of these factors are controllable and therefore present an opportunity for intervention in optimizing BMD. Unfortunately, many of these factors act subtly over a lifetime, and after significant loss of bone mass, intervention may not be particularly effective.

Heredity

Genetic factors clearly play a significant role in the determination of bone density, though the magni-

---

FACTORS AFFECTING BONE DENSITY

Factors Increasing Bone Density	Factors Decreasing Bone Density
Increased body weight	Family history of osteoporosis
Moderate exercise	
Moderate alcohol intake	Smoking
Calcium	Caffeine
Vitamin D	Excessive alcohol intake
Estrogen	
Fluoride	
Calcitonin	
Biphosphonates	

tude of this contribution remains uncertain. Studies of mother/daughter pairs have suggested that a genetic factor may explain as much as 50% to 70% of the variance of BMD.[76,77] Other studies utilizing twin pairs have found the hereditary contribution may explain as much as 80% to 90% of BMD.[32,100,114] Environmental factors have often been found to be similar between family members as well. Krall and Dawson-Hughes[67] designed a study to specifically analyze the relative contribution of environmental factors (diet, weight, activity, smoking, alcohol use) compared to genetic factors. After carefully controlling for environmental factors, 46% to 62% of bone density could be explained by heredity. Though genetic factors cannot be directly controlled, the presence of osteoporosis in family members may suggest the need to evaluate BMD and optimize controllable factors as early as possible.

Lifestyle Factors
Smoking

Several studies have demonstrated that smoking causes significant adverse effects on bone mineralization in men and women, increasing risks of vertebral fracture two- to fourfold.[3,29,66,67,83,113] An increase in hip fractures of smaller magnitude has also been demonstrated. The mechanism of this effect is uncertain. It has been demonstrated that smoking is associated with earlier menopause and depressed testosterone production, both of which may adversely affect bone mineralization. Additionally, there are many other behavioral and nutritional influences in the smoking population that may contribute to this effect. It is noteworthy that smoking has similarly been found to significantly deter bone fusion.[10,11,27,52] The mechanism for inhibition of fusion is similarly not well established, but is likely to involve early revascularization, resistance to calcitonin, and inhibition of osteoblasts. Because approximately one third of the population in the United States smokes, this is a common and preventable factor.

Alcohol

Much less clear is the effect of alcohol on bone mineralization. Studies have offered conflicting results on whether alcohol consumption is beneficial or detrimental. Alcoholics appear to have reduced bone mass and increased risk of fracture, though several other factors such as poor nutritional status may

confound this observation. Seemen et al.[113] demonstrated an increased risk of vertebral fractures in men that was related to alcohol intake. Increased risk of osteoporotic hip and forearm fractures has also been demonstrated in women with moderate alcohol consumption.[56] In contrast, Hansen et al.[53] demonstrated a decreased rate of bone loss in 121 postmenopausal women with moderate alcohol consumption followed prospectively over a 12-year period. Holbrook and Barrett-Connor[57] prospectively studied 449 men and women from an upper-middle-class area over a 15- to 18-year period and found that "moderate social drinking" was associated with an increase in bone mineral density. The mechanism by which alcohol consumption may promote bone mineralization is unclear. It has been observed that alcohol intake may correlate with increased estrogen levels.[70] It has also been found that alcohol intake induces the adrenal production of androstenedione that may be converted to estrogen.[47] A recent report demonstrated that postmenopausal women on estrogen replacement therapy who drink alcohol may have increased estradiol levels by as much as 327%.[13] The effect on postmenopausal bone loss has not yet been established. In summary, there is conflicting evidence about the role of alcohol in bone mineralization. It is possible that these contradictory studies may be secondary to an alcohol dose-dependent response on bone mineralization that has yet to be defined.

Caffeine

The few studies examining the effects of caffeine have also produced somewhat conflicting results. Some reports have suggested that caffeine consumption produces a urinary loss of calcium resulting in a negative calcium balance in humans.[81] Other investigators have not observed this association.[6,54] Daniell[29] detected an association of high caffeine intake and osteoporosis but this effect did not persist after correction for confounding factors such as weight and smoking. Similarly, Holbrook, Barrett-Connor, and Wingard[58] found a higher consumption of caffeine in women with hip fractures but the data did not reach statistical significance and confounding factors were not considered. Kiel et al.[64] studied 3170 patients as part of the Framingham study. They demonstrated that hip fractures in individuals drinking two cups of coffee occurred at the same rate as those not ingesting caffeine. However, in individuals consuming more than 2.5 cups of coffee per day, a correlation between increased hip fracture rate and coffee consumption was found. Another study by Hernandez-Avila et al.[56] examined hip fractures in middle-aged women and found a relative risk of 2.95 for individuals consuming caffeine in the fifth quintile. Though the effect of caffeine has not been fully studied in the spine, it would appear that moderate caffeine consumption is probably not associated with osteoporosis, though higher levels of caffeine consumption may be.

Exercise

It is clear that exercise is important to achieve and maintain maximal bone mass. Numerous studies have demonstrated that intensive activity is associated with increased bone mass.[18,28,49,61,71,83,90,116] Cavanaugh and Cann[16] studied the effect of brisk walking in postmenopausal women and found no effect on BMD over a 1-year period. Dalsky et al.[28] studied spine BMD in postmenopausal women who participated in an active exercise program including walking, jogging, and stair climbing. The women also received calcium supplementation to bring their total daily consumption to 1500 mg/day. BMD increased 5.2% after 9 months, and 6.1% after 22 months of training. This compared to a loss of 1.4% in BMD in the control group receiving calcium but not exercising. Unfortunately, cessation of exercise brought about an abrupt significant loss of BMD to near baseline. A prospective study of 118 children less than 14 years of age revealed significantly increased BMD in the radius, spine, and hip with increased weight-bearing physical activity.[115] However, physically inactive time, such as hours spent watching television, did not negatively affect BMD in this study. It is speculated from this data that peak bone mass may be increased by moderate activity throughout childhood. Because aging necessarily results in consistent bone loss, starting from an initially higher peak of bone mass may be an important factor in delaying the time until critically low BMD is reached.

Several studies have examined the effects of prolonged inactivity.[33,68,72] Donaldson et al.[33] studied the effect of 30 to 36 weeks of bed rest in healthy young male volunteers. They quickly developed a negative calcium balance and lost 4.2% of total body calcium during the confinement. BMD in the os calcis fell 25% to 45%. Reambulation re-established a positive

calcium balance, and recalcification appeared to occur at about the same rate as initially lost. Another study of six normal males confined to bed rest for 17 weeks found a loss of 3.9% of BMD partially recovered over 6 weeks of reambulation.[72] Krolner and Toft[68] studied loss of BMD in 34 patients confined to bed rest for treatment of low back pain. They demonstrated a 0.9% loss of BMD per week that returned nearly to normal after 4 months of reambulation.

In premenopausal women, marked exercise is often accompanied by cessation of menses.[42] This is accompanied by a marked reduction of estrogen resembling the postmenopausal state. In the absence of estrogen female athletes suffer a significant loss of bone mineralization.[61,71] Marcus et al.[80] found significant reduction of bone mass in the spines of amenorrheic long distance runners compared to age-matched nonrunner controls and menstruating long distance runners. The amenorrheic runners suffered increased stress-related fractures. Another study of matched amenorrheic and eumenorrheic athletes demonstrated significantly lower estradiol levels and 16% lower BMD of the lumbar spine.[34] When regular menses is re-established, females regain bone density. Whether this process is fully reversible has not been well established.

In male athletes, exercise may be so vigorous that significant calcium is lost in sweat, generating a negative calcium balance and loss of total body BMD. Klesges et al.[65] studied calcium balance and BMD in college basketball players. Dermal excretion of calcium was high and for those athletes with a calcium intake of less than 2000 mg/day a consistent decline of BMD was observed throughout the season. If intake was greater, or if calcium supplementation was provided, athletes demonstrated an increase of BMD throughout the training season. They concluded that exercise results in significant increase of BMD unless calcium availability is restricted.

In summary, there is ample evidence to recommend increased exercise throughout life to optimize and maintain skeletal mineralization. Extreme exercise in females may result in marked bone loss and should be avoided.

Body Weight

The PEPI trial examining the effects of estrogen/progestin collected data on the role of body mass index (BMI).[13] In the placebo group of postmenopausal women, those with high BMI had a loss of BMD over 3 years of 1.4%, compared to 4.7% in the low BMI group. This supports the clinical notion of osteoporosis preferentially affecting nonobese patients. The explanation for this observation is unclear but may relate to the role of adipose tissue in maintenance of higher estrogen levels.

Mineral and Hormonal Factors
Calcium Supplementation

The use of calcium supplementation would appear at first glance to be a well-established technique for increasing BMD. Although this is largely true, the supportive literature is often methodologically impaired and contradictory. Often studies have found effects of calcium supplementation to be greatest when the initial deficit is large, and less important when the individual is already consuming adequate levels of calcium. Unfortunately, many studies do not control for baseline calcium. The concomitant administration of vitamin D and estrogen, as well as the many other factors described previously, further complicate interpretation of data on the effect of calcium supplementation. Cumming[25] performed a meta-analysis on 49 separate observational and interventional studies concerning the effect of calcium supplementation. The majority of the studies were in postmenopausal women. He concluded that the studies demonstrated a consistent prevention of the rate of bone loss in postmenopausal women. However, when looking specifically at the spine in interventional studies, two of three studies found a decrease in vertebral bone mass of 0.78%[10,11,27,39,52,110] In three additional cross-sectional studies, a weak positive correlation was observed for increased bone density of the spine with greater calcium intake.[25]

Two studies excluded from the above meta-analysis have demonstrated reduced hip fractures and reduced vertebral fractures with calcium supplements.[58,105] Their exclusion was due to the concomitant administration of high dose vitamin D in many cases. Another study has found reduced loss of vertebral bone mass resulting from increased consumption of dairy products.[5] A study in prepubertal children by Johnston et al.[62] found a significant increase in spinal bone mass after a 3-year supplementation period with 1000 mg of calcium. This may suggest a potential to increase the peak bone mass, delaying the inevitable effects of bone loss in adulthood.

Another recent review of controlled clinical trials of calcium supplementation by Dawson-Hughes[30] has also supported the consistent reduction of bone loss in early postmenopausal women. This study also concludes that the spine is an exception, demonstrating either limited or no response to supplementation. However, a recent report from the PEPI trial carefully monitored spine BMD by DXA in a postmenopausal control group receiving no active hormonal therapy.[13] This study found that women with the highest calcium intake lost significantly less bone (–1.8%) than those with a moderate calcium intake (–3.6%) after 3 years.

Despite the many studies on the effects of calcium, several important potentially confounding factors have not been fully analyzed. Generally, the data would support ensuring the availability of calcium to maximize bone mineralization. Unfortunately, the spine in particular may be relatively refractory to the benefits of this treatment. The effect of calcium alone should be expected to be rather minimal, but may be important over a long period.

Vitamin D

Again, many confounding factors have troubled the study of the effect of vitamin D. Dawson-Hughes et al.[31] studied the effect of calcium both with and without vitamin D in postmenopausal females. Their work found the supplementation of 500 IU of vitamin D over a 1-year period to reduce the rate of spinal bone loss compared to calcium supplementation alone. In males, the addition of cholecalciferol and calcium was not found to affect bone mass. Although the effects of vitamin D are not well understood, it would seem reasonable that adequate levels should be maintained either through dietary or supplemental sources.

Hormone Replacement

Substantial evidence supports the hormonal requirements for optimal bone mineralization. The most compelling link is the accelerated loss of bone mass at the time of menopause attributed to estrogen loss due to ovarian failure. The mechanism of action has been studied in osteoblast cell culture.[37] It is known that agents that elevate cyclic adenosine monophosphate (cAMP) in osteoblasts, such as parathyroid hormone (PTH) or prostaglandins, stimulate bone resorption. In bone cell culture PTH stimulation of adenylate cyclase can be blocked by estradiol, resulting in anticatabolic effects.[44] Direct modulation by estradiol of the response of human bone cells (SaOS-2) to human PTH and PTH-related protein has been suggested. Anabolic effects of estrogen have also been demonstrated. Estradiol has been shown to stimulate osteoblast cell proliferation and matrix protein synthesis. Evidence exists for a direct effect of estrogen on bone cells in vitro.[37] Studies on avian osteoclasts have demonstrated direct binding of estradiol to osteoclasts resulting in a dose-dependent decrease in bone resorption.[92]

Several clinical studies have examined the usefulness of estrogen for prevention of postmenopausal bone loss. Ettinger, Genant, and Cann[39] studied the effects of estrogen and calcium supplementation on spinal cancellous mineralization in early postmenopausal women using QCT. This work demonstrated that bone loss was 9.0% in untreated women compared to 10.5% in those given calcium supplementation alone. The addition of 0.3 mg/day of conjugated estrogen resulted in a gain of 2.3%. This study also offered new information about effective dosage of estrogen by demonstrating that the dose of 0.3 mg/day of conjugated estrogen with calcium was effective. Earlier dose response studies by the same authors in oophorectomized females had found that 0.6 mg/day in the absence of calcium was the minimal effective dose for the prevention of bone loss.

Another study of postmenopausal bone loss examined four treatment groups including estrogen, progestin, estrogen with progestin, and control. All groups were supplemented with calcium.[45] Progestin alone did not prevent spinal bone loss (−4.58%); however, estrogen was effective in decreasing spinal bone loss (+2.10%). The combination of estrogen and progestin was no more effective than estrogen alone for the spine. Progestin did prevent bone loss in cortical skeletal bone measured in the metacarpal but not the spine.

Studies have also demonstrated that the ability of estrogen to increase BMD is clearly translated into reduction of fractures.[26] A retrospective review by Ettinger, Genant, and Cann[38] demonstrated vertebral fractures in 2.5% of estrogen treated women compared to 6.6% in an untreated control group. Riggs et al.[105] have also demonstrated lower rates of vertebral fracture in women supplemented with estrogen and calcium.

The PEPI trial was a 3-year trial studying the effect of conjugated equine estrogen alone or in combination with progesterone in 875 women.[13] This study showed a similar gain of approximately 5% of BMD in the spine and 1.7% in the hip in all estrogen treatment groups with or without progestin over a 3-year period. In contrast, the placebo patients had a 1.8% BMD loss in the spine and 1.7% BMD loss in the hip. This study did not demonstrate added benefit of progestin combinations on BMD as some other studies have. The study also did not find that smoking, body mass, ethnicity, alcohol, calcium intake, or physical activity altered the gains in BMD with hormone supplementation in the spine or the hip.

However, concerns about chronic estrogen supplementation may complicate routine use of this therapy. Estrogen stimulates mitotic activity in endometrial and breast tissue leading to malignancy. Studies have linked the use of unopposed estrogen with an increased risk of breast and uterine cancer.[15,55,97,118-120] A number of studies have demonstrated the increased risk of uterine cancer in patients using unopposed estrogen to be 2% to 15%. In absolute terms the risk increases from 1:1000 to 1:100.[55] The risk is related to dose and duration, increasing with both. A small consolation is the finding that those developing uterine cancer on estrogen have a somewhat better life expectancy than those with the same cancer not on estrogen.

The Comparative Effect on Bone Density, Endometrium, and Lipids of Continuous Hormones as Replacement Therapy (CHART) study recently reported an analysis of different doses of estrogen with or without a progestin in eight potential treatment groups in 1265 patients. This study also considered the poor compliance of estrogen therapy with cyclic progestins in postmenopausal women. The cyclic addition of progestin commonly reestablishes menses that appears to be related to poor compliance. If progestin is taken daily, menses can be avoided. This study examined the effect of different daily doses of progestin on BMD, proliferative and hyperplastic changes of the uterus, as well as lipids. The ideal agent would provide strong positive effects on BMD and lipid profiles while avoiding premalignant or malignant uterine changes.

The estrogen used was ethinyl estradiol (EE$_2$) the usual estrogen of most oral contraceptives marketed in the United States, but different from the common equine conjugated estrogen commonly used for postmenopausal women. The progestin used was norethindrone acetate (NA), also commonly used in oral contraceptives. The unopposed estrogen group demonstrated significant reduction in the rate of loss of BMD, but not a significant increase in BMD. The addition of daily norethindrone increased the BMD by 4.2% compared with a loss of 7.4% in the placebo group. The effect on BMD demonstrated a linear dose response for the combination therapies. An unacceptably high rate of endometrial hyperplasia was observed in the unopposed estrogen group, and essentially complete protection was achieved in all doses of the norethindrone combinations. All active hormonal treatment groups had a beneficial effect on their lipid profile compared to placebo. In summary, this study has demonstrated that estrogen supplementation, combined with daily rather than cyclic progestin, can increase BMD while protecting endometrium, maintaining a favorable lipid profile, and reducing vaginal bleeding to encourage maximal compliance.

A meta-analysis of the risk of breast cancer associated with the use of estrogen was performed on 25 studies concerned with this issue.[120] This analysis found no increased risk for the first 5 years of supplementation, and an increased risk of 30% after 15 years of supplementation. There also appears to be an even greater increase in the risk in those individuals with a family history of breast cancer. The authors conclude that the risk of cancer is relatively small, especially with consideration of the beneficial cardiac effects. Nevertheless, they estimate that there may be nearly 5000 cases of breast cancer and 1500 cancer deaths attributable to supplemental estrogen.[120] This number could even be two to three times greater if all postmenopausal women were using supplemental estrogen. It is interesting to note that bone mass has been proposed as a measure of cumulative exposure to estrogen to possibly reflect risk of breast cancer.[125] A recent study has demonstrated that women in the highest quartile of bone mass have a 3.5 fold increase in incidence of breast cancer.[125]

Another investigator has estimated the increased risk of breast cancer in estrogen users to be approximately twofold in long-term and high-dose users.[55] He also concluded that the relative risk is much lower in smaller doses for relatively shorter periods. The results of many studies are not uniform, some showing little if any increased risk in certain subgroups studied. The effects of the addition of progestin on breast cancer risk have not been well established. At least some studies have demonstrated a slight increased risk.

It is interesting that the largest decrease in BMD occurs in the first few years postmenopause and then levels off to a relatively slow decline. Shorter-term use of estrogen appears to have relatively minimal increased risk of malignancy. What happens when supplemental estrogen is discontinued after successfully eliminating the early phase of rapid bone loss? Lindsay et al.[74] studied this issue in 43 oophorectomized patients over an 8-year period. Patients treated with estrogen lost no bone over the first 4 postmenopausal years compared to a 10.4% loss in the untreated control. After withdrawal of their estrogen, the previously treated group experienced a 2.5% per year loss of BMD to reach the same loss as the never treated group by 8 years. This suggests that estrogen supplementation may only provide benefits as long as it is continued.

Cauley et al.[15] found that women older than 65 have a risk of breast cancer that is proportional to their BMD. Women with a one standard deviation increase in BMD had a 30% to 50% increased risk of breast cancer. It is presumed that BMD represents a surrogate measure for exposure to estrogen, and hence the higher rate of breast cancer. BMD alone is considered to be nearly as strong a risk factor for breast cancer as family history.

A literature review of the effects of estrogen supplementation on cardiac disease has found that in postmenopausal women there is a 50% reduction in cardiac disease in those taking unopposed estrogen.[7] Premenopausal women taking oral contraceptive estrogens appear to have an increased risk of cardiac events (mostly thromboembolic), particularly in those who smoke heavily. The effect of combined progestins is not well studied, but the above described PEPI trial did find favorable alterations in lipid profiles with concomitant progestin use that would suggest preservation of the protective cardiac effect.[13]

Despite the fact that estrogens clearly increase malignancy rates for breast and uterine cancer, the risk of American women dying from cardiac disease is nearly fourfold greater than dying from breast or uterine cancer combined. Henderson[55] has estimated that the beneficial effects of estrogens far outweigh the increased risks of cancer. Indeed, he has estimated that the use of 0.625 mg of unopposed conjugated estrogen for 10 years would result in an annual saving of 302 lives per 100,000 women. The rate would be even higher for women who have undergone a hysterectomy, and possibly in women using newer hormonal replacement strategies that utilize progestin combinations.

Fluoride

Fluoride has been used for at least 30 years experimentally to augment bone density. It has been found that fluoride can incorporate into the crystalline structure of bone as fluorapatite, or increase the activity of osteoblasts to encourage the formation of bone.[48] Fluoride, given over 4 years, has been demonstrated to increase the BMD of the lumbar spine by 35%.[106] Some studies have also found fluoride to be toxic in higher doses, reducing the strength of bones.[48] Fluoride, commonly available as sodium fluoride, has not been approved in the United States for the treatment of osteoporosis. However, it has been approved in at least eight European countries for this purpose.[106] Currently, fluoride may be obtained in the United States in many water supplies at a dose of 1 to 4 ppm, for the prevention of dental caries.

Unfortunately, data from clinical trials again provides rather mixed results. Riggs et al.[106] supplemented postmenopausal women with osteoporosis with fluoride and calcium and achieved significant increases in BMD but no reduction of new vertebral fractures. They also recognized an increased rate of nonvertebral fractures, raising questions about possible fragility of the fluoride stimulated bone. Mamelle et al.[79] studied 50 mg sodium fluoride supplementation in 257 patients with osteoporotic vertebral compression fractures over a 2-year period. This study demonstrated a significantly lower rate of vertebral fractures in the treatment group. Another more recent study by Pak et al.[94] studied cyclic administration of slow release sodium fluoride and calcium supplementation in a similar population, but with somewhat less severe osteoporosis. New vertebral fractures were significantly less common in the treated group, however, recurrence of spinal fractures was not reduced. There appeared to be a greater effect in subjects with less severe osteoporosis at onset of supplementation.

Bernstein et al.[9] performed comparisons of populations living in areas of high vs. low fluoride supplementation in public water supply. They demonstrated a significant reduction in vertebral fracture rate in areas with higher water supplementation of fluoride. Unfortunately, other similar population observations have not provided similar findings.[48]

Though fluoride supplementation appears promising, there is insufficient information to determine under which circumstances supplementation will be beneficial. Preliminary data suggest that there is a therapeutic dose window, avoiding ineffectively low concentrations or toxic doses. Like many therapies, earlier intervention appears more effective, and waiting until severe osteoporosis is established may be too late. Data do not appear to support routine recommendation of fluoride supplementation for the prevention or treatment of osteoporosis.

Calcitonin

Calcitonin, a polypeptide hormone secreted by the parafollicular cells of the thyroid, has been shown to bind to high infinity receptors on the osteoclasts with pronounced inhibition of activity.[17,41,89] Further evidence has suggested some stimulatory effect on osteoblasts as well.[41,59] Calcitonin has been used as an antiresorptive agent for metabolic bone disease such as Paget's and more recently for osteoporosis.

Several clinical studies have demonstrated the effectiveness of calcitonin to augment bone density by injection or intranasal spray.[78,93,101] MacIntyre et al.[78] studied calcitonin in 70 postmenopausal women with or without concomitant estrogen/progestin supplementation. Calcitonin, given subcutaneously, was as effective as estrogen in preventing bone loss. The estrogen-supplemented group treated with calcitonin showed even better protection of bone loss. Subcutaneous injection of calcitonin may cause side effects of flushing and gastrointestinal symptoms that deter its use. More recently available and approved by the FDA in 1995, intranasal preparations have also been found to be similarly effective with fewer side effects.[93,101] Overgaard et al.[93] found an 8.2% difference of BMD compared to placebo after 2 years of treatment. This study, however, did not find a similar beneficial effect in the peripheral skeleton. Calcitonin may be a good alternative to estrogen supplementation in those patients with a specific contraindication or intolerance to estrogens.

Biphosphonates

Biphosphonates are inorganic analogs of pyrophosphates that can adhere to the hydroxyapatite of bone. They represent a class of antiresorptive drugs that have been available for decades and are often used for the treatment of metabolic bone diseases such as Paget's. The biphosphonates are pyrophosphonates with several different substitutions that increase potency and reduce degradation of the various compounds. When tightly adherent to hydroxyapatite, bone becomes resistant to endogenous phosphatase activity, and therefore inhibits remodeling by osteoclasts.[43,63] Some agents similarly reduce bone formation to a lesser extent but still create a balance in favor of increasing bone mass. Certain agents such as alendronate may have relatively minimal inhibition of bone formation at doses that effectively inhibit osteoclast function.

Biphosphonates have been used successfully for the reduction of bone loss in paraplegics and patients taking long-term supraphysiological doses of steroids.[86,104] Other studies have demonstrated the successful use of etidronate in postmenopausal women showing improvement in BMD and reduction of vertebral fractures.[40,121,122]

More recently, attention has been focused on the agent alendronate (Fosomax). It is the only biphosphonate that has been approved by the FDA for the treatment of postmenopausal osteoporosis. Alendronate has a four-carbon amino side chain that creates a very high potency at a dose that does not inhibit bone mineralization as seen with etidronate. Liberman et al.[73] conducted a phase III investigation with the Osteoporosis Treatment Study Group. This study of alendronate in 994 postmenopausal women with osteoporosis, receiving 10 mg daily of alendronate for 3 years, found an increase in BMD (compared to placebo group) of 8.8% in the spine, 5.9% in the femoral neck, 7.8% in the trochanter, and 2.5% in the total body. The study showed the treatment group to have a 48% reduction in the proportion of women with new vertebral fractures, and a reduction of the progression of vertebral deformities. Alendronate was well tolerated with no greater clinical or laboratory evidence of adverse effects than with placebo. However, shortly after release of alendronate it was recognized that there was a significant increase in the incidence of serious gastrointestinal bleeding, occurring in about 34 of 450,000 patients. Current recommendations include taking the medication with a full glass of water and remaining upright for at least 30 minutes until after the first meal, and not taking it before bedtime. Though apparently promising, the exact role for alendronate is yet to be established.

CLINICAL CONSIDERATIONS
Steroid-Induced Osteoporosis

It has been well established that prolonged exposure to high-dose endogenous or exogenous steroids will result in significant loss of bone density. Several studies of patients receiving steroids for treatment of conditions such as asthma or rheumatoid arthritis have documented fracture rates of vertebral bodies to be as high as 42%.[1,75] It appears that loss of BMD is more pronounced in trabecular bone of the vertebrae than bones with a significant cortical content (femur). Studies have demonstrated significant loss of BMD reaching nearly 40% in the trabecular iliac crest or vertebral body.[102,103] When steroid excess has resolved, BMD appears to return to near normal. A study of patients cured of Cushing's syndrome for a mean of 9 years found a normal BMD in the spine and femur.[79] Another prospective study analyzed BMD before, during, and after a 2-year period of steroid treatment in the lumbar spine.[111] This study demonstrated a 15% loss of BMD while on steroid treatment and a return to baseline 16.7 months after prednisone was discontinued.

There has been significant study of the mechanisms by which steroids cause a reduction of BMD in animal and human studies. There are many contradictory findings in several of the studies. Generally the bulk of evidence seems to suggest a multifactorial interaction of steroids to reduce bone density. Studies suggest that steroids decrease the synthetic and proliferative function of osteoblasts,[96] and may increase the proliferation and activity of osteoclasts. This disturbs the balance of bone remodeling to favor incomplete replacement and eventually thinning of trabeculae resulting in loss of BMD. Other factors that may contribute to this effect include diminished intestinal absorption of calcium,[50] increased urinary excretion, and suppression of testosterone that is associated with development of

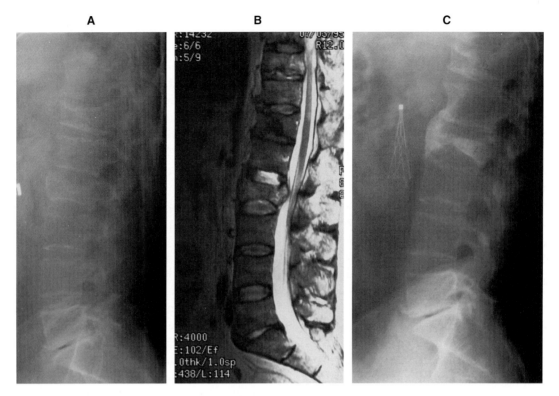

Fig. 32-5. Plain lateral radiograph **(A)** and MRI **(B)** of a 45-year-old patient dependent on steroids for asthma for many years. The patient fell from a ladder sustaining an L2 compression fracture without neurological compromise. Note also a T12 wedge compression fracture the patient had sustained earlier. The patient experienced significant pulmonary complications requiring prolonged intubation and ventilatory support after injury. The fracture was treated with bed rest for 5 weeks (during ventilatory support), followed by a TLSO for a total of 16 weeks. Excellent healing was eventually achieved. **(C)** Note the tell-tale sign of prolonged bed rest. The patient was pain-free with full neurological function.

osteoporosis.[91] Other significant interactions may include the suppression of circulating calcitonin levels, the inhibition of prostaglandin synthesis, and indirect modulation of numerous cytokines and growth factors.

Obviously, the prevention of steroid associated osteoporosis should be focused on the reduction or elimination of steroids when possible. Alternate day steroid therapy does not appear to reduce the loss of bone mass. When this is not considered feasible, measures to minimize the effects of steroids should be instituted. Supplementation of dietary calcium has been demonstrated to minimize but certainly not eliminate the significant bone loss associated with steroids. Replacement of estrogen or testosterone may also be helpful in reducing the effect of steroids. The biphosphonate agents such as Fosomax have demonstrated sustained increase in BMD compared to placebo in patients receiving steroid treatments.[104] Other factors such as vitamin D, fluoride, calcitonin, and anabolic steroids may also be useful in minimizing steroid-induced bone loss (Fig. 32-5).

Vertebral Fractures

Vertebral fractures have been found to occur in as many as 50% of white females over the age of 85.[85] Clearly the prevalence closely parallels the loss of vertebral BMD with aging with a 6:1 predilection for females. The prevalence varies significantly by region, and has been found to be as low as 2.9% in Finland and as high as 25.3% in the United States in 65 to 74-year-old females.[22] In part, the variance of these rates may be due to definition. Fractures are usually classified into three types: crush, wedge, or end plate failure. The crush fracture involves loss of height of the entire vertebral body, while the wedge fracture involves a preferential loss of ventral vertebral height. The end plate type failure may occur with relatively good preservation of both ventral and dorsal height. This results in a biconcave deformity that is thought to be due to a relative failure of the centrally weakened trabecular core compared to the somewhat stronger peripheral cortical rim.

Clear criteria for diagnosing fractures have not yet been established. Several different measurement techniques have been proposed. The most widely used technique calculates ratios of vertebral heights and compares these values to "normals." For wedge type fractures, the ventral height is compared to the dorsal height. A mild deformity can be considered a value that is within three standard deviations of normal. A "crush" fracture is measured by comparing the height with adjacent vertebrae, and an end plate failure compares the central height with the dorsal height.

Younger patients suffering vertebral fractures often experience a discrete episode of severe pain, however, older individuals may not notice the development of even severe vertebral body collapse. It has been estimated that only one third of patients with vertebral fractures seek medical treatment, and one fifth of those diagnosed will require hospital care. Unlike hip fractures, specific significant traumatic events are not generally reported for the development of vertebral fractures, occurring in 14% overall and twice as frequently in men.[22] It has long been established that hip fractures due to osteoporosis have a significant associated mortality.[23] Similarly, patients 5 years post-vertebral fracture experience a 15% excess mortality from all causes.[23] Unlike hip fractures, the excess mortality is not strongly clustered in the first few months postfracture and is not directly linked to the events of the fracture. The mortality is likely linked to comorbid conditions, such as poor nutrition and smoking, that are known to accelerate loss of BMD. Similarly, in a study of 9704 ambulatory women older than 65 years of age, Browner et al.[12] found that osteopenia is linked to nontraumatic death.

The majority of vertebral fractures occur in the midthoracic spine and result in a progressive marked kyphotic deformity when multiple vertebral bodies are involved. Acute management includes neurological evaluation to rule out spinal cord compromise and assessment for possible associated ileus. Fortunately, osteopenic fractures rarely result in neurological compromise. MRI and CT studies may be helpful for further evaluation if compromise is apparent. Brief bed rest, pain control, muscle relaxants, and early mobilization may be indicated. Orthotics may improve pain and possibly reduce deformity during healing, but this has not been well demonstrated. Serial plain radiographs throughout the time of healing may demonstrate early evidence of instability or progressive deformity throughout healing. The possibility of a metastatic pathological fracture should always be considered and biopsy performed if any doubt persists.

The rare patient that suffers neurological injury due to retropulsed or collapsed bony fragments impinging on the spinal cord or nerve roots may benefit from surgical decompression. The more common local radicular compromise may be managed expectantly if the deficit is relatively minor or the patient's general physical condition does not encourage surgical intervention. When a ventral lesion is present a ventral approach is generally indicated. Attempts to decompress the spinal cord through a standard laminectomy are likely to result in further injury. Dorsolateral transpedicular, lateral extracavitary, transthoracic, ventral thoracolumbar, or retroperitoneal approaches may be suitable choices depending on the location of the pathology. When significant instability is present, grafting and stabilization is indicated with special concerns for the osteoporotic patient discussed below.

When corpectomy is required for decompression, reconstruction with an interbody strut graft will be needed, as the osteoporotic vertebral body and end plate will not carry the load of a normal vertebral body. The graft should be "protected" and not be expected to accept the entire load of the spinal column. Instrumentation can be utilized to distribute the load to adjacent spinal elements such that no point of fixation will experience a load in excess of the ability of the osteoporotic bone to resist that load. It has often been stated that a match between the bone density of the selected graft and the vertebral body should be achieved, and that utilization of a "rigid" cortical graft may telescope into the adjacent vertebral body. While it is true that the vertebral body may not be able to resist the force transmitted by the graft, this is due to exposing the adjacent bodies to an excessive load transmitted through the graft rather than the characteristics of the graft material. The larger the effective "footprint" of the graft, the more successful the vertebral body will be at resisting a given load. For this reason a rib graft, or a tubular fibular graft with minimal cross-sectional area, would be expected to be ineffective in resisting anything but a trivial transmitted axial load. Deliberately choosing a compromised osteopenic graft from the patient's iliac crest to match the impaired mechanical attributes of the vertebral body is like supporting a sagging roof with weakened timbers to prevent its collapse. From merely a structural point of view, a steel dowel of equivalent cross-sectional area to an osteopenic iliac graft would provide far better mechanical support. While autologous iliac crest is a reasonable choice for reconstruction when it is protected from excess loads, utilizing cortical struts or a titanium cage of equal or greater cross-sectional area should be expected to provide better mechanical support. In all cases, maximizing the graft cross-sectional area is likely to significantly improve load-carrying capacity.

An interesting though not well-studied potential treatment alternative is the use of percutaneous methacrylate vertebroplasty.[20,46] This technique involves percutaneous injection of methacrylate into the collapsed and possibly adjacent vertebral bodies. It has been found to provide rapid pain relief for patients with osteoporosis, hemangiomas, or metastatic disease.[46] The main concern is the potential for the methacrylate to extravasate and cause neurological compromise. Utilizing CT guidance and real-time fluoroscopic monitoring during injection, this risk can apparently be avoided.[46] Further study of this interesting technique is certainly warranted before advocating routine use.

Fusion in the Osteopenic Patient

It is commonly stated that osteopenia is a risk factor for failed fusion of the spine. There are not good data to support this contention. Fixation of the osteopenic spine may be problematic, leading to the failure of fixation and in turn reducing fusion rate, but even this possibility has not been well established. At least one study evaluating the effects of low BMD on instrumentation and fusion failure found no differences, concluding that the use of pedicle screws for degenerative disease in grade I and II osteoporosis, with BMD as low as 40 mg/ml, was acceptable and successful.[69]

It is not uncommon for calcium stores and nutritional status of the osteopenic patient to be compromised. For this reason, it is reasonable to augment both in order to optimize fusion healing. Little is known about the potential beneficial effects of electrical stimulation on fusion. Until more data are available, one should not assume that electrical bone-growth stimulation is effective or needed in osteopenic patients any more than patients with normal bone density.

Instrumentation of the Osteopenic Spine

One must recognize that the security of spinal fixation is largely dependent on the integrity of the bone into which the anchors are affixed. This, of course, means that osteoporotic bone is not a particularly good substrate for fixation and many special concerns arise. Quite simply, as the security of each point of fixation declines, more points of fixation should be used to achieve the same overall stability. Furthermore, types of fixation that are less dependent on BMD should be used when possible. Certain techniques are particularly demanding of the integrity of the bone and should be avoided. In particular, techniques involving the placement of a single set of pedicle or vertebral body screws above and below an unstable injury are likely to result in significant rotation of the vertebral body about the screw due to the lack of resistance of the osteoporotic cancellous bone of the vertebral body. This is likely to transmit excessive loads to the intervertebral segment and result in spinal deformity. It would be best in this case to extend the construct rostrally and caudally to distribute the load on additional points of fixation.

Tests of common types of bony fixation have been performed on normal and reduced BMD spines. Coe et al.[21] compared single sublaminar hooks with pedicle screws to demonstrate that the single laminar hook provided about 50% greater resistance to pullout than the pedicle screw. This study also found that loads to failure of laminar hooks did not correlate with BMD, unlike pedicle screws, which showed significant reduction of pullout resistance with low BMD. This data strongly suggests that hook constructs may be preferable to screws in osteopenic patients. Another study compared facet–transverse process claw, lamina–transverse process claw, and various sublaminar and subpars wiring techniques in osteopenic spines.[14] Load to failure of these constructs was similar (296 to 382 newtons), though stiffness of the hook constructs was found to be greater. This study also tested single vs. double sublaminar wires and found a nonsignificant increase in the double wire configuration. Most of the failures occurred away from the site of fixation, at the isthmus of both pedicles or the pedicle body junction. This observation suggests that it is usually not the wire cutting its way out through the lamina, but failure of the arch itself. Adding a second wire may prevent a rare "cutout" but will not improve the strength of the arch and therefore should not be expected to significantly reduce failure at that point of fixation. Again there was no correlation of the hook constructs with BMD, although there was with the wire constructs. Another study of sublaminar fixation found that decortication of the lamina could reduce the pull through force to failure by nearly 60%.[24] Removal of the facets and spinous process caused no significant reduction. Decortication of the laminar arch should be minimal at most if it is strongly affecting the integrity of the construct.

Another study compared the pullout strength of a single-level pedicle–transverse process hook construct to the same construct spanning two segments.[112] This study demonstrated a 40% increase in the two-level configuration. The superiority of this configuration, though not tested specifically in osteoporotic bone, again emphasizes the potential benefits of distributing the load over multiple spinal segments.

Several factors affecting pullout strength have been studied by Zindrick et al.[126] A 6.5 mm diameter screw performed significantly better in pullout compared to a 4.5 mm screw. The pullout resistance increase is proportional to the outer diameter of the screw, suggesting that the largest possible diameter screw should be used. Though studies did not show a significant increase in pullout strength when the screw depth was increased from 50% to the ventral cortex, it did significantly increase when the ventral cortex was penetrated. Tests of cyclic loading demonstrated a 1044% increase in the number of cycles to screw loosening with the screw to the ventral cortex compared to only 50% penetration of the vertebral body. These observations suggest that to optimize pedicle fixation the largest diameter screw should be placed as deeply as considered safe. Whittenberg et al.[123] looked closely at the relationship of cyclic loading and BMD and defined different levels of BMD that could be predictably related to early screw loosening. They found significant screw loosening at an average BMD of 63 mm/cc and no loosening in spines with a mean BMD of 114 mm/cc. They concluded that at a BMD of less than 90 mm/cc, early loosening should be expected at physiological loads. Yamagata et al.[124] evaluated the relationship of BMD to axial pullout strength in several different pedicle systems, again demonstrating a remarkable reduction in osteoporotic bone with a correlation coefficient of 0.68. They also concluded that there may very

well be a BMD below which pedicle screws should only be used in conjunction with another technique to augment their fixation. Soshi et al.[117] correlated the pullout strength of pedicle screws with the Jikei osteoporosis grading scale, which is based on the plain film appearance of the vertebrae. They also found a striking reduction in pullout strength of screws in higher grades of osteoporosis partially overcome by increasing screw diameters. They too concluded that pedicle fixation could not be recommended for severe grade III osteoporosis.

In view of the above data, and the appeal or necessity for the use of pedicle screws in some cases, several techniques have been explored to augment screw fixation in osteoporotic bone. Zindrick et al.[126] demonstrated that polymethylmethacrylate (PMMA) injected into the pedicle can offer significant increase in the pullout strength in "stripped" screw holes. They demonstrated that nonpressurized PMMA could return pullout strength to nearly normal, and pressurized PMMA could increase pullout strength to nearly twice the normal level. Pfeifer, Krag, and Johnson[98] compared nonpressurized PMMA to milled and matchsticks of bone placed into the "stripped" hole. The PMMA increased pullout strength to 1.5 times the original, milled bone increased it by 70%, and "matchsticks" increased pullout strength by only 56%. Moore et al.[87] studied the use of Norian fracture grout, a calcium phosphate ceramic that initially has a paste-like consistency and sets solidly within minutes. This substance was used in a similar manner for augmentation of a "stripped" pedicle and found to provide increased resistance similar to PMMA. The substance has the advantage of being biocompatible and absorbable, though these results are preliminary and further study will be required before routine clinical application. The use of PMMA is an acceptable alternative, though with some potential risk. The risk of extravasation with neural compromise can be reduced by laminectomy and direct visualization of the thecal sac and nerve root during injection of the cement. In view of the generally successful outcomes of pedicle fixation in osteoporotic bone without such augmentation of the anchor, this technique is probably best reserved for occasional use in select situations.

Other attempts to augment the fixation of a pedicle screw in normal and osteoporotic bone have explored the use of an adjacent laminar hook. Hilibrand et al. compared the pullout resistance of a pedicle screw alone to a pedicle screw with an adjacent supralaminar hook placed in a "stripped" pedicle hole.[56a] Because the screw and hook conflict with their desired point of attachment to the rod, the hook was attached with two short Jackson connectors in an outrigger configuration. The replaced screw alone restored only 19% of the original resistance compared to 89% restoration with the screw-hook construct. The effect was most pronounced in the poorest quality bone, reaching 102%. Halvorson et al.[51] also explored these options in normal and osteoporotic human cadaveric spines. A single sublaminar hook augmentation to the pedicle screw and a two-hook claw augmentation were tested in "stripped" pedicles of varying BMD. The single hook pivoted and did not significantly increase pullout resistance, however, the two-hook claw augmentation doubled the original value. It is interesting to consider whether the pedicle screw provides any significant benefit in these cases or the laminar hooks merely replace the failed pedicle purchase. Do the hooks protect and augment the fixation of the screw or replace the fixation as it fails? In any event, a one- or two-level sublaminar claw is clearly a satisfactory fixation construct even without the pedicle screw. It is unlikely that significant structural enhancement is provided by the addition of a pedicle screw to a two-level sublaminar claw. Technically, the placement of a two-hook claw–pedicle screw construct is demanding and not possible with many instrumentation systems. It would appear that these hook augmentation studies speak strongly for the superiority of the hook constructs rather than their ability to augment the pedicle screw purchase (Fig. 32-6).

The use of adjacent laminar hooks has also been explored to protect pedicle screws from experiencing excessive bending moments experienced in short segment single level fixation. Adjacent hooks have been found to clearly reduce the bending moment and protect the screw against failure in this construct.[19] Though effective in this regard, it would be unwise to use such a short segment construct in osteoporotic spines for anything other than the lowest levels of instability with relatively good ventral column support. This may occur in degenerative disease but is not likely in ventral vertebral compression fractures. Extending the length of the construct to incorporate additional points of fixation will protect screws from both excessive bending moments and pullout.

When using pedicle fixation in osteoporotic bone the selection of the type of construct is important.

Semiconstrained pedicle constructs, though becoming rare, are not extinct. These devices are secured to the spine by forcing the plate to the lamina/facet complex under compression rather than fixing the plate or rod rigidly to the pedicle screw. These systems have a mechanism of failure that is quite distinct from rigid pedicle systems. The plate acts as a claw hammer and pulls the pedicle screw directly out of the pedicle, the most vulnerable point of an osteoporotic spine.[4] The failure mechanism of rigid pedicle fixation systems is by fracture of the proximal shaft of the screw under an excessive bending moment. Because the claw hammer effect of the semirigid fixation systems specifically exploits the weakness of osteoporotic spines, it would be best to avoid these systems entirely.

Generally, it has been established that the method of pedicle preparation to receive a screw does not significantly alter the pullout force of the screw in bone of normal density. Halvorson et al.[51] reconfirmed this observation, demonstrating that tapping, undersize tapping, and no tapping had little effect on normal bone density specimens. However, in specimens with osteoporosis there was a significant improvement in pullout force if the hole was either not tapped or tapped with a 5.5 mm tap for a 6.5 mm screw. They also demonstrated that while packing a "stripped" hole with corticocancellous bone could nearly restore the resistance to pullout, this technique was not effective in osteoporotic bone.

In summary, osteoporotic spines provide compromised points of fixation. For an equivalent force, more points of fixation will be required to distribute this force sufficiently so that no point of fixation will experience force in excess of its tolerance and result in failure. Screw purchase into cancellous bone appears to be particularly vulnerable to loss of BMD. Techniques to augment screw purchase may be needed if the use of screws is required. Alternatively, hook purchase relying more on corticated bone is more resistant to loss of BMD and may be preferable if this option exists.

CONCLUSION

Loss of BMD of the spine results in significant morbidity and mortality especially among postmenopausal women. Newer reliable techniques of identification and quantification of bone loss are becoming available and with them a renewed focus in the study and prevention of osteoporosis. Recent therapeutic developments have further encouraged

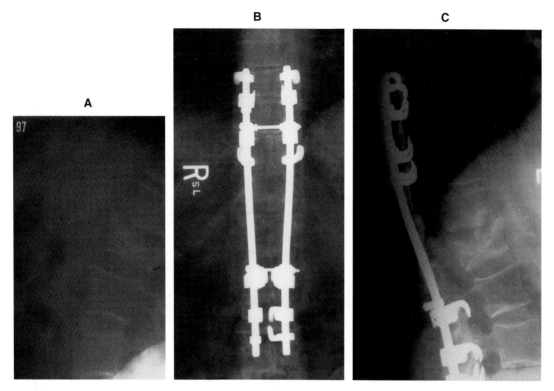

Fig. 32-6. A, Demonstration of an L1 compression fracture in a 78-year-old woman with paraparesis and marked osteoporosis. Despite multiple medical problems, including diabetes, hypertension, and cardiac disease, the patient underwent surgical decompression via a transpedicular approach due to the significant neurological compromise and canal encroachment demonstrated on MRI, myelography and CT imaging. **B** and **C,** The hook-rod fixation construct utilized 12 points of fixation avoiding screws. The procedure was tolerated well, and the patient gradually regained strength and the ability to ambulate.

this focus. We are entering an era where osteopenia should be diagnosed and addressed early to prevent the later inevitable morbid ramifications. Spine surgeons can be actively involved in the process of recognizing and preventing osteopenia. Careful consideration of the altered mechanical and biological properties of osteoporotic bone will facilitate the successful treatment of patients that have suffered loss of structural integrity of the spine.

REFERENCES

1. Adinoff AD, Hollister JR, MD. Steroid-induced fractures and bone loss in patients with asthma. N Engl J Med 309(5):265-26, 1983.
2. Albright F, Smith PH, Richardson AM. Postmenopausal osteoporosis. JAMA 116:2465-2474, 1996.
3. Aloia JF, Cohn SH, Vaswani A, Yeh JK, Yuen K, Ellis K. Risk factors for postmenopausal osteoporosis. Am J Med 78:95-100, 1985.
4. Ashman RB, Galpin RD, Corin JD, Johnston CE II. Biomechanical analysis of pedicle screw instrumentation system in a corpectomy model. Spine 14:1398-1405, 1989.
5. Baran D, Sorensen A, Grimes J, Lew R, Kraellas A, Johnson B, Roche J. Dietary modification with dairy products for preventing vertebral bone loss in premenopausal women: A three-year prospective study. J Clin Endocrinol Metab 70:264-270, 1990.
6. Barger-Lux MJ, Heaney RP, Stegman MR. Effects of moderate caffeine intake on the calcium economy of premenopausal women. Am J Clin Nutr 52:722-725, 1990.
7. Barrett-Connor E, Bush TL. Estrogen and coronary heart disease in women. JAMA 265:1861-1867, 1991.
8. Bell GH, Dunbar O, Beck JS, Gibb A. Variations in strength of vertebrae with age and their relation to osteoporosis. Calcif Tissue Res 1:75-86, 1967.
9. Bernstein DS, Sadowsky N, Hegsted DM, Guri CD, Stave FJ. Prevalence of osteoporosis in high- and low-fluoride areas in North Dakota. JAMA 198:499-508, 1966.
10. Bishop RC, Moore KA, Hadley MN. Anterior cervical interbody fusion using autogeneic and allogeneic bone graft substrate: A prospective comparative analysis. J Neurosurg 85:206-210, 1996.
11. Brown CW, Orme TJ, Richardson HD. The rate of pseudoarthrosis (surgical nonunion) in patients who are smokers and patients who are nonsmokers: A comparison study. Spine 11:942-943,1986.
12. Browner WS, Seeley DG, Vogt TM, Cummings SR. Non-trauma mortality in elderly women with low bone mineral density. Lancet 338:355-358, 1991.
13. Bush TL,Wells HB, James MK. Effects of hormone therapy on bone mineral density: Results from the postmenopausal estrogen/progestin interventions (pepi) trial. JAMA 276:1389-1396, 1996.
14. Butler TE Jr, Asher MA, Jayaraman G, Nunley PD, Robinson RG. The strength and stiffness of thoracic implant anchors in osteoporotic spines. Spine 19:1956-1962, 1994.

15. Cauley JA, Lucas FL, Kuller LH, Vogt MT, Browner WS, Cummings SR. Bone mineral density and risk of breast cancer in older woman: The study of osteoporotic fractures. JAMA 276:1404-1408, 1996.

16. Cavanaugh DJ, Cann CE. Brisk walking does not stop bone loss in postmenopausal women. Bone 9:201-204, 1988.

17. Chambers TJ, Athanasou NA, Fuller K. Effect of parathyroid hormone and calcitonin on the cytoplasmic spreading of isolated osteoclasts. J Endocrinol 102:281-286, 1984.

18. Chestnut CHI. Bone mass and exercise. Am J Med 95:345-365, 1993.

19. Chiba M, McLain RF, Yerby SA, Moseley TA, Smith TS, Benson DR. Short-segment pedicle instrumentation: Biomechanical analysis of supplemental hook fixation. Spine 21:288-294, 1996.

20. Chiras J, Sola-Martinez MT, Weill A, Rose M, Cognard C, Martin-Duverneuil N. Vertebroplasties percutanees. Rev Med Interne 16:854-859, 1995.

21. Coe JD, Warden KE, M.Biomed. Engr., Herzig MA, McAfee PC. Influence of bone mineral density on the fixation of thoracolumbar implants: A comparative study of transpedicular screws, laminar hooks, and spinous process wires. Spine 15:902-907, 1990.

22. Cooper C. Osteoporosis—An epidemiological perspective: A review. J R Soc Med 82:753-757, 1989.

23. Cooper C, Atkinson EJ, Jacobsen SJ, O'Fallon WM, Melton LJI. Population-based study of survival after osteoporotic fractures. Am J Epidemiol 137(9):1001-1005, 1993.

24. Crawford RJ, Sell PJ, Ali MS, Dove J. Segmental spinal instrumentation: A study of the mechanical properties of materials used for sublaminar fixation. Spine 14:632-635, 1989.

25. Cumming RG. Calcium intake and bone mass: A quantitative review of the evidence. Calcif Tissue Int 47:194-201, 1990.

26. Cummings SR, Kelsey JL, Nevitt MC, O'Dowd KJ. Epidemiology of osteoporosis and osteoporotic fractures. Epidemiol Rev 7:178-208, 1985.

27. Daftari TK, Whitesides TE Jr, Heller JG, Goodrich AC, McCarey BE, Hutton WC. Nicotine on the revascularization of bone graft: An experimental study in rabbits. Spine 19:904-911, 1994.

28. Dalsky GP, Stocke KS, Ehsani AA, Slatopolsky E, Lee WC, Birge SJ Jr. Weight-bearing exercise training and lumbar bone mineral content in postmenopausal women. Ann Intern Med 108:824-828, 1988.

29. Daniell HW. Osteoporosis of the slender smoker: Vertebral compression fractures and loss of metacarpal cortes in relation to postmenopausal cigarette smoking and lack of obesity. Arch Intern Med 136:298-304, 1976.

30. Dawson-Hughes B. Calcium supplementation and bone loss: A review of controlled clinical trials. Am J Clin Nutr 54:274S-280S, 1991.

31. Dawson-Hughes B, Dallal GE, Krall EA, Harris S, Sokoll LJ, Falconer G. Effect of Vitamin D supplementation on wintertime and overall bone loss in healthy postmenopausal women. Ann Intern Med 115:505-512, 1991.

32. Dequeker J, Nijs J, Verstraeten A, Geusens P, Gevers G. Genetic determinants of bone mineral content at the spine and radius: A twin study. Bone 8:207-209, 1987.

33. Donaldson CL, Hulley SB, Vogel JM, Hattner RS, Bayers JH, McMillan DE. Effect of prolonged bed rest on bone mineral. Metabolism 19:1071-1084, 1970.

34. Drinkwater BL, Nilson K, Chestnut CHI, Bremner WJ, Shainholtz S, Southworth MB. Bone mineral content of amenorrheic and eumenorrheic athletes. N Engl J Med 311:277-281,1984.

35. Eriksen EF, Hodgson SF, Eastell R, Cedel SL, O'Fallon WM, Riggs BL. Cancellous bone remodeling in Type I (postmenopausal) osteoporosis: Quantitative assessment of rates of formation, resorption, and bone loss at tissue and cellular levels. J Bone Miner Res 5:311-319, 1990.

36. Eriksen EF, Mosekilde L, Melsen F. Trabecular bone resorption depth decreased with age: Differences between normal males and females. Bone 6:141-146, 1985.

37. Ernst M, Heath JK, Schmid C, Froesch RE, Rodan GA. Evidence for a direct effect of estrogen on bone cells in vitro. J Steroid Biochem 34:279-284, 1989.

38. Ettinger B, Genant HK, Cann CE. Long-term estrogen replacement therapy prevents bone loss and fractures. Ann Intern Med 102:319-324, 1985.

39. Ettinger B, Genant HK, Cann CE. Postmenopausal bone loss is prevented by treatment with low-dosage estrogen with calcium. Ann Intern Med 106:40-45, 1987.

40. Evans RA, Somers NM, Dunstan CR, Royle H, Kos S. The effect of low-dose cyclical etidronate and calcium on bone mass in early postmenopausal women. Osteoporos Int 3:71-75, 1993.

41. Farley JR, Wergedal JE, Hall SL, Sandra H, Tarbaux NM. Calcitonin has direct effects on 3[H]-thymidine incorporation and alkaline phosphatase activity in human osteoblast-line cells. Calcif Tissue Int 48:297-301, 1991.

42. Feicht CB, Johnson TS, Martin BJ, Sparkes KE, Wagner WWJ. Secondary amenorrhea in athletes. Lancet 2:1145-1146, 1978.

43. Fleisch H, G. RRG, Francis. Diphosphonates inhibit hydroxyapatite dissolution in vitro and bone resorption in tissue culture and in vivo. Science 1675:1262-1264, 1969.

44. Fukayama S, Tashjian AH, Jr. Direct modulation by estadiol of the response of human bone cells (SaOS-2) to human parathyroid hormone (PTH) and PTH-related protein. Endocrinology 124:397-401, 1989.

45. Gallagher JC, Kable WT, Goldgar D. Effect of progestin therapy on cortical and trabecular bone: Comparison with estrogen. Am J Med 90:171-178, 1991.

46. Gangi A, Kastler BA, Dietermann J-L. Percutaneous vertebroplasty guided by a combination of CT and fluoroscopy. AJNR 15:83-86, 1994.

47. Gavaler JS, Love K, Van Thiel D, Farholt S, Gluud C, Monterio E, Galvao-Teles A, Ortega TC, Cuervas-Mons, V. An international study of the relationship between alcohol consumption and postmenopausal estradiol levels. Alcohol 1(Suppl): 327-330, 1991.

48. Gordon SL, Corbin SB. Summary of workshop on drinking water fluoride influence on hip fracture on bone health. Osteoporos Int 2:109-117, 1992.

49. Gutin B, Kasper MJ. Can vigorous exercise play a role in osteoporosis prevention? A review. Osteoporos Int 2:55-69, 1992.

50. Hahn TJ, Halstead LR, Baran DT. Effects of short term glucocorticoid administration on intestinal calcium absorption and circulating vitamin D metabolite concentrations in man. J Clin Endocrinol 52:111-115, 1981.

51. Halvorson TL, Kelley LA, Thomas KA, Whitecloud TSI, Cook SD. Effects of bone mineral density on pedical screw fixation. Spine 19:2415-2520, 1994.

52. Hanley EN, Harvell JC, Shapiro DE, Kraus DR. Use of allograft bone in cervical spine surgery. Semin Spine Surg 1:262-270, 1989.

53. Hansen MA, Overgaard K, Riis BJ, Christiansen C. Potential risk factors for development of postmenopausal osteoporosis—Examined over a 12-year period. Osteoporos Int 1:95-102, 1991.

54. Heaney RP, Recker RR. Effects of nitrogen, phosphorus, and caffeine on calcium balance in women. J Lab Clin Med 99:46-55, 1982.

55. Henderson BE. The cancer question: An overview of recent epidemiologic and retrospective data. Am J Obstet 161:1859-1864, 1989.

56. Hernandez-Avila M, Colditz GA, Stampfer MJ, Rosner B, Speizer FE, Willett WC. Caffeine, moderate alcohol intake, and risk of fractures of the hip and forearm in middle-aged women. Am J Clin Nutr 54:157-163, 1991.

56a. Hilibrand AS, Moore, DC, Graziano GP. The role of pediculolaminar fixation in compromised pedicle bone spine, volume 21, issue 4, pp 445-4351, 1996.

57. Holbrook TL, Barrett-Connor E. A prospective study of alcohol consumption and bone mineral density. Br Med J 306:1506-1509, 1993.

58. Holbrook TL, Barrett-Connor E, Wingard DL. Dietary calcium and risk of hip fracture: 14-year prospective population study. Lancet 5:1046-1049, 1988.

59. Iida-Klein A, Yee DC, Brandli DW, Mirikitani EJM, Hahn TJ. Effects of calcitonin on 3', 5'-cyclic adenosine monophosphate and calcium second messenger generation and osteoblast function in UMR 106-06 osteoblast-like cells. Endocrinology 130:381-388, 1992.

60. Jackson JA, Kleerekoper M. Osteoporosis in men: Diagnosis, pathophysiology, and prevention. Medicine 69:137-152, 1990.

61. Jacobson PC, Beaver W, Grubb SA, Taft TN, Talmage RV. Bone density in women: College athletes and older athletic women. J Orthop Res 2:328-332, 1984.

62. Johnston CCJ, Miller JZ, Slemenda CW, Reister TK, Hui S, Christian JC, Peacock, M. Calcium supplementation and increases in bone mineral density in children. N Engl J Med 327:82-87, 1992.

63. Jung A, Bisaz S, Fleisch H. The binding of pyrophosphate and two diphosphonates by hydroxyapatite crystals. Calcif Tissue Res 11:269-280, 1973.

64. Kiel DP, Felson DT, Hannan MT, Anderson JJ, Wilson PWF. Caffeine and the risk of hip fracture: The Framingham study. Am J Epidemiol 132:675-684, 1990.

65. Klesges RC, Ward KD, Shelton ML, Applegate, WB, Cantler ED, Palmieri, G, Harmon K, Davis J. Changes in bone mineral content in male athletes: Mechanisms of action and intervention effects. JAMA 276:226-230, 1996.

66. Krall EA, Dawson-Hughes B. Smoking and bone loss among postmenopausal women. J Bone Miner Res 6:331-338, 1991.

67. Krall EA, Dawson-Hughes B. Heritable and life-style determinants of bone mineral density. J Bone Miner Res 8:1-9, 1993.

68. Krolner B, Toft B. Vertebral bone loss: An unheeded side effect of therapeutic bed rest. Clin Sci 64:537-540, 1983.

69. Kumano K, Hirabayashi S. Pedicle screws and bone mineral density. Spine 19:1157-1161, 1994.

70. Laitinen K, Valimaki M. Alcohol and bone. Calcif Tissue Int 49(Suppl):S70-S73, 1991.

71. Lane NE, Bloch DA, Jones HH, Marshall WH Jr, Wood PD, Fries JF. Long-distance running, bone density, and osteoarthritis. JAMA 255:1147-1151, 1986.

72. LeBlanc AD, Schneider VS, Evans HJ, Engelbretson DA, Krebs JM. Bone mineral loss and recovery after 17 weeks of bed rest. J Bone Miner Res 5:843-850, 1990.

73. Liberman UA, Weiss SR, Broll J, Minne HW, Quan H, Bell NH, Rodrigues-Portales J, Downs RWJ, Dequeker J, Favus M, Seeman E, Recker RR, Capizzi T, Santora AC II, Lombardi A, Shah RV, Hirsch LJ, Karpf DB. Effect of oral alendronate on bone mineral density and the incidence of fractures in postmenopausal osteoporosis. N Engl J Med 333:1427-1443, 1995.

74. Lindsay R, MacLean A, Kraszewski A, Hart DM, Clark AC, Garwood J. Bone response to termination of oestrogen treatment. Lancet 1:1325-1327, 1978.

75. Luengo M, Picado C, Piera C, Guanabens N, Montserrat JM, Rivera J, Setoain J. Intestinal calcium absorption and parathyroid hormone secretion in asthmatic patients on prolonged oral or inhaled steroid treatment. Eur Respir J 4:441-444, 1991.

76. Lutz J. Bone mineral, serum calcium, and dietary intakes of mother/daughter pairs. Am J Clin Nutr 44:99-106, 1986.

77. Lutz J, Tesar R. Mother-daughter pairs: Spinal and femoral bone densities and dietary intakes. Am J Clin Nutr 52:872-877, 1990.

78. MacIntyre I, Whitehead MI, Banks LM, Stevenson JC, Wimalawansa SJ, Healy MJR. Calcitonin for prevention of postmenopausal bone loss. Lancet 1:900-902, 1988.

79. Mamelle N, Dusan R, Martin JL, Prost A, Meunier PJ, Guillaume M, Gaucher A, Zeigler G, Netter P. Risk-benefit of sodium fluoride treatment in primary vertebral osteoporosis. Lancet 2:361-363, 1988.

80. Marcus R, Cann C, Madvig P, Minkoff J, Goddard M, Bayer M, Martin M, Gaudiani L, Haskell W, Genant H. Menstrual function and bone mass in elite women distance runners. Ann Intern Med 102:158-163, 1985.

81. Massey LK, Wise KJ. The effect of dietary caffeine on urinary excretion of calcium, magnesium, sodium and potassium in healthy young females. Nutr Res 4:43-50, 1984.

82. Mazess RB. On aging bone loss. Clin Orthop 165:239-252, 1982.

83. Mazess RB, Barden HS. Bone density in premenopausal women: Effects of age, dietary intake, physical activity, smoking and birth-control pills. Am J Clin Nutr 53:132-142, 1991.

84. Meier DE, Orwoll ES, Jones JM. Marked disparity between trabecular and cortical bone loss with age in healthy men. Ann Intern Med 101:605-612, 1984.

85. Melton LJI, Lane AW, Cooper C, Eastell R, O'Fallon WM, Riggs BL. Prevalence and incidence of vertebral deformities. Osteoporos Int 3:113-119, 1993.

86. Minaire P, Berard E. Effects of disodium dichloromethylene diphosphante on bone loss in paraplegic patients. J Clin Invest 68:1086-1092, 1981.

87. Moore DC, Graziano GP, Maitra RS, Farjo LA, Goldstein SA. Calcium phosphate ceramic vs. PMMA for the augmentation of transpedicular screws. Orthop Trans 18:112-113, 1994.

88. Mosekilde L, Mosekilde L. Normal vertebral body size and compressive strength: Relations to age and to vertebral and iliac trabecular bone compressive strength. Bone 7:207-212, 1986.

89. Murrills RJ, Shane E, Lindsay R, Dempster DW. Bone resorption by isolated human osteoclasts in vitro: Effects of calcitonin. J Bone Miner Res 4:259-268, 1989.

90. Nattiv A, Agostini R, Drinkwater B, Yeager KK. The female athlete triad: The inter-relatedness of disordered eating, amenorrhea, and osteoporosis. Clin Sports Med 13:405-418, 1994.

91. Nordin BEC, Marshall DH, Francis RM, Crilly RG. The effects of sex steroid and corticosteroid hormones on bone. J Steroid Biochem 15:171-174, 1981.

92. Oursler MJ, Osdoby P, Pyfferoen J, Riggs BL, Spelsberg TC. Avian osteoclasts as estrogen target cells. Proc Natl Acad Sci USA 88:6613-6617, 1991.

93. Overgaard K, Riis BJ, Christiansen C, Hansen MA. Effect of calcitonin given intranasally on early postmenopausal bone loss. Br Med J 299:477-479, 1989.

94. Pak CYC, Sakhaee K, Adams-Huet B, Piziak V, Peterson RD, Poindexter JR. Treatment of postmenopausal osteoporosis with slow-release sodium fluoride: Final report of a randomized controlled trial. Ann Intern Med 123:401-408, 1995.

95. Parfitt AM. Bone remodeling: Relationship to the amount and structure of bone, and the pathogenesis and prevention of fractures. In Riggs BL, Melton LJI, eds. Osteoporosis: Etiology, Diagnosis, and Management. New York: Raven Press, 1988, pp 45-93.

96. Peck WA. The effects of glucocorticoids on bone cell metabolism and function. Adv Exp Med Biol 171:111-119, 1984.

97. Persson I, Adami H-O, Bergkvist L, Lindgren A, Pettersson B, Hoover R, Schairer C. Risk of endometrial cancer after treatment with oestrogens alone or in conjunction with progestogens: Results of a prospective study. Br Med J 298:147-151, 1989.

98. Pfeifer BA, Krag MH, Johnson C. Repair of failed transpedicle screw fixation. Spine 19:350-353, 1994.

99. Piziak V. Update in osteoporosis. Compr Ther 20:336-341, 1994.

100. Pocock NA, Eisman JA, Hopper JL, Yeates MG, Sambrook PN, Eberl S. Genetic determinants of bone mass in adults. J Clin Invest 80:706-710, 1987.

101. Reginster JY, Albert A, Lecart MP, Lambelin P, Denis D, Deroisy R, Fontaine MA, Franchimont P. One-year controlled randomized trial of prevention of early postmenopausal bone loss by intranasal calcitonin. Lancet 2:1481-1483, 1987.

102. Reid IR, Evans MC, Wattie DJ, Ames R, Cundy TF. Bone mineral density of the proximal femur and lumbar spine in glucocorticoid-treated asthmatic patients. Osteoporos Int 2:103-105, 1992.

103. Reid IR, Heap SW. Determinants of vertebral mineral density in patients receiving long-term glucocorticoid therapy. Arch Intern Med 150:2545-2548, 1990.

104. Reid IR, King AR, Alexander CJ, Ibbertson HK. Prevention of steroid-induced osteoporosis with (3-amino-1-hydroxypropylidene)-1, 1-bisphosphonate (APD). Lancet 1:143-146, 1988.

105. Riggs B, Lawrence, Seeman E, Hodgson SF, Taves DR, O'Fallon WM. Effect of the flouride/calcium regimen on vertebral fracture occurrence in postmenopausal osteoporosis: Comparison with conventional therapy. N Engl J Med 306:446-450, 1982.

106. Riggs BL, Hodgson SF, O'Fallon WM, Chao EYS, Wahner HW, Muhs JM, Cedel, SL, Melton LJ III. Effect of fluoride treatment in the fracture rate in postmenopausal women with osteoporosis. N Engl J Med 322:802-809, 1990.

107. Riggs BL, Melton LJI. Evidence for two distinct syndromes of involutional osteoporosis. Am J Med 75:899-901, 1983.

108. Riggs BL, Melton LJI. Involutional osteoporosis. N Engl J Med 314:1676-1686, 1986.

109. Riggs BL, Wahner HW, Dunn WL, Mazess RB, Offord KP, Melton LJ III. Differential changes in bone mineral density of the appendicular and axial skeleton with aging. J Clin Invest 67:328-335, 1981.

110. Riis B, Thomsen K, Christiansen C. Does calcium supplementation prevent postmenopausal bone loss? A double-blind, controlled clinical study. N Engl J Med 316:173-177, 1987.

111. Rizzato G, Montemurro L. The reversibility of exogenous corticosteroid-induced osteoporosis. J Bone Miner Res 17(Suppl 1):141, 1992.

112. Roach JW, Ashman RB, Allard RN. The strength of a posterior element claw at one versus two spinal levels. Spine 3:259-261, 1990.

113. Seeman E, Melton LJI, O'Fallon WM, Riggs BL. Risk factors for spinal osteoporosis in men. Am J Med 75:977-983, 1983.

114. Slemenda CW, Christian JC, Williams CJ, Norton JA, Johnston CC Jr. Genetic determinants of bone mass in adult women: A reevaluation of the twin model and the potential importance of gene interaction on heritability estimates. J Bone Miner Res 6:561-567, 1991.

115. Slemenda CW, Miller JZ, Hui SL, Reister TK, Johnston CCJ. Role of physical activity in the development of skeletal mass in children. J Bone Miner Res 6:1227-1233, 1991.

116. Snow-Harter C, Bouxsein ML, Lewis BT, Carter DR, Marcus R. Effects of resistance and endurance exercise on bone mineral status of young women: A randomized exercise intervention trial. J Bone Miner Res 7:761-769, 1992.

117. Soshi S, Shiba R, Kondo H, Murota K, MD. An experimental study on transpedicular screw fixation in relation to osteoporosis of the lumbar spine. Spine 16:1335-1341, 1991.

118. Speroff L, Rowan J, Symons J, Genant H, Wilborn W. The comparative effect on bone density, endometrium, and lipids of continuous hormones as replacement therapy (chart study): A randomized controlled trial. JAMA 276:1397-1403, 1996.

119. Stanford JL, Weiss NS, Voigt LF, Daling JR, Habel LA, Rossing MA. Combined estrogen and progestin hormone replacement therapy in relation to risk of breast cancer in middle-aged women. JAMA 274:137-142, 1995.

120. Steinberg KK, Thacker SB, Smith SJ, Stroup, DF, Zack, MM, Flanders, WD, Berkelman R. A meta-analysis of the effect of estrogen replacement therapy on the risk of breast cancer. JAMA 265:1985-1990, 1991.

121. Storm T, Thamsborg G, Steiniche T, Genant HK, Sorensen OH. Effect of intermittent cyclical etidronate therapy on bone mass and fracture rate in women with postmenopausal osteoporosis. N Engl J Med 322:1265-1271, 1990.

122. Watts NB, Harris ST, Genant HK, Wasnich RD, Miler PD, Jackson RD, Licata AA, Ross P, Woodson GC III, Yanover MJ, Mysiw WJ, Kohse L, Rao, MB, Steiger P, Richmond B, Chetnut CH III. Intermittent cyclical etidronate treatment of postmenopausal osteoporosis. N Engl J Med 323:73-79, 1990.

123. Wittenberg RH, Shea M, Swartz DE, Lee KS, White AAI, Hayes WC. Importance of bone mineral density in instrumented spine fusions. Spine 16:647-652, 1991.

124. Yamagata M, Kitahara H, Minami S, Takahashi K, Isobe K, Moriya H, Tamaki T. Mechanical stability of the pedicle screw fixation systems for the lumbar spine. Spine 17(Suppl 3):S51-S54, 1992.

125. Zhang Y, Kiel D, Kreger BE, et al. Bone mass and the risk of breast cancer among postmenopausal women. N Engl J Med 336:611-617, 1997.

126. Zindrick MR, Wiltse LL, Widell EH, Thomas JC, Holland RW, Field BT, Spencer CW. A biomechanical study of intrapeduncular screw fixation in the lumbosacral spine. Clin Orthop Rel Res 203:99-112, 1986.

33

The Pediatric Patient

Arnold H. Menezes, M.D.

The pediatric spine is not simply a scaled-down version of the adult spine. Although axiomatic, this concept is frequently forgotten in the management of pediatric spine disorders. A physician treating a child with a spinal abnormality must have an understanding of the structural features unique to the pediatric spine, the functional characteristics, and the specific pathophysiology prior to embarking on surgical management of the individual. The treating physician must have knowledge of the biomechanical characteristics of the pediatric spine and how these change with age, specifically concerning spinal instability, deformities, neoplastic disease, and trauma. The physician must select the procedure with the greatest likelihood of success in dealing with the primary pathology, while considering its potential for long-term complications. Unfortunately these two goals are not always compatible. Extensive thoracic laminectomy in a preadolescent child can lead to loss of the dorsal tension band and the possible development of progressive kyphosis.[26,57] Similarly, a dorsal thoracic spinal fusion in an infant may require the use of localized instrumentation or postoperative orthosis due to the plasticity of the immature spine.[56]

One of the most obvious differences between the adult and the pediatric spine is that the latter is actively growing. The growth velocity is highest in the infant and adolescent. In normal spinal growth, the dorsal and the ventral expansion is well balanced, as is the lateral growth. This results in lengthening of the spine with relatively little change in its gross contour. However, if a pathological condition results in asymmetrical pull, a progressive deformity will result. Likewise, the forces applied by asymmetrical growth can be used to produce progressive correction of a congenital scoliotic curvature. This is the rationale for convex hemiepiphysiodesis in congenital scoliosis.[56] However, the correction obtained depends on the magnitude and the rate of remaining growth.[6]

The "crankshaft phenomenon" is seen in skeletally immature children who undergo isolated dorsal fusion for the management of scoliosis.[57] Despite the solid construct, there may be progressive bending of the fusion mass due to continued ventral growth of the spine at the fused levels. The patients who are at most risk are those under 10 years of age at the time of the fusion. Crankshafting is less commonly seen in congenital scoliosis because of the limited growth potential remaining in many of the segments.

The pediatric spine tends to adapt to stresses much more readily than the adult spine. Thus a primary thoracic scoliotic curvature in a child is more likely to be associated with a compensatory lumbar curve that results in net balance of the head over the pelvis. Thus compensatory mechanisms play a part in the adaptability.

Adaptability is an active process. In addition, the pediatric spine is malleable and easily deformed with the application of external forces. This is a reflection of the intrinsic elasticity of the ligamentous tissues and the plasticity of the bone. Conversely, malleability regresses rapidly with age. This is observed in extensive elongation of the pars interarticularis in spondylolisthesis prior to fracture. From the point of view of trauma, the pediatric spine is able to absorb considerable energy before failure. This is because the spine is adaptable and malleable as opposed to the limited capability of the spinal cord.[5] This accounts for the low incidence of pediatric spine fractures and explains why spinal cord injury without radiographic abnormality can occur in the pediatric population.

The growth plate is the weakest link in the axial skeleton when subjected to tensile forces. Thus pediatric spine fractures are more prone to occur through the growth plate than anywhere else.[26,36] The corollary to this is that the healing potential is high and nonunion is infrequent. Likewise, an annular fragment with disc space protrusion may with traction result in a ring apophysis avulsion with a fragment of the bony end plate.

The normal thoracic spinal contour in the sagittal plane is a gentle C arc. Secondary cervical and lumbar lordotic curves are added after the development of the thoracic kyphotic curve. Transitional regions between the lordotic and the kyphotic curvatures are points of stress concentration and subject to deformation.[57] The increased incidence of burst fractures at the thoracolumbar junction is related to this stress concentration. The sagittal thoracic kyphosis stabilizes the pediatric spine against the development of coronal and rotational plane deformities.[13] With the rapid growth that takes place during the adolescent spurt, ventral spinal growth may be greater than the dorsal spinal growth, thus leading to flattening of the thoracic kyphosis. This potentially makes the spine susceptible to rotational and coronal plane deformities resulting in scoliosis. The anatomy and the embryology of the developing pediatric spine is covered in Chapters 2 and 3.

SPINAL DEFORMITY

Deformities of the pediatric spine are common and vary in their intensity from mild to severe. It must be remembered that scoliosis is multifactorial and is only a physical finding, not a disease. It is only with an accurate diagnosis that one can embark on an appropriate treatment strategy. In addition, several factors must be taken into consideration, such

Table 33-1. Classifications of Spinal Deformities

I. Scoliosis

A. Nonstructural—e.g., posture, leg discrepancy, secondary to irritative lesions
B. Structural
  1. Idiopathic
    Infantile (0-3 years)
    Juvenile (3-10 years)
    Adolescent (above 10 years)
  2. Congenital
    e.g. Defects in segmentation/formation
  3. Neuromuscular
  4. Neurofibromatosis
  5. Mesenchymal defects
    e.g. Ehlers-Danlos syndrome, Marfan's syndrome
  6. Osteochondrodystrophies
    e.g. Achondroplasia, spondyloepiphyseal dysplasia
  7. Following radiation
  8. Miscellaneous

II. Kyphosis

A. Postural
B. Scheuermann's
C. Congenital
D. After laminectomy, radiation, infection
E. Osteochondrodystrophies

III. Lordosis

A. Postural
B. Congenital
C. Neuromuscular
D. Miscellaneous

From Terminology Committee, Scoliosis Research Society. A glossary of scoliosis terms. Spine 1:57-58, 1976.

as the growth and maturation of the child, the effect of the deformity on the physiology, the flexibility and the rigidity of the deformity, and its pathological substrate.[53] Table 33-1 is a modification of the classification of spinal deformities from the Scoliosis Research Society.

Structural scoliosis is a lateral curvature of the spine that persists in the supine position, as well as on bending radiographs, demonstrating a lack of normal flexibility. Nonstructural scoliosis demonstrates lateral curvature of the spine that disappears in the supine position and has normal flexibility. It is best observed with elimination of the irritative insighting focus. Congenital scoliosis is a lateral curvature of the spine caused by anomalous vertebral development. The curves do not disappear when lying down nor is there much flexibility. As has been previously mentioned, scoliosis is classified according to whether there are primary major or secondary compensatory, or minor, curves.[57] A primary major curve is the structural curve with the least flexibility and the curve that usually comes first and is of the greatest clinical importance. The secondary curve is a compensatory one formed to balance the primary curve and is therefore more flexible and has less clinical significance.

Idiopathic Scoliosis

Idiopathic scoliosis is the most common of all spinal deformities in children, followed by Scheuermann's kyphosis.[52] Infantile or congenital idiopathic scoliosis has its onset in the first 3 years of life and is more common in males. Three percent of these can develop into severe curvatures and merit early treatment. Magnetic resonance imaging (MRI) is essential to rule out spinal and spinal cord pathology (Fig. 33-1). There are two basic groups of anomalies, those caused by a defect of formation and those caused by a defect of segmentation of one or more vertebrae.[56]

Defects of vertebral segmentation may be unilateral or bilateral. They may exist as blocked vertebrae, in which case there is bilateral failure of segmentation and very minimal scoliosis. A unilateral bar signifies complete failure of segmentation on one side with functional disc spaces in the other half. This is over several segments. This particular pathology leads to progressive scoliosis and must be corrected before 2 years of age. Unilateral bar and hemivertebra likewise requires similar attention. The rate of deterioration and the severity of the scoliosis depend on the extent of the unsegmented bar as well as the growth potential and the convexity of the spine. The only way to prevent deterioration of the deformity is to prevent further growth on the convexed side of the curvature opposite the unsegmented bar by spinal fusion. The abnormal segment does not contribute to vertical height and it is better to achieve a short, relatively straight spine that is balanced, than a spine that is longer and decompensated because of severe curvature.

Defects of formation of vertebrae may range from a mild wedging to complete absence of the vertebra, as with hemivertebra. They may affect one or more vertebrae. A hemivertebra is one of the most common causes of congenital scoliosis. This results in a laterally based wedge of bone consisting of half a vertebral body, a single pedicle, and hemilamina. There is usually an attached rib to the hemilamina resulting in an unequal number of ribs. A hemivertebra associated with a normal disc space above and below leads to longitudinal growth, as with an enlarging wedge producing a scoliosis. Two fully segmented hemivertebrae on the same side of the spine can cause a much greater growth imbalance because of the absence of full growth plates on the cavity of the curve.[26,58] Therefore early prophylactic surgical treatment is essential as soon as it is diagnosed when more than four abnormal disc spaces are present on the same side.[23] Congenital scoliosis is frequently associated with congenital anomalies in other systems, especially those formed from mesenchyme. Congenital heart disease is present in 10% of such individuals and Klippel-Feil syndrome in 25%.

Juvenile idiopathic scoliosis accounts for 11% to 15% of the scoliosis in the pediatric population. There is a relative plateau and growth of the spine between 5 and 10 years of age. The indications for surgical treatment of juvenile scoliosis are the same as for other forms of scoliosis. However, because the spine is immature, nonoperative treatment may be continued longer in children with juvenile scoliosis. Surgery may be delayed until the curve reaches 55 to 60 degrees when the spine is more mature. There is an equal distribution between males and females and the curves are equally distributed to the right and the left. Very few of these spontaneously resolve. Approximately 60% of juvenile idiopathic scoliosis cases require surgery.[6,52,56]

Adolescent idiopathic scoliosis involves curves that are detected after the onset of the pubertal growth spurt. A significant number of these probably begin during the juvenile age and the majority occur in females. Patients presenting with curves too large for bracing (over 50 degrees) or with curves over 40 degrees despite brace treatment require surgical correction.[33] It is important to keep in mind that major thoracic deformities can produce respiratory insufficiency and severe cardiopulmonary compromise.[19,52] From 1960 to 1985 the standard instrumentation for dorsal spine fusion was the Harrington rod system with rod distraction on the concavity and a compression rod on the convexity.[57] Since 1985 the Cotrel-Dubousset (CD) rod system, along with other "universal" special instrumentation systems, has been rapidly replacing the Harrington system.[10] The CD type system provides a

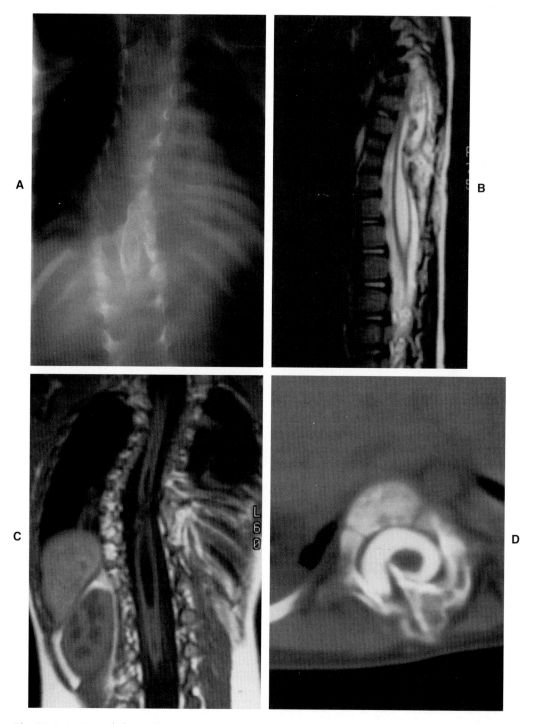

Fig. 33-1. A, Frontal thoracolumbar spine tomogram in a 3-year-old with progressive scoliosis, bladder incontinence, and a left leg smaller than the right. The scoliosis is evident. Note the midline (spinous processes) and pedicle fusion from T9 to T11 on the concavity side of the scoliosis. **B,** Midsagittal T2-weighted MRI of the thoracolumbar spine. The syrinx-filled cord is indented by a dorsal thoracic bony mass. **C,** Coronal T2-weighted MRI of the thoracolumbar spinal canal. There is a "syrinx" (actually diastematomyelia) and pedicle fusions at T9 to T11 on the left. **D,** Axial CT myelogram through plane of T10 vertebral body. Note the abnormal vertebral configuration. A dorsal midline bony spicule impales the dorsal spinal cord.

detorsional type of correction that the Harrington system does not. It appears to be more secure and a significant number of patients do not require post-operative bracing. It can be used for both single and double idiopathic curvatures.

Neuropathic Scoliosis

The neuropathic causes for scoliosis include both the upper motor neuron variety such as head injury, syringomyelia, and spinal cord tumors, as well as the lower motor neuron variety such as poliomyelitis, spinal muscular atrophy, and myelomeningocele.[56] In addition, myopathic conditions such as Duchenne type muscular dystrophy, myotonia congenita, and other forms of neuromuscular disease are included. Neuromuscular curves are usually seen early and are difficult to control with bracing. The general principles include long segment fusion over the entire curve and, at times, inclusive of the sacrum if there is pelvic obliquity. Ventral discectomy and fusion are helpful adjuncts to the dorsal surgery in selected cases. Multilevel segmental fixation is desirable for stabilization of these long fusions. The Luque technique represented an improvement over earlier function methods for spine fusion in neuromuscular scoliosis. The upper end of the fusion is usually at T2.

Pediatric Myelomeningocele

Scoliosis occurs in more than 80% of children with myelodysplasia by the tenth year of life.[25] It is well recognized that deterioration in gait, weakness, spasticity, neuro-orthopaedic deformities, and loss of urinary control and pain are common signs of a tethered cord in children with a myelomeningocele.[2,48,51] A tethered spinal cord in a repaired myelodysplastic patient is a cause for scoliosis.[57] More importantly a high lumbar myelocele repair may affect the thoracic spine quite severely. The spinal cord was untethered in 30 children with progressive loss of function in scoliosis in the series studied by McLone et al.[25] The curves of greater than 50 degrees fared poorly. However, in the majority, stabilization of the scoliosis or improvement was seen. In a large series of patients followed by Reigel et al,[39] progression of thoracic scoliosis plateaued or declined following the release of a tethered cord in children with lumbar and sacral levels. However, in children with a thoracic spinal cord level, release of the tethered cord did not halt progression of scoliosis.

Dermoid tumors at the site of a myelocele repair site are now an increasingly frequent encounter in children who presented with signs of delayed tethering.[44] An epidural and intraspinal abscess has been seen on two occasions by this author in children with myelodysplasia and sudden rapid neurological deterioration.[31]

Chiari Malformations and Scoliosis

A prospective study[32] was performed from 1985 to 1989 in children with Chiari malformations without myelodysplasia with the presence of scoliosis. Scoliosis was present in 3 of 16 individuals without syringohydromyelia.[32] Patients ranged in age from 2 to 15 years. The incidence of scoliosis was higher in patients before skeletal maturity and was 73% in the author's series. In children without syringohydromyelia, an idiopathic scoliosis is thought to be caused by abnormal brain stem dysfunction in the Chiari malformation patient, resulting in pathological vibratory responses due to dysfunction of the dorsal column pathways. This suggests that the curve may develop secondary to a disturbance of the postural reflex system. It is critical to differentiate idiopathic scoliosis from neurogenic scoliosis secondary to Chiari malformations, syringohydromyelia, or other causes of spinal cord dysfunction. This is especially so because forceful surgical correction of the scoliosis in association with syringomyelia is potentially disastrous in these patients.[53] The author's series has shown that patients under 10 years of age with scoliosis secondary to Chiari malformation and syringohydromyelia have exhibited a rapid, extensive resolution of the scoliosis following definitive surgery for the Chiari malformation. The preoperative presence of syringohydromyelia has not impaired the postoperative resolution of the scoliosis. Hematomyelia and hematobulbia were associated with persistent postdecompression scoliosis. A scoliotic curve of up to 54% has shown correction in preadolescent children following the Chiari malformation decompression-operative procedure.[32]

DIASTEMATOMYELIA

The term "diastematomyelia" was used to describe an abnormality of the spinal canal in which the dura mater was perforated by a bony spike or fibrous band to create two sleeves, each containing a portion of the spinal cord that is divided in two parts sagittally, joining together above and below the spike.[17] The bony spicule of fibrocartilaginous septum arises from the dorsal surface of the vertebral body and dorsally becomes continuous with the lamina (Fig. 33-2). Frequently the two hemicords are asymmetrical in diameter and each is associated with its own set of dorsal and ventral roots that may not be equal in number. The cleft spinal cord may be housed in a single arachnoid and dural sleeve in 50%; in the other 50%, each hemicord resides in its own distinct arachnoid-dural sleeve.[18,20] In the latter, the bone spur is invariably present and is usually located at the caudal end of the cleft. Thus the tethering effect of the spinal cord arises at several levels.[35] The first would be the fibrous medial portion of the separate dural sleeves, the next the cartilaginous or osseous septum, and in most instances there is a tight filum terminale. These structures produce traction leading to ischemia and mechanical distortion of the spinal cord and the nerve roots.

Diastematomyelia is more common in females and is associated with cutaneous abnormalities such as hypertrichosis, dimples, sinus tract, and lower limb abnormalities in 80% of individuals.[35] More often than not, the clinical history and physical findings are slowly progressive and complaints often include back and leg pain, weakness, bladder and bowel incontinence, and a foot deformity (Fig. 33-3). Of the 50 patients reported from the Hospital for Sick Children in Toronto in 1983, Humphreys, Hendrick, and Hoffman[20] found that 11 children presented with scoliosis. Eight had a tethered filum terminale in addition to the diastematomyelia. A significant number had a hairy patch, a nevus, a dermal sinus, meningocele, or a subcutaneous lipoma. The bony changes associated with the abnormality consisted of blocked vertebrae, hemivertebrae, failure of segmentation, and other areas of dysraphism. Abnormal areas of curvature and hydromyelia may occur in as much as 90% of patients with diastematomyelia.

Plain radiographs are invariably abnormal and the most pathognomonic finding is a calcified midline spur that may be identified on plain radiographs (depending on the age) or computed tomography (CT). MRI is the method of choice for definition of the anatomical features of the diastematomyelia.[3] Axial and coronal sections easily identify the associated pathology. In addition, associated lesions such as lipoma, syringohydromyelia, and dermoid and dermal sinuses are well defined by a properly accomplished MRI.[4]

The primary goal of surgery is prevention of further adverse changes. Surgical intervention consists of removal of all the areas causing a tethered effect on the spinal cord and reconstruction of the dural sac as well as the spine. Fusion segments such as a unilateral bar require fusion on the opposite side to prevent further scoliosis. In the author's opinion, an osteoplastic laminectomy is not advantageous and may be injurious considering the fact that the diastematomyelic spur may be attached to the lamina or the spinous process. Thus great care needs to be taken in removal of this bone. The bone removed during the procedure may be used for the completion of bone fusion in a segmental fashion. It is imperative that associated abnormalities be tackled at the same time.

NEURENTERIC CYSTS

The entity of neurenteric cysts has been reported under a number of confusing designations such as "enteric cysts," "teratoid cysts," "neurenteric canal remnant," "neural anomaly associated with intraspinal duplication" and "the split notochord syndrome."[29,45] This terminology differs because the various disciplines involved view the lesion from different perspectives. Neurenteric cysts form approximately 0.5% of spinal tumors. Neurenteric cysts are now being reported with increasing frequency and 50% of those reported in the literature occur in the thoracic spine.[17] These are lined by cuboidal or simple columnar epithelium with mucin droplets. They are complex malformations associated with a ventral spinal bony abnormality with the cyst being present either within the bone, intradural, or intramedullary. Neurenteric cysts are only second to neurogenic tumors (neuroblastoma, ganglioneuroma, and neurofibroma) as a cause of mass in the dorsal mediastinum in the pediatric population. Twelve percent of all mediastinal masses in any location in the young infant and child are enteric cysts.[29] They tend to lie to the right of the spine and are very likely related to the developmental process of gastric and gut rotation. These neurenteric cysts may also be present in the abdominal cavity, since the foregut structures descend from the cervicothoracic region during embryological development.

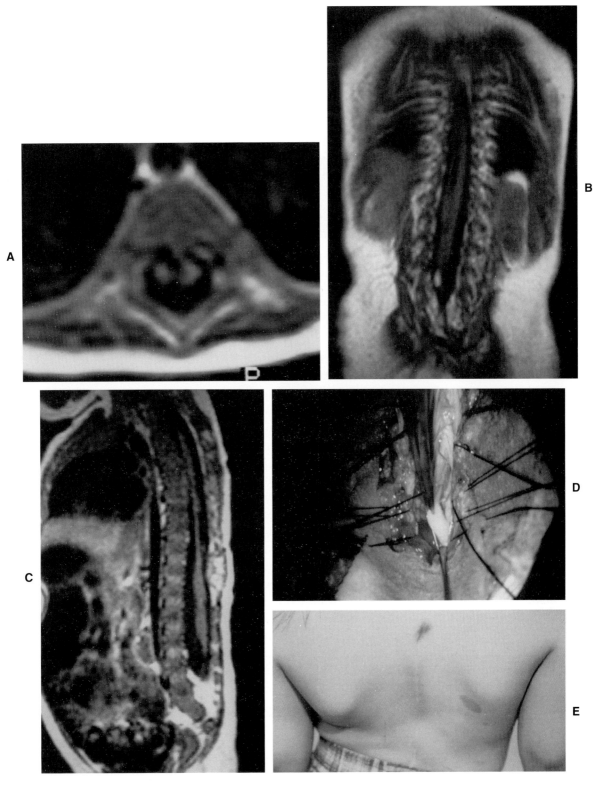

Fig. 33-2. A, Axial T1-weighted MRI through T8 vertebra reveals a diastematomyelia with ventral bone spur arising from the dorsal aspect of the vertebral body. **B,** Coronal T1-weighted MRI of thoracolumbar spine reveals the T7 to L4 diastematomyelia and lipoma in the terminal tethered cord. **C,** Midsagittal T1-weighted MRI of the thoracolumbar spine. There is an apparent widening of the abnormal lumbar spinal cord down to the sacral region. **D,** Operative photograph through the microscope. T7 to S1 osteoplastic laminectomies exposed the diastematomyelia and the lipoma in the filum terminale (white structure). **E,** The hairy midthoracic dorsal patch and a café-au-lait spot are again seen at age 4 years.

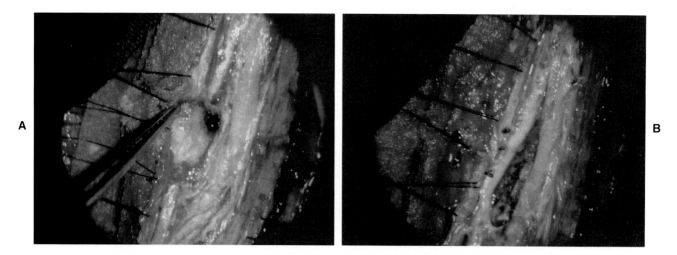

Fig. 33-3. A, Operative view of diastematomyelia with bone spur and single dural sac at T11. A 10-year-old girl had ascending level of her neurological loss from L4 to T10. Her thoracolumbar myelomeningocele was closed at birth. The bone spur arises from the dorsal vertebral body. **B,** Operative view of the diastematomyelic cords after complete resection of the bone spur.

Abdominal neurenteric cysts have little relationship to the level of the vertebral abnormalities. The latter may be missed if the cervicothoracic spine is not included in the investigation. Neurenteric cysts within the thoracic spinal canal, when connected to the dorsal mediastinal mass, may do so through a ventral vertebral defect and communicate as a fusiform dumbbell lesion, or through a small fibrous tract.[35] Fusion or malformation of the vertebral bodies at the level of the cyst occurs in approximately 50% of children with neurenteric cysts. Concurrence with intramedullary epidermoid cysts, spina bifida, spinal lipoma, syringomyelia, and myelomeningocele have been noted.[21,45] The bony anomalies and disturbances in development may lead to blocked vertebrae, hemivertebrae, splits in the vertebral body, bone spurs associated with diastematomyelia and such.[29,54] Hence it is important to obtain preoperative CT and MRI scans (Fig. 33-4).[3]

Neurenteric cysts most commonly present during the first decade of life, and depending on their location, the symptoms may be that of a mediastinal mass or from its spinal involvement. Signs and symptoms of meningitis are more common in the newborn infant and the young toddler. The most common location is the cervical canal and the upper thoracic spine. Pain in the affected region of the spine is a common prominent symptom and radicular pain or meningismus may accompany the local pain. Intermittent spinal cord compression has been ascribed to fluctuations in the size of the cyst and continued secretion of fluid by the columnar epithelium. Symptoms of meningitis have ranged from low-grade meningeal irritation secondary to cyst fluid leakage, to acute pyogenic meningitis with extensive intraspinal and intramedullary abscesses.

The goal of treatment of neurenteric cysts is surgical excision. Despite their typically ventral or ventrolateral location, the majority have been approached via a dorsal laminectomy. Simple aspiration generally allows for collapse of the cyst and excision of the majority of the lesion. However, the ventralmost dural or spinal cord attachment requires sharp microdissection. Associated anomalies such as diastematomyelia, spinal cord lipoma, and tethered spinal cord or dermoid are not uncommon and require specific attention. Likewise the mediastinal or the abdominal mass will require resection.[7,37]

EPIDERMOID AND DERMOID TUMORS

These lesions are not true neoplasms but dysembryonic malformations. Histologically both lesions are lined by stratified squamous epithelium, containing desquamated epithelial cells and keratin.[11,22] Dermoid tumors differ from epidermoid tumors in that they contain hair follicles and sebaceous glands. Dermoids are more common in children and are present in the thoracolumbar region. The major-

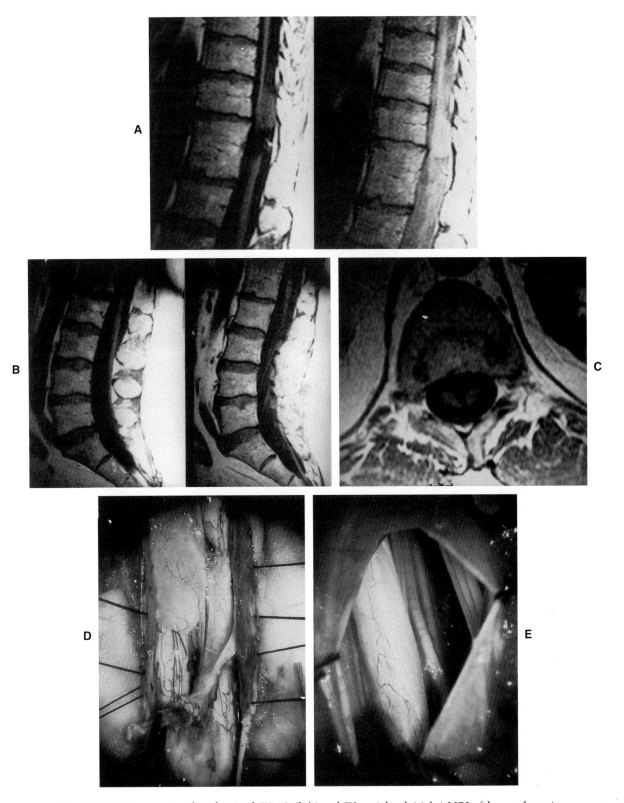

Fig. 33-4. A, Composite of midsagittal T1-10 *(left)* and T2-weighted *(right)* MRI of lower thoracic spine in a 15-year-old boy with rapidly progressive paraparesis and severe back pain. A block vertebra represents T12 to L1. The intradural extramedullary mass appears to contain fluid. **B,** Composite of midsagittal and parasagittal T1-weighted MRI of lumbar spine. Note the "tight" bowstring-like filum terminale. This is pathological. **C,** Axial T1-weighted MRI through T12 to L1 block vertebra. Note the bifid spinous process and the diplomyelia. **D,** Operative photograph after T9 to L2 laminectomies. A dermal sinus tract is present entering the dura mater at L1. Note the diplomyelic cords and a dorsal neurenteric cyst present rostral. **E,** Operative view through the microscope. The dural exposure was made after S1 laminectomy. The abnormally thick and rigid filum terminale is observed.

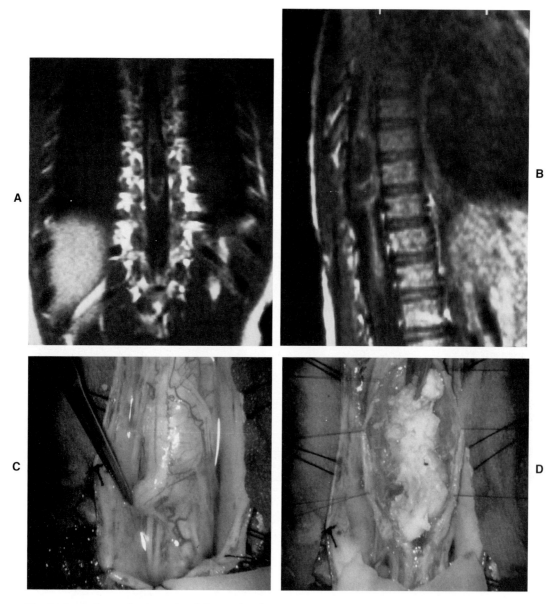

Fig. 33-5. A, Coronal T1-weighted thoracolumbar spine MRI in a 5-year-old boy with recent loss of bladder control and paraparesis. A skin tag had been excised from the middorsal region at 1 year of age. A cystic T7 to T10 intramedullary mass is seen. **B,** Midsagittal T1-weighted thoracolumbar MRI again identifies the intramedullary mass. Note the break in the surface subcutaneous fat two vertebral levels below the spinal mass. **C,** Operative photograph via the microscope. The dermal sinus tract is being grasped with the forceps. This leads to the expanded spinal cord at the T8 to T9 level. This was exposed via osteoplastic T7 to T10 laminectomies. **D,** Operative photograph exposes the intramedullary spinal cord dermoid.

ity are associated with midline cutaneous abnormalities such as port wine nevus, dermal sinus, or a hairy patch.[38] The clinical presentation is usually nonspecific unless there is a history of chronic recurring meningitis. Generally these lesions on MRI have the intensity of fat and have a high signal intensity on T2-weighted images.[3,44] Infrequently, dermoids in children may be intramedullary, making complete resection difficult (Fig. 33-5). In most instances the dermal sinus may be present on the surface with the tract leading into the spinal canal either in the interspinous location or actually through the spinous process itself.[50] Dermal sinuses may be associated with extradural lipoma.

TERATOMAS

Teratomas are lesions that contain elements of all three germinal layers. These malformations can undergo malignant change and are true neoplasms.[14,17,22] Teratomas are more frequent in the sacrococcygeal region and, following that, in the thoracic spinal canal in an epidural location. Spinal teratomas constitute 3% to 9% of intraspinal tumors in children. They are primary lesions of childhood and in one third the diagnosis is made in children younger than 5 years of age. These lesions may be present in an intradural location but are rarely intramedullary. They can be solid, cystic, or a combination. Occasionally the spinal canal is enlarged by the tumor, which may contain calcifications.

SPINAL CORD INJURY WITHOUT RADIOGRAPHIC ABNORMALITY

Spinal cord injury without radiographic abnormality (SCIWORA) describes injuries in which traumatic myelopathy occurs in the absence of demonstrable contiguous osseous or ligamentous injury.[36] It was initially theorized that transient subluxation of the spine occurred without bony fracture over ligamentous instability and elastic recoil returned the spinal column to its normal alignment. Several authors have reported this entity. This lesion compares with the acute central cord syndrome in the adult.[12,32]

The incidence of SCIWORA varies considerably, ranging between 5% to 70% of all pediatric spinal column and cord injuries. SCIWORA occurs almost exclusively in the pediatric population, with the majority of cases occurring in children less than 8 years of age. The mechanisms of neural damage include flexion, hyperextension, longitudinal distraction, and ischemia. Cervical and thoracic injuries occur with equal frequency. The neurological injuries in young children tend to be particularly severe in contrast with those found in teenagers or the occasional adult with SCIWORA. The onset of paralysis may be delayed as long as 4 days after injury and most children recall transient paresthesias, numbness, and subjective motor loss. The neurological symptoms may be trivial, and in a child with suspected spinal column injury the incident must be taken seriously so as to avoid a potentially preventable disaster. In a significant number of football and gymnastic injuries seen by this author, a burning sensation has been described by children prior to the onset of neurological devastation.

MRI has made the term "SCIWORA" inaccurate, although this is still a useful term to describe the type of injury. Fractures and instability will have already been excluded. MRI is important to identify a herniated disc, ligamentous injury, cord contusion, or epidural hematoma. It is not uncommon for children who are partially affected with neurological dysfunction to have a recurrent episode a few weeks following the initial insult. For this reason children should be braced after the initial neurological injury and kept so for 3 months so as to regain ligamentous stability. Though this is true with the cervical spine region, the same principle holds good in the thoracic region.

POSTTRAUMATIC SPINAL DEFORMITY

This problem is unique to the growing child.[34,57] It is relatively uncommon in patients who are near the end of their growth. The deformities encountered include scoliosis, kyphosis, and lordosis, each with a different etiology. The major factors that contribute to progressive spinal curvature are paralysis of the postural muscles of the spine below the level of the injury and epiphyseal damage to the growth plates, both of which interfere with the normal growth of the spine and lead to the development of scoliosis. The incidence of progressive spinal deformity in the series with pediatric spinal injury with long-term follow-ups exceeds 90%. This neuromuscular deformity requires bracing as a temporary means for delaying spinal fusion. Surgical fusion is required in the majority and will result in improved sitting balance in all cases.

SCHEUERMANN'S KYPHOSIS

This typically occurs in the juvenile between the age of 10 and 14 and is a kyphotic vertebral deformity that should be distinguished from postural kyphosis on the basis of the peculiar rigidity that occurs in Scheuermann's kyphosis.[13,28,41,57] This affects between 0.5% and 8% of healthy subjects and is second only to idiopathic scoliosis in its prevalence. The child presents with a round back appearance with or without pain. This kyphosis is not fully flexible on prone hyperextension testing. Radiographs demonstrate the classic findings of disc space narrowing, end plate irregularity, apical vertebral wedging, and sometimes hypokyphosis. Hyperextension radiographs show lack of normal flexibility.

In Scheuermann's kyphosis the primary pathological process is localized to altered areas of the growth cartilage and vertebral end plates according to a mosaic like pattern. The enchondral ossification process is altered.[41] The matrix exhibits a lower number of collagen fibers and the radiographic appearance should be interpreted as an absence of growth rather than a destructive process. Scheuermann's kyphosis presents as two forms, the more common being with the apex of the curvature localized between T7 and T9, and the so called thoracolumbar form with the apex being between T10 and T12.

In the growing child, a painful or progressive deformity should be treated. The treatment of choice is usually orthotics. In the midthoracic spine, a Milwaukee brace is used, while at the thoracolumbar junction an underarm orthosis is needed. Surgical stabilization and correction is required in 5% of children. Surgery should be reserved for adolescents with curvatures exceeding 75 degrees, children with rapidly progressive kyphosis despite treatment with bracing or casts, and adults with curves greater than 65 degrees. Spinal cord compression is extremely rare in Scheuermann's disease.

ACUTE DISC SPACE INFECTION AND DISCITIS

There is a syndrome in children distinct from vertebral osteomyelitis that is associated with intervertebral disc narrowing, fever, spinal pain, and an elevated sedimentation rate.[1,5,28,42,55] The precise cause of the disorder is speculative, although most investigators regard it as being an acute inflammatory process. Biopsies of the disc material during the active phase of the disease has produced *Staphylococcus aureus* and rarely *Diplococcus pneumoniae* and diphtheroids. In most cases biopsy specimens have been consistent with acute or chronic inflammation. Most cases have been reported in the lumbar region and very few in the thoracic region. Intravenous cephalosporin is maintained for 2 weeks followed by 4 weeks of oral antibiotics. The majority of children are braced for 14 to 18 weeks.

SPINAL NEOPLASMS

Primary vertebral neoplasms in the pediatric age group are uncommon but occur frequently enough to present a diagnostic dilemma and a therapeutic challenge.[11,30] The incidence of spinal bony tumors in a major reported series of childhood spinal lesions ranged from 4% to 15%.[3,11,14,22,30] The common aims of treatment of these primary axial neoplasms should be complete excision when feasible, preservation of neurological function, and consideration of stability in the growing spine. Spinal lesions in older patients are more frequently malignant. Those in children and adolescents are usually benign. Neurological abnormality bodes poorly because in this situation malignant lesions are more commonly seen.[15,24,27] Any child with neurological deficit and back pain warrants careful radiographic evaluation before diagnosis of herniated nucleus pulposus, Scheuermann's disease, or osteomyelitis is made.[30,47]

The prolonged natural history of benign spinal tumors in children causes a significant delay between the onset of symptoms and the achievement of a definitive diagnosis.[7,9] Localized tenderness may represent osteoid osteoma or osteoblastoma. Scoliosis or progressive tilt is indicative of nerve root irritation and may be present when these tumors compress intra- or extraforaminal segments of the vertebrae.[16,22,58,59] Neurological abnormalities relate to the size of the spinal lesion and its extension into the spinal canal. Thus myelopathy, radiculopathy, and at times plexopathy may occur, depending on the extent of the tumor into the spinal canal or extra-axially, respectively.[40,43,46]

Extradural Extramedullary Neural Crest Tumors

Tumors of the neural crest tissue are common in childhood and account for 10% to 20% of all spinal tumors.[22] This group consists primarily of ganglioneuromas and neuroblastomas.[8,11,49] The former is benign while the latter is malignant. Between these two extremes is a ganglioneuroblastoma. These tumors originate from the paravertebral sympathetic chain and as a rule involve the spinal canal by direct extension. Neuroblastomas may metastasize.

Ganglioneuromas are benign and may be found in the older child. This author has encountered ganglioglioma in a 2-year-old with paraparesis. These

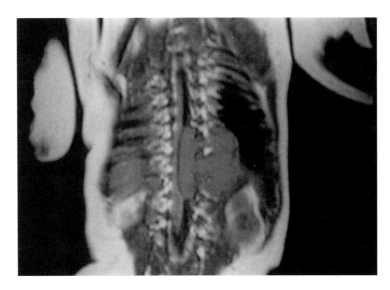

Fig. 33-6. Coronal T1-weighted MRI of the thoracolumbar spine. A large dumbbell mass is present in the extradural canal from T8 to L1 and in the extrapleural and retroperitoneal spaces. The neuroblastoma invades the spinal canal via the neural foramina.

tumors are usually well circumscribed and found in the dorsal mediastinum, but may also be located in the abdomen. They may achieve large size and require gross excision.

Ganglioneuroblastomas are believed to represent a stage in the maturation of neuroblastomas. They occur in young children and are well circumscribed. However, invasion may be present and the lesion is frequently found in the dorsal mediastinum and abdomen. The behavior is unpredictable.

Neuroblastomas are malignant tumors more common in the younger child. They are friable, fairly circumscribed masses with areas of invasion into surrounding tissue. A significant number arise from the adrenal medulla. Other locations are the sympathetic chain in the dorsal mediastinum and the retroperitoneal space. These are highly malignant tumors but have a better prognosis in children under 2 years of age. The tumor readily metastasizes and most older children show spread at the time of diagnosis. Involvement into the spinal canal is by direct extension in most cases and rarely by metastases into the spine (Fig. 33-6). These lesions are seen as paraspinal masses on plain radiographs of the chest and abdomen.[3] A visible calcification may be seen in 50% of cases. Treatment consists of surgical resection, including laminectomy. These individuals need to be followed carefully for spinal deformity.

Intramedullary Spinal Tumors

As in the adult, this consists of focal, segmental, and holocord tumors.[15,22,30] The most commonly encountered is the astrocytoma, and grade I and grade II tumors must be considered as in the adult for surgical resection. Similarly, ependymoma and ganglioglioma are surgically amenable. This author feels strongly about the possibility of osteoplastic laminectomy with replacement of lamina. Even though this does not prevent scoliosis, it assists in the surgical treatment of scoliosis at a later stage because the lamina and spinous processes are available for fixation and correction of deformity should this be necessary.

LAMINECTOMY VS. LAMINOPLASTY AND FUSION

Pediatric neurosurgeons, and especially spinal pediatric neurosurgeons, tend to expound on the benefits of osteoplastic laminectomies. This procedure should be done, when feasible. Contraindications include diastematomyelia (because of the spur), dermal sinus and lipomyelocele (because the tract is difficult to follow), and cases where the spinal cord is grossly distorted with epidural neuroblastoma or sarcoma. Extensive exposure for holocord tumors has been successfully made via osteoplastic laminoplasty. The spinous process and laminae are easily removed "en bloc" with a fine high-powered drill with a small footplate, incising the junction of the laminae with the facets on one side and then the other. Laminae may be replaced and fixed with titanium microplates. The ligamentum flavum may be left intact within the segment of dorsal bone removed. Osteoplastic laminoplasty will assist in subsequent fusion, if needed, for scoliosis or instability.

In infants and toddlers, the spinous processes may be vertically split and the laminae reflected outward to allow for excellent dural exposure. These spinous processes are then anatomically resutured.

REFERENCES

1. Alexander CJ. The etiology of juvenile spondyloarthritis (discitis). Clin Radiol 21:178-187, 1970.
2. Balasubramaniam C, Laurent JP, McCluggage C, Oshman D, Cheek WR. Tethered cord syndrome after repair of meningomyelocele. Childs Nerv Syst 6:208-211, 1990.
3. Barkovich AJ. Neoplasms of the spine. In Barkovich AJ, ed. Contemporary Neuroimaging: Pediatric Neuroimaging. New York: Raven Press, 1990, pp 273-291.
4. Barkovich A, Edwards M, Cogen P. MR evaluation of spinal dermal sinus tracts in children. Am J Neuroradiol 12:123-129, 1991.
5. Boston HC, Bianco AJ, Rhodes KH: Disc space infection in children. Orthop Clin North Am 6:953-964, 1975.
6. Bridwell KH. Idiopathic scoliosis. In Bridwell KH, DeWald RL, eds. The Textbook of Spinal Surgery. Philadelphia: JB Lippincott, 1991, pp 97-161.
7. Burk DJ Jr, Brunberg JA, Kanal E. Spinal and paraspinal neurofibromatosis: Surface coil MR imaging at 1:57. Radiology 162:797-801, 1987.
8. Dargeon HW. Neuroblastoma. J Pediatr 61:456-471, 1962.
9. Deen HG Jr, Scheithauer BW, Ebersold MJ. Clinical and pathological study of meningiomas of the first decade of life. J Neurosurg 56:317-322, 1982.
10. Denis F. Cotrel-Dubousset instrumentation in the treatment of idiopathic scoliosis. Orthop Clin North Am 19:291-312, 1988.
11. DeSousa AL, Kalsbeck JE, Mealey J Jr, Campbell RL, Hockey A. Intraspinal tumors in children. A review of 31 cases. J Neurosurg 51:437-445, 1979.
12. Dickman CA, Rekate HL, Sonntag VKH, Zabramski JM. Pediatric spinal trauma: Vertebral column and spinal cord injuries in children. Pediatr Neurosci 15:237-256, 1989.
13. Dubousset J. Three dimensional analysis of the scoliotic deformity. In Weinstein SL, ed. The Pediatric Spine: Principles and Practice. New York: Raven Press, 1994, pp 479-496.
14. Epstein FJ, Constantini S. Spinal cord tumors in childhood. In Pang D, ed. Disorders of the Pediatric Spine. New York: Raven Press, 1995, pp 371-388.
15. Epstein F, Epstein N. Surgical management of holocord intramedullary spinal cord astrocytomas in children. J Neurosurg 54:829-832, 1981.
16. Fortuna A, Nolletti A, Nardi P, Caruso R. Spinal neurinomas and meningiomas in children. Acta Neurochir 55:329-341, 1981.
17. French BN. Midline fusion defects and defects of formation. In Youmans JR, ed. Neurological Surgery, 2nd ed. Philadelphia: WB Saunders, 1982, pp 1236-1360.
18. Goldberg G, Fenelon G, Blake NS, Dowling F, Regan BF. Diastematomyelia: A critical review of the natural history and treatment. Spine 9:367-372, 1984.
19. Howell FR, Dickson RA. The deformity of idiopathic scoliosis made visible by computer graphics. J Bone Joint Surg 71(B):399-403, 1989.
20. Humphreys RP, Hendrick EB, Hoffman HJ. Diastematomyelia. Clin Neurosurg 30:436, 456, 1983.
21. James CCM, Lassman LP. Spinal Dysraphism Spina Bifida Occulta. London: Butterworths, 1972, pp 25-28, 89-97.
22. Koos W, Laubichler W, Sorgo G. Statistical studies on spinal tumors in childhood and adolescence. Neuropadiatrie 4:273-303, 1973.
23. Letts RM, Bobechko WP. Fusion of the scoliotic spine in young children. Clin Orthop 101:136-145, 1974.
24. Lo WD, Matthay KK, Kushner J. Spinal cord compression in a child with acute lymphoblastic leukemia. Am J Pediatr Hematol Oncol 7:373-382, 1985.
25. McLone DG, Herman JM, Gabriel AP, Dias L. Tethered cord as a cause of scoliosis in children with a myelomeningocele. Pediatr Neurosurg 16:8-13, 1990.
26. McMaster MJ, Ohtsuka K. The natural history of congenital scoliosis: A study of 251 patients. J Bone Joint Surg 64A:1128-1147, 1982.
27. Mellinger JF. Central nervous system involvement in childhood lymphoblastic leukemia. In Swaiman KF, Wright FS, eds. The Practice of Pediatric Neurology. St. Louis: Mosby, 1982, pp 871-880.
28. Menezes AH, Osenbach RK. Inflammatory diseases of the juvenile spine. In Pang D, ed. Disorders of the Pediatric Spine. New York: Raven Press, 1995, pp 481-492.
29. Menezes AH, Ryken TC. Craniocervical intradural neurenteric cysts. Pediatr Neurosurg 22:88-95, 1995.
30. Menezes AH, Sato Y. Primary tumors of the spine in children—Natural history and management. Pediatr Neurosurg 23:101-114, 1995.
31. Menezes AH, VanGilder JC. Spinal cord abscess. In Wilkins RH, Rengachary SS, eds. Neurosurgery. New York: McGraw-Hill, 1985, pp 1969-1972.
32. Muhonen MG, Menezes AH, Sawin PD, Weinstein SL. Scoliosis in pediatric Chiari malformations without myelodysplasia. J Neurosurg 77:69-77, 1992.
33. Nilsonne U, Lundgren KD. Long-term prognosis in idiopathic scoliosis. Acta Orthop Scand 39:456-465, 1968.
34. Osenbach RK, Menezes AH. Spinal cord injury without radiographic abnormality (SCIWORA) in children. Pediatr Neurosci 15:168-175, 1989.
35. Pang D. Split cord malformations. Part II clinical syndrome. Neurosurgery 31:481-500, 1992.
36. Pang D, Wilberger JE Jr. Spinal cord injury without radiographic abnormalities in children. J Neurosurg 57:114-129, 1982.
37. Piramoon AM, Abbassioun K. Mediastinal enterogenic cyst with spinal cord compression. J Pediatr Surg 9:543-545, 1974.
38. Powell KR, Cherry JD, Hougen T, Blinderman EE, Dunn MC. A prospective search for congenital dermal abnormalities of the craniospinal axis. J Pediatr 87:744-750, 1975.
39. Reigel DH, Tchernoukha K, Bazmi B, Kortyna R, Rotenstein D. Change in spinal curvature following release of tethered spinal cord associated with spina bifida. Pediatr Neurosurg 20:30-42, 1994.

40. Riccardi VM. Neurofibromatosis: Phenotype, Natural History and Pathogenesis, 2nd ed. Baltimore: John Hopkins University Press, 1992, pp 1-450.
41. Sachs BL, Bradford DS, Winter RB. Scheuerman's kyphosis: Long-term results of Milwaukee brace treatment. J Bone Joint Surg 69A:50-57, 1987.
42. Sartoris DJ, Moskowitz PS, Kaufman RA, Ziprkowski MN, Berger PE. Childhood diskitis: Computed tomographic findings. Radiology 149:701-707, 1983.
43. Sato Y, Waziri M, Smith W, Frey E, Yuh WT, Hanson J, Franken EA Jr. Hipple-Lindau disease: MR imaging. Radiology 166:241-246, 1988.
44. Scott RM, Wolpert SM, Barthoshesky LE, Zimbler S, Klauber GT. Dermoid tumors occurring at the site of previous myelomeningocele repair. J Neurosurg 65:779-783, 1986.
45. Smith JR. Accessory enteric formations: A classification and nomenclature. Arch Dis Child 35:87-89, 1960.
46. Solomon RA, Stein BM. Unusual spinal cord enlargement related to intramedullary neurangioblastoma. J Neurosurg 68:550-553, 1988.
47. Stein BM. Vascular malformations of the spinal cord. In Pang D, ed. Disorders of the Pediatric Spine. New York: Raven Press, 1995, pp 493-507.
48. Tamaki N, Shirataki K, Kojima N, Shouse Y, Matsumoto S. Tethered cord syndrome of delayed onset following repair of myelomeningocele. J Neurosurg 69:393-398, 1988.
49. Traggis DG, Filler RM, Druckman H, Jaffe N, Cassady JR. Prognosis for children with neuroblastoma presenting with paralysis. J Pediatr Surg 12:419-425, 1977.
50. Venger B, Laurent JP, Cheek WR. Congenital thoracic dermal tracts. In Marlin AE, ed. Concepts in Pediatric Neurosurgery. Basel: S Karger, 1989, pp 161-172.
51. Warf BC, Scott RM, Barnes PD, Hendren WH III. Tethered spinal cord in patients with anorectal and urogenital malformations. Pediatr Neurosurg 19:25-30, 1993.
52. Weinstein SL. Idiopathic scoliosis: Natural history. Spine 11:780-783, 1986.
53. Weinstein SL, Ponseti IV. Curve progression in idiopathic scoliosis: Long-term follow-up. J Bone Joint Surg 65:447-456, 1983.
54. Whiting DM, Chou SM, Lanzieri CF, Kalfas I, Hardy RW. Cervical neurenteric cyst associated with Klippel-Feil syndrome: A case report and review of the literature. Clin Neuropathol 10:285-290, 1991.
55. Wiley AM, Trueta J. The vascular anatomy of the spine and its relationship to pyogenic vertebral osteomyelitis. J Bone Joint Surg 49:796-809, 1959.
56. Winter RB. Convex anterior and posterior hemiarthrodesis and hemi-epiphyseodesis in young children with progressive congenital scoliosis. J Pediatr Orthop 1:361-366, 1981.
57. Winter RB. Congenital Deformities of the Spine. New York: Thieme-Stratton, 1983.
58. Winter RB, Moe JH, Bradford DS. Spine deformity in neurofibromatosis. A review of one hundred and two patients. J Bone Joint Surgery 61A:677-694, 1979.
59. Yaghman I. Spine changes in neurofibromatosis. Radiographics 6:261-285, 1986.

Congenital and Hereditary Anomalies

Michael L. Levy, M.D., Steven Davis, B.S., and J. Gordon McComb, M.D.

NEURAL TUBE DEFECTS

By far the most common congenital lesions involving the thoracic spine are associated with the formation of the neural tube (NT). The developmental lesions that result in abnormal midline fusion are often referred to as being dysraphic and vary from inapparent and insignificant to massive. Several different schemata are used to classify this wide variety and often complex set of malformations. However, the nomenclature is confusing and even contradictory. As all of these congenital lesions of clinical significance involve an aberration in the formation of the NT, it is suggested that the term "neural tube defects" (NTD) be used to characterize this entire group of anomalies. NTDs can be subdivided into two main groupings, those that are open and those that are closed.

Epidemiology

Open NTDs (Fig. 34-1) result from genetic factors, probably at more than one locus, interacting with environmental and dietary agents. Until recently, prevention of NTDs was not possible. However, new studies have shown a direct correlation with red blood cell folate levels in early pregnancy and the incidence of open NTDs. Increasing folic acid intake to 0.4 mg per day reduces fetal open NTDs by half in

---

**CLASSIFICATION OF CONGENITAL
AND HEREDITARY DISORDERS
OF THE THORACIC SPINE**

Neural Tube Defects (Nomenclature and Embryology)

Open
  Myelomeningocele
  Myeloschisis
Closed
  Meningocele
  Lipomatous malformations
  Congenital dermal sinus
  Diastematomyelia
  Neurenteric cyst

Cysts (Not Associated With NTD)

Arachnoid
Meningeal
Intramedullary
Miscellaneous

Vascular Lesions

Neoplasms

Intramedullary
Extramedullary

Structural Deformity of the Thoracic Spinal Column With Neurological Sequelae (Not Associated With NTDs)

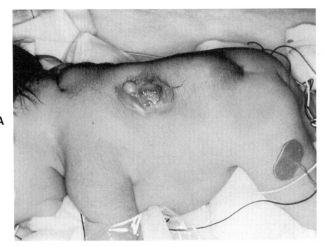 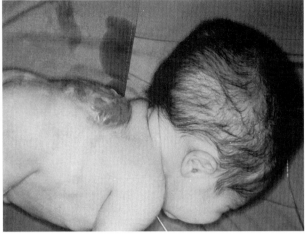

Fig. 34-1. Two photographs of 1-day-old infants with midthoracic open NTDs. Exposed neural tissue. The neural placode is visible in both. CSF is actively leaking from the lesion of the newborn in (**B**), but not in (**A**).

the population as a whole, and by over two thirds in women who previously have had a fetus with an open NTD.[35] As one half of all pregnancies in the United States are unplanned, and because open NTDs occur during the first month of gestation even before a woman knows that she is pregnant, it is currently advocated that all women of child bearing age have a daily intake of 0.4 mg of folic acid.

The incidence of infants born with open NTDs still varies considerably by locale in developed countries (currently below 0.5/1000 of live births in the United States). It continues to drop secondary to better diet (especially with increased folic acid intake) and more widespread prenatal screening. Detection of a fetus with an open spinal NTD within the first trimester was initially made possible by the work of Brock and Sutcliffe,[5] who noted that mothers carrying fetuses with an open spinal NTD had high levels of alpha-fetoprotein (AFP) in both the maternal serum and amniotic fluid. AFP, a protein made in the fetal liver, is thought to provide immunologic protection. AFP gains access to the amniotic fluid via the open spinal NTD, with a portion subsequently reaching the maternal circulation. A closed NTD does not have an elevated AFP level since the route of access is absent. Another diagnostic modality that has had a significant impact on prenatal screening has been the development and use of high-resolution fetal ultrasonography that can detect the presence of a spinal NTD.

The presence of a closed NTD can go undetected, and thus the etiology of this group of anomalies is

unknown because no information exists regarding the role of genetic, environmental, or dietary factors. The incidence of closed NTDs is undetermined, however, with better awareness and with remarkable advances in diagnostic imaging, many of these lesions that were previously missed are now being detected at birth.

Embryology

The notochord induces the overlying neural plate ectoderm to form a groove that progressively elevates, folds, and fuses in the midline via a process known as neurulation. Dorsal neural tube fusion begins midway along the neural groove during the fourth week of gestation, spreads in both a rostral and caudal direction, and is complete within a few days. The cutaneous ectoderm separates from the neural ectoderm below and subsequently fuses in the midline to form the overlying skin, while laterally located mesoderm migrates between the two separating ectoderms to form the dorsal vertebral arches and soft tissue structures. A failure of the primary spinal neurulation process leads to an open NTD, which most often occurs in the region of the posterior neuropore. The visible portion of the defect, the back mass, can be likened to the tip of an iceberg above the water, because the malformation involves the entire central nervous system (CNS). It has been postulated that the loss of cerebrospinal fluid (CSF) through the open NTD is the underlying cause of the maldevelopment found throughout the

CNS. Concomitant brain maldevelopment includes the Chiari II malformation in which the elongated cerebellar vermis, medulla, and fourth ventricle extend into the spinal canal. The brain stem is kinked and the midbrain is deformed with the aqueduct of Sylvius forked and/or stenotic in over two thirds of the cases. Interference with normal migration of cells within the cerebral hemispheres can lead to an increased number of small gyri (polymicrogyria) and clusters of neuronal and glial cells present in abnormal locations (heterotopias).

The embryology of closed NTDs is much less well understood. Most closed spinal NTDs are in the lumbosacral region, and thus do not involve the thoracic spine. The posterior neuropore is thought to mark the end of the primary NT, with the remainder of the NT, presumably the tip of the conus medullaris and filum terminale, forming from the caudal cell mass with canalization and fusion of neural elements in a process referred to as secondary neurulation. It may be during the secondary neurulation sequence that most closed dorsal NTDs occur. This, however, does not explain those meningoceles and congenital dermal sinuses in the thoracic region, where the neural tube is formed by the primary neurulation process.

Even less well understood are the ventral closed NTDs, such as split cord malformation (diastematomyelia and myelia/diplomyelia complex) and neurenteric cysts, which appear to result from abnormal interaction between the endoderm, notochord, neural plate, and the neurenteric canal. They may occur even before the process of neurulation begins. A failure of primary neurulation can explain dorsal abnormalities, be it an open or closed NTD. However, a ventral disruption in spinal cord formation is needed to produce a split cord malformation or neurenteric cyst. A theory that unifies the spectrum of this group of NTDs proposes that a disturbed mechanism occurs during gastrulation when all three germ layers are in intimate proximity. It is presumed that a second neurenteric canal becomes invested with mesenchyme to form an endomesenchymal tract that splits the notochord and neural plate, with the timing and severity determining the extent of the resultant malformation. The embryological disorder responsible for a neurenteric cyst appears to occur during gastrulation, similar to that of a split cord malformation. In fact, these NTDs can occur together. At the time of gastrulation the neurenteric canal connects with the yolk sac and amniotic cavity through the blastopore, making a temporary connection between the precursors of the gastrointestinal or respiratory tract, the spine, and spinal cord. Depending on the severity, timing, and healing process, a host of malformations can occur. Disruption of the spinal column can vary from nondiscernible to a massive combined ventral and dorsal NTD in which the vertebral bodies are divided for a number of segments with herniation of the intestinal contents through the defect. The NTD could be either open, closed, or a combination of both. Such combined ventral and dorsal lesions are quite rare and are often not compatible with viability.

OPEN NEURAL TUBE DEFECTS

A failure in the normal process of neurulation, whereby the neural plate is formed and dorsally closes to become the neural tube, results in an open NTD. The caudal portion of the neural tube closes last at the level of the posterior neuropore, corresponding to spinal cord segments L1 or L2, with a range from T11 to L4.[21] The prototype of the open spinal NTD, the myelomeningocele, is associated with widespread abnormalities throughout the CNS. The term "myelomeningocele" is preferred to "spina bifida," as spina bifida by definition refers to the mesodermal derived structures and not to those of the NT. An open NTD is one in which the neural plaque or placode is visible and represents the spinal cord that has failed to form a tube during primary neurulation. Myelomeningoceles, although more frequently located in the lumbosacral region, can also be found in a thoracic location. Myelomeningoceles can be confined just to the thoracic spine, but most involve the thoracic area as an extension of a primary lumbar lesion.[24] These lesions are generally cystic and contain CSF that will drain when the thin sac is disrupted. The neural plaque is surrounded by partially transparent dysplastic meninges and epithelium that are attached to normal skin at the periphery. Connected to the neural plaque are elongated nerve roots that are occasionally functional. Myeloschisis is an open form of spinal NTD in which the neural plaque is plastered to the ventral wall of the spinal cord, rather than being ballooned above the spinal canal, as with a myelomeningocele. Elongated nerve roots are not present in this situation, but in every other respect this is similar to that of a myelomeningocele. Closure of a myeloschisic lesion can be a significant challenge because there is less redundant skin to close the defect.

A rare form of open NTD is the hemimyelomeningocele, in which one half of the spinal cord is exposed and the other half is not. Because the two segments of the spinal cord are divided, it is also a form of split cord malformation. Because the entire CNS is involved and the incidence of hydrocephalus is high, it is the open NTD aspect that predominates. The lesions that involve the thoracic region usually have more extensive neurological deficits that render many of these infants paraplegic. These higher lesions also tend to be larger and associated with a more severe deformity of the spinal column that occurs over several segments and includes absence of the laminae and spinous processes, widening of the interpedicular distance, shortened pedicles, large transverse processes that are occasionally fused to one another, and deformed vertebral bodies that can produce a significant kyphosis.

Closure of the open spinal NTD is undertaken within the first few days of life, the main goal being to cease the leakage of CSF and cover the spinal cord with an intact epithelial barrier. If a marked kyphotic deformity is present this can be corrected at the time of closure with resection of one or more of the normal vertebral bodies. Laterally located bony protuberances from the malformed dorsal vertebral arches are also resected flush to the surrounding musculature in order to prevent breakdown of the overlying skin. A CSF diverting shunt may be placed concomitantly if hydrocephalus is already obvious, or soon thereafter if progressive.

CLOSED NEURAL TUBAL DEFECTS

Matson[24] and James and Lassman[17] were instrumental in promoting widespread recognition and clinical understanding of closed NTDs and the need for surgical treatment. Open and closed NTDs are separate entities. The disorder in embryogenesis differs for the two forms. With the open spinal NTD the failure is primary neurulation, while with a closed NTD the failure appears to result from another form of disturbance of NT formation. With but few exceptions, CNS deformities with closed NTDs are limited to the spinal cord and not associated with the Chiari II malformation and hydrocephalus. The prognosis for an infant with a closed NTD is vastly better than one with an open NTD. The child with a closed NTD has an intellectual function that is of the same distribution as the normal population, does not require a CSF diverting shunt, can ambulate because as the motor and sensory loss in the lower extremities is not marked, and bladder and bowel function are much less affected. A newborn with an open NTD has a spinal cord that is visible and often, though not necessarily, leaking CSF. In contrast, the infant with the closed NTD has no exposed neural tissue and does not drain CSF, because the lesion is fully covered with epithelialized tissue, although it may be dysplastic. Cutaneous manifestations of closed thoracic NTDs include subcutaneous lipomatous masses, myelocystoceles (Figs. 34-2 and 34-3), angiomas, pigmentary changes that vary from white to dark patches, dimples and sinuses, appendages, and hypertrichosis.

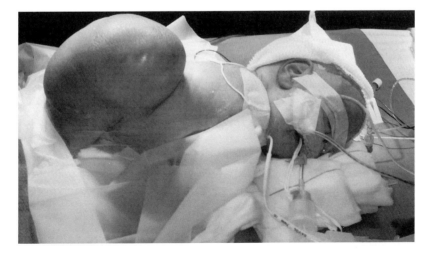

Fig. 34-2. Infant girl with a large thoracolumbar myelocystocele. A closed neural tube defect such as this has no exposed neural tissue. This lesion is fully covered with epithelialized skin.

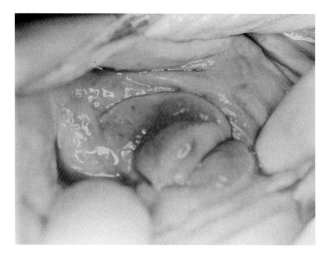

Fig. 34-3. Intraoperative photograph of a myelocystocele with the neural placode in the center. This communicates with the central canal. A separate CSF-filled space is in continuity with the lumbar subarachnoid space.

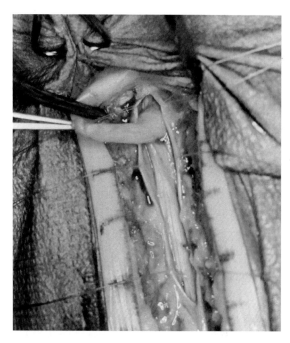

Fig. 34-4. Intraoperative photograph of a thoracolumbar lipoma that starts at the conus medullaris and extends into the filum terminale.

The large majority of closed NTDs are lipomatous malformations that involve neural elements to a varying degree and occur primarily in the lumbar or lumbosacral region (Fig. 34-4). The thoracic spinal cord usually is affected since there is usually a rostral extension of what is primarily a lumbar lesion. Although these defects with an exophytic component are detectable on fetal ultrasound, the AFP level in maternal serum or amniotic fluid is normal because the overlying cutaneous elements are fully epithelialized.

Meningocele

Because what constitutes a meningocele is subject to debate, and because meningoceles are often grouped with myelomeningoceles, it is difficult to know the true incidence.[24] Probably, all dorsal meningoceles are not "pure" in that they contain, either singly or in combination, aberrant nerve roots adherent to the inner wall of the meningocele herniation, occasional ganglion cells, and even a glial nodule that may represent a diverticulum from the central canal of the spinal cord. Even though fragmentary neural elements are beyond the confines of the spinal canal, the spinal cord is not. Because no neural tissue is visible, the sac is fully epithelialized, the Chiari II malformation absent, and the neurological examination usually normal. It appears appropriate to classify meningoceles separately from myelomeningoceles. Also the embryological abnormality does not appear to reflect the same failure of primary neurulation, as is the case of myelomeningoceles. As mentioned, meningoceles have previously been grouped with myelomeningoceles. Therefore, it is difficult to know their actual incidence. In the authors' clinical experience, they appear to be 5% or less than that of myelomeningoceles (Fig. 34-5).

The neurological examination of a child with a meningocele is normal. Because meningoceles do not have exposed neural tissue and do not leak CSF, they can be closed electively. A magnetic resonance imaging (MRI) study of the spinal cord to rule out the presence of any additional anomalies is advocated.

Surgical correction consists of resecting the herniated meninges and intraspinal exploration to make certain that the cord is untethered. This is preferable to ligating the neck of the sac. A limited laminectomy suffices and will not subsequently cause a spinal deformity. The prognosis for this group of infants is excellent, as they have no neurological deficit and are very unlikely to develop one.

Lipomatous Malformations

This category includes all closed thoracic NTDs with excessive lipomatous tissue within or attached

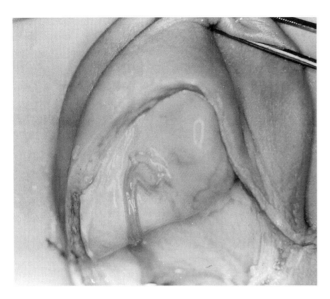

Fig. 34-5. Intraoperative photograph showing the cystic interior of a meningocele containing a diverticulum of abnormal glial tissue. The spinal cord was within the spinal canal.

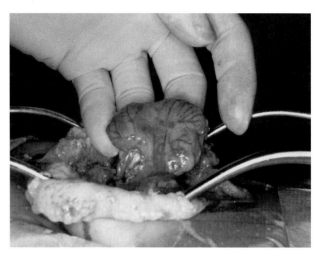

Fig. 34-6. Intraoperative photograph demonstrating an isolated loop of bowel in a teratoma found during the closure of a closed NTD and associated lipomatous malformation.

to the spinal cord. Excluded are those very rare lipomas of the spinal cord in which an actual increase in the number of adipose cells occurs, signaling a true neoplasm rather than a hamartomatous malformation. Lipomatous malformations are by far the most common form of closed spinal NTD and vary from an enlarged filum terminale containing adipose tissue to a huge fatty mass occupying much of the lower thoracolumbosacral region that contains the spinal cord and CSF. These lesions are commonly referred to as lipomyelomeningoceles, but since this group of lesions is one of a continuum with the embryological maldevelopment, clinical findings and prognosis are fairly similar. Therefore it seems more appropriate to refer to this group of closed NTDs as lipomatous malformations since the term "lipomyelomeningocele" can be misleading, implying the faulty concept that a lipomyelomeningocele is a myelomeningocele with fat, which it is definitely not. Usually the lipomatous subcutaneous mass extends through an opening in the fascia and dorsal neural arches, enters the matrix of the spinal cord, and terminates at a fatty fibral glial interface that may be asymmetrical causing the spinal cord to be rotated. Motor and sensory loss in the lower extremities is usually very asymmetrical and corresponds to the more affected side of the spinal cord.

A neurological deficit may or may not be present at birth. If present, invariably one extremity is af-

fected much more than, or even to the exclusion of, the other. As the child grows the deficit often progresses in a most asymmetrical fashion that once again corresponds to the side of the spinal cord with the greater lipomatous mass. Exactly why this occurs is unclear, as it would seem that the tethering mechanism should not favor one side so strongly. Increasing loss of sphincter function indicates bilateral involvement. However, neurological deterioration probably can result from compression of the neural elements by CSF pulsations if a cystic component is present, and more importantly by the lipomatous mass as it enters the spinal canal beneath the partial or completely intact dorsal neural arches. Since the spinal cord is tethered, growth, bending, or any factors that stretch the spinal cord probably produce minute trauma that is cumulative over many years. This may explain the progression of the neurological deficit with time.

Even when a lesion is obvious, it is best to obtain MR imaging to better define the lesion and to exclude additional abnormalities. Operative intervention is advocated early in infancy to ameliorate further loss of neurological function. Surgical correction consists of decompression and untethering of the spinal cord. Using magnified vision, a decompressive laminectomy is undertaken rostrally starting where the dorsal arches are intact. The spinal cord is meticulously separated from the lateral glial fibro-fatty interface on either side until the spinal cord is free (Fig. 34-6). An associated enlarged fatty terminale may be present caudally.

This is also divided. In some cases full untethering of the spinal cord is not possible without dividing viable nerve roots that should not be sacrificed. Most of the excess fatty tissue associated with the spinal cord is removed, with care being taken not to cause neural damage. The lateral glial fibro-fatty interface is then brought together in the midline and approximated with a running absorbable suture. This decreases the surface area via which the spinal cord can retether. Extensive surgical experience with these lesions is needed to achieve optimal surgical results without causing a new neurological deficit.

Spinal deformity is much less of a problem with this group of patients, compared with open NTD. The more severely affected patients are managed with a team approach comparable to that used for patients with a myelomeningocele.

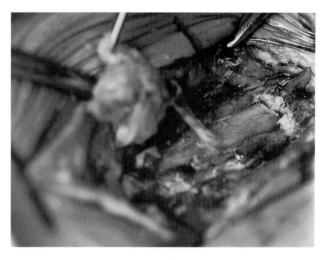

Fig. 34-7. Intraoperative photograph of a patient with a thoracic congenital dermal sinus ending in an intramedullary dermoid cyst. The tract is seen extending from the subcutaneous tissue and entering the dura mater.

Congenital Dermal Sinus

Congenital dermal sinuses are squamous epithelial line tracts that occur in or very near the midline. They are presumed to result from an abnormal persistence of adhesions of cutaneous ectoderm to the NT and thus represent an NTD. The tract can extend from just below the skin surface, or can penetrate and include the central canal of the thoracic spinal cord (Fig. 34-7). Like most NTDs, these lesions are most commonly found in the lumbar and sacral regions, with fewer than 10% involving the thoracic spine.[38] The tract may end in a fibrous band or contain one or more dermal inclusion cysts along its course. These cysts slowly enlarge by continued proliferation of squamous cells with desquamation and sebaceous secretion. The ectoderm that forms a dermoid cyst has the potential to form all layers of the skin.[22] An epidermoid cyst differs from a dermoid cyst in that it does not contain hair, sebaceous glands, or other skin appendages. Congenital inclusion cysts involving the thoracic spine are nearly always dermoid cysts. Those classified as epidermoid cysts are misdiagnosed. Although epidermoid cysts occur most frequently in the region of the cauda equina, they also can be acquired lesions in the thoracic area by implantation of cutaneous elements at the time of lumbar puncture, particularly if the needle does not contain a stylet.

A congenital dermal sinus frequently goes unnoticed until the patient presents with meningitis or an extra or intradural abscess. *Staphylococcus aureus* is the most common infecting organism, with gram-negative bacteria being more frequent with lesions in the lower spinal regions. Several other types of organisms may also be present. A sterile meningitis may occur if the cyst contents rupture into the subarachnoid space. In the absence of infection, a large cyst along the sinus tract can produce compression of surrounding neural structures. Increased resistance of CSF absorption can develop following meningitis and result in hydrocephalus. Neurological sequelae can also occur from tethering of the thoracic spinal cord by a fibrous band or neuroglial mass on its dorsal surface.[38]

On examination, the opening of the sinus may or may not be associated with other cutaneous markers and may be so small that they escape detection except with close inspection. Hairs may be observed protruding from the orifice. Debris or purulent material may drain from the site. The usual hallmarks of local infection may be present or may be completely absent with a deeper abscess or meningitis. Probing the sinus or injecting it with radiopaque contrast medium is of questionable value as a diagnostic procedure. In fact, it is contraindicated because it may incite infection or cause neural damage.

Because the tract is small, the mesoderm about the sinus usually has migrated normally during embryological development, resulting in minimal or no structural deficits to the dorsal arches. Routine radiographs of the spine may show incomplete formation of a dorsal neural arch, or the arch may be completely normal if the tract enters between the spinous processes or creates a bony passageway too small to be seen. The presence of a large dermoid cyst widens the spinal canal like any other similarly located lesion. MRI is the diagnostic modality of choice, because it best defines the anatomy. A sinus extending into the thoracic spinal cord may not be visualized unless it contains a neuroglial mass or cyst. Thus a negative imaging study does not exclude the need to explore the tract.

Treatment consists of surgically exploring the tract to its terminus and completely excising it, along with any dermal inclusions. A sinus extending to the surface of the dura mater requires an intradural exploration because the tract can continue into the subarachnoid space. If meningitis is present, surgical intervention should be delayed until the patient receives a course of appropriate antibiotic therapy. Treatment of a subcutaneous or extra- or intradural abscess may require drainage in addition to antibiotic therapy. In the presence of infection, it may be advisable to limit the procedure to drainage of purulent material and delay the removal of the remaining tract or cyst capsule until the inflammation has subsided. The most important factor influencing prognosis in these lesions is the performance of a total excision prior to infection. The vertebral bodies are normal and spinal column instability is not a problem.

Split Cord Malformations

"Diastematomyelia" is a term used to describe the malformation in which the spinal cord is split into two hemicords, each having a single set of dorsal and ventral nerve roots, and each contained within its own dural sheath (Figs. 34-8, 34-9, and 34-10). Diplomyelia, on the other hand, indicates that the two spinal cord segments are completely duplicated, with four sets of dorsal and ventral nerve roots present in a single dural sheath. Recent investigations have found that diastematomyelia and diplomyelia represent opposite ends of a continuum with few, if any, "true" examples at either end.[10,20,28] The pathological and embryological processes that result in NTDs are least understood in diastematomyelia[12] and the most likely to be associated with other abnormalities.[15,24,37] Because this group of

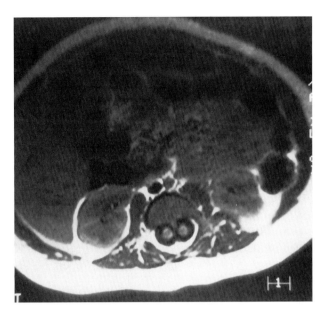

Fig. 34-8. Axial CT of a split cord malformation in a 1-year-old girl. Note the two dural sleeves encasing each spinal segment, with an associated bony spur between.

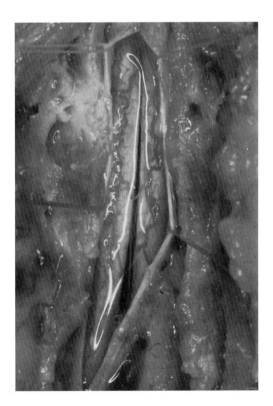

Fig. 34-9. Intraoperative photograph showing the two hemicords enclosed in a single dural sleeve. In this case there is no bone spur, but adhesions may tether the spinal cords.

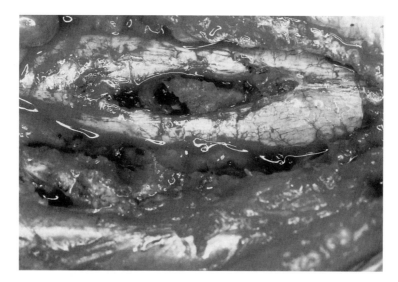

Fig. 34-10. Intraoperative photograph of a thoracic level bony spur protruding between separated spinal cord segments, each fully enclosed in dural sheath.

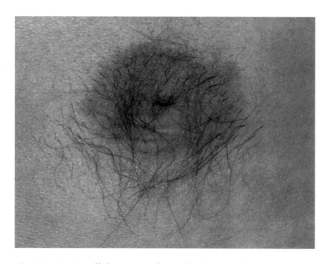

Fig. 34-11. Small hairy patch in the lower thoracic region, associated with a congenital dermal sinus and split cord malformation.

malformations appears to stem from a common embryological disorder, a strong argument has been made that the terms "diastematomyelia" and "diplomyelia" should be abandoned in favor of collectively calling these lesions "split cord malformations." The most common location for diastematomyelia is the lumbar region with the thoracic spinal cord being involved in one fourth of reported cases.[15,24] Split cord malformations differ from other NTDs in that approximately three fourths of the affected patients are female. Various cutaneous markers can be present, however, hypertrichosis

(Fig. 34-11) is frequently associated with split cord malformations. Neurological abnormalities are similar to those found with lipomatous malformations. Because segmental abnormalities of the vertebral bodies are present, including hemivertebrae, butterfly vertebrae, and block vertebrae, many patients are initially investigated for progressive scoliosis or kyphosis. Additional vertebral column structural changes include narrowed intervertebral disc spaces, a widened interpedicular space, and abnormal laminae that may be thickened or fused to adjacent segments.

Pang[28] has divided split cord malformations into two groups; the first includes those with two separate dural sheaths and the second includes those in which the split cord elements are contained within the same dural sheath. The spinal column abnormalities are generally more significant in split cord malformations in which two separate dural sheaths are present, and between which a bony or cartilaginous spur extends ventrally, dorsally, or forms a complete ventrodorsal bridge. Diagnostic evaluation includes MRI and, in selected cases, computed tomography (CT). Imaging studies also help to note the presence of any additional associated lesions, such as a neurenteric cyst.

Treatment consists of a laminectomy, at least one level above and below the area of deformity. If a bony spur is present, it should be removed until it is flush with the ventral surface of the spinal column. This is followed by resection of the surround-

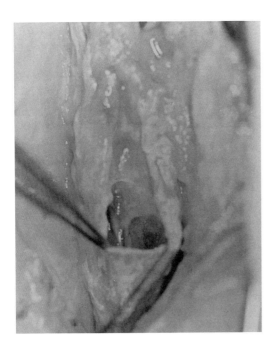

Fig. 34-12. Intraoperative exposure of a neurenteric cyst found during the untethering of a previously repaired open NTD.

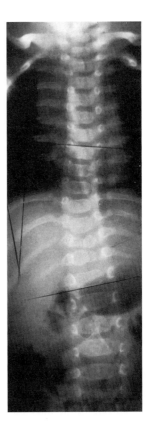

Fig. 34-13. Anteroposterior (AP) radiograph showing abnormal body segmentation associated with the neurenteric cyst in Fig. 34-12.

ing dural sleeve and lysis of any adhesions that may be present. No attempt is made to close the dura mater ventrally. The dorsal dura mater is approximated over the dorsal surface of the spinal cord. When both segments of the spinal cord are within the same dural sheath, exploration is undertaken to divide tethering fibrous adhesions to either the ventral or the dorsal surface of the spinal cord. Any additional tethering lesions, such as an enlarged filum terminale, etc., are also addressed during the same operative procedure.

Neurenteric Cysts

Neurenteric cysts may or may not be associated with other forms of closed NTDs such as split cord malformations (Figs. 34-12, 34-13, and 34-14). Those not associated with other forms of closed NTDs are the ones most likely, as a group, to involve the thoracic spine. In these lesions, endodermal tissue is displaced into the spinal canal and may or may not retain communication with an associated intrathoracic cyst or enteric duplication. The nature of the embryological abnormality that produces this defect is a matter of some debate.[12]

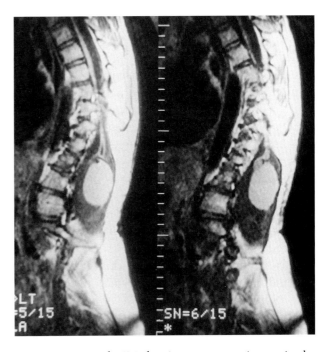

Fig. 34-14. Sagittal MRI showing a neurenteric cyst in the thoracolumbar region in a young boy who had an open NTD closed at birth. Also present is a split cord malformation.

The histology of the cysts varies. Enterogenous cysts are most likely a part of this group,[14] while it is difficult to know whether to include teratomatous cysts. In the absence of another NTD, the dorsal arches are normal and cutaneous markers absent. The ventrally located cyst may be extra- or intradural; if intradural, the cyst can be either extra- or intramedullary. The vertebrae may be normal, without a ventral defect. More frequently, however, a circular or butterfly defect is detected in the vertebral bodies. The interpedicular distance can be widened, and additional segmental abnormalities may be present, particularly if the lesion is associated with a split cord malformation. Histologically, the cysts are lined by a single layer of cuboidal epithelium similar to that found in the respiratory or gastrointestinal tract. The cysts slowly enlarge by the secretion of mucinous material that causes compression to the adjacent neural structures.

Infants who have large intrathoracic cysts may present at birth with compression of the esophagus or tracheobronchial tree. An associated neurenteric cyst within the spinal canal may come to light secondary to spinal cord compression or from aseptic meningitis. Diagnostic imaging is similar to other closed NTDs. The surgical approach is individualized, depending upon the extent of the associated malformations.

Arachnoid Cysts

Arachnoid cysts may have either an intra- or extradural location. Because their pathophysiology, clinical findings, and management are similar, it seems appropriate to consider them together (Figs. 34-15, 34-16, and 34-17). Intradural arachnoid cysts appear to result from an alteration in the arachnoid trabeculae, and extradural cysts from a congenital defect that allows the arachnoid membrane to herniate through the adjacent dura mater. With rare exception, arachnoid cysts of both types are located dorsally or dorsalaterally within the spinal canal. Although usually single, they can be multiple and are distributed fairly evenly over the thoracic spine. Extradural cysts have a pedicle that connects to the sub rachnoid space. The nature of the connection of the intradural cyst is less apparent. In virtually every case, the fluid within the arachnoid cyst has the appearance and chemical composition of that of CSF. This indicates that

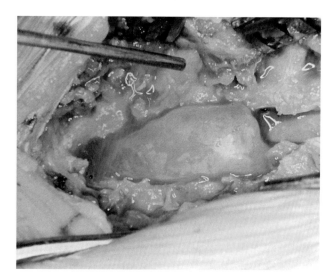

Fig. 34-15. Intraoperative photograph showing a large extradural arachnoid cyst.

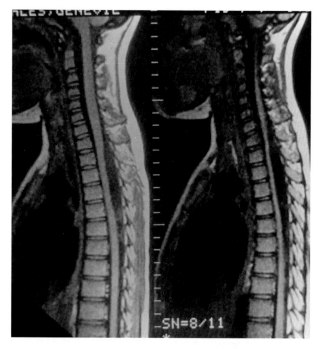

Fig. 34-16. Sagittal MRI showing an extradural arachnoid cyst compressing the thoracic spinal cord.

there must be a free communication with CSF and the subarachnoid space. Otherwise, the fluid within the cyst would have a higher protein content. One would anticipate that a loss of communication between the cyst and the subarachnoid space would cause a cyst to involute, and thus not

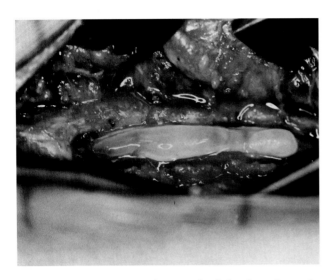

Fig. 34-17. Intraoperative photograph of the thoracic arachnoid cyst shown in Fig. 34-16, prior to fenestration.

enlarge and become symptomatic. If on myelography the cyst is not filled on first visualization, it almost always will enhance thereafter. The wall of an extradural arachnoid cyst is generally thicker than its intradural counterpart. Both contain arachnoid cells and collagen, and some contain arachnoid granulations and calcification.

Heredity rarely plays a part in the genesis of arachnoid cysts. One report exists of a familial intradural arachnoid cyst[1] and there are a few reports of familial cysts located extradurally.[4,7,31,33] The group with familial extradural arachnoid cysts, thought to represent autosomal dominance with variable penetrance, was associated with districhiasis (a double row of eyelashes) and lymphedema of the lower extremities.

The dominant symptom noted with arachnoid cysts of the thoracic region is progressive lower extremity weakness, often symmetrical, that can occasionally result in paralysis if not treated. Pain is generally not a prominent feature, although local tenderness and radiculopathy may be present. Sensory findings and sphincter disturbance are variable and usually not striking. Long tract signs are usually present. Even though symptoms may be noted for several years or longer, arachnoid cysts in the thoracic region often do not come to medical attention early. Before the advent of more sophisticated imaging techniques, patients with chronic and progressive symptoms from arachnoid cysts were often misdiagnosed as having multiple sclerosis, particularly when the extent of symptoms fluctuates.

Extradural thoracic arachnoid cysts can be associated with epiphyseal aseptic necrosis and ventral wedging of the adjacent vertebral bodies (Scheuermann's disease), leading to kyphosis.[41] A recent report has also found arachnoid cysts to be associated with open and closed spinal NTDs.[29] Some of these cysts appear to be congenital, while others may be acquired and secondary to CSF flow abnormalities associated with open NTDs.

MRI is the initial imaging modality of choice, followed if necessary by CT-myelography. Arachnoid cysts that are large enough to produce symptoms may or may not have enlarged the surrounding spinal canal. However, the presence or absence of such a finding is of limited clinical significance.

Treatment of symptomatic arachnoid cysts is surgical, since aspiration provides only temporary relief. Cysts in an extradural location are easily removed in their entirety after identifying and ligating the neck. Adequate fenestration of an intradural arachnoid cyst can be readily accomplished by removing much of its thin wall. The ventral portion, intimate with the pia mater of the surface of the spinal cord is best left intact. The prognosis for patients with these cysts is excellent and recovery dramatic if irreversible spinal cord damage has not occurred.

Perineurial Cysts

Spinal perineurial cysts, first described by Tarlov,[40] arise between the pial covering of the nerve root and the surrounding arachnoid membrane. Rarely symptomatic, these cysts are found in the region of the cauda equina and, very infrequently, in the thoracic region.

Meningeal Cysts

Meningeal cysts or diverticula are usually incidental findings on imaging studies or at autopsy. These outpouchings of the dura mater and arachnoid probably result in congenital dural defects in the region of the dorsal root ganglia. That meningeal cysts are observed in adults, and not in children, supports the contention that they slowly enlarge with time. They also appear to be influenced by a hydrostatic force generated by an erect position, because the lower their location on the spinal axis, the larger their size. Rarely do meningeal cysts produce symptoms, but if present, they are usually referable to the sacral region.[39]

Wilkins,[39] in his review of ventral and lateral thoracic meningoceles, noted that 95% are lateral. It is not known if the ventral 5% are a result of failure of normal midline closure. Approximately two thirds of thoracic meningoceles are associated with neurofibromatosis, the connecting link appearing to be regional dysplasia of the vertebral column that allows the initial outpouching of the meninges. In lateral intrathoracic meningoceles, the dura mater and arachnoid herniate through a single or, less frequently, coalescent foramina into the retropleural space of the dorsal mediastinum. The level of involvement is evenly distributed within the thoracic spine, and if a spinal deformity is present, the meningocele is located at its apex.

The meningocele is filled with CSF and slowly enlarges by eroding and displacing adjacent structures. Of those reported, approximately one third are asymptomatic, the abnormality having been noted on routine chest radiographs, one third have local back or chest pains, and the remaining one third have pulmonary or neurological symptoms. The diagnosis is established via MRI and CT–myelography. If symptomatic, the pedicle of the meningocele is ligated and the wall fenestrated.

Intramedullary Cysts

A cyst within the white matter of the thoracic spinal cord and not lined by ependyma is, by definition, termed "syringomyelia." The fluid within the cyst has a high protein concentration and is thereby xanthrochromic. This indicates a very restricted communication to the CSF and the subarachnoid space. These cysts can be associated with neoplasms, posttraumatic hematomyelia, or an occult inflammatory process (Fig. 34-18).

Dilatation of the ependymal-lined central canal is termed "hydromyelia." The fluid within this cavity has a protein content similar to CSF and is not xanthrochromic. This indicates an unrestricted communication with CSF and the subarachnoid space. With progressive dilatation of the central spinal canal, the cyst often extends beyond the limits of the ependymal lining into the white matter of the spinal cord, thereby becoming a combination of hydromyelia and syringomyelia. This occurrence is best termed "hy-

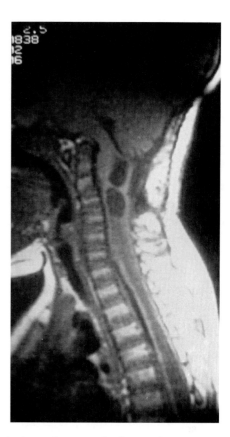

Fig. 34-18. Sagittal T1-weighted MRI showing a cervicothoracic multiloculated holocord syrinx.

drosyringomyelia." Nevertheless, the fluid in the hydrosyringomyelic cavity is crystal clear, with the protein content the same as that of CSF and the adjacent subarachnoid space, indicating nonrestricted communication. This communication most likely takes place via the central canal or through the extracellular fluid space of the spinal cord parenchyma.

The pathophysiological process that produces hydromyelia or hydrosyringomyelia, according to Williams,[42] is an intermittent pressure differential that results from restriction of normal CSF flow between the cranial and spinal compartments. A thoracic spinal cord syrinx often extends into the cervical region, and results from impairment of normal CSF flow at the cervicomedullary junction in conjunction with either a Chiari I or Chiari II malformation. Further discussion of thoracic syringomyelia is beyond the scope of this chapter, but has been well reviewed by Oakes.[27]

Miscellaneous Cysts

Intra- or extradural cysts secondary to a chronic hematoma are rarely found in conjunction with hemophilia or an arteriovenous malformation (AVM). Hemorrhage into the spinal canal most often results in an acute progressive spinal cord compression with a rapid loss of neurological function. In rare instances, the course may be chronic, allowing the hematoma to organize into a fluid-filled sac, with the etiology not apparent until the time of operation.[36,40]

Teratomatous cysts not associated with an NTD are very rare intraspinal lesions, if one excludes sacrococcygeal teratomas. Teratomatous cysts are dorsally located within the spinal canal and may represent displacement of germ cells during their migration from the yolk sac to the gonadal ridges. Those cysts usually become apparent in the second or third decade of life, when they enlarge sufficiently to compress adjacent neural structures.

VASCULAR MALFORMATIONS

Vascular malformations of the thoracic spine are developmental disorders that may go undetected for decades. Vascular lesions of the spine are correspondingly rare and take any form, be it aneurysmal, arterial, arteriovenous, or venous, with the arteriovenous form being the most common (Figs. 34-19 and 34-20). Aita[2] reports that fewer than 5% of patients with intraspinal vascular lesions have an associated cutaneous angioma of the torso, which may or may not be segmentally related. Current embryological understanding of the development of the primitive vascular network does not explain the variation in architecture, location, and depth of the metametric angiomatosis.

The vascular neurocutaneous disorder involving the spinal cord is usually known as Klippel-Trenaunay-Weber syndrome in the United States, while in Europe it is called Cobb syndrome.[18] Cobb[8] in 1915 reported a case of an 8-year-old boy with clinical evidence of lower thoracic spinal cord compression and a segmentally related cutaneous angioma. This patient was seen by Cushing, who suggested that the patient might have vascular malformation of the underlying spinal cord, an observation subsequently confirmed at operation. Cushing is also reported to have said that he observed an analogous situation involving the face and the ipsilateral cerebral hemisphere (i.e., encephalotrigeminal angiomatosis).[8] Whether the Cobb or the Klippel-Trenaunay-Weber syndrome is

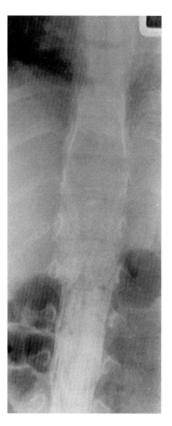

Fig. 34-19. AP radiograph showing enlargement of the thoracic spinal canal with thinning of the pedicle secondary to the presence of a large spinal cord aneurysm.

a spinal form of Sturge-Webber syndrome is subject to debate. Apparently no family history of the syndrome has been reported.

Aminoff and Edwards[3] note that spinal cord AVMs in children differ from those found in adults in several important aspects.

1. The incidence of subarachnoid hemorrhage is over 50% in children, while in adults it is about 10%.
2. The malformation tends to be more rostral along the spinal axis in children.
3. The fistulous portion of the lesion in children is more frequently located ventral to the spinal cord and can have a more extensive intramedullary course.
4. AVMs in children often have multiple feeders, some of which also supply the spinal cord.

These factors make AVMs in children more difficult to treat surgically without causing additional damage to the spinal cord. Probably no difference exists embryologically between adults and children with regard to spinal cord vascular lesions, but the

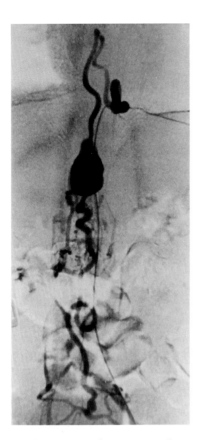

Fig. 34-20. Spinal angiogram documenting the presence of a large thoracic spinal cord aneurysm. This was successfully treated with interventional balloon occlusion of the parent artery.

high flow and pressure lead to clinical symptoms sooner.

NEOPLASMS
Intramedullary Neoplasm

Rarely is a congenital intramedullary abnormality of the thoracic spinal cord not associated with an NTD. It is exceedingly rare for intramedullary neoplasms of the spinal cord to be symptomatic at birth (Figs. 34-21, 34-22, and 34-23). In two large series of pediatric spine tumors there is no mention of tumors of the spinal cord that were symptomatic at birth.[11,24] Von Hippel-Lindau disease is a neurocutaneous syndrome that is transmitted as an autosomal dominant trait with variable penetrance and delayed expression. In von Hippel-Lindau disease, hemangioblastomas are found in the cerebellum, spinal cord, and medulla in decreasing order of frequency.[23,32] Hemangioblastomas of the spinal cord may occur in 50% of these patients,[9] although they are not necessarily symptomatic. Interestingly, there is no reported case of a segmental cutaneous angioma being associated with a spinal cord hemangioblastoma. Symptoms from hemangioblastoma are very rare in childhood, usually first appearing in young and middle-aged adults.

Neurofibromatosis is associated with an increased incidence of tumors of the entire nervous

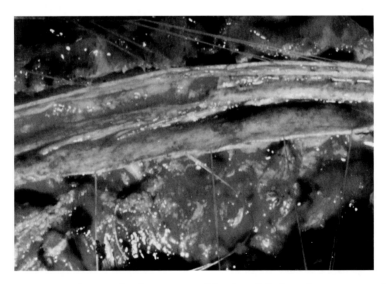

Fig. 34-21. Intraoperative photograph of an 11-year-old girl with holocord astrocytoma during resection. To the right of the middle of the picture, the astrocytoma has been removed, leaving a shell of the spinal cord.

system and its coverings, including intramedullary spinal cord neoplasms. Intramedullary spinal cord metastases (extension) have also been found following the documentation and treatment of primary CNS tumors (Fig. 34-24).

Intramedullary lipomas of the thoracic spinal cord not associated with an NTD are very rare congenital lesions that may first become manifest during rapid growth or excessive weight gain.[11] If symptomatic, they can be surgically debulked. Total removal is unnecessary and possibly hazardous. In a recent series of six patients, most had marked neurological deficits upon initial evaluation. Two patients had cervicothoracic tumors and one had a

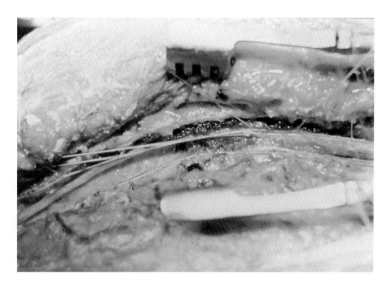

Fig. 34-22. Intraoperative photograph of a holocord astrocytoma during resection.

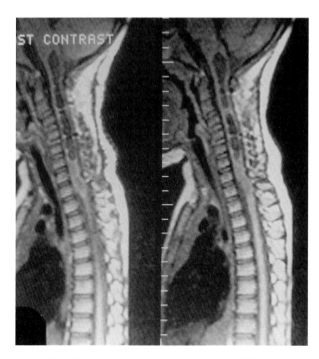

Fig. 34-23. T1-weighted sagittal post-contrast MRIs of the cervical and thoracic spine, showing the presence of multilevel and loculated syrinx associated with spinal cord astrocytoma.

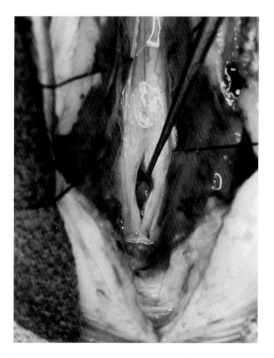

Fig. 34-24. Intraoperative photograph of an intramedullary spinal cord ependymoma.

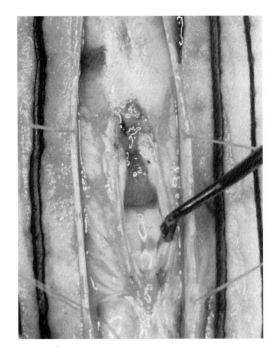

Fig. 34-25. Intraoperative photograph showing extension of a primitive neuroectodermal tumor down the central canal.

thoracic tumor. All patients underwent subtotal, decompressive resections of their lesions. Though all patients had resolution of their pain, none had improvement following surgical resection.[20]

Extramedullary Neoplasms

In adults, the majority of extramedullary intradural tumors are meningiomas and nerve sheath neoplasms. In children, the most common tumor in this location is via seeding of the subarachnoid space from an intracranial tumor, which, on occasion, can be present at birth. Occasionally spinal cord compression from subarachnoid seeding is the first manifestation of an intracranial tumor, the most common of which is a primitive neuroectodermal tumor (Fig. 34-25).

Nerve sheath tumors and meningiomas of the thoracic spinal canal are infrequently found in childhood. If they are found, neurofibromatosis should be the first consideration (Figs. 34-26 and 34-27). Neurofibromas can be solitary, multiple, or plexiform, and either intradural or extradural, or a combination of both. Pigmented plexiform neurofibromas of the neck and trunk often extend into the spinal canal, especially if there is surface extension of the lesion to

the midline.[30] In children, the intra- and extradural (dumbbell) extension of a tumor is always indicative of a neurofibroma. No report of a dumbbell-shaped meningioma in a child has yet been made.[19]

Deformity of the spine may be the first manifestation of a neurofibroma, but abnormal spinal curvature in the absence of tumor is also common in neurofibromatosis. Enlargement of a neural foramen is suggestive of a nerve sheath tumor, but this finding may be observed without the presence of tumor in neurofibromatosis.

The diagnostic imaging modality of choice is MRI, supplemented by CT and CT-myelography if necessary. If an extramedullary tumor of the thoracic spinal cord is present, imaging of the entire CNS is often advisable, as multiple tumors are frequently found if the underlying problem is neurofibromatosis. Treatment is surgical removal of tumor. The spinal cord is decompressed before removing the portion of the tumor that, if present, extends beyond the spinal canal and may require an additional surgical approach. Radiation or chemotherapy should rarely be considered. These treatments are usually reserved for those tumors that undergo malignant transformation. This is a particular risk for patients with neurofibromatosis.

Extramedullary lipomas, like their intramedullary counterparts, are rare when not part of an NTD. They enlarge very slowly and usually do not become symptomatic until adulthood.

Neuroblastoma is the most common intra-abdominal malignancy of childhood. It may be manifest at birth with thoracic spinal cord compression secondary to extension of the tumor through the neural foramina into the epidural space.[16] Treatment is laminectomy for spinal cord decompression followed by chemotherapy. The prognosis is favorable, and, contrary to most CNS tumors, the younger the patient, the better the outlook. A child with an abdominal thoracic paraspinal mass should have MRI and/or CT to rule out intraspinal extension.

Adults with spinal cord compression from malignant neoplasm have a neurological outcome that appears to be similar when comparing surgical decompression plus radiation therapy to radiation therapy alone. Thus surgical intervention is often not justified in the adult, especially since the operative procedure does not prolong survival and carries with it a risk of significant morbidity and mortality. Children, by comparison, have minimal surgical mortal-

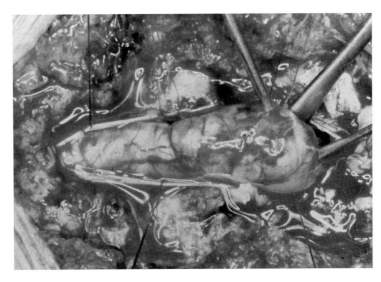

Fig. 34-26. Intraoperative photograph of a 13-year-old girl with neurofibromatosis, showing an intradural thoracic neurofibroma.

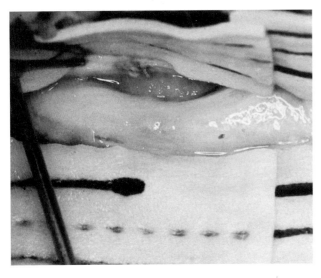

Fig. 34-27. Intraoperative photograph of a young boy with neurofibromatosis, showing meningiomas compressing the spinal cord.

ity and morbidity because the younger patient group is generally in good health at the outset and has less widespread disease. Most tumors in the pediatric age group reach the spinal canal via the intravertebral foramen from a local paravertebral neoplasm, rather than by hematogenous or lymphatic dissemination. The vertebral column destruction in children is usually minimal, reducing the need for reconstruction following tumor resection. Surgical decompression, followed by adjuvant radiation and/or chemother-

apy, results in a better outcome than radiation therapy alone in the pediatric age group with significant spinal cord compression from epidural malignant disease.[26]

NEUROLOGICAL SEQUELAE

Many neurologically significant structural deformities of the thoracic spinal column are associated with NTDs. There are, however, another group of anomalies in which multiple vertebral abnormalities are present that may be hereditary in nature. Failure of formation and segmentation of the vertebrae early in development can lead to clinical deformities that have neurological sequelae. Spinal cord compression is most often observed in structural defects that produce kyphosis, since dorsal angulation of the spine is most likely to compromise the spinal canal.[13]

Embryological segmental maldevelopment can lead to hypoplastic or absent thoracic or lumbar vertebrae.[34] The nerve roots adjacent to the bony deformity are either dysplastic or lacking in a condition referred to as segmental spinal dysgenesis. The neurological deficit distal to the segmental dysgenesis can be partial or complete. The lower extremities are often deformed. The loss of neurological function, if present, can occur secondary to rapidly increasing kyphosis from an unstable spine. Decompressive laminectomy in this situation adds to the lack of spinal stability. Thus a ventral approach is more advisable to decompress the spinal cord and stabilize the spinal column, if necessary.

The VATER association encompasses a number of congenital anomalies consisting of vertebral defects, anal atresia, tracheoesophageal fistula, radial dysplasia, renal anomalies, and congenital heart defects. The common pathogenesis for this association is unclear. Although neurological involvement is uncommon, it is observed in some cases.

In achondroplasia, spinal cord compression usually occurs either caudal or rostral to the spinal cord segment within the thoracic region. Thoracic spinal cord compression can occur in the spinal canal if this location is congenitally stenotic, particularly in the sagittal plane, secondary to stunted pedicles and further compromised by hypertrophic intervertebral discs. With aging, the stenosis can be further exacerbated by osteoarthritic spurs, disc degeneration, and thoracic kyphosis.[25]

As noted, a severe form of kyphoscoliosis in the cervical and thoracic region is commonly observed in neurofibromatosis, regardless of the presence or absence of a neurofibroma. Such marked deformities, unless aggressively treated, can lead to paralysis secondary to spinal cord compression.[6] Spinal cord compression and injury may be secondary to dysplasia of the vertebral bodies alone or associated with an eroding neurofibroma.

REFERENCES

1. Arabi B, Paternak G, Hurko O, et al. Familial intradural arachnoid cysts: Report of two cases. J Neurosurg 50:826-829, 1979.
2. Aita JA. Miscellaneous neurocutaneous diseases. In Vinkin PJ, Bruyn GW, eds. Handbook of Clinical Neurology: The Phakomatoses. New York: Elsevier, 1972; pp 772-806.
3. Aminoff MJ, Edwards MSB. Spinal arteriovenous malformations. In Edwards MSB, Hoffman HJ, eds. Cerebral Vascular Disease in Children and Adolescents. Baltimore: Williams & Wilkins, 1989, pp 321-341.
4. Bergland RM. Congenital intraspinal extradural cyst: Report of three cases in one family. J Neurosurg 28:495-499, 1968.
5. Brock DJH, Sutcliffe RG. Alpha-fetoprotein in the antenatal diagnosis of anencephaly and spina bifida. Lancet 2:197, 1972.
6. Chaglassian JH, Riseborough EG, Hall JE. Neurofibromatosis scoliosis: Natural history and results of treatment in thirty-seven cases. J Bone Joint Surg 58A:695-702, 1976.
7. Cynn K-Y. Congenital spinal extradural cyst in two siblings. AJR 101:204-215, 1967.
8. Cobb S. Haemangioma of the spinal cord associated with skin naevi of the same metamere. Ann Surg 62:641-649, 1915.
9. Cohen ME, Duffner PK. Von Hippel-Lindau disease. In Hoffman HJ, Epstein F, eds. Disorders of the Developing Ner-

vous System: Diagnosis and Treatment. Boston: Blackwell Scientific, pp 625-634, 1986.
10. Dias MS, Pang D. Split cord malformations. Neurosurg Clin North Am 6:339-358, 1995.
11. Epstein FJ, Wisoff JH. Intramedullary tumors of the spinal cord. In: McLaurin RL, Schut L, Venes JL, et al., eds. Pediatric Neurosurgery: Surgery of the Developing Nervous System. 2nd ed. Philadelphia: WB Saunders, 1989, 428-442.
12. French BN. Abnormal development of the central nervous system. In McLaurin RL, Schut L, Venes JL, et al., eds. Pediatric Neurosurgery: Surgery of the Developing Nervous System, 2nd ed. Philadelphia: WB Saunders, pp 9-34, 1989.
13. Gillespie R, Heydemann J. Congenital spinal deformities: An orthopedic perspective. In Hoffman HJ, Epstein F, eds. Disorders of the Developing Nervous System: Diagnosis and Treatment. Boston: Blackwell Scientific, pp 465-480, 1986.
14. Guilburd JN, Arieh YB, Peyser E. Spinal intradural enterogenous cyst: Report of a case. Surg Neurol 14:359-362, 1980.
15. Guthkelch AN. Diastematomyelia. In Wilkins RH, Rengachary SS, eds. Neurosurgery. New York: McGraw-Hill, pp 2058-2061, 1985.
16. Hrabovsky E, Jones B. Congenital intraspinal neuroblastoma. Am J Child 133:73-75, 1979.
17. James CCM, Lassman LP. Spinal Dysraphism: Spina Bifida Occulta. London: Butterworth, 1972.
18. Kissel P, Dureux JB. Cobb syndrome: Cutaneomeningospinal angiomatosis. In Vinkin PJ, Bruyn GW, eds. Handbook of Clinical Neurology: The Phakomatoses. New York: Elsevier, 1972, pp 429-445.
19. Klein DM. Extramedullary spinal tumors. In McLaurin RL, Schut L, Venes JL, et al., eds. Pediatric Neurosurgery: Surgery of the Developing Nervous System, 2nd ed. Philadelphia: WB Saunders,1989, pp 443-452.
20. Lee M, Rezai AR, Abbott R, et al. Intramedullary spinal cord lipomas. J Neurosurg 82:394-400, 1995.
21. Lemire RJ, Loeser JD, Leech RW, et al. Normal and abnormal Development of the Human Nervous System. Hagerstown, Md.: Harper & Row, 1975.
22. Manno NJ, Uihlein A, Kernohan JW. Intraspinal epidermoids. J Neurosurg 19:754-765, 1962.
23. Martuza RL. Neurofibromatosis and other phakomatoses. In Wilkins RH, Rengachary SS, eds. Neurosurgery. New York: McGraw-Hill, 1985, pp 511-521.
24. Matson DD. Neurosurgery of Infancy and Childhood, 2nd ed. Springfield, Ill.: Charles C Thomas, 1969.
25. Morgan DF, Young RF. Spinal neurological complications of achondroplasia: Results of surgical treatment. J Neurosurg 52:463-472, 1980.
26. Neave VCD, McComb JG. Treatment of spinal epidural metastasis in children. In Marlin AE, ed. Concepts of Pediatric Neurosurgery. Basel: S Karger, 1989, pp 153-160.
27. Oakes WJ. Chiari malformations, hydromyelia, syringomyelia. In Wilkins RH, Rengachary SS, eds. Neurosurgery. New York: McGraw-Hill, 1985, pp 2102-2124.
28. Pang D. Surgical complications of open spinal dysraphism. Neurosurg Clin North Am 6:243-257, 1995.
29. Rabb CH, McComb JG, Raffel C, et al. Spinal arachnoid cysts in the pediatric age group: An association with neural tube defects. J Neurosurg 77:369-372, 1992.
30. Riccardi VM. Von Rechlinghausen neurofibromatosis. N Engl J Med 305:1617-1626, 1981.

31. Robinow M, Johnson GF, Verhagen AD. Distichiasis-lymphedema: A hereditary syndrome of multiple congenital defects. Am J Dis Child 119:343-347, 1970.

32. Schut L, Duhaime A-C, Sutton LN. Phakomatosis: Surgical considerations. In McLaurin RL, Schut L, Venes JL, et al., eds. Pediatric Neurosurgery: Surgery of the Developing Nervous System, 2nd ed. Philadelphia: WB Saunders, 1989, pp 453-462.

33. Schwartz JF, O'Brien MS, Hoffman JC Jr. Hereditary spinal arachnoid cysts, distichiasis, and lymphedema. Am Neurol 7:340-343, 1980.

34. Scott RM, Wolpert SM, Bartoshesky LE, et al. Segmental spinal dysgenesis. Neurosurgery 22:739-744, 1988.

35. Smithells RW, Sheppard S, Schorah CJ. Possible prevention of neural tube defects by periconceptional vitamin supplementation. Lancet 1:647, 1980.

36. Stanley P, McComb JG. Chronic spinal epidural hematoma in hemophilia A in a child. Pediatr Radiol 13:241-243, 1983.

37. Ugarte N, Gonzalez-Curssi F, Sotelo-Avila C. Diastematomyelia associated with teratomas: Report of two cases. J Neurosurg 53:720-725, 1980.

38. Venger B, Laurent JP, Cheek WR. Congenital thoracic dermal sinus tract. In Marlin AE, ed. Concepts of Pediatric Neurosurgery. Basel: Karger, 1989; pp 161-172.

39. Wilkins RH. Lateral and anterior spinal meningoceles. In Wilkins RH, Rengachary SS, eds. Neurosurgery. New York: McGraw-Hill, 1985, pp 2070-2075.

40. Wilkins RH, Odom GL. Spinal intradural cysts. In Vinken PJ, Bruyn GW, eds. Handbook of Clinical Neurology. II. Tumours of the Spine and Spinal Cord. New York: Elsevier, 1976, pp 55-102.

41. Wilkins RH, Odom GL. Spinal extradural cysts. In Vinken PJ, Bruyn GW, eds. Handbook of Clinical Neurology, II: Tumours of the Spine and Spinal Cord. New York: Elsevier, 1976, pp 137-175.

42. Williams B. Simultaneous cerebral and spinal fluid pressure recordings. II. Cerebrospinal dissociation with lesions at the foramen magnum. Acta Neurochir (Wien) 59:123-142, 1981.

Overview of the Spinal Cord Injury Patient

Ranjan S. Roy, M.D., Ph.D.

Paraplegia resulting from thoracic spinal cord injury is a problem of major public health proportions in the United States. It is a catastrophic event that disrupts the quality of life of the injured and their family members and friends. The long-term sequelae of such injuries are devastating and the demands on public resources generated as a result of the disability are high. Optimal treatment includes minimizing the progression of spinal cord injury, avoiding nonneurological complications, and providing an environment that will maximize neural recovery. This chapter reviews the epidemiology, pathophysiology, and contemporary management of spinal cord injury. It also includes functional spinal cord syndromes that may result from incomplete injuries and the basis of neurological classification of spinal cord injury. Finally, promising new drugs that may alter the response to injury and improve outcome in both experimental models and patients and issues that pertain to surgical decompression and stabilization are discussed.

EPIDEMIOLOGY

The yearly incidence of spinal cord injury in the United States ranges from 28 to 50 per million with an estimated 30 to 32 per million survivors. Approximately 11,000 new cases occur each year [27] and the number of persons actually living with spinal cord injury nationally is estimated to be between 300,000 to 500,000.[34] The last decade has seen a significant rise in the prevalence of spine injured patients. Increased survivorship is largely attributed to tremendous improvements in medical, surgical, and prehospital care.

The distribution of the level of spinal cord injury at the time of admission was recently reported from a trauma center in Colorado.[34] Of 358 persons admitted between 1986 and 1989, 52% involved injury to the cervical spine, 31% to the thoracic spine, and the remainder (17%) to the lumbar and sacral segments. Within the thoracic spine, 20% suffered injury in the lower segment (T7 to T12) and 11% in the upper segment (T1 to T6). The incidence of quadraplegia from cervical injuries and paraplegia primarily from thoracic injuries are about the same and is estimated to be around 40%.

With respect to long-term outcomes, those with cervical injuries fared better than persons with more caudal lesions. Regardless of their initial Frankel class, 36% with cervical injuries improved at least one or more grade. A similar recovery was observed in only 24% of those with paraplegia or paraparesis within the same time frame.

Spinal cord injury occurs primarily in the young population with a 4:1 male to female ratio.[62] Approximately 60% occur in individuals in the 16- to

30-year age group. Most injuries are a consequence of motor vehicle accidents (50%), followed by falls (21%), acts of violence (14%), and sports-related activities (14%).[24] Although spinal cord injury patients are usually young, certain etiologies account for more injuries in some age groups than in others. Traffic accidents are fairly evenly distributed across the ages with a slight decrease in frequency with increasing age. Injuries due to falls are more commonly seen in the older population. The incidence of paraplegia and quadriplegia is fairly similar as a result of traffic accidents and falls up until the age of 60. Beyond this age, a higher proportion become quadriplegic.[62] Injuries resulting from acts of violence are most common in the 16- to 30-year age group. Cord injuries due to acts of violence are primarily the result of gunshot wounds. Violent acts are more likely to produce paraplegia. In the older population, motor vehicle injuries and falls are responsible for almost 90% of spinal cord injury.[62]

Spinal cord injury in childhood and adolescence is uncommon. The incidence is estimated to be around 5% in individuals under the age of 16.[31] A 2:1 male to female ratio exists with peak of injury being in the summer months. Traffic-related injuries account for 40% followed closely by diving and other sports-related accidents (27%). Interestingly, acts of violence are responsible for a large proportion of injuries in this age group (up to 20%) but it is unclear whether the injured are just innocent victims or active participants.[62] There are no accurate data available regarding the relative incidence of paraplegia and quadriplegia in the younger age group, although cervical traumatic instabilities resulting in quadriplegia are probably more frequent.

Multisystem trauma commonly accompanies spinal cord injury, the most frequent being long bone fractures. Visceral injuries to the chest and abdomen, fractures of the pelvis, and severe head injuries are not uncommon. Noncontiguous multiple spinal fractures occur in approximately 5% to 17% of cases;[65] failure to recognize these injuries may result in devastating spinal cord damage.

ANATOMICAL FACTOR

Forces of extreme violence are necessary to produce fracture or fracture-dislocation of the thoracic spine. This region is rigid and constitutes an integral part of the thoracic cage. Therefore less motion occurs here than in the cervical and thoracolumbar spine. The surrounding rib cage and its strong costotransverse and costovertebral ligaments provide considerable stability. Lateral bending and extension are markedly limited and the coronally oriented facet joints restrict rotation. In the upper thoracic spine (T1 to T6), each level permits four degrees of flexion and extension. The lower thoracic segments (T7 to T10) allow up to six degrees of movement, and approximately eight degrees of rotation occur at every level.[68]

Despite the stabilizing effect of the rib cage on the thoracic spine, the incidence of concomitant cord injury with fracture and dislocation ranges from 70% to 85%. Several studies quote up to 80% complete paraplegia from traumatic fractures of the upper thoracic spine.[9,10] Two important factors contribute to this unfortunate statistic. First, the thoracic spine is relatively narrow with limited space available for the spinal cord. There is considerable risk of spinal cord damage with displacement of osseous elements or disc herniation. Second, the blood supply is relatively sparse,[25] especially in the midthoracic cord between T4 and T8, which receives only one radicular artery located at about T7.

PATHOLOGICAL FACTORS AND MECHANISMS OF INJURY

Damage to the spinal cord often results in partial or complete loss of motor, sensory, and reflex function below the level of injury. Traumatic fractures are the most common cause but infection, tumor, and vascular compromise are also etiological factors. Under age 40, traumatic injury is twice as common as nontraumatic causes; over age 40, cancer exceeds trauma-induced cord injury by a ratio of 4:1.[29,62]

Bohlman[9,10] extensively reviewed the various types of thoracic fractures in a series of 218 patients with paralysis. Because of the limited rotational ability and normal anatomical kyphosis of the thoracic spine, most bony fractures occur in flexion with varying degrees of axial loading. Flexion-compression (wedge compression) fractures are the most commonly encountered. Other mechanisms include axial loading or burst fracture, sagittal slice fracture, and ventral, or rarely, dorsal dislocation with varying degrees of ligamentous disruption. Spinal cord injury ranges from incomplete with a less devastating outcome to complete with resultant paraplegia. The retropulsed material is usually comminuted bone, although traumatic herniated disc can also produce neural compression. Epidural venous bleeding may also contribute to neural compromise.

Trauma is responsible for the majority of thoracic spinal cord injuries. Cord compression is also seen with neoplasms of the thoracic spinal canal, including epidural metastatic tumors. Pyogenic or tuberculous infection with spread into the epidural space accounts for a small minority of cases. This may involve mechanical compression by the abscess, although a vascular mechanism has been postulated. It is believed that venous compression and thrombophlebitis of the epidural space and spinal cord eventually result in cord infarction.[46] Finally, interference with the vascular supply of the spinal cord in chest injuries, in operative surgery, and in aortography can also produce lesions in the thoracic spinal cord.

PATHOPHYSIOLOGY OF ACUTE SPINAL CORD INJURY

Acute trauma to the spinal cord results in the mechanical disruption of axons. Generally, it does not cause total transection of the spinal cord even though the functional loss may be complete.[52] Mechanical trauma to the cord is an irreversible process and is referred to as the primary injury. The mechanism is believed to be acute compression or laceration of the spinal cord by bone or disc during fractures of the thoracic spine.[63] The primary injury then triggers a cascade of events, all of which constitute secondary injury. Secondary injury is characterized by a sequence of morphological, physiological, and biochemical changes. Experimental studies with pharmacological agents have suggested that secondary spinal cord injury can be modified.[13,17,74] If untreated, secondary injury will spread in a bidirectional manner away from the site of the initial primary injury.

Immediately following a traumatic insult, microscopic appearance of the contused site reveals little evidence of injury. Within 1 hour of injury, microscopic changes become visible, first in the gray matter. Some sections of gray matter show petechial hemorrhage whereas other areas show patches of necrotic hemorrhage, edema, and extravasated blood. By 3 hours, necrotic patches become confluent and a picture of central hemorrhagic necrosis with cavitation develops.[4,8,26] Pathological changes to the adjacent white matter follow shortly thereafter.

Morphological studies of injured spinal cords reveal major changes within the microvasculature.[26,63] Endothelial damage is evident along with intravasculature clotting, both of which lead to an alteration in blood flow. Most studies document hypoperfusion adjacent to the site of contusion whereas others note posttraumatic hyperemia. Hypoperfusion appears to accompany severe spinal cord injury and hyperemia is seen in spinal cords subjected to less severe insults. The functional significance of this observation remains unclear.

Blood flow measurements in spinal cords subjected to severe trauma indicate a major reduction of blood flow.[7,38,44,54,61] There is a difference in the degree of hypoperfusion in the gray and white matter. In the white matter, blood flow falls to approximately 50% of its preinjury value within 2 to 3 hours.[61] In contrast, a similar decrease occurs within 1 hour in gray matter. Because gray matter experiences ischemia earlier than white matter, it is not surprising that pathological changes are first witnessed in gray matter.

Many mechanisms have been proposed to explain secondary injury. These include posttraumatic falls in blood flow,[7,38,44,54,61] release of neurotransmitters and toxic byproducts,[2,21,42,48,57] extracellular ionic shifts,[55,71,75] and metabolic derangements,[3,16,50] calcium influx into traumatized axons[72] with subsequent activation of proteases and phospholipases,[5] activation of lysosomal enzymes,[19] and generation of oxygen free radicals.[22,23] These mechanisms may act in concert to enhance cellular autodestruction shortly after injury. Despite the abundance of data, the temporal sequence beginning with the initial event and culminating with cell death is unknown. It seems certain, however, that biochemical or blood-flow alterations precede gross morphological changes.

MANAGEMENT OF SPINAL CORD INJURY

Care of the patient with thoracic injury is designed to minimize further injury to the spinal cord and to provide an environment that will maximize recovery of function. The recognition of spinal cord injury, immobilization of the injured spine during transfer, and rapid treatment of the problem can influence the final recovery of spinal cord injury patients.

In the emergency room, details of the accident should be sought to determine the mechanism of vertebral injury. A careful systemic examination is then conducted, followed by detailed neurological testing. One must be alert to the possibility of anesthesia below the level of injury because it may mask significant injuries to the chest, abdomen, pelvis, or lower extremities. The goal of the initial neurological examination is to determine the level of injury and whether it is complete or partial. Serial neurological examination provides insight into the "completeness" of the injury and prognosis for future recovery. Persistence of complete injuries after the initial trauma has a less favorable outcome than patients with incomplete injuries.

A number of factors may make the initial neurological assessment incomplete or unreliable. An altered level of consciousness secondary to drugs, alcohol, hypotension, or associated head injury can lead to false interpretation. Injuries to the trunk and peripheral nerves can also confuse the neurological picture. Spinal shock interferes with the evaluation of spinal cord function. The determination of the "completeness" of the injury can be ascertained only with serial testing after resolution of spinal shock (see below).

High-dose methylprednisolone (30 mg/kg loading dose followed by 5.4 mg/kg/hour for 23 hours) is now generally given to patients with spinal cord injury either in the field or the emergency room. It is recommended that the drug be administered within 8 hours of the injury.[13] The effect of steroids appears to correlate with the initial severity of injury. The improvement in neurological recovery is thought to be greater in patients with paraparesis than in those with paraplegia.

Patients with acute spinal cord injury are prone to many disturbances and complications. These are secondary to both direct and indirect effects of the disordered physiology as a result of the injury. These changes can lead to early death unless they are understood and controlled. A major cause of deterioration in patients with mechanical spinal cord injury is superimposed ischemia. The finding of neurogenic shock, characterized by systemic hypotension and bradycardia, must be attended to immediately. Adequate volume expansion supplemented with the judicious use of pressor agents to maintain normotension may avoid conversion of an incomplete or reversible lesion to one that fails to respond to therapy. Interruption of the corticospinal fibers may impede pulmonary function as a result of intercostal muscle denervation with a subsequent decrease in pulmonary excursion. Frequent pulmonary function tests and arterial blood gases may alert the physician to an impending hypoxic insult.

Sympathetic denervation will result in the loss of thermal regulation, allowing for the development of hypothermia with potentially disastrous cardiovascular consequences. Loss of bladder control after such injuries requires meticulous attention to a bladder drainage system. A massively distended bladder may never recover sufficient tone to function adequately even in the face of spinal cord recovery. Intermittent catheterization every 6 hours in the acute phase helps to avoid complications of bladder overdistension and urinary stasis. This technique is preferred over the use of an indwelling catheter because of a lower incidence of urinary tract infections. Finally, careful attention to skin care in the spinal cord injured patient is of paramount importance. With the loss of skin sensation, and perhaps of motor function preventing voluntary changes in position, the patient is prone to developing pressure sores and decubitus ulcers. Precautions must be taken to prevent skin damage. Mechanical kinetic therapy beds have been used in an effort to minimize skin compression with possible necrosis. Log-rolling of the patient every 2 to 3 hours and padding bony prominences are also effective measures for prevention of skin damage.

Another potentially catastrophic complication of immobilization in these patients is the development of deep vein thrombosis and subsequent pulmonary embolism. Pulmonary embolism is one of the most common causes of sudden death in the spinal cord injury patient. Various measures have been utilized in an attempt to reduce this potential, including compression stockings, sequential pneumatic compression devices, subcutaneous heparin injections, and kinetic therapy beds.

Spinal cord injury patients obtain tremendous benefit from early aggressive treatment directed by a multidisciplinary rehabilitation team. Early use of rehabilitation appears to have a favorable influence on patient outcome.

SYNDROMES OF SPINAL CORD TRAUMA

The extent of spinal cord injury relates most directly to the force applied to the cord at the time of impact. Some patients suffer severe cord damage despite stable fractures whereas others experience little neurological deficit even in the face of gross instability. In general, the more severe the spinal column disruption, the greater the potential for spinal cord injury. Vascular consequences of the initial impact, both hemorrhagic and ischemic, may also contribute significantly to the ultimate clinical picture.

Complete Lesion

Spinal cord injuries are classified as either complete or incomplete. The most severe consequence of trauma is the complete loss of all functional activity below the level of the lesion. Frequently, if not always, high thoracic cord injury is associated with sympathetic spinal shock. While in this state, there is no motor, sensory, or monosynaptic reflex function distal to the lesion. Spinal shock may have a variable time period, although it usually lasts less than 24 hours. During this period, one cannot classify a patient as having a complete spinal cord injury. The patient may still make an excellent neurological recovery as spinal shock begins to resolve.

Resolution of spinal shock is heralded by return of the bulbocavernosus reflex, a function of the spinal cord itself. It is elicited by genital stimulation or a tug on the Foley catheter and produces a reflex contraction of the anal sphincter. If no motor or sensory recovery is noted within 24 to 48 hours of the injury, the paralysis and sensory loss is more likely to be complete. As the time period increases further from the acute event, the chance for return of function diminishes even more.

Complete cord injury may occur as a consequence of true anatomical disruption of the cord, physiological disruption of neural function because of compression or ischemia, or a combination of both. On rare occasion, a clinical picture of complete transverse myelopathy may be seen that spontaneously resolves within 24 to 72 hours after the injury. Such an occurrence might relate to transient physiological dysfunction and has been considered to be a concussion of the spinal cord. Another explanation for the recovery may simply be resolution of spinal shock.

Incomplete Syndromes

Patients with thoracic injury and with some sparing of neurological function distal to the lesion are classified as having an incomplete or partial spinal cord injury. The prognosis for future neurological recovery is much better than in patients with complete injury. Progressive deterioration of a partial injury to a complete status can result with persistent cord compression by bone fragments, extruded disc material, hematoma or spinal instability. Specific syndromes of incomplete injury may occur, depending upon the degree and location of the injury.

Anterior Cord Syndrome

There are three common syndromes of incomplete spinal cord injury. All have in common some sparing of cord function below the injury level but with variable prognosis regarding future recovery. The most common incomplete lesion is ventral cord syndrome. Although seen more often with cervical injury, it often accompanies thoracic compression or flexion fractures. One observes an alteration of spinal cord function served by the ventral two thirds of the spinal cord. This includes dysfunction of the corticospinal tracts and the ventrolateral spinothalamic systems. Clinically, there is loss of voluntary motor activity and light touch, sharp/dull discrimination, and temperature sensation distal to the lesion. Reflex activity below the lesion is absent acutely, although one may see extensor plantar responses. The usual cause of ventral cord syndrome is direct trauma to the ventral and lateral cord. However, ischemic injury due to compromise of the anterior spinal artery, which supplies the ventral two thirds of the cord, may also add to the pathology. Dorsal column function, which includes deep pressure sensation and proprioception, is preserved. The prognosis for recovery is poor. Only 10% to 20% of patients will recover significant functional motor strength in the lower extremities.

Central Cord Syndrome

A less common partial injury is central cord syndrome. The injury lies in the central gray matter but it may spread into adjacent white matter tracts. Underlying pathological substrates include edema and hemorrhagic contusion to the center of the cord, mechanical disruption, ischemia, or a combination of the above. Clinical presentation is variable. Motor deficit in the lower extremities can range from relative preservation to profound or even complete paralysis. Sensory loss is also variable both in the legs and the perineum. Deep tendon reflexes in the lower extremities are generally preserved and may show signs of an upper motor neuron pattern. Patients with this syndrome have a variable recovery pattern. It ranges from almost complete recovery to profound and permanent residual deficit. Up to 50% of patients will have enough motor recovery to become ambulatory even though there may be a component of spasticity. Bladder function is restored in about half of the patients even though they may have an increase in frequency and urgency.

Brown-Sequard Syndrome

Brown-Sequard syndrome can be produced by penetrating thoracic injuries in which half the cord is injured and the other half remains intact. This is most commonly seen with stab wounds of the back, although, rarely, blunt spinal cord trauma with lateral cord compression can produce some of the findings. Classically, there is ipsilateral weakness of one leg with good sensation and contralateral loss of sensation with good motor strength in the other leg. Functional recovery is more favorable in patients with this incomplete syndrome than in those with ventral cord or central cord syndrome.

CLASSIFICATION SCHEMES

It is impossible to overstate the importance of establishing a uniform standard for assessment and classification of spinal cord injuries. Accurate and early clinical evaluation of neurological function is essential in determining the severity of the initial injury. Serial testing using a reliable method of assessment is crucial in documenting spontaneous neurological changes. It further enables clinicians

and researchers to perform statistical analysis and meaningful comparisons of groups of patients with different severity of injury or with different treatment protocols. Finally, adoption of a consistent and reliable quantitative measure of cord function allows for comparisons in collaborative multicenter studies.

Multiple classification schemes have been published to measure the severity of trauma to the spinal cord.[18,53,58,64] The early schemes relied heavily on anatomical and pathological criteria whereas more recent schemes depend more on functional neurological damage. Motor, sensory, reflex, and sphincter functions are assessed in all patients soon after the injury and repeat examination is performed to determine neurological recovery or deterioration.

Frankel Scale

The first grading system widely used among neurosurgeons was one devised by Frankel et al.[30] This classification places the patient into one of five functional categories (see box). Complete injuries are differentiated from incomplete injuries and patients with partial function are further subdivided into categories based more on motor rather than sensory capabilities. There are two major limitations of the Frankel grading scheme. First, a significant improvement or deterioration in neurological function may go unnoticed unless the change is great enough to be placed into a different category. A second limitation is the inter-observer variability in grading incomplete motor function into "motor useless" (Frankel C) and "motor useful" (Frankel D) categories, because what constitutes "useful" requires subjective judgment. In spite of the limitations, this classification has been widely used in

---

FRANKEL SCALE

A No motor or sensory function below the lesion level
B No motor but some sensory preservation below the lesion
C Motor function present but useless
D Useful motor function present in the lower limbs
E Normal motor and sensory function

spinal cord injury to evaluate long-term outcome of patients and drug treatment protocols.

Attempts have recently been made to move away from methods that assess functional capabilities and toward scoring systems. Use of vague descriptive words such as "motor useful," "motor useless," and "significant" does not provide a real sense of the patient's neurological status. Furthermore, patients with similar functional capabilities are often grouped into the same category despite obvious differences in neurological examination. Analysis of outcome results for a particular treatment effect is also diminished with functional classification. A number of authors have advocated the use of scoring systems to document neurological recovery or deterioration.[13,49,58] In most of the classification systems, numerical grading is performed on the basis of both motor and sensory examination.

ASIA/IMSOP Impairment Scale

In 1990 the American Spinal Injury Association (ASIA) and the International Medical Society of Paraplegia (IMSOP) published their standard for neurological and functional classification of spinal cord injury[49] (Fig. 35-1). Although based on the original Frankel classification, the new protocol stipulated a much more detailed neurological examination. A systemic protocol for scoring both motor and sensory function above and below the level of injury is followed. Motor examination is conducted in ten key muscles on each side of the body. Selection of the muscles routinely tested is based on the consistent nature of their innervation. Muscle strength is graded on a six-point scale as follows: 0—total paralysis, 1—palpable or visible contraction, 2—active movement with gravity eliminated, 3—active movement against gravity, 4—active movement against moderate resistance, and 5—active movement against full resistance. Sensory response to both light touch and pinprick is tested in 28 segmental dermatomes bilaterally and graded as 0 if absent, 1 if impaired, and 2 if normal. Motor score can therefore range from a minimum of 0 to a maximum of 100 (10 muscle groups tested bilaterally and graded on 0 to 5 scale) while sensory score varies from 0 to 224 (28 dermatomes graded from 0 to 2 bilaterally and separately for light touch and pinprick).

As in the Frankel system, The ASIA/IMSOP classification also contains five grades of impairment

---

ASIA/IMSOP IMPAIRMENT SCALE*

Grade A-complete	No motor or sensory function is preserved in the sacral segments S4 and S5.
Grade B-incomplete	Sensory but not motor function is preserved below the neurological level and extends through the sacral segments S4 to S5.
Grade C-incomplete	Motor function is preserved below the neurological level, and the majority of key muscles below the neurological level have a muscle grade less than 3.
Grade D-incomplete	Motor function is preserved below the neurological level, and the majority of key muscles below the neurological level have a muscle grade greater than or equal to 3.
Grade E-normal	Motor and sensory function are normal.

*Classification of spinal cord injury based on the International Standards for Neurological and Functional Classification of Spinal Cord Injury by the American Spinal Injury Association (ASIA) and the International Medical Society of Paraplegia (IMSOP).

(see box). The functional capabilities of patients with grades A, B, and E are the same in both classifications. However, the ASIA system defines more precisely the terms "useless" and "useful" in Frankel's grade C and D, respectively: in grade C, muscle strength is less than 3 below the level of injury and in grade D, strength is equal to or greater than 3 caudal to the lesion.

The ASIA standard is unique in that it uses changes of summed neurological scores (i.e., the difference between admission and follow-up scores) to assess improvement or deterioration. It also developed the concept of percentage recovery (i.e., the change score divided by the extent of neurological loss on admission). This system is sufficiently sensitive to detect modest or even transient changes in neurological function. Consequently, improvement or deterioration in cord function can be detected by a change in the numerical score, even if this does not result in a change in the patient's functional status. In clinical trials, detection of subtle neurological change are of obvious importance. Clinical testing determines whether a treatment may be ef-

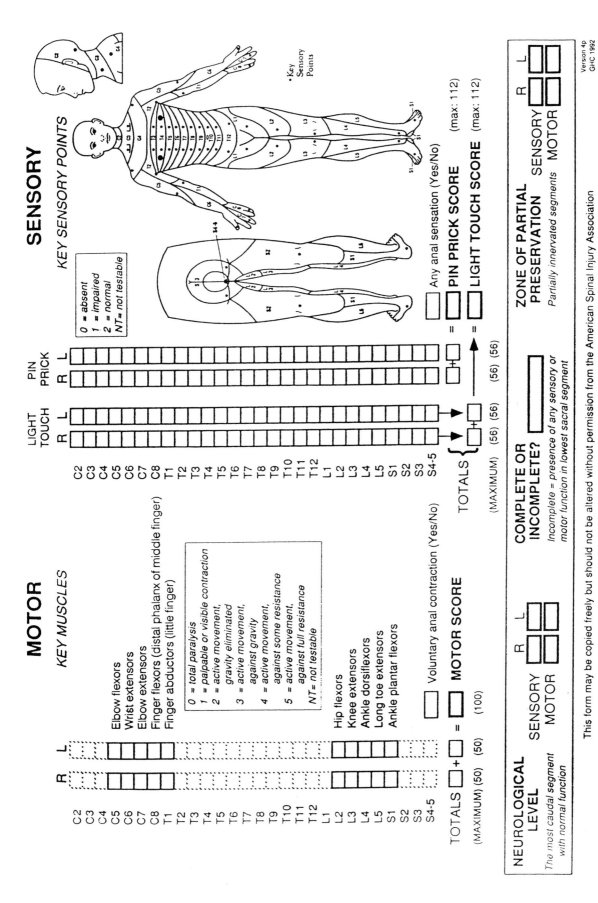

Fig. 35-1. Neurological classification of spinal cord injury (ASIA/IMSOP). This diagram contains the principal information about motor, sensory, and sphincter function necessary for accurate classification and scoring of acute spinal cord injuries. The 10 key muscles to be tested for the motor examination are shown on the left, along with the MRC grading system, and the 28 dermatomes to be tested on each side for the sensory examination are shown on the right. The system for recording the neurological level(s), the completeness of the injury, and the zone of partial preservation (in complete injuries) are shown at the bottom.

fective, but not whether it is optimal. A higher dose or a different timing and length of the treatment period may result in even more beneficial effects. In this regard, the ASIA method of analysis is well designed to detect minute changes, which may result from treatment, providing insight into ways to further improve treatment effects.

PHARMACOLOGICAL TREATMENTS

A critical hypothesis of acute spinal cord injury research is that preservation of surviving axons from further damage provides the best chance for recovery from injury. Acutely injured spinal cords undergo progressive pathological changes. The recognition that acute injury is naturally progressive led investigators to design therapeutic interventions to prevent or reduce the extent of secondary damage. Among the many treatment modalities, one that has seen some success is treatment with pharmacological drugs shortly after injury.

Two drugs that have been extensively studied are the glucocorticoid hormone methylprednisolone, and the opiate receptor blocker naloxone. Both were able to alter the injury response and improve neurological outcome of animals subjected to spinal cord injury.[23,73,74,76] Methylprednisolone had a positive effect on both functional recovery and histological appearance of injured spinal cords.[74,76] Others, however, did not find steroids to be effective. Differences in methodology, treatment protocols, steroid preparations, and dosages may account for some of the discrepancy. Dexamethasone, a relatively weak inhibitor of lipid peroxidation, and low doses of methylprednisolone (<15 mg/kg) provided minimal protection against experimental cord injury. On the other hand, methylprednisolone at doses of 30 mg/kg was neuroprotective.[76] The beneficial effects of high-dose methylprednisolone are attributed to its ability to scavenge free radicals and maximally inhibit lipid peroxidation, and less likely to its anti-inflammatory or antiedema properties.[41]

Along this line, a new class of steroids, tirilazad mesylate, has been developed. These compounds are even more potent inhibitors of lipid peroxidation but do not possess the glucocorticoid effect of methylprednisolone. In cat spinal cord injury models, tirilazad enhanced local motor function when given within 4 hours after the injury but was not protective when administered 8 hours following impact.[1] Multicenter clinical trials are underway in the United States to determine the effects of tirilazad in acute spinal cord injury.

High doses of naloxone (>2 mg/kg) have been reported to improve posttraumatic blood flow and functional outcome in injured spinal cords. Other opiate antagonists, namely nalmefene and thyrotropin-releasing hormone (TRH), are even more effective than naloxone. The mechanism by which naloxone has its effect is not entirely understood. Laboratory investigations have demonstrated release of opiate-like substances in the blood of cats subjected to spinal cord injury.[28] Because of their peripheral vasodilatory effect, opiates were held responsible for the systemic hypotension and decreased perfusion of injured cords. Naloxone, by blocking opiate receptors, led to an improvement in mean systemic pressure, which also ameliorated the trauma-induced hypotension. Others have proposed that naloxone increases cardiac output without causing a significant increase in systemic pressure. More recent investigations by Wallace and Tator[66,67] challenged the previous positive results obtained with naloxone. They reported no improvement in cardiac output, spinal cord blood flow, or functional outcome after spinal cord injury. However, simply raising the blood pressure and cardiac output with fluids and pressors improved spinal cord blood flow.

Based on the observation that methylprednisolone improved recovery in animals, the National Acute Spinal Cord Injury Study (NASCIS) group conducted a multicenter double-blind randomized trial in human spinal cord injury.[12,15] Between 1979 and 1984, NASCIS 1 randomized 330 patients and compared the effect of high-dose (1000 mg bolus followed by 1000 mg/day for 10 days) vs. low-dose (100 mg bolus followed by 100 mg/day for 10 days) methylprednisolone started within 48 hours of spinal cord injury. Neurological examination was conducted at the time of admission with follow-up examination at 6 weeks, 6 months, and 1 year after injury. Recovery was defined as the difference between admission and follow-up motor and sensory scores. At 6 months and 1 year after injury, no significant difference was seen in motor and sensory recovery between the two groups. In addition, a higher rate of wound infection accompanied the high-dose group, perhaps due to immunosuppression from prolonged steroid treatment.

NASCIS 1 was criticized for three reasons.[73] First, the treatment groups were not compared against placebo, therefore one could not conclude that low-dose steroid had no effect on functional recovery. Second, the high dose of methylprednisolone used in the study was suboptimal. A 70 kg person receiving 1000 mg of the drug per day, as in the NASCIS 1 study, is equivalent to a dose of 15 mg/kg. New evidence from animal studies suggested an optimal dose of 30 mg/kg for methylprednisolone to effectively inhibit lipid peroxidation, increase posttraumatic blood flow, and improve motor function. Third, experimental studies indicated that the drug should be administered within a few hours of injury to have maximal effect. In contrast, the treatment protocol for NASCIS 1 allowed for drug delivery as late as 48 hours after injury. Thus much damage would have already occurred prior to drug therapy.

Important lessons learned from NASCIS 1, including earlier treatment with a higher dose and comparison of results against a placebo group, were incorporated into NASCIS 2. The study started in 1985 and randomized 487 patients to one of three groups: treatment with methylprednisolone (30 mg/kg bolus followed by 5.4 mg/kg/hour for 23 hours), naloxone (5.4 mg/kg/hour for 23 hours), and placebo.[13] Bolus and maintenance doses of drugs were derived from dose-response testing in animals. To avoid the complication of prolonged steroid therapy, the study chose a treatment duration of 24 hours. The conclusion of the study was that high-dose methylprednisolone, if given within 8 hours after injury, significantly improved motor and sensory recovery at 6 weeks, 6 months, and 1 year postinjury. Improvement in motor scores was consistent with up to two Frankel grade category changes for both "plegic" and "paretic" patients. Patients receiving naloxone or methylprednisolone after 8 hours of injury did not differ in their scores from the placebo group.

A more recent clinical trial in human spinal cord injury was reported with Gangliosides in combination with low-dose steroids. Gangliosides are sialic acid containing glycosphingolipids found in high concentrations in synaptic regions of nervous tissue. In animal studies, Gangliosides attenuated retrograde axonal degeneration and facilitated neuronal sprouting and development.[11] In humans, Gangliosides improved recovery of motor function

when given within 48 to 72 hours after injury and following treatment with low-dose steroids.[32,33] However, a recent experimental study recommended against the use of steroids and Gangliosides concomitantly. The result showed that Gangliosides actually antagonized the neuroprotective effect of steroids.[20] The validity of the use of Gangliosides in human spinal cord injury is at present questionable.

Generation of oxygen-free radicals by injured cells is now thought to be an important secondary injury mechanism.[43] Superoxide free radicals are produced by the univalent reduction of molecular oxygen. This free radical and subsequent derived oxygen species are highly reactive and attack lipids and proteins. Superoxide dismutase, catalase and other antioxidants effectively reduce posttraumatic changes and promote function and survival in experimental studies of various organ systems. Among the potential sources of free radicals that may contribute to posttraumatic myelopathy (arachidonic acid metabolism, polymorphonuclear cell infiltration, and mitochondrial dysfunction), one that is becoming increasingly popular is the enzyme xanthine oxidase.

The in vivo form of the enzyme, xanthine dehydrogenase, is not able to produce superoxide.[56] Under ischemic conditions, it converts to xanthine oxidase, which has the ability to produce free radicals in the presence of oxygen and xanthine derived from ATP catabolism.[59] Such conversion has been documented in human head injury and acutely injured spinal cords.[70] Endothelial cells are a rich source of xanthine oxidase.[51] The high concentration in endothelial cells is consistent with the microvasculature as being the trigger for posttraumatic hypoperfusion and subsequent secondary damage. A recent study evaluated the role of xanthine oxidase in rat spinal cord injury using allopurinol to specifically inhibit the enzyme. The results suggested a strong neuroprotective effect with allopurinol, suggesting that xanthine oxidase–derived free radicals contribute significantly to secondary damage.[60] To date, allopurinol has not been studied in human spinal cord injury.

A multitude of drugs have been reported to produce beneficial effects in animal impact injury models. These have included a number of antioxidants, neurotransmitter receptor blockers, cyclo-oxygenase inhibitors, protease inhibitors, calcium channel blockers, modulators of intracellular messengers, and others.[73] The demonstration of postinjury treatment being neuroprotective by such diverse drugs lends support to the concept that primary injury initiates a cascade of endogenous mechanisms that can be manipulated at multiple levels. Thus far, methylprednisolone has been the only drug to have an impact on the treatment of human spinal cord injury. Other promising drugs have yet to be evaluated in a clinical setting.

A novel treatment for acutely traumatized spinal cords is the use of pedicled omental onlay graft at the site of injury.[36,37] The rationale for this procedure is based on the sequelae of spinal cord trauma, that is, cord swelling and local ischemia, and the omentum's ability to absorb extraordinary amounts of vasogenic edema fluid and to revascularize traumatized spinal cords. In previous studies, Goldsmith had shown the formation of vascular connections between omentum and the cerebral surface with a consequent increase in blood flow, sufficient to prevent infarction following occlusion of the middle cerebral artery.[36] Revascularization was also confirmed at the omental-spinal cord interface and in deep spinal cord tissue in normal and in traumatized spinal cords. The omentum also prevents the formation of scar tissue at the site of injury. The hypothesis is that omentum decreases fibroblastic proliferation by reducing the level of fibrinogen in vasogenic edema fluid, which is believed to initiate scar formation. Alternatively, omental tissue may possess antifibrotic activity. Despite such convincing evidence from animal studies and limited human studies, the use of omentum in acute spinal cord injury remains in the experimental phase.

SURGICAL CONSIDERATIONS

There is considerable controversy as to the role of surgery in the management of thoracic spinal cord injuries and spinal fractures. Historically, injuries have been treated with bed rest, postural reduction, and cast immobilization.[30] More recently, surgical management of spinal injuries has been advocated. This has been in large part due to the poor outcomes associated with nonoperative therapy, such as late neurological deterioration, persistent and progressive kyphosis, chronic and severe pain, and poor return to employment.[40] Furthermore, operative treatment decreases hospital stay and overall medical costs and permits early physical rehabilitation. Finally, surgical intervention reduces the rate of systemic medical complications such as pneumonia, urinary tract infections, deep vein thrombosis, pulmonary embolus, and skin necrosis.[14,69] These complications readily develop in patients not mobilized quickly following injury.

Surgical indications include restoration and realignment of the spinal column and decompression of neurological structures to enhance neural recovery.[69] The need for surgical stabilization often parallels the degree of spinal instability, but not all neurological decompression requires simultaneous stabilization. Stable spine fractures in the absence of neurological compromise can often be managed by nonoperative means. External bracing, such as with the thoracolumbosacral orthosis (TLSO), usually maintains good alignment until bony healing takes place. Operative stabilization is used only for injuries that are intrinsically unstable and cannot be adequately treated without surgical fixation. For example, patients with flexion-compression injury and loss of vertebral body height greater than 50% or kyphotic angulation of more than 10 to 12 degrees may be suitable candidates for surgery.[47] Similarly, axial loading burst fractures with disruption of both the ventral and middle columns may be more effectively immobilized by internal fixation. Complex fractures with significant rotational and translational components are invariably unstable and will require surgical intervention. Even though operative management is advocated for unstable fractures, there is still controversy with regard to the optimal technique of stabilization (i.e., ventral vs. dorsal vs. combined approaches).

Acute spinal cord injury is often associated with spinal cord compression. It is logical to think that removal of the offending agent might restore at least some spinal cord function. However, one must remember that a variety of factors in addition to the physical compression are at work in promoting injury. Thus neural recovery may not occur despite early and aggressive surgical intervention. The indications for surgical decompression are not clear cut. Progressive deterioration in the presence of spinal canal compromise by retropulsed bone, disc material, or epidural hematoma is an indication for decompressive surgery. A number of clinical studies also support surgical intervention in patients with incomplete spinal cord injuries.[6,10] Patients with functionally complete cord injuries rarely benefit from surgery, although some authors continue to believe that early aggressive surgery in even these patients is warranted.[35,45,69]

Traditionally, management for decompression in patients with vertebral body fractures involved laminectomy with no attempt at decompression of the ventral lesion. It was soon realized that laminectomy offered no advantage in terms of neurological recovery and, in fact, patients had a higher rate of late deformity, chronic pain, and progressive neural compromise. Laminectomy was thus discarded as a surgical technique for decompression of ventrally located pathology. Newer approaches have been devised to directly decompress neural elements and re-establish the size of the canal. Among these include transpedicular, transfacet pedicle-sparing, costotransversectomy, lateral extracavitary, and ventral or ventrolateral approaches. Each procedure has advantages and disadvantages and treatment considerations should be individualized. The approach taken should be dictated by the patient's age and medical condition, associated injuries, and perhaps most important of all, the surgeon's familiarity with the surgical technique.

Even more controversial is the timing of surgical decompression. Early intervention (less than 24 hours after injury) to remove a compressive lesion would inherently be expected to enhance functional recovery. Proponents of this theory believe that early decompression will decrease the spread of secondary injury that occurs after spinal cord trauma. Anecdotal experiences of a number of surgeons reflect some neurological improvement after immediate surgery. There is experimental evidence to support that decompression within the first 24 hours of injury significantly improves neural recovery.[39] Other studies, however, have not found significant neural recovery following surgical intervention. The data on this subject matter are not at all conclusive.

CONCLUSION

There are a number of reasons for the dramatic improvement in the overall care of patients with thoracic spinal cord injuries. A great deal of research has been done on the topic of spinal cord injury pathophysiology in the last 20 years. This has enabled researchers to develop drugs to be given shortly after injury in order to limit injury spread. Future developments in the area of neural protec-

tion and axonal regeneration will undoubtedly provide additional treatment options. There is now a more uniform method of classifying patients with complete or incomplete functional cord syndromes. This allows for a much more precise estimation of the long-term recovery potential in these unfortunate patients. Furthermore, universal classification permits controlled comparisons of various drug treatments and also better communication among spinal cord injury centers involved with clinical studies. Refinements in the medical care of cord injured patients has decreased the catastrophic complications that may occur and has led to a significant increase in long-term survival. Surgical intervention and timing of surgery remain controversial and recommendations range from no surgery to early aggressive surgical treatment. A large-scale prospective randomized clinical trial will be required to shed light on this controversy.

REFERENCES

1. Anderson DK, Hall ED, Braughler JM, et al. Effect of delayed administration of U74006F (tirilazad mesylate) on recovery of locomotor function after experimental spinal cord injury. J Neurotrauma 8:187-192, 1991.
2. Anderson DK, Means ED. Iron-induced lipid peroxidation in spinal cord: Protection with mannitol and methylprednisolone. J Free Radiol Biol Med 1:59-64, 1985.
3. Anderson DK, Means ED, Waters TR, et al. Spinal cord energy metabolism following compression trauma to the feline spinal cord. J Neurosurg 53:375-380, 1980.
4. Balentine JS. Pathology of experimental spinal cord trauma. Lab Inves 39:236-253, 1978.
5. Banik NL, Hogan EL, Powers JM, et al. Degradation of cytoskeletal proteins in experimental spinal injury. Neurochem Res 7:1465-1475, 1982.
6. Benzel EC, Larson SJ. Functional recovery after decompressive operation for thoracic and lumbar spine fractures. Neurosurgery 19:772-778, 1986.
7. Bingham WG, Goldman H, Friedman SJ, et al. Blood flow in normal and injured monkey spinal cord. J Neurosurg 43:162-171, 1975.
8. Blight AR. Cellular morphology of chronic spinal cord injury in the cat: Analysis of myelinated axons by line sampling. Neuroscience 10:521-543, 1983.
9. Bohlman HH. Treatment of fractures and dislocations of the thoracic and lumbar spine. J Bone Joint Surg 67A:165-169, 1985.
10. Bohlman HH, Freehafer A, Dejak J. The results of treatment of acute injuries of the upper thoracic spine with paralysis. J Bone Joint Surg 67A:360-369, 1985.
11. Bose B, Osterholm JL, Kalia M. Ganglioside-induced regeneration and re-establishment of axonal continuity in spinal cord transected rats. Neurosci Lett 63:165-169, 1986.
12. Bracken MB, Collins WF, Freeman DF, et al. Efficacy of methylprednisolone in acute spinal cord injury. J Am Med Assoc 251:45-52, 1984.
13. Bracken MB, Shepard MJ, Lcollins WF, et al. A randomized controlled trial of methylprednisolone or naloxone in the

treatment of acute spinal cord injury: Results of the second National Acute Spinal Cord Injury. New Engl J Med 322:1405-1411, 1990.

14. Bracken MD, Shepard MJ, Collins WF, et al. Methylprednisolone or naloxone treatment after acute spinal cord injury: One-year follow-up data. Results of the Second National Acute Spinal Cord Injury. J Neurosurg 76:23-31, 1992.

15. Bracken MB, Shepard MJ, Hellenbrand KG, et al. Methylprednisolone and neurological function one year after spinal cord injury. J Neurosurg 63:704-713, 1985.

16. Braughler JM, Hall ED. Lactate and pyruvate metabolism in the injured cat spinal cord before and after a single large intravenous dose of methylprednisolone. J Neurosurg 59:256-261, 1983.

17. Braughler JM, Hall ED, Means ED, et al. Evaluation of an intensive methylprednisolone sodium succinate dosing regimen in experimental spinal cord injury. J Neurosurg 67:102-105, 1987.

18. Chehrazi B, Wagner FC, Collins WF, et al. A scale for evaluation of spinal cord injury. J Neurosurg 54:310-315, 1981.

19. Clendenon NR, Allen N, Ito T, et al. Response of lysosomal hydrolases of dog spinal cord and cerebrospinal fluid to experimental trauma. Neurology 28:78-84, 1978.

20. Constantini S, Young W. The effects of methylprednisolone and the ganglioside GM1 on acute spinal cord injury in rats. J Neurosurg 80:97-111, 1994.

21. Demediuk P, Saunders RD, Anderson DK, et al. Membrane lipid changes in laminectomized and traumatized spinal cord. Proc Natl Acad Sci USA 82:7071-7075, 1985.

22. Demopoulos HB, Flamm ES, Pietronigro DD, et al. The free radical pathology and the microcirculation in the major central nervous system disorders. Acta Physiol Scand 492:91-119, 1980.

23. Demopoulos HB, Flamm ES, Seligman MC, et al. Further studies on free radical pathology in the major central nervous system disorders: Effect of very high doses of methylprednisolone on the functional outcome, morphology and chemistry of experimental spinal cord impact injury. Can J Physiol Pharmacol 60:1415-1424, 1982.

24. DeVivo ML, Richards JS, Stover SL, et al. Spinal cord injury: Rehabilitation adds life to years. West J Med 154:602-606, 1991.

25. Dommisse GF. The blood supply of the spinal cord: A critical vascular zone in spinal surgery. J Bone Joint Surg. 56:225-235, 1974.

26. Ducker TB, Kindt GW, Kempe LG. Pathological findings in acute experimental spinal cord trauma. J Neurosurg 35:700-708, 1971.

27. Dunn HK. Anterior spine stabilization and decompression for thoracolumbar injuries. Orthop Clin North Am 17:113-119, 1986.

28. Faden AI, Jacobs TP, Holaday JW. Opiate antagonist improves neurological recovery after spinal injury. Science 211:493-494, 1981.

29. Fine PR, Kuhlemeier KV, DeVivo MJ, et al. Spinal cord injury: An epidemiologic perspective. Paraplegia 17:237-250, 1979.

30. Frankel HL, Hancock DO, Hyslop G, et al. The value of postural reduction in the initial management of closed injuries of the spine with paraplegia and tetraplegia. Paraplegia 7:179-192, 1969.

31. Gaufin LM, Goodman SJ. Cervical spine injuries in infants. J Neurosurg 42:179-184, 1975.

32. Geisler FH, Dorsey FC, Coleman WP. Recovery of motor function after spinal cord injury—A randomized, placebo

controlled trial with GM-1 ganglioside. N Engl J Med 324:1829-1838, 1991.

33. Geisler FH, Dorsey FC, Coleman WP. GM-1 ganglioside in human spinal cord injury. J Neurotrauma 9S:517-530, 1992.

34. Gerhart KA. Spinal cord injury outcomes in a population-based sample. J Trauma 31:1529-1535, 1991.

35. Gertzbeim SD. Scoliosis Research Society: Multicenter spine fracture study. Spine 17:525-540, 1992.

36. Goldsmith HS, Duckett S, Chen WF. Spinal cord vascularization by intact omentum. Am J Surg 129:262-265, 1975.

37. Goldsmith HS, Steward E, Duckett S. Early application of pedicled omentum to the acutely traumatized spinal cord. Paraplegia 23:100-112, 1985.

38. Griffiths IR. Spinal cord blood flow after acute experimental cord injury in dogs. J Neurol Sci 27:247-259, 1976.

39. Guha A, Tator CH, Endrenyi L, et al. Decompression of the spinal cord improves recovery after acute experimental spinal cord compression injury. Paraplegia 25:324-329, 1987.

40. Haid RW, Kopitnik TA. Thoracic fractures: Classification and the relevance of instrumentation. Clinical Neurosurgery, vol 37. Baltimore: Williams & Wilkins, 1990, pp 213-233.

41. Hall ED, Braughler JM. Glucocorticoid mechanisms in acute spinal injury: A review and therapeutic rationale. Surg Neurol 18:320-327, 1982.

42. Hall ED, Braughler JM. Role of lipid peroxidation in posttraumatic spinal cord degeneration. CNS Trauma 3:281-294, 1986.

43. Hall ED, Braughler JM, McCall JM. Antioxidant effects in brain and spinal cord injury. J Neurotrauma 9:S165-S172, 1992.

44. Hall ED, Wolf DL. A pharmacological analysis of the pathophysiologic mechanisms of post traumatic spinal cord ischemia. J Neurosurg 64:951-961, 1986.

45. Hansebout RR. The neurosurgical management of cord injuries. In Bloch RF, Basbaum M, eds. Management of Spinal Cord Injuries. Baltimore: Williams & Wilkins, 1986, pp 1-27.

46. Hlavin ML, Kaminski MD, Ross JS, et al. Spinal epidural abscess: A ten-year perspective. Neurosurgery 27:177-184, 1990.

47. Hollowell JP, Maiman DJ. Management of thoracic and thoracolumbar spine trauma. In Rea G, Miller C, eds. Spinal Trauma: Current Evaluation and Management. American Association of Neurological Surgeons, 1993, pp 127-156.

48. Hsu CY, Halushka PV, Hogan EL, et al. Alterations of thromboxane and prostacyclin levels in experimental spinal cord injury. Neurology 35:1003-1009, 1985.

49. International Standards for Neurological and Functional Classification of Spinal Cord Injury. Revised 1992. American Spinal Injury Association, International Medical Society of Paraplegia—ASIA/ IMSOP, 1992.

50. Ito T, Allen N, Yashon D. A mitochondrial lesion in experimental spinal cord trauma. J Neurosurg 48:434-442, 1978.

51. Jarasch E, Grund C, Bruder G, et al. Localization of xanthine oxidase in mammary-gland epithelium and capillary endothelium. Cell 25:67-82, 1981.

52. Kakulas BA. Pathology of spinal injuries. Cent Nerv Syst Trauma 1:117-129, 1984.

53. Klose KJ, Green BA, Smith RS, et al. University of Miami Neuro-spinal index: A quantitative method for determining spinal cord function. Paraplegia 18:331-336, 1980.

54. Kobrine AI, Doyle TF, Martins AN. Local spinal cord blood flow in experimental traumatic myelopathy. J Neurosurg 42:144-149, 1975.

55. Lewin MG, Hansebout RR, Pappius HM. Chemical characteristics of traumatic spinal cord edema in cats. Effects of steroids on potassium depletion. J Neurosurg 56:106-113, 1974.

56. McCord JM, Roy RS. The pathophysiology of superoxide: Roles in inflammation and ischemia. Can J Physiol Biochem 60:1346-1352, 1982.

57. Osterholm JL. The pathophysiological response in spinal cord injury. J Neurosurg 40:5-33, 1974.

58. Piepmeier JM, Collins WF. Recovery of function following spinal cord injury. In Frankel HL, ed. Handbook of Clinical Neurology, vol 17. Spinal Cord Trauma. New York: Elsevier Science Publishers, 1992, pp 421-433.

59. Roy RS, McCord JM. Superoxide and Ischemia: Conversion of xanthine dehydrogenase to xanthine oxidase. In Greenwald R, Cohen G, eds. Oxy Radicals and Their Scavenger Systems, vol II. Cellular and Molecular Aspects. New York: Elsevier Science Publishers, 1983, pp 145-153.

60. Roy RS, Young W, Zagzag D, et al. Allopurinol minimized pathologic changes in spinal cord injury. J Neurosurg 80:388, 1994.

61. Senter HJ, Venes JL. Altered blood flow and secondary injury in experimental spinal cord trauma. J Neurosurg 49:569-578, 1978.

62. Stover SL, Fine PR. Spinal Cord Injury: The Facts and Figures. Birmingham: University of Alabama Press, 1986.

63. Tator CH, Fehlings MG. Review of the secondary injury theory of acute spinal cord trauma with emphasis on vascular mechanisms. J Neurosurg 75:15-26, 1991.

64. Tator CH, Rowed DW, Schwartz ML. Sunnybrook cord injury scales for assessing neurological injury and neurological recovery. In Tator CH, ed. Early Management of Acute Spinal Cord Injury. New York: Raven Press, 1982, pp 7-24.

65. Tearse DS, Keene JS, Drummond DS. Management of non-contiguous vertebral fractures. Paraplegia 25:100-105, 1987.

66. Wallace CM, Tator CH. Failure of naloxone to improve spinal cord blood flow and cardiac output after spinal cord injury. Neurosurgery 18:428-432, 1986.

67. Wallace CM, Tator CH, Gentles WM. Failure of blood transfusion or naloxone to improve clinical recovery after experimental spinal cord injury. Surg Neurol 28:269-276, 1987.

68. White AA, Panjabi MM. Clinical Biomechanics of the Spine. Philadelphia: JB Lippincott, 1978.

69. Wilberger JE. Acute spinal cord injury. In Menezes AH, Sonntag VKH, Benzel EC, Cahill DW, McCormick P, Papadopoulos SM, eds. Principles of Spinal Surgery. New York: McGraw-Hill, 1996, pp 753-767.

70. Xu J, Beckman JS, Hogan EL, et al. Xanthine oxidase in experimental spinal cord injury. J Neurotrauma 8:11-18, 1993.

71. Young W. Blood flow, metabolic and neurophysiologic mechanisms in spinal cord injury. In Becker D, Povlishock JT, eds. Central Nervous System Trauma Status Report. Bethesda, Md.: NIH, NINCDS, 1985, pp 463-473.

72. Young W. Calcium paradox in neural injury: A hypothesis. CNS Trauma 3:235-251, 1986.

73. Young W. Medical treatments of acute spinal cord injury. J Neurol Neurosurg Psychiatry 55:635-639, 1992.

74. Young W, Bracken MB. The second national acute spinal cord injury study. J Neurotrauma 9:S429-S451, 1992.

75. Young W, Koreh I. Potassium and calcium changes in injured spinal cords. Brain Res 365:42-53, 1986.

76. Young W, Ransohoff J. Acute spinal cord injuries: Experimental therapy, pathophysiological mechanisms, and recovery of function. In Sherk HH, Dunn EJ, Eismont FJ, Fielding JW, Long DM, Ono K, Penning L, Raynor R, eds. The Cervical Spine. Philadelphia: JB Lippincott, 1989, pp 464-497.

Acute Care of the Spinal Cord Injury Patient

George H. Lum, M.D., Geoffrey Shiu-Feng Ling, M.D., Ph.D., and Seth M. Zeidman, M.D.

Each year, some 10,000 Americans will sustain an injury to the spinal cord, resulting in paraplegia or quadriplegia.[16] The most common etiologies of injury to the spinal cord are motor vehicle accidents, sport and recreational accidents, and work-related accidents. These three categories account for approximately 77% of all causes of spinal cord injury.[32] Fractures of the thoracic spine occur less frequently overall, in comparison to fractures of the cervical and thoracolumbar regions. This is due to the inherent stiffness of the thoracic spine and support from the rib cage. Fractures of the thoracic spine are most commonly due to falls and gunshot wounds.[6]

The trauma most commonly occurs in young adults. The mean age of patients sustaining spinal cord injuries is 34.5 years, with a median of 27 years.[32] These are people in the prime of their productive years. Therefore the psychological and physical impact on these patients, and the economic impact on society, is enormous. Johnson, Brooks, and Whiteneck[15] estimated the annual expenditure for spinal cord injury patients to be $3.4 billion.

The immediate goals for the treatment of spinal cord injury are to halt any ongoing damage, to preserve and restore neurological function, to prevent possible secondary injuries to the spinal cord, and to prevent possible medical complications. Very often this requires care in an intensive care unit (ICU).

INITIAL MANAGEMENT

The emergency management of the spinal cord injury patient, as with any trauma patient, begins with the "ABCs." A secure airway is of paramount importance. If intubation is required, and the cervical spine has not been cleared, nasotracheal intubation with fiberoptic guidance is preferred. In the field, nasotracheal or orotracheal intubation can be performed safely with immobilization of the spine, along with in-line traction.[26] Hypotension raises the issue of neurogenic spinal shock vs. hypovolemia as the etiology. Any obvious bleeding should be addressed. The presence of tachycardia makes hypovolemia much more likely, in which case intravenous fluids may be indicated.

Any neurological complaints or findings should raise the index of suspicion of spinal injury. The patient should be appropriately immobilized and then a complete radiographic spine series obtained. Plain radiographs remain the mainstay of the initial imaging. Abnormalities on the plain radiographs may require further imaging evaluation. For evaluation of the bony spine, computed tomography (CT) is the study of choice, whereas magnetic resonance imaging (MRI) is indicated for the evaluation of the spinal cord itself, including the presence of edema or hemorrhage.[5] Intervertebral and paravertebral soft tissue pathology is also more clearly seen with an MRI.

A frequent finding on the initial imaging survey for thoracic trauma is the presence of a pleural effusion. This is usually a traumatic hemothorax. This occurs in 36% of patients with a thoracic spine injury.[8] In 24% of cases, the hemothorax is not visualized on the initial chest radiograph, but is identified on repeat radiographs.[19] The presence of a hemothorax often requires drainage by tube thoracostomy.

PHARMACOLOGICAL THERAPY

Many agents and modalities have been used for the acute treatment of spinal cord injury. Currently, the only drug that has been shown to improve neurological outcome in spinal cord injury is methylprednisolone.[5] In the second National Acute Spinal Cord Injury Study, methylprednisolone was shown to significantly improve neurological function. Patients received 30 mg/kg of methylprednisolone as an initial bolus, which was then followed with 5.4 mg/kg of methylprednisolone per hour for 23 hours. These patients were followed for 6 months, at which time they had improved sensory and motor function, compared with the placebo group. However, when the methylprednisolone was not begun within 8 hours of injury, efficacy was not observed.

The modality of spinal cord cooling has been used in animal studies and human trials. Hansebout[13] cooled the dura mater and the spinal cord in 10 spinal cord injury patients to 6° C. Both mortality and neurological improvement were better than expected, compared with historical controls. His review of the literature revealed a total of 52 patients so treated. The mortality was 17%, and another 17% were able to ambulate at a higher level than expected from the literature on spinal cord injury. The therapeutic effectiveness of this modality has not been proven in a prospective controlled manner.

An agent that has shown promise for the treatment of spinal cord injury is monosialotetrahexosyl-ganglioside (GM-1). A pilot study with 16 patients demonstrated a statistically significant difference in neurological improvement at 1 year in patients given GM-1 vs. placebo.[9] Currently, a prospective randomized trial with this drug is ongoing.[27]

A number of other agents, such as thyrotropin-releasing hormone (TRH), NMDA-receptor antagonists, and arachidonic acid inhibitors are being evaluated in ongoing research.

NEUROLOGICAL ISSUES

After initial stabilization, a complete neurological assessment must be performed in any patient with suspected spinal cord injury. In addition, the neurological examination must be repeated serially. The level of spinal cord injury is the lowest spinal cord segment with intact motor and sensory function.[7] In a complete spinal cord lesion, there is absence of all motor and sensory function. There is decreased motor tone in muscles below the injury in the peripheral musculature. In an incomplete spinal cord lesion, some neurological pathways are intact. Common patterns of incomplete spinal cord injury include Brown-Sequard syndrome, central cord syndrome, ventral cord syndrome, and the dorsal cord syndrome.[22] These patterns arise from anatomical relationships and vascular supply.

Brown-Sequard syndrome is caused by a unilateral hemisection injury to the spinal cord. The findings include ipsilateral paralysis, ipsilateral loss of touch/vibration/proprioception, and contralateral loss of pain and temperature sensation.[22]

Central cord syndrome is characterized by loss of motor and sensory function of the upper extremities that is out of proportion to the lower extremity function loss. Ventral cord syndrome is thought by some to be due to the interruption of the blood supply from the anterior spinal artery. This is manifested by the loss of pain and temperature sensation along with weakness below the level of injury. Proprioception and gross touch is preserved. Conversely, dorsal cord syndrome results in loss of proprioception and preserved motor and pain sensation (gross) and temperature.[22]

Prognostically, the presence of an incomplete lesion carries a much higher likelihood of some improvement in function. Patients who present with a complete lesion are not likely to have significant improvement in neurological function.[7]

In the acute period following the injury, there may be some temporary loss of spinal reflex activity below the level of injury. This is known as "spinal shock."[3] This is manifested by the absence of spinal reflexes, such as deep tendon reflexes, the bulbocavernosus reflex, and the anal wink. However, with high spinal cord injuries, the most distal reflexes, such as the bulbocavernosus reflex and anal wink may be preserved. Reflexes above the level of injury may be affected. This is termed the "Schiff-Sherrington phenomenon."[3] The loss of autonomic reflexes results in hypotension due to pooling of venous blood in the lower extremities. Visceral organs, such as the colon, bladder, and small bowel, may be affected, resulting in an ileus and urinary retention. Resolution of the deficit occurs in a caudal to rostral direction. However, some deficits may remain permanently.

CARDIOVASCULAR ISSUES

The cardiovascular effects of spinal cord injury are due to autonomic dysfunction. The cardiovascular response depends on the level of spinal cord injury. The sympathetic pathways exit the spinal cord from T1 to L2, whereas the parasympathetic pathways arise from the brain stem and S2 to S4.[30] The sympathetic fibers to the heart arise from T1 to T3. The initial response to acute spinal cord injury is hypertension, which is followed within minutes with hypotension.[21] This is due to the loss of peripheral vascular tone. If the level of injury is above T3, hypotension is accompanied by bradycardia. This is known as "neurogenic shock." The EKG may show a left ventricular strain pattern.[22]

Initial management is via fluid resuscitation, because diffuse vasodilation results in peripheral venous pooling. Vasopressors may subsequently be needed for their vasoconstriction and chronotropic effects. Agents such as dopamine, dobutamine, and phenylephrine may also be used. Optimal management usually requires continuous invasive hemodynamic monitoring with an arterial line and a pulmonary artery catheter. Mackenzie et al.[20] noted that cardiac output was optimized with pulmonary capillary wedge pressures up to 18 mm Hg. Bradycardia is usually responsive to atropine, with repeated doses administered as needed.

RESPIRATORY ISSUES

Patients with thoracic spinal cord injury retain function of the diaphragm and the accessory muscles of respiration because their neural input is from the cervical spine. However, intercostal muscles and abdominal wall muscle function is lost. Therefore these patients are often not ventilator dependent and may often be extubated as soon as possible. The primary finding is a decreased cough. Tidal breathing at rest should not be a problem. However, the ability to increase ventilation is impaired. In pa-

PULMONARY FUNCTION IN THORACIC SPINAL CORD INJURY PATIENTS	
FVC	69% of predicted
TLC	82% of predicted
FRC	86% of predicted
MVV	61% of predicted
PIP	79% of predicted
PEP	98% of predicted

tients with lesions below T3, pulmonary function testing shows the pattern depicted in the accompanying box.[2] The predominant respiratory complication is atelectasis and pneumonia due to an impaired ability to clear secretions.[25] Aggressive pulmonary toilet is necessary to prevent the development of these complications. Chest percussion and drainage, bronchodilators when indicated, and patient instruction by respiratory therapy are invaluable in this setting. In quadriplegics, early bronchoscopy for segmental collapse has been shown to decrease infection and time on the ventilator.[21] However, this has not been shown in thoracic spinal cord injury.

Thromboembolic disease is a major cause of morbidity and mortality in spinal cord injury. These patients are at significantly increased risk for development of thromboembolic disease due to prolonged immobility. This risk is further increased if there is associated trauma with significant vascular injury. The incidence of thromboembolic disease, including deep venous thrombosis (DVT) and pulmonary embolus (PE), may be as high as 70% in spinal cord injury.[14] Many drugs and modalities have been used individually or in combination for the prevention of DVT. In this population of patients, certain agents have been found to be ineffective (e.g., aspirin). Oral Coumadin is effective in preventing DVT, however the level of anticoagulation required is associated with an unacceptable risk of bleeding complications.

In 1992 a summary statement by the American College of Chest Physicians with regard to DVT prophylaxis in spinal cord injury, recommended that:

1. All patients with a spinal cord injury should receive prophylaxis;
2. Initial prophylaxis should be with intermittent compression devices (ICDs);

3. Anticoagulation should be added after the first 72 hours because the risk of postinjury bleeding is decreased, whereas the risk of development of DVT significantly increases at day 3 postinjury;

4. Acceptable anticoagulation regimens are heparin 5000 U subcutaneously twice a day, or Coumadin with an international normalized ratio (INR) goal of 2 to 3;

5. An inferior vena cava filter should be placed for all patients with a contraindication for anticoagulation (e.g., active bleeding, multiple surgeries); and

6. When patient is started on physical therapy requiring periods without ICDs, the heparin dose needs to be increased to 10,000 to 15,000 U twice a day.[31]

Prophylactic vena cava filters have been shown to be safe and effective in the prevention of pulmonary thromboembolism in high-risk patients. This group of patients includes those with injuries such as lower extremity long bone fractures or pelvic fractures in addition to their spinal cord injury.[28]

TUBE THORACOSTOMIES

The spinal cord injury patient often requires a tube thoracostomy for several reasons. There may be a traumatic hemothorax that requires drainage, or surgical intervention may necessitate a thoracotomy.

Once the tube thoracostomy has been placed, the drainage output must be followed closely for the amount and the character of the fluid. If bleeding continues at a rate of greater than 200 ml per hour after the initial drainage, an exploratory thoracotomy may be indicated.[23] Likewise, if a residual undrained blood clot is greater than 30% of the hemothorax, a thoracotomy is required. If there has been any penetrating trauma to the chest, prophylactic antibiotics are indicated.[19]

Initially, after placement or return from the operating room the tube should be placed on 20 cm H_2O suction.[19] When drainage has decreased to less than 100 ml over a 24-hour period, the tube can be clamped or placed on H_2O seal. If there is no significant reaccumulation of fluid on chest radiographs after 12 to 24 hours and no pneumothorax, the tube can be pulled.

GASTROINTESTINAL ISSUES

All of the major abdominal organs receive their innervation from the thoracic and upper lumbar spine. The muscles of the abdominal wall are innervated by T7 to T12. The stomach, small bowel, liver, pancreas, and proximal two thirds of the colon are innervated via T5 to L2. Therefore injury of the thoracic spine is often accompanied by abdominal complications. The most common complication is gastrointestinal atony with an ileus in up to 36% of spinal cord injuries.[1] This is often observed acutely in the setting of spinal shock. Therefore a nasogastric tube should be placed in the acute setting of spinal cord injury to decompress the stomach. Enteral feedings should be initiated as soon as motility returns, usually in 2 to 3 weeks. Metoclopramide may be given to promote gastrointestinal motility.[22] Other agents that may improve motility are erythromycin and cisapride.

Prophylaxis for an upper gastrointestinal hemorrhage should be administered to all patients with a spinal cord injury. The incidence of stress-induced peptic ulcer disease is as high as 29% in some series[1] where no prophylaxis was given. This may be due in part to unblocked parasympathetic activity in this patient population. H_2 blockers, antacids, or sucralfate can be used with equal efficacy. With H_2 blockers and antacids, gastric pH should be checked every 4 hours initially with a goal of pH greater than 4.[21] Studies where patients routinely received gastrointestinal prophylaxis demonstrated significantly lower incidences of peptic ulcers.[10]

Pancreatitis has been described in association with spinal cord injury,[10] with an incidence of 1.5%. The mechanism is believed to be due to overstimulation of the sphincter of Odi from unchecked parasympathetic outflow. Standard treatment is bowel rest and supportive care.

The presence of an abdominal complication is fairly common. In situations where abdominal wall tone or visceral sensation are lost, however, the usual signs may be obscure. The patient may not complain of any pain, and there may be no guarding or rigidity. Therefore vigilance and awareness of the possible complications must be maintained.

GENITOURINARY ISSUES

During the acute phase of spinal cord injury, when spinal shock may be active, bladder tone is diminished. A Foley catheter should be inserted immediately and left in place for 5 to 7 days.[11] This serves to drain the bladder and as a means to follow volume status and the adequacy of renal perfusion. In patients with injuries above T7, after the phase of spinal shock, autonomic dysreflexia may occur. This is manifest by sweating, skin flushing, and hypertension. It can be caused by bladder distension or instrumentation. Treatment is to ensure adequate bladder drainage. Phenoxybenzamine can be used if the problem persists.[29]

Once the patient has been stabilized, a urological evaluation of function is appropriate. The level and extent of injury will have an impact on prognosis. An upper motor neuron injury eventually results in a hyperreflexic bladder, while a lower motor neuron injury results in an areflexic bladder. The ultimate goal is to remove the permanent indwelling catheter and proceed to bladder training or intermittent catheterization.

INFECTIOUS ISSUES

The incidence of primary wound infections is much higher after spinal surgery than after cranial surgery (2.75% for spinal surgery vs. 0.49% for cranial surgery).[17] In the same study, antibiotic prophylaxis was shown to decrease the infection rate from 5% to less than 2%. The most common organisms are *Staphylococcus aureus*, *Staphylococcus epidermidis*, *Streptococci*, and, on occasion, gram-negative rods. Resistant patterns differ according to the individual institutions. If a wound infection is suspected, appropriate cultures should be obtained immediately. Antibiotics should be initiated as soon as cultures have been sent. Initial coverage with Vancomycin is appropriate. Antipseudomonal coverage should be added if the patient has been in the hospital for any significant period of time (e.g., Ceftazidime and Gentamycin). This can be tailored when culture results become available.

Nosocomial infections can become an issue very quickly in a neuro ICU. Overall, the incidence of nosocomial infections is lower than in the medical or ICUs, but the incidence is still significant. The most common nosocomial infection in the neuro ICU is a urinary tract infection. The risk for bacteriuria is 3% to 10% for each day that an indwelling bladder catheter is in place.[17] Gram-negative enteric organisms are most common. Therefore antibiotic coverage should be directed toward this until culture results and sensitivities become available.

Pneumonia is the second most common nosocomial infection in a neuro ICU. The incidence is up to 20% in this patient population.[17] The mechanism is usually due to the aspiration of oropharyngeal contents. Endotracheal intubation is the greatest risk factor for the development of pneumonia. The presence of a nasogastric tube also predisposes the patient to this complication. Gram-negative rods are the most common organisms. Antibiotic coverage should begin with a combination of drugs such as Ceftazidime or a semisynthetic penicillin, such as Piperacillin, along with an aminoglycoside. This provides excellent gram-negative coverage, including *Pseudomonas*.

Very often, the patient admitted to the neuro ICU has one or more central venous catheters for diagnostic monitoring and intravenous access. These are the third most common source of nosocomial infections.[17] Skin flora are the most common organisms. Therefore initial antibiotic coverage should be with Vancomycin or an equivalent drug.

NUTRITION ISSUES

Enteral nutrition should begin as soon as the ileus is resolved. In the interim, nutritional support with total parenteral nutrition (TPN) should begin as soon as possible. The nutritional needs of the spinal cord injury patient vary greatly from the acute postinjury period to the more chronic rehabilitation and recovery period. The normal response to a systemic stress, such as trauma or surgery, is peripheral protein mobilization.[18] ICU patients should receive at least 1 gm/kg/day of protein, and 1.5 to 2.0 gm/kg/day are needed for those who are more critically ill and under higher stress.[4] A reasonable approach is to begin with a protein supplementation of 1.5 gm/kg/day. A 24-hour urinary urea nitrogen is then needed to determine nitrogen balance. The protein intake can be adjusted subsequently.

The calorie needs for ICU patients range from 25 kcal/kg/day for mildly ill patients up to 50 kcal/kg/day in severely ill patients (such as burn or septic patients).[4] Spinal cord injury patients appear to have a decreased energy requirement compared with standard prediction formulas such as the Harris-Benedict equations. The level of spinal cord injury significantly affects the daily energy expenditures.

In a study by Mollinger et al.[24] high cervical injury resulted in a daily energy expenditure of 19 kcal/kg whereas injuries below T10 resulted in energy expenditures of 35.8 kcal/kg/day in a patient actively undergoing rehabilitation. Precise recommendations for caloric needs are not available for all levels of spinal cord injury. Kolpek et al.[18] recommend a caloric level of 80% of the Harris-Benedict prediction for quadriplegic patients.[29] Low thoracic spine paraplegic patients should probably receive the full Harris-Benedict predicted amount.

The thoracic spine injury patient should not have any problems with eating or swallowing, unless a concomitant injury has occurred elsewhere. They should be allowed to eat as soon as the ileus has resolved and a pancreatitis is not present.

ANESTHESIA

The greatest concern with regard to the induction and administration of anesthesia in patients with spinal cord injury is hemodynamic/autonomic instability.[22] The patient must be adequately volume resuscitated before the administration of any anesthetic agents. This prevents hypovolemia complicating the picture when blood pressure and heart rate swings become manifest. A pulmonary artery catheter can be very useful in assisting with the management of this situation. The pulmonary capillary wedge pressure should be pushed to 18 mm Hg if necessary to ensure adequate filling pressures.[20] If hypotension occurs, a direct vasoconstricting agent, such as phenylephrine should be used. If bradycardia develops, atropine or isoproterenol can be used. If adrenergic excess becomes a problem, then a beta blocker or hydralazine can be used to treat the hypertension.

During induction, a nondepolarizing muscle relaxant such as vecuronium or pancuronium should be used. A word of caution: Denervated muscle can be extremely sensitive to acetylcholine, whereas a depolarizing agent such as succinylcholine may precipitate a hyperkalemic crisis with persistent twitches.[12]

REFERENCES

1. Albert TJ, Levine MJ, Balderston RA, et al. Gastrointestinal complications in spinal cord injury. Spine 16(Suppl 10):S522-S525, 1991.
2. Aldrich TK, Rochester DF. The Lungs and Neuromuscular Diseases. In Murray JF, Nadel JA, eds. Textbook of Respiratory Medicine, 2nd ed. Philadelphia: WB Saunders, 1994.
3. Atkinson PP, Atkinson JLD. Spinal shock. Mayo Clin Proc 71:384-389, 1996.
4. Berger R. Nutritional support and modulation in the ICU. In Pulmonary and Critical Care Update Mosby-Year Book 11:1-12, 1996.
5. Bracken MB, Shepard MJ, Collins WF, et al. A randomized, controlled trial of methylprednisolone or naloxone in the treatment of acute spinal cord injury. N Engl J Med 322:1405-1411, 1990.
6. Burney RE, Maio RF, Maynard F, et al. Incidence, characteristics, and outcomes of spinal cord injury at trauma centers in North America. Arch Surg 128:596-599, 1992.
7. Chehrazi B, Wagner FC, Collins WF, et al. A scale for evaluation of spinal cord injury. J Neurosurg 54:310-315, 1981.
8. El Khoury GY, Whitten CG. Trauma to the upper thoracic spine: Anatomy, biomechanics, and unique imaging features. AJR 160:95-102, 1993
9. Geisler FH, Dorsey FC, Coleman WP. Recovery of motor function after spinal cord injury: A randomized, placebo-controlled trial with GM-1 ganglioside. N Engl J Med 324:1829-1838, 1991.
10. Gore RM, Mintzer RA, Calenoff L. Gastrointestinal complications of spinal cord injury. Spine 6:538-544, 1981.
11. Graham SD. Present urological treatment of spinal cord injury patients. J Urol 126:1-4, 1981.
12. Gronert GA, Theye RA. Pathophysiology of hyperkalemia induced by succinylcholine. Anesthesiology 43:89, 1975.
13. Hansebout RR, Tanner JA, Romero-Sierra C. Current status of spinal cord cooling in the treatment of acute spinal cord injury. Spine 9:508-511, 1984.
14. Hull RD. Venous thromboembolism in spinal cord injury patients. Chest 102(Suppl 6):658S-663S, 1992.
15. Johnson RL, Brooks CA, Whiteneck GG. Cost of traumatic spinal cord injury in a population-based registry. Spinal Cord 34:470-480, 1996.
16. Kelly BJ, Luce JM. Spinal cord trauma. Handbook of Clinical Neurology 61:1929-1938.
17. Kim YS, Pons VG. Infections in the neurosurgical intensive care unit. Neurosurg Clin N Am 5:741-754, 1994.
18. Kolpek JH, Ott LG, Record KE, et al. Comparison of urinary nitrogen excretion and measured energy expenditure in spinal cord injury and nonsteroid-treated severe head trauma patients. JPEN 13:277-280, 1989.
19. Light RW. Chylothorax, hemothorax, and fibrothorax. In Murray JF, Nadel JA, eds. Textbook of Respiratory Medicine, 2nd ed. Philadelphia: WB Saunders, 1994.
20. Mackenzie CF, Shin B, Krishnaprasad D, et al. Assessment of cardiac and respiratory function during surgery on patients with acute quadriplegia. J Neurosurg 62:843-849, 1985.
21. McBride DQ, Rodts GE. Intensive care of patients with spinal trauma. Neurosurg Clin N Am 5:755-766, 1994.
22. McVicar JP, Luce JM. Management of spinal cord injury in the critical care setting. Crit Care Clin 2:747-758, 1986.
23. Miller KS, Sahn SA. Chest tubes: Indications, technique, management and complications. Chest 91:258-263, 1987.
24. Mollinger LA, Spurr GB, El Ghatit AZ, et al. Daily energy expenditure and basal metabolic rates of beta patients with spinal cord injury. Arch Phys Med Rehabil 66:420-426, 1985.
25. Reines HD, Harris RC. Pulmonary complications of acute spinal cord injuries. Neurosurgery 21:193-196, 1987.

26. Rhee KJ, Green W, Holcroft JW, et al. Oral intubation in the multiply injured patient: The risk of exacerbating spinal cord damage. Ann Emerg Med 19:511, 1990.

27. Rhoney DH, Luer MS, Hughes M, et al. New pharmacologic approaches to acute spinal cord injury. Pharmacotherapy 16:382-392, 1996.

28. Rogers F, Shackford SR, Wilson J, et al. Prophylactic vena cava filter insertion in severely injured trauma patients: Indications and preliminary results. Trauma 35:637-642, 1993.

29. Scott MB, Morrow JW. Phenoxybenzamine in neurogenic bladder dysfunction after spinal cord injury. I. Voiding dysfunction. J Urol 119:480-486, 1978.

30. Snell RS. Clinical Neuroanatomy for Medical Students. Boston: Little Brown, 1980.

31. Summary and recommendations. Deep vein thrombosis in spinal cord injury. Chest 102(Suppl 6):633S-635S, 1992.

32. Tator CH, Duncan EG, Edmonds VE, et al. Changes in epidemiology of acute spinal cord injury from 1947 to 1981. Surg Neurol 40:207-215, 1993.

CHAPTER 37

Trauma

Edward C. Benzel, M.D., and Charles B. Stillerman, M.D.

IMAGING AND DIAGNOSIS

The imaging diagnosis of spinal instability and pathological anatomy relies heavily on the plain radiograph (anteroposterior [AP] and lateral radiographs). Computed tomography (CT), however, plays a significant role, particularly when dorsal bony element disruption is in question.[14] Magnetic resonance imaging (MRI) is particularly useful for the definition of soft tissue injury and for the definition of neural element compromise.

These techniques are commonly employed clinically for the assessment of the posttraumatic patient. Hence they play a major role in the clinical decision-making process.

INJURY TYPE DEFINITION

The anatomy of the thoracic spine is relatively similar at each segmental level. Therefore thoracic injuries are not as varied as are injuries that are located elsewhere in the spinal column.

Denis' description of several fracture types[7] is currently the most widely utilized (Table 37-1). As opposed to the definition scheme of Denis,[7] the injury types that are described below are based on mechanism of injury[1] (Table 37-2). The difference between the two schemes is subtle. It is most evident regarding the difference between ventral wedge compression and burst fractures. The presence or absence of retropulsed bone and/or disc fragments in the spinal canal is the criteria in the Denis scheme for fracture type definition.[7] This is not employed in the description based on mechanism of injury. However, Denis' three-column concepts are usually used for stability and instability determination (see below).

Injury type is altered by the position and orientation of the force application (force vector) in relation to the instantaneous axis of rotation (IAR). This affects the type and extent of injury by affecting the bending moment. An alteration of the IAR, therefore, can significantly affect the bending moment and, in turn, the injury extent and type.

Table 37-1. Basic Modes of Failure of the Three Columns in the Four Types of Spinal Injuries*

| Type of Fracture | Column | | |
	Ventral	Middle	Dorsal
Compression	Compression	None	None or severe distraction
Burst	Compression	Compression	None
Seat-belt type	None or compression	Distraction	Distraction
Fracture-dislocation	Compression rotation shear	Distraction rotation shear	Distraction rotation shear

*From Denis F. The three-column spine and its significance in the classification of acute thoracolumbar spine injuries. Spine 8:817-831, 1983.

Table 37-2. Quantitation of Acute Instability for Subaxial Cervical, Thoracic, and Lumbar Injuries* (Point System†)

Loss of integrity of ventral (and middle) column‡	2
Loss of integrity of dorsal column(s)‡	2
Acute resting translational deformity§	2
Acute resting angulation deformity§	2
Acute dynamic translation deformity exaggeration‖	2
Acute dynamic angulation deformity exaggeration ‖	2
Neural element injury¶	3
Acute disc narrowing at level of suspected pathology	1
Dangerous loading anticipated	1

*With permission from Benzel EC. Biomechanics of Spine Stabilization: Principle and Clinical Practice. New York: McGraw-Hill, 1995, p. 26.
†Five points or more implies the presence of overt instability; two to four points implies the presence of limited instability.
‡By clinical examination, MRI, CT, or radiograph. One point only may be allotted if incomplete evidence exists; for example, only MRI evidence of posterior ligamentous injury (i.e., evidence of only interspinous ligament injury on T2-weighted images).
§From static resting anteroposterior and lateral spine radiographs. It must be the result of an acute clinical process. Tolerance for this criteria is variable with respect to surgeon and clinical circumstances. Guidelines as per White and Panjabi.
‖ From dynamic (flexion and extension) spine radiographs. Only recommended after other mechanisms of instability assessment have been exhausted and then only by an experienced clinician. Usually only indicated in cervical region. Must be the result of an acute clinical process. Tolerance for this criteria is variable with respect to surgeon's opinion and clinical circumstances. Guidelines as per White and Panjabi.
¶Three points for cauda equina, 2 points for spinal cord, or 1 point for isolated nerve root neurological deficit. *The presence of neural element injury indicates that a significant spinal deformation occurred at the time of impact, implying that structural integrity may well have been disturbed.*

The magnitude and characteristics of the failure-producing force and the configuration of the injured spinal level significantly influence the management scheme. Therefore they are used as criteria for injury type definition. This scheme limits the incidence of burst fracture, as compared to that associated with the scheme of Denis.[7]

INJURY TYPES AND MECHANISMS OF INJURY
Ventral Wedge Compression Fractures

Ventral wedge compression fractures result from an axial load and a ventrally oriented bending moment to failure. In other words, an axial load is eccentrically placed, ventral to the IAR (Fig. 37-1). This results in a flexion deformity.[3,10-13,19] The relatively flexed posture of the thoracic spine at the moment of impact increases the incidence of this injury type. An eccentric load application is, therefore, encouraged by the kyphotic posture, whether it is secondary to a "natural" kyphosis or to a superimposed flexion (Fig. 37-2).

Burst Fractures

If a true axial load to failure is applied to the thoracic spine, a wedging of the resultant vertebral

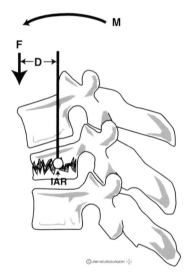

Fig. 37-1. A depiction of the injury force vector causing a ventral wedge compression fracture. F = applied force vector; D = length of moment arm (from IAR to the plane of F); M = bending moment.[1]

body fracture is unlikely, since a bending moment is not applied. Thus, a symmetrical compression of the vertebral body results and is termed a "burst fracture."[3,5,6,10-15] This is uncommon in the thoracic spine because of the kyphotic posture assumed in this region. This "pancaking" of the vertebral body

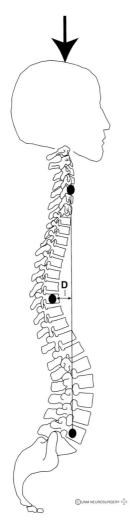

Fig. 37-2. A kyphotic posture (as is present in the thoracic spine) increases the length of the natural moment arm *(D)* and thus the magnitude of the bending moment resulting from an eccentrically placed (with respect to the thoracic spine IAR) axial load *(arrows)*. Dots = IARs.[1]

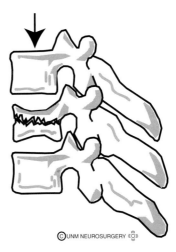

Fig. 37-3. The mechanism of injury of a burst fracture; true axial loading without a bending moment (i.e., D = 0).[1]

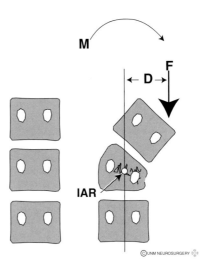

Fig. 37-4. Eccentrically applied loads cause bending of the spine. The bending occurs toward the side of the eccentrically applied load *(F, large arrow)* with respect to the IAR. If failure of the vertebral body occurs, it will be oriented in the same direction (concave side of the curve). D = length of moment arm (from IAR to the plane of *F*); M = bending moment.[1]

often causes a retropulsion of bony fragments into the spinal canal and dural sac compression (as per Denis).[7,9] It is a manifestation of an axial load that is not eccentrically placed with regard to the IAR (Fig. 37-3).

Lateral Wedge Compression Fractures

Most vertebral body fractures consist of more than one injury. Wedge compression and burst fractures are rarely pure. Although these injuries are common, coronal plane deformities often simultaneously occur. Anteroposterior (AP) radiographs often demonstrate as asymmetrical loss of height of the vertebral body (lat-

eral wedge compression fracture) (Figs. 37-4 and 37-5). However, they can also occur as isolated injuries.

The mechanism of injury of the lateral wedge compression fracture may be secondary to a "buckling" of the spine. This buckling results in the application of an effective lateral bending moment[1] (Fig. 37-6).

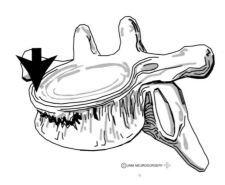

Fig. 37-5. The mechanism of injury of a combination ventral and lateral wedge compression fracture. Eccentrically applied load is shown (arrow).[1]

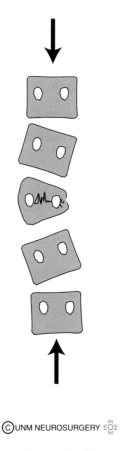

©UNM NEUROSURGERY

Fig. 37-6. A depiction of spine "buckling" secondary to axial load application as an etiology of a wedge compression fracture.[1]

Flexion-Distraction (Chance) Fractures

A distraction component in thoracic spine fractures is uncommon. The mechanism of injury is such that this injury is most common in the thoracolumbar and lumbar regions. This is because of the fact that a distraction component of trauma is rarely applied to the thoracic spine. If a lap belt is worn without a shoulder harness by a person involved in a deceleration motor vehicle accident, particularly if the lap belt is "worn high," a thoracic injury could occur. Distraction and flexion of the thoracic spine results.[3,4,8,16,17] Unrestricted distraction and forward flexion results in an isolated flexion bending moment. This injury was initially described by Chance[4] and thus commonly bears his name.[2] It may be broken down into two basic types: (1) a diastasis (fracture cleavage) through the pedicles and (2) a fracture through the vertebral end plate[1] (Fig. 37-7). Additionally, some classification schemes describe a third type, which consists of both osseous and ligamentous disruption.[1,2]

Dorsal Element Fractures

The majority of the failure-producing axial load force vectors in the thoracic spine are oriented in a plane that is ventral or ventrolateral to the IAR. If, indeed, these vectors are oriented dorsal to the IAR (i.e., an extension component to the injury), an excessive compressive force is applied to the dorsal elements at the effected spinal level. This increases the chance of dorsal element failure (Fig. 37-8).

Dorsal element fractures are uncommon as isolated entities in the thoracic spine (Fig. 37-8, *C*). This is opposed to the cervical region, where the spine's orientation acts in concert with the small vertebral body size and facet to create dorsal element disruption. The lumbar spine, however, has a lower incidence of dorsal element fractures because of the more massive nature of the vertebrae and the somewhat sagittal orientation of the facet joints.

A rotatory component of the injury may cause dorsal element injury by forcing opposing inferior and superior articulating facet joints against each other with such force that failure occurs. This is much more common in the lumbar region where the facet joints are sagittally oriented.

Ligamentous Injuries

Isolated ligamentous injuries of the thoracic spine are uncommon. They occur more commonly in the cervical region, due in part to its substantial flexibility.

Facet Dislocation

Facet dislocation occasionally occurs in the thoracic region. This is most common in the upper thoracic

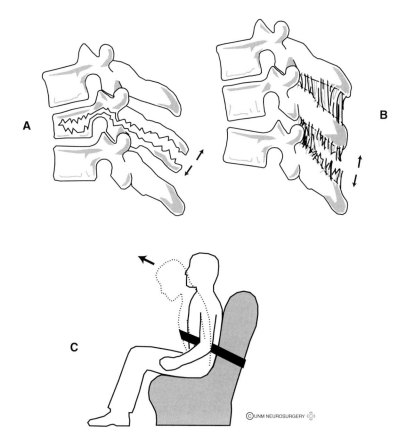

Fig. 37-7. Two fundamental Chance (flexion-distraction) fracture types. **A,** A diastasis fracture through the pedicles and vertebral body. **B,** A fracture through the vertebral end plate or disc. **C,** The mechanism of injury is depicted. Note that a "high belt" mechanism is required to cause a thoracic spine Chance fracture.[1]

region where flexion bending moment application is not uncommon. Facet dislocations are most often bilateral and usually associated with high-grade or complete spinal cord injuries. Spinal cord injury results from the limited space available for the spinal cord in this region. Additionally, the blood supply in various thoracic areas (the watershed zone) is tenuous, making the spinal cord particularly susceptible to injury from mechanical forces. Facet dislocation is created by a limitation of rotation in this region (by the rib cage, etc.). A true flexion moment application most commonly results in bilateral facet dislocation.

MANAGEMENT STRATEGIES

Management strategy determination for trauma is not significantly different than for other pathological processes, such as tumor or infection. As usual, the process must take into consideration any indications for surgery. This includes a consideration

for both neural element decompression and spinal stabilization. Also, if a significant spinal deformity is present, its correction must be considered. Operation selection and complexity are obviously affected by these three considerations. Additionally, the patient's overall medical condition, physiological age, and the surgeon's familiarity with the various surgical options influence surgical planning.

Neural element decompression is often the most important consideration. Neurological recovery, or the prevention of neurological deterioration, is of prime importance. Thus the determination of the method of neural element decompression must obligatorily dictate the method of spinal stabilization or deformity correction employed. In fact, in most cases the method of neural element decompression should be an independent decision. The method of spinal stabilization or deformity correction employed should therefore be dictated by the underlying pathology and by the decompression operation to be employed.

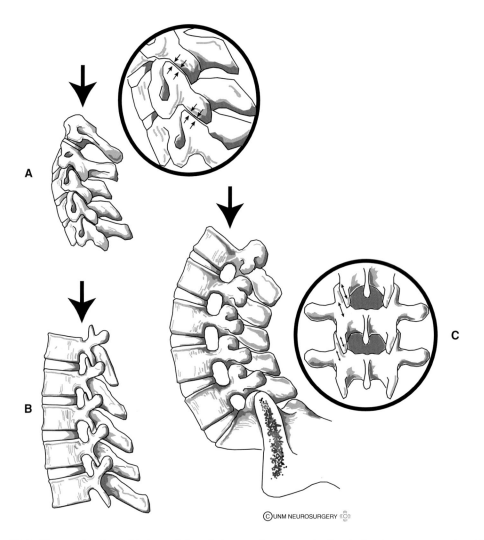

Fig. 37-8. The mechanism of injury of dorsal element fractures. **A,** Cervical spine extension forcibly approximates the facet joints and/or the laminae. The inset depicts this in greater magnification. Short arrows depict the opposing forces that can lead to facet fracture during excessive axial loading while in the extended posture. **B,** The thoracic spine would have to be in extreme relative extension in order for axially applied loads to cause isolated dorsal element fractures. This is due to the "natural" thoracic kyphosis that would have to be overcome by extreme extension during axial loading. **C,** In the lumbar region, the facet joints are able to slide past each other during extension and axial loading (*inset, arrows*), thus minimizing the chance for facet fracture by this mechanism.[1]

Neural Element Decompression

As a rule, ventral lesions should be decompressed from a ventral orientation and dorsal lesions should be decompressed from a dorsal orientation. The presence of an incomplete neurological deficit with spinal canal compromise requires neural element decompression. Dorsal operations usually pose only minor problems for the spine surgeon. An exception is the upper thoracic spine, where a dorsal decom-pression in the face of an unstable spine presents problems with subsequent spinal stabilization.

Ventral mass lesions can obviously pose formida-ble problems. The choices of operative approaches are several. They include (1) ventral approaches to the upper thoracic spine through the thoracic inlet or upper mediastinum and (2) ventrolateral and lat-eral approaches to the mid- and lower thoracic re-gions. The upper thoracic region is a "no-man's land" regarding ventral thoracic spine exposure.

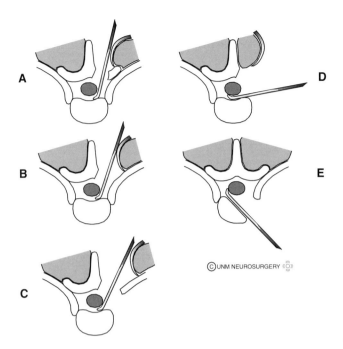

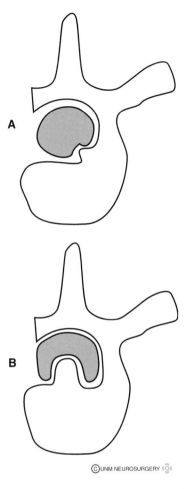

Fig. 37-9. A depiction of the optimal surgical exposures of the thoracic spine. **A,** Dorsal transpedicle. **B,** Transfacet pedicle-sparing. **C,** Costotransversectomy. **D,** Lateral (extracavitary, transcavitary, or extrapleural). **E,** Ventrolateral (transpleural, thoracoabdominal, or extrapleural). The curette in each illustration is situated to demonstrate the ventral dural sac access acquired.

Fig. 37-10. A, During true lateral exposures of the spine, a partial ventral decompression can result in an overhanging of the dura mater and spinal cord, thus obscuring the view of the pathology, as depicted. This can pose significant risk to neural elements and lead to excessive intraoperative blood loss. **B,** True central lesions may be a relative contraindication to lateral exposures for the same reason.

Ventrolateral exposures include the thoracotomy, thoracoabdominal, and extrapleural thoracotomy approaches. The lateral approaches include the lateral extracavitary, the lateral intracavitary, and the extrapleural thoracotomy. These are discussed in Chapters 9 and 10.

The choice of the optimal surgical exposure is dictated in part by surgeon bias. The precise location of the lesion, however, also plays a role in this decision-making process (Fig. 37-9). A truly ventral lesion should most often be attacked via a ventrolateral approach rather than a lateral approach. The overhanging dura mater and spinal cord can make a lateral approach potentially dangerous (Fig. 37-10). On the other hand, a more laterally located lesion is perhaps optimally approached via a lateral approach.

In summary, the location of the lesion with respect to the dural sac should dictate the orientation of the decompression operation (see Fig. 37-9). The specific operative decompression procedure should then be dictated by the confines of the region, surgeon abilities, and surgeon bias. A consideration for the type of stabilization technology to be employed should also enter into the decision-making process.

Spinal Stabilization

The indication for the placement of a spinal implant is dictated by the presence and extent of spinal instability. Multiple schemes have been employed for this purpose, such as the scheme of White and Panjabi,[18] which has been modified to be applicable to all regions of the spine.[1] These schemes are fundamentally based on the three-column theory of Denis.[7]

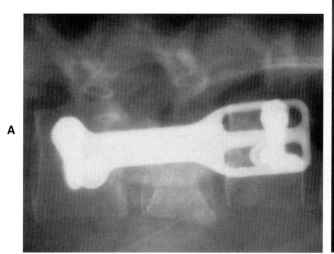
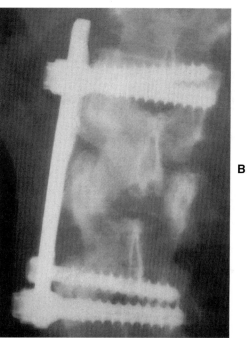

Fig. 37-11. A ventral implant, as depicted, can be employed in cases where dorsal instability is not present.

True column injury and instability dictates the type of stabilization technique employed. As a general rule, a single-column injury or instability usually does not require surgical stabilization. If a single column is injured, it is almost always the ventral or dorsal column. Because other columns are not injured, the injury to the affected column is, by the nature of the injury, not severe.

Two-column injury usually involves the ventral and middle columns. If significant spinal canal compromise and/or neurological deficit is present, decompression may be necessary. Because dorsal column stability is present, ventral implant placement alone, or only the placement of an interbody fusion mass, may suffice for surgical stability acquisition (Fig. 37-11).

However, if three-column injury has been incurred, or surgically created, a circumferential injury to the integrity of the spine exists. Ventral instrumentation, which is usually short segment in nature, may be insufficient to account for the lost dorsal stability (dorsal column injury). Therefore, failure of the construct may be expected. This being the case, dorsal instrumentation is most often indicated in cases of three-column spinal instability. These constructs are usually lengthy, and generally attach to the spine from three segments above to two segments below the injury. This obviously dictates that a ventral decompression and a dorsal implant be placed, which complicates the surgical procedure in many cases.

Occasionally, both ventral and dorsal implant placement procedures are indicated. These situations include those in which significant spinal instability is present or when multiple spinal levels are involved (Fig. 37-12).

Deformity Correction

Deformity correction is a consideration when significant spinal deformity creates a pathological relationship between the neural elements and their surrounding bony and soft tissue confines or predisposes to further progression of deformity, with or without neural element compression.

Sagittal plane deformities may be managed by ventral short segment techniques (Fig. 37-13). These are clearly less effective than longer dorsal techniques, due to the obligatorily shorter bending moment through which they work.

Longer dorsal techniques employ longer moment arms and are thus able to apply significant leverage

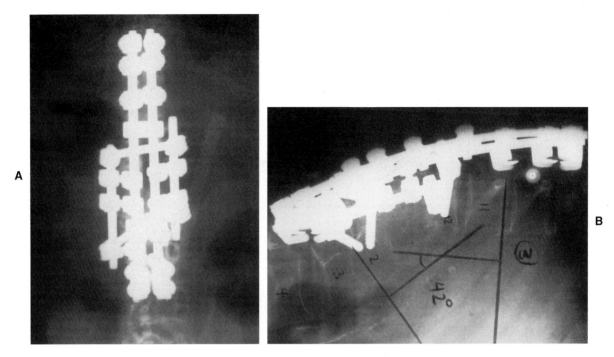

Fig. 37-12. Occasionally, if both dorsal and ventral instability are present (three-column injury), both dorsal and ventral spinal implants may be appropriately placed. Significant three-column instability may dictate this complex approach. The crossfixation of the ventral and dorsal components of the implant, as depicted, may add to the rigidity and rotational stability. AP (**A**) and lateral (**B**) views are depicted.

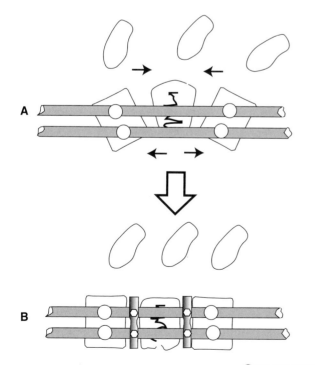

Fig. 37-13. An intrinsic implant bending moment can be applied via short segment ventral instrumentation. **A,** The forces applied to reduce a kyphotic deformity are depicted. **B,** Rigid crossfixation can be employed for maintenance of correction. Remember, the short moment arm of this short construct limits its efficacy for deformity reduction.[1]

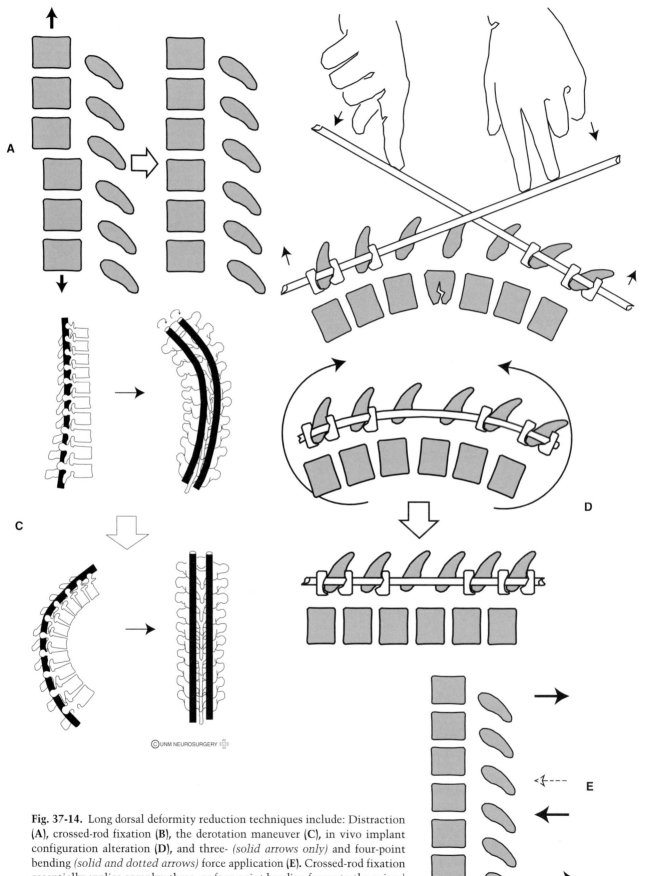

Fig. 37-14. Long dorsal deformity reduction techniques include: Distraction (**A**), crossed-rod fixation (**B**), the derotation maneuver (**C**), in vivo implant configuration alteration (**D**), and three- *(solid arrows only)* and four-point bending *(solid and dotted arrows)* force application (**E**). Crossed-rod fixation essentially applies complex three- or four-point bending forces to the spine.[1]

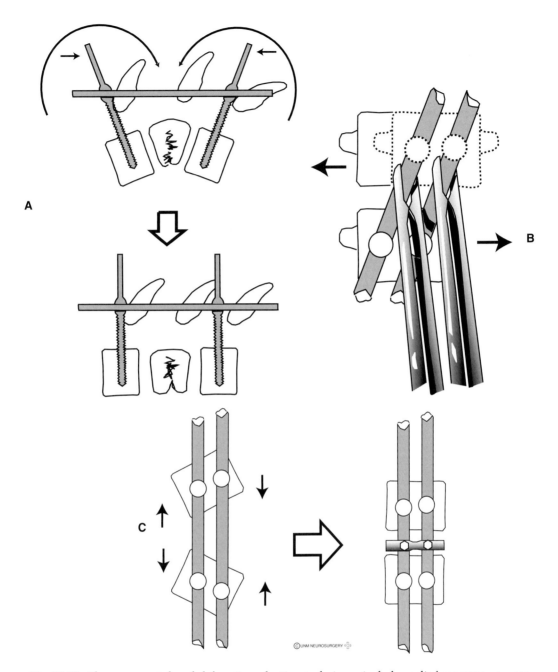

Fig. 37-15. Short segment dorsal deformity reduction techniques include applied moment arm cantilever beam fixation (**A**), short segment parallelogram deformity reduction (**B**), and intrinsic implant bending moment application techniques (**C**).[1] In *B* the configuration is changed from the translated position *(dotted vertebral body)* to the aligned position *(solid vertebral body).*

to the spine. Distraction, the crossed-rod technique, the derotation maneuver, in vivo implant contouring, and three- and four-point bending fixation application are all applicable in the thoracic spine (Fig. 37-14). Short segment techniques may occasionally be useful in the dorsal thoracic spine as well. These include the applied moment arm cantilever beam fixation technique and the short segment parallelogram deformity reduction technique (Fig. 37-15). The choice of the optimal technique in each situation must be individualized.

REFERENCES

1. Benzel EC. Biomechanics of Spine Stabilization: Principles and Clinical Practice. New York: McGraw-Hill, 1995.
2. Benzel EC, Haid RD Jr, Stillerman C, et al. Traumatic thoracolumbar instability. Perspect Neurosurg 7:109-129, 1996.
3. Bucholz RW, Gill K. Classification of injuries to the thoracolumbar spine. Orthop Clin North Am 17:67-83, 1986.
4. Chance GQ. Note on a type of flexion fracture of the spine. Br J Radiol 21:452-453, 1998.
5. Cope R, Kilcoyne RF, Gaines RW. The thoracolumbar burst fracture with intact posterior elements. Implications for neurologic deficit and stability. Neuro-Orthopedics 7:83-87, 1989.
6. Court-Brown CM, Gertzbein SD. The management of burst fractures of the fifth lumbar vertebrae. Spine 12:308-312, 1987.
7. Denis F. The three-column spine and its significance in the classification of acute thoracolumbar spine injuries. Spine 8:817-831, 1983.
8. Gertzbein SD, Court-Brown CM. Flexion-distraction injuries of the lumbar spine. Clin Orthop 227:52-60, 1988.
9. Hashimoto T, Kaneda K, Abumi K. Relationship between traumatic spinal canal and neurologic deficits in thoracolumbar burst fractures. Spine 13:1268-1272, 1988.
10. Holdsworth FW. Fractures, dislocations and fracture dislocations of the spine. J Bone Joint Surg 52A:1534-1551, 1970.
11. Jelsma RK, Kirsch PT, Rice JF, et al. The radiographic description of thoracolumbar fractures. Surg Neurol 18:230-236, 1982.
12. Keene JS. Radiographic evaluation of thoracolumbar fractures. Clin Orthop 189:58-64, 1984.
13. Kelly RP, Whitesides TE Jr. Treatment of lumbodorsal fracture-dislocations. Ann Surg 167:705-717, 1968.
14. McAfee PC, Yuan HA, Frederickson BE, et al. The value of computed tomography in thoracolumbar fractures. J Bone Joint Surg 65A:461-473, 1983.
15. McEnvoy RD, Bradford DS. The management of burst fractures of the thoracic and lumbar spine. Experience in 53 patients. Spine 10:631-637, 1985.
16. Rennie W, Mitchell N. Flexion distraction fractures of the thoracolumbar spine. J Bone Joint Surg 55A:386-390, 1973.
17. Smith SW, Kaufer H. Patterns and mechanisms of lumbar injuries associated with lap seat belts. J Bone Joint Surg 51A:239-254, 1969.
18. White AA, Panjabi MM. Clinical Biomechanics of the Spine, 2nd ed. Philadelphia: JB Lippincott, 1990, pp 30-342.
19. Whitesides TE Jr. Traumatic kyphosis of the thoracolumbar spine. Clin Orthop 128:78-92, 1977.

Metabolic Diseases

Benjamin T. White, M.D., and John A. Wilson, M.D.

Metabolic diseases of the spine may be defined as disease processes that have their pathological effect on the spine via mechanisms of disturbed homeostasis. These processes are most often systemic, with varied effects on other organ systems. The diagnosis and understanding of these conditions is an important aspect of a spine surgeon's practice. Patients with complaints of progressive or persistent back pain are often referred to a specialist without a clear diagnosis. Therefore it is vitally important for the physician treating spinal disorders to have a good understanding of metabolic disturbances that can lead to spinal symptoms.

BONE PHYSIOLOGY
Structure of Bone

From a mechanical standpoint, bone provides the basic framework for motion and protection. These functions require a rigid structure, a high strength-to-weight ratio, and an ability to adapt to a variety of stresses. Bone has the ability to alter its mass and shape over time in order to adapt itself to physical stresses. Bone remodeling is the process by which old bone is reabsorbed and new bone is created. Metabolic derangements that disturb this process can lead to faulty bone remodeling, and thus to bone disease.

Providing mechanical structure is only one of the functions of bone. Bone acts as a mineral store and is intimately involved in both calcium and phosphorus metabolism. Trabecular, or spongy, bone provides the high surface area necessary for the metabolic interaction between the mineral stores in calcified bone and the body's extracellular fluid compartment. It is also a site of hematopoiesis. The compact, or cancellous, bone component provides more of the structural strength of the individual bone. Cancellous bone is made up of concentric rings with alternating fiber orientation that gives it its strength. Both cancellous and trabecular bone are composed of the same materials in similar structural arrangements. Either can be remodeled to the other as changing stress demands.

Extracellular Elements

The composition of bone consists of an organic substrate made of structural proteins and an inorganic mineral matrix. Structural proteins make up approximately 25% of the bone mass. The inorganic mineral matrix accounts for another 50% of bone mass. The remaining mass of a bone consists of water. The organic substrate of bone is made up of a network of collagen and ground substance. The collagen of bone is type I. It is fibrous and high in glycine, with the unique capacity to become calcified. The ground substance of bone is composed of mucoproteins and hexosamine and glycuronic polymers. It is similar in composition to the ground substance of other connective tissues.[45] The mineral portion of bone is hydroxyapatite: $Ca_{10}(PO_4)_6(OH)_2$. Other moities can be substituted for the hydroxyl or the phosphorus group in hydroxyapatite. This can be important for both diagnostic and therapeutic reasons.

Cellular Elements

Osteocyte

The cellular elements of bone are responsible for all bone remodeling, and are closely tied to calcium metabolism. Osteocytes are the principal cell of mature bone. They reside in lacunae surrounded by mineralized bone. They maintain contact with the nutrient blood vessels, the periosteum, and other osteocytes by means of long canicular processes. Osteocytes are thought to have important roles in calcium homeostasis and maintaining local ionic environment of mature bone. The canicular system has an enormous surface area that provides an excellent junction between mineralized bone and the osteocyte.

Osteoblast

Osteoblasts are the basic bone-forming cells. They are mature cells that do not divide. Osteoblasts produce and secrete unmineralized matrix that is called osteoid. They also participate closely in the mineralization process. Osteoblasts participate in the control of calcium and phosphorus metabolism in bone. They have extracellular receptors for parathyroid hormone and 1,25-dihydroxy vitamin D_3. Both of these hormones are important in the regulation of calcium metabolism. There is evidence that osteoblasts are also involved in the induction of bone resorption by osteoclasts.

Osteoclasts

Osteoclasts are multinucleated giant cells intimately involved with bone resorption. Evidence supports the theory that these cells are derived from mononuclear cells that originate in the bone marrow. Osteoclasts are large cells with a ruffled border, and are usually found in resorption pits or Howship's lacunae. Osteoclasts produce a variety of dehydrogenases and proteases that act to degrade both the mineral and protein components of mature bone. Osteoclasts respond to hormonal influences that induce bone resorption, such as 1,25-dihydroxy vitamin D_3, parathyroid hormone, prostaglandin E_2, and calcitonin. However, they lack receptors for these substances and their response is believed to be mediated by other cell types, such as osteoblasts.[55]

Calcium Metabolism

The principal considerations of calcium metabolism are absorption from the gut, transport in the circulation, deposition and removal from the bone, and urinary and fecal excretion. Calcium absorption is an energy-dependent, highly regulated process that occurs primarily in the upper small bowel. Absorption in all portions of the gut is increased by 1,25-dihydroxy vitamin D_3. Calcium's absorption is closely regulated. Net calcium absorption is the difference between gastrointestinal absorption and fecal excretion. True calcium absorption is expressed as a percentage of dietary intake. In a normal adult approximately 40% of dietary calcium is absorbed.

Calcium is transferred in the circulation in two states, ionic and bound or ultrafiltratable. Approximately 4.5 mg/dl of serum calcium is ionic. The rest (usually 50% to 60% of total serum calcium) is bound to serum proteins and complex organic acids. Seventy-five percent of total binding is accounted for by albumin, the most important of the calcium binding proteins. Ionic calcium concentrations are highly regulated and remain constant, despite changes in serum protein and total calcium concentrations. Mechanisms responsible for this tight regulation involve peptide hormones.

The kidneys play a central role in calcium metabolism. Ultrafiltratable serum calcium is freely filterable by the glomerulus and is avidly resorbed by proximal and distal tubules. In a normal adult, about 95% of calcium filtered by the glomerulus is resorbed. The bulk of calcium resorption is closely tied to sodium resorption in the proximal tubule and the loop of Henle. The remainder of calcium resorption (30%) is sodium independent and occurs in the more distal tubule and collecting duct. The sodium-independent resorptive process is increased by parathyroid hormone, increased serum phosphorus concentrations, and metabolic alkalosis.

The storage and release of calcium in bone makes up the remainder of the calcium metabolic cycle. Conventionally, the predominant influence of bone on calcium levels was thought to be the variations in the rate of bone resorption. More recent evidence supports a distinction between the two functions of the cell populations of bone.[69,70] The remodeling system made up of osteoblasts and osteoclasts is responsible for bone turnover, but is not directly responsible for serum calcium levels. As resorption increases so does bone deposition, so that any level of bone resorption calcium concentrations may remain normal.

The second cellular system of bone is made up of the osteocyte and the bone syncytium. This system is the junction between the serum and the calcium and phosphorus stored in bone. This system is believed to be most important in the regulation of serum ionic calcium and phosphorus levels.

Hormonal Control

The hormonal control of calcium metabolism is closely related to the control of bone mineralization and resorption. Therefore it is important in the treatment of the subject of metabolic diseases of the spine to discuss the actions of the hormones related to calcium metabolism.

Vitamin D₃

Vitamin D, or cholecalciferol, is a naturally occurring derivative of cholesterol. The human body can produce vitamin D by ultraviolet radiation of 7-dihydroxy cholesterol in the skin. Environmental conditions and daily sun exposure are therefore important determinants of vitamin D production. Dietary sources of vitamin D include fortified products such as milk, and natural sources such as fish oils and animal liver. Vitamin D that is absorbed in the gut is first hydroxylated in the liver to yield a transport form of vitamin D, 25-hydroxy vitamin D_3. Transport in the serum is via protein binding with special globulins. Excess vitamin D is stored in adipose tissue. In the kidney, 25-hydroxy vitamin D_3 is hydroxylated to 1,25-dihydroxy vitamin D_3, its active metabolite. This hydroxylation is under a negative feedback control of vitamin D. This leads to a decrease in 1-hydroxylation in the presence of vitamin D excess, and an increase in 1-hydroxylation with a vitamin D deficiency. 1-hydroxylation is also stimulated by parathyroid hormone.

The active metabolite of vitamin D, 1,25-dihydroxy vitamin D_3, has its effects on three primary target organs: the gut, kidney, and bone. Vitamin D_3 has its primary effect in up-regulating active calcium absorption in the gut. It acts at the intestinal epithelium as a steroid hormone, up-regulating production of membrane proteins associated with the energy-dependent absorption of calcium.

The actions of vitamin D_3 in bone are complex and not completely understood. At physiological levels, it increases serum calcium levels via unclear mechanisms. This increase is dependent on parathyroid hormone. Both mineralization and osteoid formation are inhibited in the vitamin D deficient state. This suggests that vitamin D plays a significant role in the regulation of both osteoid formation and mineralization, although mechanisms that mediate this are still being studied.

Vitamin D also has calcium conserving effects on the kidneys. 1,25-dihydroxy vitamin D_3 increases absorption in the distal tubule and collecting ducts, and acts to increase phosphate resorption in the more proximal tubule.

Parathyroid Hormone

Parathyroid hormone (PTH) is a peptide hormone produced by the parathyroid glands. PTH consists of 84 amino acids, cleaved from a larger precursor called proPTH. PTH has a short half-life, being quickly cleared to leave an inactive C-terminal fragment with a much longer half-life. It is the C-terminal fragment that is assayed in most PTH assays. PTH secretion is increased by low plasma ionic calcium concentrations and decreased by high plasma ionic calcium concentrations. There are multiple mechanisms that affect changes in levels of PTH secretion. Increased cleavage of stores of proPTH allows for rapid increases in PTH. This allows for rapid temporal changes in PTH levels. Increased production of proPTH and eventual gland hyperplasia with increasing numbers of hormone-producing parathyroid cells provide mechanisms for increasing PTH over days to years in response to chronically low serum calcium levels.

PTH has its most significant effect on the bone and the kidney. These target organs have a complex response to PTH. The end result, however, is an increase in serum ionized calcium. This response is quite rapid, but via complex mechanisms can be sustained over an indefinite time.

PTH has direct effects on osteoclasts, increasing resorptive activity of existing cells and recruiting additional progenitor cells to proliferate into new osteoclasts. PTH also has effects on osteoblasts. Of note, receptors for PTH have been found on osteoblasts, but not osteoclasts. This suggests that changes observed in osteoclastic actions might be mediated via the osteoblast. In humans, PTH causes an increase in a number of osteoblasts associated with bone remodeling units, but a decrease in osteoid apposition and mineralization.[59]

PTH has complex actions on the nephron that are important in calcium metabolism. The most rapid change observed in response to PTH is an increase in urinary phosphate. This effect is observed within minutes of the administration of PTH. PTH also acts to increase calcium absorption in the distal nephron. The physiological result of PTH on the kidney is to increase serum calcium with a net increase in phosphate excretion.

Calcitonin

Calcitonin is the other peptide hormone with a direct influence over serum calcium levels. Its functions oppose that of PTH and it is secreted in response to high levels of serum ionized calcium. Calcitonin is produced by the parafollicular, or C, cells of the thyroid gland. It is a 32-amino acid polypeptide and exists as a single molecule or as a dimer. Other factors that stimulate calcitonin release include certain gastrointestinal hormones, such as gastrin.

Calcitonin's actions prompt movement of calcium and phosphorus ions into bone. The mechanism behind this movement is not clear and is not entirely explained by inhibition of bone resorption. However, calcitonin does inhibit bone resorption by two mechanisms. First, calcitonin inhibits individual osteoclasts, and second, it inhibits the differentiation of progenitor cells into osteoclasts. Calcitonin has effects on the excretion of calcium in the kidney. Renal calcium excretion is increased by calcitonin in direct opposition to the action of PTH.

Calcitonin participates in a complex system with PTH to regulate serum ionized calcium concentrations. Some researchers believe that calcitonin represents a specialized feedback system that prevents transient increases in serum calcium, caused by increases in dietary calcium intake. This allows calcium absorbed from dietary sources to be stored rather than being lost in urine, as the unopposed PTH system would tend to cause.

Components of Bone

Structure of mature bone can be divided into two anatomical forms, cortical and trabecular. Cortical bone usually makes up 80% of bone volume and trabecular bone makes up the remaining 20%. In the spine, however, trabecular bone makes up about two thirds of the bone volume, whereas cortical bone makes up about one third of the remaining bone volume. The basic structure of a mature bone is defined by the process of remodeling. The remodeling process leaves bone made up of mature osteons of differing ages. These osteons are welded together at cement planes formed by the system of remodeling.

Cortical bone is made up of a series of concentric laminae. These laminae contain a series of osteons of different ages. The osteons and related structures are also referred to as the Haversian system. Each osteon has a central canal, termed the "Haversian canal." It contains nutrient vessels, lymphatics, and connective tissue. The central canals of osteons are connected to their neighbors via small transverse Volkmann's canals. The typical osteon is about 200 μm in diameter and runs nearly parallel to the long axis of the bone. In the laminae of mineralized osteoid around the central canal, osteocytes are contained in spaces termed "lacunae." These osteocytes are connected to the Haversian canal and to each other via a complex system of canaliculi.

Layers of bone oriented along lines of stress make up trabecular bone. Trabecular bone is lined by small cuboidal cells termed the "endosteum." The space between the trabecula are filled with either fat or marrow. The individual trabeculae form a complex three-dimensional network that is recognized as trabecular bone. Other than this trabecular network, the ultrastructure of trabecular bone is identical to that found in cortical bone.

Bone Formation and Growth

Bone formation in the mature bone is appositional (i.e., new bone is formed only on existing bone surfaces). The process of de novo formation and growth in children is different and considered only briefly here for completeness.

In the child, bone formation and growth can be divided into two categories: (1) intramembranous ossification and (2) endochondral ossification. Intramembranous ossification is a formation of local bone on the substrate of local collection of fibrous tissue. This bone lacks the regular arrangement of collagen fibers that marks lamellar bone. It is usually short-lived and progressively replaced by lamellar bone by the process of remodeling. The skull, mandible, scapula, and pelvis develop via intramembranous ossification.

All long bones and the vertebral bodies develop via endochondral ossification. A cartilaginous model is transformed by osseous development into immature bone. This process is complicated, and is the result of three separate areas of growth—the periosteal collar, the growth plate, and the epiphyses. All of these processes produce woven bone as a first product. This is subsequently remodeled to lamellar bone.

Bone Remodeling

The primary physiological process of interest in studying metabolic diseases of the bone is the process of bone remodeling. This process is basic to the physiology of bone and its ability to adapt to changing loads, resisting the high-frequency, low-impact stress that would otherwise cause a static structure to fail. In the normal adult, maximum bone mass is obtained during the third decade. During most of adult life, there is nearly a perfect match between bone resorption and bone formation. The fine balance between resorption and formation is quite important, particularly in diseases such as osteoporosis. Understanding physiological processes that govern each of the steps of bone formation, osteoid production, and mineralization is basic to understanding the pathology observed in metabolic bone disorders.

The concept of quantitized units of bone remodeling is helpful in understanding bone physiology and those disease processes that result in abnormal bone physiology. The basic multicellular unit (BMU) is the quantitized unit of remodeling. Each BMU will eventually become a mature osteon. The osteon is a physiological unit made up of a central canal (Haversian canal) with nutrient vessels, lymphatics, and nerves. The cells of the osteon are primarily the osteocyte, which can be found in individual lacunae surrounded by mineralized bone. The individual osteon has obvious structural functions as bone, but it also has complex physiological functions in maintaining homeostasis.

The BMU is the basic unit of bone remodeling. It removes a quantum of bone through osteoclastic activity and replaces it, through the activity of osteoblasts, with an equal amount of newly formed lamellar bone. The cellular elements that make up the BMU are the resorptive osteoclast, followed by the osteoid-producing osteoblast. Also included are supportive structures, such as nutrient vessels and lymphatics. The BMU in action is a cylinder with the processes of resorption and formation extending longitudinally. Any single cross-section of the BMU is a snapshot in time of the processes that all cross-sections encounter during the life of the BMU. Fig. 38-1 is a schematic description of a functional BMU demonstrating the complete cycle of remodeling described here.

The length of time from formation of a new BMU to completion of bone formation is variable, depending on the length of the resorption cavity carved out by the osteocytes. The length of time for any particular cross-section of the BMU to undergo the complete remodeling process is on the order of 120 days.[55]

The entire process of bone remodeling can be broken down into six stages: (1) activation, (2) bone resorption, (3) reversal, (4) bone formation, (5) mineralization, and (6) quiescence.[55]

The initial event in the formation of a BMU is the recruitment of osteoclasts from the stem cell population found in the bone marrow. The activation process, which precedes any actual resorption of bone, takes approximately 3 days. The mechanisms regulating the activation of osteoclasts before the formation of BMUs is thought to be one of the primary steps in control of the remodeling of bone. Although it is not entirely clear what triggers activation of a BMU, it is known that it is under tight hormonal control. PTH and 1,25-dihydroxy vitamin D_3 are both hormones that can increase the number of active BMUs.

Once osteoclasts begin resorbing bone they form a so-called cutting cone that is about 200 µm in diameter and 300 µm long. It is this process by which the new osteon is created. Existing osteons can be partially or totally incorporated by the new resorption cavity. This gives mature bone the appearance of multiple osteons of various ages overlaid on top of each other. The cutting cone of a BMU precedes into the existing bone about 40 to 50 µm per day. The cutting cone tends to proceed down the long

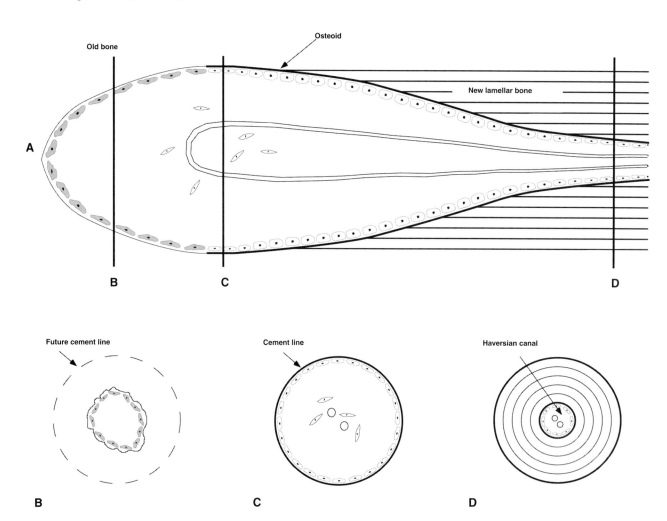

Fig. 38-1. A, Schematic diagram of a section along the long axis of a complete BMU. Note the cutting cone lined with osteoclasts and the concentric narrowing of the central canal as new lamellar bone is laid down by osteoblasts. **B,** A cross-section through the cutting cone of the BMU. Osteocytes progressively enlarge the cavity to the level of the future cement line. **C,** A cross-section at the time of quiescence demonstrating the flattened lining of osteoblasts, stromal cells, and nutrient vessels. **D,** A cross-section through a now mature osteon demonstrating the lining of small flat cells, a small central Haversian canal, and the concentric laminae of newly formed bone.

shaft of the bone for a variable distance, perhaps a centimeter or more.

Between resorption and new bone formation is a resting period that lasts several days. This period is known as reversal. The cement line of a mature osteon marks the bone surface during this period. The period of reversal varies considerably in length, depending on the lag between resorption and new bone formation.

Osteoblasts are recruited and the bone formation process begins. Bone matrix is produced in concentric laminae, slowly refilling the cavity left by the osteoclastic activity. The average closure rate of a cross-section of a BMU is on the order of 1 to 2 µm per day. This, however, seems to slow during the later process of bone formation. The osteon is not completely closed, leaving a 40 to 50 µm canal, the Haversian canal, with nutrient vessels that supply the osteocytes, osteoclasts, and other supportive cells.

Mineral is deposited in the bone matrix between and within the collagen fibers. This process follows matrix formation after a lag of about 10 days. Approximately 60% of osteoid is mineralized in the first 24 hours, and thereafter, the remaining osteoid is mineralized in a decreasing rate over the following 6 months.[21,55]

The period after complete mineralization of the newly formed osteoid is termed the "quiescent phase." The osteoclasts disappear and the remaining cells are mature osteocytes descending from the osteoblasts. The nutrient capillaries with lymphatics and nerves remain in the Haversian canal. Newly encased osteocytes maintain metabolic contact with each other and the Haversian canal by fine processes, the canaliculi.

Application to the Spine

The spine is composed of 24 individual vertebrae and the sacrum. The individual vertebrae are made up of a vertebral body attached to the dorsal elements by the pedicles. The vertebral body is formed by endochondral ossification, and is largely ossified by birth. Dorsal elements are formed by intramembranous ossification. During growth, the vertebral body has an epiphysis, just as do long bones; the physiology of vertebral bone is essentially the same as that found in other long bones. However, periosteal expansion of the width of the epiphysis is more important for growth of the vertebrae than in the appendicular skeleton. The remodeling process of the new bone laid down by periosteal expansion yields vertical trabeculae. This trabecular bone is the major component of the vertebral body.

In the extraspinal skeleton, the ratio of cortical to trabecular bone is approximately 4:1. In contrast, the volumetric ratio of cortical to trabecular bone in the spine is about 1:2. This is important, because under normal physiological conditions, trabecular bone is about eight times more metabolically active than cortical bone.

BONE PATHOLOGY

It is useful to segregate bone pathology into three pathological processes: osteoporosis, osteomalacia, and osteitis fibrosa cystica.[70] Although attempting to compartmentalize all metabolic pathologies into one of these groups is counterproductive, it is useful to relate components of them to pathological processes that are well understood at both the microscopic and physiological level. Metabolic disease of bone will often display elements of each of the three basic pathological processes.

This brief examination of basic features of bone pathology is not an attempt to serve as a reference on the topic. The pathologies encompassed by metabolic diseases of bone are broad and a complete treatment is a subject unto itself. This section attempts to briefly describe the three basic pathologies and provide useful information to help clarify the specific entities discussed later.

Osteoporosis

The usual meaning of "osteoporosis" in modern medical practice is a decrease in overall bone volume. "Diminished bone mass" is not a good definition of osteoporosis, because conditions that produce a loss of mineralization of bone can yield significant decreases in bone mass without changes in bone volume. Thus osteoporosis is a result of a decrease in both mineralized and unmineralized bone. In other respects the cellular component and the ultrastructure of osteoporotic bone appears similar to healthy bone on microscopic examination. However, there are qualitative as well as quantitative changes in bone physiology in osteoporosis. Histologically, these changes are not evident on routine examination. Therefore histological examination of osteoporotic bone is often of little help. An exception is the exclusion of osteomalacia and osteitis fibrosa cystica as comorbid conditions existing contemporaneously with osteoporosis.

Osteomalacia

The basic pathophysiological mechanism of osteomalacia is the abnormal mineralization of formed osteoid. Histologically, this translates into increased volumes of unmineralized osteoid tissue. Osteoid seams are increased in surface area and width, not because of increased birth rate of new BMUs, but because of the increased lag time to complete mineralization. The osteoid matrix observed with osteomalacia is also abnormal. There are often small islands of partially calcified osteoid, in contrast to normal osteoid that is completely unmineralized. The osteoblasts of osteomalacia are also characteristic. The wide osteoid seams of the incompletely calcified lamellar bone are covered with flat terminal osteoblasts, with evidence of impaired function.

Paget's disease, fluorosis, and osteitis fibrosa cystica can also have widened osteoid seams. The primary difference between these conditions and osteomalacia is that these conditions produce woven bone, whereas osteomalacia produces well-formed lamellar osteoid. There is also no evidence of osteoblastic dysfunction in these conditions, as is seen in osteomalacia.

Osteitis Fibrosa Cystica

Osteitis fibrosa cystica is not an inflammatory condition as its name might imply. It is the pathological result of hyperparathyroidism. The term "osteitis fibrosa" is old and some prefer not to use it. It is, however, the classic description of the pathology seen in patients with hyperparathyroidism.

The histological hallmark of osteitis fibrosa cystica is the increased surface area of osteoclastic activity. The number of BMUs is increased, as well as the turnover time of each BMU. Individual osteoclastic activity is actually decreased in hyperparathyroid states. This leads to a prolongation of BMU turnover. In mild or early hyperparathyroidism, histological examination may simply show an increase in the number of normally configured BMUs. In severe cases, these BMUs may become so numerous that their lumens become confluent, forming large osteoclast-lined cavities. The resorbed bone in these conditions is replaced with woven bone, compared with the normal lamellar bone. There can also be large areas of marrow fibrosis and fibrous tissue observed in the Haversian canals.

The cysts observed in osteitis fibrosa cystica occur in two varieties. True cysts are unusually large resorption cavities that are filled with a proteinaceous fluid. Pseudocysts consist of masses of osteoclasts, partially mineralized osteoid, and fibrous tissue. These pseudocysts are the classic "brown tumor" of severe hyperparathyroidism that can resemble giant cell tumors. Both varieties of cysts can cause significant bone deformation.

CLINICAL ASSESSMENT

The clinical assessment of a patient with spinal abnormality, in whom a metabolic disorder of bone is suspected, has several important elements: history, physical examination, laboratory examination, radiographic examination, and more rarely, histological examination. The information gained from these elements should help confirm or exclude the presence of a metabolic disorder of the spine and aid in its diagnosis as well as form the basis for assessment of treatment.

History

A thorough history is the first step in evaluating metabolic disorders of the spine. Often there may be no presenting complaint because in many of these patients an abnormality will have been incidentally discovered on a radiograph. However, the history may still yield valuable clues to the diagnosis. Past and present illnesses should be identified, as well as a complete medication history. Medications may be particularly important, because they are related to certain iatrogenic causes of metabolic bone disorders (i.e., thiazide diuretics, lithium, corticosteroid treatment). Family history and menstrual history should be obtained. The social history can be of particular importance, especially as it relates to occupational exposure, activity level, nutrition, and social habits such as tobacco and alcohol use.

In those patients who are symptomatic, the presenting symptom is very likely related to pain, but fracture, deformity, or neurological dysfunction also may be associated features. Pain is such a common complaint in these disorders that it deserves special mention. Because no nerve endings have been found within bone it has been suggested that all bone pain comes from the periosteum, which has a rich supply of nerve endings.[19] It is clear, however, that expanding lesions of the bone may cause pain long before the periosteum has become involved. This bone pain may be mediated by autonomic nerves within the bone, providing a basis for the usual nature of the pain, which can be deep and throbbing. The more severe lancinating pain associated with vertebral collapse or cortical buckling is likely explained by periosteal involvement. Other causes of pain may be related to spinal deformity and its mechanical effects on the muscular and ligamentous structures supporting the spine or from direct pressure on neural structures. Thus the nature and location of pain can be of great importance in determining its etiology.

In patients presenting with fracture or deformity, the nature of any inciting event must be carefully discerned. The force of any injury or impact load will have significant bearing on the subsequent workup of the patient. Specifically, the implications of a spinal fracture occurring with low energy forces being applied to the spine should raise questions about the structural integrity of the spine.

Laboratory Evaluation

Routine serum and urine tests may be performed on all patients suspected of having a metabolic bone disorder. Hematological, renal, and liver function are screened by the appropriate tests. A complete blood count should reveal most hematological disorders. Creatinine can be used to screen for renal function, although creatinine clearance provides a more accurate assessment if there is any question. Hepatic function is measured by alkaline phosphatase and gamma-glutamyl transpeptidase. If alkaline phosphatase is elevated, fractionation may be useful. Basic fluid and electrolyte measurements are necessary, and if malabsorption is suspected a serum carotene level may be used as a screening test. Based on results of these routine tests, further evaluation may be indicated for direct measurement of PTH and/or vitamin D levels. If serum calcium is low, vitamin D and vitamin D_3 levels should be measured. With hypercalcemia, primary or secondary hyperparathyroidism is suspected and PTH and vitamin D levels should be tested.

There are several additional tests that can help delineate bone metabolism. Twenty-four–hour urinary measurement of calcium and phosphorus can determine calcium and phosphorus balance and help direct treatment. The measurement of osteocalcin can also indicate the rate of bone turnover. This protein is synthesized by osteoblasts and is released from bone during bone resorption. High levels suggest a rapid turnover of bone with active formation and resorption.[70] Serum protein electrophoresis and, if indicated, urine protein electrophoresis may be performed to rule out myeloma.

Radiographic Evaluation

Despite the rapid expansion in imaging technology, plain anteroposterior and lateral radiographs remain the cornerstone of imaging evaluation in metabolic disorders of the spine.

Plain radiographs of the thoracic and lumbar spine are indicated in all metabolic bone disorders that affect the spine. In osteoporosis, vertebral bodies are the most common skeletal elements at risk

for fracture. Thus radiographs, in addition to helping confirm the diagnosis, can assess vertebral status at the beginning of treatment and give a baseline for comparison throughout treatment. In Paget's disease plain radiographs of the involved site are often diagnostic. Characteristic changes in the shape of the vertebral bodies can help distinguish osteomalacia from more common osteoporotic compression.

Plain radiographs do have significant limitations in terms of quantitative analysis. They are not particularly sensitive to changes in bone mineralization; at least 30% of bone tissue must be lost to be noticed on a standard radiograph.[70] Changes in radiolucency of bone are related to bone mineralization. Loss of bone mineralization is common to all three types of metabolic bone disease. Therefore using the term "osteoporosis" to describe the radiographic appearance can be confusing. The appropriate terminology is not agreed upon, but "osteopenia" is commonly used. A less confusing and more descriptive term might simply be "increased radiolucency."[70]

Bone densitometry measurements have been accomplished via a number of techniques. Single photon absorptiometry (SPA) and dual photon absorptiometry (DPA) have been used in quantitatively evaluating bone density. SPA provides a measure of density per area of cortical bone. However, its use is limited to the radius of the bone and there is poor correlation between the bone mineral content of the peripheral and axial skeleton. DPA has been developed more recently. It measures the attenuation of radiation of two different energies. DPA requires specialized, dedicated equipment, but is able to provide accurate bone density measurements of the spine.

Quantitative computed tomography (CT) is accomplished by performing a CT of the vertebrae with quantitative readings. It is compared to the known density of solutions in calibration phantoms. This method is fairly accurate, provides density as a measure of bone volume, and is readily available at many institutions. It does involve more radiation exposure for the patient than SPA or DPA, but uses approximately one tenth the radiation of a standard CT scan.

Isotope scanning most commonly uses technetium-based isotope agents. These agents reflect new bone formation and may bind to immature collagen as well. Positive scans are observed with fractures, areas of increased bone turnover, and in osteomalacia.[70] Its relative lack of specificity limits its usefulness in metabolic bone disorders.

Other diagnostic tests such as myelography, CT, and magnetic resonance imaging (MRI) are primarily reserved for the rare instances when there are signs or symptoms of neurological involvement. MRI in particular may be quite sensitive in identifying subtle changes in bone structure. However, its expense precludes its use as a screening test. As further experience is gained with MRI spectroscopy it may ultimately play a greater role in evaluating bone physiology.

Bone Biopsy

Transiliac bone biopsy is rarely performed, but can be useful in establishing the diagnoses of osteomalacia and occult malignancy, or in differentiating between osteomalacia and osteitis fibrosa cystica in chronic dialysis patients. Practically speaking, it has little utility over other noninvasive methods of investigation. From a research and educational standpoint it may facilitate diagnosis and further understanding of the disease process and response to treatment. It can easily be performed in an ambulatory setting with a very low morbidity. Usually tetracycline is administered preoperatively in two divided dosing regimens. This can then be used as a marker of the dynamic properties of bone. Pathological examination of undecalcified sections requires special equipment for cutting the sections, but is desirable.

CLINICAL FEATURES AND TREATMENT
Osteoporosis

Osteoporosis is a disease characterized by decreased bone mass, micro-architectural deterioration of bone leading to bone fragility, and an increase in fracture rates.[15] The definition of osteoporosis is not without difficulty because the processes that lead to symptomatic osteoporosis are similar to the processes of normal aging.

The loss of bone mass is an inevitable aspect of the human aging process. The amount of bone loss has been correlated with risk of fracture, both in extremities and in the spine.[42,79] The term "osteoporosis," in common medical usage, has come to represent this decrease in bone density observed most often in postmenopausal women. It is debated if the clinical syndrome described here represents a true disease or is part of the spectrum of normal aging. Persons with atraumatic vertebral fractures have significantly less bone than age-matched controls. However, other members of the population with similar bone mass may not have fractures.

The relationship between bone mass and fracture risk is complex. The mechanisms leading to fractures are multifactorial. Not only bone mass, but also bone quality and risk of falls play major roles. The risk of falls in the population of patients at risk for osteoporosis is significant, and factors influencing fall rates are numerous, including age, vision, and environmental factors, such as presence of steps in the house.

Experimental studies seem to support bone mass as providing significant contribution to overall bone strength. In vitro studies demonstrate bone mass as having a strong correlation with fracture threshold (with a correlation coefficient of 0.6 to 0.8)

Bone mass loss in postmenopausal women deserves special mention. There is strong evidence that gonadal failure at the time of menopause is associated with significant acceleration of bone mass loss. Mechanisms behind this have been investigated vigorously. The loss of the major portion of the circulating estrogens at menopause leads to an increased sensitivity of bone to PTH. The normal homeostatic mechanisms keep serum calcium concentrations normal despite increases in other markers of bone turnover. The resultant decrease in PTH has the secondary effect of decreasing production of 1,25-dihydroxy vitamin D_3, leading to less efficient absorption of dietary calcium. Thus the increased sensitivity to PTH has the overall effect of maintaining serum calcium at the expense of bone, instead of the use of dietary calcium. This effect seems to be most pronounced in the 4 to 8 years after menopause.

Although the mechanisms of bone loss may not be pathologic in nature, their end result is. There is a clear clinical picture of fractures, bone pain, and loss of height associated with osteoporosis. The components of this clinical presentation seem to be integrally linked to the loss of bone mass and to a lesser extent to degradation of bone quality. The threshold at which loss of bone density and quality predisposes an individual to osteoporotic fractures has not been precisely quantified.

Clinical Presentation

The typical patient with osteoporosis is asymptomatic and undiagnosed until an acute fracture requires medical attention. The diagnosis is occasionally made in the asymptomatic patient by incidental findings of compression fractures on plain radiographs such as a chest radiograph. The diagnosis of a decrease in bone mass is unpredictable on plain films. It is important to keep in mind that although most women undergo the metabolic changes thought to lead to osteoporosis at menopause, only 10% to 20% of women develop symptomatic osteoporosis.

Osteoporosis can lead to a variety of fractures, including vertebral fractures. Spine fractures in osteoporosis are usually compression fractures, with the loss of vertebral body height, typically more ventrally than dorsally. Figs. 38-2 and 38-3 demonstrate compression fractures in the thoracic spines of elderly patients. Although kyphotic deformities can be significant, neural injury is rare. The overall loss of bone volume associated with this condition allows the vertical collapse of the vertebral body without significant lateral or dorsal expansion. If

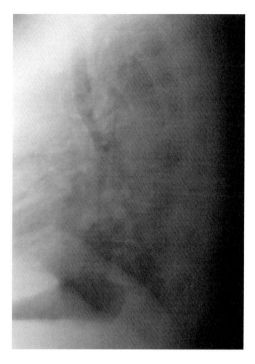

Fig. 38-2. Lateral plain radiograph of the thoracic spine demonstrating a severe midthoracic osteoporotic compression fracture in an elderly woman. There is nearly complete loss of height of the affected vertebral body with a kyphotic deformity.

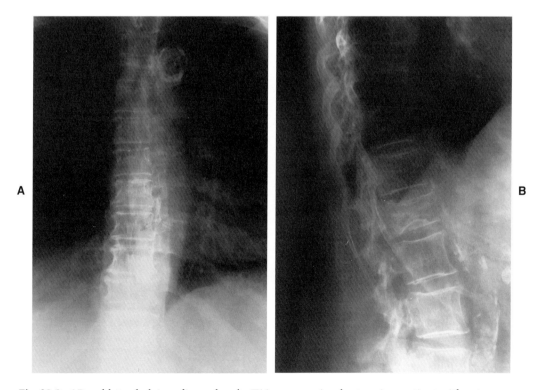

Fig. 38-3. AP and lateral plain radiographs of a T11 compression fracture in a patient with osteoporosis. The vertebral bodies appear osteopenic and there is a 30% to 40% loss of height of T11.

the volume of bone material were preserved, the compression fracture would invariably lead to circumferential expansion of the collapsed vertebrae, and neurological compression would be the expected result. These fractures are often precipitated by a fall, but it is not uncommon for trivial trauma such as bending or light lifting to lead to such compression fractures. Patients present with intense back pain without neurological deficit. There are few cases of neurological deficit reported in the literature associated with an osteoporotic compression fracture. An apparent osteoporotic fracture presenting with neurological symptoms should trigger an exhaustive search for other pathology, such as metastatic disease.

Epidemiology

The population in which osteoporosis becomes symptomatic is defined by a variety of factors. Bone mass and quality, propensity for falls, and numerous environmental variables are all important. The typical osteoporotic fracture patient is a fair skinned, postmenopausal female. In general, the age, sex, and race determinants of bone mass translate directly into fracture risk. Hip fractures, for which the best population data exists, are far more common in women and in whites, but increase exponentially with age in all ethnic groups. They reach a peak of 30 per 1000 in white women over 85 years of age.[44]

A large list of risk factors have been found to be associated with bone density and osteoporosis-related fractures. Genetic factors are sure to play a role. Sorting out the genetic contribution to osteoporosis is complicated by the large number of environmental factors, such as occupation, fluoride content of water, exercise, and exposure to sunlight, that are involved. The box below lists both modifi-

---

CONDITIONS ASSOCIATED WITH OSTEOPOROSIS

Gastric surgery
Thiazide diuretic use
Corticosteroid use
Hyperthyroidism
Calcium deficiency
Vitamin D deficiency
Type II diabetes mellitus

---

able and nonmodifiable risk factors. Other associations are listed in the box above.

Laboratory and Radiographic Evaluation

As a starting point, initial tests should consist of a complete blood count, erythrocyte sedimentation rate, serum glucose, serum creatinine and creatinine clearance, serum protein electrophoresis, and serum calcium and phosphorus levels. In addition to diagnosis and assessing the effects of treatment, these studies may also help exclude other bone disorders such as myeloma.

Radiographic evaluation is primarily directed by the patient's symptoms and physical examination. The role of screening radiographs or bone density measurements in asymptomatic postmenopausal women is controversial. Currently, public health initiatives may be best directed at modifiable risk factors in the population at risk.

Treatment

Calcium and Vitamin D Therapy. Calcium supplementation has been studied extensively. Absorption of calcium in the elderly is significantly decreased compared with younger control subjects. These changes are secondary to changes in vitamin D metabolism and a decreased absorption of the mineral. There is good evidence that increased calcium intake can lead to slowed loss of bone mass or even increases in bone mass.[10]

Translation of decreased bone resorption to a decrease in fracture rates has been more difficult. A prospective population analysis demonstrated a correlation between dietary intake of calcium (by diet questionnaire) and hip fracture rates.[38] Other investigations have failed to reproduce this result.[64]

RISK FACTORS FOR DEVELOPMENT OF SYMPTOMATIC OSTEOPOROSIS

Premature menopause
Short stature
Smoking
Prior pregnancy
Caucasian race
Heavy alcohol use
Sedentary lifestyle

The current recommended daily amounts of calcium for the postmenopausal woman is 800 mg. There is some evidence from studies focused on calcium supplementation and bone mass that higher levels of calcium intake are beneficial. One thousand to 1200 mg of elemental calcium per day may be a more appropriate target for postmenopausal women.

Changes in vitamin D metabolism may also contribute to the negative calcium balance observed in the osteoporotic patient. There is a decrease in vitamin D absorption in the aging population. This, coupled with a decrease in sun exposure, can lead to a relative vitamin D deficiency. Ten percent of hip fractures contain pathological evidence of osteomalacia. These findings suggest that vitamin D supplementation is likely needed in the osteoporotic patient population. It is common clinical practice for patients on calcium supplementation to also receive vitamin D supplements. Preparations that combine elemental calcium and modest supplements of vitamin D are commercially available.

Estrogen/Progestin Replacement. Estrogen replacement along with calcium supplementation has become the standard regime for prevention and treatment of symptomatic osteoporosis. Estrogen therapy is most useful for the prevention of high turnover osteoporosis, such as that observed in the immediate postmenopausal patient. There is a large body of scientific work regarding the effects of estrogen on postmenopausal women.[48,49] Most of these studies reach similar conclusions. Estrogens seem to reduce bone remodeling to premenopausal levels. This effect continues while the patient continues the estrogen replacement, and is quickly reversed when that replacement is stopped.

The mechanism of action of estrogen replacement on osteoporosis is still open for debate. There is evidence that estrogen replacement increases serum 1,25-dihydroxy vitamin D_3 and, via this mechanism, improves dietary absorption of calcium.[31] Estrogen also seems to directly decrease bone resorption.[35,76] Some believe that this is the primary mechanism by which estrogen has its protective effects.[13] Estrogen receptors have also been found in cells of osteoblastic origin, although the significance of this is not clear.[26,47] Secondary mechanisms linking estrogen receptors to the mechanisms of bone loss in the postmenopausal state are yet to be worked out. Another proposed mechanism

is based on the association of estrogen deficiency in rats with increased production of prostaglandin E. Prostaglandin E has been found to stimulate bone resorption via osteoclasts.[29]

Estrogens have been shown clinically useful in slowing loss of bone and may actually increase bone mass.[13,53] Prospective trials have demonstrated benefit not only in increases in bone mass, but also in decreased incidence of osteoporotic fractures.[27] Estrogen therapy seems to be most useful in the immediate postmenopausal period. It has, however, been demonstrated to be of utility in older women with established osteoporosis.[13,50]

The optimal duration of estrogen therapy for the prevention and treatment of osteoporosis is not completely agreed upon. When estrogen therapy is discontinued, there is an accelerated bone loss mirroring that observed at natural menopause.[73] Some authors believe that estrogen therapy should be initiated at menopause and continued indefinitely.[12,28]

Direct complications of estrogen therapy are few, but extraskeletal effects deserve mention. The incidence of endometrial carcinoma is increased in women taking estrogen replacement.[77] This increase is eliminated by the concurrent administration of progestins. Studies also find a moderate increase in the incidence of breast cancer in populations of women taking estrogen replacement.[1] There appears to be a significant cardiac protective effect provided by estrogen replacement in the postmenopausal woman. A 25% to 50% reduction in cardiovascular mortality can be expected in populations of women taking estrogen replacement.[85] It is also thought that estrogen replacement may confer cerebrovascular benefits, although this has yet to be conclusively demonstrated. All of these facts make decisions regarding initiation of estrogen replacement ones that must be considered on an individual basis. Currently, large prospective studies are underway to help delineate the risks and benefits of estrogen replacement. What is clear is that estrogen has significant effects on calcium and bone metabolism that decrease detrimental resorption in the postmenopausal woman.

Exercise. Low activity levels are a risk factor for development of osteoporosis. This has led to the idea of treatment and prevention practices that include a regular exercise routine. Experimental evidence suggests that skeletal loading incites osteoblast function and bone growth. Studies in osteoporotic patients demonstrate increases in bone mass with moderate to vigorous exercise regimens. These effects, however, are local to the area of the body exposed to the stress of exercise, and benefits continue only as long as the activity is maintained. There is evidence that a regular program of exercise with calcium supplementation in osteoporotic women can significantly increase bone mass in the vertebral column.[16] This increase continues only with continuation of the exercise regimen. There is a return to baseline bone mass about 12 months after cessation of exercise, even with continued calcium supplementation.

Calcitonin. Calcitonin, as discussed previously, is a hormone primarily concerned with calcium homeostasis. Its action of inhibiting osteoclastic resorption of bone sparked interest in its potential uses in metabolic diseases such as Paget's disease and osteoporosis. Calcitonin, because of its mechanism of action, is most useful in high turnover osteoporosis. Postmenopausal, steroid-associated, and postoophorectomy osteoporosis are examples of high turnover states.

Clinical data documenting the utility of calcitonin therapy in the osteoporotic patient have been produced. In a 1-year randomized trial, Reginster, Albert, and Lecart[74] demonstrated the protective effect of calcitonin in the immediate postmenopausal patient. Prospective randomized studies followed that demonstrated the utility of calcitonin in postmenopausal, steroid-associated, and postoophorectomy patients.[4] There is also evidence that certain regimens of calcitonin can promote increases in bone mass.[66]

Calcitonin also has a well-documented analgesic effect separate from its skeletal effect.[4] Unlike the skeletal effect that is dose responsive within a certain range, the analgesic properties of calcitonin are not dose related. The analgesia is thought to occur secondary to central actions, perhaps involving the opioid system. This is supported by the finding that intrathecal and subarachnoid calcitonin has been found to be effective for pain relief.[30]

Calcitonin is a well-tolerated drug with few adverse reactions. Eight to ten percent of patients report mild gastrointestinal symptoms, and 2% to 5% have a dermatological hypersensitivity. There are no reports of serious drug interactions

Other Treatments. Other medical therapies are available to combat bone loss from the various causes of osteoporosis. The bisphosphonates appear quite promising. These are a group of compounds that are analogs of pyrophosphates. Bisphosphonates bind to mineralized bone and are thought to function by direct inhibition of the action of mature osteoclasts.[78,81] This is thought to decrease the rate at which bone remodeling units are formed, as well as the depth of resorption of each BMU.[87] Prospective trials of intermittent cyclic administration of bisphosphonates demonstrate an increase in bone mass and a decrease in spinal fracture rates.[88,89]

Sodium fluoride has been utilized in the setting of osteoporosis as a bone-loss prevention therapy. It appears to be a direct stimulant of osteoblastic activity.[45] Treatment with sodium fluoride must be accompanied by calcium supplementation to avoid osteomalacia. Sodium fluoride increases bone mineral density but there are conflicting data about the effects on fracture rates. Currently, sodium fluoride is not used extensively.

Observational studies have noted a decrease in fracture rates and protection from bone loss in patients taking thiazide diuretics over a prolonged period.[64] Thiazide therapy decreases urinary calcium secretion. Thiazide has some associated risks. Studies evaluating a fracture prevention regimen are not available.

Osteomalacia

Osteomalacia and rickets are disorders of mineralization of formed osteoid. In children, rickets appear when defects in mineralization lead to failure of primary ossification of cartilage during endochondral ossification. In adults, the mineralization phase of remodeling is slowed or arrested. The result is poorly ossified osteoid and resultant osteomalacia. In children, both of these processes are possible and rickets can be seen with superimposed osteomalacia. In adults, whose epiphyseal plates have fused, rickets cannot exist and osteomalacia is observed in isolation. The classic form and most common cause of osteomalacia and rickets is associated with a deficiency of active forms of vitamin D. Less common causes include renal disease, malabsorption syndromes, and rare genetic conditions.

The etiologies of osteomalacia are numerous. Most involve the absorption and metabolism of vitamin D, but other conditions that affect bone mineralization yield the pathology of osteomalacia. The accompanying box lists possible causes of osteomalacia.

CAUSES OF OSTEOMALACIA

Vitamin D deficiency
Gastrectomy
Small bowel disease
Chronic pancreatic insufficiency
Hereditary disorders of vitamin D deficiency
Acquired disorders of vitamin D deficiency
   Anticonvulsant therapy
   Chronic renal failure
Chronic metabolic acidosis
Phosphate deficiency
Tumor associated
   Mesenchymal tumors
   Prostatic carcinoma
Fanconi's syndrome
Aluminum intoxication
Parenteral alimentation

Pathology

The common pathophysiological process involved in all forms of osteomalacia is the defect in mineralization of formed osteoid. However, there is good evidence that not only is osteoid improperly mineralized, but the actual rate of osteoid formation is decreased and the osteoid matrix formed by the osteoblast is defective.[18,90]

The role of phosphorus metabolism in osteomalacia deserves mention. Hypophosphatemia has been shown in experimental models to impair not only mineralization but also osteoid matrix formation. Decreased phosphorus levels can directly suppress osteoblast function.[70,71] Vitamin D deficiency can directly and indirectly affect serum phosphorus concentrations. 1, 25-dihydroxy vitamin D_3 deficiency directly affects the proximal tubule in the kidney, allowing increased excretion of phosphorus. The PTH system is also involved in the decrease in phosphorus observed with osteomalacia. Serum calcium concentrations are decreased in vitamin D deficiency. This leads to increased productions of PTH. PTH has a direct effect on the renal tubule (fostering phosphorus excretion).

Clinical Presentation

Osteomalacia is clinically characterized by softening and deformation of the skeleton. In rickets, the pathology occurs in the vertebrae as well as in the long bones, but the rate of longitudinal growth makes the clinical findings more prominent in the long bones. Spinal involvement observed with rickets can be subtle (e.g., a slight kyphotic curvature of the whole spine, which is reducible, and is worse with sitting). This deformity is rarely painful. In contrast, adults with osteomalacia nearly uniformly present with low back pain. The spinal deformity can become quite impressive. Severe kyphosis is often accompanied by scoliosis and rotational deformities. Abnormal curvatures of the sacrum may also be present. Compressive fractures of the thoracic spine are uncommon, except when osteomalacia is accompanied by superimposed osteoporosis. Patients often complain of extraspinal pain, notably in the ribs, pelvis, and extremities. These locations are locally tender to palpation and can be misdiagnosed as arthritis. Characteristically, attendant muscle weakness observed with osteomalacia can yield a wide-based waddling gait. Patients are predisposed to femoral neck fractures, and may present with pain from a callous at a poorly healed fracture site.

Radiographic and Laboratory Evaluation

Plain radiographs of the spine observed with osteomalacia reveal demineralization and loss of the transverse trabecular pattern. Cortical surfaces become indistinct close to the partially mineralized osteoid, due to secondary hyperparathyroidism. The characteristic Looser zones are bands of radiolucency that abut the cortex in an axis perpendicular to the long axis of the bone in question. Looser zones are seen primarily in advanced cases of osteomalacia and represent incomplete fractures with accumulation of unmineralized osteoid. The other characteristic finding on plain radiographs is the codfish spine, where the intervertebral discs bulge into the soft vertebral bodies as demonstrated in Fig. 38-4.

Generally, in osteomalacia serum calcium levels are slightly decreased. Profoundly low serum calcium levels are unusual, due to the secondary increases in PTH excretion. Serum phosphorus levels are also below normal. Alkaline phosphatase is found to be elevated. Fecal calcium determination yields elevated calcium levels, whereas urinary calcium is often decreased. Evidence of secondary hyperparathyroidism is often observed in laboratory studies. More elaborate laboratory analyses, such as calcium balance studies, can be performed, but are

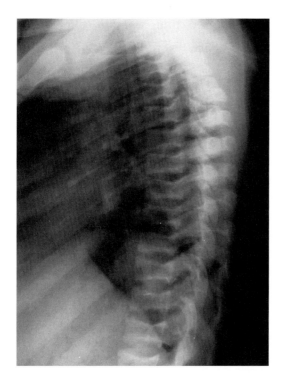

Fig. 38-4. Lateral plain radiograph of the thoracic spine demonstrating the so-called codfish spine seen in osteomalacia. The intervertebral discs protrude into the adjacent vertebral bodies through the softened end plates.

rarely necessary. Associated findings include aminoaciduria and low serum bicarbonate.

The diagnosis of osteomalacia can be difficult. It often presents with only vague complaints and the results of radiographic and laboratory evaluations may be equivocal. Transiliac bone biopsy may be necessary in certain patients.

Treatment

Surgical treatment of osteomalacia is rarely indicated. Most forms of this disease respond rapidly to adequate vitamin D administration. Certain forms such as chronic renal disease or chronic liver disease require 25-hydroxy vitamin D_3 and phosphorus administration as well. Correction of other underlying metabolic abnormalities, such as chronic metabolic acidosis, may also be necessary.

Hyperparathyroidism

Primary hyperparathyroidism is a disorder that results from an inappropriate increase in the production of PTH by the parathyroid glands. The most common pathology associated with hyperparathyroidism is a single benign adenoma. Less frequently observed are multiple adenomas and multiglandular hyperplasia. Carcinoma of the parathyroid is very rare. Primary hyperparathyroidism is often a surgical disease because excision of the offending adenoma can effect a cure.

PTH affects calcium metabolism via two primary mechanisms. Total renal resorption of calcium is increased by the actions of PTH, and resorption of calcium from mineralized bone is also increased by complex mechanisms mediated by PTH. Thus the biochemical hallmark of hyperparathyroidism is the increased serum calcium levels. The clinical features of this disease are caused by increases in serum calcium and the direct effects produced by chronic increases in PTH.

Reported incidences of hyperparathyroidism range from 26 to 146 per 100,000.[9,34,36,62] The incidence increases with age, and is most common in postmenopausal women. The clinical presentation of hyperparathyroidism has changed substantially with the advent of accurate and readily available serum chemical evaluations. The classic presentation of a patient with renal stones, fractures, and ectopic calcifications is rarely seen in modern practice. The typical patient diagnosed with hyperparathyroidism today is found serendipitously by an increased serum calcium level found on electrolyte screening evaluations. Most of these patients are asymptomatic.

Clinical features associated with hyperparathyroidism include chronic constipation, mental depression, neuromuscular dysfunction, recurrent pancreatitis, peptic ulcer disease, and unexplained or premature osteopenia.

Evaluation

A careful history should be taken from patients suspected of hyperparathyroidism. Family history of hyperparathyroidism, multiple endocrine neoplasia, and a history of childhood head and neck exposure to ionizing radiation favor the diagnosis of hyperparathyroidism. A medication history should also be obtained, because chronic thiazide and lithium use can lead to hypercalcemia.

Laboratory evaluation of serum calcium and PTH levels are the mainstay of modern diagnosis of hyperparathyroidism. Total serum calcium is usually the first laboratory study. An elevated serum calcium should be repeated, and a concomitant serum albumin determination is made to correct total calcium for protein binding. In some instances, an ionized calcium level should be drawn to help clarify a borderline total calcium, after albumin correction. Once a confirmed increase in serum calcium is found, other diagnostic tests should be ordered. A serum phosphorus and PTH level should be determined. A variety of immunoassays for PTH are available routinely, and should suffice except in patients with impaired renal function, in which the inactive C-terminal portion of PTH accumulates. In such patients, determinations of the midportion of PTH are available and should be made. An increase in serum calcium with a decrease in phosphorus and an increased PTH level are most consistent with the diagnosis of asymptomatic hyperparathyroidism, and confirmatory of symptomatic hyperparathyroidism.

The utility of other diagnostic modalities is not as clear. In many patients who are asymptomatic, bone densitometry measurements can be useful in determining need for surgical treatment of hyperparathyroidism. There are many studies demonstrating a decrease in bone mass in patients with hyperparathyroidism.[57,68,75,83] These measurements may overstate bone loss because they measure mineralized bone, and with the increase in bone turnover observed in hyperparathyroidism, a larger portion of total bone is unmineralized matrix. In patients with underlying osteoporosis the increased bone turnover seen with hyperparathyroidism can exacerbate bone loss.

Pathology

The pathological hallmark of hyperparathyroidism is osteitis fibrosa cystica, although both osteopenia and osteomalacia may also be observed with hyperparathyroidism. Osteitis fibrosa cystica yields pathological evidence of bone disease long before radiographic and clinical evidence appears. Currently, most patients do not have severe bone disease at initial diagnosis. Those who do tend to have severe, rapidly progressive hyperparathyroidism.

Application to the Spine

Involvement of the spine in hyperparathyroidism is inconsistent. In many cases, even with profound disease, spinal involvement is minor whereas in others

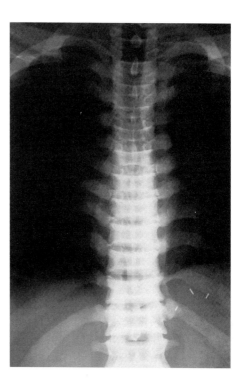

Fig. 38-5. Plain radiograph of the thoracic spine in a patient with hyperparathyroidism demonstrating the "rugger jersey" spine. New bone formation at the periosteal surface and a decrease in trabeculae give this characteristic appearance.

it can be the dominant skeletal feature. Loss of vertebral height, kyphosis, and back pain can be prominent features. As with the other clinical features of untreated hyperparathyroidism, these are decreasing in frequency in current clinical presentations.

The risks of long bone and vertebral fractures in hyperparathyroidism are still under debate. There is conflicting evidence over whether fracture rates in the axial skeleton are increased. Some studies have found increased vertebral fracture rates.[17,54] A prospective study by Wilson et al.[91] followed patients with asymptomatic hyperparathyroidism whose bone densities were not severely decreased. They found no increase in vertebral fracture rates in this population. They concluded that in the asymptomatic population, mild hyperparathyroidism posed no increased risk of vertebral compression fractures.

Clinical manifestations of spinal disease related to hyperparathyroidism include loss of vertebral height, kyphosis, pain, and vertebral collapse in severe cases. The subperiosteal bone deposition and loss of the normal trabecular architecture can yield a radiographic pattern known as the "rugger jersey" spine (Fig. 38-5).

Certain features of hyperparathyroidism differentiate it from the clinical spectrum observed in spinal disease caused by other metabolic diseases. In hyperparathyroidism spinal involvement is continuous in progression and distributed regularly throughout the spine. All areas of the spine may be affected progressively as with osteomalacia. This is in contrast to the pattern of spinal disease seen in osteoporosis where intermittent exacerbation and noncontiguous involvement of the spine is the rule.

Treatment

The principal treatment of primary hyperparathyroidism is surgery. Parathyroid exploration and excision of adenoma is the treatment of choice for primary hyperparathyroidism. In experienced hands, success rates are better than 90%, with low morbidity and mortality.[20] There appears to be a subgroup of asymptomatic persons with mild hyperparathyroidism who do not require neck exploration. Some authors have attempted to define the populations of patients safe to follow with expectant management.[20,22] Clear indications for surgical treatment of hyperparathyroidism include manifestations of typical symptoms, serum calcium levels greater than 1 mg/dl above normal over time, a decrease in renal function, a decrease in bone mass less than two standard deviations below age- and sex-matched means, and sustained increases in 24-hour urinary calcium excretions (>400 mg per 24 hours).

Renal Osteodystrophy and Dialysis-Related Spondyloarthropathy

Renal osteodystrophy and dialysis-related spondyloarthropathy (DRSA) are related entities that have the potential to affect the vertebral columns of patients with renal disease. Biochemical and hormonal abnormalities associated with renal failure interact to produce spine disease. The onset of renal osteodystrophy is insidious. The biochemical damage of this disease can be far advanced before clinical symptoms arise. DRSA is also a product of renal failure in patients requiring chronic dialysis. It is a rapidly progressive syndrome of joint and bone erosion that is observed most often in the cervical spine. Serious spinal cord compression can result. Several fatal cases of cervical spinal cord compression related to DRSA have been reported in the literature.[2]

Pathology

The pathological processes produced by renal osteodystrophy can be roughly divided into three categories: (1) osteitis fibrosa cystica, (2) osteomalacia, and (3) adynamic bone disease.[32,41] Many patients display mixed disease. They therefore have components of more than one of the pathological processes. This yields a heterogeneous mix of disease in patients who go on to present with clinical syndromes associated with renal osteodystrophy.

Osteitis Fibrosa Cystica. Osteitis fibrosa cystica is the most common pathological change observed in patients with renal osteodystrophy. As described previously, osteitis fibrosa cystica is characterized by fibrosis of marrow spaces and an increased rate of remodeling. In renal osteodystrophy this is primarily caused by secondary hyperparathyroidism, locally-produced cytokines, and a deficiency of 1,25-dihydroxy vitamin D_3. The secondary hyperparathyroidism observed in patients with renal failure is mediated by multiple factors, such as hyperphosphatemia. Increased phosphorus levels in patients with decreased renal function cause a direct decrease in serum ionized calcium. In response the parathyroid glands secrete more PTH. This acts to increase ionized calcium and increase phosphate excretion. However, other mechanisms by which increased serum phosphorus levels may induce hyperparathyroidism are not quite this simple. Increased serum phosphorus levels may interfere with vitamin D metabolism, and dietary phosphorus content may play a more complicated role in the control of PTH secretion.[51,52]

Vitamin D metabolism and its derangement in renal failure are thought to play an important role in secondary hyperparathyroidism observed in patients with chronic renal failure. A decrease in production of 1,25-dihydroxy vitamin D_3 leads to a decrease in intestinal absorption of calcium and also increases skeletal resistance to the calcemic actions of parathyroid hormone. Thus to maintain ionized calcium levels the parathyroid glands are forced to chronically raise PTH levels.

The hallmark hyperparathyroidism observed in renal patients is the common pathway leading to osteitis fibrosa cystica. Hypocalcemia produced by various mechanisms associated with renal failure can lead to an increase in the steady-state levels of PTH. There are other mechanisms by which oversecretion of PTH is maintained. The peripheral skeleton's resistance to PTH is increased in chronic renal failure.

There are also intrinsic abnormalities of parathyroid function in these patients. It has been demonstrated in the chronically uremic renal failure patient that increased levels of calcium are required to suppress PTH secretion.[11] Vitamin D_3 has also been implicated directly in effects on the parathyroid gland, promoting hyperparathyroidism.[32]

Osteomalacia. Osteomalacia is a pathology commonly seen in patients with renal failure. Pathological details are described above, and are quite similar in this variety of the disease process. Osteomalacia in patients with renal failure is characterized by low rates of bone turnover, and an accumulation of unmineralized osteoid secondary to a defect in mineralization. Deficiency of vitamin D_3 and its active metabolites is routinely observed in patients with renal failure. It is believed, however, that this is not the primary pathophysiology associated with osteomalacia in renal failure. Most osteomalacia in renal failure is thought to be due to aluminum intoxication. Such intoxication can cause defects in mineralization and increased osteoid synthesis by the osteoblasts. Over the long term, aluminum intoxication also seems to produce a decrease in the differentiation of osteoblasts from marrow precursors.[41] Iron has also been implicated in the etiology of the osteomalacia seen in renal failure.

The accumulation of unmineralized osteoid in patients with renal failure–associated osteomalacia yields a significant decrease in bone strength. Pain and deformity are common. Osteomalacia in renal failure has decreased in incidence in recent years.[43,61] This may be due to the decreasing use of aluminum-containing phosphate binders and aluminum-containing dialysis fluids since their contribution to renal osteodystrophy has been recognized.

Adynamic Bone Disease. Adynamic bone disease is an entity associated with chronic dialysis. Its hallmark is a marked decrease in bone turnover. Bone biopsy reveals an acellular field with a paucity of BMUs. This pathology is seen in patients with end-stage renal disease without the secondary hyperparathyroidism. These patients are often maintained on ambulatory peritoneal dialysis and have significant calcium and vitamin D supplementation.[14] Low PTH levels are thought to play a significant role in the genesis of adynamic bone disease. Increased levels of PTH may be necessary to maintain normal levels of bone turnover in patients with end-stage renal disease. Higher levels of calcium, either via supplementation or higher transfer of cal-

cium via the peritoneal dialysis, may act to suppress PTH production in these patients.

Adynamic bone disease may also occur in patients with normal parathyroid function. In these patients, it is hypothesized that bone growth suppressors may have increased expression, or perhaps the necessary bone growth promoters are not expressed adequately. Certain interleukins are known to be bone-growth suppressors. End-stage renal disease may stimulate release of these interleukins.[23,24]

Adynamic bone disease is associated with an increase in fracture rates and serum calcium lability as the pool of metabolically active calcium in bone is decreased by the paucity of active BMUs.[37]

Dialysis-Related Spondyloarthropathy. Dialysis-related spondyloarthropathy (DRSA) is a destructive, erosive process of joints in patients on long-term hemodialysis. Although there are many theories regarding the pathogenesis of DRSA, the most current focus on a unusual type of amyloid deposit in the articular cartilage, periosteum, joint capsule, synovium, and associated ligaments in chronic hemodialysis patients. This protein has been identified as beta-2 microglobulin that is associated with class 1 of the major histocompatibility class proteins. Beta-2 microglobulin is seen in increased amounts in the serum of patients receiving chronic hemodialysis.[8,84] Two causes have been proposed. Plasma beta-2 microglobulin is not well cleared by current dialysis membranes. This allows the protein to accumulate. The second possibility is that immune activation by dialysis membranes may lead to increased production of beta-2 microglobulins.[86] The vertebral joints may be predisposed to DRSA by the other mechanisms of renal osteodystrophy. Severe secondary hyperparathyroidism occurs in 80% of patients with DRSA,[7] and causes softening of subchondral bone.[46,58,65] Other changes noted in the vertebral columns of patients with DRSA include vertebral body corner erosions, erosions of the end plate cartilage and bone, articular facet erosions with spondylolisthesis, and even vertebral body collapse.[3]

Clinical Features

Many patients with renal osteodystrophy have extraspinal manifestations such as fractures, deformities, and pain. Spinal involvement is common, with back pain being the most common presenting symptom. Because both renal osteodystrophy and DRSA may occur and interact, differentiating their contributions to clinical manifestations can be difficult. Back and neck pain are by far the most frequent clinical complaints. Frank DRSA often also presents with a rapidly progressive deformity. The lower cervical spine is the most frequently involved, and neurological sequelae are infrequent, but can occur.[56] Myelopathy and radiculopathy have been reported in 20% of patients presenting with DRSA.[2,65] Patients with progressive DRSA may present with acute cord compromise and profound neurological deficit.[19] There is a report in the literature of two patients presenting with sudden death from severe canal compromise associated with DRSA.[2]

Patients with DRSA are those with long histories of dialysis, an average of 10.2 years in one series.[56] Patients also often have involvement of other joints, particularly the wrists and hands. Symptoms and deformity can be rapidly progressive in DRSA. This can help differentiate true DRSA from other pathology such as chronic degenerative arthritis and calcium pyrophosphate crystal deposition disease.

Radiographic Evaluation

Radiographic evaluation of the spine in patients with pathology related to renal disease reveals several distinctive patterns. In renal osteodystrophy, increased bone resorption, most commonly observed in the extraspinal locations, is observed in patients with hyperparathyroidism along with subperiosteal bone resorption in vertebral bodies or the so-called rugger jersey sign. Fig. 38-6 depicts a woman maintained on chronic peritoneal dialysis. Marked osteoporosis and evidence of hyperparathyroidism combine to produce the pathology. Renal osteodystrophy is characterized by such mixed clinical presentations.

Vertebral rim erosions, periarticular cystic radiolucencies, and progressive kyphotic deformities are the hallmarks of progressive DRSA. The cervical spine is the most common spinal location involved with DRSA, with nearly 65% involving C5 to C6 and C6 to C7 levels.[56] Although the findings of renal osteodystrophy and DRSA can be discrete, these entities are often present together, and radiographic evaluations regularly demonstrate the findings of both pathologies.

MRI provides excellent resolution of soft tissues and neural structures, and can be very helpful in clinical decision making. Fig. 38-7 depicts a classic

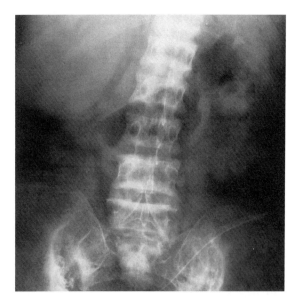

Fig. 38-6. Plain anteroposterior radiograph of the lumbar spine in a patient maintained on chronic peritoneal dialysis. Marked osteopenia and sclerosis of the end plates give the "rugger jersey" appearance. This is most likely due the secondary hyperparathyroidism seen in patients with chronic renal failure.

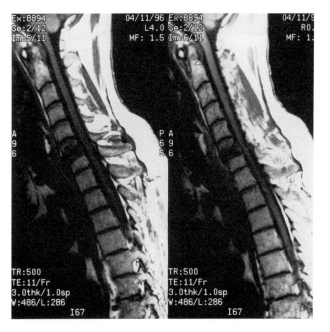

Fig. 38-7. Sagittal MRI of the crevicothoracic spine demonstrating the typical low signal on T1-weighted sequences seen in DRSA. There is significant erosion of C7 and some ventral listhesis of C7. The spinal canal is largely unaffected in this example.

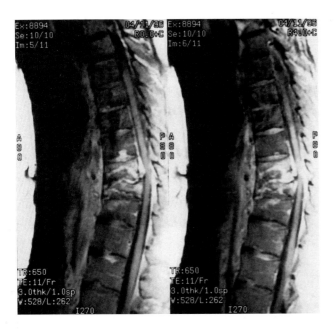

Fig. 38-8. Sagittal MRI of the thoracic spine demonstrating an erosive and destructive lesion in a patient on chronic hemodialysis. Although the differential includes osteomyelitis, subsequent surgery for progressive myelopathy revealed DRSA.

lesion of DRSA at the cervicothoracic junction. DRSA usually displays decreased signal characteristics of the affected tissue and bone on T2-weighted images, distinguishing it from osteomyelitis.[56] However, patients can present with MRI findings that are indistinguishable from osteomyelitis and disc space infection.[19] Needle biopsies or other invasive procedures may be necessary to differentiate between the two. A good example of this is seen in Fig. 38-8 in a patient who had a progressive thoracic myelopathy requiring surgery. The pathological diagnosis was DRSA at the time of surgery.

Treatment

Both renal osteodystrophy and DRSA are difficult entities to treat effectively. Both have significant potential for morbidity in advanced stages. The chronic changes in bone associated with DRSA are difficult, if not impossible, to reverse. Therefore early preventive measures aimed at preserving bone mass and quality are the mainstays of treatment. The restriction of phosphorus intake and calcium supplementation with monitoring of PTH levels are the first-line strategies in controlling the metabolic derangements observed with DRSA. Currently, aluminum-containing dialysis compounds are routinely avoided. Vitamin D supplementation should be undertaken with care. In refractory cases of hyperparathyroidism, parathyroidectomy can be considered.

There is some evidence that the composition of the dialysis membrane can have an effect of the onset of DRSA. The deposition of amyloid is thought to have an immunological basis, possibly from an immunological activation by a bioincompatible dialysis membrane. Certain types of dialysis membranes (i.e., cuprophane) are associated with increased plasma levels of beta-2 microglobulin and possible development of DRSA.

The initial management of the patient presenting with spinal disease related to renal failure and/or dialysis is immobilization. This has obvious risks of increasing bone loss secondary to inactivity. Many patients have mechanical symptoms of back pain and will see improvement with time and conservative management such as a well-fitted orthosis. There is a subset of patients with severe disease that will have intractable pain and/or neurological involvement from progressive DRSA. These patients may need surgery.

Dialysis-dependent patients are difficult surgical patients. The decision to operate on patients with DRSA must be carefully weighed against the risks of what is often a substantial surgery to a patient who is prone to medical complications.

Patients who undergo operation for neurological symptoms of DRSA usually need decompression and stabilization. Although there is little literature about operating on these patients, it would seem prudent to supplement fusion with immobilization, such as with a halo vest or with internal fixation. A ventral approach for vertebral body collapse in the cervical spine is usually indicated because this allows for excellent spinal cord decompression in most cases.[19] After decompression, ventral fusion and internal fixation should be attempted. In patients with significant dorsal pathology, consideration must be given to dorsal fusion as well. In the thoracic spine, ventrolateral decompression with a short segment ventral reconstruction and stabilization has been used successfully by the authors.

Paget's Disease

Paget's disease was first described in 1877 by Sir James Paget.[67] An understanding of Paget's disease is dependent upon an understanding of the metabolic mechanics of bone turnover. This disease is a focal progressive abnormality resulting in replacement of normal bone with new bone having abnormal shape and architecture. This progression can be broken down into three phases. First is a phase of increased osteoclastic resorption. This is followed by a period of continued increased absorption balanced by an increase in formation of bone. This newly formed bone is abnormal in architecture, with a haphazard matrix of cortical and trabecular bone. A final phase is seen when there is little cellular activity.

Epidemiology

Paget's disease is relatively common, with 3% to 6% of the population older than 45 years of age exhibiting radiographic evidence of the disease.[40] It is rare in the young, almost never observed in patients younger than the age of 30. The prevalence of Paget's disease continues to increase with increasing age, with a slight female predominance. Most patients are asymptomatic and never require treatment.

Etiology

The precise etiology of Paget's disease is unknown. Immunofluorescent studies suggest the presence of antigenic material related to the measles virus in pagetic osteoblasts.[6] This would suggest a viral etiology, and although this has not been conclusively proven, it is the best hypothesis to date.

Clinical Features

The most common presenting complaint in Paget's disease is bone pain and deformity. Back pain from lumbar spine involvement is one of the most common initial complaints. Involvement of the skull is also common, with patients noting increasing hat size, tinnitus, vertigo, or headache from encroachment on the cranial nerves. Pathological fractures are also a presenting feature. They can occur both secondary to bone loss and to the disorganized nature of replacement bone in Paget's disease.

In adults, the most common deformity of the extremities is seen in the tibia. Ventral bowing of the tibia associated with warmth from the increased blood flow in the region is regularly encountered in patients with Paget's disease. In some patients, the increases in blood flow to involved pagetic bone and surrounding tissue can be so substantial that high-output cardiac failure can ensue in severe cases.

Malignant degeneration of pagetic lesions is also a known complication of this disease. About 1% of patients with Paget's disease will have malignant degeneration at some point during the course of their disease. The most common malignancy is osteogenic sarcoma. The spine is an uncommon site for malignant degeneration, the limbs being the most common site.

Spinal involvement of Paget's disease is common. Most patients have radiographic evidence of one or more involved vertebrae. The lumbar spine is the most common site of vertebral involvement (60% of patients). The thoracic spine is the next most common site (45% of patients). Cervical spine involvement is less common (about 15% of patients).[60] Although many spinal lesions are asymptomatic, the usual symptom caused by spine involvement is low back pain.

Other spinal involvement includes invasion of the intervertebral disc space. Disc space invasion by pagetic tissue is not necessarily symptomatic, and is seen in perhaps 10% of patients with spinal involvement from Paget's disease.[33] Most cases of neurological dysfunction in Paget's disease of the spine are produced by stenosis syndromes. Spinal canal diameter is compromised by expanding vertebral bodies. This can cause either a slowly progressive syndrome or, rarely, profound neurological deficit after minor trauma. Other less common manifestations of Paget's disease in the spine include sarcomatous degeneration, epidural hematoma, extramedullary hematopoiesis, and ossification of the epidural fat.[80]

Paget's disease can produce neurological involvement in a number of ways. Cranial nerves can be compressed in their foramina at the skull base, as previously mentioned. The most common neurological symptoms, however, are caused by compression of the spinal cord and cauda equina. Basilar impression and spastic quadriparesis have also been reported from cervical spine involvement, but this is quite uncommon.

Vascular compromise is another theory proposed to explain neurological deficits associated with Paget's disease of the spine. It is hypothesized that the intensely vascular pagetic bone results in a steal phenomenon from the spinal cord and other neural structures. Reduction of this steal is thought to be responsible for improvement in patients treated medically without evidence of structural compression or without improvement in patients treated for structural compression.[25]

Radiographic Findings

The radiographic findings in established Paget's disease are characteristic and diagnostic. During the osteolytic period of Paget's disease there is a radiolucent appearance in long bones and in the skull. Long bones demonstrate a V-shaped line clearly delimiting normal bone from pagetic bone. Well-defined decalcified lesions are present in radiographs of the skull. Vertebral osteolysis is rarely displayed so prominently on plain radiographs. Vertebral bodies demonstrate thickened cortex and coarse trabeculations. They also enlarge, especially in ventrodorsal diameter, and assume a more square overall shape (Figs. 38-9 and 38-10). Compression fractures are not infrequently observed. Fig. 38-9 depicts a compressive lesion of L3 in a patient with Paget's disease. Adjacent vertebral bodies are sometimes involved and several adjacent pagetic vertebrae can yield a kyphotic deformity.

Laboratory Findings

An elevated alkaline phosphatase level is characteristic of Paget's disease, and reflects the amount of osteoclastic activity in the disease. Urine hydroxyproline, a marker of bone activity, is also elevated. Urine calcium levels in patients with Paget's disease are typically normal. An exception to this is the immobilized patient and patients with associated hyperparathyroidism. Both serum alkaline phosphatase and urine hydroxyproline are useful markers of disease. They can be used to monitor disease progression as biochemical markers of response of Paget's disease to medical treatment.

Treatment

Medical treatment of Paget's disease has improved markedly from just a few years ago. Potent antiresorptive agents are available that offer control of Paget's disease by lowering levels of bone resorp-

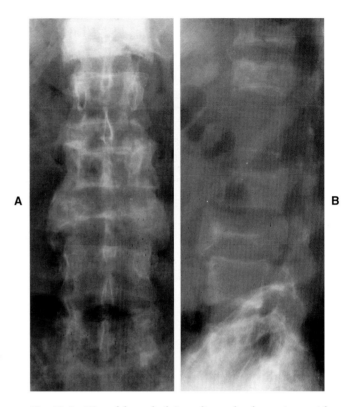

Fig. 38-9. AP and lateral plain radiograph of a patient with Paget's disease with spinal involvement. These films demonstrate an expansile lesion of the lumbar spine with sclerosis at T11, T12, L2, and L3. There is a compression deformity of L3 as well.

tion. The bisphosphonates have superseded calcitonin in recent years as the first-line therapy for Paget's disease.[40] The bisphosphonates are pyrophosphate analogs that are potent inhibitors of osteoclastic activity. Etidronate, pamidronate, and, recently, alendronate are available for treatment of Paget's disease in the United States.

The indications for initiating treatment of Paget's include pain, neural compression, pathological fractures, or impending fractures. Additional indications include progressive bony deformity and heart failure.

Salmon calcitonin, described earlier in the discussion of osteoporosis, is a potent inhibitor of osteoclastic activity. However, it produces shorter duration of remission of Paget's disease than do the bisphosphonates.[39] Mithramycin is a cytotoxic antibiotic that is directly toxic to osteoblasts and other bone marrow cell lines. It has been used in treatment of Paget's disease but most believe it is too toxic for general use.

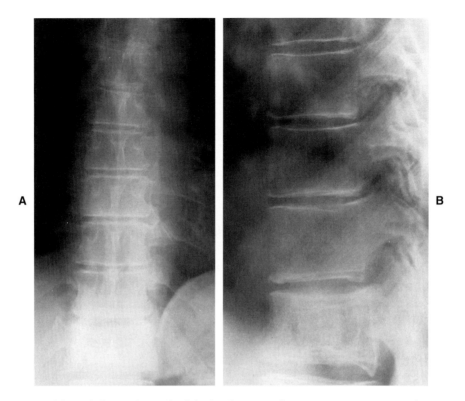

Fig. 38-10. AP and lateral plain radiograph of the lumbar spine demonstrating pagetic involvement of T11 *(last pictured vertebra)*. Findings include increased density of T11 with enlarged vertical trabeculae producing a striated appearance. The vertebral body is slightly enlarged in ventrodorsal and mediolateral dimensions.

Surgical treatment for Paget's disease of the spine usually involves decompressive procedures for stenosis. The reported experience for stenosis for Paget's disease requiring spinal decompression is limited to case reports and small series. Proposed indications for surgery include progressive neurological deficit, fixed acute neurological deficit, and pain unresponsive to traditional medical therapy. There is still debate over indication for surgery in this population.[25,80] Complication from spinal surgery in the pagetic patient is not uncommon. Blood loss can be a significant problem, and can lead to coagulopathies. Some authors treat Paget's disease patients requiring surgery with one of the antiresorptive agents preoperatively in an attempt to reduce the vascularity of the bone to help decrease intraoperative blood loss. Postoperative spinal instability in patients who have been operated on for pagetic involvement of the spine can also be seen. Further procedures, including extensive spinal stabilization, may be required in these patients.

Storage Diseases

The various storage diseases based on inherited biochemical deficiencies are not truly metabolic diseases. A short discussion of the mucopolysaccharidoses is included to provide an idea of how other biochemical derangements can yield significant pathology of the spine. Many of the conditions described below are chronic and degenerative in nature. They can be frustrating entities for parents, patients, and clinicians. A spine surgeon's involvement in the care of these patients may be important, because presentation with significant neurological compromise is possible.

The mucopolysaccharidoses are a group of loosely related disorders of inherited enzyme deficiency. The pathophysiology of all of these disorders relates to a derangement in the metabolism and breakdown of glycosaminoglycans. Glycosaminoglycans are found in all connective tissues of the body and hence disorders of their breakdown yield accumulations of these substances throughout

CURRENT CLASSIFICATION OF THE MUCOPOLYSACCHARIDOSES

Type	Eponym	Enzyme Deficiency
MPS IH	Hurler	Iduronidase
MPS IS	Scheie	Iduronidase
MPS I H/S	Hurler-Scheie	Iduronidase
MPS II	Hunter	Iduronate sulphate sulphatase
MPS III A	Sanfilippo	Heparan-N-sulphatase
MPS III B		N-acetylglucosaminidase
MPS III C		Acetyl-CoA-glucosaminidase acetyltransferase
MPS III D		N-acetylglucosamine-6-sulphatase
MPS IV A	Morquio	Galactosamine-6-sulphatase
MPS IV B		β-galactosidase
MPS VI	Maroteaux-Lamy	N-acetylgalactosamine-4-sulphatase
MPS VII	Sly	β-glucuronidase

multiple organ systems. The current classification used in describing the mucopolysaccharidoses and their related enzyme deficiencies is presented in the accompanying box.[92] Detailed accounts of the biochemistry of the mucopolysaccharidoses are readily available and are beyond the scope of this chapter.

Spinal involvement in the mucopolysaccharidoses is variable. There are spinal manifestations of those conditions that are most likely to be encountered in a practice that has occasion to see these patients. The need for spinal surgery in these patients is uncommon, but there are cases where it is indicated.

Hunter's Syndrome

MPS II, or Hunter's syndrome, is an iduronidase deficiency with variable penetrance. Variations in the severity of this disease are quite impressive. In some, death in early infancy from a progressive cardiomyopathy is the rule, where others are near-normal appearing adults.[92] In the severely affected patient the clinical picture is dominated by cardiac manifestations and upper airway obstructive problems. Spinal problems in this population are predominantly observed in more mildly affected patients who reach adulthood. These adults have a high incidence of lumbar spondylolisthesis and can have compromise of the lower spinal nerve roots requiring decompressive procedures. Radiographic findings of the spines of MPS I patients have some distinctive features. Caudal thoracic vertebrae often will display concave dorsal and ventral surfaces. Ventral-inferior beaking of lumbar vertebrae is also seen. Patients may have multiple levels with this abnormality.[82]

Hurler's Syndrome

MPS IH, or Hurler's syndrome, also has features of interest to the spine surgeon. In general, manifestations are similar to Hunter's syndrome, but changes are less severe. As with the other mucopolysaccharidoses, a slow degenerative course is to be expected with severely affected patients declining to a vegetative existence by their mid- to late teens. In more mildly affected patients cervical myelopathy secondary to both dural and ligamentum flavum hypertrophy is the rule by the late teens.

Morquio's Syndrome

Morquio's syndrome (MPS IV A), is the mucopolysaccharidosis of most concern to the spine surgeon. Most patients have normal intelligence and the clinical syndrome is dominated by severe bone dysplasia. One of the most serious complications of Morquio's is the cervical myelopathy associated with atlantoaxial instability that invariably accompanies this syndrome.[63] Progressive myelopathy and even an incidence of sudden death from high spinal cord injury have been reported associated with the cervical dysplasias seen with this disease.[92]

Atlantoaxial instability in Morquio's is a product of hypoplasia of the dens and general ligamentous laxity of the cervical spine. Because of the grave consequences of upper cervical cord damage, many clinicians perform routine MRI evaluation of the upper cervical spine in these patients. Operative intervention with both ventral and dorsal cervical decompression and stabilization procedures has been described in patients with Morquio's.[72,92]

Maroteaux-Lamy Syndrome

Maroteaux-Lamy syndrome or MPS VI is a very rare form of the mucopolysaccharidoses. This syndrome, unlike the other mucopolysaccharidoses, does not directly affect the central nervous system. The primary features are related to the progressive narrowing of airways that inexorably leads to cor pulmonale and an early death from heart failure. It is mentioned here because of the cervical and thoracic myelopathy that has been reported in these patients secondary to meningeal hypertrophy.[5]

REFERENCES

1. Adami HO. Long-term consequences of estrogen and estrogen-progestin replacement. Cancer Causes Control 3:83-90, 1992.
2. Allard JC, Artze ME, Porter G. Fatal destructive cervical spondyloarthropathy in two patients on long-term dialysis. Am J Kidney Dis 19:81-85, 1992.
3. Athanasou NA, Ayers D, Rainey AJ, Oliver DO, Duthie RB. Joint and systemic distribution of dialysis amyloid. QJM 78:205-214, 1991.
4. Avioli LV. Calcitonin therapy in osteoporotic syndromes. Rheum Dis Clin North Am 20:777-785, 1994.
5. Banna M, Hollenberg R. Compressive menigeal hypertrophy in mucopolysaccharidoses. AJNR 8:385-386, 1987.
6. Revel A. Basle M, Pouplard A, Kouyoumdjian S, Filman R, Lepatezour. Viral antigens in osteoclasts from Paget's Disease of Bone. Lancet 2:344-346, 1980.
7. Bindi P, Chanard J. Destructive spondyloarthropathy in dialysis patients: An overview. Nephron 55:104-109, 1990.
8. Blumberg A, Burgi W. Behavior of beta-2 -microglobulin in patients with chronic renal failure undergoing hemodialysis, hemodiafiltration, and continuous ambulatory peritoneal dialysis. Clin Nephrol 27:245-249, 1987.
9. Boonstra CE, Jackson CE. Hyperparathyroidism detected by routine serum calcium analysis. Ann Intern Med 63:468-474, 1965.
10. Breslau NA. Calcium, estrogen, and progestin in the treatment of osteoporosis. Rheum Dis Clin North Am 20:691-726, 1994.
11. Brown EM, Wilson RE, Eastman RC, Pallotta J, Marynick SP. Abnormal regulation of parathyroid hormone release by calcium in secondary hyperparathyroidism due to chronic renal failure. J Clin Endocrinol Metab 54:172-179, 1982.
12. Cauley JA, Seeley DG, Ensrud K, Ettinger B, Black D, Cummings SR. Estrogen replacement therapy and fractures in older women. Study of osteoporotic fractures research group. Ann Intern Med 122: 9-16, 1995.
13. Civitelli R, et al. Effects of one-year treatment with estrogens on bone mass, intestinal calcium absorption, and 25-hydroxyvitamin D-1a-hydroxylase reserve in postmenopausal osteoporosis. Calcif Tissue Int 42:77-86, 1988.
14. Coburn JW. Mineral metabolism and renal bone disease: Effects of CAPD versus hemodialysis. Kidney Int 40(Suppl): S92-S100, 1993.
15. Consensus development conference: Prophyaxis and treatment of osteoporosis. Osteoporos Int 1:114-117, 1991.
16. Dalsky GP, Stocke KS, Dhsani AA. Weight-bearing exercise training and lumbar bone mineral content in postmenopausal women. Ann Intern Med 108:824, 1988.
17. Dauphine RT, Riggs BL, Scholz DA. Back pain and vertebral crush fractures. An unemphasized mode of presentation for primary hyperparathyroidism. Ann Intern Med 83:365-367, 1975.
18. David DS. Mineral and bone homeostasis in renal failure: Pathophysiology and management. In David DS, ed. Calcium Metabolism in Renal Failure and Nephrolithiasis. New York: John Wiley & Sons, 1977.
19. Davidson GS, Montanera WJ, Fleming JF, Gentili F. Amyloid destructive spondyloarthropathy causing cord compression: related to chronic renal failure and dialysis. Neurosurgery 33:519-522, 1993.
20. Davies M. Primary hyperparathyroidism: Aggressive or conservative treatment. Clin Endocrinol 36:325-332, 1992.
21. Debnam JW, Staple TW. Trephine bone biopsy by radiologists. Radiology 116:607-609, 1975.
22. Deftos LJ, Parthemore JG, Stabile B. Management of primary hyperparathyroidism. Annu Rev Med 44:19-26, 1993.
23. Descamps-Latscha B. The immune system in end-stage renal disease. Curr Opin Nephrol Hypertens 2:883-891, 1993.
24. Descamps-Latscha B, Herbelin A. Long-term dialysis and cellular immunity: A critical survey. Kidney Int 41(Suppl):S135-S142, 1993.
25. Douglas DL, Duckworth T, Kanis JA. Spinal cord dysfunction in Paget's disease of bone. J Bone Joint Surg 63B:495-503, 1981.
26. Erikssen EF, Colvard DS, Berg NJ. Evidence of estrogen receptors in normal human osteoblast-like cells. Science 241:84, 1988.
27. Ettinger B, Genant HK, Cann CE. Long-term estrogen replacement therapy prevents bone loss and fractures. Ann Intern Med 102:319-324, 1985.
28. Ettinger B, Grady D. The waning effect of postmenopausal estrogen therapy on osteoporosis. N Engl J Med 329:1192, 1993.
29. Feyen JHM, Raisz LG. Prostagladin production by calvariae from sham operated and oophorectomized rats: Effect of 17-b-estradiol in vivo. Endocrinology 121:819, 1987.
30. Fiore CE, Castorina F, Malatino LS. Antalgic activity of calcitonin: Effectiveness of the epidermal and subarachnoid routes in man. Br J Clin Pharmacol 3:257, 1983.
31. Gallagher JC, Riggs BL, DeLuca HF. Effect of estrogen of calcium absorption and serum vitamin D metabolites in postmenopausal osteoporosis. J Clin Endocrinol Metab 51:1359-1364, 1980.
32. Gonzalez EA, Martin KJ. Renal osteodystrophy: Pathogenesis and management. Nephrol Dial Transplant 10(Suppl 3): 13-21, 1995.
33. Hadjipavlou A, Lander P, Srolovitz H. Pagetic arthritis: pathophysiology and management. Clin Orthop 208:15-19, 1986.
34. Harrop JS, Bailey JE, Woodhead JS. Incidence of hypercalcaemia and primary hyperparathyroidism in relation to the biochemical profile. J Clin Pathol 35:395-400, 1982.
35. Heaney RH, Recker RR, Saville PD. Menopausal changes in bone remodeling. J Lab Clin Med 92:964-970, 1978.
36. Heath H, Hodgson SF, Kennedy MA. Primary hyperparathyroidism: Incidence, morbidity and potential economic impact in a community. N Engl J Med 302:189-193, 1980.
37. Hercz G, Sherrard DJ, Chan W, Pei Y. Aplastic osteodystrophy: follow-up after 5 years. J Am Soc Nephrol 5:851, 1994.

38. Holbrook TL, Barrett-Connor E, Wingard DL. Dietary calcium and risk of hip fracture: 14-year prospective population study. Lancet 2:1046-1049, 1988.

39. Hosking DL, Mevnier PJ, Ringe JD, Reginster JY, Gennari C. Advances in the management of Paget's disease of bone. Drugs 40:829-840, 1990.

40. Hosking D, Meunier PJ, Ringe JD, Reginster JY, Gennari C. Paget's disease of bone: Diagnosis and management. Br Med J 312:491-494, 1996.

41. Hruska KA, Teitelbaum SL. Renal osteodystrophy. N Engl J Med 333:166-174, 1995.

42 Hui SL, Slemenda CW, Johnston CC. Baseline measurement of bone mass predicts fracture in white women. Ann Intern Med 111:355-361, 1989.

43. Hutchison AJ, Whitehouse RW. Correlation of bone histology with parathyroid hormone, vitamin D₃, and radiology in end-stage renal disease. Kidney Int 44:1160-1166, 1993.

44. Jacobsen S, Goldberg J, Miles T. Hip fracture incidence among the old and very old: A population-based study. Am J Public Health 80:871-873, 1990.

45. Kane WJ. Osteoporosis, osteomalacia, and Paget's disease. In Frymoyer JW, ed. The Adult Spine: Principles and Practice. New York: Raven Press, 1991, pp 637-659.

46. Kerr R, Bjorkengren A, Bielecki A. Destructive spondyloarthropathy in hemodialysis patients. Skeletal Radiol 17:176-180, 1988.

47. Komm BS, Terpening CM, Benz DJ. Estrogen binding, receptor mRNA, and biologic response in osteoblast-like osteosarcoma cells. Science 241:81, 1988.

48. Lindsay R. Estrogens, bone mass and osteoporotic fracture. Am J Med 91:10S-13S, 1991.

49. Lindsay R. Hormone replacement therapy for prevention and treatment of osteoporosis. Am J Med 95:37S-39S, 1993.

50. Lindsay R, Tohme J. Estrogen treatment of patients with established postmenopausal osteoporosis. Obstet Gynecol 76:290-295, 1990.

51. Lopez-Hilker S, Gakeran T, Chan YL, Rapp N, Martin KJ, Slatopolsky E. Hypocalcemia may not be essential for the development of secondary hyperparathyroidism in chronic renal failure. J Clin Invest 78:1097-1102, 1986.

52. Lopez-Hilker S, Dusso AS, Rapp NS, Martin KJ, Slatopolsky E. Phosphorus restriction reverses hyperparathyroidism in uremia independent of changes in calcium and calcitrol. Am J Physiol 259:F432-F437, 1990.

53. Lufkin EG, Wahner HW, O'Fallon WM, Hodgson SF, Kotowicz MA, Lane AW, Judd HL, Caplan RH, Riggs BL. Treatment of postmenopausal osteoporosis with transdermal estrogen. Ann Intern Med 117:1-9, 1992.

54. Martin P, Bergmann P, Gillet C, Fuss M, Kinnaert P, Corvilarin J, van Geertruyden J. Partially reversible osteopaenia after surgery for primary hyperparathyroidism. Arch Intern Med 146:689-691, 1986.

55. Martin RB, Burr DB. Structure, Function, and Adaptation of Compact Bone. New York: Raven Press, 1989, p 275.

56. Maruyama H, Gejyo F, Arakawa M. Clinical studies of destructive spondyloarthropathy in long-term hemodialysis patients. Nephron 61:37-44, 1992.

57. Mautalen C, Reyes HR, Ghiringhelli G, Fromm G. Cortical bone mineral content in primary hyperparathyroidism: Changes after parathyroidectomy. Acta Endocrinol 111:494-497, 1986.

58. McCarthy JT, Dahlberg PJ, Kriegshauser JS, Valente RM, Swee PG, O'Duffy JD, Kurtz SB, Johnson WJ. Erosive spondyloarthropathy in long-term dialysis patients: Relationship to severe hyperparathyroidism. Mayo Clin Proc 63:446-452, 1988.

59. Meunier PJ, Bressot C, Edouard C. Dynamics of bone remodelling in primary hyperparathyroidism: Histomorphometric data. In Copp DH, Talmage RV, eds. Endocrinology of Calcium Metabolism. Amsterdam: Excerpta, 1978.

60. Meunier PJ, Salson C, Mathiev L, Chapuy MC, Delmas P, Alexandre C, Charhon S. Skeletal distribution and biochemical parameters of Paget's disease. Clin Orthop 217:37-44, 1987.

61. Moriniere P, Cohen-Solal M, Belbrik S, Boudailliez B, Marie A. Westeel PF, Renaud H, Fievet H, Lalau JD. Disappearance of aluminic bone disease in a long term asymptomatic dialysis population restricting Al(OH)3 intake: Emergence of an idiopathic adynamic bone disease not related to aluminum. Nephron 53:93-101, 1989.

62. Mundy GR, Cove DH, Fisken R. Primary hyperparathyroidism: Changes in the pattern of clinical presentation. Lancet 1:1317-1320, 1980.

63. Nelson J, Thomas PS. Clinical findings in 12 patients with MPS IV A (Morquio's disease). Clin Genet 33:126-130, 1988.

64. Nevitt MC. Epidemiology of osteoporosis. Rheum Dis Clin North Am 20:535-559, 1994.

65. Orzincolo C, Bedani PL, Sertellari PN, Cardona P, Trotta F, Gilli P. Destructive spondyloarthropathy and radiographic follow up in hemodialysis patients. Skeletal Radiol 19:483-487, 1990.

66. Overgaard K, Hansen MA, Nielsen MA, Riis BJ, Christiansen C. Discontinuous calcitonin treatment of established osteoporosis—Effects of withdrawal of treatment. Am J Med 89:1, 1990.

67. Paget J. On a form of chronic inflammation of one (osteitis deformans). Clin Orthop 49:3-16, 1966.

68. Pak CYC, Stewart A, Kaplan R, Bone H, Notz C, Browne R. Photon absorptiometric analysis of bone density in primary hyperparathyroidism. Lancet 2:7-8, 1975.

69 Parfitt AM. Equilibrium and disequilibrium hypercalcemia: New light on an old concept. Metab Bone Dis Rel Res 1:279-293, 1979.

70. Parfitt AM, Duncan H. Metabolic bone disease affecting the spine. In Rothman RH, Simeone FA, eds. The Spine. Philadelphia: WB Saunders, 1982, pp 775-905.

71. Parfitt AM, Kleerekoper M. The divalent ion homeostatic system: Physiology and metabolism of calcium, phosphorus, magnesium and bone. In Maxwell M, Kleeman CR, eds. Clinical Disorders of Fluid and Electrolyte Metabolism. New York: McGraw-Hill, 1979, pp 947-1152.

72. Piccirilli CB, Chadduck WM. Cervical dyphotic myelopathy in a child with Morquio syndrome. Childs Nerv Syst 12:114-116, 1996.

73. Quigley ME, Martin PL, Burnier AM, Brooks P. Estrogen therapy arrests bone loss in elderly women. Am J Obstet Gynecol 156:1516, 1987.

74. Reginster JY, Albert A, Lecart MP. One-year controlled randomized trial in prevention of early postmenopausal bone loss by intranasal calcitonin. Lancet 2:1481, 1987.

75. Richardson ML, Pozzi-Mucelli RS, Kanter AS, Kolb FO, Ettinger B. Bone mineral changes in primary hyperparathyroidism. Skeletal Radiol 15:85-95, 1986.

76. Riggs BL, Jowsey J, Goldsmith RS, Kelly PJ, Hoffman DL, Arnaud CD. Short- and long-term effects of estrogen and synthetic anobolic hormones in postmenopausal osteoporosis. J Clin Invest 51:1649-1663, 1972.

77. Riggs BL, Melton LJ. The prevention and treatment of osteoporosis. N Engl J Med 327:620, 1992.

78. Rooijen NV. Extracellular and intracellular action of clodronate in osteolytic diseases? A hypothesis. Calcif Tissue Int 52:107, 1993.

79. Ross PD, Davis JW, Vogel JM, Wasnich RD. A critical review of bone mass and the risk of fractures in osteoporosis. Calcif Tissue Int 46:149-161, 1990.

80. Ryan MD and Taylor TKF, Spinal manifestations of Paget's disease. Aust N Z J Surg 62:33-38, 1992.

81. Sato M, Grasser W, Endo N, Akins R, Simmons H, Thompson DD, Golub E, Rodan GA. Bisphosphonate action: Alendronate localizaton in rat bone and effects on osteoclast ultrastructure. J Clin Invest 88:2095, 1991.

82. Schmidt H, Ullrich K, von Lengerke HJ, Kleine M, Bramswig J. Radiological findings in patients with mucopolysaccharidosis I H/S (Hurler-Scheie syndrome). Pediatr Radiol 17:409-414, 1987.

83. Seeman E, Wahner HW, Offord KP, Kumar R, Johnson WJ, Riggs BL. Differential effects of endocrine dysfunction on the axial and appendicular skeleton. J Clin Invest 69:1302-1309, 1982.

84. Sethi D, Gower PE. Dialysis arthropathy, beta-2-microglobulin and the effect of dialyser membrane. Nephrol Dial Transplant 3:768-772, 1988.

85. Stampfer MJ, Colditz GA, Willett WC. Postmenopausal estrogen therapy and cardiovascular disease: Ten year follow-up from the Nurses' Health Study. N Engl J Med 325:756, 1991.

86. Stolpen AH. Case of the Season: Spondyloarthropathy of renal dialysis. Semin Roentgenol 28:96-100, 1993.

87. Storm T. Changes in bone histomorphometry after long-term treatment with intermittent, cyclic etidronate for postmenopausal osteoporosis. J Bone Miner Res 8:199, 1993.

88. Storm T, Thamsborg G, Steiniche T. Effect of intermittent cyclical etidronate therapy on bone mass and fracture rate in women with postmenopausal osteoporosis. N Engl J Med 322:1265, 1990.

89. Watts NB, Harris ST, Genant HK, Wasnich RD, Miller PD, Jakcson RD, Licata AA, Ross P, Woodson GC, Yanover MJ. Intermittent cyclical etidronate treatment of postmenopausal osteoporosis. N Engl J Med 323:73, 1990.

90. Westerman MP, Greenfield GB, Wong PWK. Fish vertebrae, homocystinuria, and sickle cell anemia. JAMA 230:261-262, 1974.

91. Wilson RJ, et al. Mild asymptomatic primary hyperparathyroidism is not a risk factor for vertebral fractures. Ann Intern Med 109:959-962, 1988.

92. Wraith JE. The mucopolysaccharidoses: A clinical review and guide to management. Arch Dis Child 72: 263-267, 1995.

Spinal Infections

Eldan Eichbaum, M.D., Paul Matz, M.D., and Bruce M. McCormack, M.D.

Thoracic spinal infections occur relatively infrequently, but in recent years their incidence has increased in connection with a resurgence of tuberculosis, increased use of intravenous drugs, and an aging population.[18,71,81,107,117,123,140] The three major categories of infections are vertebral osteomyelitis, spinal epidural abscess, and discitis. These entities are frequently intertwined, and are interpreted as the same disease process. However, for the purpose of clarity they are discussed separately. Spinal subdural abscesses and intramedullary abscesses are extremely rare and are not discussed in this chapter.

Because spinal infections are difficult to diagnose and have an insidious onset and indolent course, the diagnosis is usually delayed. Patients may present late in the course of the disease with impending paralysis, overt spinal instability, or sepsis, and may die despite treatment. The spectrum of management varies from simply the use of intravenous antibiotics to circumferential surgery with arthrodesis and spinal instrumentation. Because of anatomical differences, thoracic spondylitis requires surgical and medical management that differs significantly from the management of cervical and lumbar disease.

This chapter addresses the definition, epidemiology, diagnosis, and prevention of thoracic spinal infections, as well as their management, with an emphasis on surgical approaches to the thoracic spine. Postoperative spinal infections occurring in patients with or without instrumentation are also reviewed.

PYOGENIC INFECTIONS
Vertebral Osteomyelitis
Epidemiology

Vertebral osteomyelitis, or spondylodiscitis, is the most common form of spinal infection in adults.[10] It refers to an infection of the vertebral body, pedicles, and dorsal elements, or combinations thereof. Vertebral osteomyelitis is almost always associated with discitis, and is frequently associated with spinal epidural abscesses.[11,28,32,99,105,133,139] Of all cases of pyogenic vertebral osteomyelitis, more than 95% involve the vertebral body, and less than 5% involve the dorsal elements.[4,18,36] The incidence is approximately 1 per 100,000 to 250,000 population,[18,33,41] with thoracic spine involvement ranging from 10% to 60%.*

Risk factors for spondylodiscitis stem mainly from an attenuated host immune response. They include diabetes mellitus, advanced age, chronic alcoholism, steroid use, rheumatoid arthritis, and chemotherapy-induced myelosuppression.[10,14,18,19,32,37,39,51,71,81,105,124,126] More recently, intravenous drug use has emerged as an important risk factor. The rise in intravenous drug use and in the use of urinary tract manipulations (e.g., cystoscopy) is thought to be responsible, in part, for the increased incidence of infectious spondylitis.[40,67,81,98,107,123,126,140] Sources of infections are identified in approximately 70% of cases. They include skin infections, soft tissue infections, and urinary tract

---

*References 10, 16, 18, 19, 32, 37, 39, 41, 46, 56, 57, 79, 88, 107, 114, 126, 141.

infections and manipulations. Less common are dental abscesses, endocarditis, pneumonia, and pharyngitis.[14,16,18,32,33,37,46,79,105,124,126,140,141]

The mean age of occurrence is during the sixth or seventh decade of life.[10,16,19,39,46,51,71,81,105,107,114,124,140] Patients who have a compromised immune system tend to be older, whereas intravenous drug users tend to be younger.[67,125,126] Men are more frequently affected than women, with most studies demonstrating at least a 2:1 ratio.[10,37,79,81,105,107,124,126]

Pathophysiology

Vertebral osteomyelitis is believed to occur by one of three mechanisms: hematogenous spread, contiguous spread, or direct inoculation.[14,18,89,124,126,141,145] It is rare to have a contiguous source of spread in the thoracic spine. However, possible sources include retropharyngeal abscess, pleural empyema, or perinephric abscess.[119,135] Direct inoculation of bacteria may occur after a diagnostic needle biopsy (e.g., discography, cultures) or after surgery.[13,129] The risk of discitis after discectomy is approximately 1%.[18,58,106]

Hematogenous spread is believed to be the most common route of infection.[14,39,89,126,141] In adults, the vertebrae are the most common sites of hematogenously acquired osteomyelitis.[10,51,126,141] The preponderance of axial skeletal involvement in hematogenous vertebral osteomyelitis is thought to be due to the persistence of rich cellular bone marrow, the lack of true epiphyseal growth, and the presence of a sluggish, voluminous blood supply in the adult vertebrae.[2,126] This environment is conducive to bacterial growth.

Hematogenous spread of microbes may occur through an arterial or venous route. Pyogenic microemboli arterially disseminate into the metaphyseal end-arteries and lodge in the vertebral subchondral end plate.[12,110,113,126,143] Septic infarction ensues, followed by infection with direct spread into the avascular disc space. Eventually, suppuration into the prevertebral and epidural spaces occurs. The predictable involvement of adjacent segments of contiguous vertebrae is consistent with the arterial supply of the axial skeleton.[113,122,126] During embryogenesis, one sclerotome contributes to the formation of two adjacent segments of vertebral bodies, including the intervening disc space. The main artery supplying the vertebral bodies is the posterior spinal artery, which enters the intervertebral foramen, splits to form equatorial arteries, and supplies the lower portion of the rostral vertebrae and the upper portion of the caudal vertebrae.[113,122,126]

Spondylodiscitis is less frequently a result of venous dissemination than of arterial dissemination.[126,143] Batson's vertebral veins are the venous conduit to the vertebral column. This extensive valveless venous plexus intimately surrounds and drains the entire vertebral column. Batson[12] demonstrated that a single injection of contrast agent through a penile vein concentrated in the thoracolumbar vertebral column and reached as high as the intracranial sinuses when Valsalva maneuvers were performed. Sources of vertebral osteomyelitis by venous dissemination include urinary tract infections, urinary tract manipulations (e.g., cystoscopy), and intravenous drug injection.[39,79,98,124,125]

The mechanism of neurological compromise in vertebral osteomyelitis and epidural abscess is caused by either direct spinal cord compression or vascular compromise, or by both events. Vascular ischemia may occur after direct compression of the vessel or from toxic effects on the spinal cord vasculature from epidural suppuration. Arterial and venous thrombosis ensue, with subsequent spinal cord infarction. This vascular mechanism of neurological injury may be even more devastating than a compressive mechanism, because spinal cord infarction frequently occurs rapidly and unpredictably and is irreversible.[11,18,26,65]

Vertebral osteomyelitis is a destructive process that predominantly affects the vertebral body and intervertebral disc space. Progressive destruction of the vertebral body may lead to spinal instability, manifested by localized back pain and progressive kyphotic deformity (Fig. 39-1). Usually, this phenomenon occurs over a period of weeks to months and hence is termed "glacial instability." In general, the thoracic spine is relatively protected from instability owing to the support of the rib cage. The combination of ribs, costovertebral ligaments, and costotransverse ligaments increase the stability of the thoracic spine twofold to threefold.[7]

Diagnosis

The diagnosis of vertebral osteomyelitis, epidural abscess, and/or discitis may be suggested by a constellation of findings from the clinical history, examination, laboratory results, and radiographic findings. Absolute confirmation depends on the results of culture and histological findings.

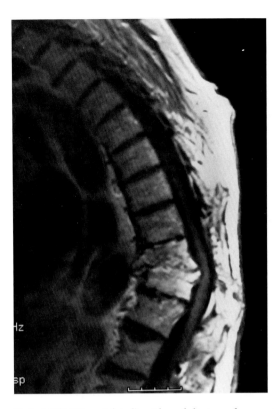

Fig. 39-1. MRI (T1-weighted) with gadolinium demonstrating staphylococcal thoracic osteomyelitis with ventral column destruction and kyphotic deformity.

The hallmark symptom of vertebral osteomyelitis is back pain, occurring in approximately 92% to 100% of patients.* This pain is usually exacerbated with movement. The mean duration of symptoms is approximately 7 weeks, but may be as long as several years.[10,18,41,81,98,114,124] The cardinal physical finding is severe tenderness with spinal palpation over the involved region, with associated muscle spasm(s). Only 50% of patients have a fever.[18,98,105,124,140] Neurological deficits affect up to 65% of patients[10,18,37, 51,57,79,81,105,114,126] and more often occur in conjunction with lesions in the cervical and thoracic region.[37,81,126] In general, patients who present earlier often have neurological deficits and more advanced disease. Occasionally, patients have evidence of a primary focus, such as a cutaneous infection(s).

Leukocytosis occurs in approximately one half of patients and is more frequently found in patients who present with acute symptoms.[10,18,81,105,107,124,140] The erythrocyte sedimentation rate (ESR) is an extremely sensitive diagnostic assay, but is not specific. It is usually elevated to three to five times the normal value of <20 mm per hour. Although the numerical value is not a sensitive indicator of disease severity, rises or falls in the ESR are useful for assessing response to therapy. Adequacy of treatment after antibiotic therapy may be indicated by a two-thirds decrease in the ESR.[105,126] This decrease may take several months and even longer to normalize. In rare cases, the ESR may not decrease significantly after adequate treatment.

Patients who are candidates for nonoperative therapy often require a bacteriological diagnosis. The specimen for culture may come from a needle biopsy of the involved vertebra, disc, or epidural space, a recent separate infectious focus, or blood.[14,124] A bacterial diagnosis may be difficult to obtain. The negative culture rate for fine-needle biopsy is as high as 30%, and is 14% in open biopsies.[14,18,126] Use of computed tomography (CT) or fluoroscopic guidance is helpful when inserting needles for biopsies.[14] Reasons for negative cultures include poor placement of the needle, insufficient sample, or the prior initiation of antibiotic therapy. Blood cultures are positive in approximately 50%, and cerebrospinal fluid (CSF) cultures are positive in approximately 15% of cases.[18,33,65,124,126]

Microbiology

For diagnostic purposes, cultures may be obtained from the involved vertebra, a preexisting infected anatomical site, or blood. Positive blood cultures range from 20% to 100%, with most studies demonstrating bacterial growth in approximately 50%.[10,18,19,33,41,98,105,107,124,140] Bacterial identification on cultures is greatly reduced when antibiotics are given before a specimen is obtained for culture.

Staphylococcus aureus is by far the most common infective organism in pyogenic vertebral osteomyelitis. It is found in approximately 50% to 80% of cases, with other gram-positive organisms being recovered less frequently.[10,18,19,32,33,39,41,98,105,107,114,124,126] Factors that contribute to this high rate of *S. aureus* infections include its ubiquitous nature, its propensity to form abscesses, and its ability to infect both immunocompetent and immunosuppressed patients. Gram-negative organisms, such as *Escherichia coli* and *Pseudomonas aeruginosa* are the second most common organisms in most studies.[14,32,39,79,81,105,114,124,126]

---

*References 10, 16, 18, 32, 33, 41, 46, 81, 105, 107, 114, 124, 126, 140.

*References 10, 18, 41, 79, 81, 105, 107, 114, 124, 126, 140.

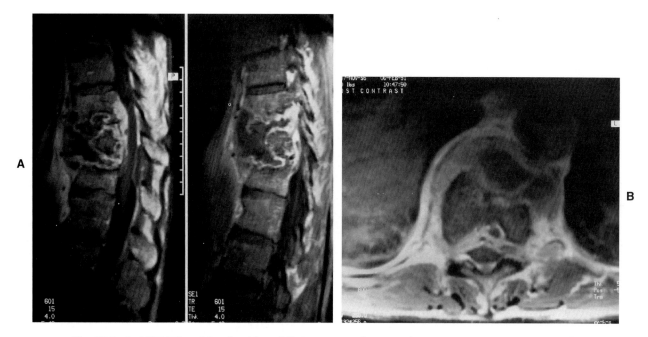

Fig. 39-2. A, MRI (T1-weighted) with gadolinium, sagittal views, demonstrating T9 to T11 coccid-ioidomycosis with extensive heterogeneously enhancing vertebral body destruction, prevertebral and epidural suppuration with spinal cord compression. **B,** MRI (T1-weighted) with gadolinium, axial view, demonstrating vertebral destruction, enhancing prevertebral and epidural mass with cord compression.

E. coli is more frequently associated with patients who have had urinary tract manipulations and infections, whereas *P. aeruginosa* is found more frequently in intravenous drug users.[17,77,126,131] In the vast majority of hematogenous vertebral osteomyelitis, a single organism is cultured. When multiple organisms are found, a contiguous infection is the more likely source of spread.[126]

Imaging

Magnetic resonance imaging (MRI) is the imaging modality of choice, but plain radiographs, CT, and radionuclide bone scans all contribute useful diagnostic information. Plain film radiographs are usually normal for the first 8 to 10 days. The earliest finding is disc space narrowing, which occurs at 1 to 3 weeks.[38,104,121] This is due to digestion of the nucleus pulposis from the acute inflammatory response.[14] The adjacent rostral and caudal vertebral bodies show decreased radiodensity and bone destruction at 6 to 8 weeks. Frequently, there is prevertebral soft tissue swelling.[14,121] Kyphosis may result if there is significant destruction of bone. Reactive new bone formation is initiated at 12 weeks, as shown by increased radiodensity. This

almost always leads to radiographic evidence of intervertebral fusion at 6 to 24 months.[14,33]

A technetium-99 bone scan is a sensitive indicator of early disease, but it lacks specificity.[38,91] When combined with gallium scintigraphy, such scans are highly sensitive (>93%), specific (100%), and accurate (94%).[91] CT shows changes in the bone earlier than do plain radiographs, and better demonstrates paravertebral abscesses, soft tissue masses, and intradiscal air.

MRI has become the study of choice in evaluating spinal infections and inflammatory diseases.[14,21,91,121] The ability to distinguish soft tissues, the sensitivity to disease, its noninvasive nature, and its multiplanar capability are among the reasons for this standing.[133,134] The sensitivity of MRI is 96%, with a specificity of 93% and an accuracy of 94%.[25,91] Characteristic findings include narrowed disc space and low signal intensity in the adjacent vertebral bodies on T1-weighted sequences, reflecting increased extracellular fluid within the bone marrow.[91,104,133,139] Subligamentous or epidural soft tissue masses and cortical bone erosion are frequently seen. Intravenous gadolinium enhances the infected disc, bone, and epidural abscess or granulation tissue (Fig. 39-2). T2-weighted sequences show high signal in the

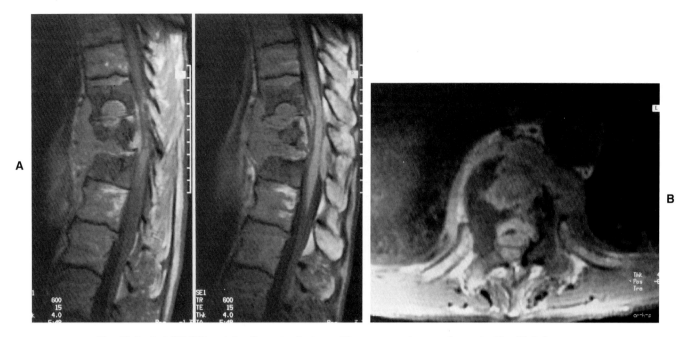

Fig. 39-3. A, MRI (T2-weighted), sagittal views. The same patient as shown in Fig. 39-2 demonstrating a typical hyperintense disc space, prevertebral and epidural lesions. **B,** MRI (T2-weighted), axial view.

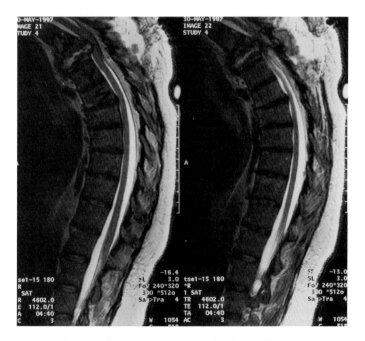

Fig. 39-4. MRI (T2-weighted) of a patient with salmonella T2 to T3 osteomyelitis.

involved disc space and vertebral bodies (Figs. 39-3 and 39-4). Effacement of the nuclear cleft, typically seen as an area of decreased signal in the middle of the disc, may be noted.[133]

The radiographic differential diagnosis of pyogenic spondylitis includes granulomatous spondylitis, intervertebral osteochondrosis, calcium pyrophosphate crystal deposition disease, renal osteodystrophy, and axial neuropathy.[104,133] Rarely, severe degenerative disc disease is accompanied by secondary spinal changes that can also simulate infection.[104,133]

Spinal Epidural Abscess
Epidemiology

Spinal epidural abscess has been discussed historically as a distinct entity from vertebral osteomyelitis. The association of these two disease processes had been reported to range from 5% to 45%.[11,27,28,124] With the introduction of MRI, it is now recognized that most spinal epidural abscesses are ventral to the spinal cord dura and are associated with spondylodiscitis.[8,34,133]

The incidence of spinal epidural abscess has been reported to range from 0.2 to two patients per 10,000 hospital admissions.[11,18,27,64,100,115] Thoracic spinal involvement ranges from 25% to 50%.[11,18,28,65,100] Before MRI was introduced, investigations erroneously indicated a predilection for the dorsal spinal canal.[11] A more recent study with MRI demonstrated that 50% of spinal epidural abscesses were ventral, 36% were circumferential, and 14% were dorsal.[65]

The mean age of patients at diagnosis is the sixth decade. Men predominate, with an approximate ratio of 1.5:1.[11,26-28,65,87,100] The risk factors associated with spinal epidural abscess are the same as those associated with vertebral osteomyelitis and include diabetes, intravenous drug use, and immunosuppressive states.[11,26-28,65] Sixty to eighty percent of patients have at least one identifiable chronic disease state or incident that increases their risk for spinal epidural abscess.[11,26,27,65]

Pathophysiology

Epidural abscess without spondylodiscitis is believed to develop as a result of bacteremic spread from infectious foci, including parenteral injections, with spread to the vertebral column by venous dissemination.[12] Cervical and upper thoracic epidural abscesses develop in intravenous drug users after injections into the upper extremities.[100] The thoracic and lumbar regions are more frequently seeded by pelvic or lower extremity infectious foci.

Diagnosis

More than 90% of patients have spinal pain and tenderness.[11,26,64,65] Radiculopathy occurs in 10% to 70% of patients, and objective neurological deficit occurs in up to 90%.[11,26,27,65,87,100] Up to 76% of patients have fever.[11,26,27,65,87,100]

The classic clinical presentation of a spinal epidural abscess consists of spinal ache followed by radicular pain, then weakness, and ultimately paralysis.[64,112] The interval from one stage to the next is highly variable. One study quantitated the mean time period between each stage as follows: spinal pain led to nerve root pain in 3 days; nerve root pain advanced to weakness in 4.5 days; and weakness progressed to paralysis in 24 hours.[11] Spinal epidural abscess is even more difficult to diagnose in a patient who has preexisting encephalopathy or paralysis. Ascending neurological deficits should alert the clinician to a spinal epidural abscess in a paraplegic or quadriplegic patient.

Some investigators have divided the patients into acute and chronic groups, based upon the duration of their symptoms. The acute group has symptoms for less than 2 weeks, the majority of whom have symptoms for less than 1 week. In contrast, the chronic group has symptoms for longer than 2 weeks, with a mean of 6 weeks.[11,26,65,100] On presentation, patients in the acute group typically have a higher mean temperature and a higher probability of having a neurological deficit.[11,26,65]

White blood cell and ESR values are similar to the values noted in patients with pyogenic vertebral osteomyelitis.[11,26,28,65] Examination of the CSF usually reveals a parameningeal infection with elevated protein, leukocytosis, and normal glucose values.[11,65,98]

Whether to perform a lumbar puncture is a major dilemma when contemplating the diagnosis of spinal epidural abscess. Passing a spinal needle into the abscess and subsequent inadvertent introduction of this material into the subarachnoid space could further complicate the course of the disease. With the introduction of MRI, the need for lumbar puncture to aid in the differential diagnosis of infectious processes of the spine has decreased immensely. In fact, use of a lumbar puncture is not usually recommended unless there is radiographic documentation that no abscess exists. In the event that an emergency lumbar puncture is required for either diagnosis or myelography, and if MRI capabilities are not available, the lumbar puncture should be performed with extreme caution. In this situation, a C1 to C2 puncture is preferred, because the risk of contaminating the subarachnoid space is much less at C1 to C2 than at other spinal levels. If a C1 to C2 puncture is not possible, either because of the patient's anatomy or the physician's inexperience, then careful insertion of the spinal needle in the lumbar region, with frequent aspirations of its contents, is recommended.

Microbiology

S. aureus is by far the most common infective organism, occurring in 50% to 90% of cases.[11,26,28,65,100] The greatest yield is from operative cultures, which are positive in 80% to 100% of cases.[26,65] The infecting organism may be isolated from blood cultures in 40% to 70% of cases,[26,28,65] whereas the yield for CSF cultures is only 15%.[65]

Imaging

MRI is the imaging modality of choice for the reasons discussed earlier in the section on spondylodiscitis. Specifically for spinal epidural abscess, the multiplanar capabilities of MRI can rapidly reveal the full rostral and caudal extent of the lesion in the spinal canal, including involvement of the bone and soft tissue. A spinal epidural abscess on T1-weighted images appears as an isodense (with vertebral marrow) extradural mass with or without compression of the thecal sac[104,134] (see Fig. 39-2). On the first echo study, the signal intensity exhibited by an epidural abscess may be higher than that exhibited by CSF, presumably because of the higher protein content of the abscess.[133] On T2-weighted images, the abscess may be completely silhouetted by the high signal from CSF.[133] Gadolinium enhancement on T1-weighted images should show homogeneously or rim-enhancing lesions.[99,133] The differentiation between pus and granulation tissue is not very reliable, but typically ring enhancement with an isodense center suggests frank pus, whereas homogeneous enhancement signifies granulation tissue.

Plain radiographs are not reliable in detecting epidural abscesses. Occasionally, they demonstrate bone destruction with epidural abscesses, when associated with spondylodiscitis.[18,27,65] CT-myelography is very sensitive, but requires intrathecal insertion of contrast agent. It does not readily demonstrate the extent of the lesion. Radionuclide studies are of little utility unless osteomyelitis is also present.[18]

Childhood Discitis

Isolated discitis occurs only rarely and is thought to be primarily a childhood disease, occurring more frequently in young children.[18,53,70] Because the in-

tervertebral disc is well vascularized until the late teenage years, it is more likely to be a target for pyogenic infections.[18,113,122] Some investigators think childhood discitis is an inflammatory condition because blood and disc cultures often yield negative results and because, in some children, the condition has a self-limiting course.[18,53,103] Hematogenous vertebral osteomyelitis rarely occurs in children. In adults, the disc is avascular and becomes involved secondarily through subchondral end plate extension. If it is not associated with vertebral osteomyelitis, discitis in adults occurs most often in patients after lumbar disc surgery.[18,62] Thoracic disc surgery is relatively rare and the incidence of postoperative discitis is negligible.

Back pain without a radicular component that has persisted for 2 to 4 weeks is the most common symptom. Children frequently refuse to sit, stand, or walk.[18,142] Paraspinous and point tenderness are common, but weakness is rarely present.[18,103] Although the white blood cell count may be normal, often the ESR is elevated. Blood cultures frequently yield negative findings.[18] Radiographic studies are described in previous sections of this chapter. Follow-up plain radiographs often demonstrate fused or "block" vertebrae.[70]

GRANULOMATOUS AND FUNGAL SPONDYLITIS
Tuberculous Vertebral Osteomyelitis

Although tuberculosis (TB) is a disease found predominantly in developing nations, pulmonary tuberculosis as well as its spinal counterpart, Pott's disease, have recently had a resurgence in the United States.[49,101,117] This renascence is mainly attributable to larger numbers of homeless people, crowding in prisons, a rise in immigration from countries that have a high prevalence of TB, the emergence of drug-resistant strains, and poor compliance with medication.[15,49,117] Spinal tuberculosis occurs in approximately 1% of patients who have tuberculosis.[101,102,117]

Tuberculous vertebral osteomyelitis typically occurs in the thoracic/thoracolumbar region.[15,101,117] Most cases involve the ventral spinal column, but dorsal element involvement in TB and fungal osteomyelitis is more common than in pyogenic infections.[18,69] Pott's disease is more indolent than pyogenic osteomyelitis and is usually diagnosed after significant bone destruction. Most patients present with chronic mid- to low back pain, lower extremity radiculopathy, and occasionally with paraparesis/myelopathy. The white blood cell count typically is not elevated. The ESR is usually elevated, although not to the extent of pyogenic infections. Tuberculin skin testing (Mantoux test) usually yields positive findings, but false negative results may be obtained in anergic patients, possibly as a result of malnutrition, immunocompromised states, renal failure, overwhelming TB, or old age.[15,49] Therefore in addition to TB skin testing, a simultaneous anergy panel is required to rule out poor reaction due to anergy.

In TB of the spine, three radiographic patterns of involvement have been described.[15,35] In the paradiscal pattern, the most common pattern, mycobacteria invade the well-oxygenated vertebral metaphysis, spread through the interconnected arterioles to adjacent vertebral bodies, and classically spare the poorly vascularized disc space. The disc space may become involved in late or extensive disease after erosion through the cartilaginous end plate.

Ventral lesions are the second described pattern. These lesions develop beneath the anterior longitudinal ligament and may spread to involve several vertebrae. Subsequent bone devascularization occurs by elevation of the periosteum, leading to necrosis and abscess formation.[15] The end result may be spinal deformity, although rare in the United States in the modern era. The least common are central lesions. They may appear as vertebral plana with significant spinal deformity.

Plain radiographs may not reveal disc space narrowing until 2 to 3 years after the onset of the disease process. Loss of radiographic subchondral vertebral density is similar to pyogenic disease, but reactive new bone formation is often mild or absent.[14,49,53] Occasionally, bone destruction with concurrent bone regeneration is observed. A large soft tissue mass, typically in the thoracic region, may form with calcifications that can be found on plain radiographs and CT.[69,104] MRI of tuberculous spondylitis is very similar to that of pyogenic spondylitis. Minor differences may aid in differentiating the two radiographically. For instance, tuberculous spondylitis usually involves more vertebral levels, and its signal intensity in the involved vertebral bodies is less homogeneous.[9] Differential diagnoses include pyogenic, fungal, or atypical infections (Brucella), as well as malignancy. In general, malignancy spares the disc space, early TB may spare the disc space and but pyogenic or late TB osteomyelitis rarely spares the disc space.[5,104]

Fungal Vertebral Osteomyelitis

Fungal infections are rare and can be very difficult to treat. Many reported cases are related to, or are complications of, medical advances, such as iatrogenic immunosuppression, invasive monitoring, hyperalimentation, medical success in chronic diseases, and increasing numbers of operative procedures.[22,24,37,47,49,74] Fungal infections are also more frequently found in areas of the country where the organisms are endemic and in patients who have AIDS. The clinical and radiographic findings are similar to tuberculous infections, but fungal infections rarely involve the epidural space.[49,104]

Candida spinal infections are usually chronic, frequently developing months after *Candida* sepsis. The histology and microbiology are critical.

In aspergillus spinal infections, the primary site of infection is usually pulmonary or gastrointestinal.[24,49,60] There are characteristic dense new areas of bone formation with concurrent lytic lesions on imaging studies. Paravertebral abscesses are rare, and serum antibodies or serum antigens are present in one half of patients.[18]

Coccidioides immitis is a dimorphic fungus endemic to the southwest United States and to Central and South America. Disseminated coccidioidomycosis involves the spine in approximately 20% of cases, most commonly in the thoracic and thoracolumbar regions[18,49] (see Figs. 39-2 and 39-3). Tissue diagnosis may be assisted by a serum complement fixation antibody titer. Other fungal infections include blastomycosis and torulopsis.

Brucellosis is caused by a nonencapsulated gram-negative aerobic bacillus. Even though it is not a fungus or mycobacteria, it deserves mention because it may be confused with either organism and is difficult to diagnose.[18,49] The incidence is very low in the United States but significant in Turkey and the Middle East.[18,138] Ingestion of infected milk or raw meat are important sources of infection.[80] Diagnosis is made with an agglutination test.[18,49,138] Other atypical bacterial infections include actinomycosis and nocardiosis.

MANAGEMENT

The management of patients with thoracic spinal infections differs from the management of those patients with cervical or lumbar disease because of the unique anatomy of the region. The thoracic spinal canal is narrow and has a tenuous blood supply when compared to the cervical and lumbar regions. As a result, paraplegia may develop rapidly and unpredictably in patients with thoracic spine infections despite appropriate antibiotic treatment. For this reason, urgent surgery is indicated for those patients with symptomatic spinal cord compression or significant disease in the spinal canal on imaging studies. Secondly, the thoracic spine is rigidly supported by the rib cage. Biomechanical studies indicate that the rib cage and its costotransverse and costovertebral ligamentous attachments increase stability two- or threefold.[7] Hence infectious lesions are less likely to destabilize the thoracic spine compared to the cervical or lumbar spine. When instability does occur, surgical stabilization can often be accomplished simply with interbody bone grafting without spinal instrumentation. Finally, the presence of the rib cage and the close proximity of the heart, lungs, and great vessels require specialized surgical approaches.

Nonoperative Management

Patients with thoracic osteomyelitis who are neurologically intact may be treated with intravenous antibiotics and external bracing.[10,18,19,33,93,95,105,106] Spinal epidural abscesses have been treated successfully with intravenous antibiotics alone, but this treatment is recommended only for selected patients,[28,61,78,84,100] and those patients must have frequent and vigilant neurological examinations with rapid access to MRI. MRI permits frequent and accurate assessments of the lesion and emergency evaluations for patients who have acute neurological decline.

Many studies done in East Asia and Africa on Pott's disease have examined medical management with or without bracing, as well as medical management with bed rest vs. surgery. In general, most patients do well with all forms of medical management.[93,95,117]

Children with isolated spontaneous discitis often have complete resolution of their symptoms with bracing and no antibiotic treatment.[70,103] Patients with positive blood or disc cultures should be treated for at least 2 weeks with intravenous antibiotics. Some investigators recommend antistaphylococcal therapy if cultures yield negative findings.[18,23,130]

Antimicrobial Therapy

Four to six weeks of antimicrobial therapy is indicated for all spinal infections. A longer course is recommended when patients have a poor clinical response or if the ESR has not decreased to at least one half of the pretreatment value.[18,105,124,126] Enteral antibiotics are often recommended for 2 weeks to several months after completion of the intravenous regimen. Staphylococcal infections are generally treated with high-dose semisynthetic penicillins (i.e., nafcillin), or cephalosporins (i.e., cefazolin) if the patient is mildly allergic to penicillins.[125,126,127] Detailed drug regimens are described elsewhere.[42,83,125,127]

Longer courses of therapy may be required for infections caused by actinomyces, brucella, and tuberculosis. Actinomyces is treated with 6 weeks of intravenous penicillin, followed by months of oral penicillin. Brucella is treated with 3 months of trimethoprim/sulfisoxazole or tetracycline with rifampin. Pott's disease requires a four-drug regimen in geographical areas with a significant incidence of isoniazid (INH) resistance.[49,117,125] This regimen consists of INH, rifampin, ethambutol, and pyrazinamide. Ethambutol is usually dropped when cultures demonstrate nonresistant organisms, but pyrazinamide is continued for 8 weeks.[125] A 12-month course is recommended for patients with Pott's disease.

Empiric intravenous antibiotic treatment is started in patients with sepsis and in all patients after appropriate cultures have been taken. Broad spectrum antibiotics should be given, including gram-positive (especially methicillin-resistant *S. aureus*) and gram-negative coverage. Antifungal and antituberculous coverage should be initiated in high-risk patients.

Tuberculosis skin testing should be performed in all patients with vertebral osteomyelitis, especially in patients who are immunocompromised, who come from countries where tuberculosis is endemic, or who have pulmonary infections. Although a positive test aids in diagnosis, a negative result is not unusual. Patients of advanced age and immunocompromised patients are often anergic.

Bracing

External bracing aids in pain relief and promotes bony healing by immobilizing the spinal segments that are infected. Spinal deformity is minimized. In general, patients are braced for at least 6 weeks and often longer. A thoracolumbosacral orthosis (TLSO) is used for mid- to lower thoracic spine stabilization. A neck extension may be added to this brace for upper thoracic stabilization.

Operative Management

Surgical decision making and operative procedures for vertebral osteomyelitis and epidural abscesses, whether they are pyogenic, fungal, or tuberculous, are similar. Therefore their management is discussed uniformly.

Surgery is indicated for significant pyogenic and tuberculous infections in the thoracic spine with infected tissue or bone in the spinal canal because abrupt neurological deterioration may occur with medical management alone.[1,10,32,37,66,97] Even though spinal epidural abscesses have been treated successfully with medical management alone, many surgeons recommend immediate drainage of all spinal epidural abscesses. This is because there has been a significant population of patients who have had acute neurological decline despite appropriate antibiotic therapy and vigilant neurological examinations.[26-28,65,100,115] The acute neurological decline frequently occurs without warning and typically is irreversible. Although Pott's disease can be successfully treated medically, the best results are observed in patients treated with ventral surgical debridement, with arthrodesis combined with chemotherapy.[94,96,97,101,117] These patients are mobilized earlier, have faster pain relief and neurological recovery, and less frequently develop kyphosis compared to medically managed patients. Therefore patients with Pott's disease and significant osseous involvement should be treated with ventral surgery if adequate surgical, anesthetic, and nursing expertise are available.[97,101,117]

Indications for urgent surgery include progressive neurological deficit, significant osseous involvement with deformity, sepsis with a large phlegmonous mass, or vertebral destruction without bacteriologi-

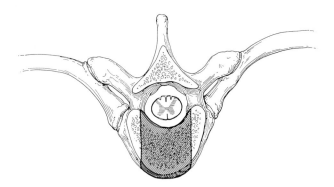

Fig. 39-5. Ventral approach by median sternotomy for upper thoracic lesions, demonstrating the excellent ventral and middle column exposure. (Reproduced with permission of Barrow Neurologic Institute, Phoenix, Ariz., USA from Ronderos JF, Sonntag VKH. Approaches to the thoracic spine. Tech Neurosurg 1:222-229, 1996.)

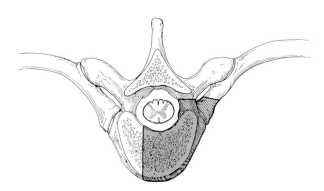

Fig. 39-6. Ventral approach via thoracotomy for mid- to lower thoracic lesions. The shaded region demonstrates the bone removal. (Reproduced with permission of Barrow Neurologic Institute, Phoenix, Ariz., USA from Ronderos JF, Sonntag VKH. Approaches to the thoracic spine. Tech Neurosurg 1:222-229, 1996.)

cal diagnosis.[10,32,37,41,56,79,81,105] Delayed surgical intervention is performed if medical management fails.

The anatomy of the chest cavity and the proximity of the heart and lungs require specialized surgical approaches to the thoracic spine. Surgical approaches can be divided into three major categories: ventral, dorsolateral, and dorsal. These approaches may be used alone or in combination with each other, either at the same time or in a staged procedure.[10,32,37,39,44,79,81,105] The operative approach is determined by the pathological process (i.e., neural compression, direction of canal compromise, and instability) and the patient's medical condition. No one surgical approach is preferred in all cases and the surgeon should be familiar with all approaches. Ventral approaches are sternotomy for upper thoracic

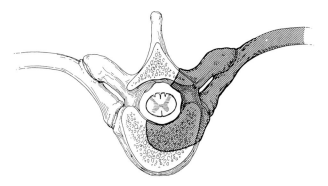

Fig. 39-7. Lateral extracavitary approach demonstrating removal of the rib, transverse process, and vertebral body. Despite a dorsal incision, this approach allows for significant exposure of the ventrolateral dura. (Reproduced with permission of Barrow Neurologic Institute, Phoenix, Ariz., USA from Ronderos JF, Sonntag VKH. Approaches to the thoracic spine. Tech Neurosurg 1:222-229, 1996.)

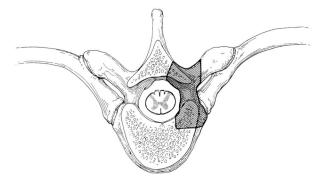

Fig. 39-9. Transpedicular approach demonstrating the bone removal of the lamina, transverse process, and pedicle. The costotransversectomy approach is identical to the transpedicular approach except the rib head and transverse process are removed. (Reproduced with permission of Barrow Neurologic Institute, Phoenix, Ariz., USA from Ronderos JF, Sonntag VKH. Approaches to the thoracic spine. Tech Neurosurg 1:222-229, 1996.)

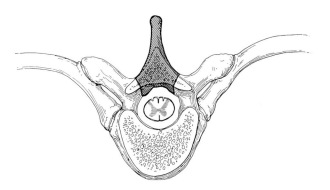

Fig. 39-8. Standard laminectomy demonstrating dorsal bone removal. (Reproduced with permission of Barrow Neurologic Institute, Phoenix, Ariz., USA from Ronderos JF, Sonntag VKH. Approaches to the thoracic spine. Tech Neurosurg 1:222-229, 1996.)

lesions (T1 to T3) (Fig. 39-5), thoracotomy for the mid- to lower thoracic spine (T3 to T12) (Fig. 39-6), thoracoabdominal approaches for (T12 to L2), and, more recently, thoracoscopic spinal surgery (T4 to T10). The lateral extracavitary approach is a dorsolateral exposure of the spine (Fig. 39-7) for lesions between T3 to T12. Dorsal spinal exposures are laminectomy, transpedicular, and costotransversectomy (Figs. 39-8 and 39-9).

Regardless of surgical approach, basic surgical tenets are similar. Cultures are obtained and antibiotics administered only after the intraoperative cultures are obtained. Resection of all involved bone and soft tissue should be performed in attempts to eradicate as much infectious material as possible. Adequate debridement is indicated by firm bleeding bone in the rostral and caudal extent of the resec-

tion cavity. Healthy bone found at the limits of the infection provides structural support and blood supply for interbody bone grafts and thereby optimizes spinal alignment and bony healing. Epidural and paraspinous phlegmons are often decompressed from the spinal cord using microsurgical technique. Attempts to correct spinal deformity and stabilize the spinal column should be made by using optimally sized bone grafts, and internal fixation when indicated. The wound is closed after thorough antibiotic irrigation.

Ventral Approaches

The major advantages of the ventral approaches to the thoracic spine are improved visualization for spinal cord decompression and interbody bone grafting.[6,66] The major disadvantage is the magnitude of surgery involved and associated medical complications. Pulmonary complications are the most common and include atelectasis and pneumonia. However, empyema, hemothorax, chylothorax, and pulmonary injury may also occur. Other complications include vascular injury and traumatic thoracic neuralgia.[6,86] A postoperative thoracostomy tube is required. Adequate preoperative pulmonary and cardiovascular assessments are required to decrease perioperative and postoperative complications.[6,86] The ventral approach is, therefore, less desirable for the older patient or patients with significant pulmonary disease.

There are several ventral approaches to the thoracic spine depending upon the anatomical levels of the spinal column affected: C7 to T2, T2 to T6, T6 to T12, and T6 to L3.[111] Lesions at C7 to T2 are best approached by combining an upper neck or sternal split technique, with the incision paralleling the ventral aspect of the sternocleidomastoid muscle and an upper sternotomy to T4 (see Fig. 39-5).[6] The innominate artery is encircled and retracted caudally, and the carotid sheath is retracted laterally. The pharynx, thyroid, and esophagus are gently retracted medially. The recurrent laryngeal nerve and thoracic duct are localized, if possible, and preserved. The approach provides a direct ventral exposure to the cervicothoracic spine.

Lesions from T2 to T6 are best approached from a right dorsolateral thoracotomy because the heart limits exposure of the spine on the left. Lesions at T6 to T12 are approached through a left dorsolateral thoracotomy because aortic mobilization is easier to perform than mobilization of the vena cava (see Fig. 39-6). The patient is positioned in a lateral position, with an axillary roll to prevent brachial plexus injury. The incision is made over the rib(s) corresponding to one or two levels above the level of involvement, and the ribs may be excised for use as either a free bone graft or left as a vascularized pedicle graft. After entrance of the thoracic cavity, the parietal pleura is incised at the diseased levels and segmental vessels are ligated. Segmental vessels supply blood to the thoracic spinal cord from radicular branches that enter the neural foramina and anastomose with the anterior spinal artery. Segmental arteries should be ligated close to the aorta in order to preserve collateral blood flow to radicular vessels from the intercostal arteries located near the neural-foramina. For this reason, electrocautery should be used cautiously in the region of the neuralforamina to avoid injuring these anastomosing vessels.[6] The artery of Adamkiewicz is a radicular vessel that provides the major blood supply to the mid- and lower spinal cord. This vessel arises from segmental vessels anywhere from T7 to L2, but most frequently on the left between T8 to T10.[6] Preoperative spinal angiography may be indicated for patients with lesions in this region to identify this vessel and plan surgical treatment to avoid injury to this vessel.

For lesions of the lower thoracic spine extending to L2, the diaphragm is incised to expose the thoracolumbar junction.[6] The incision is made at the tenth rib, and the diaphragm is divided and retracted for spinal exposure. Mobilization and retraction of retroperitoneal structures are performed with particular attention to the kidney and ureter.

After thoracotomy, exposure of the spine is performed by mobilizing the parietal pleura off the appropriate vertebral body and rib. The rib head is removed to expose the pedicle, which is an important anatomical landmark to identify the location of the spinal cord. The pedicle is removed and the spinal cord is directly visualized. Vertebrectomy and spinal reconstruction are then performed. The thoracotomy closure is performed in the usual manner with one or two thoracostomy tubes in place.

Thoracoscopic surgery has been used in some specialized centers to perform ventral vertebrectomy(ies), drainage of paravertebral abscesses, interbody grafting, and instrumentation in patients with spondylodiscitis.[31,85] The technique is performed endoscopically by using specialized elongated instruments. Briefly, four port sites are drawn on the lateral thorax with the patient placed in the lateral decubitus position.[31,85] The small-port incisions permit the performance of spinal dissection while minimizing disturbance to the thoracic wall. This procedure causes less morbidity than thoracotomy,[31,85] but it also has disadvantages. The procedures are technically demanding, lengthy, and there is some risk of conversion to open thoracotomy.[31] Contraindications include poor tolerance to single-lung collapse or extensive adhesions from previous surgery or illness.[31,85]

Dorsolateral Approaches

The lateral extracavitary approach was first described in 1900 for the treatment of Pott's disease.[90] With recent modifications, the approach can provide excellent exposure to all levels of the thoracic spine below T2.[55,75] This approach permits ventral spinal cord decompression with good visualization of the ventrolateral thecal sac through a dorsal incision (see Fig. 39-7).[55,75] When combined with laminectomy, circumferential spinal cord decompression can be performed. Dorsal instrumentation may be performed concurrently through the same incision. The dorsolateral approach does not violate the chest cavity and, in general, has less surgical morbidity than ventral approaches. It is an appropriate operation for aged or physically debilitated patients who may not tolerate ventral surgery. Critics of this approach cite that ventral dural exposure is good, but not optimal, particularly on the side contralateral to the surgical approach. Interbody strut grafting may be difficult and ventral instrumentation is rarely possible. The patient is placed in the prone position, and a "hockey-stick" or paramedian incision is used. The hockey-stick incision describes a midline incision in which the most caudal portion of the incision is curved 45 degrees off the midline for 6 to 8 cm. A midline incision provides access to the dorsal spinal elements for circumferential decompression or dorsal instrumentation.[55] If midline exposure is not required, a paramedian incision centered over the lateral aspect of the paraspinal muscles can be used. A hockeystick incision is often preferred at T1 to T7 because the origin of the rhomboid and trapezius musculature may be detached and reapproximated on the midline. Paramedian incisions incise the belly of these muscles and result in more postoperative shoulder dysfunction.

If a midline incision is used, the surgeon uses finger dissection to develop the plane between the superficial fascia and muscles and the deep paraspinal muscles. The superficial fascia and muscles are mobilized and reflected laterally off the paraspinal muscles as a myocutaneous flap. This maneuver is facilitated by the lateral exposure provided by a hockey-stick incision and thereby exposes the rib cage and lateral border of the paraspinous muscles.[55] The paraspinous muscles are mobilized off the underlying ribs and transverse processes. The appropriate spinal level is determined with radiographs. One or more ribs and their ligamentous attachments to the spine are exposed and removed without violating the pleura.[55] The transverse process is removed. Each associated neurovascular bundle is isolated, and the intercostal musculature is peeled away from the parietal pleura. The tagged intercostal nerve root is used as a guide to the location of the foramina.[55] The pedicle is removed to expose the dura mater and the nerve root is usually sacrificed proximal to the dorsal root ganglion to facilitate exposure. As mentioned in the section on thoracotomy, preoperative identification of the location of the artery of Adamkiewicz and preservation of radicular vessels are important. This avoids interruption of the blood supply to the thoracic spinal cord. This concern is important with the lateral extracavitary approach because this approach requires significantly more dissection in the region of the neural foramina, past the point of collateral arterial supply.

The lateral side of the vertebral body is exposed with blunt finger dissection. Segmental vessels are identified and ligated as they course around the midvertebral body. The rami communicantes are transected from the ventral root to permit ventral retraction of the sympathetic chain away from the body. A malleable retractor is used to retract the tissues ventral and lateral to the vertebral body and the paraspinous muscles are retracted with Penrose drains. The vertebrectomy is performed. The lamina and contralateral pedicle can be removed if circumferential decompression is indicated. Interbody and supplemental dorsal onlay grafts may be used for spinal fusion.[32] Pleural tears, if present, are repaired, and a layered closure is performed.

Dorsal Approaches

Dorsal surgical approaches to the thoracic spine from medial to lateral orientation include laminectomy, transpedicular, and costotransversectomy procedures. The principal indication for laminectomy is to remove a dorsal epidural abscess or to obtain a diagnosis of dorsal element osteomyelitis. Laminectomy is contraindicated if there is ventral spinal cord compression.

Transpedicular and costotransversectomy approaches provide progressively more lateral exposure. These approaches have the advantage of avoiding the morbidity of ventral surgical approaches, but effect spinal canal decompression indirectly and, therefore, less completely and reliably. In addition, interbody grafting is difficult and often may not be possible. If interbody grafting is not performed, vertebral collapse may cause recurrent spinal cord compression or spinal deformity. This later complication may be avoided with the use of concurrent dorsal instrumentation.[114]

Laminectomy (see Fig. 39-8) and transpedicular approaches are performed through a standard dorsal midline incision. Removal of the lamina exposes the dorsal thecal sac. The pedicle and ipsilateral facet joint are removed with a drill, while protecting the spinal cord with a small, malleable, metal retractor. This maneuver exposes the lateral thecal sac and exiting nerve root. The nerve root may be sacrificed to provide additional exposure for partial vertebrectomy. A bilateral transpedicular approach can be used to perform more complete vertebrectomy (Fig. 39-10). Costotransversectomy (see Fig. 39-9) is performed though a midline or paramedian

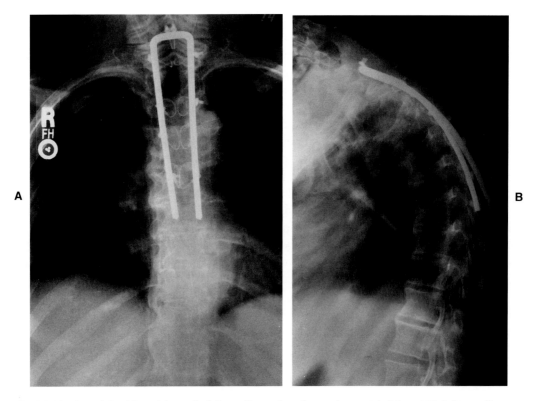

Fig. 39-10. **A** and **B**, AP and lateral plain radiographs of a patient with T2 to T3 Salmonella osteomyelitis after bilateral costotransversectomies with iliac crest bone graft. The patient was paraparetic preoperatively and ambulatory postoperatively.

incision. The proximal rib and transverse process are removed in addition to the pedicle and facet joint to provide additional lateral exposure.

Bone Graft

Most surgeons believe that placement of an interbody bone graft may be performed if most of the infected bone and soft tissue is resected and bleeding bone is exposed in the rostral and caudal extent of the lesion.[10,16,32,39,51,56,79,81,88,105] A smaller number of surgeons defer bone grafting to a staged procedure after the patient has received antibiotic treatment to sterilize the infection. Autogenous grafts are preferred to allografts,[10,16,32,39,51,56,79,81,88,105] but when autogenous grafts are not available, allografts have been used with success.[32,53] Autogenous bone grafts include tricortical iliac crest, vascularized rib or fibula, and free rib or fibula. Tricortical iliac crest graft is the autologous donor site of choice. Its cortical structure provides immediate stability, while its cancellous component promotes early union.[14,39,73] Advantages of rib grafts include their accessibility and a high content of bone morphogenic protein. A

disadvantage is that rib grafts have a greater possibility of graft cutout with resultant kyphosis.[73,128]

Spinal Instrumentation

Spinal instrumentation developed for the treatment of spinal deformity and traumatic instability is now often used in patients with spinal infections. Spinal instrumentation improves neurological outcome and minimizes spinal deformity in patients with spinal instability, regardless of etiology. One investigator, reporting on 292 instrumented fusions, noted a 3% overall complication rate, a 2% reoperation rate, a 99% arthrodesis rate, and no neurological complications.[132]

In the past, placement of hardware in a patient who had an infection was strongly discouraged. More recent studies have demonstrated the safe and effective use of both bone grafts and spinal instrumentation in the face of an active infection.[20,30,31,114,116,132] These studies report excellent long-term fusion rates and low postoperative infection rates. One investigator retrospectively reviewed 17 patients with pyogenic vertebral osteomyelitis treated by vertebral resection, arthrodesis, and instrumentation. He reported an 11% instrument failure rate and one wound dehiscence.[116] Another investigation reported on a series of 20 patients with pyogenic or tuberculous vertebral osteomyelitis.[32] Primary reconstruction with bone grafts was performed in 20 patients, of whom 15 had internal fixation. Seventeen patients were clinically improved and 18 had radiographic evidence of fusion. There were no postoperative wound infections.[32]

Dorsal instrumentation is more rigid than ventral instrumentation, and may be used to span multiple spinal segments. Hooks and rods are most commonly used in the thoracic spine. If the instrumentation is extended into the cervical spine, sublaminar wires or lateral mass screws may be used. Occasionally, pedicle screw fixation is sometimes possible in the upper thoracic (T1 to T4) and lower thoracic (T10 to T12) spine. Disadvantages of dorsal spinal instrumentation are that these procedures immobilize multiple spinal segments and are associated with significant soft tissue dissection, blood loss, and prolonged operative procedure times. Dorsal instrumentation requires extensive spinal exposure and risks bacterial contamination of other spinal segments. Multiple studies have shown good results for treatment of spondylitis with circumferential surgery using dorsal instrumentation, performed either as a single- or two-stage procedure.[10,32,44,56,88,117]

In general, ventral instrumentation is biomechanically less rigid than dorsal instrumentation, but newer thoracolumbar plates have demonstrated excellent stiffness and an extended fatigue life in biomechanical studies.[29] Ventral instrumentation is usually used for partial, single-level, and, on occasion, two-level vertebrectomies.[31,85] It is contraindicated if overt spinal instability, marked deformity, or multiple spinal segments are involved.

Bracing is indicated for those patients treated with surgery in whom interbody grafting or onlay fusions have been performed, regardless of whether spinal instrumentation is used.

POSTOPERATIVE SPINAL INFECTIONS

The incidence of postoperative infection after discectomy is approximately 1%.[18,58,63,106] When a fusion is added to this procedure, the incidence may rise to 8%.[68,146] Most data on infection after noninstru-

mented arthrodesis are from the scoliosis literature. These reports demonstrate an incidence of infections ranging from 1% to 4.6%.[43,54,92,109] The incidence of infection after dorsally instrumented spinal fusions ranges from 0% to 13%.[3,59,72,76,82,111,132,136] One study reviewing 452 patients treated consecutively with instrumented spinal fusion reported 17 infections for an incidence of 3.8%. In those patients with infection, the mean operative time was 5.3 hours, mean blood loss was 960 ml, and the average time to presentation was 26 days.[76]

Old age, malnutrition, diabetes mellitus, chronic steroid use, synchronous remote infections, prolonged preoperative hospitalization, smoking, radiation therapy, and immunosuppression increase the risk for wound infection.[63,144]

Wound infections are separated into two anatomical groups, superficial and deep. Superficial wound infections are confined to the dermis and subcutaneous tissue. Patients present with back pain and a tender erythematous wound with purulent drainage. The wound edges may dehisce. The usual treatment is to open and debride the wound. Any evidence of subfascial involvement requires further imaging studies and possibly operative exploration to rule out a deep wound infection. Wound cultures are obtained and oral antibiotics are begun. The wound may be packed with surgical dressing and typically wet-to-dry dressings are used to promote granulation tissue and healing by secondary intention.

Deep wound infections extend below the dorsal spinal fascia. Patients typically present with back pain that is disproportionate to physical examination findings. The wound may appear normal.[63,72,76,144] Often fever is not present. The white blood cell count may be mildly elevated, but the ESR is uniformly elevated.[63,76,118,144] *S. aureus* and gram-negative rods are the most common infective organisms.[72,76,111,144] Wound cultures may be nondiagnostic. One study of patients with infected wounds and spinal implants reported nondiagnostic cultures in 45% of patients with early infections (1 week postoperative) compared to a 70% rate in patients with late infections (6 weeks postoperative).[144] MRI and CT are useful in making a diagnosis, but may be inconclusive. Abscess may be difficult to differentiate from routine postoperative fluid collection in the operative field by CT and MRI. Artifact from metallic implants may obscure visualization. If a deep wound infection is suspected, surgical exploration is indicated to make a definitive diagnosis. Treatment is surgical exploration, debridement, and thorough antibiotic irrigation with a pulse irrigator.[48,76,144] A course of postoperative parenteral antibiotics is given, and if there is osteomyelitis a 6-week treatment regimen is recommended. Bracing is indicated if there is significant back pain or osteomyelitis.

The management of patients with deep wound infections and spinal implants deserves special mention. Salvaging spinal implants in infected wounds is particularly important for patients with traumatic instability and in those patients in whom spinal stability is critically dependent upon the implant. This occurs in patients with metastatic disease of the spine treated with vertebrectomy and instrumentation. Metallic implants may be retained in almost all instances, but methylmethacrylate must be removed to eradicate infection. Gram-negative infections are the most problematic. In patients in whom infection cannot be eradicated, antibiotics can be administered to suppress infection until there is spinal arthrodesis and the implant can be safely removed. Infection can almost always be cleared with antibiotics after removal of the implant.[18] For those patients with metastatic disease of the spine, suppressive antibiotic treatment may be lifelong. A chronic infection with cutaneous fistula may develop.

It may be safest to remove the implant to eradicate infection. This is the best treatment for patients with instrumented fusions for degenerative disease, in whom the implant augments fusion rates but is not critical for spinal stability. Infected implants are also removed in those infected patients who have undergone spinal fusions in the remote past. Most of these patients have gone on to develop arthrodesis, but some will have pseudarthrosis. The presence of infection has been associated with a threefold increase in pseudarthrosis.[136,137] One study reported a pseudarthrosis rate of 30% in patients with late infection.[63] If pseudarthrosis is present, it can be treated after eradication of infection with antibiotics.

Recently described techniques have produced excellent results in salvaging spinal implants in infected wounds.[48,52,76,144] A closed wound suction-irrigation system is inserted after wound debridement and antibiotic irrigation. Catheters are placed deep and superficial to the dorsal fascia, but not in close proximity to exposed neural elements. The catheters are then brought out through separate skin stab incisions and the wound is closed in layers with either nonabsorbable sutures or steel wires. Retention sutures are recommended. Postoperatively, the patient receives continuous irrigation of antibiotic solution at 25 ml to 50 ml per hour through the catheters. Wall suction or hemovac containers draw the fluid out of the wound into reservoirs.[48,76,144] Solutions that have been used include nafcillin (1 gm/l normal saline solution) and vancomycin (500 mg/l normal saline solution).[76] The drains are removed after 5 to 7 days. The patient is then treated with 6 weeks of intravenous antibiotics followed by enteral antibiotics. Others have successfully treated implant infection with repeated wound irrigation and antibiotic-impregnated polymethylmethacrylate beads affixed to metal wires placed in the deep and superficial tissue compartments.[52]

The identification and assessment of individuals undergoing elective surgery who are at high risk for infectious complications is helpful. Risk may be reduced by improving the patient's medical condition. Nutritional supplementation is provided to patients with malnutrition or absorptive deficiencies. Internal medicine consultations are valuable for helping to identify and correct hormone and nutritional deficiencies and treat chronic skin or urinary tract infections.

The organism inoculum usually comes from the patient or the operating room environment or personnel.[63] In order to reduce exposure, patients should bathe the night before the procedure, and the operative field should be prepared in a sterile manner. The operating room personnel, as well as operating room traffic, should be kept to a minimum. Strict sterile technique should be practiced. Gentle handling of the tissues, precise use of the cautery, and periodic release of retractors will aid in decreasing the risk of infection. Prolonged tissue retraction causes ischemia and devitalization of the underlying muscle and soft tissue, which is a nidus for infection. Devitalized tissues at the wound edges should be debrided, and the wound copiously irrigated with antibiotic solution. The authors routinely use 3 l of antibiotic solution with a pulsed irrigator in all instrumented fusions. Prophylactic intravenous antibiotics should be administered 30 to 60 minutes preoperatively. This has been shown to reduce the risk of spinal surgery–related infections when tissue levels are adequate.[43,68,72,108] The antibiotics are often continued for 24 hours after the procedure. In healthy patients undergoing elective surgery, a first-generation cephalosporin is the drug of choice, whereas broader coverage is required for higher-risk patients.[63]

CONCLUSION

Thoracic spinal infections may cause paraplegia, painful spinal deformity, and death. Immediate medical attention is required. Most are pyogenic, hematogenously borne, and occur in the vertebral body and intervertebral disc space. Epidural abscess may occur with or without bony infection. Tuberculous and fungal infection occur less frequently. Spinal infections may have an insidious onset and indolent course and are often difficult to diagnose. The combination of back pain with an elevated ESR is typical. MRI is the imaging modality of choice, and is usually diagnostic.

The mainstay of treatment is antibiotic therapy. Nonoperative management may be attempted in patients who are neurologically normal and have a bacterial diagnosis. Operative management is otherwise recommended, particularly in patients with symptomatic spinal cord compression or significant disease in the spinal canal. The operative approach is determined by the pathological process (i.e., neural compression, direction of canal compromise, and instability) and the patient's medical condition. The anatomy of the chest cavity and the proximity of the heart and lungs require specialized surgical approaches to the thoracic spine that can be divided into three major categories: ventral, dorsolateral, and dorsal. Surgical treatment is aimed at eradicating as much infectious material as possible, decompressing the spinal cord and stabilizing the spinal column using interbody bone grafts and, in some cases, spinal instrumentation.

Postoperative thoracic spinal infections are rare and can be successfully treated with antibiotics. Specialized surgical techniques are available to salvage spinal implants.

REFERENCES

1. Abramovitz JL, Batson RA, Yablon JS. Vertebral osteomyelitis: The surgical management of neurologic complications. Spine 11:418-420, 1986.
2. Adatepe MH, Parnell OM, Isaacs GH. Hematogenous pyogenic vertebral osteomyelitis: Diagnostic value of radionuclide bone imaging. J Nucl Med 27:1680-1685, 1986.
3. Allen BL, Ferguson RL. The Galveston experience with L-rod instrumentation for adolescent idiopathic scoliosis. Clin Orthop 229:59-69, 1988.
4. An HS, Munk R. Osteomyelitis of the posterior elements of the cervical spine in an infant. Orthopedics 16:618-620, 1993.
5. An HS, Vaccaro AR, Dolinskas CA, Cotler JM, Balderston RA, Bauerle R. Differentiation between spinal tumors and infections with magnetic resonance imaging. Spine 16:S334-S338, 1991.
6. Anderson TM, Mansour KA, Miller JI. Thoracic approaches to anterior spinal operations: Anterior thoracic approaches. Ann Thorac Surg 55:1447-1452, 1993.
7. Andriacchi T, Schultz A, Belytschko T. A model for studies of mechanical interaction between the human spine and the rib cage. J Biomech 7:497-506, 1974.
8. Angtuaco EJ, McConnel JR, Chaddack WM, Flanigan S. MR imaging of spinal epidural sepsis. AJNR 8:879-883, 1987.
9. Arizono T, Oga M, Shiota E, Honda K, Sugioka Y. Differentiation of vertebral osteomyelitis and tuberculous spondylitis by magnetic resonance imaging. Intern Orthop 19:319-322, 1995.
10. Arnold PM, Baek PN, Bernardi RJ, Luck EA, Larson SJ. Surgical management of nontuberculous thoracic and lumbar vertebral osteomyelitis: Report of 33 cases. Surg Neurol 47:551-561, 1997.
11. Baker AS, Ojeman R, Swartz MN, Richardson EP. Spinal epidural abscess. N Engl J Med 293:464-468, 1975.
12. Batson OV. The function of vertebral veins and their role in the spread of metastases. Ann Surg 112:138-149, 1940.
13. Bhatoe HS, Gill HS, Kumar N, Biswas S. Post lumbar puncture discitis and vertebral collapse. Postgrad Med J 70:882-884, 1994.
14. Blumberg K, Balderston R. Presentation and treatment of pyogenic vertebral osteomyelitis. Semin Spine Surg 2:283-294, 1990.
15. Boachie-Adjei O, Squillante RG. Tuberculosis of the spine. Orthop Clin North Am 27:95-103, 1996.
16. Cahill D, Love L, Rechtine G. Pyogenic osteomyelitis of the spine in the elderly. J Neurosurg 74:878-886, 1991.
17. Calderone RR, Larsen JM. Overview and classification of spinal infections. Orthop Clin North Am 27:1-8, 1996.
18. Carey ME. Infections of the spine and the spinal cord. In Youmans JR, ed. Neurological Surgery: A Comprehensive Reference Guide to the Diagnosis and Management of Neurosurgical Problems, 4th ed. Philadelphia: WB Saunders, 1996, pp 3270-3304.
19. Carragee E. Pyogenic vertebral osteomyelitis. J Bone Joint Surg 79A:874-880, 1997.
20. Carragee EJ. Instrumentation of the infected and unstable spine: A review of 17 cases from the thoracic and lumbar spine with pyogenic infections. J Spinal Disord 10:317-324, 1997.
21. Carragee EJ. The clinical use of magnetic resonance imaging in pyogenic vertebral osteomyelitis. Spine 22:780-785, 1997.
22. Cortet B, Richard R, Deprez X, Lucet L, Flipo RM, Le Loet X, Duquesnoy B, Delcambre B. Aspergillus spondylodiscitis: Successful conservative treatment in 9 cases. J Rheumatol 21:1287-1291, 1993.
23. Cushing AH. Discitis in children. Clin Infect Dis 17:1-6, 1993.
24. D'Horre K, Hoogmartens M. Vertebral aspergillosis: A case report and review of the literature. Acta Orthop Belg 59:306-314, 1993.

25. Dagirmanjian A, Schils J, McHenry M, Modic MT. MR imaging of vertebral osteomyelitis revisited. AJR 167:1539-1543, 1996.

26. Danner RL, Hartman BJ. Update of spinal epidural abscess: 35 cases and review of the literature. Rev Infect Dis 9:265-274, 1987.

27. Darouiche RO, Hamill RJ, Greenberg SB, Weathers SW, Musher DM. Bacterial spinal epidural abscess. Medicine 71:369-385, 1992.

28. Del Curling O Jr, Gower D, McWhorter JM. Changing concepts in spinal epidural abscess: A report of 29 cases. Neurosurgery 27:185-192, 1990.

29. Dick JC, Brodke DS, Zdeblick TA, Bartel BD, Kunz DN, Rapoff AJ. Anterior instrumentation of the thoracolumbar spine. Spine 22:744-750, 1997.

30. Dickman C, Fessler R, MacMilan M, Haid R. Transpedicular screw-rod fixation of the lumbar spine: Operative technique and outcome in 104 cases. J Neurosurg 77:860-870, 1992.

31. Dickman CA, Rosenthal D, Karahalios DG, Paramore CG, Mican CA, Apostolides PJ, Lorenz R, Sonntag VKH. Thoracic vertebrectomy and reconstruction using a microsurgical thorascopic approach. Neurosurgery 38:279-293, 1996.

32. Dietze DD Jr, Fessler RG, Jacob RP. Primary reconstruction for spinal infections. J Neurosurg 86:981-989, 1997.

33. Digby JM, Kersley JB. Pyogenic non-tuberculous spinal infection: An analysis of thirty cases. J Bone Joint Surg 61B:47-55, 1979.

34. Donovan-Post NJ, Bowen BC, Sze G. Magnetic resonance imaging of spinal infection. Rheum Dis Clin North Am 17:773-794, 1991.

35. Doub HP, Bagley CE. The roentgen signs of tuberculosis of the spine. Am J Roentgenol 27:827-837, 1932.

36. Ehara S, Khurana JS, Kattapuram SV. Pyogenic vertebral osteomyelitis of the posterior elements. Skeletal Radiol 18:175-178, 1989.

37. Eismont F, Bohlman H, Soni P, Goldberg V, Freehafer A. Pyogenic and fungal vertebral osteomyelitis with paralysis. J Bone Joint Surg 65A:19-29, 1983.

38. Elgazzar AH, Abdel-Dayem AM, Clark JD, Maxon HR III. Multimodality imaging of osteomyelitis. Eur J Nucl Med 22:1043-1063, 1995.

39. Emery S, Chan D, Woodward H. Treatment of hematogenous pyogenic vertebral osteomyelitis with anterior debridement and primary bone grafting. Spine 14:284-291, 1989.

40. Endress C, Guyot D, Fata J, Salciccioli G. Cervical osteomyelitis due to IV heroin use: Radioglogic findings in 14 patients. AJR 155:333-335, 1990.

41. Fang D, Cheung K, Dos Remedios I, Lee Y, Leong J. Pyogenic vertebral osteomyelitis: Treatment by anterios spinal debridement and fusion. J Spinal Disord 7:173-180, 1994.

42. Fitzgerald RH Jr, Thompson RL. Cephalosporin antibiotics in the prevention and treatment of musculoskeletal sepsis. J Bone Joint Surg 65A:1201-1205, 1983.

43. Fogelberg EV, Zitzman EK, Stinchfield FE. Prophylactic penicillin in orthopedic surgery. J Bone Joint Surg 52:95-98, 1970.

44. Fountain S. A single-stage combined surgical approach for vertebral resections. J Bone Joint Surg 61A:1011-17, 1979.

45. Fountain SS. A single-stage combined surgical approach for vertebral resections. J Bone Joint Surg 61A:1011-1017, 1979.

46. Fredrickson B, Hansen Y, Olans R. Management and outcome of pyogenic vertebral osteomyelitis. Clin Orthop Rel Res 131:160-167, 1978.

47. Friedman BC, Simon GL. Candida vertebral osteomyelitis: Report of three cases and a review of the literature. Diagn Microbiol Infect Dis 8:831-836, 1987.

48. Garrido E, Rosenwasser RH. Experience with the suction-irrigation technique in the management of spinal epidural infection. Neurosurgery 12:678-679, 1983.

49. Garvey TA, Eismont FJ. Tuberculous and fungal osteomyelitis of the spine. Semin Spine Surg 2:295-308, 1990.

50. Genster HG, Andersen MJF. Spinal osteomyelitis complicating urinary tract infection. J Urol 107:109-111, 1972.

51. Gepstein R, Folman Y, Lidor C, Barchilon V, Catz A, Hallel T. Management of pyogenic vertebral osteomyelitis with spinal cord compression in the elderly. Paraplegia 30:795-798, 1992.

52. Glassman SD, Dimar JR, Puno RM, Johnson JR. Salvage of instrumented lumbar fusions complicated by surgical wound infection. Spine 21:2163-2169, 1996.

53. Glassman SD, Shields CB, Menlo JC, Johnson JR, Puno RM. Pyogenic infections of the spine. J Ky Med Assoc 90:374-379, 1992.

54. Goldstein LA. Treatment of idiopathic scoliosis by Harrington instrumentation and fusion with fresh autogenous iliac bone grafts. J Bone Joint Surg 51:209-222, 1969.

55. Graham AW, MacMillan M, Fessler RG. Lateral extracavitary approach to the thoracic and thoracolumbar spine. Orthopedics 20:605-610, 1997.

56. Graziano G, Sidhu K. Salvage reconstruction in acute and late sequelae from pyogenic thoracolumbar infection. J Spinal Disord 6:199-207, 1993.

57. Griffiths HED, Jones DM. Pyogenic infection of the spine. J Bone Joint Surg 53B:383-391, 1971.

58. Griffiths HJ. Orthopedic complications. Radiol Clin North Am 33:401-410, 1995.

59. Gurr KR, McAfee PC. Cottrell-Dubousset instrumentation in adults: A preliminary report. Spine 13:510-520, 1988.

60. Hanley E Jr, Phillips E. Profiles of patients who get spine infections and the type of infections that have a predilection for the spine. Semin Spine Surg 2:257-267, 1990.

61. Hannigan WC, Asner NG, Elwood PW. Magnetic resonance imaging and the nonoperative treatment of spinal epidural abscess. Surg Neurol 34:408-413, 1990.

62. Harris LF, Haws FP. Disc space infection. Ala Med 63:12-14, 1994.

63. Heller JG, Garfin SR. Postoperative infection of the spine. Semin Spine Surg 2:268-282, 1990.

64. Heusner AP. Nontuberculous spinal epidural infections. N Engl J Med 239:845-854, 1948.

65. Hlavin ML, Kaminski HJ, Ross JS, Ganz E. Spinal epidural abscess: a ten year perspective. Neurosurgery 27:177-184, 1990.

66. Hodgson AR, Stock FE. Anterior spine fusion for the treatment of tuberculosis of the spine. J Bone Joint Surg 42A:295-310, 1960.

67. Holztman R, Bishko F. Osteomyelitis in heroin addicts. Ann Intern Med 75:693-696, 1971.

68. Horwitz NH, Curtain JA. Prophylactic antibiotics and wound infections following laminectomy for lumbar disc herniation: A retrospective study. J Neurosurg 43: 727-731, 1975.

69. Jain R, Sawhney S, Berry M. Computed tomography of vertebral tuberculosis: patterns of bone destruction. Clin Radiol 47:196-199, 1993.

70. Jansen BRH, Hart W, Schreuder O. Acta Orthop Scand 64:33-36, 1993.

71. Jensen AG, Espersen F, Skinhoj P, Rosdahl VT, Frimodt-Moller N. Increasing frequency of vertebral osteomyelitis following staphlycoccus aureus bacteremia in Denmark 1980-1990. J Infect 34:113-118, 1997.

72. Keller RB, Pappas AM. Infection after spinal fusion using internal fixation instrumentation. Orthop Clin North Am 3:99-111, 1972.

73. Kemp HBS, Jackson JW, Cook J. Anterior fusion of the spine for infective lesions in adults. J Bone Joint Surg 55B:713-734, 1973.

74. Lafont A, Olive A, Gelman M, Roca-Burniols J, Cots R, Carbonell J. Candida albicans spondylodiscitis and vertebral osteomyelitis in patients with intravenous heroin drug addiction: Report of three new cases. J Rheumatol 21:953-956, 1994.

75. Larson SJ, Holst RA, Hemmy DC, Sances A Jr. Lateral extracavitary approach to traumatic lesions of the thoracic and lumbar spine. J Neurosurg 45:628-637, 1976.

76. Levi ADO, Dickman CA, Sonntag VKH. Management of postoperative infections after spinal instrumentation. J Neurosurg 86:975-980, 1997.

77. Lewis R, Sherwood G, Altner P. Spinal pseudomonas chondro-osteomyelitis in heroin users. N Engl J Med 286:1303-1305, 1972.

78. Leys D, Lesoin F, Pasquier F, Rousseaux M, Jomin M, Petit H. Decreased morbidity from acute bacterial spinal epidural abscesses using computed tomography and neurosurgical treatment in selected patients. Ann Neurol 17:350-355, 1985.

79. Liebergall M, Chaminsky G, Lowe J, Robin G, Floman Y. Pyogenic vertebral osteomyelitis with paralysis: Prognosis and treatment. Clin Orthop Rel Res 269:142-149, 1991.

80. Lifesco RM, Harder E, McCorkell SJ. Spinal brucellosis. J Bone Joint Surg 67:345-351, 1985.

81. Lifeso RM. Pyogenic spinal sepsis in adults. Spine 15:1265-1271, 1990.

82. Lonstein J, Winter R, Moe J. Wound infection with Harrington instrumentation and spine fusion for scoliosis. Clin Orthop Rel Res 96:222-223, 1973.

83. Mader JT, Norden C, Nelson JD, Calandra GB. Evaluation of new anti-infective drugs for the treatment of osteomyelitis in adults. Clin Infect Dis 15(Suppl 1):S155-S161, 1992.

84. Malmpalam TJ, Rosegay H, Andrews BT, Rosenblum ML, Pitts LH. Nonoperative treatment of spinal epidural infections. J Neurosurg 71:208-210, 1989.

85. McAfee PC, Regan JR, Zdeblick T, Zuckerman J, Picetti GD III, Heim S, Geis WP, Fedder IL. The incidence of complications in endoscopic anterior thoracolumbar spinal reconstructive surgery. Spine 20:1624-1632, 1995.

86. McDonnell MF, Glassman SD, Dimar JR, Puno RM, Johnson JR. Perioperative complications of anterior procedures on the spine. J Bone Joint Surg 78A:839-847, 1996.

87. McGee-Collett M, Johnston IH. Spinal epidural abscess: Presentation and treatment. Med J Aust 155:14-17, 1991.

88. McGuire RA, Eismont, FJ. The fate of autogenous bone graft in surgically treated pyogenic vertebral osteomyelitis. J Spinal Disord 7:206-215, 1994.

89. McLaurin RL. Spinal suppuration. Clin Neurosurg 14:314-336, 1966.

90. Menard V. Etude pratique sur le mal de Pott. Masson et Cie, 1900.

91. Modic MT, Feiglin DH, Piraini DW, Boumphrey F, Weinstein MA, Duchesneau PM, Rehm S. Vertebral osteomyelitis: Assessment using MR. Radiology 157:157-166, 1985.

92. Moe JH, Gustilo RB. Treatment of scoliosis. J Bone Joint Surg 46:292-312, 1964.

93. Medical Research Council. Working party on tuberculosis of the spine: A controlled trial of ambulant outpatient treatment and inpatient rest in bed in the management of tuberculosis of the spine in young Korean patients on standard chemotherapy. First report. J Bone Joint Surg 55:6778-6797, 1973.

94. MRC. Working party on tuberculosis of the spine: A controlled trial of anterior spinal surgery and debridement in the surgical management of tuberculosis of the spine in patients on standard chemotherapy: A study in Hong Kong. Br J Surg 61:853-866, 1974.

95. MRC. Working party on tuberculosis of the spine. A five-year assessment on controlled trials of inpatient and outpatient treatment and of plaster-of-Paris jackets for tuberculosis of the spine in children on standard therapy: Studies in Masan and Pusan, Korea. J Bone Joint Surg 58:399-411, 1976.

96. MRC. Working party on tuberculosis of the spine. A five-year assessment of controlled trials of ambulatory treatment, debridement, and anterior spine fusion in the management of tuberculosis of the spine: Studies in Bulawayo (Rhodesia) and in Hong Kong. J Bone Joint Surg 60:163-177, 1978.

97. MRC. Working party on tuberculosis of the spine: A ten-year assessment of a controlled trial comparing debridement and anterior spinal fusion in management of tuberculosis of the spine in patients of standard chemotherapy in Hong Kong. J Bone Joint Surg 65:393-398, 1982.

98. Musher DM, Thorsteinsson SB, Minuth JN, Luchi RJ. Vertebral osteomyelitis. Arch Intern Med 136:105-110, 1976.

99. Numaguchi Y, Rigamonti D, Rothman MI, Sato S, Mihara F, Sadato N. Spinal epidural abscess: Evaluation with gadolinium-enhanced MR imaging. Radiographics 13:545-559, 1993.

100. Nussbaum ES, Rigamonti D, Standiford H, Numaguchi Y, Wolf AL, Robinson WL. Spinal epidural abscess: A report of 40 cases and review. Surg Neurol 38:225-231, 1992.

101. Nussbaum ES, Rockswold GL, Bergman TA, Erickson DL, Seljeskog EL. Spinal tuberculosis: A diagnostic and management challenge. J Neurosurg 83:243-247, 1995.

102. Omari B, Robertson JM, Nelson RJ, Chiu LC. Pott's disease: A resurgent challenge to the thoracic surgeon. Chest 95:145-150, 1989.

103. Onofrio BM. Intervertebral discitis: Incidence, diagnosis, and management. Clin Neurosurg 27:481-516, 1980.

104. Osborn AG. Nonneoplastic disorders of the spine and spinal cord. In Osborn AG, ed. Diagnostic Neuroradiology. St. Louis: Mosby, 1994, pp 820-875.

105. Osenbach R, Hitchon P, Menezes A. Diagnosis and management of pyogenic vertebral osteomyelitis in adults. Surg Neurol 33:266-275, 1990.

106. Ozuna RM, Deiamarter RB. Pyogenic vertebral osteomyelitis and postsurgical disc space infections. Orthop Clin North Am 27:87-94, 1996.

107. Patzakis M, Santi R, Wilkins J, Moore T, Harvey P. Analysis of 61 cases of vertebral osteomyelitis. Clin Orthop Rel Res 264:178-183, 1991.

108. Pavel A, Smith RL, Ballard A. Prophylactic antibiotics in clean orthopedic surgery. J Bone Joint Surg 56A:777-782, 1974.

109. Pavon SJ, Manning C. Posterior spinal fusion for scoliosis due to anterior poliomyelitis. J Bone Joint Surg 52:420-431, 1970.

110. Perronne C, Saba J, Behloul Z, Salmon-Ceron D, Leport C, Vilde JL, Kahn MF. Pyogenic and tuberculous spondylodiscitis (vertebral osteomyelitis) in 80 adult patients. Clin Infect Dis 19:746-750, 1994.

111. Perry JW, Montgomerie JZ, Swank S, Gilmore DS, Maeder K. Wound infections following spinal fusion with posterior segmental spinal instrumentation. Clin Infect Dis 24:558-561, 1997.

112. Rankin RM, Flothow PG. Pyogenic infection of the spinal epidural space. West J Surg Obstet Gynecol 54:320-323, 1946.

113. Ratcliffe JF. Anatomic basis for the pathogenesis and radiologic features of vertebral osteomyelitis and its differentiation from childhood discitis. Acta Radiol Diagn 26:137-143, 1985.

114. Rath S, Neff U, Schneider O, Richter H. Neurosurgical management of thoracic and lumbar vertebral osteomyelitis and discitis in adults: A review of 43 patients consecutively surgically treated patients. Neurosurgery 38:926-933, 1996.

115. Rea GL, McGregor JM, Miller CA, Miner ME. Surgical treatment of the spontaneous spinal epidural abscess. Surg Neurol 37:274-279, 1992.

116. Redfern R, Miles J, Banks A, Dervin E. Stabilisation of the infected spine. J Neurol Neurosurg Psychiatry 51:803-807, 1988.

117. Rezai A, Lee M, Cooper PR, Errico TJ, Koslow M. Modern management of spinal tuberculosis. Neurosurgery 36:87-97, 1995.

118. Richards BS. Delayed infections following posterior spinal instrumentation for the treatment of idiopathic scoliosis. J Bone Joint Surg 77:524-529, 1995.

119. Ring D, Vaccaro AR, Scuderi G, Green D. Vertebral osteomyelitis after blunt traumatic esophageal rupture. Spine 20:98-101, 1995.

120. Ronderos JF, Sonntag VKH. Approaches to the thoracic spine. Tech Neurosurg 1:222-229, 1996.

121. Rothman SLG. The diagnosis of infections of the spine by modern imaging techniques. Orthop Clin North Am 27:15-31, 1996.

122. Rudert M, Tillmann B. Lymph and blood supply of the human intervertebral disc. Acta Orthop Scand 64:37-40, 1993.

123. Sapico FL. Microbiology and antimicrobial therapy of spinal infections. Orthop Clin North Am 27:9-13, 1996.

124. Sapico F, Montgomerie J. Pyogenic vertebral osteomyelitis: report of nine cases and review of the literature. Rev Infect Dis 1:754-776, 1979.

125. Sapico FL, Montgomerie JZ. Vertebral osteomyelitis in intravenous drug abusers: Report of three cases and review of the literature. Rev Infect Dis 2:196-206, 1980.

126. Sapico F, Montgomerie J. Vertebral osteomyelitis. Infect Dis Clin North Am 4:539-550, 1990.

127. Savoia M. An overview of antibiotics useful in the treatment of bacterial, mycobacterial, and fungal osteomyelitis. Semin Spine Surg 2:309-321, 1990.

128. Sawin PD, Traynelis VD, Menezes AH. A comparison analysis of fusion rates and donor site morbidity for autogenic rib and iliac crest bone grafts in posterior cervical fusions. J Neurosurg 88:255-65, 1998.

129. Schultz KP, Assheuer J. Discitis after procedures on the intervertebral disc. Spine 19:1172-1177, 1994.

130. Scoles PV, Quinn TP. Intervertebral discitis in children and adolescents. Clin Orthop 162:31-36, 1982.

131. Selby R, Pillay K. Osteomyelitis and disc infection secondary to pseudomonas aeruginosa in heroin addiction: Case report. J Neurosurg 37:463-466, 1972.

132. Shapiro SA, Snyder W. Spinal instrumentation with a low complication rate. Surg Neurol 48:566-574, 1997.

133. Sharif HS. Role of MR imaging in the management of spinal infections. AJR 158:1333-1345, 1992.

134. Smith AS. MR of infectious and inflammatory diseases of the spine. Crit Rev Diagn Imaging 32:165-189, 1991.

135. Sullivan PJ, Currie D, Collins JV, Johnstone DJ, Morgan A. Vertebral osteomyelitis presenting with pleuritic chest pain and bilateral pleural effusions. Thorax 47:395-396, 1992.

136. Swank SM, Lonstein JE, Moe JH. Surgical treatment of adult scoliosis. J Bone Joint Surg 63:268-287, 1981.

137. Tamborino JM, Ambruss EN, Moe JH. Harrington instrumentation in the correction of scoliosis. J Bone Joint Surg 46:313-323, 1964.

138. Tekkok IH, Berker M, Ozcan O, Ozgen T, Alarlin Z. Brucellosis of the spine. Neurosurgery 33:838-844, 1993.

139. Thrush A, Enzmann D. MR imaging of infectious spondylitis. AJNR 11:1171-1180, 1990.

140. Torda A, Gottlieb T, Bradbury R. Pyogenic vertebral osteomyelitis: Analysis of 20 cases and review. Clin Infect Dis 20:320-328, 1995.

141. Waldvogel F, Medoff G, Swartz M. Osteomyelitis: A review of clinical features, therapeutic considerations and unusual aspects. N Engl J Med 282:198-206, 260-266, 316-322, 1970.

142. Wenger DR, Bobechko WP, Gilday DL. The spectrum of intervertebral disc-space infection in children. J Bone Joint Surg 60A:100-108, 1978.

143. Wiley A, Trueta J. The vascular anatomy of the spine and its relationship to pyogenic vertebral osteomyelitis. J Bone Joint Surg 41B:796-809, 1959.

144. Wimmer C, Gluch H. Management of postoperative wound infection in posterior spinal fusion with instrumentation. J Spinal Disord 9:505-508, 1996.

145. Winters JL, Cahen I. Acute hematogenous osteomyelitis: A review of sixty-six cases. J Bone Joint Surg 42A:691-704, 1960.

146. Wright RL. Septic Complications of Neurosurgical Spinal Procedures. Springfield, Ill.: Thomas, 1970, pp 6-88.

Degenerative and Noninfectious Inflammatory Diseases

David G. Malone, M.D., John R. Caruso, M.D., and Nevan G. Baldwin, M.D.

Several inflammatory and degenerative conditions involve the thoracic spine. Some affect the thoracic spine as their major disease manifestation, while others affect the thoracic spine only rarely. The seronegative spondyloarthropathies are a group of inflammatory conditions with several commonalities. They share a predilection for spinal and sacroiliac inflammation, but involvement at sites other than the spine is common. Peripheral arthritis, extra-articular inflammatory foci such as uveitis, and aortitis commonly occur with the spondyloarthropathies. Enthesopathy (the tendency for inflammation at bony insertions of tendons and fascia) is a prominent feature of seronegative spondyloarthropathies and it occurs in the periphery as well as in the spine.

The seronegative spondyloarthropathies tend to occur in young males. Additionally, there is a strong association between the seronegative spondyloarthropathies and the class I antigen HLA-B27.[2,6] The seronegative spondyloarthropathies affecting the thoracic spine include ankylosing spondylitis, Reiter's syndrome, psoriatic arthritis, and colitic arthritis. Other inflammatory or degenerative conditions affecting the thoracic spine include diffuse idiopathic skeletal hyperostosis (DISH), Scheuermann's disease, rheumatoid arthritis, ossification of the posterior longitudinal ligament (OPLL), and Forestier's disease.

INFLAMMATORY SPINAL PAIN

The clinical picture in patients with spinal pain of inflammatory etiology is often highly suggestive of the diagnosis (Table 40-1). The history usually includes pain that is worse on arising in the morning and that lessens with activity. This is a feature that distinguishes inflammatory back pain patients from those with mechanical back pain. Mechanical pain typically worsens with activity. Radicular pain or stenosis type symptoms may occur rarely.[37,55] A positive family history of arthritis may further increase suspicion of an inflammatory process causing spinal pain.

Physical examination of patients with inflammatory spinal pain may reveal pain on palpation of the sacroiliac joints, restriction of spinal motion, and signs of peripheral joint inflammation. Changes in spinal curvature, particularly increased thoracic kyphosis with lessened lumbar lordosis, increase the likelihood of an underlying inflammatory spinal disease. The workup of patients with a suspected inflammatory disease involving the spine should begin with plain radiographs of the spine and sacroiliac joints. A sedimentation rate and rheumatoid factor should also be obtained.

There is a strong correlation between the spondyloarthropathies and the presence of the antigen HLA-B27.[2,5] If the symptoms and/or examination are strongly suggestive, a test for this antigen may be obtained. However, it must be stressed that this

Table 40-1. Comparison of Features of Degenerative and Inflammatory Diseases of the Thoracic Spine

	AS	Reiter's	Psoriatic	Colitic	DISH	Rheumatoid	Scheuermann's	OPLL
Sex	M>F	M>F	F>M	M=F	M>F	F>M	M=F	M=F
Onset	<30	<30	Any	<50	Any	Peds	40–50	40–50
HLA B-27	90%	90%	20%	5%	–	–	–	–
Osteopenia	+	+/−	+/−	+/−	NO	+	+	+/−
Facet fusion	+	–	–	–	–	–	–	–
Sacroiliitis	+	+	+	+	–	−/+	–	–

AS = ankylosing spondylitis; DISH = diffuse idiopathic skeletal hyperostosis; OPLL = ossification of the posterior longitudinal ligament.
Modified from Calin A. Ankylosing spondylitis and the spondyloarthropathies. In Schumacher HR, ed. Primer on Rheumatologic Diseases, 9th ed. Atlanta: Arthritis Foundation, 1988, pp 142-147.

test does not confirm the diagnosis of inflammatory spondyloarthropathy and it is usually not cost-effective because the diagnosis is made clinically. Randomly selected patients possessing the HLA-B27 antigen have a less than 10% chance of developing disease.[9]

Offspring of patients with seronegative spondyloarthropathy have only a 10% to 20% chance of developing disease.[9] Seronegative spondyloarthropathy may occur when a patient with the HLA-B27 or another cross-reacting antigen is exposed to an arthritic trigger of any form.[2,9,46] Several infectious pathogens have been proposed as potential arthritic triggers. Infections caused by *Klebsiella, Mycoplasma, Chlamydia trachomatis, Salmonella, Campylobacter,* and *Yersinia* have all been postulated to be arthritic triggers.[9]

ANKYLOSING SPONDYLITIS

Ankylosing spondylitis (AS) is a seronegative arthropathy having a strong association with the class I antigen HLA-B27.[6,9] It has a 3:1 male preponderance and occurs in 0.2% of Caucasians. The usual age of onset is between puberty and 35 years, with a peak in the mid-twenties. The disease is usually less severe in females than in males.[26]

Symptoms of AS begin with stiffness in the lower back. Back pain in AS usually improves with exercise. This is in contrast to the back pain of degenerative conditions, in which exercise exacerbates the pain. On physical examination, flattening of the lumbar spine with increased thoracic kyphosis may be found.

Radiographic evidence of sacroiliitis is one of the diagnostic criteria for the disease and it is usually seen bilaterally.[20] Sacroiliitis does not have to be se-

vere for the diagnosis of AS to be made.[9] Squaring of vertebrae occurs early in the disease from enthesopathy, bony fusion of apophyseal joints occurs later, and ligamentous ossification is also seen on plain radiographs [9,52] (Fig. 40-1).

In advanced cases of AS, the radiographic appearance is that of the classical "bamboo spine." AS is associated with osteopenia demonstrable by either plain radiographs or bone mineral density analysis.[13,14] Laboratory evaluation may reveal elevation of the sedimentation rate. However, the sedimentation rate, acute phase proteins, and protease inhibitors do not correlate with clinical activity of the disease.[57]

Extra-articular manifestations of AS are also common. Organ and soft tissue involvement can be severe. Ventral uveitis is evident in 25% of AS patients, aortitis or heart block in 5%, renal amyloidosis in 4%, and pulmonary fibrosis in 1%.

Neurological complications occur in 5% of patients with AS. These usually result from the associated spinal problems such as atlantoaxial subluxation and cervical spine fractures.[2,55] Cauda equina syndrome can also result from changes at the thoracolumbar junction or in the lumbar spine.[2,55] Thoracic spine fractures occur in patients with AS, and due to the ankylosed nature of the spine these often occur through the disc space.[61]

Minor trauma often leads to spinal fracture in AS patients. These fractures are often unstable and lead to a neurological deficit. Evaluation for suspected fracture should be performed in AS patients after minor trauma or even if there is a complaint of spontaneous back pain associated with a grating sensation.[61]

Both AS and DISH have been reported to exist in the same patient. Differentiation between these two diseases may be difficult early in the clinical

A   B   C

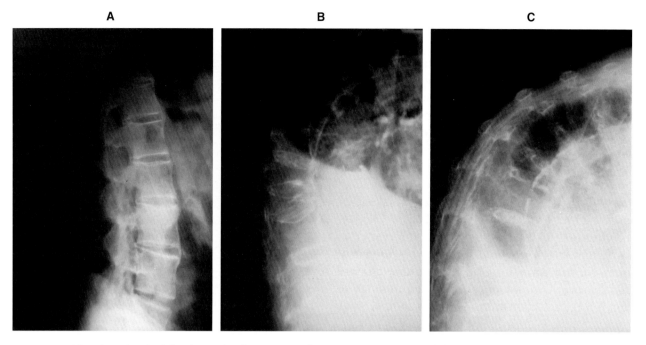

Fig. 40-1. A, AS of the thoracolumbar junction demonstrating squaring of the vertebrae. **B** and **C,** AS of the thoracic spine demonstrating squaring of the vertebrae, fusion across the disc space, increased thoracic kyphosis, and osteopenia.

course of the disease.[38] Early diagnosis for AS patients lessens the risk of progressive spinal deformity.[9] Because humans spend approximately one third of their lives sleeping, AS patients should be advised to sleep without a pillow to maintain less kyphosis in the thoracic spine while sleeping. This will allow the progressive autofusion of the spine to occur with a smaller degree of deformity. Physical therapy, swimming, and sleeping on a firm mattress are all helpful adjuncts to therapy.[2]

Spondylodiscitis and postfracture pseudarthrosis are both common complications of AS. Spondylodiscitis usually occurs early in the course of the disease and may involve multiple spinal levels simultaneously.[41] It can be distinguished from infectious discitis by an absence of paraspinal soft tissue involvement. Pseudarthrosis after spine fracture in AS is also seen.[41,50] Pseudarthrosis most commonly occurs in the lower thoracic segments and at the thoracolumbar junction. It is commonly found adjacent to a region with solid fusion of multiple segments above and below the pseudarthrosis.[41,49] In some cases, it may be indistinguishable from spondylodiscitis.

DIFFUSE IDIOPATHIC SKELETAL HYPEROSTOSIS

DISH has been described using a variety of names, including spondylitis ossificans ligamentosa, spon-

---

SYNONYMS FOR INFLAMMATORY AND DEGENERATIVE DISEASES OF THE SPINE

DISH

Spondylitis ossificans ligamentosa
Spondylosis hyperostotica
Physiological vertebral ligamentous calcification
Generalized juxta-articular ossification of vertebral ligaments
Spondylitis deformans
Vertebral osteophytosis
Senile ankylosing hyperostosis

Scheuermann's Disease

Intervertebral osteochondrosis

Ankylosing Spondylitis

Bekhterev's disease
Marie-Strumpell disease
Rheumatoid spondylitis

Ankylosing Hyperostosis

Forestier's disease

---

dylosis hyperostotica, physiological vertebral ligamentous calcification, and senile ankylosing hyperostosis of the spine, among others (see box). DISH occurs in all regions of the spine, with the thoracic spine being involved in 97% of patients with DISH, followed by the lumbar spine at 90%, and the cervical spine with involvement in 78% of patients with DISH.[54] In the thoracic spine DISH most frequently involves the seventh through eleventh vertebral bodies, with ossification more exuberant on the right lateral side of the vertebral body.

Radiographic criteria are used to diagnose DISH. There is no laboratory test with which to confirm the diagnosis. Radiologically DISH is diagnosed by three criteria. The first criteria is flowing calcification and ossification along the ventrolateral aspect of at least four contiguous vertebral bodies. The second criteria is relative preservation of intervertebral disc height in the involved area and the absence of extensive radiographic evidence of degenerative disc disease. The last criterion is the absence of apophyseal joint bony ankylosis and sacroiliac joint erosion, sclerosis, or intra-articular osseous fusion[54] (Fig. 40-2). Those patients who do not meet all three criteria may have early DISH and may meet all of these criteria if followed over time.

The clinical symptoms of DISH include spinal stiffness and middle or low back pain that appears on arising in the morning and dissipates within an hour of activity.[54] This pain is usually relieved by mild analgesics or heat treatments. Physical examination usually reveals little change in spinal motion, but finger joint nodules may be present.[56]

The incidence of DISH is around 6% to 12% of autopsy specimens in the United States.[10,42] It is associated with increasing age, male sex, obesity, diabetes mellitus, and gout.[42] DISH may coexist with other rheumatological diseases, and 40% to 50% of patients with DISH will also have OPLL.[54,62] DISH is not associated with osteoporosis.[54] Diagnosis of DISH may be made from thoracic radiographs or chest radiographs.[42] Hyperostosis of ribs occurs with a 21% incidence in patients with DISH, leading to decreased chest expansion.[27,48]

Although the etiology of DISH is unknown, some evidence suggests that abnormal metabolism of vitamin A may be a factor in the development of DISH. Low-dose isotretinoin, a vitamin A derivative, has been shown to cause the development of skeletal hyperostosis that is radiographically and clinically similar to DISH.[59] Spine fractures have been reported after minor trauma in DISH patients with frequent delay in diagnosis and permanent neurological deficit.[10,23]

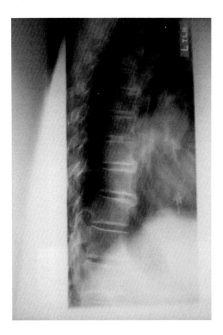

Fig. 40-2. DISH of the thoracic spine with flowing calcification of four contiguous vertebrae, relative preservation of disc space height, and absence of facet joint ankylosis.

Fractures in DISH tend to occur where the bone is thinnest. This may be through the mid-portion of the vertebral body, the intervertebral disc space, or between the ankylosed segment and the next motion level.[10,23] Neurological deficit is more closely related to the number of ankylosed spinal segments than to whether the patient suffered a high- or low-energy injury. In one study, eight of nine patients with complete spinal cord injury had 16 or more contiguously ankylosed vertebrae.[23]

REITER'S SYNDROME

Reiter's syndrome is defined by the clinical triad of urethritis, conjunctivitis, and arthritis. It has a 9:1 male preponderance, and is probably the most common cause of peripheral arthritis in young men. There is a strong association between HLA-B27–positive patients with a history of *C. trachomatis* infection and Reiter's syndrome.

Spinal involvement may occur in patients with Reiter's syndrome. Sacroiliac region pain or low back pain may be the only symptoms of spinal involvement. Radiographic evidence of sacroiliitis, usually unilateral, is found in 20% of Reiter's patients. Only rarely is spinal involvement above the sacroiliac joint present, though some patients with persistent disease have been reported to develop complete spinal fusion.[2]

PSORIATIC ARTHRITIS

Psoriatic arthritis is a seronegative arthropathy that occurs in less than 5% of patients with cutaneous psoriasis. HLA-B27 occurs with increased frequency in patients with axial disease, and 20% of patients with psoriatic arthritis have sacroiliitis and spondylitis.[2] Psoriatic arthritis may affect any level of the spine.[9] Up to 40% of patients with psoriatic arthritis have clinical or radiological spinal disease.[21]

Psoriatic arthritis results in asymmetrically distributed marginal and paramarginal syndesmophytes, an absence of ligamentous ossification, and sparing of the apophyseal joints. Marginal syndesmophytes are thin, vertically-oriented ossifications occurring at the outer margin of the annulus fibrosis with no disc space narrowing. Paramarginal syndesmophytes are vertical ossifications occurring in a vertical fashion away from the edge of the vertebrae, as compared with osteophytes that are horizontally oriented, usually thicker, and associated with disc space narrowing.[21,47] Long-term follow-up in patients with psoriatic arthritis shows that despite radiologic progression of spinal disease, there is usually little progression of clinical symptoms or loss of spinal motion. The sparing of spinal motion may be explained by the pattern of ossification of the spine in psoriatic spondyloarthropathy.[21]

SCHEUERMANN'S DISEASE

Scheuermann's disease is also known as intervertebral osteochondrosis. It occurs in the thoracic spine in the region of the thoracic kyphosis and may affect the lumbar spine as well. It is a common cause of juvenile kyphosis, and is an underdiagnosed cause of back pain.[15] The degenerative changes in Scheuermann's disease are thought to be secondary changes caused by rupture of the intervertebral discs through vertebral body end plates.[33] Intervertebral discs normally contain a relatively high amount of intradiscal oncotic pressure. This pressure can lead to focal penetration of the end plate, resulting in Schmorl's nodes.

In Scheuermann's disease, thoracic kyphosis is exaggerated due to two principal factors: a direct dis-

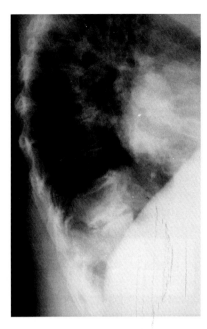

Fig. 40-3. Scheuermann's disease of the thoracic spine with three wedged vertebral bodies 5 degrees kyphosed and Schmorl's nodes in the ventral third of the vertebral bodies.

proportionate loss of ventral vertebral body height and narrowing of the disc interspaces. These factors lead to increased thoracic kyphotic deformity and eventual bony fusion in the region of disc degeneration.[4] Schmorl's nodes and irregularities of the vertebral end plates are also evident in these patients.

Scheuermann's disease is of juvenile onset with radiographic appearance of the disease occurring in the early teen years. Wedged vertebral bodies with 5 degrees of angulation at three or more levels resulting in a thoracic kyphosis of greater than 45 degrees, combined with Schmorl's nodes confirms the diagnosis radiographically. Schmorl's nodes usually occur at the ventral portion of the end plate, compared with the usual Schmorl's node that occurs in the center of the end plate[1] (Fig. 40-3).

RHEUMATOID ARTHRITIS

Rheumatoid arthritis most commonly affects the cervical spine. Involvement of subcervical spinal regions in rheumatoid arthritis patients is observed in only 1% to 5%.[35,39] Osteoporosis of the spine is seen commonly in rheumatoid arthritis, and sacroiliitis may be seen in up to 17% of patients.[22] The term "rheumatoid spondylitis" has been used synonymously with AS but should be confined to description of those patients having rheumatoid arthritis with spinal involvement.[25]

Radiographically, rheumatoid spondylitis may be distinguished from degenerative spondylosis by the blurred, ill-defined margins of the vertebral body end plates. Erosion of the facet joints is also seen with rheumatoid spondylitis and there is also usually an obvious clinical picture of severe articular disease. Both degenerative and rheumatoid disease may result in osteophyte formation.[25]

Three distinct lesions are seen in rheumatoid spondylosis when the thoracic region is involved by the disease process: rheumatoid discitis, facet joint erosion, and inflammatory involvement of the costotransverse joints.[25] These lesions decrease stability of the spine, leading to spondylolisthesis or degenerative scoliosis.[25] Subluxation of the upper thoracic spine in patients with rheumatoid arthritis has been reported by Redlund-Johnell and Larsen.[53] In this series, upper thoracic spinal cord compression was reported in six patients due to subluxation. All of the patients had either spontaneous or iatrogenic fusion in either the cervical spine or the occipitocervical junction that may have contributed to thoracic instability by increasing the stress borne by the upper thoracic region.[53]

Radiographic imaging of the upper thoracic region is frequently difficult in rheumatoid arthritis patients due to the stiffness of the shoulder joints. Conventional radiography is unsuccessful in over 50% of such patients. The use of magnetic resonance imaging (MRI) or planar tomography is required to image the upper thoracic region in most rheumatoid arthritis patients.[53]

Involvement of rheumatoid arthritis in the spine affects the vertebral bodies, the dorsal elements, and the spinal canal. Destruction of thoracic vertebral bodies by rheumatoid granulomas has been reported in rheumatoid arthritis patients despite the fact that no synovial joint exists in the center of the vertebral body.[3,18,36] The costovertebral and costotransverse joints of the thoracic spine are diarthrodial (synovial capsule present) joints. They may become inflamed due to the rheumatoid arthritis, and spontaneous fusion can occur similar to the process more commonly seen in AS.[12] Intraspinal rheumatoid nodules have been reported as a cause of radiculopathy, and intradural rheumatoid granulations have been reported rarely as a cause of thoracic spinal cord compression.[17,35]

OSSIFICATION OF THE POSTERIOR LONGITUDINAL LIGAMENT

Ossification of the posterior longitudinal ligament (OPLL) is seen worldwide with a highly variable prevalence. It occurs in 3.7% of the Japanese population aged older than 50 years, and has a prevalence of 0.12% in the European population. OPLL may coexist with several rheumatological diseases such as DISH, spondylosis, AS, and calcification of the ligamentum flavum.[62] Forty to fifty percent of patients with DISH have OPLL.[62] Possible etiological factors for OPLL and DISH include endocrinological factors and retinoids. Patients with DISH have a higher incidence of obesity, type II diabetes, and impaired glucose tolerance. Long-term treatment with isotretinoin has a high incidence of calcification of ligaments and extraspinal tendons.[62]

FORESTIER'S DISEASE

Ankylosing hyperostosis, otherwise known as Forestier's disease, may be thought of as the ventral counterpart of OPLL. Forestier's disease most commonly occurs in the thoracic spine, followed in frequency by involvement in the lumbar and cervical spine. Because spinal structural integrity is pre-

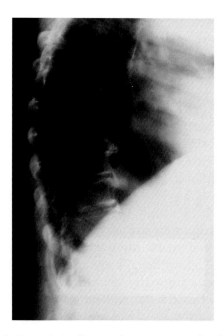

Fig. 40-4. Forestier's disease demonstrating focal ventral ankylosis, intact disc height, intact vertebral end plates, and no involvement of the facet joints.

served, joints are not involved, and neural tissues are generally unaffected, clinical symptoms are uncommon in Forestier's disease. Radiographic findings include focal ventral ankylosis, intact disc height, intact vertebral end plates, and ventral ankylosis (Fig. 40-4). Forestier's disease is differentiated from AS by lack of involvement of the facet joints. It can be distinguished from OPLL by ossification of the anterior, rather than the posterior, longitudinal ligament.[4]

COLITIC ARTHRITIS

The inflammatory bowel diseases (Crohn's disease and ulcerative colitis) may be associated with peripheral or axial arthritis. Sacroiliitis, with or without higher spinal levels of spondylitis, occurs in 10% of patients with inflammatory bowel disease. In those with spinal involvement, about 50% also have the HLA-B27 antigen.[2]

MEDICAL TREATMENT

If a diagnosis of inflammatory spine disease is entertained, consultation with a rheumatologist may be warranted. Drug therapy may be useful in many cases. In mild cases, treatment with salicylates or ibuprofen is usually adequate. Additionally, drugs such as indomethacin, tolmetin, sulindac, piroxicam, and naproxen are often required. Phenylbutazone and antimetabolites such as methotrexate and azathioprine are usually effective but should be limited to patients with severe disease. Systemic corticosteroids and spinal injections of corticosteroids are of limited benefit.[2] Treatment with sulfasalazine has been shown to be effective in the treatment of extraspinal symptoms of AS.[31]

MORTALITY

Some studies have concluded that life expectancy is not decreased in patients with AS.[11,30] Other studies have shown decreased life expectancy in AS patients, including those who underwent radiation therapy for treatment of their disease as well as those who did not receive radiation.[51] Causes of excess mortality cited in AS patients include gastrointestinal diseases, trauma, respiratory disease, renal disease, and circulatory diseases.[51]

Rheumatoid arthritis patients clearly have a decreased life expectancy, with high rates of morbidity as well. Common causes of death in rheumatoid arthritis patients include sepsis, infection, myocardial infarction, rheumatoid lung disease, C1 to C2 subluxation with neurological impairment, and vasculitis.[16,45] Patients with RA who have extra-articular expression of the disease are at greater risk than those without extra-articular expression. Extra-articular expression is associated with circulating immune complexes. Positive detection of these complexes by cryoglobulin formation is predictive of excess mortality.[16]

SURGICAL THERAPY

There are three general indications for surgical intervention in degenerative or inflammatory afflictions of the thoracic spine: spinal instability, unacceptable and/or progressive deformity, and the presence of a progressive or potentially reversible neurological deficit. Many of the degenerative and inflammatory conditions result in increased kyphosis of the thoracic region with accompanying tissue changes causing increased brittleness of the spine. Increased operative mortalities have been reported in patients with AS undergoing operative therapy for fracture stabilization. The operative mortality has been reported to be as high as 50% for cervical spine fracture stabilization in the older literature, while the mortality for conservative treatment in the same population of patients is around 25%.[19] The major cause of death in these patients was respiratory complications.[19]

Before the advent of spinal instrumentation systems for the thoracic spine, all thoracic fractures in AS patients were treated nonsurgically with postural reduction and immobilization.[28] These treatments resulted in a very high rate of fusion, and some current authors recommend conservative treatment for thoracic fractures in DISH.[43] Frequently in AS or DISH, three-column injury to the thoracic spine has occurred via a hyperextension mechanism of injury, thereby leaving these patients unstable and prone to neurological deterioration.[8,19,28] Epidural hematoma as a cause of neurological deterioration has been reported as a unique complication of patients with AS and spinal fracture.[19,28] Clear indications for surgical intervention include progressive neurological deterioration and an incomplete deficit that fails to improve.[19,28]

Instability of the spine due to multicolumn injury remains another indication for surgery.[8] Universal spinal instrumentation has been used in cases of thoracic spine fracture in patients with DISH with good results.[8] Kyphosis of more than 40 degrees of angulation is considered abnormal in the thoracic spine, but this alone does not necessitate operative intervention.[32] Patients are surgical candidates for deformity correction if there is sufficient angulation to cause neurological deficit, unremitting pain, or interference with daily life activities. The final decision to embark on surgical therapy depends upon whether the patient and surgeon agree that the risk of surgical mortality (up to 10%), in addition to the higher-than-normal surgical morbidity, is worth the potential benefit.

Operations to Reduce Deformity

Osteotomies have been performed to correct kyphotic spinal curvature in AS and other degenerative and inflammatory conditions. For thoracic kyphosis, osteotomies are usually performed in the lumbar region to create a compensatory lumbar lordosis.[7,24,34,44,58] In younger patients who are otherwise in good health, it is reasonable to consider a combined ventral and dorsal procedure to mobilize fused thoracic segments, realign the spine, and place instrumentation to maintain the correction until bony union occurs.

The Smith-Peterson Ventral Opening Wedge

The wedge osteotomy of this operation is performed from a dorsal approach, usually at the L2 to L3 level. Only one level is chosen for osteotomy. This is due to published evidence that osteotomy at multiple levels results in most of the reduction still occurring at one level.[44]

The operation begins with removal of the dorsal elements. The spinous process of L2, the rostral margin of the L3 lamina, and all of the L2 lamina and transverse processes are resected. The L2 pedicles and the L2 to L3 facet complexes are then removed to the base of the L2 vertebral body. At this point, cancellous bone is removed from the L2 body through the exposed pedicles bilaterally, the dura is stripped from the dorsal portion of the vertebral body, and the cortical bone of the L2 body is sectioned dorsally and laterally with a small osteotome. All bony material is saved for grafting. At this point in the procedure, a rectangular opening exists with the thecal sac, and the L1 and L2 nerve roots are visible.

With the spine essentially destabilized by the dorsal element removal and wedge osteotomy, reduction is performed. The desired reduction is obtained by elevating the patient's legs and lower lumbar spine by extending the operating table. A cracking sound is often heard and felt as this closes the dorsal wedge.[7,44,60] As the wedge closes dorsally, the ventral surface of the vertebral body fractures and opens up, giving the procedure the name "ventral opening wedge osteotomy." Instrumentation is then inserted to maintain reduction, and bone graft placed in a dorsolateral position to obtain fusion.

Dangers with the opening wedge are rupture of calcified ventral great vessels from elongation of the spine and sudden fracture of the ventral vertebral body surface, as well as cauda equina damage from stretch and compression.[29,44] Another common complication is intestinal ileus caused by stretch of the superior mesenteric artery over the third portion of the duodenum. This may lead to emesis with aspiration pneumonia, and can be prevented by placing a nasogastric tube to suction until the ileus resolves.[58]

Closing Wedge Osteotomy

The Smith-Peterson ventral opening wedge has a mortality of 10%, is uncontrolled, and uses substantial force. Jaffray, Becker, and Eisenstein[29] has devised a procedure utilizing a dorsal closing wedge osteotomy combined with dorsal instrumentation that is more controlled, safer, and provides rigid three-dimensional fixation. The operative approach is similar to that performed for the ventral opening wedge. The same amount and location of bony dissection is performed. The difference between the two procedures lies in the use of pedicle screws to compress across the osteotomy while deformity reduction takes place simultaneously. This prevents elongation of the spine and allows slower, more controlled closure of the osteotomy.[29]

Ventral Approaches to the Thoracic Spine

Dorsal fusions have been used for the treatment of thoracic kyphosis, but have been problematic. Pseudarthrosis and loss of correction have been reported in as many as 40% of Scheuermann's disease patients undergoing surgical treatment via a dorsal approach.[32] Kostuik[32] has devised a method of direct operation on the involved region of thoracic kyphosis using a thoracotomy approach, ventral vertebrectomy, and ventral grafting with instrumentation. Results of this procedure are reportedly superior to those obtained with dorsal approaches.[32]

Kostuik's technique involves a thoracotomy incision two levels above the level of maximum curvature. The thoracic vertebral bodies are resected, decompressing the thecal sac and sparing the ventral most portion of the vertebral bodies. Screws are then placed bicortically into the vertebral bodies above and below, and distraction rods are placed. Distraction is applied to the construct while manual pressure is added dorsally to obtain deformity reduction. Iliac crest or rib struts are then placed and the instrumentation construct is placed in compression and tightened.[32]

Malone et al.[40] have developed a method of simultaneous ventral and dorsal instrumentation and fusion in the thoracic spine through a combined dorsal and lateral extracavitary approach. This technique involves a dorsal curvilinear incision with dissection of the paraspinous musculature from both the medial and lateral directions. This mobilizes the erector column such that the spine can be approached dorsally in the midline as well as from a lateral direction.

The lateral view allows for direct access to vertebral body pathology and for the placement of bone screws in the bodies above and below the vertebrectomy site. These screws are then placed in distraction and manual dorsal pressure is applied to obtain deformity reduction. Iliac crest and/or rib struts are then placed into the vertebrectomy site and the instrumentation is placed in compression with a single rod connecting the vertebral body screws. Conventional dorsal instrumentation is then placed and distraction forces are applied to the dorsal spine. Crossmembers are used to link the two dorsal rods together and to link one dorsal rod (on the side having the ventral hardware) to the ventral rod. No operative mortality has occurred in either Kostuik's or Benzel's series of patients.[32,40]

CONCLUSION

A variety of degenerative and inflammatory conditions affect the thoracic spine. The seronegative spondyloarthropathies represent a major component of these conditions. Most patients with these conditions can be managed nonoperatively. Operation is sometimes necessary for fracture stabiliza-

tion, deformity reduction, or to address lesions causing neurological deficits. Operation on these patients generally carries increased operative morbidity and mortality when compared with that of the general population.

REFERENCES

1. An HS, Balderston RA. Juvenile kyphosis. In Rothman RH, Simeone FA, eds. The Spine. Philadelphia: WB Saunders, 1992, pp 485-499.
2. Arnett FC. Seronegative spondyloarthropathies. Bull Rheum Dis 38:1-12, 1987.
3. Baggenstoss AH, Bicknell WH, Ward LE. Rheumatiod granulomatous nodules as destructive lesions of vertebrae. J Bone Joint Surg 34A:601-609, 1952.
4. Benzel EC. Degenerative and inflammatory diseases of the spine. In Benzel EC, ed. Biomechanics of Spinal Stabilization. New York: McGraw-Hill, 1995, pp. 41-53.
5. Blackburn WD, Alarcon GS, Ball GV. Evaluation of patients with back pain of a suspected inflammatory nature. Am J Med 85:766-770, 1988.
6. Brewerton DA, Hart FD, Nichols A, Cafferey M, James DC, Sturrock RD. Ankylosing spondylitis and HL-A 27. Lancet 1:904-907, 1973.
7. Briggs H, Keats S, Schlisinger PT. Wedge osteotomy of the spine with bilateral intervertebral foraminotomy. J Bone Joint Surg 29:1075-1082, 1947.
8. Burkus JK, Denis F. Hyperextension injuries of the thoracic spine in diffuse idiopathic skeletal hyperostosis. J Bone Joint Surg 76A:237-243, 1994.
9. Calin A. Ankylosing spondylitis and the spondyloarthropathies. In Schumacher HR, ed. Primer on Rheumatologic Diseases, 9th ed. Atlanta: Arthritis Foundation, 1988, pp 142-147.
10. Callahan EP, Aguillera H. Complications following minor trauma in a patient with diffuse idiopathic skeletal hyperostosis. Ann Emerg Med 22:1067-1069, 1993.
11. Carette S, Graham D, Little H, Rubenstein J, Rosen P. The natural disease course of ankylosing spondylitis. Arthritis Rheum 26:186-190, 1983.
12. Cohen MJ, Ezekiel J, Persellin RH. Costovertebral and costotransverse joint involvement in rheumatiod arthritis. Ann Rheum Dis 37:473-475, 1978.
13. Collie DA, Smith GW, Merrick MV. 99mTc-MDP scintography in ankylosing spondylitis. Clin Radiol 48:392-397, 1993.
14. Devogelaer JP, Maldague B, Malghem J, Deuchaisnes CN. Appendicular and vertibral bone mass in ankylosing spondylitis. Arthritis Rheum 35:1062-1067, 1992.
15. Dillin WH, Watkins RG. Back pain in children and adolescents. In Rothman RH, Simeone FA, eds. The Spine. Philadelphia: WB Saunders, 1992, pp 231-259.
16. Erhardt CC, Mumford PA, Venables PJ, Maini RN. Factors predicting a poor life prognosis in rheumatoid arthritis: An eight year prospective study. Ann Rheum Dis 48:7-13, 1989.
17. Friedman H. Intraspinal rheumatiod nodule causing nerve root compression. J Neurosurg 32:689-691, 1970.
18. Glay A, Rona G. Nodular rheumatoid vertebral lesions versus ankylosing spondylitis. Campian Med Ass J 94:631-638, 1965.
19. Graham B, Peteghem PK. Fractures of the spine in ankylosing spondylitis. Spine 14:803-807, 1989.
20. Gran JT, Husby G, Hordvik M. Spinal ankylosing spondylitis: A variant form of ankylosing spondylitis or a distinct disease entity? Ann Rheum Dis 44:368-371, 1985.

21. Hanly JG, Russell ML, Gladman DD. Psoriatic spondyloarthorpathy: A long term prospective study. Ann Rheum Dis 47:386-393, 1988.

22. Helliwell PS, Zebouni LN, Porter G, Wright V. A clinical and radiological study of back pain in rheumatoid arthritis. Br J Rheum 32:216-221, 1993.

23. Hendrix RW, Melany M, Miller F, Rogers LF. Fracture of the spine in patients with ankylosis due to different skeletal hyperostosis: Clinical and imaging findings. Am J Roentgenol 162:899-904, 1994.

24. Herbert JJ. Vertebral osteotomy for kyphosis, especially in Marie-Strumpell arthritis. J Bone Joint Surg 41A:291-302, 1959.

25. Heywood AW, Meyers OL. Rheumatoid arthritis of the thoracic and lumbar spine. J Bone Joint Surg 68B:362-367, 1986.

26. Hill HF, Hill AG, Bodmer JG. Clinical diagnosis of ankylosing spondylitis in women and relation to the presence of HLA-B27. Ann Rheum Dis 35:267-270, 1976.

27. Huang GS, Park YH, Taylor JA, Sartoris DJ, Seragini F, Pathria MN, Resnick D. Hyperostosis of ribs: Association with vertebral ossification. J Rheumatol 20:2073-2076, 1993.

28. Hunter T, Dubo H. Spinal fractures complicating ankylosing spondylitis. Ann Intern Med 88:546-549, 1978.

29. Jaffray D, Becker V, Eisenstein S. Closing wedge osteotomy with transpedicular fixation in ankylosing spondylitis. Clin Orthop 279:122-126, 1992.

30. Kaprove RE, Little AH, Graham DC, Rosen PS. Ankylosing spondylitis survival in men with and without radiotherapy. Arthritis Rheum 23:57-61, 1980.

31. Kirwan J, Edwards A, Huitfeldt B, Thompson P, Currey H. The course of established ankylosing spondylitis and the effects of sulfasalazine over 3 years. Br J Rheum 32:729-733, 1993.

32. Kostuik JP. Anterior Kostuik-Harrington distraction systems for the treatment of kyphotic deformities. Spine 15:169-180, 1990.

33. Kramer J. Intervertebral Disc Disease: Causes, Diagnosis, Treatment, and Prophylaxis, 2nd ed. Stuttgart and New York: George Theime-Verlag, 1990, pp 14-47.

34. Law WA. Surgical treatment of the rheumatic diseases. J Bone Joint Surg 34B:215-225, 1952.

35. Linquist PR, McDonnell DE. Rheumatiod cyst causing extradural compression. J Bone Joint Surg 52A:1235-1240, 1970.

36. Lorber A, Pearson CM, Rene RM. Osteolytic vertebral lesions as a manifestation of rheumatoid arthritis and related disorders. 514-532

37. Luken MG, Patel DV, Ellman MH. Symptomatic spinal stenosis associated with ankylosing spondylitis. Neurosurgery 11:703-705,1982.

38. Maertens M, Mielants H, Verstraete K, Veys EM. Simultaneous occurrence of diffuse idiopathic skelatal hyperostosis and ankylosing spondylitis in the same patient. J Rheumatol 19:1978-1983, 1992.

39. Magnes B, Hauge T. Rheumatiod arthritis contributing to lumbar spinal stenosis. Scand J Rheumatol 7:215-217, 1978.

40. Malone DG, Benzel EC, Baldwin NG, Adams MS, McCormack BM, Caruso JR. The outrigger attachment for vertebrectomy with posterior instrumentation [abstract]. Rocky Mountain Neurosurgery Society Meeting. Sun Valley, Idaho: June 18-21, 1995.

41. Martel W. Spinal pseudoarthrosis. Arthritis Rheum 21:485-490, 1978.

42. Mata S, Hill RO, Joseph L, Kaplan P, Dussalt R, Watts CS, Fitzcharles MA, Shiroky JB, Fortin PR, Esdaile JM. Chest radiographs as a screening test for diffuse idiopathic skeletal hyperostosis. J Rheumatol 20:1905-1910, 1993.

43. McKenzie MK, Barthal E, Pay NT. A hyperextension injury of the thoracic spine in association with diffuse idiopathic skeletal hyperostosis. Orthopedics 14:895-898, 1991.

44. McMaster MJ, Coventry MB. Spinal osteotomy in ankylosing spondylitis. Mayo Clin Proc 48:476-486, 1973.

45. Mitchell DM, Spitz PW, Young DY, Bloch DA, McShane DJ, Fries JF. Survival, prognosis, and causes of death in rheumatoid arthritis. Arthritis Rheum 29:706-714 1986.

46. Moll JM, Haslock I, Macrae IF, Wright V. Associations between ankylosing spondylitis, psoriatic arthritis, Reiter's disease, the intestinal arthropathies, and Bechet's syndrome. Medicine 53:343-363, 1974.

47. Park YH, Huang GS, Taylor JA, Marcelis S, Kramer J, Pathria MN, Clopton P, Resnick D. Patterns of vertibral ossification and pelvic abnormalities in paralysis: A study of 200 patients. Radiology 188:561-565, 1993.

48. Pascual E, Castellano JA, Lopez E. Costovertebral joint changes in ankylosing spondylitis with thoracic pain. Br J Rheumatol 31:413-415, 1992.

49. Pastershank SP, Resinck D. Pseudoarthrosis in ankylosing spondylitis. Can J Radiol 31:234-235, 1980.

50. Peh WC, Ho TK, Chan FL. Case report: Pseudoarthrosis complicating ankylosing spondylitis-appearances on magnetic resonance imaging. Clin Radiol 47:359-361, 1993.

51. Radford EP, Doll R, Smith PG. Mortality among patients with ankylosing spondylitis not given x-ray therapy. N Engl J Med 297:572-576, 1977.

52. Ralston SH, Urquhart GD, Brzeski M, Sturrock RD. A new method for the radiological assessment of vertebral squaring in ankylosing spondylitis. Ann Rheum Dis 51:330-333, 1991.

53. Redlund-Johnell L, Larsson EM. Subluxation of the upper thoracic spine in rheumatiod arthritis. Skeletal Radiol 22:105-108, 1993.

54. Resnick D, Shapiro RF, Wiesner KB, Ninwyama G, Utsinger PD, Shaul SR. Diffuse idiopathic skeletal hyperostosis. Semin Arthritis Rheum 7:153-187, 1978.

55. Russell ML, Gordon DA, Ogryzlo MA, McPhedran RS. The cauda equina syndrome of ankylosing spondylitis. Ann Intern Med 78:551-554, 1973.

56. Schlapbach P, Beyeler C, Gerber NJ, Van Der Linden S, Burg U, Fuchs WA, Ehrengruber H. The prevalence of palpable finger joint nodules in diffuse idiopathic skelatal hyperostosis. A controlled study. Br J Rheum 31:531-534, 1992.

57. Sheehan NJ, Slavin BM, Donovan MP, Mount JN, Mathews JA. Lack of correlation between clinical disease activity and erythrocyte sedimentation rate, acute phase proteins or protease inhibitors in ankylosing spondylitis. Br J Rheum 25:171-174, 1986.

58. Simmons EH. Kyphotic deformity of the spine in ankylosing spondylitis. Clin Orthop 128:65-77, 1977.

59. Tangrea JA, Kilcoyne RF, Taylor PR, Helsel WE, Adrianza ME, Hartman AM, Edwards BK, Peck GL. Skelatal hyperostosis in patients receiving chronic, very low-dose isotretinoin. Arch Dermatol 128:921-925, 1992.

60. Thomasen E. Vertebral osteotomy for correction of kyphosis in ankylosing spondylitis. Clin Orthop 194:142-152, 1985.

61. Thorngren KG, Liedberg E, Aspelin P. Fractures of the thoracic and lumbar spine in ankylosing spondylitis. Arch Orthop Trauma Surg 98:101-107, 1981.

62. Trojan DA, Pouchot J, Pokrupa R, Ford RM, Adamsbaum C, Hill RO, Esdaile JM. Diagnosis and treatment of ossification of the posterior longitudinal ligament of the spine: Report of eight cases and literature review. Am J Med 92:296-306, 1992.

Complications

41

Medical and Perioperative Complications

Edward S. Connolly, M.D., and Bryan Payne, M.D.

Surgery of the thoracic spine has evolved rapidly over the past several decades. Advances in spinal instrumentation, as well as surgical technique, have enhanced the spine surgeon's ability to effectively treat complex lesions. However, complications from this enhanced treatment have risen in parallel. A priority that should be in the mind of every surgeon is the prevention and early recognition and treatment of complications arising from surgery. This includes not only complications involving the spine and spinal cord but also those arising from the wide variety of surgical approaches used to reach the thoracic spine. Germane to this discussion is an understanding of the anatomy of the thorax and the unique anatomy of the thoracic spine and spinal cord. Complications herein are broadly divided into three groups: neurological complications, spinal instability, and soft tissue complications arising from the surgical exposure.

ANATOMY OF THE THORACIC SPINE

The thoracic spine differs in several significant ways from the cervical and lumbar spine. The morphology of the vertebrae represents a spectrum of gradation from the smaller cervical vertebrae to the large weight-bearing lumbar vertebrae. The anteroposterior diameter of the thoracic spinal canal is significantly decreased in relation to spinal cord di-

ameter. This disparity, in conjunction with the relatively poor vascular supply of the thoracic spinal cord, makes the thoracic spinal cord very susceptible to compression and ischemic insults, particularly from T4 to T9.[9] Unique to the thoracic spine are the costovertebral joints and the costotransverse joints. The costovertebral joints are synovial joints formed by the heads of the ribs and the lateral masses of the corresponding vertebrae and the vertebrae above. The costotransverse joints connect the tubercles of the ribs where they articulate with the transverse processes of the corresponding vertebrae. In conjunction with the sternum, the ribs significantly enhance the overall stability[1] of the thoracic spine and provide resistance to deformation during trauma.

The dorsal height of the vertebrae is relatively greater than the ventral height. Therefore a physiological kyphosis of the thoracic spine exists. The normal range of motion of the thoracic spine is limited by its anatomical and geometric relationships. The distinctly coronal orientation of the facet joints allows significant axial rotation. Compared with the cervical and lumbar regions, the range of flexion, extension, and lateral bending is relatively limited. Because the laminae are broad and overlap, hyperextension is prevented.[39] The anatomy of the thoracic spinal cord is unique in several ways. As mentioned above, the arterial blood supply in the midthoracic region (T3 to T7) is relatively tenuous.[9] In this region, the anterior spinal artery is often narrowed such that unidirectional flow is the rule. Therefore it often does not function as an anastomotic vessel if the proximal radicular artery is sacrificed.

The lumbar spinal cord enlargement (L3 to S3) is located in the caudal thoracic and proximal lumbar spine. Its primary blood supply is via the artery of Adamkiewicz, which arises between T7 and L4 85% of the time and on the left side 60% to 80% of the time.[9] Interruption of this major radicular artery may lead to ischemia of the lumbar spinal cord enlargement, and therefore should be vigorously avoided.

The rostral thoracic spinal cord is relatively protected by a rich vascular anastomotic network, including the multiple anterior and posterior radicular arteries that arise from the subclavian artery and its branches.

COMPLICATIONS RELATED TO EXPOSURE

The relative indications for the variety of approaches to the thoracic spine depend on the specific pathological disease process and the level of occurrence. The ventral approaches provide excellent exposure of the vertebral bodies over extended levels. The additional risks and complications of thoracotomy, however, are evident. The upper and lower extremes of the thoracic spine are reached with greater difficulty, owing to the diaphragm below and the great vessels, esophagus, trachea, and mediastinum at more rostral levels (T1 to T3). The costotransversectomy approach provides access to the pedicle, transverse process, intervertebral disc, and vertebral body, but because the length of exposure along the spine and the view of the midline are limited, this approach may best be reserved for focal lateral lesions. The midline dorsal approach provides excellent access to the dorsal elements and spinal cord along the length of the thoracic spine.

Supraclavicular Approach

The lower cervical and upper thoracic vertebrae may be reached via a supraclavicular approach. The most caudal vertebra that may be exposed can be determined by observing the level of the upper margin of the manubrium and clavicle on a plain lateral radiograph. The approach may be from either side, but the right side is preferred to avoid the thoracic duct.

While potential complications of this approach are numerous, they can be minimized with careful surgical technique. Perforations of the esophagus should be immediately primarily repaired. If a perforation occurs and is not recognized intraoperatively, the patient usually presents several days later with dysphagia, cervical swelling, and signs of sepsis. After the retroesophageal abscess is urgently drained and debrided, the defect can be repaired.

If the pleura is entered during the procedure, a pneumothorax may develop. If only the pleura has been entered and the lung has not been injured, the wound is closed while the anesthesiologist keeps the lung fully expanded. A large pneumothorax or tension pneumothorax predicates the placement of a tube thoracostomy, and a postoperative chest radiograph is indicated.

Injuries to the thoracic duct should be corrected by ligation, both proximal and distal to the duct injury, to avoid a postoperative chylous effusion, which is difficult to treat. Serial aspirations of a chylous effusion usually lead to eventual resolution. Although the thoracic duct is usually located on the left, a right-sided duct or bilateral ducts are occasionally encountered.[17] Large effusions that are symptomatic and appear early are unlikely to close spontaneously. Surgical ligation of the leak with oversewing of adjacent tissues is the preferred method of repair; however, when this method is inadequate, direct ligation of the thoracic duct, proximal to the leak, is usually effective.[31]

The recurrent laryngeal nerves and phrenic nerve may be injured by retraction, causing postoperative hoarseness (laryngeal nerve) and ipsilateral diaphragm dysfunction (phrenic nerve). To prevent retraction injury, the visualization and mobilization of these nerves is often necessary.

Because vascular injuries may occur due to the complex vascular anatomy of the thoracic inlet, usually the simplest remedy is to ligate the thyrocervical trunk. In general, to avoid entering the common carotid artery or the jugular vein, blunt dissection should be commonly used. Vascular injuries should be repaired primarily, if possible.

Ventral (Transthoracic) Exposure
Sternum Splitting

The upper thoracic three or four vertebrae may be reached from a sternal splitting approach.[7] This approach is applicable for a wide variety of lesions, including decompression of the spinal cord and the rare herniated intravertebral disc, tumors, and spinal deformity. The sternal splitting thoracotomy is the most common approach employed by cardiothoracic surgeons. Its risks are well documented. The incision extends from several centimeters caudal to the jugular notch to several centimeters past the xiphoid process. The manubrium and sternum are divided in the midline. The sternum is separated with a specialized sternal spreader placed near the midportion of the sternum. More rostral placement may lead to a brachial plexus stretch injury.[37] The mediastinal structures, esophagus, and great vessels must be retracted carefully to avoid intraoperative injury. Because the surgeon is operating in a deep hole, decompressive procedures of the spine must be carried out with great care. The depth of the wound is due somewhat to the kyphosis of the upper thoracic spine.[27] The operating microscope provides improved illumination and magnification of the operative field.

Multiple postoperative complications can occur. Wound infections after median sternotomy can be extremely serious, even life-threatening. Early signs and symptoms are those of an occult, nonspecific infection, such as fever and leukocytosis. Specific indicators include chest pain, sternal instability, and wound drainage, either serosanguineous or purulent. Management is by surgical debridement augmented with antibiotics. Debridement of the wound is mandatory and may include resection of the entire sternum and collagenous structures.[27]

High output of air, blood, or serosanguineous fluid from a chest tube postoperatively betrays an intrathoracic pulmonary, vascular, or mediastinal injury. If output is initially very high or does not resolve within several days, operative intervention is required. The surgical approach is limited caudally by the aortic arch. Injuries to the great vessels require urgent vascular repair. The approach is usually made on the right side of the trachea and esophagus, as in the supraclavicular approach.

Anterolateral Approach

The transthoracic approach to the thoracic spine, usually through a dorsolateral thoracotomy, has become the most common approach to ventral lesions of the spine. Similar to other ventral and lateral approaches (e.g., median sternotomy, thoracoabdominal), postoperative medical complications are significantly increased. In most cases, the complications are related to the exposure rather than the spinal procedure itself. Hypotension may occur due to postoperative unrecognized blood loss or to heart failure, dysrhythmias, or insufficient intraoperative fluid resuscitation. Patients who require transthoracic spinal procedures are often older, debilitated, or have metastatic cancer. Intraoperative intensive care monitoring, which may include central venous catheterization as well as pulmonary artery catheterization, is essential. Mechanical ventilation is often required postoperatively or may be reinstituted several days after surgery due to pulmonary edema, atelectasis, pneumonitis, pneumonia, or respiratory insufficiency.

The side of approach chosen is occasionally dictated by the location of the lesion. If not, approaching from the left is generally preferable, particularly in the mid- and lower thoracic spine. Injury to the vena cava is significantly more difficult to remedy than injury to the aorta. In the upper thoracic spine, to avoid the left-lying heart and mediastinum, a right-sided approach may be preferred, but this is only a relative consideration. The rostral two or three levels of the thoracic spine are difficult to approach via a dorsolateral thoracotomy because of the short ribs, obstructing scapula, and anatomically busy thoracic outlet. A median sternotomy is generally more appropriate.

During the ventral approach to the thoracolumbar spine, the diaphragm is usually transected. To minimize degeneration of the diaphragm, one should incise the diaphragm as close to the periphery as possible, leaving enough tissue to allow tight closure to prevent hiatal hernia. A significant hernia can be detected postoperatively by a chest radiograph. Patients who have a significant hiatal hernia may present with respiratory embarrassment.

Specific complications after dorsolateral thoracotomy are related to the anatomy of the approach. Because the pleural space is violated during the procedure, a tube thoracostomy connected to a water seal is left in place. Postoperative bleeding of 100 to 200 ml/hr for more than 6 hours or persistent loss at a lesser rate requires operative re-exploration. Air leaks occasionally occur if the visceral pleura is inadvertently entered during the procedure. Most air leaks can be detected intraoperatively by filling the thoracic cavity with saline and hyperinflating the lung, after which the presence of bubbles will betray the leak. These leaks generally resolve within

2 to 3 days; however, if a leak does not resolve, administering a pleural sclerosing agent usually leads to closure. Uncommonly, a leak requires operative intervention.

Another potentially significant complication is a cerebrospinal fluid (CSF) pleural fistula. This has also been reported after laminectomy.[12] Patients with indolent symptoms of spinal headache should be treated with lumbar subarachnoid external drainage. Definitive diagnosis may be difficult, owing to pleural absorption of CSF, but if a tube thoracostomy is in place, fluid may be analyzed in the laboratory for the presence of beta-2 transferrin.[3]

Acute changes in neurological status after surgery or after removal of a chest tube could be caused by pneumocephalus from air entering the subarachnoid space from the fistula. This requires urgent intervention with chest tube placement and definitive repair. If an indolent leak does not resolve with spinal fluid diversion, a myelogram may provide a definitive diagnosis and the location of the leak before surgical repair.

Empyema may occur in the presence of a thoracostomy tube or following its removal. If the chest tube is in place, the diagnosis is simplified by the presence of purulent drainage from the tube, and continued suction and parenteral antibiotics generally clear the infection. If the thoracostomy tube has been removed, a high index of suspicion must be maintained, and fever, leukocytosis, chest pain, tachycardia, or signs of sepsis should raise the question of empyema. If empyema is present, reinstitution of closed tube thoracostomy is indicated with parenteral antibiotics. Chest computed tomography (CT) clearly demonstrates even small empyemas. Chronic empyema requires operative decortication.

Injury to the long thoracic nerve may occur during a high dorsolateral thoracotomy. The degree of serratus anterior denervation is dependent upon the level of injury and completeness of the lesion, but tends to be self-limited, with resolution of the "winged scapula" appearance over time if the nerve was not transected during surgery.

Dorsal Approach

Laminectomy for exposure of the dorsal elements and dorsal spinal cord is an excellent approach because the length of incision is not limited and wide visualization is possible. Complications of this approach are similar to those observed in the cervical spine. Dural tears should be repaired primarily. Large rents may require grafting. Small lateral tears may usually be repaired by using a dorsal durotomy to pass a suture (with a small piece of muscle or fat attached at its end) from within the dural sac to the outside.[24] Postoperative leaks can usually be managed with lumbar external drainage. Rarely, reoperation may be necessary.[19]

NEUROLOGICAL COMPLICATIONS

Neurological deterioration may occur preoperatively, during surgery, or in the postoperative period. In patients who have extrinsic mass lesions, such as herniated intervertebral discs or tumors, progressive neurological loss is an indication for urgent, if not emergent, decompression of the spinal cord. Laminectomy for a ventral mass is unwise.[2,5,16,22,32,35] Improvement is sporadic, and postoperative deterioration is far too common. Ventral mass lesions should generally be exposed from a ventral approach. If preoperative progression of neurological deficit is due to chronic mass effect on the spinal cord, postoperative improvement is common. However, if progression is due to acute ischemia, postoperative improvement is rare.

In cases of ruptured intravertebral discs in the upper thoracic spine, a T1 to T3 limited lateral unilateral laminectomy may often be appropriate because a more lateral protrusion appears to be more common in the upper thoracic spine than at lower levels, and spinal cord decompression may be possible from a dorsal approach.[20,21]

Experience in scoliosis surgery has shown that both overdistraction of the thoracic spine and inadequate decompression of the ventral kyphotic bony deformity can lead to intraoperative neurological complications.[23] Postoperative neurological deficits mandate urgent radiographic evaluation and usually require reoperation to remove the cause of overdistraction, such as a persistent compressive lesion or instrumentation placed during the original operation. Patients who awaken from surgery with a severe neurological deficit can be expected to fare worse than those with a milder progressive deficit treated in a timely fashion.

In the postoperative period, neurological deterioration may occur from a variety of causes, such as vascular compromise and delayed deterioration from overdistraction or compression by spinal instrumentation. In the early postoperative period, the presence of an epidural hematoma may be indicated by a progressive neurological deficit. Although epidural hematoma is an uncommonly reported complication in thoracic spine surgery, experience from the cervical and lumbar regions infers that early decompression is mandatory.[29,33] In many operations on the thoracic spine, the vertebral canal is significantly compromised or the spinal cord is edematous. The blood supply to the spinal cord, therefore, is reduced, secondary to edema or compression. Perioperative hypotension should be avoided, because low blood pressure may result in further spinal cord ischemia.

A significant number of patients undergoing instrumentation of the dorsal spine develop neurological sequelae. As noted previously, overdistraction most commonly occurs with corrective scoliosis surgery,[23] but it also occurs when compression and distraction rod systems are used for stabilization.[25] The monitoring of somatosensory-evoked potentials may be helpful whenever significant forces are to be applied intraoperatively to the thoracic spine or when dorsal instrumentation or wires are to be placed near the spinal cord. Changes in the somatosensory-evoked potentials that are temporally related to distraction of the spine dictates that the distraction be released. Postoperative neurological deterioration from the preoperative state is an absolute indication for urgent return to the operating room to remove the offending instrumentation if emergent studies fail to reveal another treatment explanation.[25]

The passage of sublaminar wires should be carefully employed or avoided, if possible, in the thoracic spine due to the relatively high percentage of the canal being occupied by the spinal cord. A neurological complication rate of 1.8% with passage of sublaminar wires has been reported by the Scoliosis Research Society Morbidity and Mortality Committee.[34] If sublaminar wires are needed, the following three requirements should minimize the risk: (1) the intralaminar space must be opened adequately, because the width of the lamina determines the minimum depth through which the wire must pass within the canal (tempered with the knowledge that removing portions of the lamina also weakens the construct); (2) the surgeon must be experienced with passing sublaminar wires (compli-

cation rates decrease with increased experience); and (3) if an acute spinal cord injury has caused spinal cord edema (which increases the volume of spinal cord within the spinal canal and reduces the space available for wire passage), one should avoid passing sublaminar wire in the area of acute injury or delay the procedure until the edema has resolved.[18,38] The introduction of softer cable systems may be expected to lower the incidence of associated spinal cord injury.

INFECTIONS

Epidural abscesses usually present themselves days to weeks after surgery. The presentation is generally dramatic, with the patient complaining of excruciating back pain and exhibiting signs of sepsis and variable neurological dysfunction.[4,13] The degree of neurological loss and recovery are directly related to the timeliness of the decompression. Therefore rapid diagnosis and timely surgical intervention are mandatory. Magnetic resonance imaging (MRI) clearly delineates the location and extent of the abscess and is therefore the diagnostic modality of choice. The surgical approach is dictated by the location of the abscess.

Discitis is more likely to present in an indolent fashion, with back pain being the primary complaint. Plain radiographs are unlikely to demonstrate discitis until late in its course when surgical management becomes more complex. The erythrocyte sedimentation rate, which should be near normal by 6 to 8 weeks postoperatively, as well as the C-reactive protein level, are generally significantly elevated.[6,28] MRI is the diagnostic modality of choice.[26] Conservative therapy after culture is the general rule, with bed rest and parenteral antibiotics for 6 weeks followed by enteral antibiotics for 2 to 3 months. Because it may herald the onset of an epidural abscess, any evidence of neurological compromise is an indication for urgent surgical debridement.

COMPLICATIONS ASSOCIATED WITH STABILITY

Iatrogenic spondylolysis that becomes symptomatic in the immediate or delayed postoperative period may occur after thoracolumbar dorsal fusion.[10,15,30,36] Overdistraction and aggressive laminotomies to allow deep seating of the laminar hook are thought to be responsible. Focal postoperative pain at the caudal hook site is the usual presenting symptom. Plain radiographs may demonstrate the pars defect, adjacent to the caudal laminar hook. The defect may be grossly unstable. This may be observed with flexion and extension views. Depending on the clinical situation, correction requires either extension of the fusion or removal of the instrumentation with a shorter fusion crossing the spondylolysis.

Lamina hook and rod compression and distraction fixation systems have been associated with a variety of mechanical complications. The instrumentation, most commonly the rostral hook, may dislodge.[14] Inadequate contouring of the rods to conform to the sagittal kyphosis is often associated with slippage of the hooks because an excessive force is applied away from the intended distractive or compressive force. Excessive distraction or compression, as well as poor hook placement, may also lead to hook slippage. Much less commonly, the caudal end of the construct may dislodge. Hook dislodgment should be suspected when loss of correction or progressive deformity is encountered. If the hook dislodges before a solid fusion mass has formed, reoperation with replacement of the hook is indicated. If any doubt exists that the cause of the dislodgment has not been corrected, the hook should be placed at a more rostral level. The rod also may slip when adequate fixation is not obtained. The necessity of surgical correction depends on loss of structural integrity of the construct determined by serial radiographic examinations and flexion and extension radiographs.

With ventral thoracic spine procedures in which bone grafts have been placed after corpectomy, the graft may dislodge or penetrate into the end plates. Careful contouring of the graft so that it lies flush against the adjoining vertebral bodies is important. A compressive force should be acting on the graft, both to help prevent dislodgment and to promote arthrodesis. Pseudarthrosis as well as the aforementioned complications are more likely to occur in osteoporotic patients. Pain and loss of correction are the usual presentations.

Ventral screw fixation systems are prone to the same failures in the thoracic spine as elsewhere. If a clinical fusion does not occur, the screws often fracture and pull out, or, less likely, the plate may fracture. Also, if undue stress is placed on a ventral construct because of significant unaddressed dorsal spine disease, instrumentation failure may occur before a solid arthrodesis is in place.

Of interest, dorsal iliac bone grafts taken for nontraumatic reconstructive procedures are twice as likely to cause chronic graft-site pain as grafts taken for traumatic spine procedures.[11]

POST-THORACOTOMY PAIN

Many patients who undergo thoracotomy have pain that persists past the immediate postoperative period. Severe pain is unusual, but the prevalence of moderate pain is high. Over half of the patients who underwent a thoracotomy reported pain at the thoracotomy site 1 year after surgery.[8] This number decreases to 30% after 3 years. The majority of patients consider the pain mild, but a sizable minority report their pain as mildly to moderately disabling, and 5% to 10% of post-thoracotomy patients require treatment for pain.[8] Conservative treatment is advocated initially. Because lasting, rapid relief is uncommon, nonnarcotic analgesics are preferred to narcotics. In the more severe cases, the pain that often follows a dermatomal distribution or pain that occurs at the incision site only is thought to be due to the intercostal nerves having been damaged at the time of surgery. Contributing factors are either direct trauma or retraction injury to the nerve. Removing a rib at the time of surgery increases the risk of chronic pain postoperatively. If conservative measures fail, intercostal nerve blocks may be effective.

CONCLUSION

Avoiding complications and promptly diagnosing and treating them when they do occur are integral to a satisfactory outcome after thoracic spine surgery.

Spine surgeons must be cognizant of all potential complications of thoracic spine surgery, not only neurological complications and spinal instability but also complications arising from the surgical approaches performed themselves or by thoracic or general surgeons.

REFERENCES

1. Andriacchi TP, Schultz A, Belytschko T, Galante J. A model for studies of mechanical interactions between the human spine and rib cage. J Biomech 7:497-507, 1974.

2. Arce CA, Dohrmann GJ. Thoracic disc herniation. Improved diagnosis with computed tomographic scanning and a review of the literature. Surg Neurol 23:356-361, 1985.

3. Assietti R, Kibble MB, Bakay RAE. Iatrogenic cerebrospinal fluid fistula to the pleural cavity: Care report and literature review. Neurosurgery 33:1104-1108, 1993.

4. Baker AS, Ojemann RG, Schwartz MN, Richardson EP. Spinal epidural abscess. N Engl J Med 293:463-468, 1975.

5. Barnett GH, Hardy RW, Little JR, Bay JW, Sypert GW. Thoracic spinal canal stenosis. J Neurosurg 66:338-344, 1987.

6. Bircher MD, Tasker T, Crawshaw C, Mulholland RC. Discitis following lumbar surgery. Spine 13:98-102, 1988.

7. Cauchoix J, Binet JP. Anterior surgical approaches to the spine. Ann R Coll Surg Engl 27:237-243, 1957.

8. Dajczman E, Gordon A, Kreisman H, Wolkove N. Long-term postthoracotomy pain. Chest 99:270-274, 1991.

9. Domissee GF. The blood supply of the spinal cord. A critical vascular zone in spinal surgery. J Bone Joint Surg 56B:225-235, 1974.

10. Fernyhough JC, Schimandle JH, Levine AM. Iatrogenic spondylolysis complicating distal laminar hook placement. Spine 16:849-850, 1991.

11. Fernyhough JC, Schimandle JJ, Weigel MC, Edwards CC, Levine AM. Chronic donor site pain complicating bone graft harvesting from the posterior iliac crest for spinal fusion. Spine 17:1474-1480, 1992.

12. Gupta SM, Frias J, Garg A, Herrera NE. Aberrant cerebrospinal fluid pathway. Detection by scintigraphy. Clin Nucl Med 11:593-594, 1986.

13. Hancock DO. A study of 49 patients with acute spinal extradural abscess. Paraplegia 10:285-288, 1973.

14. Harrington PR. Technical details in relation to the successful use of instrumentation in scoliosis. Orthop Clin North Am 3:49-67, 1972.

15. Harris RI, Wiley JJ. Acquired spondylolysis as a sequel to spine fusion. J Bone Joint Surg 45A:1159-1170, 1963.

16. Hulme A. The surgical approach to thoracic intervertebral disc protrusions. J Neurol Neurosurg Psychiatry 23:133-137, 1960.

17. Johnson RM, Murphy MJ, Southwick WD. Surgical approaches to the spine. In Rothman RH, Simeone FA, eds. Spine. Philadelphia: WB Saunders Co., 1992.

18. King AG. Complications in segmental spinal instrumentation. In Luque ER, ed. Segmental Spinal Instrumentation. Thorofare, N.J.: Slack, 1984, pp 301-330.

19. Kitchel SH, Eismont FJ, Green BA. Closed subarachnoid drainage for management of cerebrospinal fluid leakage after an operation on the spine. J Bone Joint Surg 71A:984-987, 1989.

20. Kumar R, Buckley TF. First thoracic disc protrusion. Spine 11:499-501, 1986.

21. Kumar R, Cowie RA. Second thoracic disc protrusion. Spine 17:120-121, 1992.

22. Larson SJ, Holst RA, Hemmy DC, Sances A Jr. Lateral extracavitary approach to traumatic lesions of the thoracic and lumbar spine. J Neurosurg 45:628-637, 1976.

23. MacEwen GD, Burnell WP, Sriram K. Acute neurological complications in the treatment of scoliosis. J Bone Joint Surg 57A:404-408, 1975.

24. Mayfield FH, Kurokawa K. Watertight closure of spinal dura mater. Technical note. J Neurosurg 43:639-640, 1975.

25. McAfee PC, Bohlman HH. Complications following Harrington instrumentation for fractures of the thoracolumbar spine. J Bone Joint Surg 67A:672-685, 1985.

26. Modic MT, Feiglin DH, Piraino DW, Boumphrey F, Weinstein MA, Duchesneau PM, Rehm S. Vertebral osteomyelitis: Assessment using MRI. Radiology 157:157-166, 1985.

27. Pairolero PC, Arnold PG. Management of recalcitrant median sternotomy wounds. J Thorac Cardiovasc Surg 88:357-364, 1984.

28. Puranen J, Mäkelä J, Lähde S. Postoperative intervertebral discitis. Acta Orthop Scand 55:461-465, 1984.

29. Reynolds AF. Epidural bleeding in anterior discectomy [letter]. J Neurosurg 50:126, 1979.

30. Rombold C. Spondylolysis: A complication of spine fusion. J Bone Joint Surg 47A:1237-1242, 1965.

31. Rubin JW. Chylothorax complicating intrathoracic operations. In Cordell AR, Ellison RG, eds. Complications of Intrathoracic Surgery. Boston: Little Brown, 1979, pp 359-362.

32. Russell T. Thoracic intervertebral disc protrusion: Experience of 67 cases and review of the literature. [review] Br J Neurosurg 3:153-160, 1989.

33. Sang H, Wilson CB. Postoperative epidural hematoma as a complication of anterior cervical discectomy. J Neurosurg 49:288-291, 1978.

34. Scoliosis Research Society. Morbidity & Mortality Committee Report, Park Ridge, Ill.: Scoliosis Research Society, 1987.

35. Sekhar LN, Janetta PJ. Thoracic disc herniation: Operative approaches and results. Neurosurgery 12:303-305, 1983.

36. Tietjen R, Morgenstern JM. Spondylolisthesis following surgical fusion for scoliosis: A case report. Clin Orthop 117:176-178, 1976.

37. Vander Salm TJ, Cereda J-M, Cutler BS. Brachial plexus injury following median sternotomy. J Thorac Cardiovasc Surg 80:447-452, 1980.

38. Weber SC, Benson DR. A comparison of segmental fixation and Harrington instrumentation in the management of unstable thoracolumbar spine fractures. [abstract]. Orthop Trans 9:36, 1985.

39. White AA III, Punjabi MM. Clinical Biomechanics of the Spine. Philadelphia: JB Lippincott, 1978, p 240.

Complications of Decompressive Spinal Surgery

Sait Naderi, M.D., Mehmet Zileli, M.D., and Edward C. Benzel, M.D.

Decompressive procedures of the thoracic spine are indicated to remove bone, disc material, or other mass lesions compressing neural structures in order to either relieve an incomplete neurological deficit or to prevent progression of a neurological lesion. The localization and type of pathological condition dictates the choice of treatment. A decompressive procedure can be performed using a ventral, lateral, or dorsal approach. Complications observed after decompressive thoracic spine surgery are either general (e.g., dural tears) or approach-specific (e.g., pulmonary) complications.[3,4,7,9] Recently many of these procedures are being performed endoscopically. Endoscopic approaches pose unique challenges.[8] This chapter reviews the predominant complications of decompressive thoracic spine surgery, their prevention, and their management (see box).

NERVE ROOT AND SPINAL CORD INJURY

Neural structures may be injured during decompressive procedures. However, neural injuries rarely occur after thoracic spine surgery. They can occur from direct trauma (e.g., laceration of the neural structures), or indirectly, due to interruption of the vascular supply of the neural structures (i.e., anterior spinal artery). Indirect injuries are less common.

COMPLICATIONS OF DECOMPRESSIVE THORACIC SPINE SURGERY

Neural Injury
Nerve root and spinal cord injury
Dural tears and CSF fistulas
Deformity
Iatrogenic compression
Infection
Ischemia
Hemorrhage
Nonneurosurgical procedure-related complications (e.g., pulmonary or vascular complications)
Medical complications

Neurological complications may be categorized on the basis of (1) neural compression as a result of delayed nonsurgical care, (2) neural compression related to patient positioning during surgery, (3) intraoperative trauma, and (4) intraoperative or postoperative bleeding.

The degree of injury is related to the degree and duration of compression. The spinal cord tolerates compression less than nerve roots, and peripheral nerve roots tolerate compression better than intradural nerve roots. Neural injury may result from inadvertent contusion, laceration, electrocauterization, or traction. Occasionally, an incomplete neural injury may increase during a decompressive procedure. It may result from intolerance of the spinal cord to additional surgical trauma.

Indirect neural injury may occur during correction of scoliosis. Direct injury is more likely during re-exploration operations.

Although the injury of thoracic nerve roots is not as problematic as injury of lumbar nerve roots, one should make every attempt to preserve them. Traction, laceration, or thermal burns of the nerve root may cause injury. The improper use of surgical instrumentation may also cause nerve root and/or spinal cord injury. A prudent tactic to avoid neural and dural injury is to begin the laminectomy at a normal level and extend the laminectomy from this level to the pathological level.

DURAL TEARS AND CEREBROSPINAL FLUID LEAKS

Dural tears can occur during both ventral and dorsal operations. Factors affecting an increased incidence of dural tears include (1) the relative experience of the surgeon, (2) failure to attend to the basic principles of surgical technique, (3) previous surgery, and (4) the altered anatomy.

Following intraoperative dural tearing, the operative site commonly fills with cerebrospinal fluid (CSF). To visualize the tear, the affected region should be covered with cotton and suction performed. The repair of the torn dura mater can then be performed. If this is not possible, it should be covered with Gelfoam and the patient's head should be tilted down. After completion of the operation, the dura should be closed in a watertight manner, if possible.

The use of magnification and enhanced lighting by a head light can improve the surgeon's visualization. Once a rongeur is used, one should be certain that the depth of the rongeur lip is less than the space underneath the lamina or spinous process. If it is not, the bone may be thinned first with a drill and then removed with a series of small curettes.

Improper use of a high-speed drill may also cause a dural tear. To avoid dural injury, the dura mater should be protected. The selection of the proper drill bit is also important. In a critical area, the use of a diamond drill bit may be prudent.

Finally, dissection in the presence of bleeding during decompression may predispose to dural injury. A dural tear and CSF fistula should be repaired as soon as possible by means of direct repair. Dural

grafting with either muscle or fascia may provide other options. Lumbar drainage is advocated by some in the initial postoperative period.

POSTSURGERY THORACIC SPINE DEFORMITY

A postsurgical thoracic spine deformity most commonly occurs after dorsal surgical procedures. Spinal deformities after ventral spinal procedures are unusual because these operations are commonly combined with fusion and instrumentation.

Dorsal and lateral approaches for decompression of tumors and other pathological processes can be performed by means of laminectomy, costotransversectomy, or the lateral extracavitary approach. A spinal deformity after laminectomy in adults is rare, whereas it is more common in children (especially in patients with spinal cord tumor). The rate of deformity after decompressive procedures for malignant spine tumors in childhood has been reported to be 33% to 78%.[5] Kyphosis is the most common. The occurrence of scoliosis is less common.

Postlaminectomy kyphosis is due, in part, to the disruption of the facet joints and dorsal ligaments. The dorsal ligaments are the most important dorsal spinal stabilizers against tensile forces. Gravity normally exerts a flexion bending moment on the thoracic spine. Dorsal ligaments resist this flexion moment. An extensive laminectomy leads to loss of dorsal stability, and in turn, the flexion moment produces kyphosis. The most important factor in the development of a kyphosis is the integrity of the facet joints. A total bilateral removal of the facet joint may lead to an angulation at that level, whereas a unilateral removal of the facets may lead to an angular kyphosis associated with a sharp scoliosis.

The presence of postlaminectomy deformity may be aggravated by radiation therapy. Underlying tumors (e.g., osteoid osteoma, neurofibromatosis) may also be associated with the development of deformity.

Yasuoka et al.[10] reported the results of laminectomies performed at the Mayo Clinic between 1965 and 1974. They reported a 46% incidence of deformity in patients under age 15, whereas it was only 6% in patients aged 15 to 25. In the same series, postlaminectomy deformity was observed in 100% of the patients after cervical or cervicothoracic laminectomy, in 36% after thoracic laminectomy, and in none of patients with lumbar laminectomies.

A child younger than the age of 10 with high thoracic paresis may have a collapsing paralytic scoliosis after surgery. The deformity is commonly progressive. The best treatment of postlaminectomy deformity is its prevention by the preservation of facet joint integrity and, if necessary, instrumentation and fusion during the first intervention. However, when a kyphosis develops, early bracing should be instituted. For a progressive kyphosis, however, the use of spinal fusion and instrumentation is usually indicated.

In contrast to laminectomy, a thoracic microdiscectomy using costotransversectomy seems not to lead to deformity.[2] Hence a prophylactic fusion is not recommended by some authors after costotransversectomy and microdiscectomy unless clinical evidence of instability exists or unless there is structural loss of other spinal elements (e.g., prior laminectomy or facetectomy).

FOREIGN AND FOREIGN-LIKE BODY COMPRESSION

Fat grafts, Gelfoam, Surgicel, and other substances used to shield the dura mater from scar tissue may cause iatrogenic compression of the dural sac. Therefore the use of such materials should be minimized.[1]

POSTOPERATIVE INFECTIONS

The increased complexity of spinal surgery and its combination with instrumentation has resulted in longer operative times. This, in turn, increases the incidence of postoperative infections.

Postoperative infection after decompressive thoracic spine surgery is relatively uncommon. A 0.7% to 5% rate of local infection after elective laminectomy has been observed.[6] This includes superficial or deep wound infections, postoperative discitis, postoperative vertebral osteomyelitis, and epidural abscess.

Superficial Wound Infection

Infections above the fascia are known as superficial infections. Their true incidence is not known. Although they are not as serious as deep wound infections, they can cause prolonged hospitalization. Many factors, including excessive local tissue trauma, overaggressive tissue retraction, the presence of necrotic tissue in the wound upon closure, and host factors such as diabetes, alcoholism, previous local irradiation, as well as obesity may predispose to this complication.

Superficial infections usually become symptomatic within days of surgery. Symptoms and signs include pain, tenderness, the presence of erythema, and a warm and edematous wound. Symptomatic manifestations of infection such as fever and leukocytosis may not always exist. The predominant etiological agents include the patient's own epidermal organisms, such as *Staphylococcus epidermidis* and *Staphylococcus aureus.*

Superficial wound infections may respond well to appropriate antibiotic therapy; however, open debridement may be necessary.

Deep Infections

Deep infections following spinal surgery include discitis, epidural abscess, and vertebral osteomyelitis. Fortunately, their incidence is low, increasing with the complexity of the procedure. The incidence of infection after discectomy is less than 1%, whereas after spinal fusion without instrumentation the rate increases to 5%. The risk of infection after instrumentation is about 7% (range, 1.3% to 12%).[6]

Some endogenous or exogenous factors may also affect the risk of postoperative infection. These include the use of aseptic techniques, rough tissue handling, retained necrotic tissue, excessive blood loss, postoperative wound hematoma, prolonged operation time, foreign material (methylmethacrylate or metallic instrumentation), excessive operating room traffic, the contamination of the wound with the patient's skin flora, advanced age, chronic malnutrition, immunosuppression, steroid therapy, prolonged preoperative hospitalization and postoperative immobilization, and the presence of remote infection (e.g., pulmonary or urinary tract infection, decubitus ulceration).

Organisms and Prophylaxis

Most postoperative superficial or deep infections are caused by coagulase positive *S. aureus.* Other organisms include *S. epidermidis, Staphylococcus albus, beta-hemolytic streptococcus, Escherichia coli, Pseudomonas aeruginosa,* and *Klebsiella.*

The use of prophylactic antibiotics reduces the risk of postoperative infection. A proper antibiotic should cover prevalent organisms. For elective spinal surgery, preoperative intravenous antibiotic therapy is usually recommended. The use of a surgical drain dictates the use of postoperative antibiotic for a longer time frame.

Diagnosis and Treatment

The diagnosis of superficial infection is relatively easy. The diagnosis of deep infections, however, is often difficult. Postoperative deep infections generally cause a leukocytosis and an elevated erythrocyte sedimentation rate. They also cause severe back pain and tenderness that are aggravated by motion. Imaging studies usually corroborate infection. The diagnosis can be confirmed with needle biopsy. The surgical treatment consists of aggressive open wound re-exploration, debridement, irrigation, and drainage. Additional strategies include immobilization and antibiotic therapy.

Re-exploration of discitis is usually not necessary. However, postoperative vertebral osteomyelitis may dictate a re-exploration. The indications for surgery for vertebral osteomyelitis may include progressive neurological deficit, abscess formation, progressive spinal deformity, and refractory infections.

ISCHEMIA

An important source of spinal decompression failure is spinal cord ischemia. Ischemia may be due to the ligation of segmental intercostal arteries (including the artery of Adamkiewicz), compression, spasm, or ligation of the anterior spinal artery.

Spinal cord ischemia is rare, and in most cases, irreversible. Therefore spinal angiography may be considered before any critical decompressive thoracic spine surgery in which primal rodicular artery may be sacrificed.

HEMORRHAGE

Hemorrhage in the immediate postoperative period is one of the most important complications of spinal surgery. It may occur with both ventral and dorsal approaches. It may be avoidable if the surgeon pays meticulous attention to hemostasis during the operation.

Hemorrhage may be bony or epidural venous plexus in origin. It can also result from tumor remnants. Bony bleeding can be controlled by bone wax, whereas bleeding from venous plexus may be controlled using Gelfoam or Surgicel. Bleeding from small vessels, however, is controlled by bipolar electrocoagulation. A drain may be considered in cases in which there is an increased risk of hematoma.

NON-NEUROSURGICAL COMPLICATIONS OF VENTRAL SPINAL SURGERY

The most commonly reported postoperative complication of ventral thoracic spine surgery is pulmonary complications, including atelectasis, pneumothorax, hemothorax, and adult respiratory distress syndrome. Perforation of the esophagus, injury of the recurrent laryngeal nerve, Horner's syndrome, and injury of the vertebral artery are the most well-known complications of approaches to the upper thoracic spine. Congestive heart failure or pulmonary edema may occur if fluid replacement is excessive.

Major vessel complications are rare. However, bleeding from intercostal arteries may occur. This may also lead to spinal cord ischemia.

A thoracoabdominal approach may dictate the incision of the diaphragm. It can result in the injury of the phrenic nerve, and in turn, reduced postoperative respiratory reserve.

MEDICAL COMPLICATIONS

As expected the incidence of complications in the elderly is higher than in younger patients. Gastrointestinal, cardiac, pulmonary, deep venous thrombosis, and urinary complications are more common in aged patients. A careful preoperative patient evaluation may reduce the incidence of these complications. In elective cases, the patient's operation should be postponed until medical stability is achieved.

CONCLUSION

The complexity of procedures performed on the spine has greatly increased over the last decade. This, however, has led to a commensurate increase in the number of complications. Spine surgeons should know how to diagnose and treat these problems appropriately.

REFERENCES

1. Alander DH, Stauffer ES. Gelfoam-induced acute quadriparesis after cervical decompression and fusion. Spine 20:970-971, 1995.
2. Broc GG, Crawford NR, Sonntag VKH, Dickman CA. Biomechanical effects of transthoracic microdiscectomy. Spine 22:605-612, 1997.
3. Gill K, Frymoyer JW. The management of treatment failures after decompressive surgery. Surgical alternatives and results. In Frymoyer JW, ed. The Adult Spine: Principles and Practice. New York: Raven Press, 1991, pp 1849-1870.
4. Grimes PF, Vaccaro AR, Garfin SR. Treatment complications of thoracolumbar spine trauma. Semin Spine Surg 7:141-151, 1995.
5. Lonstein JE. Postlaminectomy deformities: Thoracic and lumbar spine. In Bridwell KH, DeWald RL, eds. The Textbook of Spinal Surgery. Philadelphia: Lippincott-Raven, 1997, pp 1055-1075.
6. Massie JB, Heller JG, Abitol JJ, McPherson D, Garfin SR. Postoperative posterior spinal wound infections. Clin Orthop 284:99-107, 1992.
7. McAfee PC, Bohlman HH, Yuan HA. Anterior decompression of traumatic thoracolumbar fractures with incomplete neurological deficit using a retroperitoneal approach. J Bone Joint Surg 67A:89-104, 1985.
8. McAfee PC, Regan JR, Zdeblick T, Zuckerman J, Picetti GD, Heim S, Geis WP, Feder IL. The incidence of complications in endoscopic anterior thoracolumbar spinal reconstructive surgery. A prospective multicenter study comprising first 100 consecutive cases. Spine 20:1624-1632, 1995.
9. Payne DH, Fischgrund JS, Herkowitz HN. Decompression procedures of the thoracolumbar spine. Semin Spine Surg 7:128-136, 1995.
10. Yasuoka S, Peterson HA, Laws ER Jr, MacCarty CS. Pathogenesis and prophylaxis of postlaminectomy deformity of the spine after multiple level laminectomy: Difference between children and adults. Neurosurgery 9:145-154, 1981.

Complications of Spinal Stabilization and Fusion

David M. McKalip, M.D., Bruce Chozik, M.D., and Richard M. Toselli, M.D.

Stabilization and fusion of the thoracic spine require the application of complex hardware in a dynamic environment that has been adversely affected by various pathological processes. Because of this, many unique complications arise. However, clinical experience and basic research over the last two decades have allowed the identification of pathological processes and risk factors that may lead to associated complications. Surgical technique has been refined to avoid many complications in certain settings, and algorithms have been developed to manage complications when they arise. This chapter considers neurological and infectious complications, instrumentation and graft failures, and postoperative deformity and pain associated with thoracic spinal stabilization and fusion.

The goal of thoracic spinal stabilization and fusion should be to re-establish a clinically functional spine. An ideal operation should provide correction of deformities while fixating compromised areas until fusion occurs. In the perfect operation, instrumentation that avoids injury to supporting structures and neural tissues is easily applied and remains secure until fusion occurs. Bone grafts should heal completely without allowing the formation of pseudarthrosis in the fusion bed. The ideal operation allows for patient recovery without infection or postoperative neurological deficits, and provides for long-term correction of deformities without pain. No thoracic

spinal instrumentation and fusion paradigm can be completely free of the risk of complication.

INSTRUMENTATION SYSTEMS

Instrumentation used for fusion and stabilization of the thoracic spine is highly variable. There is no current randomized prospective study comparing different systems for instrumentation and fusion of the thoracic spine for their worth or complication rate. Many of the past studies have included management of lumbar pathology. Thus the analysis of complications arising solely from surgical management of the thoracic spine is presently imperfect.

The classification of thoracic spinal instrumentation systems is difficult because of the many variations used. Systems can be broadly categorized as either ventral or dorsal. The dorsal group has been further classified as pedicle, hook-rod, and rod-wire (cable).[25] Pedicle systems include those that use pedicle screws, even if they also use wires and/or hooks. The universal systems (e.g., Cotrel-Dubousset [CD], Texas Scottish Rite Hospital [TSRH], and Isola) may fit into this group when used with pedicle screws. However, they may also fall into the hook-rod group when used without screws. The Harrington compression and distraction system is similar in this regard. Luque devices, also termed "segmental spinal instrumentation" (SSI), include

621

Luque rectangles and L rods with sublaminar or spinous process wires. Ventral systems include screw-cable, screw-plate, and screw-rod devices.

Another classification scheme describes a system as segmental or nonsegmental, indicating whether a system uses only two (nonsegmental) or multiple (segmental) fixation points. For clarity in this chapter, the ventral and dorsal classification scheme is used.

A meta-analysis of surgical management of thoracolumbar fractures using this classification included data on complications.[25] The authors found no significant difference in the incidence of overall complications between systems. However, the incidence of instrument failure and removal was higher with hook-rod systems, compared with ventral, pedicle, and Luque systems. The Luque systems had a significantly greater incidence of wound complications compared with other devices.

INFECTION

A postoperative infection carries with it a great financial cost and often more than doubles the length of hospitalization.[44] For instance, with Harrington instrumentation of the thoracolumbar spine, an average of 2.5 additional spinal reconstructive surgeries are required in patients with wound infections.[81] The most common site of postoperative infection is the subcutaneous tissue. However, the more serious infections occur in the deep tissues (below fascia), and may involve the instrumentation.

Direct contamination accounts for most infections. However, they may also be due to hematogenous spread to the operative site. Most wound infections are due to *Staphylococcus aureus*. Other causative organisms include beta-hemolytic streptococcus, *Escherichia coli*, and *Pseudomonas*, *Klebsiella*, and *Proteus* species.[39,73,97]

The risk factors (Table 43-1) associated with infections are related to intraoperative and systemic factors. Intraoperative sources for infection can be minimized by observing the basic techniques of wound closure as described by Halsted.[86] These include (1) gentle handling of tissues, (2) sharp anatomical dissection, (3) use of fine sutures, (4) meticulous hemostasis, and (5) removal of foreign bodies, hematoma, and necrotic tissue. The length of surgery can increase the number of bacteria in the wound from 10^2 per gram of tissue at 2.2 hours to 10^5 at 5.7 hours. Although some authors re-

Table 43-1. Risk Factors for Infection

Host	Increased age
	Malnutrition
	Morbid obesity
	Poorly controlled diabetes
	Steroid therapy
	Immunosuppression
	Remote infection
Local	High operations room traffic
	Open operation room doors
	Lack of operations rom air filter and exchange 25×/hour
	Lack of careful scrub technique and clean surgical clothing
	Lack of careful skin preparation and drape
	Failure to follow Halsted's principles of wound closure

Adapted from Heller JG. Postoperative infections of the spine. In Rothman RH, Simeone FA, eds. The Spine. Philadelphia: WB Saunders, 1992, pp 1817-1838

port an increased incidence of postoperative wound infections with 10^5 or more bacteria per gram of tissue,[99] other studies have not correlated length of time of surgery with incidence of postoperative infections.[54,88] Minimizing operating room traffic may also decrease the rate of infection.[75,88]

Systemic illness such as diabetes mellitus, rheumatoid arthritis, renal and liver failure, malnutrition, immune deficiency, and alcohol abuse increase the risk of infection. Instrumentation procedures should be delayed in patients with active preoperative infections, especially in the lungs, skin, and genitourinary tract.

Prophylactic antibiotics significantly decrease the rate of postoperative wound infections after instrumentation.[54,75,88,95] Lonstein et al.[75] reduced the incidence of infectious complications after Harrington instrumentation and fusion from 9.3% to 2.8% with the use of prophylactic antibiotics. When used, the antibiotic should have antistaphylococcal activity (such as cefazolin) and be delivered within 2 hours before skin incision to allow maximal tissue and bone penetration at the time of possible contamination.[10,17] If there is a locally high incidence of methicillin-resistant staphylococcal organisms, vancomycin should be considered for prophylaxis.[84] Arpin-Sypert and Sypert[3] advocate leaving the patient on intravenous antibiotics until drains are removed (if they are used). Antibiotic irrigation can dilute organism number but may not reduce woundbeta infection rate.

Table 43-2. Incidence of Infection Associated With Specific Spinal Instrumentation Systems

Pedicle screw and plate	0.7-6%
Universal	0-13%
TSRH[96]	10%
Hook-rod and Harrington distraction and compression	0-12.5%
Luque[25]/SSI[16]	12.5%/1.2-5.1%
Ventral	0-6.2%

All data as reviewed by Chozik and Toselli,[16] Dickman,[25] and Richardson.[98]

The reported infection rates from various types of instrumentation are shown in Table 43-2. Instrumentation significantly increases the risk of infection, compared with fusion without instrumentation. Infection rates following spinal fusion were 0.9% to 4.6%, compared with 0% to 35% with fusion and instrumentation.[47] Variability among surgeons and reporting techniques prevents defining which instrumentation technique is associated with the lowest incidence of infection based on this literature. The 1994 meta-analysis by Dickman et al.[25] showed an increased rate of infection with Luque instrumentation.

Management of an infection, once it has occurred, varies based on the site of the infection and the status of the patient's spinal stability and degree of fusion. The infection may occur in the wound, possibly extending below the fascia and to the fusion site. Deeper infections may occur in the form of discitis, vertebral osteomyelitis, or epidural abscess. The instrumentation and graft material may be involved with the infection as well.

Wound infections are usually visible on inspection, and may present with fever, erythema, swelling, fluctuantes, pain, and tenderness. Drainage may occur. The erthrocyte sedimentation rate (ESR) is usually elevated, although leukocytosis may not occur. If no purulent collection is palpated, the infection may be amenable to intravenous antibiotics alone. However, the presence of subcutaneous purulence necessitates reopening the wound. If the degree of infection appears extensive, the wound may require debridement in the operating room, where the fascia can be opened if needed. Removal of purulent and necrotic material until bleeding, healthy tissue is evident is required. Infection extending to the fusion site may require removal of loose bone fragments or graft involved in purulent material.[47] Many surgeons advocate leaving instrumentation and bone graft in place to allow for fusion of the spine and to prevent instability, which could lead to further pseudarthroses and infection.[40] After debridement, the wound may be closed over a drain or may be left open for wet-to-dry dressings and gradual granulation and reepithelialization of the wound.

Cultures should be taken, either by needle aspiration of a cellulitic wound or at the time of incision and debridement. Broad-spectrum antibiotics should be modified based on the culture and sensitivity results from the wound culture.

Discitis may occur if the disc space was entered in the course of a ventral or dorsolateral fusion of the thoracic spine. It generally presents with back pain and an elevated ESR. The appearance of disc space destruction on plain radiographs may not be present for weeks to months. However, sequential gallium-67 scans may be valuable regarding the detection of early discitis.[40] A gallium-67 bone scan may differentiate inflammatory and infectious processes from normal postoperative changes detected by technetium-99 scanning. Diagnosis of the offending organism may be accomplished by direct needle aspiration in the lumbar spine, but may prove difficult in the thoracic spine.

The treatment of isolated discitis is usually nonoperative, requiring the long-term administration of antibiotics. However, if the discitis is accompanied by a paraspinal abscess or extensive vertebral osteomyelitis and involvement of the bone graft or fusion, open operative management may be required. The advent of thoracic endoscopic spine procedures may allow diagnosis and treatment without a major operation.[94]

The presence of an epidural abscess after instrumentation and fusion may also require open surgical drainage and possible decompression of the spinal cord. As mentioned above, the decision regarding removal of instrumentation and/or graft material at the time of operation depends on the degree of infectious involvement of the site and consideration of the patient's spinal stability.

NEUROLOGICAL INJURY

Intraoperative injury to the spinal cord or nerve roots may arise due to either mechanical trauma or vascular insult. The incidence and type of injury varies, based on the instrumentation system (Table 43-3) and operation used, but there are common

Table 43-3. Incidence of Neurological Injury Associated With Various Instrumentation Systems Used in the Thoracic (and Lumbar) Spine

Pedicle screw and plate	0-7%
Universal—TSRH[16,98]	0%
Universal—CD	0-1.5%
Hook-rod and Harrington distraction and compression	0-28%
Luque (SSI)	1-17%
Ventral	0-6.3%/(Z-plate 0%)[119]

All data as reviewed by Chozik and Toselli,[16] except by Zdelblick,[123] and by Richardson.[98]

pathways of injury during stabilization and fusion that may account for neurological injury.

Factors associated with intraoperative neurological injury are (1) direct injury to the spinal cord or nerve roots during surgical exposure, (2) inadequate space for placement of instrumentation into the spinal canal, (3) inaccurate anatomic placement of instrumentation, (4) traction of spinal cord or nerve roots, and (5) injury to vascular supply of the spinal cord and nerve roots.

Mechanical trauma may occur at the time of surgical exposure. During subperiosteal dissection, the surgical instruments used may penetrate into the spinal canal or foramen. A patient with a congenital, traumatic, or surgical defect, such as a laminectomy or foraminotomy, is at higher risk for this specific complication. Preoperative imaging with plain radiographs, computed tomography (CT), or magnetic resonance imaging (MRI), and a careful review of previous operative documentation should alert the surgeon of the potential for this complication. Failure to adequately dissect soft tissue from dural structures may lead to accidental injury of dura mater, nerve root, or spinal cord when using rongeurs (i.e., Leksell, Kerrison). High-speed air drills may slip during usage, damaging dural and/or neural elements. This may be avoided by aiming the drill bit away from endangered structures, avoiding excessive pressure on the drill, and protecting structures with metallic instruments (such as a malleable ribbon retractor) when possible. Penetration may be avoided by bracing the hand on the patient's body or another stable structure during dissection. Dural leaks that occur during surgery can be repaired primarily when indicated. If this is not possible or desired, placement of a lumbar drain and maintenance of the patient in a recumbent position postoperatively may decompress the thecal sac and allow primary healing of the dural tear.

Neurological Injury Occurring With Dorsal Instrumentation

Placement of dorsal hardware carries the risk of directly injuring underlying spinal roots, spinal cord, or dura mater. This may occur at the time of operation due to inadequate space to accommodate instrumentation and neural structures (sublaminar wires or hooks), or because of inaccurate placement in or around bony structures (pedicle screws).

Luque and Hook-Rod Systems

Lack of adequate space for placement of instrumentation may lead to neurological injury when placing sublaminar wires or hooks. An acquired or congenitally narrowed spinal canal is associated with an increased risk of neurological injury.[48]

Although some have suggested that thoracic sublaminar hooks should be used only in the presence of complete myelopathy or below T11,[4] steps can be taken to extend their use to neurologically intact patients at higher thoracic spine levels. Adequate preparation of the surgical bed can avoid penetration of sublaminar hooks into the spinal canal and possible spinal cord compression. This includes assuring that the hook is apposed to the undersurface of the lamina and placed laterally. Stripping of ligamentum flavum from the lamina is nearly always necessary for this. Furthermore, the lamina must be inspected for its strength and ability to support a hook.

The use of doubled 18- or 20-gauge wires instead of the usual 16-gauge wire may decrease the risk of neurological injury.[64] Based on a cadaver study, Goll et al.[43] recommend that during sublaminar wire passage the wire tip should be bent as little as possible (<45 degrees), and the radius of the curvature of the wire should be as large as possible to allow for easy passage. The wire is bent 45 degrees around the lamina, wrapping twice around the dorsal aspect of the lamina. Wires passed centrally were less likely to penetrate into the foramen and removal of the spinous process decreased depth of penetration by allowing a more central passage. Rods secured with the wire should be precisely contoured to allow them to rest directly on the lamina, avoiding migration of the wire into the spinal canal. The introduction of soft spinal cables may significantly reduce the complications seen with wire passage.

Removal of sublaminar wires may also place a patient at risk for neurological injury. Nicastro et al.[92] noted that removal of double and single wire from cadaver spines led to a greater than 25% compression of the thecal sac during removal of 27% of the wires. They recommended avoiding winding the wire on a wire extractor because it produced the most erratic pathway of the wire in the spinal canal. Use of a wire extraction guide resulted in the least amount of thecal compression. Before removal, the wires should be cut as close to the lamina as possible to minimize the course of the wire through the spinal canal. Double wires, when untwisted, should be pulled out separately.

Pedicle Screws

The placement of pedicle screws requires precise localization of the target trajectory to ensure that the screw remains in the pedicle. Otherwise, the screw may break through the pedicle, causing damage to the nerve root. The reported incidence of placement of pedicle screws outside the desired pedicle ranges from 1.2% to 28.8%.[67,117] However, the incidence of neurological injury after pedicle screw-plate fixation is 0% to 7% in the thoracolumbar and lumbar spine.[15,26,72,74,76,100] Thus neurological injury associated with these complications is low despite possible instrument failure, inaccurate screw placement, or vertebral body penetration. In fact, the reported incidence of instrumentation failure with pedicle screws was found to be 7% in a recent large evaluation of pedicle screws for thoracic, lumbar, and sacral spinal fusions. However, the rate of neurological injuries in this group of patients was less than 0.5%.[122]

Detailed knowledge of pedicle anatomy at each level of the spine, as well as the use of intraoperative imaging techniques, can minimize the risks of improper placement of pedicle screws. Intraoperative computer-assisted image guidance may minimize the risk of misplacement.[93] However, the use of an intraoperative image intensifier does not guarantee accurate screw placement.[33,114] Insertion of screws just lateral to the superior articular process, at a point met by a line bisecting the transverse process, produces a high rate of accuracy for screw placement in the pedicle. Screws placed slightly laterally and rostrally in the pedicle are less likely to damage neural elements.[117]

Pedicle dimensions vary and must be considered before screw insertion. Angles of insertion greater than 15 degrees above T12 result in spinal canal encroachment unless the entry point is more lateral than usual.[42] In addition to entry point and angle of insertion, the width of the pedicle isthmus is another key parameter in correct pedicle screw placement. A narrow isthmus reduces the margin of error for the angle of insertion and entry point. This is reflected by the low incidence of penetration of the medial cortex of the pedicle by screws placed in the lower lumbar spine, where pedicle isthmus widths are greatest.[42]

On postoperative CT scans, Gertbein and Robbins[42] assessed the accuracy of pedicle screw placement in 40 consecutive patients treated with the AO fixateur interne. Eighty-one percent of screws penetrated less than or equal to 2.0 mm beyond the medial border of the pedicle, whereas 9% and 6% of screws penetrated 2.1 to 4.0 mm and 4.1 to 8.0 mm, respectively, into the spinal canal. Twenty-five percent of patients in the latter group developed signs of nerve root irritation that spontaneously resolved. Because the epidural and subarachnoid spaces are each approximately 2 mm in depth from T10 to L4, 90% of screws were placed within a theoretically safe zone.

Neurological and Other Complications With Ventral Instrumentation

Many of the complications associated with placement of ventral instrumentation are related to the process of the approach itself. The transthoracic approach to the spine may require resection of a rib to allow exposure. It is important that the resected rib not be too low, lest the surgeon be limited in working in an upward direction on the spine. Resecting the rib above the lesion allows for an easier dissection.[113] Care must be taken to avoid injury to the intercostal nerve and artery and underlying parietal pleura. The intercostal neurovascular complex may be protected by working on the rostral surface of the rib. Should damage to the vasculature occur, electrocautery, direct pressure, or suture ties should allow for control of bleeding. Adhesions of the parietal pleura to the visceral pleura may lead to injury to the underlying lung during rib resection. Care must be taken to directly visualize such adhesions and to lyse them. A tube thoracostomy may be required if the pleura has been compromised during the case and cannot be repaired easily. Obtaining a postoperative chest radiograph is essential to rule out pneumo- and hemothorax. Cohen and McAfee[18] advocate obtaining this radiograph in the operating room so that a tube thoracostomy can be placed before the patient awakens from anesthesia, should it be necessary. They also recommend filling the thoracic cavity with irrigant and performing a Valsalva maneuver to check for air leaks. The most common pulmonary complication usually associated with transthoracic approaches to the spine appears to be atelectasis of the contralateral lung secondary to patient position.

When approaching the lower thoracic spine or thoracolumbar junction, the diaphragm may need to be incised to allow exposure. Tags can be placed to allow for accurate reapproximation of the diaphragm at the end of the procedure. A complete diaphragmatic repair is necessary to avoid a hiatal hernia or postoperative atelectasis.[18] McAfee et al.[82] states that by approaching the thoracolumbar junction at T11 with an extrapleural, retroperitoneal approach, the diaphragm need not be resected, thus avoiding the possible complications of that maneuver. If the iliopsoas muscle is to be retracted, the genitofemoral nerve (arising at L1 and L2) should be visualized to avoid injury.

After the lung has been retracted and the spine exposed, the great vessels of the thorax are encountered. Care must be taken when dissecting these structures from the spine to avoid excessive bleeding or irreversible vascular damage. If approaching from the left, the thoracic aorta presents on the ventrolateral portion of the spine, beginning at T4 retropleurally. Nine sets of segmental vessels (from T3 to T12) typically arise from the aorta and pass retropleurally over the midportion of the vertebral bodies, becoming the intercostal arteries distally. Damage to these segmental vessels can lead to excessive bleeding. If approaching from the right side, the major vascular structure visualized is the azygous vein, ascending from the L1 to L2 level to empty into the superior vena cava at about T4. The hemiazygous vein ascends from the left thoracolumbar junction and crosses to the right at about

T9. The segmental vessels are also present over the middle of the vertebral body.

As they pass from the vertebral bodies, the segmental arteries provide a radicular artery at each nerve root. However, only a few of these arteries contribute to spinal cord blood supply in the thoracic spine. The anterior spinal artery receives contributions from the radicular arteries, chiefly at T4 or T5, and the artery of Adamkiewicz. The latter artery typically arises between T8 and L2 (85%), but may arise from T5 to T12 (15%), and is located on the left 80% of the time.[43]

The transthoracic approach may require the sacrifice of segmental vessels over several vertebral levels to expose the spine. If one of the segmental vessels taken also supplies the spinal cord at T4 or T5 or via the artery of Adamkiewicz, the spinal cord may be placed at risk for infarction. The incidence of spinal cord injury from unilateral disruption of unnamed segmental vessels is reportedly very low.[104] Only one case of vascular infarction out of 412 ventral approaches for tuberculosis occurred in one series.[53] Controversy exists over the necessity for preoperative angiographic localization of arteries supplying the spinal cord[31,36,61,63] because the angiography itself may induce a spinal cord infarction, and the outcome from taking a named artery itself is not clear. When the segmental vessels are to be taken, they should be ligated near the midportion of the vertebral body[21] to avoid damaging the aorta and to prevent disruption of collateral flow to the spinal cord.

Ventral instrumentation hardware itself may cause vascular or neurological injury. When placing screws through the vertebral body, care must be taken to avoid overpenetration through the body into the opposite thoracic cavity. This could result in the injury of great vessels and subsequent hemorrhage. The planning of the final placement of the instrumentation is also critical to avoid direct contact of metallic and vascular structures. This can lead to erosion through vessels. Screws should be placed parallel to the posterior longitudinal ligament to avoid penetration into the spinal canal. These rules apply to both the Kaneda and Z-plate systems. When placing the plate portion of the Kaneda system, the spike on the plate must not be seated in disc space. This may lead to postoperative slippage of the plate, possibly into the spinal canal.

Management of Immediate Postoperative Neurological Deficits

If the patient displays a new postoperative deficit upon awakening from an instrumentation procedure, prompt evaluation and possible reoperation are indicated. The goal of the workup should be to rule out correctable causes of the deficit. Compression of the spinal cord may arise from hematoma or slipped instrumentation or graft as well as from remnants of disc, fractured bone, or tumor. Spinal cord traction from overcorrection of deformities may also occur. Postoperative plain radiography, CT-myelography, and MRI (if metallic instrumentation permits) assists with diagnosis.

Some authors advocate early removal of instrumentation in those patients with complete neurological deficits.[115] Patients undergoing Luque instrumentation for correction of scoliosis may experience postoperative paraplegia due to spinal cord ischemia. Performing a Stagnara wake-up test in the operating room after instrumentation, but before closing, may allow for earlier detection of those patients with neurological deterioration due to this problem.[112]

Overdistraction with Harrington rods, or other dorsal rodding systems, may lead to disruption of the anterior and posterior longitudinal ligaments, possibly leading to disc herniation or migration of fractured bone into the spinal cord.[51]

If postoperative imaging reveals spinal cord compression from any mechanism, rapid return to the operating room may enable complete correction of the neurological deficits. If hematoma is present, identification of the arterial or venous bleeding site is essential. Placement of a drain should be considered. Postoperative epidural hematomas after screw fixation due to epidural bleeding after penetration of the pedicular cortex have been reported.[33]

INSTRUMENTATION FAILURE

In their meta-analysis of fixation of thoracolumbar spine fractures, Dickman et al.[25] defined several categories related to the failure of instrumentation. These can be summarized as (1) breakage or bending of a rod, plate, screw, hook, or wire, (2) loss of fixation or attachment of device components from bone or from the longitudinal member (i.e., hardware dislodging from bone, stripping bone, slipping on rods),

Table 43-4. Rates of Instrumentation Failure as Reported in the Literature

Pedicle screw and plate	0.8-28.8%
Universal instrumentation	0-3%
Hook-rod and Harrington distraction and compression	6.2-27%
Luque/SSI	3.8-8.0%
Ventral	Kaneda 0-8%
	Zielke 0-33%
	Z-plate 0%[119]

Meta-analysis of instrumentation failure by Dickman[25] found a significantly higher rate for hook-rod systems.
All data as reviewed by Chozik and Toselli[16] except Zdeblick.[125]

and (3) fracture of bony components of the host-device junction, including intraoperative pedicle fracture or breakout, penetration of ventral cortex of the vertebral body, or lamina fracture from a hook or sublaminar wire.

Instrumentation failure can result in inadequate fusion and possible pseudarthrosis formation, mechanical pain, and neurological and vascular injury. However, it may also be asymptomatic, discovered only radiographically. In addition, failure of instrumentation, or incorrect initial placement of instrumentation, may result in failure to adequately correct a preoperative deformity or in the formation of a progressive postoperative deformity. Any of these complications may require revision or removal of hardware and/or graft material. The instrumentation failure rates of various systems are shown in Table 43-4.

Instrumentation Failure With Dorsal Systems

The 1994 meta-analysis of fixation of thoracolumbar fractures by Dickman et al.[25] found a significantly greater incidence of loss of fixation (9.5% vs. 5.3% weighted proportions) and removal of hardware (9.7% vs. 4.0%) in the hook-rod instrumentation group, compared with the pedicle group, respectively. Furthermore, fusion rates were significantly lower in the hook-rod system, compared with the pedicle group (96.9% vs. 99.4%, respectively). However, there was no difference in the incidence of pain or functional outcomes between groups.

Harrington Distraction and Compression Instrumentation

The incidence of hook migration or rod fracture for Harrington instrumentation of the thoracic and lumbar spine is reported to be 6.2% to 27%.[2,8,19,26,38,41,58,121] Spine injury may remove some of the counterforce needed to keep laminae in the hooks of distraction rods.[56,57] The most common site of implant failure is the bone-metal junction of the rostral hook and lamina, due to hook cutout[81] perhaps due to the gradual resorption and remodeling of bone that occurs with movement.[8] Lack of rotational control may also lead to distal hook dislodgment. Proximal hook dislodgment may occur if less than 1 cm of rod is left beyond the hook.[21]

Rod fracture with the Harrington system occurs most commonly at the ratchet-shaft junction, where the rod undergoes a 25% decrease in cross-sectional area. This results in stress concentration that may surpass the fatigue limit of the rod.[13,20,96] Rod fracture is most likely to occur between 18 to 72 months postoperatively, and is significantly associated with pseudarthrosis,[30] which occurs in 0% to 13% of patients with thoracic and lumbar fractures treated with Harrington instrumentation.[19,26,38,41,58]

Cross-linking rods together decreases the incidence of hook displacement. Placement of the ratchet-shaft junction as close to the hook as possible minimizes the moment arm and decreases stress on the rod.[20] Distraction rods with concomitant bone grafts have a significantly lower rate of rod fracture than ungrafted rods.[32]

Osteoporosis predisposes to hook cutout due to fractures of laminae and pedicles.[46] Therefore an orthotic support should be worn in osteoporotic patients postoperatively.

Universal Instrumentation

Hook loosening and screw and rod breakage occur rarely with CD instrumentation. A significant rate of pedicle hook placement outside the intended pedicle is reported with CD instrumentation, but is rarely associated with instability. The distance between the tines of the pedicle hook is smaller than the transverse diameter of the typical thoracic pedicle, which makes it difficult to determine when the hood is situated in proper position. Furthermore, the manipulation involved in threading the rod through the hooks may cause unrecognized minor displacement of the pedicle hooks. The reported incidence of pseudarthrosis with CD instrumentation is 0% to 1.5%[35,84,91] (some using pedicle screws).

Benzel, Kesterson, and Marchand[7] found no instances of instrumentation failure, dislodgment, postoperative instability, or pseudarthrosis among 28 patients with thoracic and lumbar fractures stabilized with TSRH instrumentation over a 9-month follow-up period. However, when used for correction of adolescent idiopathic scoliosis in 103 patients, three patients experienced a lower hook dislodgment over a follow-up period of at least 2 years.[98]

Pedicle Screws

The addition of pedicle screws to instrumentation systems has improved the fusion rate compared with systems using hooks and rods alone.[25] However, failures may occur and are etiologically related to three factors: (1) excessive preload forces introduced at the time of surgery,[6] (2) limitations caused by the size and orientation of the pedicles,[6] and (3) excessive flexion and axial loading, particularly in the lower-thoracic and upper lumbar regions.[50]

Screw bending during operative placement weakens the screw structurally. Minimizing excessive force on screws during placement can minimize risk of screw bending or breakage.[90]

The largest fully-threaded screw that can be safely accommodated by a pedicle should be used to increase resistance to breakage and pullout.[125] Screws with a diameter of 6.5 mm are significantly stronger than 4.5 mm screws.[125]

Gurr and McAfee[46] report a 3% incidence of 5 mm CD pedicle screws bending at the upper thread-shank junction, although all patients achieved a stable fusion. They now recommend using 6 mm pedicle screws. Because of the desire for larger screws, the mid- and upper thoracic pedicles have been viewed as suboptimal locations for screw placement because of their smaller size.[110,111] Pedicle morphology and size varies based on age, gender, and race.[55] Generally, the transverse diameter of the thoracic pedicle measures a minimum of 4.5 to 5 mm at T4 and increases to 7.8 mm at T12.[110,124]

The biomechanics of most of the thoracic spine differs from that occurring in the thoracolumbar junction, where the natural kyphosis converts to lordosis and the ribs become deficient as a stabilizing agent.[62] Thus the instrumentation failures associated with each of these regions may also differ.

Much of the data related to instrumentation failure of pedicle screws are based on the management of lumbar[23,76,79,83,110,117,126] or thoracolumbar pathology.[22,33,72,85,102] Mid- and upper thoracic use of pedicle screws has been described in the management of idiopathic scoliosis[108,109] and thoracic spine fractures,[101] as described below.

In the thoracolumbar, lumbar, and lumbosacral spine, the reported incidence of screw breakage is 0.8% to 24.6%. It occurs most commonly at the thoracolumbar junction.[22,23,33,72,76,79,83,100,102,116,126] In pedicle screw-plate systems, more commonly used in the lumbar spine, the rigid fixation of the screws to plates may predispose to screw breakage due to the lack of micromotion.[79] Screw breakage or bending typically occurs at the junction of the uppermost thread and collar,[83] and has a higher incidence in patients undergoing major reductions and multilevel fusions.[23,83] It more often occurs in the most rostral screws in multilevel fusions and the distal screws in single-level fusions.[79] Pseudarthrosis may lead to screw breakage before full fusion, and late breakage (after fusion) can be related to renewed spinal mobility.[15,23,76,100] Late pedicle screw breakage or bending may be avoided by removal of the plate when fusion has occurred.[100]

Screw bending or breakage occurs most frequently at the thoracolumbar junction because compressive forces act more ventrally.[15] Krag[67] suggests extending segmental pedicle fixation to two levels above the fracture to avoid implant failure for thoracolumbar fractures. Also, severe comminution of the ventral vertebral column under a plated segment places severe stresses on pedicle screws and can lead to rapid fatigue failure. For the treatment of thoracolumbar fractures with dorsal plates in the presence of ventral-column compromise, a supplementary ventral arthrodesis is recommended.[118]

Pedicle screws should be correctly positioned in relation to the plate or rod. To avoid unidirectional torque that can cause screw weakening, pedicle erosion or fracture, and excessive vertebral tilt, nut tightening should be performed when screws are set in a position 90 degrees in relation to a plate.[106,126] From a practical standpoint, this is rarely obtained because a deviation of at least 5 degrees in the sagittal and transverse screw angles usually exists at all levels.[79] With rigid plates, it is often difficult to obtain proper contour in order to achieve a screw-plate angle of 90 degrees at all levels. The use of variable-angled screws in such universal systems as the Isola

and TSRH systems may avoid this problem in the thoracic spine.

In lumbar and thoracolumbar series, screw bending or breakage was most likely to occur within 24 months of instrumentation insertion[83] and reoperation was required in up to 68% of cases in one series where this occurred.[126] In a 1991 survivorship analysis of pedicle screw systems, McAfee, Weiland, and Carlow[83] found a 16% probability of screw bending or breakage within 24 months of surgery, vs. less than a 2% chance after 24 months.

In the thoracic spine, it may be that the added support of the rib cage prevents excessive axial or flexion loading on screws and screw-rod or screw-plate junctions. When pedicle screws were used with the CD system for correction of idiopathic scoliosis of the thoracic spine, no breakages were reported.[108,109] Twenty-four patients who underwent segmental spinal instrumentation using pedicle screws only, with the highest vertebrae instrumented reported to be T3, were followed for at least 2 years. Each patient received an average of 7.1 screws and had an average of 8.2 segments fused. Although there were no breakages, 13 screws (3%) were malpositioned, but no neurological complications were reported. Roy-Camille, Saillant, and Mazel[101] reported on 40 patients who underwent fixation of thoracic spinal fractures using a pedicle screw-plate system. They reported no incidences of screw bending or breakage or malpositions, but the reporting on specific complications and patient demographics was incomplete.

Screw loosening is unusual, occurring in 0% to 2.2% of cases of pedicle screw-plate instrumentation of the lumbar spine.[76,83,100] Screw loosening often is indicative of a fusion defect. It is caused by inhibition of bone formation and remodeling of dead bone induced by movement between screw threads and bone, and appears as a lucence around the screw. Screw pullout strength is greater in fully-threaded screws. A linear correlation exists between screw pullout strength and bone mineral density.[120,125] Nut loosening, which occurs in up to 56% of pedicle screw-plate procedures, is a cause of loss of reduction.[23,33]

Sublaminar Wires

Overall, implant failure is reported in 3.8% to 8.0% of patients undergoing segmental spinal instrumentation with Luque systems.[71,77] Migration of sublaminar wires can cause L-shaped rods to rotate and lead to prominence of the rod tip below the skin.[2,71] Rod rotation occurs more often in short-instrumented segments and is less likely when the instrumentation spans several segments and the rods are contoured in the sagittal plane.[64] The use of a square rod also prevents this complication.[71]

The reported incidence of wire breakage with Luque systems used for thoracic and lumbar fractures is 8.3%.[24] Wire breakage is a cause of progressive deformity and late neurological deterioration.[9] When wires break early after surgery, it is usually due to the use of wire of insufficient strength or improper technique during tightening.[64] Proper technique includes avoiding kinks and square knots, which decrease the strength of wire by 25%. Furthermore, wire should not be twisted to approximate the rod to the lamina.[64] The risk of wire breakage is increased when quarter-inch rods are used, due to their stiffness, and occurs most commonly at the ends of the implant, especially at the rostral wire, due to flexion bending.[64] However, quarter-inch rods are recommended when severe loading occurs, as in fractures and kyphosis, despite an increased risk of wire breakage.[64]

Late wire failure is caused by repeated cyclical loads at the most proximal or distal ends of the double L construct.[9] The presence of broken wires should alert the physician to a pseudarthrosis. If fusion does not occur, implant failure can occur due to cyclical loading of the wires. The breakage of a single wire predisposes to additional wire fractures and recurrent deformity. Also, sliding of wires on rods is an important cause of late collapse of fracture sites with Luque instrumentation.[37]

The reported incidence of pseudarthrosis with SSI is between 1% and 6%.[71,77] The pseudarthrosis rate is higher in fusions of the spine from T12 to the sacrum when postoperative bracing is not used, predominantly due to wire breakage, compared with fusions at higher levels.[69] Rod fracture is usually indicative of pseudarthrosis. Excessive intraoperative contouring also increases the likelihood of rod fracture.

Instrumentation Failure With Ventral Systems

As with most thoracic stabilization and fusion procedures there are few well-controlled, randomized studies that compare outcomes from various ventral instrumentation systems. Many reports give the incidence of complications in their series, but such studies must be considered carefully given their limitations.

Dickman et al.[25] reported an incidence of 6.2% and 8.4% for ventral rod/plate or screw fractures, respectively, in their 1994 meta-analysis of thoracic and lumbar instrumentation. However, the incidence of complications secondary to this is not clear, and instrumentation revision rates and actual loss of fixation were not reported in the original papers.

Kostiuk[66] reported a 12% incidence of screw breakage using the ventral Kostiuk-Harrington instrumentation for the treatment of various kyphotic deformities. Among 100 patients with burst fractures, four developed nonunion, two of whom had severe dorsal column comminution. In the case of dorsal column comminution or instability, second stage dorsal instrumentation is recommended.

The reported incidence of pseudarthrosis in thoracic and lumbar fractures treated with Kaneda instrumentation is 0% to 8.9%; the use of a transverse fixator reduces the pseudarthrosis rate.[59,60] No adverse sequelae have been reported when the spike of the vertebral plate is inserted in the disc space.[59] Similarly, no cases of implant failure have been reported with Kaneda instrumentation.[59]

The reported incidence of pseudarthrosis in thoracic and lumbar fractures treated with Zielke instrumentation is 33%.[60] Zielke instrumentation, with its two small threaded rods, does not eliminate the instability between the vertebrae above and below the injured segment.

Dunn[28] reported a 6.2% incidence of pseudarthrosis with Dunn instrumentation spanning a single level above and below the level of thoracic and lumbar fractures. Kostiuk[65] reports a 50% incidence of pseudarthrosis in the treatment of thoracic and lumbar fractures with narrow AO plates.

Vertebral body fractures can occur intraoperatively in the presence of osteoporotic bone. The use of bone cement in osteoporotic vertebral bodies is recommended.[66]

Zdeblick[123] reported no instrumentation failures in 68 Z-plate placements with short follow-up. Ensuring placement into the opposite bony cortex should prevent most of these complications.

SPINAL DEFORMITY

One goal of instrumentation and fusion of the spine is to prevent or correct spinal deformities. One also endeavors to ensure that no deformity is introduced by the application of instrumentation (for instance, flat back syndrome in the lumbar spine). However, spinal deformities may fail to be adequately corrected at the time of surgery, may occur early after surgery, or may appear in the late postoperative period. The causes are many, and are related to the timing of the occurrence of the deformity.

Abnormal kyphosis is the most common postoperative deformity of the thoracic spine and is considered pathological if the curvature approaches greater than 50 degrees and there are symptoms associated with the curvature. Division or removal of costovertebral articulations or supporting ligaments or joints, or ventral decompressive surgery, may lead to instability. These must all be considered when selecting the appropriate instrumentation and fusion paradigm.

Perioperative Deformity

The failure to adequately correct a deformity during an operation may occur from improper application of instrumentation, limitations imposed by the deformity, or use of an inappropriate instrumentation system or operative approach to the problem at hand. The latter is more common and may occur if the surgeon fails to understand the underlying biomechanical pathology of the diseased spine to be instrumented and fused. These principles and the indications for the various approaches are described elsewhere in this book, but a few generalizations may be made.

When determining the appropriate instrumentation and operative approach, the integrity of each of three columns of the spine must be considered: ventral, middle, and dorsal.[24,62] In the thoracic spine, the application of long dorsal implants with fixation via hooks or screws and fusion over a short segment is adequate for most forms of instability. Although short segment stabilization may be desired in some cases to prevent long-term complications, the thoracic spine often requires a long lever arm to achieve the force necessary for correction.[6] However, in cases of ventral and middle column disease, a ventral screw-plate construct and strut graft may be required to correct the initial deformity and assure long-term stability.

Postoperative Deformity

Deformities occurring immediately postoperatively or early after the operation may occur due to failure of instrumentation or load-bearing grafts, or fracture of associated bone. The same factors leading to a failure to correct a deformity can also cause an early postoperative deformity, namely, an inappropriate instrumentation paradigm for the pathology. A late deformity often indicates that a pseudarthrosis has weakened the instrumentation to a point of failure.

Dorsal Constructs

Universal Instrumentation. McLain, Sparling, and Benson[85] report a 19% incidence of early (1 to 6 months) failure of CD short segment pedicle screw instrumentation for the management of thoracolumbar fractures. Their definition of failure included an increase in kyphosis of at least 10 degrees. Their patients all wore customized TLSO braces for 6 months postoperatively. They noted a nonstatistical correlation of progressive kyphosis with failure to treat ventral instability and prestressing of screws occurring with in situ contouring of rods. Seven of the 10 failed patients experienced bent or broken screws.

Others have reported that the loss of correction of the angle of deformity in thoracic and lumbar fractures stabilized with CD instrumentation ranges from 0 to 3.6 degrees, whereas the loss of reduction of retropulsed bone fragments varies from 0 to 0.9 mm.[34,84,91] Despite an initially satisfactory correction of the kyphosis due to thoracic and lumbar fractures, a significant loss of correction is often apparent at follow-up.[22,74,102] Most patients with loss of correction of posttraumatic kyphotic angles achieve a solid fusion, however. After thoracic and lumbar fractures, this loss of correction occurs frequently at the level of the upper disc space, which is usually disrupted and overdistracted at the time of reduction.[74] It is not known if inability to maintain complete postoperative correction of traumatic kyphosis is clinically significant.

In the management of adolescent idiopathic scoliosis, the use of pedicle screws appears to offer better maintenance of correction than hook-rod systems alone. After a minimum of 2 years follow-up, Suk et al.[109] reported a 6% loss of correction in 31 patients managed with hooks alone, vs. a 1% loss in those managed with pedicle screws in a segmental fashion. Richards et al.[98] report an average 14% loss of scoliosis correction in patients managed with the TSRH system using hooks alone. Of the 103 patients reported, two required repeat operation for loss of correction, one due to the crankshaft phenomenon. The crankshaft phenomenon describes a progressive postoperative increase in the scoliotic deformity after dorsal spinal fusion.[27] It is thought to occur in fused patients who are skeletally immature and experience continued ventral growth after a dorsal fusion. It is suggested that ventral fusion in high-risk patients should be done at the time of dorsal fusion to prevent this.[68]

Luque or Segmental Spinal Instrumentation (SSI). If the length of instrumentation is too short, kyphosis can occur above an immobilized segment, after the placement of Luque rods. It is believed that, at the junction of a mobile and immobile segment, stress can cause ligament weakening that is exacerbated by unnecessary muscle stripping and ligament removal.[64]

The reported loss of correction of nontraumatic scoliotic and kyphotic curves with SSI ranges from 1 to 6 degrees.[49,50,77] After thoracic and lumbar fractures, Aebi et al.[2] report loss of reduction and unsatisfactory correction in 57% of patients treated with SSI, suggesting it to be an unreliable construct for the stabilization of thoracic and lumbar fractures when used alone. Leatherman et al.[71] recommend supplementation of SSI with a ventral arthrodesis in the case of vertebral body fractures with greater than 50% loss of height and in the presence of angular deformities between T8 and L3 to avoid late vertebral collapse, although this is controversial.

When anatomical curves are lost in the thoracic spine, complications can result. Flattening of the thoracolumbar spine is a cause of the flat back syndrome, abnormalities of gait and posture, and pain.[89] A progressive loss of vital capacity has been reported in patients with thoracic fusions.[76]

Ventral Constructs

Postoperative deformity after ventral surgery typically is manifested as kyphosis. However, if concomitant dorsal instability is present and untreated, subluxation can occur. Asymmetrical placement of a strut graft after decompression can also lead to scoliosis. Deformity usually results from inadequate ventral column support after decompression, instrumentation or graft failure, pseudarthrosis and nonunion, or from inappropriate management of a concomitant dorsal instability. Pseudarthrosis and

nonunion rates for various ventral systems were described earlier.

Kaneda, Abumi, and Fujiya[60] report an average loss of correction of 2 degrees with fractures at T12 to L2, and no loss of correction with fractures of L3 and L4, using Kaneda instrumentation. Zdeblick[123] noted no progressive deformities following Z-plate application, however, follow-up is short and specific indications are not reported. Patients with failure of ventral systems rarely require repeat ventral exposure and can usually be managed with dorsal instrumentation and fusion.[18]

GRAFT FAILURES

Bone graft failures can manifest as a loss of integrity of the graft or as a lack of fusion. The former is more likely to occur early, before expected fusion. The latter usually presents in the late postoperative course.

Pseudarthrosis

When fusion does not occur, a pseudarthrosis forms in the fusion bed. Pseudarthrosis has been defined as the failure of a solid fusion 1 year after operation.[107] The rates of pseudarthrosis associated with various instrumentation strategies were described earlier. Failure of a fusion mass to form may be due to inadequate instrumentation or external bracing to support the spine. If this is the case, constant motion in the graft bed may prevent fusion. This often manifests itself as instrumentation failure, because most systems are designed to serve as temporary internal fixators while fusion occurs, and are not meant to tolerate continuous, lifelong stress. Patients with underlying metabolic abnormalities[107] or who smoke cigarettes[12] are also at increased risk for pseudarthrosis.

Not all pseudarthrosis is preventable, but attention to certain principles should minimize the risk. As mentioned, internal and external fixation must support most of the load until fusion occurs. Surfaces to be used for fusion must be meticulously prepared to provide sufficient surface area of decorticated host bone and a rich vascular supply. The best choice for graft material has been argued in the literature, but the surgeon should at the least ensure that an adequate amount of material is used in the graft.

Pseudarthrosis can present with pain, loss of correction and failed instrumentation. However, its diagnosis may not be readily apparent radiographically if instrumentation failure has not occurred. Plain radiographs, CT, MRI, or tomography have been used, but can routinely miss pseudarthrosis.[107] Tomograms and dynamic studies such as flexion-extension radiographs may prove more useful. Steinman and Herkowitz[107] outline five criteria for diagnosing pseudarthrosis: (1) lack of trabecular bone continuity from one end of the fusion to the other, (2) collapse of graft height with a gap present between vertebral end plate and the bone graft, (3) shift in position of the graft after expected healing was to have occurred, (4) loss of fixation through dislodgment or fractures of the rods, screws, or hooks after expected healing was to have occurred, and (5) unexplained pain occurring in the area of fusion. On flexion-extension lateral radiographs, 4 mm of motion or 10 degrees or more of angular motion suggest development of pseudarthrosis.

Surgical management of a symptomatic spinal pseudarthrosis may involve removal of overlying instrumentation, takedown of nonfused graft, decortication, and replacement of graft and instrumentation. A ventral operation may be required in some patients with dorsal failure and vice versa with ventral failures, possibly in two stages.[107]

Mechanical Failures

Bone grafts face risks of mechanical failure, especially when placed as a load-bearing component. This is most typical of ventral strut grafts, which must bear a significant amount of compressive load in the thoracic spine, particularly at the more caudal levels. If they are improperly placed, or when used in an inappropriate situation, they may fracture, collapse, or extrude. Various graft material may offer distinct advantages in grafting, however, no statistically powerful, prospective study has evaluated the mechanical stability of these grafts in patients.

The rib is a convenient autograft for ventral thoracic procedures, but should be limited to short segments due to relative weakness compared to other sources.[34] Meding and Stambough[87] compared autologous iliac crest, fibula, and rib to fibular allograft ventral strut grafts in 52 patients and found no difference in rates of graft extrusion or early failures.

Although the number of patients studied was too small to reach statistical significance, the only early fracture of a graft occurred in autologous iliac crest within 2 days due to a noncompliant patient walking. Butterman, Glazer, and Bradford[14] reviewed the use of ventral strut grafts in the thoracolumbar spine and found no difference between graft materials. These materials included allograft (some frozen) rib, iliac crest, fibula, tibia, and femoral cortical rings, and autologous iliac crest, rib, and fibula. Some grafts were supplemented with allograft or autologous cancellous bone. The incidence of fracture, dislodgment, or extrusion of ventral strut grafts was 0% to 3%. The high variability of the management methods makes such comparisons difficult to interpret. These studies have yet to be fully analyzed in a peer-review format.

In the authors' experience, avoiding mechanical failure of bony grafts occurs best by careful consideration of the pathological process at hand. Cases of combined ventral and dorsal column instability treated with ventral strut and plate alone have a high risk of early failure if a dorsal stabilization is also not performed.[11] When placing fibular strut grafts, the status of the host bone should be carefully evaluated to ensure that the graft does not piston into the surrounding vertebrae when faced with high compressive loads. Again, supplementary dorsal instrumentation may be required to avoid this.

PAIN

Pain after thoracic instrumentation and fusion may be mechanically due to instrumentation or due to postoperative deformity. With all systems, painful bursae can form under the skin if the implant protrudes. This can occur after rod rotation to a point where skin is tented. Similarly, the cut ends of wires may rotate into a vertical position under the skin and cause discomfort.

After Harrington instrumentation, the reported incidence of pain is 2.5% to 34%.[2,8,19,26,38,121] The causes of pain after Harrington instrumentation include direct irritation by the implant, pseudarthrosis, angular deformity, and nonanatomical reduction. Postoperative pain correlates with the initial degree of angular deformity postoperatively and not with the average initial and final angles of deformity. Gertzbein, MacMichael, and Tile[41] observed pain in 13 of 14 patients with an unsatisfactory postoperative alignment, whereas 12 of 13 patients with anatomical reduction had no pain. Aebi et al.[2] found that in more than two thirds of patients with persistent postoperative pain, anatomical reduction was not achieved.

Harrington instrumentation requires the fusion of at least two intact vertebrae above and below the injured vertebra. Consequently, a minimum of five vertebral bodies and four motion segments of the spine are fused. Every fused segment in the lumbar spine contributes to stiffness. The incidence of lumbar rigidity and pain increases with descending lower hook level.[1] Rod removal may be necessary because of excessive stiffness.[8] Pain after universal instrumentation is due to either direct irritation by the implant or the loss of anatomical curves. The reported incidence is 0% to 33%.[7,84,91] Hooks placed beyond the extent of the fusion can increase the incidence of pain, which usually resolves with implant removal.[7]

Up to 10% of patients experience mechanical discomfort after placement of pedicle screw-plate systems. A limited osteosynthesis with the use of a plaster cast postoperatively to prevent kyphosis has been employed to decrease stiffness.[72]

CONCLUSION

As with all operations, thoracic spinal stabilization and fusion carries the risk of complications. Common complications fall into the categories of infection, neurological injury, instrumentation and graft failure, spinal deformity, and pain. There is a variety of ventral, dorsal, segmental, and nonsegmental spinal stabilization systems. Each carries with it unique complication risks but there is little data identifying any one system as less prone to overall complications and poor patient outcome than another.

The placement of foreign bodies (instrumentation and nonautologous bone graft) increases the risk of postoperative infection. Simple cellulitis, subcutaneous phlegmon, deep or epidural abscesses, discitis, or osteomyelitis may ensue. Management ranges from the delivery of intravenous antibiotics to reoperation and possible removal of hardware, with subsequent reoperation for stabilization and fusion. The risk of infection can be minimized by observing careful operative technique, the delivery of perioperative antibiotics, and the delay of opera-

tion on patients with remote infection, when possible. Although no conclusive studies are available, the use of Luque rods may carry a higher incidence of infection.[25]

Neurological injuries can occur from the direct injury of the spinal cord or nerve roots from the operative approach or instrumentation itself. Vascular injury during ventral procedures may also compromise spinal cord perfusion with subsequent ischemia and infarction possible. Traction on nerve roots or the spinal cord during deformity correction may also lead to neurological injury. Careful preparation of instrumentation placement sites, assuring adequate space for instrumentation components, knowledge of the anatomy of the spine and surrounding structures, and attention to surgical technique and exposure should minimize complications. Again, no single instrumentation system seems superior to any other in avoiding neurological injury based on the data available.

Instrumentation failure can occur due to breaking or bending of hardware, loss of instrumentation fixation or attachment, or fracture of bony components of the host-device junction. This can lead to inadequate fusion, pseudarthrosis formation, mechanical pain, neurological or vascular injury, failure to correct a spinal deformity, or loss of correction of a deformity. Reoperation for revision or removal of hardware is often necessary. Overall, pedicle screw systems seem to offer a higher rate of fusion compared with hook-rod and ventral devices.[25] However, this conclusion is based on a meta-analysis of existing literature.

Postoperative spinal deformities may occur independently of overt instrumentation or graft failure. However these most frequently arise due to improper use or application of an instrumentation system or operative approach, or limitations imposed by the deformity. Deformities may manifest as a failure to correct the initial deformity, the progression of a deformity, or the appearance of a late postoperative deformity. Neurological compromise may occur, and reoperation to correct or prevent further progression of such deformities may be necessary.

A graft failure can present as a pseudarthrosis or overt mechanical failure of implanted material. Pseudarthrosis is likely to manifest late in the postoperative course and may present as pain, spinal deformity, or instrumentation failure. Failure to provide adequate internal fixation with instrumentation, lack of proper external bracing, inadequate preparation of bony surfaces for junction with the graft, and inadequate amount of graft material may increase the risk for pseudarthrosis. Diagnosis can be difficult and management may require reoperation. A mechanical failure may occur if a graft is load-bearing, as is often the case with ventral struts. Attention to adequate support of the spine around a load-bearing graft should minimize such failures.

Postoperative pain may occur due to mechanical irritation by instrumentation hardware, the presence of underlying pseudarthrosis, or spinal deformity. Evaluation of specific patient presentations with particular attention to these factors may lead to management with nonsurgical methods or reoperation.

No well-controlled, randomized, prospective studies are available to adequately analyze the factors associated with poor outcomes after thoracic spinal stabilization and fusion. This, coupled with the wide variety of operative techniques and instrumentation systems, prevents the clear identification of complication rates, risk factors, long-term outcomes, or the optimum operative intervention for a given presentation. The formulation of strategies to best avoid and manage these complications thus relies on the less than perfect data available, the clinical judgment of the surgeon, and an assessment of patients on a case-by-case basis.

REFERENCES

1. Aaro S, Ohlen G. The effect of Harrington instrumentation on the sagittal configuration and mobility of the spine in scoliosis. Spine 8:570-575, 1983.
2. Aebi M, Etter C, Kehl T, Thalgott J. The internal fixation system: A new treatment of thoracolumbar fractures and other spinal disorders. Clin Orthop 227:30-43, 1988.
3. Arpin-Sypert EJ, Sypert GW. Septic Ccomplications of spinal surgery. In Tarlov EC, ed. Complications of Spinal Surgery. Park Ridge, Ill.: American Association of Neurological Surgeons, 1991, pp 29-40.
4. Bennett GJ. Cotrel-Dubosset instrumentation for thoracolumbar instability. In Hitchon PW, Traynelis VC, Rengachary SS, eds. Techniques in Spinal Fusion and Stabilization. New York: Thieme Medical Publishers, 1995, pp 209-212.
5. Benzel EC. Short segment fixation of the thoracic and lumbar spine. In Benzel EC, ed. Spinal Instrumentation. Park Ridge, Ill.: American Association of Neurological Surgeons, 1994, pp 111-124.
6. Benzel EC, Baldwin NG. Crossed-screw fixation of the unstable thoracic and lumbar spine. J Neurosurg 82:11-16, 1995.
7. Benzel EC, Kesterson L, Marchand EP. Texas Scottish Rite Hospital rod instrumentation for thoracic and lumbar spine trauma. J Neurosurg 75:382-387, 1991.
8. Benzel EC, Larson SJ. Operative stabilization of the post-traumatic thoracic and lumbar spine: A comparative analysis of the Harrington distraction rod and the modified Weiss spring. Neurosurgery 19:378-385,1986.
9. Bernard TN, Johnston CE, Roberts JM, Burke SW. Late complications due to wire breakage in segmental spinal instrumentation. J Bone Joint Surg 65A:1339-1345, 1983.
10. Boscardin JB, Ringus JC, Feingold DJ, Ruda SC. Human intradiscal levels with cefazolin. Spine 17(Suppl 6):S145-S148, 1992.
11. Bridwell KH, Lenke LG, McEnery KW, Baldus C, Blanke K. Anterior fresh frozen structural allografts in the thoracic and lumbar spine. Spine 20:1410-1418, 1995.
12. Brown CW, Orme TJ, Richardson HD. The rate of pseudoarthrosis (surgical nonunion) in patients who are smokers and patients who are nonsmokers: A comparison study. Spine 11:942-943, 1986.
13. Brunski JB, Hill DC, Meskowitz A. Stresses in a Harrington distraction rod: Their origin and relationship to fatigue fractures in vivo. J Biomech Eng 105:101-107, 1983.
14. Buttermann GR, Glazer PA, Bradford DS. The use of bone allografts in the spine. Clin Orthop 324:75-85, 1996.
15. Carl AL, Tromanhauser SG, Roger DJ. Pedicle screw instrumentation for thoracolumbar burst fractures and fracture-dislocations. Spine 17:S317-S324, 1992.
16. Chozick B, Toselli R. Complications of spinal instrumentation. In Benzel EC, ed. Spinal Instrumentation. Park Ridge, Ill.: American Association of Neurological Surgeons, 1994, pp 257-274.
17. Classen DC, Evans RC, Pestotnik SL, et al. The timing of prophylactic administration of antibiotics and the risk of surgical-wound infection. N Engl J Med 326:281-286, 1992.
18. Cohen MG, McAfee PC. Kaneda anterior spinal instrumentation. In Hitchon PW, Traynelis VC, Rengachary SS, eds. Techniques in Spinal Fusion and Stabilization. New York: Thieme Medical Publishers, 1995, pp 264-278.
19. Convery FR, Minteer MA, Smith RW, Emerson SM. Fracture-dislocation of the dorsal-lumbar spine acute operative stabilization by Harrington instrumentation. Spine 3:160-166, 1978.
20. Cook SD, Barrack RL, Georgette FS, Whitecloud TS, Burke SW, Skinner HB, Renz EA. An analysis of failed Harrington rods. Spine 10:313-316, 1985.
21. Cotler JM, Simpson JM, An HS. Principles, indications, and complications of spinal instrumentation. In An HS, Cotler JM, eds. Spinal Instrumentation. Baltimore: Williams & Wilkins, 1992, pp 435-456.
22. Daniaux H, Seykora P, Genelin A, Lang T, Kathrein A. Application of posterior plating and modifications in thoracolumbar spine injuries: Indications, techniques and results. Spine 16:S125-S133, 1991.
23. Davne SH, Myers DL. Complications of lumbar spinal fusion with transpedicular instrumentation. Spine 17:S184-S189, 1992.
24. Denis F. The three-column spine and its significance in the classification of acute thoracolumbar spine injuries. Spine 8:817, 1983.
25. Dickman CA, Yahiro MA, Lu HTC, Melkerson MN. Surgical treatment alternatives for fixation of unstable fractures of the thoracic and lumbar spine. Spine 19:S2266-S2273, 1994.
26. Dickson JH, Harrington PR, Erwin WD. Results of reduction and stabilization of the severely fractured thoracic and lumbar spine. J Bone Joint Surg 60A:799-805, 1978.

27. Dubousset J, Herring JA, Shufflebarger H. The crankshaft phenomenon. J Pediatr Orthop 9:541-550, 1989.

28. Dunn HK. Anterior stabilization of thoracolumbar injuries. Clin Orthop 189:116-124, 1984.

29. Edwards CC, Levine AM. Early rod-sleeve stabilization of the injured thoracic and lumbar spine. Orthop Clin North Am 17:121-145, 1986.

30. Edwards CC, Levine AM. Complications associated with posterior instrumentation in the treatment of thoracic and lumbar injuries. In Garfin SR, ed. Complications of Spine Surgery. Baltimore: Williams & Wilkins, 1989, pp 164-199.

31. Efsen F. Spinal cord lesions as a complication of abdominal aortography. Acta Radiol 4:47-58, 1966.

32. Erwin WD, Dickson JH, Harrington PR. Clinical review of patients with broken Harrington rods. J Bone Joint Surg 62A:1302-1307, 1980.

33. Esses Sl, Botsford DJ, Wright T, Bednar D, Bailey S. Operative treatment of spinal fractures with the AO internal fixator. Spine 16:S146-S150, 1991.

34. Fang HSY, Ong GB, Hodgson AR. Anterior spinal fusion: The operative approaches. Clin Orthop 35:16, 1964.

35. Farcy JP, Weidenbaum M, Michelsen CB, Hoeltzel DA, Athanasiou KA. A comparative biomechanical study of spinal fixation using CotrelDubousset instrumentation. Spine 12:877-881, 1987.

36. Feigleson HH, Ravin HA. Transverse myelitis following selective bronchial arteriography. Radiology 85:663-665, 1965.

37. Ferguson RL, Allen BL. The evolution of segmental spinal instrumentation in the treatment of unstable thoracolumbar spine fractures. Orthop Trans 7:14-15, 1983.

38. Flesch JR, Leider LL, Erickson DL, Chou SN, Bradford DS. Harrington instrumentation and spine fusion for unstable fractures and fracture-dislocations of the thoracic and lumbar spine. J Bone Joint Surg 59A:143-153, 1977.

39. Fogelberg EV, Zitzmann EK, Stinchfield FE. Prophylactic penicillin in orthopaedic surgery. J Bone Joint Surg 52A:95-98, 1970.

40. Gepstein R, Eismont FJ. Postoperative spine infections. In Garfin SR, ed. Complications of Spine Surgery. Baltimore: Williams & Wilkins, 1989, pp 302-322.

41. Gertzbein SD, MacMichael D, Tile M. Harrington instrumentation as a method of fixation in fractures of the spine. A critical analysis of deficiencies. J Bone Joint Surg 64B:526-529, 1982.

42. Gertzbein SD, Robbins SE. Accuracy of pedicular screw placement in vivo. Spine 15:11-14, 1990.

43. Goll SR, Balderston RA, Stambough JL, Booth RE, Cohn JC, Pickens GT. Depth of intraspinal wire penetration during passage of sublaminar wires. Spine 13:503-509, 1988.

44. Green JW, Wenzel RP. Postoperative wound infection: A controlled study of the increased duration of hospital stay and direct cost of hospitalization. Ann Surg 185:264-268, 1977.

45. Greenberg MS. Spinal cord vasculature. In Greenberg MS, ed. Handbook of Neurosurgery. Lakeland: Greenberg Graphics, 1991, pp 96-97.

46. Gurr KR, McAfee PC. Cotrel-Dubousset instrumentation in adults: A preliminary report. Spine 13:510-520, 1988.

47. Heller JG. Postoperative infections of the spine. In Rothman RH, Simeone FA, eds. The Spine. Philadelphia: WB Saunders, 1992, pp 1817-1838.

48. Herring JA, Fitch R, Wenger DR, Roach J, Cook J, Candace F. Segmental spinal instrumentation—A review of early results and complications. Orthop Trans 8:172, 1984.

49. Herring JA, Wenger DR. Early complications of segmental spinal instrumentation. Orthop Trans 6:22, 1982.

50. Herring JA, Wenger DR. Segmental spinal instrumentation. A preliminary report of 40 consecutive cases. Spine 7:285-298, 1982.

51. Hitchon PW. Harrington distraction rods for thoracic and lumbar fractures. In Hitchon PW, Traynelis VC, Rengachary SS, eds. Techniques in Spinal Fusion and Stabilization. New York: Thieme Medical Publishers, 1995, pp 204-208.

52. Hitchon PW, Follett KA. Transpedicular screw fixation of the thoracic and lumbar spine. In Hitchon PW, Traynelis VC, Rengachary SS, eds. Techniques in Spinal Fusion and Stabilization. New York: Thieme Medical Publishers, 1995, pp 240-247.

53. Hodgson AR, Stock FE, Fang HSY. Anterior spinal fusion: The operative approach and pathological findings in 412 patients with Pott's disease of the spine. Br J Surg 48:172-178, 1960.

54. Horowitz NH, Curtin JA. Prophylactic antibiotics and wound infections following laminectomy for lumbar disc herniation. J Neurosurg 43:727-731, 1975.

55. Hou S, Hu R, Shi Y. Pedicle morphology of the lower thoracic and lumbar spine in a Chinese population. Spine 18:1850-1855, 1993.

56. Jacobs RR, Casey MP. Surgical management of thoracolumbar spinal injuries: General principles and controversial considerations. Clin Orthop 189:22-35, 1984.

57. Jacobs RR, Nordwall A, Nachemson A. Reduction, stability, and strength provided by internal fixation systems for thoracolumbar spinal injury. Clin Orthop 171:300-308, 1982.

58. Jelsma RK, Kirsch PT, Jelsma LF, Ramsey WC, Rice JF. Surgical treatment of thoracolumbar fractures. Surg Neurol 18:156-166, 1982.

59. Kaneda K. Anterior approach and Kaneda instrumentation for lesions of the thoracic and lumbar spine. In Bridwell KH, Dewald RL, eds. Textbook of Spinal Surgery. Philadelphia: JB Lippincott, 1991, pp 959-990.

60. Kaneda K, Abumi K, Fujiya M. Burst fractures with neurological deficits of the thoracolumbar-lumbar spine. Results of anterior decompression and stabilization with anterior instrumentation. Spine 9:788-795, 1984.

61. Keim HA, Hilal SK. Spinal angiography in scoliosis patients. J Bone Joint Surg 53A:904-912, 1971.

62. Kern MB, Malone DG, Benzel EC. Evaluation and surgical management of thoracic and lumbar instability. Contemp Neurosurg 18:1-8, 1996.

63. Killian DA, Foster JH. Spinal cord injury as a complication of contrast angiography. Surgery 59:969-981, 1966.

64. King AG. Complications in segmental spinal instrumentation. In Luque ER, ed. Segmental Spinal Instrumentation. Thorofare, N.J.: Slack, 1984, pp 303-305.

65. Kostiuk JP. Anterior fixation for fractures of the thoracic and lumbar spine with or without neurological involvement. Clin Orthop 89:103-115, 1984.

66. Kostiuk JP. Anterior KostiukHarrington distraction systems for the treatment of kyphotic deformities. Spine 15:169-180, 1990.

67. Krag MH. Biomechanics of thoracolumbar spinal fixation: A review. Spine 16:S84-S99, 1991.

68. Lapinsky AS, Richards BS. Preventing the crankshaft phenomenon by combining anterior fusion with posterior instrumentation. Spine 20:1392-1398, 1995.

69. Lavallee S, Sautot P, Troccaz J, Cinquin P, Merloz P. Computer-assisted spine surgery: A technique for accurate transpedicular screw fixation using CT data and a 3-D optical localizer. J Imaging Guid Surg 1:65-73, 1995.

70. Lauerman WC, Bradford DS, Transfeldt EE, Ogilvie JW. Management of pseudarthrosis after arthrodesis of the spine for idiopathic scoliosis. J Bone Joint Surg 73A:222-236, 1991.

71. Leatherman KD, Johnson JR, Holt RT, Broadstone P. A clinical assessment of 357 cases of segmental spinal instrumentation. In Luque ER, ed. Segmental Spinal Instrumentation. Thorofare, N.J.: Slack, 1984, pp 165-184.

72. Lesoin F, Bouasakao N, Cama A, Lozes G, Combelles G, Jomin M. Posttraumatic fixation of the thoracolumbar spine using Roy-Camille plates. Surg Neurol 18:167-173, 1982.

73. Lindholm TS, Pylkkanen P. Discitis following removal of intervertebral disc. Spine 7:618-622, 1982.

74. Lindsey RW, Dick W. The Fixateur Interne in the reduction and stabilization of thoracolumbar spine fractures in patients with neurological deficit. Spine 16:S140-S145, 1991.

75. Lonstein JE, Winter RB, Moe JH, Gaines D. Wound infection with Harrington instrumentation and spine fusion for scoliosis. Clin Orthop 96:222-233, 1973.

76. Louis R. Fusion of the lumbar and sacral spine by internal fixation with screw plates. Clin Orthop 203:18-33, 1986.

77. Luque ER. Segmental spinal instrumentation for correction of scoliosis. Clin Orthop 163:192-198, 1982.

78. Luque ER. Interpeduncular segmental fixation. Clin Orthop 203:54-58, 1986.

79. Matsuzaki H, Tokuhashi Y, Matsumoto F, Hoshino M, Kiuchi T, Toriyama S. Problems and solutions of pedicle screw plate fixation of lumbar spine. Spine 15:1159-1165, 1990.

80. McAfee PC. Complications of anterior approaches to the thoracolumbar spine. Clin Orthop 306:110-119, 1994.

81. McAfee PC, Bohlman HH. Complications following Harrington instrumentation for fractures of the thoracolumbar spine. J Bone Joint Surg 67A:672-686, 1985.

82. McAfee PC, Bohlman HH, Yuan HA. Anterior decompression of traumatic thoracolumbar fractures with incomplete neural deficit using a retroperiotoneal approach. J Bone Joint Surg 67A:89-104, 1985.

83. McAfee PC, Weiland DJ, Carlow JJ. Survivorship analysis of pedicle spinal instrumentation. Spine 16:S422-427, 1991.

84. McBride GG. CotrelDubousset rods in spinal fractures. Paraplegia 27:440-449, 1989.

85. McLain RF, Sparling E, Benson DR. Early failure of short-segment pedicle instrumentation for thoracic fractures. J Bone Joint Surg 75A:162-167, 1993.

86. Meakins JL. Guidelines for prevention of surgical site infection. In Meakins JL, ed. Surgical Infections—Diagnosis and Treatment. New York: Scientific American, 1994, pp 127-138.

87. Meding JB, Stambough JL. Critical analysis of strut grafts in anterior spinal fusions. J Spinal Disord 6:166-174, 1993.

88. Moe JH. Complications of scoliosis treatment. Clin Orthop 53:21-30, 1967.

89. Moe JH, Denis F. The iatrogenic loss of lumbar lordosis. Orthop Trans 1:131, 1977.

90. Moran JM, Berg WS, Berry JL, Geiger JM, Steffee AD. Transpedicular screw fixation. J Orthop Res 7:107-114, 1989.

91. Moreland DB, Egnatchik JG, Bennett GJ. Cotrel-Dubousset instrumentation for the treatment of thoracolumbar fractures. Neurosurgery 27:69-73, 1990.

92. Nicastro JF, Hartjen CA, Traina J, Lancaster JM. Intraspinal pathways taken by sublaminar wires during removal. J Bone Joint Surg 68A:1206-1209, 1986.

93. Nolte LP, Visarius H, Arm E, Langlotz F, Schwarzenbach O, Zamorano L. Computer-aided fixation of spinal implants. J Imaging Guid Surg 1:88-93, 1995.

94. Parker LM, McAfee PC, Fedder IL, Weis JC, Geis WP. Minimally invasive surgical techniques to treat spine infections. Orthop Clin North Am 27:183-199, 1996.

95. Pavel A, Smith RC, Ballard CA, Larsen IJ. Prophylactic antibiotics in clean orthopedic surgery. J Bone Joint Surg 56A:777-782, 1974.

96. Peterson RE. Stress Concentration Factors. New York: John Wiley and Sons, 1976.

97. Pilgaard S. Discitis (closed space infection) following removal of lumbar intervertebral disc. J Bone Joint Surg 51A:713-716, 1969.

98. Richards BS, Herring JA, Johnston CE, Birch JG, Roach JW. Treatment of adolescent idiopathic scoliosis using Texas Scottish Rite Hospital instrumentation. Spine 19:1598-1605, 1994.

99. Ropson MC, Duke WF, Krizek TJ. Rapid bacterial screening in the treatment of civilian wounds. J Surg Res 14:426-430, 1973.

100. Roy-Camille R, Saillant G. Internal fixation of the lumbar spine with pedicle screw plating. Clin Orthop 203:717, 1986.

101. Roy-Camille R, Saillant G, Mazel CH. Plating of thoracic, thoracolumbar, and lumbar injuries with pedicle screw plates. Orthop Clin North Am 17:147-159, 1986.

102. Sasso RC, Cotler HB, Reuben JD. Posterior fixation of thoracic and lumbar spine fractures using DC plates and pedicle screws. Spine 16:S134-S139,1991.

103. Schofferman J, Schofferman L, Zucherman J, Hsu K, White A. Metabolic bone disease in lumbar pseudarthrosis. Spine 15:687-689, 1989.

104. Stambough JL, Simeone FA. Vascular complications in spine surgery. In Garfin SR, ed. Complications of Spine Surgery. Baltimore: William & Wilkins, 1989, pp 110-126.

105. Stambough JL, Simeone FA. Vascular complications in spine surgery. In Rothman RH, Simeone RA, eds. The Spine. Philadelphia: WB Saunders, 1992, pp 1877-1885.

106. Steffee AD, Biscup RS, Sitkowski DJ. Segmental spine plates with pedicle screw fixation a new internal fixation device for disorders of the lumbar and thoracolumbar spine. Clin Orthop 203:45-53,1986.

107. Steinman JC, Herkowitz HN. Pseudarthrosis of the spine. Clin Orthop 284:80-90, 1992.

108. Suk SI, Lee CK, Min HJ, Cho KH, Oh JH. Comparison of Cotrel-Dubousset pedicle screws and hooks in the treatment of idiopathic scoliosis. Int Orthop 18:341-346, 1994.

109. Suk S-I, Choon KL, Kim W-J, Chung Y-J, Park Y-B. Segmental pedicle screw fixation in the treatment of thoracic idiopathic scoliosis. Spine 20:1399-1405, 1995.

110. Vaccaro AR, Rizzolo SJ, Allardyce TJ, Ramsey M, Salvo J, Balderston RA, Cotler JM. Placement of pedicle screws in the thoracic spine. Part I: Morphometric analysis of the thoracic vertebrae. J Bone Joint Surg 77A:1193-1199, 1995.

111. Vaccaro AR, Rizzolo SJ, Balderston RA, Allardyce TJ, Gardin SR, Dolinskas C, An HS. Placement of pedicle screws in the thoracic spine. II. An anatomical and radiographic assessment. J Bone Joint Surg 77A:1200-1206, 1995.

112. Vauzelle D, Stagnara P, Jouvinroux P. Functional monitoring of spinal cord activity during spinal surgery. Clin Orthop 93:173-178, 1973.

113. Watkins RG. Cervical, thoracic, and lumbar complications—Anterior approach. In Garfin SR, ed. Complications of Spine Surgery. Baltimore: Williams & Wilkins, 1989, pp 211-247.

114. Weinstein JN, Spratt KF, Spengler D, Brick C. Spinal pedicle fixation: Reliability and validity of roentgenogram based assessment and surgical factors on successful screw placement. Proceedings of the 23rd annual meeting of the Scoliosis Research Society. Baltimore, Md.: September 29-October 2, 1988.

115. Wenger DR, Mubarak SJ. Managing complications of posterior spinal instrumentation and fusion. In Garfin SR, ed. Complications of Spine Surgery. Baltimore: Williams & Wilkins, 1989, pp 127-143.

116. West JL, Bradford DS, Ogilvie JW. Steffee instrumentation: Two year results. Scoliosis Research Society. Orthop Trans 13:112, 1989

117. West JL, Ogilvie JW, Bradford DS. Complications of the variable screw plate pedicle screw fixation. Spine 16:576-579, 1991.

118. Whitecloud TS III, Butler JC, Cohen JL, et al. Complications with the variable spinal plating system. Spine 14:472-476, 1989.

119. Wittenberg RH, Lee K-S, Shea M, White AA, Hayes WC. Effect of screw diameter, insertion technique, and bone cement augmentation of pedicular screw fixation strength. Clin Orthop 296:278-287, 1993.

120. Yamagata M, Kitahara H, Minami S, Takahashi K, Isobe K, Moriya H,Tamaki T. Mechanical stability of the pedicle screw fixation systems for the lumbar spine. Spine 17:S51-S54, 1992.

121. Yosipovitch Z, Robin GC, Makin M. Open reduction of unstable thoracolumbar spinal injuries and fixation with Harrington rods. J Bone Joint Surg 59A:1003-1015, 1977.

122. Yuan HA, Garfin SR, Dickman CA, Mardjetko SM. A historical cohort study of pedicle screw fixation in thoracic, lumbar, and sacral spinal fusions. Spine 19:S2279-S2296, 1994.

123. Zdeblick TA. Z-Plate anterior thoracolumbar instrumentation. In Hitchon PW, Traynelis VC, Rengachary SS, eds. Techniques in Spinal Fusion and Stabilization. New York: Thieme Medical Publishers, 1995, pp 279-289.

124. Zindrick MR, Wiltse LL, Doornik A, Widell EH, Knight GW, Patwardhan AG, Thomas JC, Rothman SL, Fields BT. Analysis of the morphometric characteristics of the thoracic and lumbar pedicles. Spine 12:160-166, 1987.

125. Zindrick MR, Wiltse LL, Widell EH, Thomas JC, Holland WR, Field T, Spencer CW. Biomechanical study of interpedicular screw fixation in the lumbosacral spine. Clin Orthop 203:99-111, 1986.

126. Zucherman J, Hsu K, White A, Wynne G. Early results of spinal fusion using variable spine plating system. Spine 13:570-579, 1988.

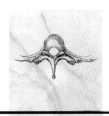

Index